Chronic Kidney Disease, Dialysis, and Transplantation

A Companion to Brenner and Rector's The Kidney

FOURTH EDITION

Jonathan Himmelfarb, MD
Professor of Medicine
Director, Kidney Research Institute
Co-Director, Center for Dialysis Innovation
Joseph W. Eschbach MD Endowed Chair for Kidney Research
Department of Medicine, Division of Nephrology
University of Washington

T. Alp Ikizler, MD
Director, Division of Nephrology
Catherine McLaughlin-Hakim Chair in Vascular Biology
Professor of Medicine
Department of Medicine, Vanderbilt University
Medical Center
Nashville, Tennessee

ELSEVIER

ELSEVIER

1600 John F. Kennedy Blvd.
Ste 1800
Philadelphia, PA 19103-2899

CHRONIC KIDNEY DISEASE, DIALYSIS, AND TRANSPLANTATION, FOURTH EDITION

ISBN: 978-0-323-52978-5

International Standard Book Number: 978-0-323-52978-5

Content Strategist: Nancy Duffy
Senior Content Development Manager: Kathryn DeFrancesco
Content Development Specialist: Meghan Andress
Publishing Services Manager: Julie Eddy
Book Production Specialist: Carol O'Connell
Design Direction: Bridget Hoette

Printed in the United States of America

Last digit is the print number: 9 8 7 6 5 4 3 2 1

To Deb, Sarah, Rachel, and Joshua, for their love, support, and guidance.

–JH

To Mine, Omer, and Irem, for their patience, support, and understanding.

–TAI

PREFACE

This fourth edition of *Chronic Kidney Disease, Dialysis, and Transplantation*, a companion to *Brenner and Rector's The Kidney*, was conceived to bring the latest information available across a broad swath of disease conditions to the fingertips of the reader. Since the previous edition much has changed in our knowledge about epidemiology, pathogenesis, diagnosis, and treatment of kidney disorders. Our goal was to create a useful vehicle for the dissemination of this knowledge to busy clinicians, scientists, educators, and students of the kidney. Chapters are designed to be state of the art and comprehensive, but not so encyclopedic as to be burdensome to the reader. While chapters can be read individually, sections of the book are thoughtfully organized to provide a systematic approach to understanding the kidney. To accomplish these goals, we were fortunate to assemble an outstanding group of authors and associate editors who are leading content experts and excellent writers. We have also tried to ensure that each chapter is well illustrated with figures and tables conveying critical information that is visually accessible to readers. Every chapter in this edition of *Chronic Kidney Disease, Dialysis, and Transplantation* has been thoroughly revised to be up to date, while at the same time containing canonical knowledge that stands the test of time. New chapters have been added to increase coverage of 'hot topics' such as Genetic Causes of Chronic Kidney Disease, Ethical Challenges and the Role of Palliative Care in Kidney Disease, and Home Dialysis.

We wish to thank Barry M. Brenner for his confidence in our editorial capabilities, and the Elsevier staff, including Nancy Duffy, Dolores Meloni, Maureen Iannuzzi, Meghan Andress, and Carol O'Connell for their efforts and skill in pulling together publication of this book in an authoritative and timely manner. The section editors (Drs. Tuttle, Mehrotra, Bloom, and Waikar) were instrumental in working closely with each of the authors to carefully edit all the content for accuracy and clarity of presentation. We owe them a great debt of gratitude for the high level of intellect and knowledge they applied to this project. Above all we wish to thank the authors of each chapter who took time away from their otherwise busy lives to work tirelessly to make this text as useful and valuable as possible. We hope the readers learn from and enjoy their work as much as we have done.

SECTION EDITORS

Roy D. Bloom, MD
Professor of Medicine
University of Pennsylvania;
Medical Director
Penn Kidney Pancreas Transplant Program
Philadelphia, Pennsylvania

Rajnish Mehrotra, MD
Professor of Medicine
Section Head, Nephrology
Harborview Medical Center
University of Washington
Seattle, Washington

Katherine R. Tuttle, MD, FASN, FACP
Executive Director for Research
Providence Health Care;
Regional Co-Principal Investigator, Clinical Professor of Medicine
Institute of Translational Health Sciences
University of Washington
Spokane, Washington

Sushrut S. Waikar, MD, MPH
Constantine L. Hampers, MD Distinguished Chair in Renal Medicine
Director of Translational Research and Ambulatory Services, Renal Division
Brigham and Women's Hospital
Associate Professor of Medicine
Harvard Medical School
Boston, Massachusetts

LIST OF CONTRIBUTORS

Sophoclis Alexopoulos, MD, FACS
Associate Professor
Department of Surgery
Vanderbilt University Medical Center
Nashville, Tennessee

Tarek Alhamed, MD, MS
Medical Director, Kidney and Pancreas Transplant Program
Assistant Professor
Washington University School of Medicine
St. Louis, Missouri

Radica Z. Alicic, MD, FHM, FACP
Providence Health Care
University of Washington School of Medicine
Spokane, Washington

Amatur Amarah, MD
John H. Stroger, Jr., Hospital of Cook County
Chicago, Illinois

Shubha Ananthakrishnan, MD
Associate Clinical Professor
Department of Internal Medicine
University of California, Davis School of Medicine;
Medical Director
Southgate Dialysis Clinic;
Medical Director
University Home Dialysis Clinic
Sacramento, California

Matthew J. Arduino, MS, DrPH
Senior Advisor for Environmental Hygiene and Infection Prevention
Division of Healthcare Quality Promotion
Centers for Disease Control and Prevention
Atlanta, Georgia

Deborah S. Rosenthal Asher, PhD
Memory and Psychological Services, Inc.
Brecksville, Ohio

David Axelrod, MD, MBA
Surgical Director of Kidney, Pancreas, and Living Donor Transplant
Division of Transplant and Hepatobiliary Surgery
University of Iowa
Iowa City, Iowa

Rasheed Abiodun Balogun, MBBS, FACP
Professor of Medicine
Division of Nephrology
Department of Medicine
University of Virginia
Charlottesville, Virginia

Joanne M. Bargman, MD, FRCPS
Division of Nephrology
Department of Medicine
University Health Network
Toronto, Ontario, Canada

Gerald A. Beathard, MD, PhD, FASN
Clinical Professor of Medicine
University of Texas Medical Branch
Galveston, Texas

Monica C. Beaulieu, MD, FRCPC, MHA
St. Paul's Hospital;
University of British Columbia
Vancouver, British Columbia, Canada

Justin M. Belcher, MD, PhD
Instructor
Department of Internal Medicine
Section of Nephrology
Yale University School of Medicine
New Haven, Connecticut;
Instructor
Department of Internal Medicine
Section of Nephrology
VA Connecticut Healthcare System
West Haven, Connecticut

Jeffrey S. Berns, MD
Renal, Electrolyte, and Hypertension Division
Hospital of the University of Pennsylvania
Philadelphia, Pennsylvania

Scott D. Bieber, DO
Department of Medicine
University of Washington
Seattle, Washington

Roy D. Bloom, MD
Professor of Medicine
University of Pennsylvania;
Medical Director
Penn Kidney Pancreas Transplant Program
Philadelphia, Pennsylvania

Emily A. Blumberg, MD
Professor of Medicine
Perelman School of Medicine
Infectious Diseases Division
Department of Medicine
Hospital of the University of Pennsylvania
Philadelphia, Pennsylvania

Brendan Bowman, MD
Assistant Professor of Medicine
Division of Nephrology
University of Virginia Health System
Charlottesville, Virginia

Juan J. Carrero, PhD, MBA
Associate Professor
Department of Medical Epidemiology and Biostatics
Karolinska Institutet
Stockholm, Sweden

Esteban Cedillo-Couvert, MD
South Texas Renal Care Group
San Antonio, Texas

Christopher T. Chan, MD
Director of Nephrology
University Health Network
Toronto, Ontario, Canada

Anil Chandraker, MD, FRCP
Associate Professor
Transplantation Research Center
Renal Division
Brigham and Women's Hospital
Harvard Medical School
Boston, Massachusetts

Tushar Chopra, MD, MBBS, FASN
Assistant Professor of Medicine
Department of Medicine
Division of Nephrology
University of Virginia
Charlottesville, Virginia

Gabriela Cobo, MD, PhD
Department of Education and Research
Hospital Eugenio Espejo
Quito, Equador

Lewis M. Cohen, MD
Professor of Psychiatry
University of Massachusetts-Baystate;
Consultation Psychiatrist
Baystate Medical Center
Springfield, Massachusetts

Allan J. Collins, MD
Director
Chronic Disease Research Group
Minneapolis Medical Research Foundation;
Professor
Department of Medicine
University of Minnesota
Minneapolis, Minnesota

Beatrice P. Concepcion, MD
Assistant Professor of Medicine
Division of Nephrology
Vanderbilt University
Nashville, Tennessee

Michael J. Connor Jr., MD
Associate Professor of Medicine
Emory University
Atlanta, Georgia

Josef Coresh, MD, MHS, PhD
Professor of Epidemiology, Biostatistics & Medicine Johns Hopkins University
Director, George W. Comstock Center for Public Health Research and Prevention
Director, Cardiovascular Epidemiology Training Program
Baltimore, Maryland

Daniel Cukor, PhD
Department of Psychiatry
SUNY Downstate Medical Center
Brooklyn, New York

Solomon Dawson, MD
Nephrology Fellow
Renal, Electrolyte, and Hypertension Division
Hospital of the University of Pennsylvania
Philadelphia, Pennsylvania

Ian de Boer, MD, MS
Professor of Medicine
Adjunct Professor of Epidemiology
Division of Nephrology
University of Washington
Seattle, Washington

Michelle Denburg, MD, MS
Assistant Professor
Pediatrics and Epidemiology
The Children's Hospital of Philadelphia
Perelman School of Medicine at the University of Pennsylvania
Philadelphia, Pennsylvania

Thomas A. Depner, MD
Professor Emeritus
Department of Internal Medicine
University of California, Davis School of Medicine
Sacramento, California

Vikas R. Dharnidharka, MD, MPH
Professor and Chief
Division of Pediatric Nephrology
Washington University School of Medicine
St Louis Children's Hospital
St Louis, Missouri

Michael J. Germain, MD
Professor of Medicine
University of Massachusetts-Baystate;
Nephrologist
Baystate Medical Center
Springfield, Massachusetts

John S. Gill, MD, FRCPC, MS, FAST
Professor of Medicine
Division of Nephrology
University of British Columbia
Vancouver, British Columbia

Simin Goral, MD
Professor of Medicine
Perelman School of Medicine
Renal, Electrolyte, and Hypertension Division
Department of Medicine
Hospital of the University of Pennsylvania
Philadelphia, Pennsylvania

Monica Grafals, MD, MPH
Associate Professor
Clinical Practice, Medicine-Renal Med Diseases/Hypertension
University of Colorado, Anschutz Campus
Aurora, Colorado

Judi M. Graham, MBBChBAO
St. Paul's Hospital;
Vancouver General Hospital
Vancouver, British Columbia, Canada

Gentzon Hall, MD, PhD
Assistant Professor of Medicine
Duke Molecular Physiology Institute
Duke University School of Medicine
Durham, North Carolina

Olof Heimbürger, MD, PhD
Senior Consultant
Patient Area Endocrinology and Renal Medicine
Karolinska University Hospital;
Associate Professor
Department of Clinical Science, Intervention and Technology
Karolinska Institutet
Stockholm, Sweden

Sangeeta R. Hingorani, MD, MPH
Division of Nephrology, Department of Pediatrics
Seattle Children's Hospital and University of Washington
Seattle, Washington

Joanna Q. Hudson, PharmD
Professor
Departments of Clinical Pharmacy & Translational Science and Medicine (Nephrology)
The University of Tennessee Health Science Center
Memphis, Tennessee

Lesley A. Inker, MD, MS
Division of Nephrology
Tufts Medical Center
Boston, Massachusetts

Magdalena Jankowska, MD, PhD
Department of Nephrology Transplantology, and Internal Medicine
Medical University of Gdańsk
Gdańsk, Poland

Emily J. Johnson, PhD
Providence Health Care
Spokane, Washington

Olwyn Johnston, MB, MRCPI, MD, MHSc
Clinical Associate Professor of Medicine
Division of Nephrology
University of British Columbia
Vancouver, British Columbia

Clare B. Jones, MB, ChB
Clinical Fellow
Nephrology
University Health Newtowrk
Toronto, Ontario, Canada

Anna Jovanovich, MD
University of Colorado School of Medicine
Division of Renal Disease and Hypertension
Aurora, Colorado

Philip Kam-Tao Li, MD, FRCP, FACP
Consultant and Honorary Professor
Prince of Wales Hospital
The Chinese University of Hong Kong
Hong Kong, China

Seth J. Karp, MD
Professor and Chairman
Department of Surgery
Vanderbilt University Medical Center
Nashville, Tennessee

Jessica Kendrick, MD, MPH
University of Colorado School of Medicine
Division of Renal Disease and Hypertension
Aurora, Colorado

Paul L. Kimmel, MD, MACP
Department of Medicine
George Washington University Medical Center
Washington, DC

Derk C.F. Klatte, MD
Leiden University Medical Center
Leiden, The Netherlands

Greg Knoll, MD, MSc, FRCPC
Head, Division of Nephrology
University of Ottawa and the Ottawa Hospital
Ottawa, Canada

Michael A. Kraus, MD
Professor of Clinical Medicine
Department of Nephrology
Indiana University
Indianapolis, Indiana;
Senior Medical Advisor
NxStage Kidney Care
Lawrence, Massachusetts

James P. Lash, MD
The University of Illinois at Chicago
Division of Nephrology, Department of Medicine
Chicago, Illinois

Krista L. Lentine, MD, PhD
Professor of Medicine, Director of Living Donation
Center for Abdominal Transplantation
Saint Louis University School of Medicine
St. Louis, Missouri

Andrew S. Levey, MD
Division of Nephrology
Tufts Medical Center
Boston, Massachusetts

Adeera Levin, MD, FRCPC
St. Paul's Hospital;
University of British Columbia
Vancouver, British Columbia, Canada

Philip Kam-Tao Li, MD, FRCP, FACP
Consultant and Honorary Professor
Prince of Wales Hospital
The Chinese University of Hong Kong
Hong Kong, China

Mary Ann Lim, MD
Assistant Professor of Clinical Medicine
PENN Transplant Institute
Renal, Electrolyte, and Hypertension Division
Perelman School of Medicine
Philadelphia, Pennsylvania

Bengt Lindhom, MD, PhD
Adjunct Professor
Division of Renal Medicine and Baxter Novum, Department of Clinical Science, Intervention, and Technology
Karolinska Institutet
Stockholm, Sweden

Kathleen Liu, MD, PhD, MAS
Professor
Departments of Medicine and Anesthesia
University of California, San Francisco
San Francisco, California

Helen MacLaughlin, BSc, PhD
Department of Nutrition and Dietitics
King's College Hospital
London, United Kingdom

Nicola Marsh, BSc, MSc
Department of Nutrition and Dietetics
King's College Hospital
London, United Kingdom

Lea Matsuoka, MD, FACS
Associate Professor
Department of Surgery
Vanderbilt University Medical Center
Nashville, Tennessee

Habib Mawad, MD, FRCPC
Clinical Assistant Professor
University of Montreal
Postdoctoral Fellow
University of British Columbia
Vancouver, British Columbia

Rajnish Mehrotra, MD, MS
Professor of Medicine
Section Head, Nephrology
Harborview Medical Center
University of Washington
Seattle, Washington

Sharon Moe, MD
Stuart A. Kleit Professor of Medicine and Director, Division of Nephrology
Department of Medicine, Division of Nephrology
Indiana University School of Medicine
Indianapolis, Indiana

Nadar Najafian, MD
Lecturer on Medicine
Renal Division
Harvard Medical School
Boston, Massachusetts;
Director, Clinical Research
Alnylam Pharmaceuticals
Cambridge, Massachusetts

Melissa Nataatmadja, MBBS, MPH&TM, FRACP
St. Paul's Hospital;
Vancouver General Hospital
Vancouver, British Columbia, Canada

Duc B. Nguyen, MD
Service Fellow
Division of Healthcare Quality Promotion
Centers for Disease Control and Prevention
Atlanta, Georgia

Mark Douglas Okusa, MD, FASN
Professor of Medicine
Chief, Division of Nephrology
University of Virginia
Charlottesville, Virginia

Matthew J. Oliver, MD, MHS
Department of Medicine
University of Toronto
Toronto, Ontario, Canada

Paul M. Palevsky, MD
Professor of Medicine
University of Pittsburgh;
Chief, Renal Section
VA Pittsburgh Healthcare System
Pittsburgh, Pennsylvania

Chirag R. Parikh, MD, PhD
Director, Division of Nephology
Ronald Peterson Professor of Medicine
Johns Hopkins School of Medicine
Baltimore, Maryland

Priti R. Patel, MD, MPH
Medical Officer
Division of Healthcare Quality Promotion
Centers for Disease Control and Prevention
Atlanta, Georgia

Anna C. Porter, MD
The University of Illinois at Chicago
Division of Nephrology, Department of Medicine
Chicago, Illinois

Robert R. Quinn, MD, PhD
Departments of Medicine & Community Health Sciences
University of Calgary
Calgary, Canada

Leonardo V. Riella, MD, PhD
Assistant Professor of Medicine, Associate Physician
Medicine
Brigham and Women's Hospital
Harvard Medical School
Boston, Massachusetts

Eugene P. Rhee, MD
Nephrology Division
Massachusetts General Hospital
Boston, Massachusetts

Matthew B. Rivara, MD
Clinical Assistant Professor
Division of Nephrology
University of Washington;
Investigator
Kidney Research Institute
Seattle, Washington

Mitchell H. Rosner, MD
Professor of Medicine
Division of Nephrology
University of Virginia Health System
Charlottesville, Virginia

Maria-Eleni Roumelioti, MD
Research Assistant Professor
Division of Nephrology
Department of Internal Medicine
University of New Mexico
Albuquerque, New Mexico

Athanasios K. Roumeliotis, MD
Nephrology
Toronto General Hospital
Toronto, Ontario, Canada

Mark J. Sarnak, MD, MS
Chief, Division of Nephrology
Tufts Medical Center
Boston, Massachusetts

Deirdre Sawinski, MD
Assistant Professor of Medicine
Perelman School of Medicine
Renal, Electrolyte, and Hypertension Division
Department of Medicine
Hospital of the University of Pennsylvania
Philadelphia, Pennsylvania

Heidi Schaefer, MD
Associate Professor of Medicine
Division of Nephrology
Vanderbilt University
Nashville, Tennessee

Tariq Shafi, MBBS, MHS
Associate Professor of Medicine
Division of Nephrology
The Johns Hopkins University School of Medicine
Baltimore, Maryland

Neil Sheerin, MBBS, PhD, FRCP
Professor of Nephrology
Newcastle University
Newcastle upon Tyne, United Kingdom

Edward D. Siew, MD, MSCI
Associate Professor of Medicine
Division of Nephrology and Hypertension
Vanderbilt University Medical Center;
Tennessee Valley Health Systems
Nashville Veterans Affairs Hospital
Nashville, Tennessee

Anand Srivastava, MD, MPH
Assistant Professor of Medicine
Center for Translational Metabolism and Health
Institute for Public Health and Medicine
Division of Nephrology and Hypertension
Northwestern University Feinberg School of Medicine
Chicago, Illinois

Michelle C. Starr, MD, MPH
Division of Nephrology, Department of Pediatrics
Seattle Children's Hospital and University of Washington
Seattle, Washington

Peter Stenvinkel, MD, PhD
Professor
Division of Renal Medicine, Department of Clinical Science, Intervention, and Technology
Karolinska Institutet
Stockholm, Sweden

Wendy L. St. Peter, PharmD
Professor
Department of Pharmaceutical Care and Health Systems
University of Minnesota
College of Pharmacy
Minneapolis, Minnesota

Cheuk-Chun Szeto, MD, FRCP
Professor
Department of Medicine and Therapeutics
The Chinese University of Hong Kong
Shatin, Hong Kong, China

Ashita J. Tolwani, MD, MS
Professor of Medicine
University of Alabama at Birmingham
Birmingham, Alabama

Emilie Trinh, MD
Division of Nephrology
McGill University Health Center
Montreal, Quebec, Canada

Katherine R. Tuttle, MD, FACP, FASN, FNKF
Executive Director for Research
Providence Health Care;
Regional Co-Principal Investigator, Clinical Professor of Medicine
Institute of Translational Health Sciences
University of Washington
Spokane, Washington

Mark L. Unruh, MD, MS
Professor and Chair
Department of Internal Medicine
University of New Mexico
Albuquerque, New Mexico

John P. Vella, MD, FACP, FRCP, FASN, FAST
Director of Nephrology & Transplantation
Department of Medicine
Maine Medical Canter
Portland, Maine;
Associate Professor of Medicine
Tufts University School of Medicine
Boston, Massachusetts

Sushrut S. Waikar, MD, MPH
Constantine L. Hampers, MD Distinguished Chair in Renal Medicine
Director of Translational Research and Ambulatory Services, Renal Division
Brigham and Women's Hospital
Associate Professor of Medicine
Harvard Medical School
Boston, Massachusetts

Angela Yee-Moon Wang, MD, PhD
Hon. Associate Professor
Associate Consultant
Department of Medicine
University of Hong Kong, Queen Mary Hospital
Hong Kong, China

Monnie Wasse, MD, MPH, FASN
Director, Interventional Nephrology
Professor of Medicine
Department of Medicine
Rush University Medical Center
Chicago, Illinois

Lori Wazny, BSc, PharmD
Extended Practice Pharmacist
Manitoba Renal Program
Health Sciences Centre
Winnipeg, Manitoba, Canada

Daniel E. Weiner, MD, MS
Nephrologist
Tufts Medical Center;
Associate Professor of Medicine
Tufts University School of Medicine
Boston, Massachusetts

Eric Weinhandl, PhD, MS
Adjunct Assistant Professor
Department of Pharmaceutical Care and Health Systems
University of Minnesota
Minneapolis, Minnesota;
Clinical Epidemiologist
NxStage Medical
Lawrence, Massachusetts

Jessica W. Weiss, MD, MCR
Oregon Health & Science University
Portland, Oregon

James B. Wetmore, MD, MS
Associate Professor of Medicine
University of Minnesota School of Medicine;
Staff Nephrologist
Division of Nephrology
Hennepin County Medical Center
Minneapolis, Minnesota

Tiffany C. Wong, MD
Nephrology Fellow
Renal, Electrolyte, and Hypertension Division
Hospital of the University of Pennsylvania
Philadelphia, Pennsylvania

Tyler B. Woodell, MD
Oregon Health & Science University
Portland, Oregon

Hong Xu, MD
Department of Medical Epidemiology and Biostatics
Karolinska Institutet
Stockholm, Sweden

Jane Y. Yeun, MD
Clinical Professor
Department of Internal Medicine
University of California, Davis School of Medicine
Sacramento, California;
Staff Nephrologist
Sacramento Veterans Administration Medical Center
Department of Medicine
Mather, California

Nadia Zalunardo, MD, SM, FRCPC
Vancouver General Hospital;
University of British Columbia
Vancouver, British Columbia, Canada

CONTENTS

SECTION I

Chronic Kidney Disease

1

Chronic Kidney Disease: Definition, Epidemiology, Cost, and Outcomes

Tariq Shafi, MBBS, MHS, and Josef Coresh, MD, MHS, PhD

OUTLINE

Chronic kidney disease (CKD) is a global public health problem. CKD is defined based on the presence of kidney damage or reduced glomerular filtration rate (GFR), which is considered the best overall index of kidney function.[1,2] CKD staging is based on its cause, the GFR level, and degree of albuminuria. The past 20 years have seen significant improvement in recognition of the incidence, prevalence, and complications of CKD due in major part to the standardized definition and staging of CKD in 2002. The global adoption of this approach to CKD, with its emphasis on routine and automated estimation of GFR (eGFR) from serum creatinine, has improved recognition of CKD in many populations and settings where it was previously underrecognized. Increased awareness of CKD and uniform classification criteria also has led to a better understanding of the burden of illnesses that accompany CKD, an increased focus on developing methods to slow CKD progression, and a stronger emphasis on early recognition and prevention of complications associated with CKD. Fig. 1.1 shows a conceptual diagram emphasizing the importance of looking at both progression of CKD itself, from normal to damaged without reduced GFR, to reduced GFR, to kidney failure and death (horizontal progression), as well as risk for complications that can lead to mortality. Complications outside the kidney, particularly cardiac and metabolic complications are important as they often lead to death before the onset of kidney replacement therapy (KRT) with dialysis or transplantation.

Acknowledgment: The authors thank Eugenia Shing Yu Wong, BSc, for assistance with making figures and editing the chapter.

In the following sections, we will review the epidemiology, cost, and outcomes of CKD, emphasizing advances in knowledge over the past decade.

DEFINITION AND STAGING OF CHRONIC KIDNEY DISEASE

CKD is a general term for a number of heterogeneous disorders that result in sustained kidney damage with implications for the health of the individual. The initial decline of kidney function is asymptomatic and clinical manifestations of kidney failure occur late in the course of the disease. Definitions of kidney disease therefore include measures of function (e.g., GFR) and measures of damage (e.g., proteinuria, anatomical abnormalities).

Definition

Before the Kidney Disease Outcomes Quality Index (KDOQI) guidelines in 2002, there were numerous definitions of CKD in use. Many of these definitions were not well understood by patients and the lay public due to the use of word *renal* and its Latin and Greek roots. Hsu and Chertow enumerated the different names used for CKD from abstracts submitted to the American Society of Nephrology (ASN) meetings in 1998 and 1999 as well as from articles indexed in Medline.[3] They noted 23 different terms used to describe states of reduced GFR along with a number of different and overlapping definitions of kidney failure using serum creatinine, creatinine clearance, or GFR. Considering these and other factors, the 2002 KDOQI working group decided on using the word *kidney* instead of *renal* and developed an operational uniform

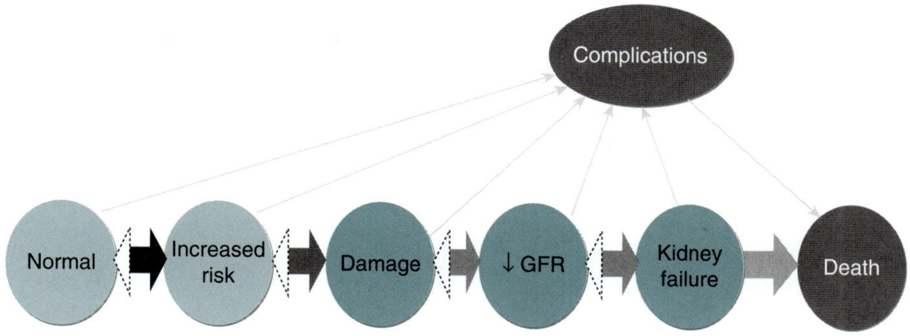

FIG. 1.1 Conceptual model of renal decline. (From Levey AS, de Jong PE, Coresh J, et al. The definition, classification, and prognosis of chronic kidney disease: a KDIGO Controversies Conference report. *Kidney Int.* 2011;80(1):17-28.)

TABLE 1.1A Definition of Chronic Kidney Disease

Criteria (either one of the following for > 3 months)
1. Markers of Kidney Damage (One or More):
• Albuminuria (AER ≥30 mg/24 h; ACR ≥30 mg/g [≥3 mg/mmol])
• Urine sediment abnormalities
• Electrolyte and other abnormalities due to tubular disorders
• Abnormalities detected by histology
• Structural abnormalities detected by imaging
• History of kidney transplantation
2. Decreased GFR
• GFR <60 mL/min/1.73 m^2 (GFR categories G3a-G5)

ACR, Albumin-to-creatinine ratio; *AER*, albumin excretion rate; *GFR*, glomerular filtration rate.
From Kidney Disease: Improving Global Outcomes (KDIGO) CKD Work Group. *KDIGO 2012 Clinical Practice Guideline for the Evaluation and Management of Chronic Kidney Disease;* 2013.

definition of CKD that was endorsed by multiple subsequent workgroups, including the KDIGO 2012 workgroup[4] despite some challenges.[5,6]

CKD is defined as abnormalities of kidney structure of function, present for >3 months, with implications for health. The 2012 Kidney Disease: Improving Global Outcomes (KDIGO) group provides a clear CKD definition (Table 1.1A) and its operational criteria (Table 1.1B).[2,7] The key elements of this definition include chronicity (>3 months), presence of kidney damage, decreased GFR, and implications for health. The chronicity component of the definition (>3 months) is arbitrarily defined to distinguish CKD from acute kidney injury (AKI). The chronicity component, implies but does not necessitate, irreversibility. Presence of kidney damage can be inferred by the presence of albuminuria, abnormal urinary sediment such as hematuria or casts, functional disorders such renal tubular acidosis or nephrogenic diabetes insipidus, pathological abnormalities detected on kidney biopsy such as immunoglobulin (Ig)A nepthropathy, or structural abnormalities of the kidney such as polycystic kidney disease. Decreased GFR is a manifestation of kidney damage from underlying renal pathology. The KDIGO 2012 guidelines kept the GFR at the <60 mL/min/1.73 m^2 threshold for definition of CKD. The threshold of <60 mL/min/1.73 m^2 was selected as it can be reliably assessed by eGFR from serum creatinine and is also a threshold below which the risk for complications of CKD increases. The CKD definition component for implications on health emphasizes that presence of CKD associates with the risk for a number of outcomes including some that were not recognized as CKD complications before the 2002 KDOQI guidelines.

Staging

The 2002 KDOQI guidelines defined a five-stage system for classification of CKD based on GFR and the 2012 KDIGO guidelines updated this staging to include the cause of CKD and the degree of albuminuria (staging by cause, GFR, and albuminuria [CGA]). The guidelines reemphasized staging by cause of CKD to remind clinicians that CKD is not a diagnosis in itself and that determination of cause is important for prognosis and treatment. The cause of the kidney disease can be assigned based on known anatomical of pathological abnormalities such as IgA nephropathy, polycystic kidney disease, vasculitis, and so on. The GFR and albuminuria categories are described in Fig. 1.2. Note that a low GFR in the G2 category, without evidence of kidney damage, is not considered CKD. KDIGO guidelines also subdivided CKD stage 3 into two categories, a and b, recognizing that the risk for complications and death in G3b CKD (eGFR 30 to 44 mL/min/1.73 m^2) is markedly higher than in G3a CKD (eGFR 45 to 59 mL/min/1.73 m^2) with the same level of albuminuria.[8,9] The guidelines also emphasize the use of albuminuria over proteinuria. Urinary protein comprises of numerous proteins including albumin, light chains, and other proteins. The concentration of these proteins can vary and standardization of measuring urine protein is difficult as there is always a variable mixture of proteins being measured. Urine albumin measurement also is difficult to standardize; however, efforts are ongoing to improve its standardization.[10-12] The guidelines suggest that urinary albumin excretion >2200 mg/day (>2200 mg/g creatinine) should be considered as nephrotic-range proteinuria, roughly corresponding to urinary protein excretion >3500 mg/day. The guidelines recognized that the use of only three categories for albuminuria

TABLE 1.1B Criteria for Definition of Chronic Kidney Disease.

Criteria	Comment
1. Duration >3 months, based on documentation or inference	**Duration is necessary to distinguish chronic from acute kidney diseases** • Clinical evaluation will often enable documentation or inference of duration • Documentation of duration is usually not declared in epidemiologic studies
2. GFR <60 mL/min/1.73 m^2 (GFR categories G3a-G5)	**GFR is the best overall index of kidney function in health and disease** • The normal GFR in young adults is approximately 125 mL/min/1.73m^2; GFR <15 mL/min/1.73 m^2 (GFR category G5) is defined as kidney failure • Decreased GFR can be detected by current estimating equations for GFR based on SCr or cystatin C but not by SCr or cystatin C alone • Decreased eGFR can be confirmed by measured GFR, if required
	Albuminuria as a marker of kidney damage [increased glomerular permeability], urine AER ≥30 mg/24 h, approximately equivalent to urine ACR ≥30 mg/g (≥3 mg/mmol) • The normal urine ACR in young adults is >10 mg/g (>1 mg/mmol) • Urine ACR 30-300 mg/g (3–30 mg/mmol; category A2) generally corresponds to "microalbuminuria," now referred to as "moderately increased" • Urine ACR ≥300 mg/g (≥30 mg/mmol; category A3) generally corresponds to "macroalbuminuria," now termed "severely increased" • Urine ACR <2200 mg/g (220 mg/mmol) may be accompanied by signs and symptoms of nephrotic syndrome (e.g., low serum albumin, edema, and high serum cholesterol) • Threshold value corresponds approximately to urine reagent strip values of trace or +, depending on urine concentration. • High urine ACR can be confirmed by urine albumin excretion in a timed urine collection expressed as AER
	Urinary sediment abnormalities as markers of kidney damage • Isolated nonvisible (microscopic) hematuria with abnormal RBC morphology (anisocytosis) in GBM disorders • RBC casts in proliferative glomerulonephritis • WBC casts in pyelonephritis or interstitial nephritis • Oval fat bodies or fatty casts in diseases with proteinuria • Granular casts and renal tubular epithelial cells in many parenchymal diseases (nonspecific)
	Renal tubular disorders • Renal tubular acidosis • Nephrogenic diabetes insipidus • Renal potassium wasting • Renal magnesium wasting • Fanconi syndrome • Non-albumin proteinuria • Cystinuria
	Pathologic abnormalities detected by histology or inferred (examples of causes) • Glomerular diseases (diabetes, autoimmune diseases, systemic infections, drugs, neoplasia) • Vascular diseases (atherosclerosis, hypertension, ischemia, vasculitis, thrombotic microangiopathy) • Tubulointerstitial diseases (urinary tract infections, stones, obstruction, drug toxicity) • Cystic and congenital diseases
	Structural abnormalities as markers of kidney damage detected by imaging (ultrasound, computed tomography and magnetic resonance with or without contrast, isotope scans, angiography) • Polycystic kidneys • Dysplastic kidneys • Hydronephrosis due to obstruction • Cortical scarring due to infarcts, pyelonephritis, or associated with vesicoureteral reflux • Renal masses or enlarged kidneys due to infiltrative diseases • Renal artery stenosis • Small and hyperechoic kidneys (common in more severe CKD due to many
	History of kidney transplantation • Kidney biopsies in most kidney transplant recipients have histopathologic abnormalities even if GFR is >60 mL/min/1.73 m^2 (GFR categories G1-G2) and ACR is <30 mg/g (<3 mg/mmol) • Kidney transplant recipients have an increased risk for mortality and kidney failure compared to populations without kidney disease • Kidney transplant recipients routinely receive subspecialty care

ACR, Albumin-to-creatinine ratio; *AER,* albumin excretion rate; *CKD,* chronic kidney disease; *eGFR,* estimated glomerular filtration rate; *GBM,* glomerular basement membrane; *GFR,* glomerular filtration rate; *RBC,* red blood cell; *SCr,* serum creatinine; *WBC,* white blood cell.

From Kidney Disease: Improving Global Outcomes (KDIGO) CKD Work Group. *KDIGO 2012 Clinical Practice Guideline for the Evaluation and Management of Chronic Kidney Disease*; 2013.

Prognosis of CKD by GFR and Albuminuria Categories: KDIGO 2012

GFR categories (ml/min/ 1.73 m²) Description and range			Persistent albuminuria categories Description and range		
			A1	A2	A3
			Normal to mildly increased	Moderately increased	Severely increased
			<30 mg/g <3 mg/mmol	30–300 mg/g 3–30 mg/mmol	>300 mg/g >30 mg/mmol
G1	Normal or high	≥90			
G2	Mildly decreased	60–89			
G3a	Mildly to moderately decreased	45–59			
G3b	Moderately to severely decreased	30–44			
G4	Severely decreased	15–29			
G5	Kidney failure	<15			

FIG. 1.2 Chronic kidney disease staging. *Dark gray,* low risk (if no other markers of kidney disease, no CKD); *light gray,* moderately increased risk; *light green,* high risk; *dark green,* very high risk. Protein to creatinine ratio (PCR) categories of <150 mg/g, 150-500mg/g, >500 mg/g are approximately equivalent to the albuminuria categories of A1-A3. (From Kidney Disease: Improving Global Outcomes (KDIGO) CKD Work Group. *KDIGO 2012 Clinical Practice Guideline for the Evaluation and Management of Chronic Kidney Disease*; 2013.)

may represent oversimplification and specialized clinical nephrology settings may need to further subdivide A3 albuminuria (>300 mg/d) into further subcategories. The use of the term *microalbuminuria* was discouraged as it implies that the size of albumin molecules rather than the rate of excretion is smaller, which is misleading.

Strengths and Limitations of the Current Chronic Kidney Disease Classification System

Strengths

The KDOQI classification system for CKD has been widely adopted. Its operational simplicity of allowing CKD to be defined based on serum creatinine or proteinuria even when the cause of CKD or its full characterization are uncertain enabled a great expansion of CKD research leading to increased recognition of CKD as a major health issue. Using eGFR and albuminuria as central CKD markers allowed for the use of much larger data sets demonstrating a wide range of complications and risks associated with CKD. Early work focused on cross-sectional complications[1] and cardiovascular risk.[13,14] Later, global collaborations, partly formed in response to challenges to the staging system, allowed for recognition of the broad validity of the independent contributions of GFR and albuminuria levels to risk.[8,15] This in turn suggested a risk-based staging system with GFR and albuminuria as two key markers.[15] Risk algorithms have been developed and validated globally for incidence of KRT (also called end-stage renal replacement therapy [RRT]) in CKD and potential kidney donors.[16,17] The definition and staging are based on GFR, determined in any method including measurement or estimation from creatinine, cystatin C, or other markers. This has allowed clinical practice to easily incorporate improvements including the global standardization of serum creatinine measurements to gold standard traceable methods and the improved GFR estimation formulas from serum creatinine and cystatin C. This eased the incorporation of a growing literature showing that eGFR by cystatin C is an even stronger risk predictor for cardiovascular disease (CVD) and mortality, but not KRT, than estimates from serum creatinine.[18 19] The KDIGO guidelines[2] recommend that evaluation of eGFR, in addition to cause and albuminuria, include evaluation of chronicity by repeat testing, use of serum creatinine, and a GFR estimating equation for an initial assessment with additional tests, such as cystatin C or a clearance measurement, for confirmatory testing in specific circumstances where GFR estimation based on serum creatinine is less accurate. They recommend that clinical laboratories use assays with calibration traceable to international standard reference materials and specify the equation used to estimate GFR. In adults, the 2009 CKD Epidemiologic Prognosis Initiative (CKD-EPI) creatinine equation is recommended but an alternative equation is acceptable if it has been shown to improve accuracy of GFR estimates. It is also recommended that serum creatinine concentrations be reported to the nearest 100th of a whole number when expressed in mg/dL. They suggest using cystatin C in adults with estimated GFR from creatinine of 45 to 59 mL/min/1.73 m^2 who do not have other markers of kidney damage when confirmation of CKD is required. Thus overall the guidelines provide a clear methodology for uniform evaluation and staging of CKD.

Automated reporting of eGFR with serum creatinine greatly increased the recognition of CKD and facilitated addressing it clinically. Serum creatinine is tested widely. Arguably, the only reason to measure serum creatinine is to assess GFR.[20] Automated reporting of estimated GFR overcomes the difficulty of determining the severity of kidney disease with serum creatinine due to the log-linear relationship between serum creatinine levels and measured GFR and multiple non-GFR determinants of serum creatinine concentration. There is widespread agreement that CKD classification has raised awareness of the full spectrum of CKD and its wide range of complications. The challenge and controversy is that increased awareness is also pointing a brighter spotlight on gaps in the knowledge base, particularly with regard to efficacy, cost-effectiveness, and thresholds for interventions. Changing the practice from excluding severe CKD patients from trials to including CKD patients and focusing on testing efficacy in this high-risk population may be one of the most important outcomes of a clear and simple classification system centered on uniform reporting of the key markers of kidney damage (albuminuria) and function (eGFR). Finally, kidney disease has evolved from being viewed as a subspecialty issue to a global health issue,[21] including a roadmap for closing the gaps in care, research, and policy.[22]

Limitations

The current classification system also has its limitations and these have been actively debated.[5,23-25] There is inherent error and variability in the measurement of GFR and albuminuria. In addition, there are limitations in the accuracy and precision of the estimating equations used to predict GFR. The creatinine estimating equations suffer the limitations imposed by serum creatinine as an endogenous marker of GFR and are not reliable at extremes of body weight as well as when patients' creatinine metabolism is not in steady state, such as in AKI. There has been criticism of estimating GFR; suggestions for using different equations to estimate GFR; concerns about defining CKD based on a single eGFR cutoff rather than age-specific cutoffs; and defining CKD stages 1 and 2 based on persistent microalbuminuria without significant proteinuria as having a "disease."[26] Application of the CKD definitions to the population provides a useful indicator of the implications of the definition. However, it has also clearly pointed out that a large number of individuals meeting the CKD definition, particularly among many older individuals, will never require dialysis or transplantation. Some fear that these individuals may undergo unnecessary diagnostic testing,[23] whereas others suggest the potential benefit of alerting physicians to optimize existing therapies and avoiding nephrotoxic medications.[24] General screening for CKD using eGFR has not been directly demonstrated to be cost-effective.[27] The National Kidney Foundation's Kidney Early Evaluation Program (KEEP) uses a targeted screening protocol based on the presence of hypertension, diabetes, CVD, and first-degree relatives on KRT based on cost-effectiveness in high-risk groups.[28-30] Finally, the presence of CKD has been misinterpreted as indicating a need for referral to a nephrologist despite guideline suggestions that only a subset of patients require specialty care. The 2012 KDIGO guidelines clarify nephrology referral is only needed for progressive disease, GFR <30 mL/min/1.73 m^2, albuminuria >300 mg/g, or other refractory conditions.[2,31]

Future Directions

The concept of defining and classifying CKD based on estimated GFR, albuminuria, and cause of CKD when known has been transformative in the field. However, an imprecise understanding of the cause of CKD and its progression in the majority of patients is a chief limitation. The current classification system addresses major common pathways in CKD. One of its strengths has been not requiring a precise knowledge of CKD etiology. However, efforts to better understand CKD etiology at the molecular and genetic basis could lead to new effective treatments possibly targeted to specific subpopulations of patients. This can be complementary, rather than competitive with the integrative approach of the current CKD definition and staging. Finally, there is still a paucity of clinical trials for CKD prevention and treatment. The current staging system and increased recognition of the importance of CKD is helping with the design of new trials. Developing more powerful biomarkers and surrogate measures of CKD outcomes and integrating them into CKD staging would lead to further progress.

EPIDEMIOLOGY OF CHRONIC KIDNEY DISEASE

Epidemiological descriptions of CKD have advanced greatly over the past decade. Prevalence estimates are becoming more widespread globally, although the methodological rigor of studies varies. Incidence studies have described a range of risk factors but use a range of definitions of CKD progression and incidence. Substantial progress has been made in studying risks associated with CKD through global consortia. In addition, registries of the incidence and prevalence of kidney failure treated with KRT and associated complications and costs have been in existence for decades in most developed countries. The United States Renal Data System (USRDS) now provides comprehensive descriptions of both end-stage renal disease (ESRD) and CKD incidence and prevalence. In addition, the system has expanded to cover treatment and outcomes in the administrative data.[32] The Centers for Disease Control and Prevention (CDC) also has developed a project to provide surveillance for CKD using a wide range of parameters and data sources that will be tracked continuously (https://nccd.cdc.gov/ckd/). Finally, the Global Burden of Disease Study examines CKD as a cause of death, low GFR, and recently added albuminuria as a risk factor for death and disability.[33]

Etiology of Chronic Kidney Disease

CKD can result from a variety of different pathological processes that are discussed in detail elsewhere in this book. From an epidemiological perspective, it is important to recognize that etiologies of CKD as determined by ESRD registries are limited for a number of reasons. First and foremost, in the vast majority of patients with CKD and ESRD, tissue diagnosis by kidney biopsy is not available and the cause is assumed based on the presence and severity of comorbidities, such as diabetes and hypertension. Second, ESRD patients are disease "survivors" who initiate KRT and thus reflect the slowly progressive forms of CKD. Initiation of KRTs is also determined by physician practice characteristics, availability of resources, and societal and cultural norms. Finally, registry data are dependent on completion of regulatory forms such as Form 2728 in the United States. Exact cause of CKD, even if known, may not be captured on these forms. Finally, efforts to better understand CKD etiology at the molecular and genetic basis could be transformative if they led to new effective treatments possibly targeted to specific subpopulations of patients.

Cause of CKD is now formally a part of the CKD staging system to acknowledge the importance of etiology in treatment. However, the most common assigned causes are diabetes and hypertension. In both conditions, the precise pathogenesis and factors leading to more rapid progression of disease are not fully understood. The discovery of the *APOL1* genetic susceptibility locus leading to much of the increased risk beyond environmental factors in kidney disease among populations of African descent provides the most dramatic example of a better etiological understanding of CKD.[34-41] Separate chapters address specific subgroups of CKD by known and presumed etiology and its implications for treatment and prevention.

Prevalence and Incidence of Chronic Kidney Disease

Prevalence estimates for CKD provide a useful measure of the burden of disease by stage. Early work on the burden of kidney failure treated with dialysis or transplantation pointed out the large costs to patients, and society of this most severe stage of CKD and its epidemic increase. Subsequent work demonstrated that the full spectrum of CKD goes well beyond "predialysis" with over 10% of the population affected with CKD based on kidney damage or decreased kidney function with adverse consequences to their health. Understanding the variation across time, geography, and risk factors is important for grasping the full implications for public health. Incidence is important to understand as it is more directly linked to changes in risk factors. Likewise, mortality and complications are important to quantify, particularly as reduction in mortality will lead to increases in prevalence through longer disease duration.

Prevalence of Chronic Kidney Disease

The most definitive prevalence estimates for CKD are based on population-based surveys with rigorous sampling and laboratory methods. The 2002 KDOQI definition of CKD was accompanied by population based estimates for the United States.[1,42] This early work struggled with and brought attention to many of the complexities needed for valid estimates, including the need for understanding creatinine and albuminuria measurement and variability. These methods have now been applied in a number of settings providing a global estimate of CKD prevalence.

United States CKD Prevalence: Estimates by guidelines working groups, the USRDS, and the CDC still center on the analysis of the National Health and Nutrition Examination Surveys (NHANES).[43-45] The NHANES are cross-sectional, multistage, stratified, clustered probability samples of the US civilian noninstitutionalized population conducted by the National Center of Health Statistics (NCHS), a branch of the CDC. The NHANES were conducted from 1988 to 1994 in two phases (1988 to 1991 and 1991 to 1994) and starting in 1999 to 2000 in 2-year phases until the present.

Initial prevalence estimates from NHANES were based on participants who were older than 20 years of age and did not have a missing serum creatinine concentration. Serum creatinine in NHANES was measured using the kinetic rate Jaffe method and the creatinine values were initially calibrated to the Cleveland Clinic Research Laboratory and subsequently to reference methods.[46-49] Albuminuria was assessed using a spot urine sample and calculation of urine albumin to creatinine ratios. Estimates of persistence of albuminuria were based on a sample of 1241 patients in NHANES 1988 to 1994 who underwent repeat measurements; this showed that although severely increased albuminuria (A3 >300 mg/g) measured on one occasion nearly always indicated persistent albuminuria, moderately increased albuminuria (A2 30 to 300 mg/g) only corresponded to an elevated level of repeat measurement in 50% to 75% of the participants. As a result, modeling the lack of persistent results in lower prevalence of albuminuria and CKD, analysis of CKD trends over time are not influenced by persistence issues since they usually assume persistence is unchanged over time. The CKD stages were based on the KDOQI classification system and showed an increase in prevalence from 1988 to 2004 (Fig. 1.3).[50]

Prevalence estimates for the US population have been updated using the CKD-EPI creatinine equation.[51] The CKD-EPI equation results in a shift to the right in GFR values at eGFR ≥45 mL/min/1.73 m^2; below that level, the GFR distribution remains largely unchanged. The overall prevalence of CKD in adults in the United States in 1996 to 2006 was 11.5% (95% confidence interval [CI], 10.6 to 12.4) which translates to 23.2 (95% CI, 21.3 to 25.) million people in the United States with CKD. This estimate is somewhat lower than the estimated 13.1% based on the MDRD (Modification of Diet in Renal Disease) study equation. The prevalence of CKD stages 1 to 4 based on the CKD-EPI equation were 2.24% (stage 1), 2.56% (stage 2), 6.32% (stage 3), and 0.4% (stage 4). Compared with the prevalence estimates based on MDRD

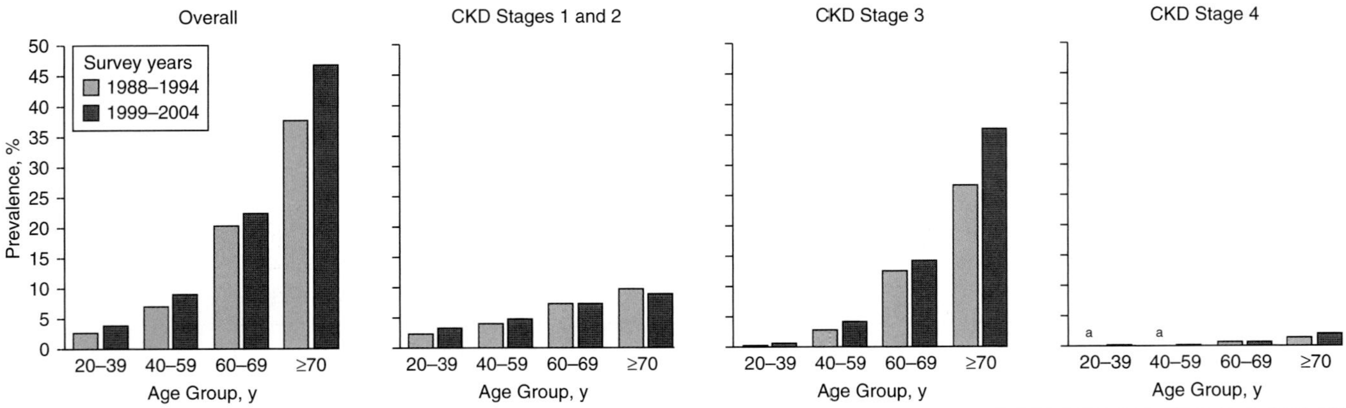

NHANES indicates National Health and Nutrition Examination Surveys.
[a]There were no cases in 1988–1994.

FIG. 1.3 Prevalence of chronic kidney cisease (CKD) stages by age group in NHANES 1988-1993 and 1999-2004. (From Coresh J, Selvin E, Stevens LA, et al. Prevalence of chronic kidney disease in the United States. *JAMA*. 2007;298(17):2038-2047.)

equation, the CKD-EPI equation eGFR leads to a lower prevalence of CKD estimates in women (compared with men) and in whites (compared with blacks). As a result, the prevalence of stage 3 to 4 CKD is not statistically higher in women than in men and in whites than in blacks as was the case when using prevalence estimates based on MDRD study eGFR. Using the CKD-EPI equation, the prevalence estimates of CKD for those older than 70 years of age are similar estimates calculated from the MDRD equation.

In contrast to the lower estimate of CKD prevalence provided by using the CKD-EPI equation to estimate GFR, many recent estimates are higher because they have chosen not to explicitly model the lack of persistence of albuminuria. The argument in favor of using single measures of eGFR and albuminuria is that most epidemiological studies only have a single visit. Therefore estimates that better approximate the CKD population and meet the 3-month persistence criterion to define CKD require samples with more than one visit, which often are only available on a relatively small subsample of each study.

Fig. 1.4A shows the prevalence of CKD stages by eGFR and albuminuria categories measured on a single occasion combining data from multiple years to increase the sample size. The total US CKD prevalence in 2011 to 2014 was 14.9% based on eGFR and albuminuria at a single visit. Cells are colored based on KDIGO risk categories, which show that risk increases with both lower eGFR and higher albuminuria. In fact, risk associations usually are based on one-time measures so the prevalence estimates given indeed correspond to higher-risk groups. The total prevalence of CKD across moderately high-risk, high-risk, and very high-risk has not shown a large increase since the mid-2000s (Fig. 1.4B). Murphy et al.[45] updated the analysis of trends in NHANES CKD prevalence data in the United States. They focused on CKD stage G3+ (eGFR <60 mL/min/1.73 m^2). They found that both CKD prevalence overall and CKD stage G3+ rose until 2003 to 2004, but have plateaued since. Analysis of subgroups shown in Fig. 1.5 reveals that much of this trend was driven by participants older than 60 years of age, where the prevalence of CKD stage G3+ is high. For example, among patients 65 to 79 years of age, the prevalence increased from 19.4% (95% CI, 17% to 21.8%) in 1988 to 1994 to 25.1% (95% CI, 20.7% to 29.5%) in 2003 to 2004 and then decreased to 21.7% (95% CI, 18% to 25.4%) in 2011 to 2012. Patterns were similar in other subgroups, with the notable exception of non-Hispanic blacks and individuals with diabetes, where the increase in the adjusted prevalence of CKD stage G3+ continued. It is worth noting that diabetics are older than nondiabetics, so although the adjusted prevalence of CKD stage G3+ is approximately 8%, the crude prevalence is 19% with a total CKD prevalence of 40%. A detailed examination of CKD among adults with diabetes in NHANES showed that this increase in low eGFR was counterbalanced by a decrease in the prevalence of albuminuria leading to an overall stable prevalence of CKD among diabetics in the United states.[52] They showed that the decreased prevalence of albuminuria was concurrent with higher use of glucose-lowering medications, renin–angiotensin–aldosterone inhibitors and statins, and lower hemoglobin A_{1c}, systolic blood pressure, and low-density lipoprotein cholesterol. This suggests that more aggressive treatment of diabetes and CKD risk factors may be leading to the lower prevalence of albuminuria among individuals with diabetes. In fact, the decreasing prevalence of albuminuria was observed only among adults younger than 65 years of age and non-Hispanic whites, where medication use was higher and risk factor control was better. Finally, the 2016 USRDS Annual Data Report (ADR)[53] shows that when an additional 2 years of NHANES data are added, the prevalence estimate increased slightly with a most recent estimate of 14.8 in 2011 to 2014 compared with 14% in 1999 to 2004 and a lower 12% in 1988 to 1994 (Fig. 1.6). Therefore the reassuring picture of plateauing CKD prevalence in the United States is mitigated by the plateau being at a high prevalence and uncertainty about the future trends among high-risk subgroups.

GFR categories (ml/min/1.73 m²)				Albuminuria categories: A1 Normal to mildly increased <30 mg/g <3mg/mmol	A2 Moderately increased 30–300mg/g 3–30mg/mmol	A3 Severely increased >300 mg/g >30mg/mmol	
G1	Normal to high	≥90		54.7	4.3	0.4	59.5
G2	Mildly decreased	60–89		30.4	2.6	0.3	33.3
G3a	Mildly to moderately decreased	45–59		3.9	0.9	0.2	5.0
G3b	Moderately to severely decreased	30–44		1.0	0.5	0.2	1.7
G4	Severely decreased	15–29		0.1	0.1	0.2	0.4
G5	Kidney failure	<15		<0.001	0.001	0.01	0.012
				90.1	8.4	1.3	100

A

Risk Category		1999–2002		2003–2006		2007–2014		2011–2014
Low risk		86.1%		85.5%		86.5%		85.1%
Moderately high risk	13.9%	10.4%	14.5%	10.6%	13.5%	9.6%	14.9%	10.8%
High risk		2.2%		2.7%		2.5%		2.6%
Very high risk		1.3%		1.2%		1.4%		1.5%

B

FIG. 1.4 (A) Prevalence of chronic kidney disease by KDIGO 2012 risk categories (2011-2014). Values represent percentages of the NHANES 2011–2014 cohort in each risk category. (B) Prevalence of chronic kidney disease in the United States based on NHANES (1999–2014). (A, Adapted from United States Renal Data System. 2016 USRDS annual data report: Volume 1 Table 1.1. Epidemiology of kidney disease in the United States. National Institutes of Health, National Institute of Diabetes and Digestive and Kidney Diseases, Bethesda, MD, 2016. B, Data source: National Health and Nutrition Examination Survey (NHANES), 1999–2002, 2003–2006, 2007–2010 & 2011–2014 participants aged 20 and older. Single-sample estimates of eGFR and ACR; eGFR calculated using the CKD-EPI equation. From US Renal Data System. 2016 USRDS annual data report: Volume 1 Table 1.1. Epidemiology of kidney disease in the United States. National Institutes of Health, National Institute of Diabetes and Digestive and Kidney Diseases, Bethesda, MD, 2016.)

In particular, even if CKD prevalence stabilized among diabetics, the full effect of the obesity epidemic on diabetes and its consequences will take time to fully materialize.

CKD prevalence information in the United States is also available through claims data for services provided to healthcare beneficiaries. Lack of a universal healthcare system in the United States limits the ability to obtain this data. Although prevalence estimates from population-based samples, such as NHANES, are more standardized and representative for estimating disease prevalence, review of claims-based data allows for an estimation of provider assessment of CKD, estimation of costs associated with CKD care, as well as a larger sample size. The 2016 USRDS ADR provides useful data.[53] Prevalence estimates of CKD based on claims data from Medicare (≥65 years of age) rose from 3% in 2000 to 10% in 2014 (Fig. 1.7). However, these data reflect trends in recognition and coding of CKD as much as the disease itself, as even the current prevalence estimates are more than threefold lower than estimates in NHANES at this age range. Testing for albuminuria among Medicare patients age ≥65 years of age is increasing but is still only 40% in diabetes and 20% in hypertension without diabetes.[53] This is also consistent with the low rates of awareness of CKD. Overall, only approximately 10% of NHANES participants with CKD reported awareness of having weak or failing kidneys; even at stage G4 CKD, this rate is <50%, although this is an increase from <40%.[53] Overall, CKD remains largely unrecognized, and consequently metabolic complications of CKD are unlikely to be identified and/or treated.

European CKD Prevalence: Studies of CKD burden in Europe were recently reviewed and their results aggregated.[54,55] Overall, the results support a high prevalence of CKD similar to that of the United States. However, the review

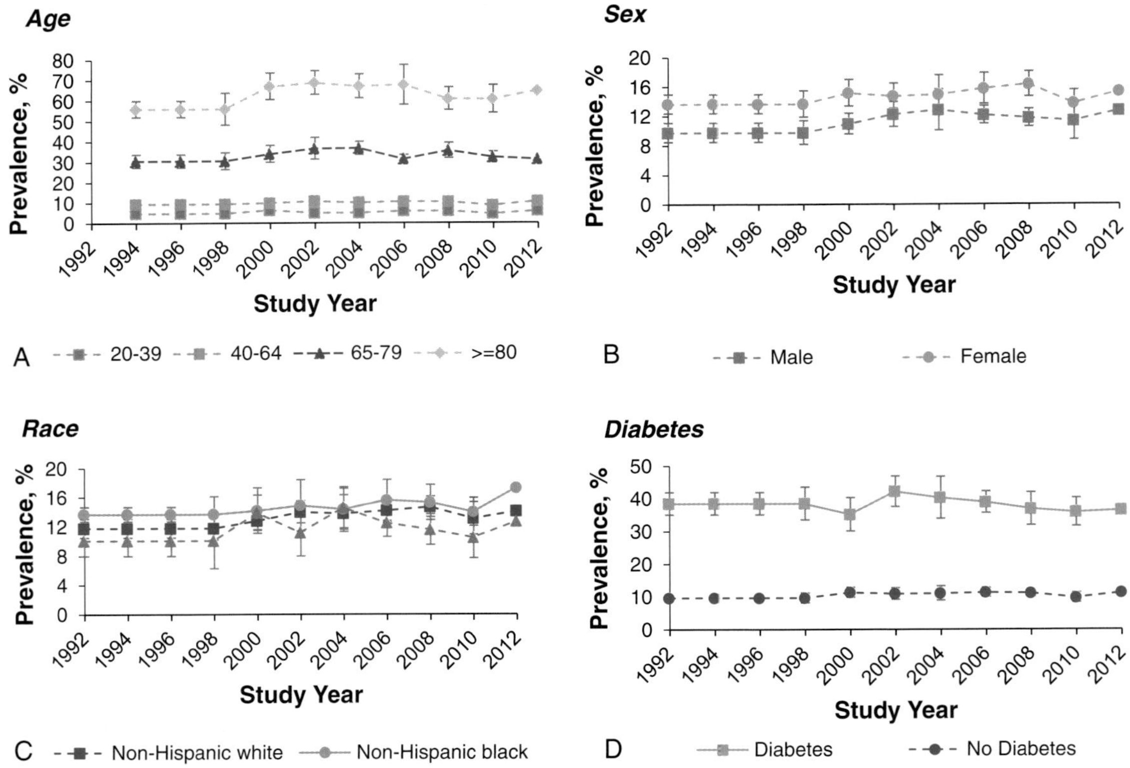

FIG. 1.5 Adjusted prevalence of CKD stages 3 and 4 (estimated glomerular filtration rate of 15 to 59 mL/min/1.73 m^2 calculated with chronic kidney cisease epidemiology collaboration equation) in US adults by (A) age, (B) sex, (C) race/ethnicity, and (D) presence or absence of diabetes, NHANES 1988–1994 through 2011–2012. Each subgroup is adjusted for the other 3 subgroup variables (e.g., age-specific prevalence is adjusted for sex, race/ethnicity, and diabetes status). *NHANES,* National Health and Nutrition Examination Survey. (Adapted from Murphy D, McCulloch CE, Lin F, et al. Trends in prevalence of chronic kidney disease in the United States. *Ann Intern Med.* 2016;165(7):473-481.)

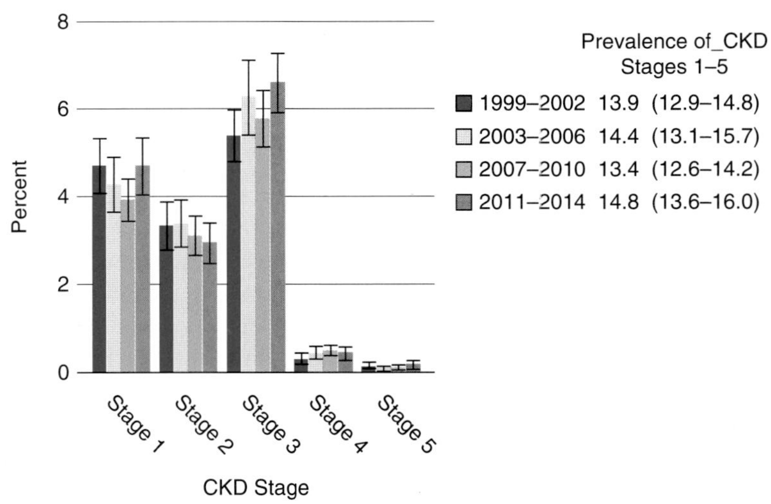

FIG. 1.6 Prevalence of CKD by stage among NHANES participants, 1999–2014. (Data source: National Health and Nutrition Examination Survey (NHANES), 1999–2002, 2003–2006, 2007–2010 & 2011–2014 participants aged 20 & older. Whisker lines indicate 95% confidence intervals. Abbreviation: CKD, chronic kidney disease. From US Renal Data System, 2016 USRDS annual data report: Volume 1. Fig. 1.1. Epidemiology of kidney disease in the United States. National Institutes of Health. National Institute of Diabetes and Digestive and Kidney Disease, Bethesda, MD, 2016.)

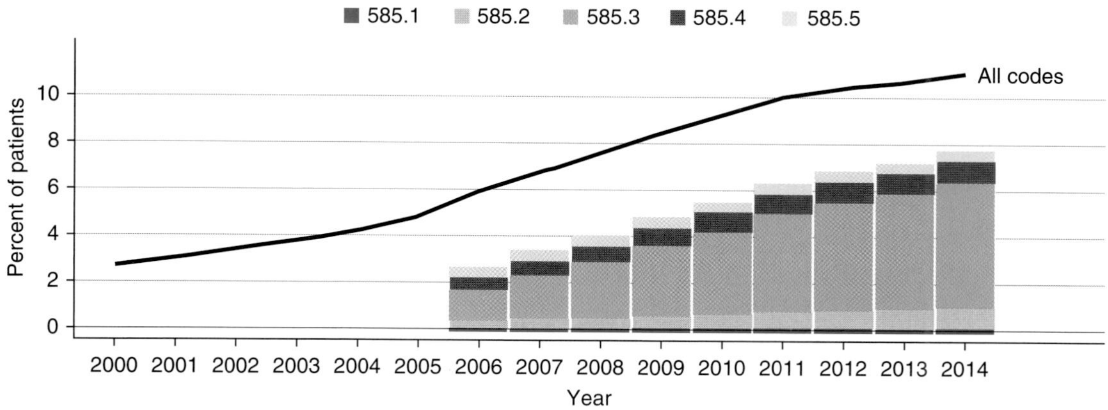

FIG. 1.7 Trends in prevalence of recognized CKD, overall and by CKD stage, among Medicare patients (aged 65+ years), 2000–2014. (Data source: National Health and Nutrition Examination Survey (NHANES), 1999–2002, 2003–2006, 2007–2010 & 2011–2014 participants aged 20 & older. Whisker lines indicate 95% confidence intervals. From US Renal Data System, 2016 USRDS annual data report: Volume 1. Figure i.4. Epidemiology of kidney disease in the United States. National Institutes of Health. National Institute of Diabetes and Digestive and Kidney Disease, Bethesda, MD, 2016.)

pointed out marked variation in prevalence across countries, from 3.3% in Norway to 17.3% in northwest Germany. However, the studies represent a very limited geography when data are focused solely on high-quality studies. Much of the variation persisted despite stratification by diabetes and hypertension and attempts to standardize definitions and assays. It is unclear how much of the variation is explained and how much is due to residual methodological variation.[56] The majority of studies did not report the sampling frame used and response rates varied from 10% to 87%. Further variation was seen in the creatinine assay (67% Jaffe and 13% enzymatic with 29% calibrated to isotope dilution mass spectrometry), the equation used to estimate GFR (52% CKD-EPI and 75% MDRD), definition of CKD (92% used eGFR<60), inclusion of urinary markers (in 60% of studies), and reporting of 95% CIs (39% of studies). The 2013 KDIGO guidelines keep the same definition of CKD but few of the studies to date incorporate the updated staging, which includes CGA as parallel measures.

Global CKD Prevalence: Estimates are now available from two metaanalyses[57,58] whose results were remarkably similar, although both note major limitations and methodological heterogeneity in the studies reviewed. A metaanalysis of 44 country prevalence studies, estimated the worldwide prevalence of CKD at 13.4% (95% CI, 11.7% to 15.1%).[58] A metaanalysis of 33 prevalence studies estimated worldwide prevalence of CKD by sex at 10.4% in men (95% CI, 9.3% to 11.9%) and 11.8% in women (95% CI, 11.2% to 12.6%).[57] Interestingly, prevalence estimates were about 15% higher in low- and middle-income countries than in high-income countries. Prevalence data in low- and middle-income countries were expanded by a study of convenience samples from 12 countries in six world regions.[59] They found a prevalence of 14.3% (95% CI, 14% to 14.5%) in general populations and 36.1% (95% CI, 34.7% to 37.6%) in high-risk populations. This study also confirmed that awareness of CKD remains very low (6% in the general populations and 10% in high-risk populations).[60]

Data from Asia are still limited but some studies provide interesting insights. In China, a large cross-sectional population-based study similar in design to NHANES estimated an overall 10.8% prevalence of CKD corresponding to 119 million people.[60] Interestingly, in China the prevalence of low GFR (1.7%; 95% CI, 1.5 to 1.9) was a smaller fraction than that of albuminuria (9.4%; 95% CI, 8.9 to 10). Furthermore, an analysis of 35 million patients hospitalized in tertiary (class 3) Chinese hospitals, which typically have over 500 beds and provide specialist health services, from 2010 to 2015 shows that the percentage of hospitalizations with CKD related to diabetes now exceeds the percentage related to glomerular nephritis.[61]

The Global Burden of Disease project estimated increasing prevalence of CKD over the past decade based on a complex Bayesian model integrating multiple sources of data globally with the caveat that the data completion index of decreased low GFR was poor.[62,63] They estimated that the aging of the global population completely accounted for the CKD rise. This is in contrast with other vascular diseases that have declined after age standardization. The 2016 estimated global prevalence among adults ≥20 years of age based on a Bayesian model summarizing the literature is 5.5% for low GFR (<60 mL/min/1.7 m^2), 0.1% for ESRD, 8.2% albuminuria, and 13.7% total CKD prevalence.[64]

Methodological limitations: Although the mounting evidence now makes it clear that the prevalence of CKD in the United States, Europe, and globally is high and the quality of the studies is improving, methodological limitations still leave uncertainty. Only a minority of studies use population-based random samples, standardized laboratory methods, and the latest staging of CKD. Trends in prevalence are particularly hard to study as populations change slowly and even small changes in creatinine calibration influence prevalence estimates meaningfully. For example, a 0.04 mg/dL higher mean serum creatinine due to calibration issues can contribute to meaningful changes (5% lower eGFR, 23% higher stage G3 CKD, and 12% higher overall CKD prevalence estimate for the United States).[50]

Incidence of Chronic Kidney Disease

Incidence of CKD is difficult to ascertain precisely as it requires establishment of a cohort without CKD at baseline with serial measurements of estimated GFR and albuminuria over a long period of time. Therefore generalizable databases comparing CKD incidence estimates over time and geography are limited. Most studies focusing on CKD incidence are studies of risk factors where the associations are of primary interest and absolute risk is of secondary interest. A number of the studies also require some measure of progression in addition to incidence.

KDIGO defines CKD progression as a decline in GFR staging category (GFR or albuminuria). A certain drop in eGFR is defined as a 25% or greater drop in eGFR from baseline.[53] Subsequent work showed that percent decline in eGFR is strongly and exponentially (log hazard ratio increases linearly with percent decline) associated with the risk for ESRD.[65] For defining CKD progression as a surrogate outcome for ESRD, 30% and 40% declines were evaluated in detail and shown that particularly if the decline is confirmed by a repeat visit, declines of this magnitude were very predictive. The most important caveat in using changes in estimated GFR to define CKD progression is the presence of acute effects on GFR (e.g., hemodynamic effects by blood pressure or angiotensin converting inhibitor use), which can alter the meaning of a GFR change. This is particularly worrisome when an acute decrement in GFR is thought to offer long-term protection for the kidney. It is noteworthy that even moderate acute effects (>1 to 2 mL/min/1.73 m^2) can invalidate the use of change in GFR as a surrogate for ESRD risk, although the larger the decrement used, the more robust the surrogacy.[66] Incidence of albuminuria is even more difficult to establish due to high biological variability and poorer standardization of measurements. Making progress in understanding the significance of changes in albuminuria, their relationship to risk, and their strengths and limitations as surrogates for ESRD is of great importance as albuminuria often is used to test early efficacy of treatments but its use as a definite surrogate outcome is debated.[67-70]

Examples of studies that focus on estimated GFR and incidence provide some useful data. CKD incidence was examined in the 2585 participants of the Framingham cohort who attended both a baseline examination from 1978 to 1982 and a follow-up examination from 1998 to 2001, and were free of kidney disease at baseline. CKD was defined as eGFR (by MDRD equation) in the fifth or lower percentile (≤59.25 mL/min/1.73 m^2 in women; ≤64.25 mL/min/1.73 m^2 in men). CKD developed in 9.4% of participants over the follow-up period and was associated with baseline GFR, diabetes, hypertension, and smoking.[71] In a later pair of Framingham heart study examinations, albuminuria (defined as albumin to creatinine ratio ≥17 mg/g in men or ≥25 mg/g in women) developed in 10% of participants who did not have albuminuria over the 9.5 years.[72] Although some of the incidence may be due to biological variability, incidence of albuminuria was associated with older age, baseline diabetes, smoking, and baseline log urine albumin-to-creatinine ratio (UACR) and negatively associated with female sex and high-density lipoprotein cholesterol. Incident CKD was examined in the ARIC (Atherosclerosis Risk in Communities) study participants, including 3859 African American and 10,661 white adults 45 to 64 years of age without severe kidney dysfunction at baseline in 1987 to 1989. Incident CKD was defined as hospitalization or death with kidney disease or increase in serum creatinine level of 0.4 mg/dL. During median follow-up of 14 years, CKD developed in 1060 individuals (incidence per 1000 person-years: 5.5 overall; 8.8 in African Americans, and 4.4 in whites).[73] ARIC also showed that patients with incident CKD are less likely to come to repeat visits. In the CARDIA (Coronary Artery Risk Development in Young Adults) study, eGFR by creatinine and cystatin C and UACR were measured at scheduled examinations and used to define CKD incidence and relate it to race and *APOL1* genetic susceptibility. An early study reported higher incidence based on eGFR of <60 and 25% decline in African Americans.[74] For albuminuria, the incidence rate per 1000 person-years (95% CI) over 15 years was 15 (11 to 22) for *APOL1* high-risk blacks, 8 (6 to 9) for APOL1 low-risk blacks, and 4 (3 to 5) for whites.[37] A higher incidence of CKD defined by GFR estimated from cystatin C <60 mL/min/1.73 m^2 and declining by ≥1 mL/min/1.73 m^2 was also found among African Americans and Hispanics in MESA (Multi-Ethnic Study of Atherosclerosis).[75] The differences between whites and low-risk blacks were explained by baseline risk factors. In a 10-year prospective cohort study of 104,523 Korean men and 52,854 Korean women, aged 35 to 59 years who attended Korea Medical Insurance Corporation health examinations and who did not have proteinuria at baseline, incident proteinuria developed in 3951 men (3.8%) and 1527 women (2.9%) and the associated risk factors were diabetes, male gender, and obesity.[76]

A complementary approach to incidence is to examine the rate of decline in eGFR as a slope or GFR trajectory. This is particularly effective in high-risk populations such as patients with CKD or diabetes[77] but has been applied to general population studies as well.[37,38,78] GFR estimated by cystatin C shows a greater decline with age than estimates from serum creatinine.[79] It is also worth noting that slope estimates over longer periods of time and at lower GFR are associated with greater risk.[65]

Prevalence and Incidence of Kidney Failure

Advanced CKD, stage G5 (eGFR <15 mL/min/1.73 m^2), is referred to as having kidney failure but only a subset of these cases are treated with KRT. Patients who start KRT are referred to as having reached ESRD or end-stage kidney disease (ESKD). However, the term *kidney replacement therapy,* which includes hemodialysis, peritoneal dialysis, and kidney transplantation, has the advantage of avoiding the negative and poorly defined connotations of "end-stage." The use of the term *ESRD* in the United States dates back to 1972 when Congress passed legislation authorizing the End-Stage Renal

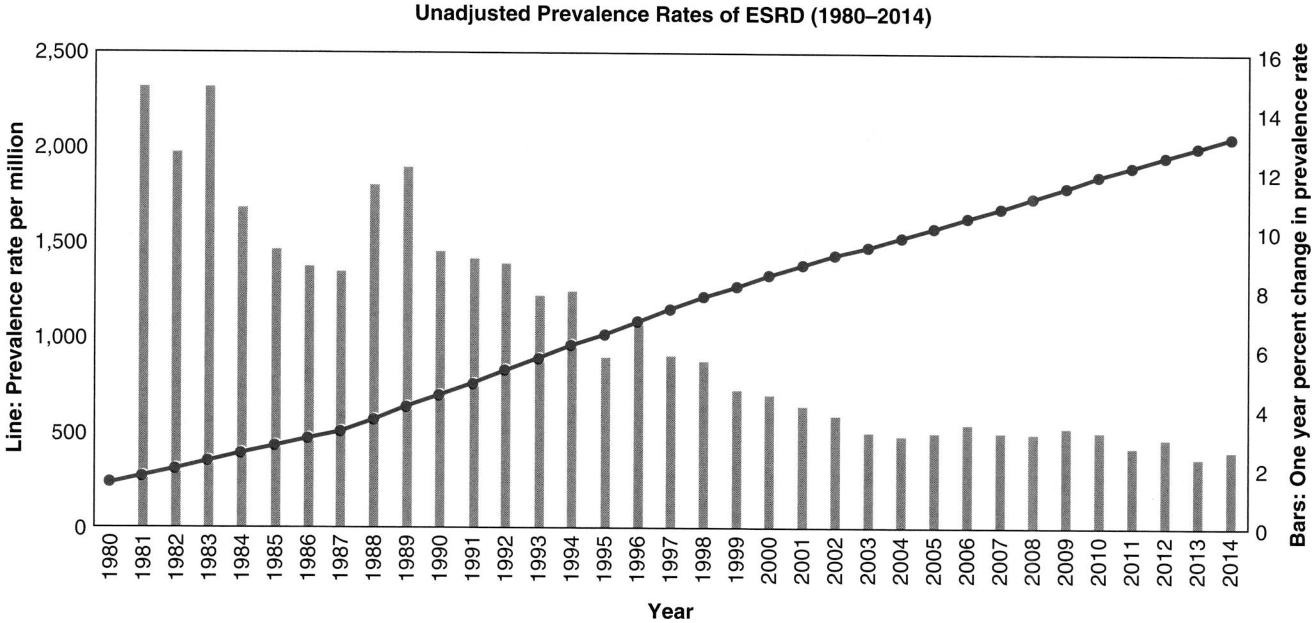

FIG. 1.8 Unadjusted prevalence rates of ESRD in the United States (1980–2014). Patients with unknown age, race dropped. (Data from US Renal Data System. *2014 USRDS annual data report: Epidemiology of kidney disease in the United States*. National Institutes of Health, National Institute of Diabetes and Digestive and Kidney Diseases, Bethesda, MD, 2014, and US Renal Data System. *2016 USRDS annual data report: Epidemiology of kidney disease in the United States*. National Institutes of Health, National Institute of Diabetes and Digestive and Kidney Diseases, Bethesda, MD, 2016.)

Disease (ESRD) program under Medicare (Section 299I of Public Law 92-603). Coverage for ESRD, considered a "rare" disease at the time, was authorized for all individuals regardless of their age if they would otherwise be eligible for social security benefits. In the United States, The USRDS collects, analyzes, and distributes information about ESRD. The USRDS is funded by the National Institute of Diabetes and Digestive and Kidney Diseases (NIDDK) in conjunction with the Centers for Medicare & Medicaid Services (CMS). The USRDS has become an excellent resource for providing precise data on ESRD in the United States, as well as summaries from international registries, and publishes an ADR summarizing its findings. The 2016 ADR includes data up until 2014. The most up-to-date data are available at www.usrds.org.

It is important to note that many patients experience a slow decline in GFR and can avoid dialysis for a long period of time. Many others succumb to complications of CKD and CVD without ever starting dialysis. Deaths often outnumber incident dialysis cases with the ratio increasing with age and lower kidney function.[80-82] Thus ESRD defined as kidney failure treated with dialysis or transplantation reflects not only incidence but also availability and acceptance into the dialysis or transplantation programs that vary over time and place. Prevalence estimates further include survival on dialysis or transplantation.

Prevalence of Treated Kidney Failure

In the United States, ESRD at its inception was expected to plateau at 40,000 prevalent patients, a number that was reached over 30 years ago. At the end of 2014, there were 678,383 prevalent dialysis and transplant patients receiving treatment for ESRD for an unadjusted prevalence of 2067 per million in the US population. The unadjusted prevalence rate of ESRD continues to rise in the United States (Fig. 1.8) despite a plateau in incidence. The crude prevalence rise was 2.6% from 2013 and 34% from 2004 to 2014; whereas the adjusted prevalence rose 1.1% and 12% during the same time, indicating that much of the increase was due to changing demographics of the US population. The prevalence of ESRD has increased the most among persons ≥75 years of age, exceeding 6000 per million population, reflecting a doubling since 1996. This prevalence is now nearly equal to that for 65- to 74-year-olds, but numerically the largest single age group receiving RRT is still those aged 45 to 64 years. Prevalent ESRD rates continue to reflect the race and ethnic disparities observed with incident ESRD. In 2014 prevalence of ESRD adjusted for age and sex was 5004 per million population in African Americans, 2691 per million population in Native Americans, 1831 per million population among Asians, and 1194 per million population among whites. Diabetes continues to be the leading assigned cause for prevalent ESRD patients (604 per million population) followed by hypertension and glomerulonephritis. In the United States, hemodialysis is the dominant therapy (63% of all prevalent ESRD cases and 88% of incident cases), with 6.9% of ESRD cases being treated with peritoneal dialysis, and 29.6% with a functioning kidney transplant in 2014. Among hemodialysis cases, 88% used in-center hemodialysis, and 1.8% used home hemodialysis.

Globally, our understanding of KRT is based on a combination of registry data and estimates based on models where data are limited. Liyanage et al.[83] estimated that in 2010, 2.6 million

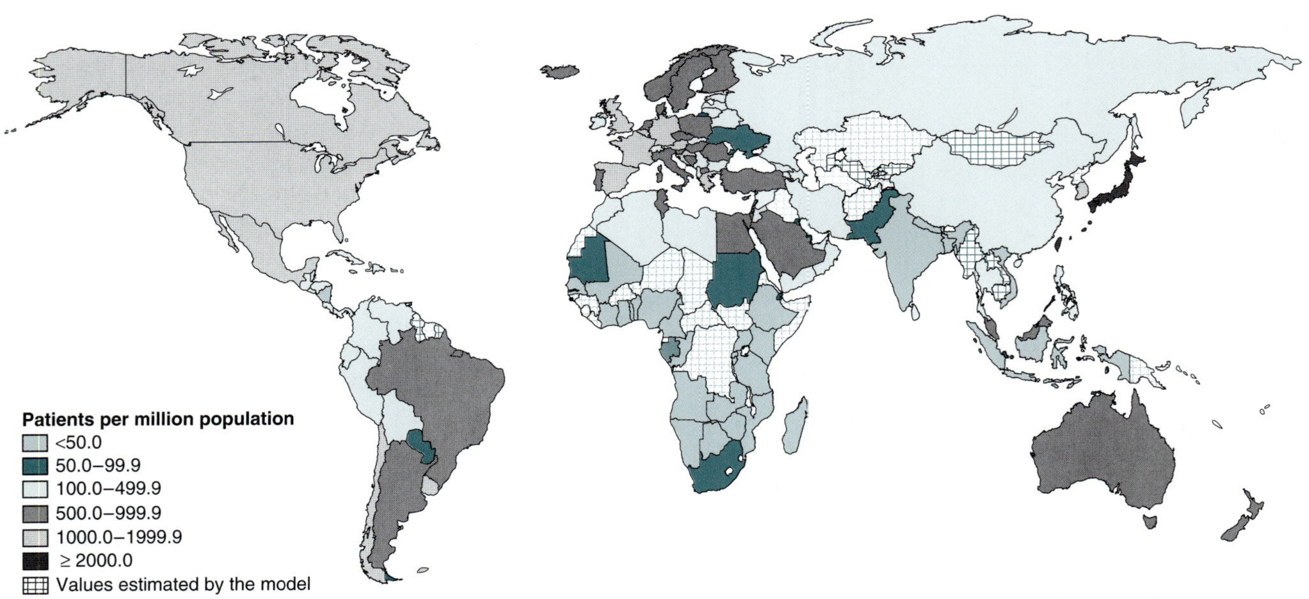

FIG. 1.9 Patients receiving renal replacement therapy in 2010. (From Liyanage T, Ninomiya T, Jha V, et al. Worldwide access to treatment for end-stage kidney disease: A systematic review. *Lancet.* 2015;385(9981):1975-1982.)

people received KRT worldwide; whereas the number of patients needing KRT is between 4.9 and 9.7 million. Prevalence rates of KRT are highest in North America, Europe, and high-income Asian countries including Taiwan and Japan (Fig. 1.9), but Asia already has the highest number of patients on RRT because of its large population (Fig. 1.10). Liyanage et al. confirmed the very strong relationship between KRT prevalence and per-capita income (Fig. 1.11). This relationship is stronger than the relationship to the prevalence of diabetes, suggesting availability and affordability of KRT is still rate-limiting in many settings globally. As a result, Liyanage et al. projected that with rising global incomes, worldwide use of RRT is projected to more than double to 5.4 million people by 2030, with the most growth in Asia (1 million to a projected 2.2 million) and most rapid relative increase projected in Latin America.

In a complete registry data on KRT, among 3 million urban insured employees in Nanjing,[84] trends from 2005 to 2014 revealed that although RRT incidence rates decreased, survival improved, prevalence increased, and importantly, the base urban insured population doubled. Hence, they conclude that there is a real threat of ESRD confronting China during its process of healthcare transition. In India, MDS (Million Death Study),[85] which used an enhanced verbal autopsy tool between 2001 and 2013, found 2.9% of deaths were due to renal failure in 2010 to 2013 among 15- to 69-year-olds, an increase of 50% from 2001 to 2003. Diabetes was the largest factor leading to renal failure deaths. This is likely an underestimate given the nonspecific nature of renal symptoms.

Incidence of Treated Kidney Failure

In the United States, 120,688 individuals reached ESRD in 2014, reflecting an age, race, and sex-adjusted incidence of 354 per million population. Adjusted incidence rates rose dramatically until 2000, plateaued for the subsequent decade, and have declined or stayed stable since (Fig. 1.12). Several factors play a role in the rising incidence of ESRD, but perhaps the most important reason is liberalization of criteria for accepting patients for RRT. With aging and increased population burden of diabetes, hypertension, and obesity, the absolute numbers of patients initiating RRT continues to increase even as adjusted incidence rates decline. Similarly, US incidence rates have declined among those ≥65 years of age, but the aging of the population results in the ESRD population being older as well.

Globally, the incidence of KRT is dominated by increasing access to dialysis in developing middle-income countries where the burden of CKD is high and KRT rates are strongly linked to gross national income and are projected to increase as incomes rise.[83]

COSTS OF CHRONIC KIDNEY DISEASE

The KDOQI classification and the new CKD diagnostic billing codes introduced in 2006 have allowed for improved enumeration of costs. Costs for CKD care can be divided into costs for CKD patients not on KRT and KRT costs. It is important to note that most available data are limited to healthcare insurance claims, and little information is available on the nonmedical costs of CKD and its complications.[86]

Chronic Kidney Disease (Not on Kidney Replacement Therapy) Costs

The 2016 USRDS ADR reports the economic effects of CKD using the Medicare 5% sample. Since approximately 98% of US adults ≥65 years of age qualify for Medicare, these data are representative of US adults ≥65. Important caveats to the data are the growth of Medicare managed-care plans with capitated payments without specific billing data. The data on the rising costs associated with CKD also should be considered with the increasing ascertainment of CKD in mind; in Medicare beneficiaries ≥65 of age, claims-based identification of CKD was 1.7% in 1995, 3.8% in 2003, and 11.1% in 2014.

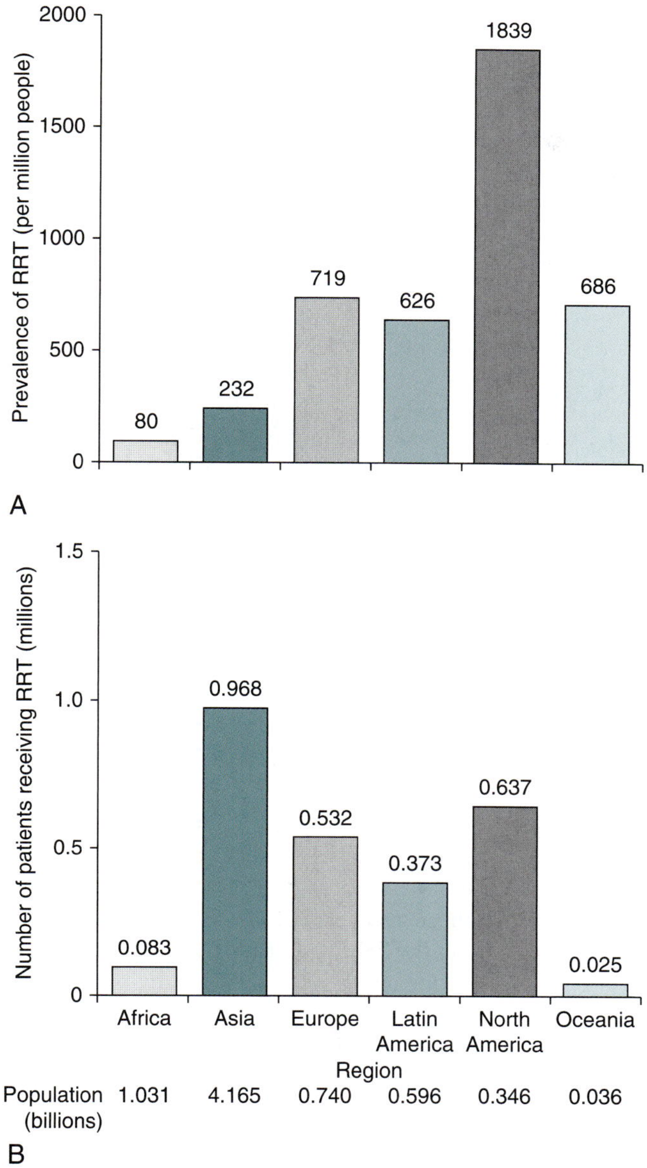

FIG. 1.10 Worldwide prevalence by (A) number of patients and (B) number receiving renal replacement therapy (RRT). (From Liyanage T, Ninomiya T, Jha V, et al. Worldwide access to treatment for end-stage kidney disease: A systematic review. *Lancet*. 2015;385(9981):1975-1982.)

CKD is an important cost multiplier in the Medicare population. In 2014 Medicare expenditures for CKD patients (not including ESRD) were \$52.9 billion. The CKD expenditures exceeded Medicare spending on ESRD, which was \$30.9 billion in 2014. The total costs for care of Medicare beneficiaries ≥65 years of age with CKD, congestive heart failure, and diabetes mellitus are described in Fig. 1.13. Patients with CKD comprise 10.8% of the CKD population but account for 20.8% of the total Medicare non-ESRD spending. Fig. 1.14 describes the per-person per-year (PPPY) costs for Medicare beneficiaries with CKD (but not ESRD), highlighting the cost multiplier effect of CKD. The major component of the PPPY costs include inpatient hospitalizations (34%) and physician/supplier services (23%).

End-Stage Renal Disease Costs

Costs of RRT include expenses of the dialysis treatment (peritoneal or hemodialysis); creation of access for dialysis treatment; hospitalizations due to cardiovascular, infectious, and access-related complications; transplant-related costs including costs of organ procurement, surgery, and immunosuppression; as well as costs of medications used for treatment of anemia (erythropoietin supplementation agents and iron) and hyperparathyroidism (vitamin D analogs). The high disease burden of this population contributes to high utilization of healthcare resources.

In 2014 ESRD costs as determined by Medicare spending were \$32.8 billion or 7.2% of the Medicare budget. Although the overall ESRD costs continue to increase, the PPPY costs have remained flat for the last several years. The increase in total costs reflects an increase in the total number of patients treated for ESRD. Fig. 1.15 describes the trends in PPPY cost for treatment of ESRD over the past decade.

OUTCOMES OF CHRONIC KIDNEY DISEASE

CKD is progressive disorder associated with a myriad concurrent complications and elevated risk for future outcomes. Some of these complications are directly consequences of loss of kidney function such as volume overload, hyperkalemia, hyperphosphatemia, metabolic acidosis, secondary hyperparathyroidism, as well as anemia and hypertension. Many complications are also the result of treatment of causes of CKD as in the case of

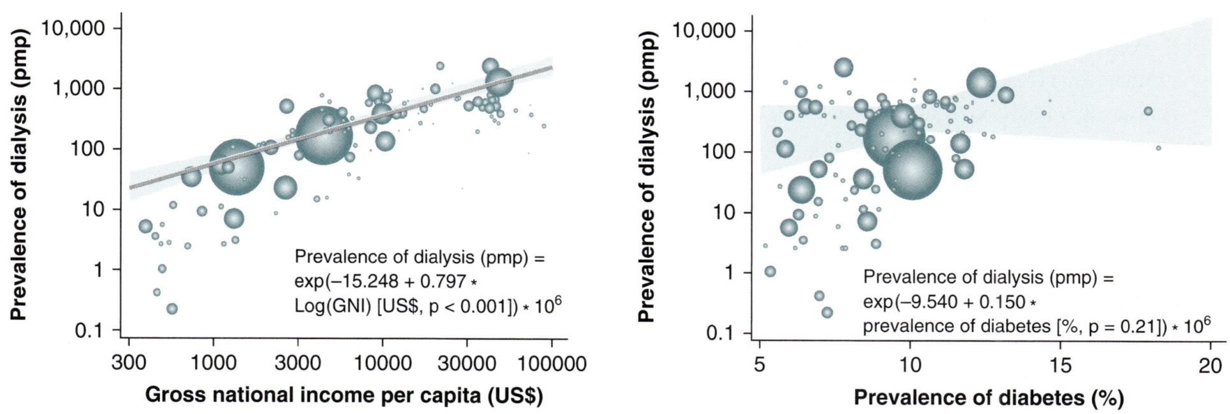

FIG. 1.11 Association between prevalence of dialysis in 123 countries and (gross national income per capita *(left)*, prevalence of diabetes *(right)*. (From Liyanage T, Ninomiya T, Jha V, et al. Worldwide access to treatment for end-stage kidney disease: A systematic review. *Lancet*. 2015;385(9981):1975-1982.)

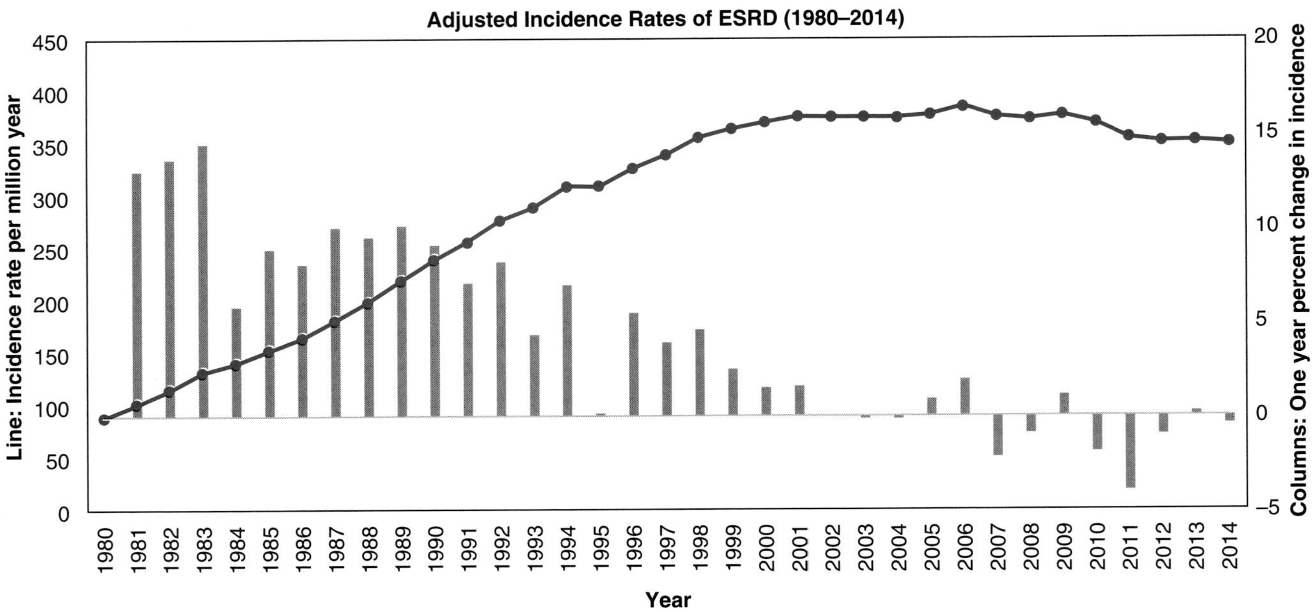

FIG. 1.12 Adjusted Incident Rates of ESRD in the United States (1980–2014). Adjusted for age, sex, race, and ethnicity. Patients with unknown age, race dropped. (Data from US Renal Data System. *2014 USRDS annual data report: Epidemiology of kidney disease in the United States*. National Institutes of Health, National Institute of Diabetes and Digestive and Kidney Diseases, Bethesda, MD, 2014, and US Renal Data System. *2016 USRDS annual data report: Epidemiology of kidney disease in the United States*. National Institutes of Health, National Institute of Diabetes and Digestive and Kidney Diseases, Bethesda, MD, 2016.)

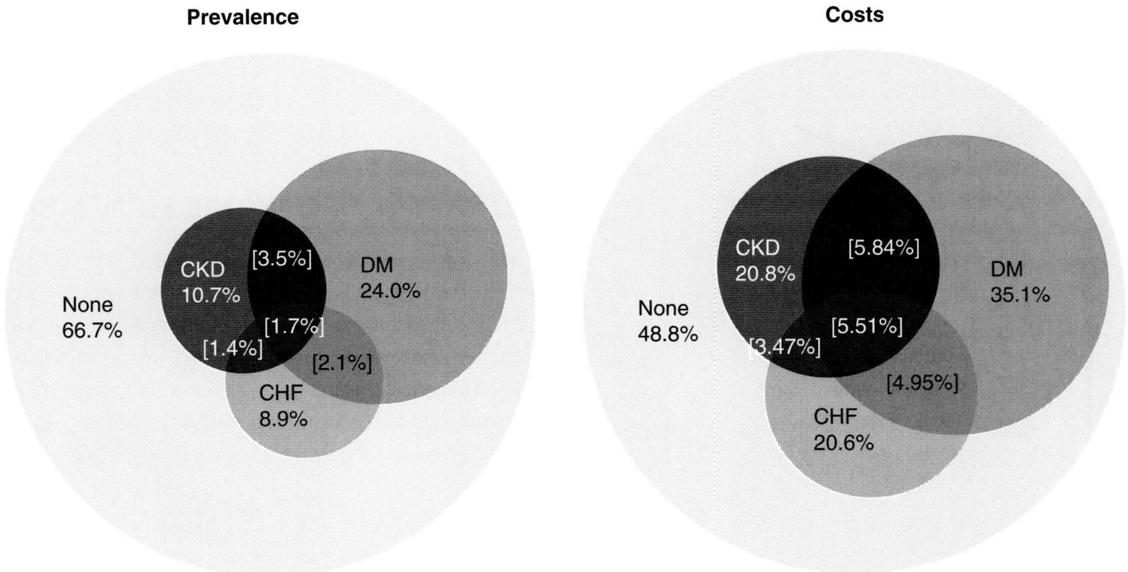

FIG. 1.13 Prevalence and cost of Medicare beneficiaries aged 65 and older by outcome in 2014. Percentages include the bracketed subsets. *CHF,* Congestive heart failure; *CKD,* chronic kidney disease; *DM,* diabetes mellitus. (Adapted from US Renal Data System, 2016 USRDS annual data report: Volume 1, Table 6.1 Epidemiology of kidney disease in the United States. National Institutes of Health. National Institute of Diabetes and Digestive and Kidney Disease, Bethesda, MD, 2016.)

chemotherapy for glomerulonephritis. Future outcomes whose risk is elevated include the most direct outcome of kidney failure and the need for KRT but equally important are an elevated risk for death and CVD and an increasing recognition that CKD-associated risks extend broadly.

It is important to note that markers of severity such as eGFR and albuminuria have a different importance for different outcomes. In addition, risk for different outcomes will depend on a range of other covariates including some that are not CKD measures such as age, sex, and others that relate to CKD but have a strong additional effect such as hypertension and heart failure. Communicating a full picture of prognosis in CKD without making a system that is too complex to be useful is a major challenge. Discussion of all these complications

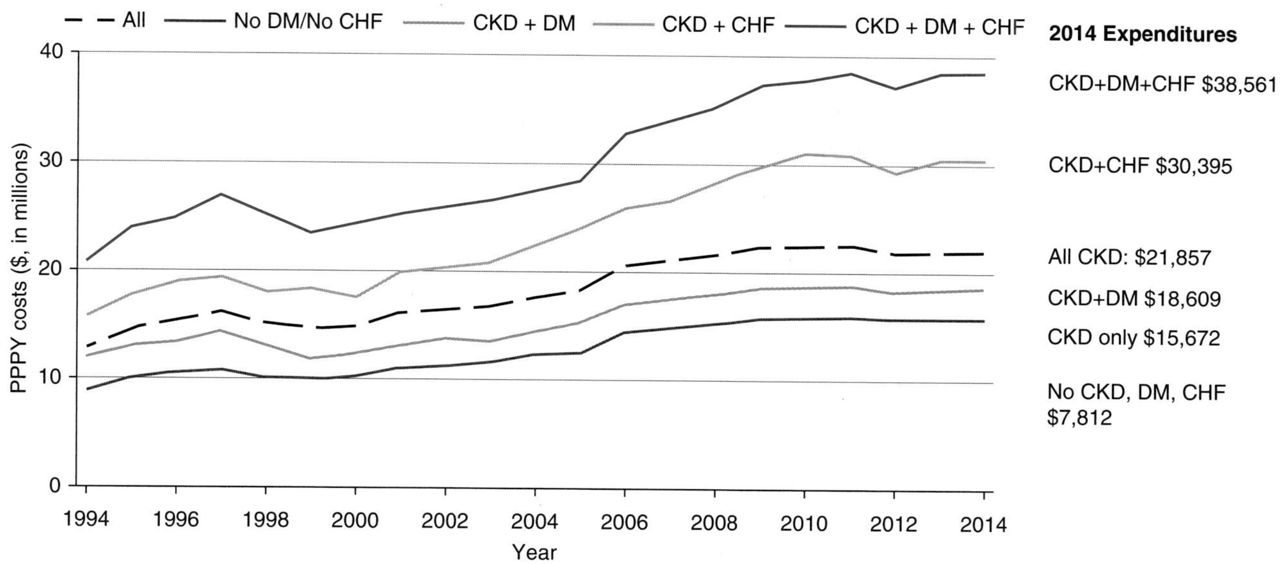

FIG. 1.14 Per-person per-year Medicare Parts A, B, and D fee-for-service spending for CKD patients aged 65 and older, by outcome. *CHF,* Congestive heart failure; *CKD,* chronic kidney disease; *DM,* diabetes mellitus; *ESRD,* end-stage renal disease; *PPPY,* per person per year. (From US Renal Data System, 2016 USRDS annual data report: Volume 1, Figure 6.5. Epidemiology of kidney disease in the United States. National Institutes of Health. National Institute of Diabetes and Digestive and Kidney Disease, Bethesda, MD, 2016.)

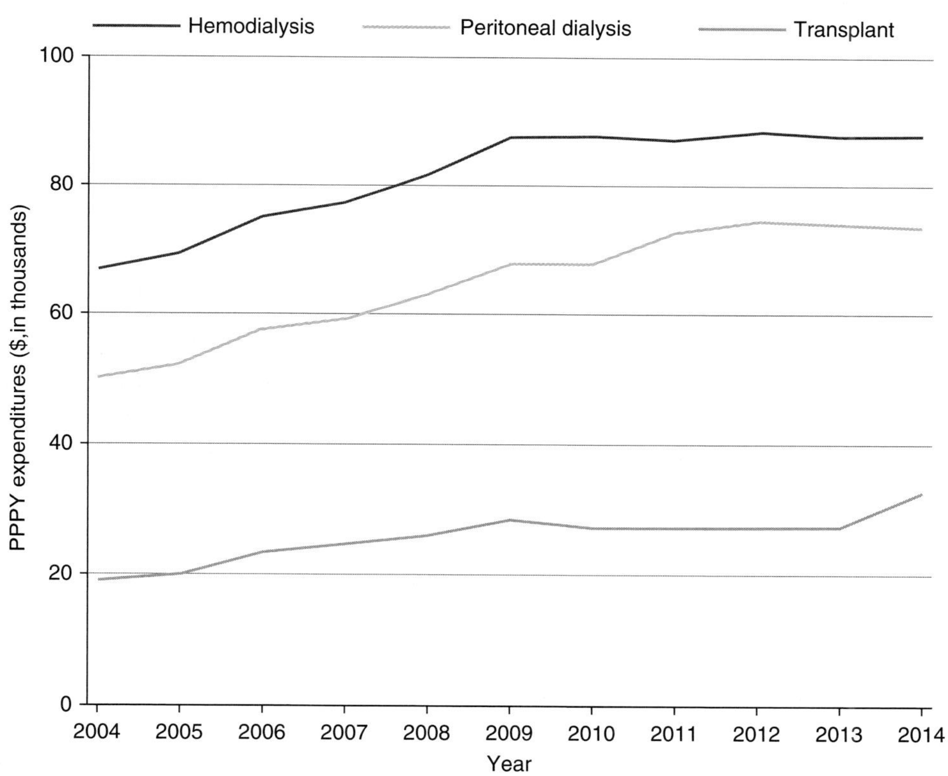

FIG. 1.15 Total Medicare ESRD expenditures per person per year, by modality, 2004–2014. *ESRD,* End-stage renal disease; *PPPY,* per person per year. (From US Renal Data System, 2016 USRDS annual data report: Volume 2, Figure 11.5. Epidemiology of kidney disease in the United States. National Institutes of Health. National Institute of Diabetes and Digestive and Kidney Disease, Bethesda, MD, 2016.)

is beyond the scope of this chapter. Instead, we focus on the epidemiological associations between CKD (not on dialysis), CVD, and related morbidity and mortality including the potential prognostic role of albuminuria. We then provide an overview of morbidity and mortality associated with ESRD.

Outcomes Before Kidney Replacement Therapy

Large epidemiological studies have demonstrated the increased risk for mortality with reduced level of GFR and presence of albuminuria. To address concerns about whether the definition of CKD is associated with risk at all ages and

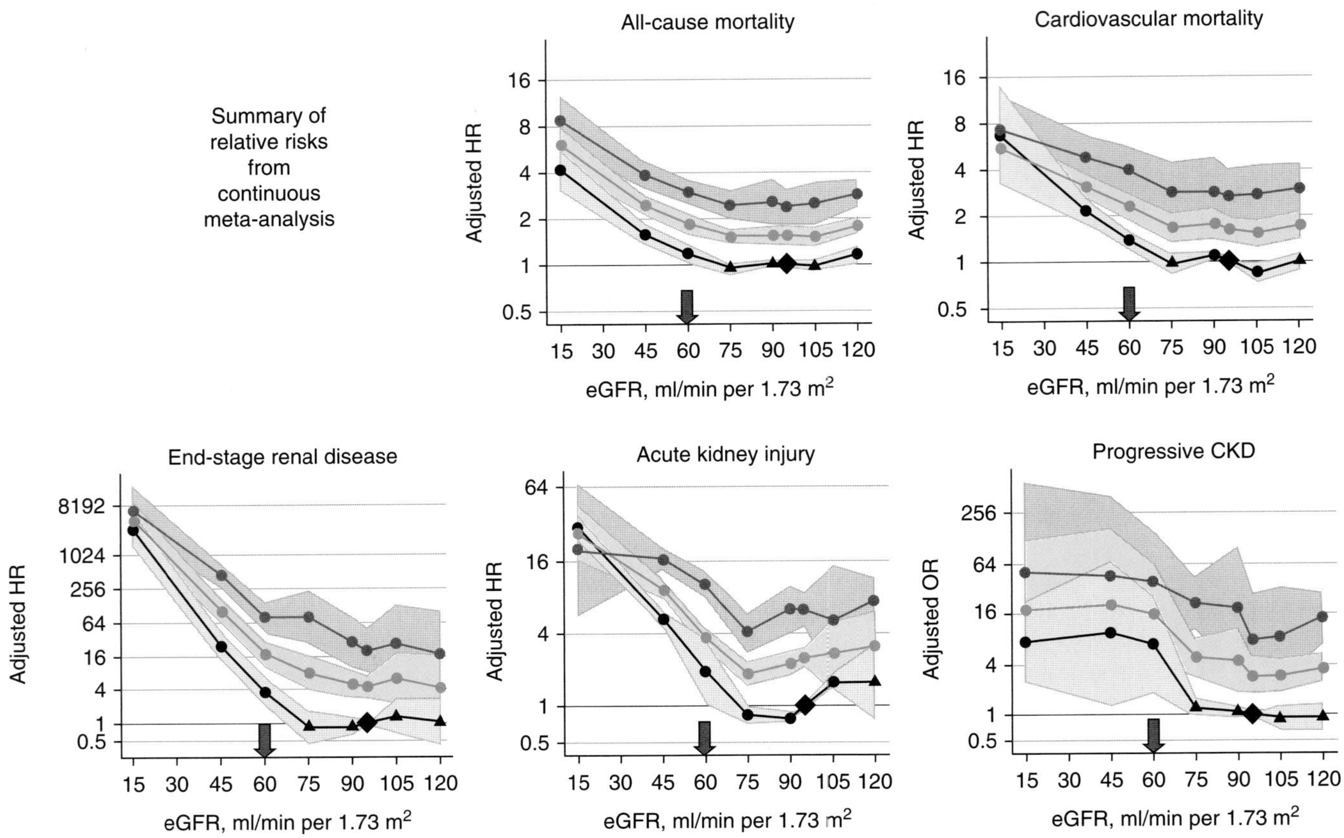

FIG. 1.16 Relative risks of multiple outcomes based on continuous meta-analysis. The three lines represent: urine ACR of <30 mg/g or dipstick negative and trace (black), urine ACR 30–299 mg/g or dipstick 1+ positive (green), and urine ACR ≥300 mg/g or dipstick ≥ 2+ positive (gray). All results are adjusted for covariates and compared with reference point of eGFR of 95 ml/min per 1.73m^2 and ACR of <30 mg/g or dipstick negative (diamond). Each point represents the pooled relative risk from a meta-analysis. Solid circles indicate statistical significance compared with the reference point (P = 0.05); triangles indicate nonsignificance. Arrows indicate eGFR of 60 ml/min per 1.73m^2, threshold value of eGFR for the current definition of chronic kidney disease (CKD). *HR,* Hazards ratio; *OR,* odds ratio. (From Levey AS, de Jong PE, Coresh J, et al. The definition, classification, and prognosis of chronic kidney disease: a KDIGO Controversies Conference report. *Kidney Int.* 2011;80(1):17-28.)

to solidify the role of albuminuria as a risk factor, a KDIGO controversies conference in 2009 assembled as much of the world's prospective data as possible. This led to the formation of the CKD Prognosis Consortium, which facilitates individual-level metaanalyses to advance CKD research. Fig. 1.16 shows an early publication that established that the risk for five examined complications was related exponentially (linear on the log relative hazard) to decreased GFR at levels below approximately 75 mL/min/1.73 m^2. Above this level, associations were flatter and a rise in risk has been reported at high eGFR. However, for all outcomes, eGFR of <60 mL/min/1.73 m^2 was associated with statistically significantly increased risk. In addition, at a higher level of albuminuria (red indicating >300 mg/g and green 30 to 299 mg/g), risk was higher than at a lower level of albuminuria (<30 mg/g). In fact, risk was lower at even lower levels of albuminuria within the normal range. The strong linear (log hazard ratio increased linearly with log albumin-to-creatinine ratio) association of albuminuria with risk was similar across a wide range of GFR, with the possible exception of very low GFR. This supported the two key dimensions of staging formalized in the 2013 KDIGO guidelines.

An important aspect of the mortality associated with CKD is the effect of age. Early studies raised the concern that although the risk for ESRD increased with lower GFR at all ages, the risk for mortality increased with age even faster, such that the threshold eGFR where the risk for ESRD exceeded risk for mortality became ever lower at older ages.[87] The effect of older participants being less likely to initiate RRT is only beginning to be understood.[88] However, a metaanalysis from the CKD Prognosis Consortium showed that both low eGFR and albuminuria were important risk predictors at all ages.[89] In fact, although relative hazards of mortality associated with lower GFR and albuminuria decreased with older age, the attributable risk increased. Furthermore, the relative hazards of ESRD were similar across the age range, although absolute risks declined at old age. This supported a staging system that uses the same principles for all ages but tailors treatments to age and other patient-specific risks and benefits.

A 2003 American Heart Association summary statement concluded that CKD appears to be an independent risk factor for CVD and reinforced the National Kidney Foundation guidelines for early recognition and treatment of CKD as well as screening individuals with CVD for the presence of CKD.[13] Subsequently, data supporting this association increased. It is

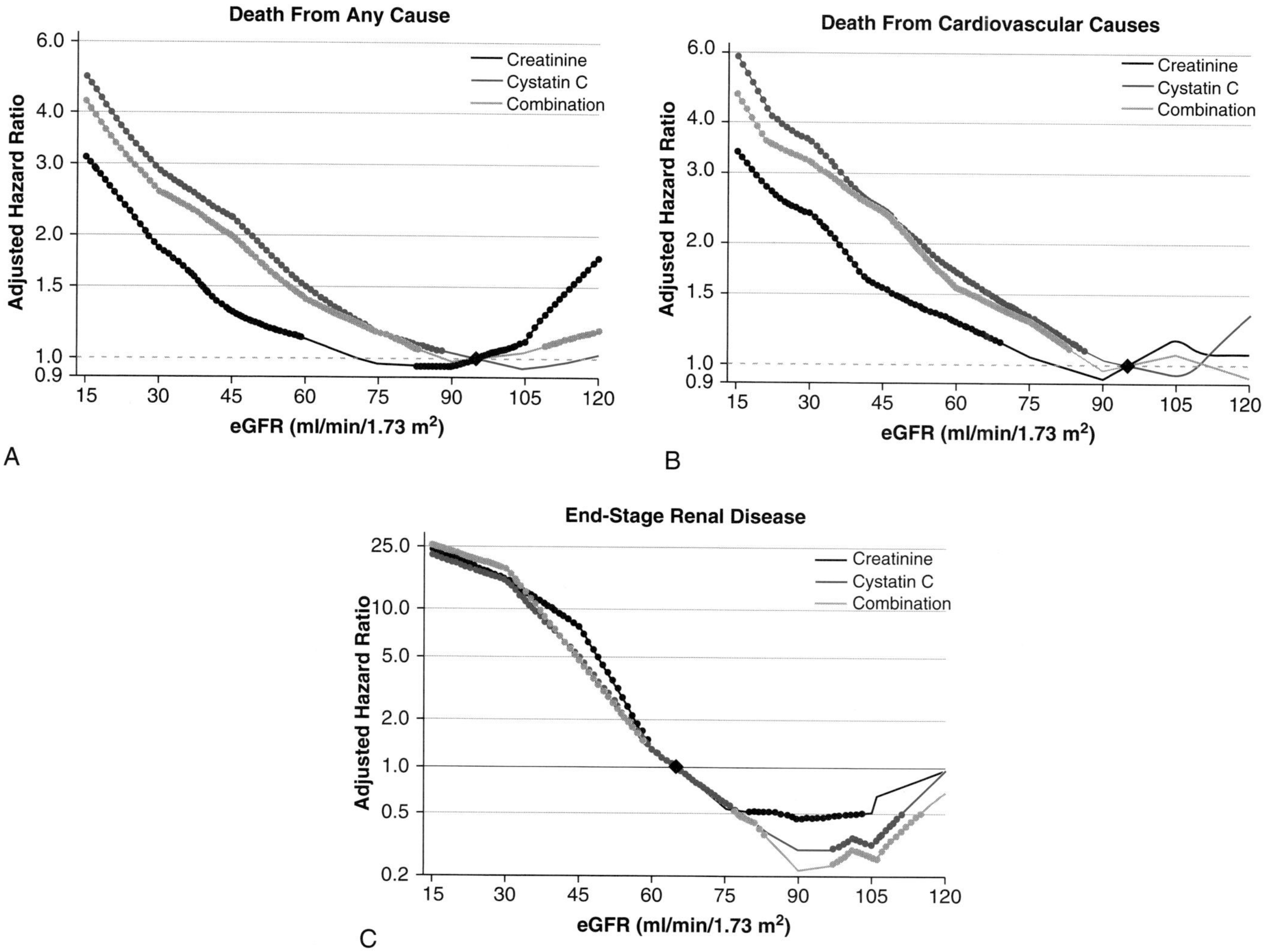

FIG. 1.17 Adjusted hazard ratios by eGFR and (A) death from any cause, (B) death from cardiovascular causes, (C) end-stage renal disease. Lines indicate measurement of eGFR by creatinine, cystatin C, or both. (From Shlipak MG, Matsushita K, Ärnlöv J, et al. Cystatin C versus creatinine in determining risk based on kidney function. *N Engl J Med.* 2013;369(10):932-943.)

also clear that compared with serum creatinine, using cystatin C as a marker of GFR results in stronger associations with the risk for mortality and CVD but not ESRD[18,19] (Fig. 1.17).

Concurrent complications of CKD likely explain the progressive increase in risk for future events. Metabolic abnormalities including anemia, acidosis, hypophosphatemia, hypoalbuminemia, hyperparathyroidism, and hypertension all increase with low GFR.[9] Associations of these abnormalities with albuminuria were much weaker than for GFR and nonexistent for hyperphosphatemia. In addition to these abnormalities, fluid retention and cardiac dysfunction are common with CKD.[2]

The 2016 USRDS ADR shows that hospitalizations in diagnosed CKD patients who are eligible for Medicare are more than twice as high as for those without CKD, adjusted for age, sex, and race.[53] Rates have been declining in both groups. The excess risk is seen across a wide range of hospitalization codes (congestive heart failure, atherosclerotic heart disease, and infections).

Data are not summarized for all outcomes. However, it is worth noting that presence of CKD is also a risk factor for development of AKI. In a study comparing 1746 hospitalized members of Kaiser Permanente who developed dialysis requiring AKI with 600,820 hospitalized members who did not, the adjusted risk for AKI was 2-fold, 6-fold, 29-fold, and 40-fold higher for those with baseline eGFR of 45 to 59, 30 to 44, 15 to 29, and <15 mL/min/1.73 m^2, respectively, compared with those with eGFR ≥60 mL/min/1.73 m^2.[90] Risk data on medication toxicity and other preventable outcomes are growing.

Global Burden of Disease estimates indicate that CKD is an important contributor to mortality and disability-adjusted life years (DALYs). Data on CKD, low GFR, and albuminuria are limited so the results rely on modeling assumptions but are interesting. Among the leading causes of global DALYs, CKD's rank rose to 22nd in 2016 from 24th in 2006 and 30th in 1990.[91] In the past decade, CKD has seen a 20% increase in DALYs, 6.8% rise in DALY rate, and −3% in age-standardized DALYs, indicating the rise is due to a growing and aging global population. In comparison, ischemic heart disease (IHD) and cerebrovascular disease were ranked the top two causes of global DALYs in 2016, but their age-adjusted DALYs decreased by 12% and 19%, showing an improvement that is lacking in CKD. Cerebrovascular disease or IHD were the leading cause of all-age DALYs for males in almost all Global Burden of Disease regions. Among a handful of exceptions was Nicaragua where CKD was the leading cause of DALYs for males in 2016.

Both Sexes, All Ages, 2016, Deaths per 100,000

	Low SDI	Low Mid SDI	Mid SDI	High Mid SDI	High SDI	SE & E Asia & Oceania	C & E Europe & C Asia	HI	Latin Am & Caribbean	MENA	S Asia	Sub-Sah Africa	Earth
High blood pressure	1	1	1	1	1	1	1	1	1	1	1	4	1
Smoking	11	3	2	2	2	2	4	2	4	5	4	13	2
High fasting plasma glucose	8	2	3	5	3	3	6	3	2	2	2	10	3
High body mass index	12	8	4	4	4	6	3	4	3	3	7	12	4
High total cholesterol	14	6	6	3	5	5	2	5	5	4	6	17	5
Ambient particulate matter	5	4	5	7	9	4	9	9	8	6	3	7	6
Alcohol use	13	13	8	6	7	8	5	7	6	25	17	11	7
Household air pollution	2	5	12	21	35	10	22	36	17	16	5	5	8
Impaired kidney function	16	11	9	10	6	12	11	6	7	7	10	16	9
Low whole grains	17	15	10	8	8	9	7	8	24	8	19	14	10
Low fruit	15	10	11	12	13	11	10	13	12	13	9	15	11
High sodium	22	20	7	11	10	7	12	10	13	14	16	23	12
Low nuts and seeds	19	12	13	9	11	13	8	11	9	9	12	19	13
Low birth weight & short gestation	3	7	21	25	32	24	25	32	16	11	11	1	14

FIG. 1.18 Ranking of risk factors for deaths by world region and globally (earth) in 2016. Risk factors ranking for deaths in 2016 per 100,000 among the following regions defined by development and geography. *E,* East; *HI,* high-income; *Latin Am,* Latin American; *MENA,* Middle East and North Africa; *S,* South; *SDI,* Socio-demographic Index; *SE,* Southeast; *Sub-Sah,* Sub-Saharan. (Data from courtesy of the Theo Vos, Institute for Health Metrics Research, based on data from Collaborators GBDRF. Global, regional, and national comparative risk assessment of 84 behavioural, environmental and occupational, and metabolic risks or clusters of risks, 1990-2016: a systematic analysis for the Global Burden of Disease Study 2016. *Lancet.* 2017;390(10100):1345-1422.)

GFR was added to the Global Burden of Disease metabolic risk factor analyses in 2015,[33] and albuminuria, summarized as kidney dysfunction, was incorporated into publications starting in 2017,[92] which refer to impaired kidney function as the combination of both low GFR and albuminuria. Although data are limited and methods are still evolving, the combination of low GFR and albuminuria is estimated to be the ninth risk factor for deaths globally and is ranked even higher among high-income countries and in Latin America and the Caribbean region (Fig. 1.18).[92] Because low GFR is most prevalent at older ages, the rank for low GFR and albuminuria for DALYs was somewhat lower at 13th in men and 11th in women in 2016, but this rose from 19th in both men and women in 1990. The map of DALYs lost due to low GFR shows the enormous burden in Latin America and Mexico (Fig. 1.19). The DALYs per 100,000 are also estimated to be high in Asia and Africa, but lower in North America and Europe despite a similar prevalence, presumably due to older age and better outcomes.

Outcomes on Kidney Replacement Therapy

Since 1996, the adjusted mortality rates of ESRD have decreased by 32% for dialysis patients and 44% for transplant recipients. A brief summary is provided here with details in separate chapters. The absolute mortality rates remain quite high. For patients reaching ESRD in 2009, 1-year age, sex, race/ethnicity, and cause of ESRD-adjusted mortality was 22.6% for hemodialysis, 12.8% for peritoneal dialysis, 7.7% for deceased donor transplant, and 2.9% for living donor transplant. The corresponding 5-year mortality was 58.5% for hemodialysis, 48.6% for peritoneal dialysis, 24.3% for deceased donor transplant, and 15.4% for living donor transplant. Of particular concern in relation to the pre-ESRD course is the high risk for death in hemodialysis patients during the initial months of hemodialysis. Specifically, among patients ≥65 years of age, the mortality rate peaks at 62 deaths per 100 patient-years at month 2 and then falls to 29.7 per 100 patient-years by month 12. For patients treated with peritoneal dialysis, this early spike is not seen. These differences may be due to differences in patient selection for dialysis modalities and predialysis care. CVD is the leading cause of death in dialysis patient; among patients with a known cause of death, 54% of all deaths are due to CVD and 38.7% of all deaths are due to arrhythmias and cardiac arrest (Fig. 1.20).

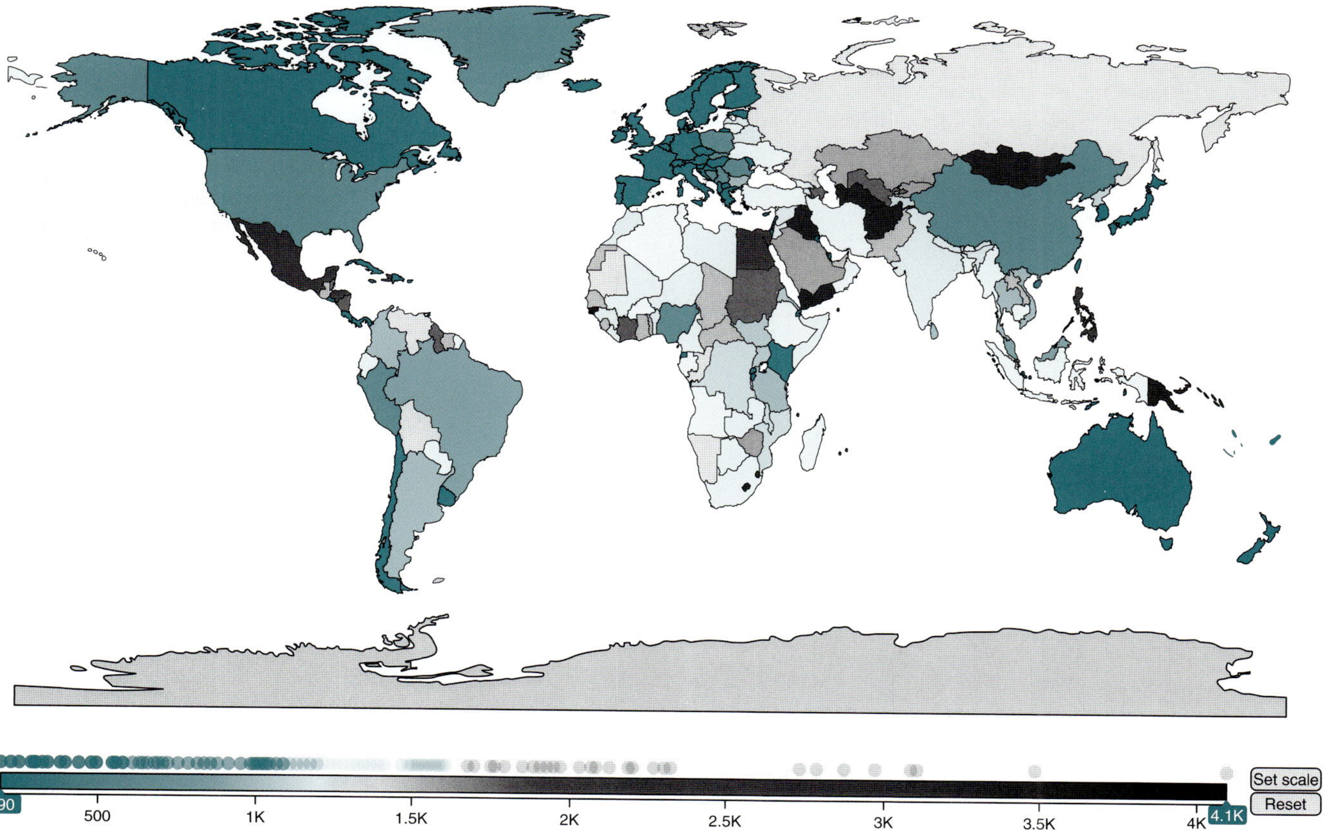

FIG. 1.19 Higher burden of impaired kidney function attributable disability-adjusted life years (DALYs) per 100,000 by country 2016. (Data from courtesy of Institute for Health Metric based on data presented in Collaborators GBDRF. Global, regional, and national comparative risk assessment of 84 behavioural, environmental and occupational, and metabolic risks or clusters of risks, 1990-2016: a systematic analysis for the Global Burden of Disease Study 2016. *Lancet.* 2017;390(10100):1345-1422.)

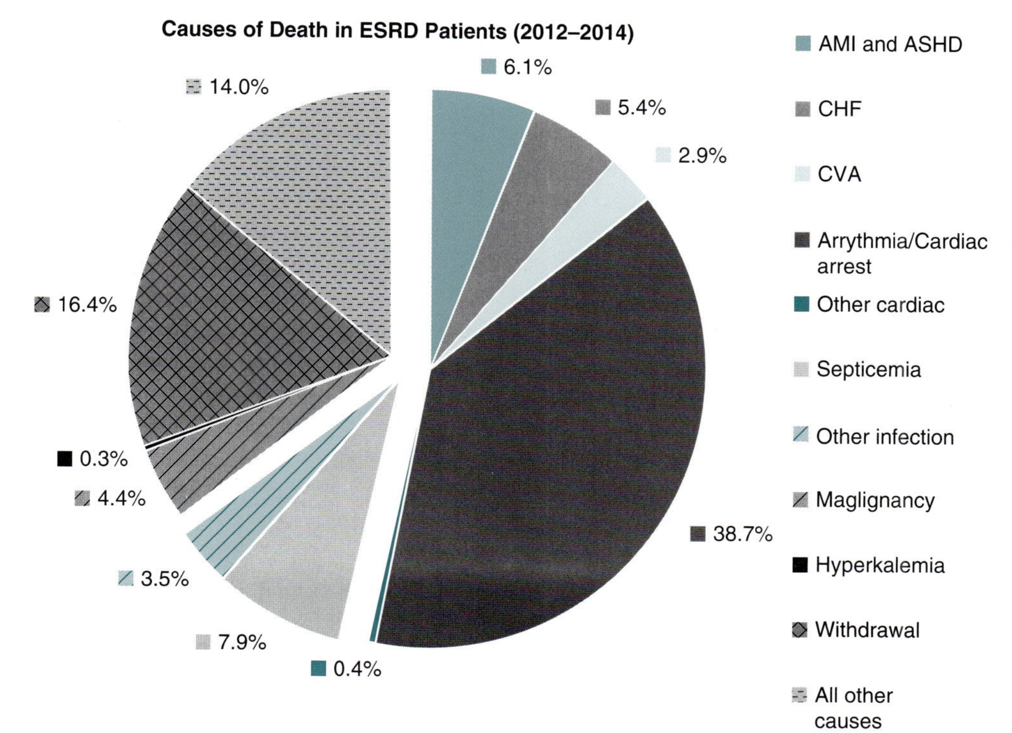

FIG. 1.20 Causes of death in ESRD patients (2012–2014). Separated by cardiovascular, infectious, and other causes of death. (Adapted from United States Renal Data System, 2016 USRDS annual data report: Volume 2, Figure i.21. Epidemiology of kidney disease in the United States. National Institutes of Health. National Institute of Diabetes and Digestive and Kidney Disease, Bethesda, MD, 2016.)

CONCLUSION

The past two decades have seen a major change in the understanding of the epidemiology of CKD, driven to a major extent by a standardized definition of CKD proposed in 2002 paired with a focus on estimated GFR and albuminuria as strong and easily measured staging factors. The burden of CKD is now well recognized and its growing global importance for a wide range of outcomes is beginning to be addressed. Concerted efforts are needed to identify mechanisms of kidney injury and disease progression and to test new paradigms of prevention and treatment at the individual and population level to improve outcomes in patients with CKD and ESRD.

A full list of references is available at www.expertconsult.com.

2

Measurement and Estimation of Kidney Function

Lesley A. Inker, MD, MS, and Andrew S. Levey, MD

OUTLINE

The kidney performs specialized functions to maintain constancy of the internal composition of the body fluids. These functions include excretion of waste products, regulation of extracellular fluid volume and composition, production and catabolism of hormones, and regulation of acid–base balance. The normal kidney can adapt to wide variations in intake and in extrarenal loss of fluid and electrolytes through regulation of glomerular filtration and tubular reasbsorption and secretion. In this chapter, we focus on measurement and estimation of glomerular filtration rate (GFR) as an index of overall kidney function. The rationale is that GFR is a property of the kidney, has a large range, and is affected by physiological, pharmacological, and pathological conditions. Furthermore, GFR decline is associated with many physiological and clinical consequences and is correlated with decline in other functions. Decreased GFR is one criterion in the definition and staging of acute and chronic kidney diseases, and GFR estimating equations are recommended for routine use for kidney function assessment in clinical practice.[1-3]

GLOMERULAR FILTRATION

Determinants of Glomerular Filtration Rate

The human kidney contains approximately 1 million glomeruli,[4,5] each approximately 150 to 200 microns in diameter. The total surface area provided for glomerular filtration approximates one square meter.[6] Approximately 180 liters per day (or 125 mL/min) of tubular fluid are produced from renal plasma flow (RPF) by the process of ultrafiltration, driven by the high hydrostatic pressure across the glomerular capillaries and facilitated by the hydraulic permeability of the glomerular capillary wall, which is one to two orders of magnitude greater than other capillaries.[7]

The glomerular filtration barrier is both size- and charge-dependent. Solutes with molecular weights lower than 10,000 daltons freely pass the glomerular capillary wall.[8-10] Large plasma proteins are excluded from the filtrate as a consequence of the structure of the glomerular capillary wall.

The GFR is dependent on the number of nephrons (N) and the single-nephron glomerular filtration rate (SNGFR), as described here:

$$GFR = N \times SNGFR \quad \textbf{(Eq. 1)}$$

In normal individuals and in patients with kidney disease, in whom nephron number may be reduced, regulation of GFR occurs via regulation of SNGFR.

$$SNGFR = K_f\,(\Delta P - \Delta\pi) \quad \textbf{(Eq. 2)}$$

where

ΔP = the difference between the net transcapillary hydraulic pressure favoring filtration

$\Delta\pi$ = net oncotic pressure opposing filtration

K_f = the ultrafiltration coefficient, a composite measure of the surface area and permeability characteristics of the glomerular ultrafiltration barrier

ΔP is determined by the difference between the glomerular capillary hydraulic pressure and that in the earliest proximal tubule. $\Delta\pi$ is determined by the glomerular oncotic pressure alone as the ultrafiltrate is virtually protein-free. Absent from this equation is the RPF rate. Alterations in RPF affect SNGFR largely by influencing ΔP and $\Delta\pi$.

Variability of Glomerular Filtration Rate

Normal values show considerable variation among individuals, principally due to differences in age, sex, and body size. Hence measured values of GFR are typically adjusted for body size and compared with normative values.[11] A compilation of inulin clearance measurements in young adults shows the mean value in men to be 131 mL/min/1.73 m^2, and in women to be 120 mL/min/1.73 m^2 (Fig. 2.1),[2,11] with considerable variation among individuals and over time. Some of these same factors also contribute to variation in GFR in patients with kidney disease.

1. *Sex and Body Size.* The GFR is related to glomerular surface area and kidney size. Measured values for GFR are conventionally factored by 1.73 m^2, the mean body surface area (BSA) of men and women 25 years of age. Nonetheless, as described previously, BSA-adjusted values for GFR are approximately 8% higher in young men than in women of the same age. The appropriateness of the use of BSA as the factor by which GFR is adjusted for body size is uncertain.[12] Some have suggested that extracellular volume is a more appropriate index given that the purpose of GFR is to regulate body fluid composition.[13] Adjustment for body size may be of particular importance in obesity, in which GFR is increased, but the increase in body size appears to be proportionately greater than the increase in GFR, potentially leading to a reduction in BSA-adjusted GFR.[14]
2. *Age.* Both cross-sectional and longitudinal studies show a decline in GFR of approximately 10 mL/min/1.73 m^2 per decade after the age of 30 years, such that during the 50 years from age 30 to age 80, GFR declines by almost 40%, from approximately 130 to 80 mL/min/1.73m^2.[11,15,16] Age-related decline in GFR has been traditionally interpreted as normal; however, other data suggest that there is considerable variation,[15-17] and recent data suggest that lower GFR in the elderly is associated with increased risk for mortality, which suggests that it is related to disease or other factors rather than normal.[18] This is an area of ongoing debate.[19-22]
3. *Pregnancy.* A marked increase in GFR occurs during pregnancy due to an increase in RPF and a decrease in plasma oncotic pressure.[10] GFR may increase up to 50% during the first trimester, persist at that level until term, and then return to normal approximately 4 to 8 weeks after the end of pregnancy. Pregnancy-induced hyperfiltration also

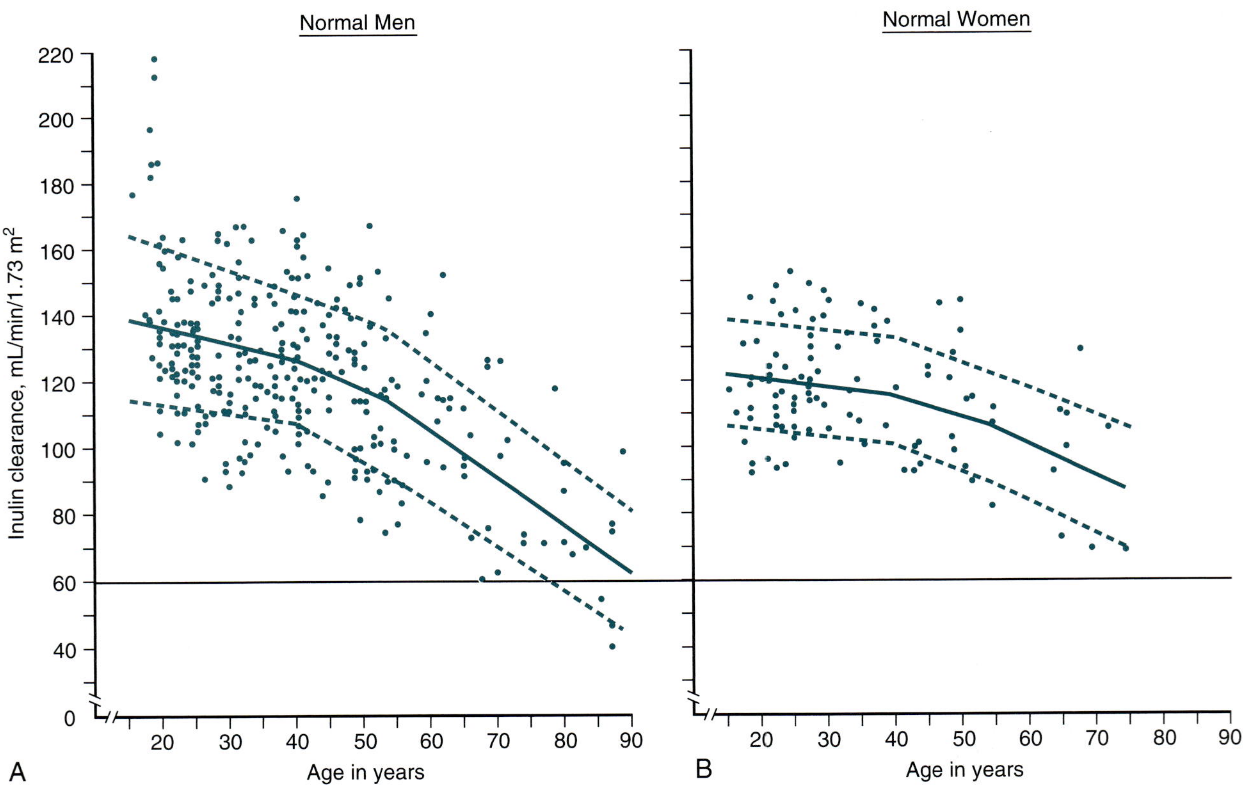

FIG. 2.1 Normal values for GFR in men and women. Normal values for inulin clearance are shown for men (A) and women (B) of various ages, with the GFR measured as the urinary clearance of inulin. A GFR value of 60 mL per minute per 1.73 m^2 is the threshold for the definition of chronic kidney disease. Solid lines represent the mean value of GFR per decade of age, and dashed lines represent the value 1 standard deviation from the mean value of GFR per decade of age.[11] (From Wesson LG. Renal hemodynamics in physiological states. In: Wesson LG, ed. *Physiology of the Human Kidney.* New York: Grune and Stratton; 1969:96–108.)

occurs in women with preexisting chronic kidney disease, and the percentage increase appears proportionate to the prepregnancy level of GFR.

4. *Protein Intake.* The effect of protein intake on the GFR varies according to the duration of protein feeding (habitual protein intake vs. meat meals or amino acid infusions) and type of protein (animal vs. vegetable or soya protein sources; essential vs. nonessential amino acids).[23] After a meat meal, GFR and RPF rise within an hour and remain elevated for several hours. Similar increases in GFR and RPF were noted in participants fed a high-, medium-, or low-protein diet for 2 weeks. Some studies suggest a greater response to animal than vegetable protein in habitual diets and in response to protein loads. Conversely, long-term malnutrition is associated with reduced kidney size, suggesting structural and hemodynamic alterations. It had been proposed that protein-induced hyperfiltration represents "renal reserve capacity," which is lost before the reduction in baseline GFR associated with kidney disease. However, it has now been shown conclusively that changes in GFR occur in response to changes in habitual protein intake or meat meals in patients with kidney disease and reduced GFR and in animals with experimental kidney disease.[23]
5. *Diurnal Variation.* GFR is approximately 10% higher in the afternoon than in the middle of the night, which may be related to the variation in protein intake or hydration during the day, or to transient reductions in GFR associated with exercise.
6. *Race and Ethnicity.* There are few studies of measured GFR in healthy populations other than Caucasians. In two studies in India, mean measured GFR in kidney donor candidates was lower than prior studies in Caucasians and did not improve after amino acid infusion, which was attributed to their vegetarian diet.[24,25] In another study in Pakistan, the observed age-associated measured GFR was lower than in prior studies in Caucasians, and lower protein intake was related to lower observed GFR.[26] A recent study comparing US blacks with whites demonstrated no significant difference in measured GFR.[27]
7. *Antihypertensive Therapy.* The level of GFR remains relatively constant throughout a wide range of blood pressure. Nonetheless, antihypertensive therapy can be associated with reductions in GFR, due, in part, to the effect of lowering blood pressure and, in part, to specific effects of classes of antihypertensive agents.[28] It has long been known that marked reduction in GFR can complicate treatment in patients with severe hypertension and acute or chronic kidney disease,[29] an effect thought to be due to loss or reset of autoregulation due to sclerosis of the renal vasculature from hypertensive injury.[30] The effects of antihypertensive therapy are discussed in Chapter 4.

Reductions in GFR in acute and chronic kidney disease may result from a decline in the SNGFR from hemodynamic alterations associated with diseases of other organ systems or from a decrease in the nephron number as a consequence of kidney disease. It is hypothesized that a decrease in nephron number is often associated with an increase in SNGFR (hyperfiltration in remnant nephrons).[31] As a result, there may be substantial kidney damage before GFR decreases. As discussed in Chapter 3, hyperfiltration is hypothesized to be a major contributor to the development and progression of kidney disease, particularly in diabetes. However, as neither nephron number nor SNGFR can be measured in humans, there is much uncertainty about the causes and consequences of hyperfiltration.[32]

MEASUREMENT OF GLOMERULAR FILTRATION RATE

The GFR cannot be measured directly. Instead, it is assessed from clearance measurements or estimated from plasma concentrations of filtration markers: exogenous or endogenous solutes eliminated from body fluids primarily by glomerular filtration.

Physiology of Urinary Clearance and the Measurement of GFR

The "gold standard" for the measurement of GFR is the urinary clearance of an ideal filtration marker. The requirements for an ideal filtration marker are:[2]

1. It is freely filtered at the glomerulus. It passes from glomerular capillary blood into the Bowman space unhindered by its size, charge, or binding to plasma proteins.
2. It is not altered during its passage through the nephron. It is not reabsorbed, secreted, synthesized, or metabolized by the tubules.
3. It is physiologically inert. It does not alter the function of the kidney.

The clearance of a solute is defined as the rate at which it is cleared from the plasma per unit concentration. The clearance of solute "x" (Cx) is given by the following equation:

$$Cx = Ax/Px \quad \textbf{(Eq. 3)}$$

where Ax is the amount of x eliminated from the plasma per unit time and Px is the average plasma concentration. Hence, Cx is expressed in units of volume per time and can be calculated without reference to the route of elimination. For a solute that is cleared by urinary excretion, the clearance formula may be rewritten as follows:

$$Cx = Ux \times V/Px \quad \textbf{(Eq. 4)}$$

where Ux is the urinary concentration of x and V is the urine flow rate. The term Ux × V represents the urinary excretion rate of x. If solute x is freely filtered at the glomerulus, then urinary excretion represents the net effects of glomerular filtration, tubular reabsorption, and secretion as follows:

$$Ux \times V = GFR \times Px - TRx + TSx \quad \textbf{(Eq. 5)}$$

where GFR × Px is the filtered load, and TRx and TSx are the rates of tubular reabsorption and secretion of x, respectively. By rearrangement, GFR can be related to urinary clearance:

$$GFR = (Ux \times V - TRx + TSx)/Px \quad \textbf{(Eq. 6)}$$

$$GFR = Cx - TRx/Px + TSx/Px \quad \textbf{(Eq. 7)}$$

where TRx/Px and TSx/Px are the clearances of solute x due to reabsorption (CTRx) and secretion (CTSx), respectively. If solute x is an ideal filtration marker, then GFR can be assessed from urinary clearance of x.

$$GFR = Cx \quad \textbf{(Eq. 8)}$$

True GFR versus Measured GFR

As described later, most filtration markers deviate from ideal behavior and clearance measurements are difficult to perform; thus values for measured GFR often contain an element of error, which differentiates it from the physiological or "true" GFR. True GFR, like other physiological properties that cannot be observed directly, can be modeled using the observed measured GFR and estimates of its error. Measurement error is related to both the specific filtration marker used and the clearance method and can be quantified in terms of bias and precision. Bias generally reflects systematic differences from the ideal filtration marker in renal handling, extrarenal metabolism, or assay of the filtration marker. Imprecision generally reflects random error in performance of the clearance procedure or assay of the filtration marker. Precision is assessed by repeated measurement over a short time and under standard conditions to minimize biological variation. Bias is assessed by comparison to an ideal filtration marker and standardized clearance method. Later, we will discuss clearance methods and filtration markers for assessment of GFR.

Clearance Methods

1. *Urinary clearance.* Urinary clearance is the most direct method for measurement of GFR. Urine concentration of the filtration marker is assayed in a timed urine sample during which the plasma concentration is assayed. GFR is computed according to eq. 4. This procedure is applicable for both exogenous and endogenous filtration markers.

For an exogenous filtration marker, multiple (two to four) timed urine collections, each of approximately 20 to 30 minutes, are performed after administration of the marker, and the results are averaged. The classic method of Homer Smith includes fasting conditions in the morning, using a continuous intravenous infusion of the marker, multiple clearance periods requiring repetitive blood and urine collections over 3 hours, oral water loading to stimulate diuresis, bladder catheterization to ensure complete urine collection, and careful timing of blood sampling at the midpoint of the urine collection.

As an alternative to continuous intravenous infusion, the exogenous filtration marker may be administered via bolus intravenous injection. This method requires additional blood samples to compute the average plasma concentration as it declines (see later). Subcutaneous bolus administration of the marker allows for slow release of the marker into the circulation, providing more constant plasma levels compared with intravenous bolus.[33] Spontaneous voiding is used in the majority of research studies and clinical practices.

For an endogenous filtration marker, the urinary collection period may be prolonged to avoid the requirement for water loading, and a single plasma sample obtained either at the beginning or the end of the collection period may be assumed to represent the average plasma concentration. A 24-hour urine collection is the method most commonly used in clinical practice, but it is subject to errors in timing and collection of the urine specimen.

2. *Plasma clearance.* As an alternative to urinary clearance, GFR can be calculated from plasma clearance after a bolus intravenous injection of an exogenous filtration marker computed from eq. 3, where Ax is the amount of the marker administered and Px is computed from the entire area under the disappearance curve or from 1-compartment or 2-compartment analysis of the slope of the plasma disappearance plot (Fig. 2.2).[34]

Advantages of this method include the lack of requirement for urinary collection, which is particularly important in populations wherein bladder emptying may be impaired, such as the elderly or children with urinary tract abnormalities. In principle, plasma clearance methods would have greater precision than urinary clearance methods because they eliminate errors in timing of urine collection and incomplete bladder emptying. This has not been extensively tested.

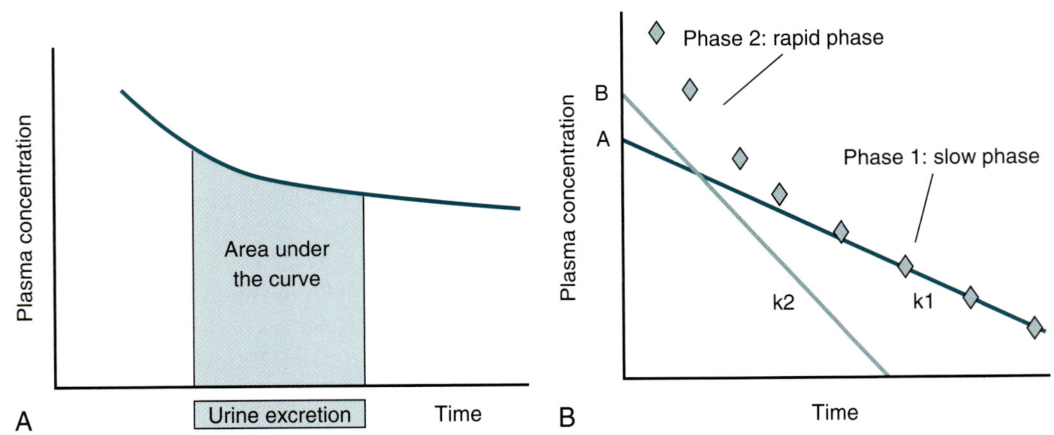

FIG. 2.2 Urinary and plasma clearance calculations after a bolus infusion of an exogneous filtration marker. (A) Urinary clearance. (B) Plasma clearance.

However, there are also several disadvantages to plasma clearance.[35] First, there is a relatively long time (~5 hours) required to determine the disappearance curve, with an even longer time required in people with very low GFR (8 to 10 hours). Shorter time periods may lead to overestimation of GFR throughout the GFR range. Second, expansion of the extracellular fluid compartment in edematous conditions causes a prolongation of the first compartment of the two-compartment curve and an overestimation of GFR. Third, extrarenal elimination of the filtration marker leads to an overestimation of urinary clearance, which would be more apparent at lower GFR.

3. *Nuclear and other imaging.* Measurement of GFR by external counting or imaging over the kidneys and bladder using an exogenous isotopic marker is another alternative to urinary clearance.[36] Studies have been done in conjunction with dynamic kidney imaging using ^{99m}Tc-diethylenetriamine pentaacetic acid (DTPA), comparing the percent kidney (and bladder) uptake at a defined time after injection to simultaneously measured GFR by other techniques. Several studies indicate low correlation of 99mTc-DTPA dynamic renal imaging with simultaneous urinary or plasma clearance, especially in people with normal and elevated GFR, reflecting both bias and imprecision.[37,38] It is premature to recommend external counting or imaging techniques for routine clinical purposes. The main value of dynamic renal imaging would appear to be in determining the function of each of the two kidneys or for use in individuals already undergoing imaging procedures, rather than as a primary method of measuring GFR.

Recently there has been consideration of magnetic resonance imaging (MRI) for measurement of GFR. Several techniques have been evaluated, including assessment of signal intensity within abdominal organs, measurement of the extraction fraction of the agent, and monitoring of tracer intrarenal kinetics. A recent study highlights a potential advantage of dynamic contrast enhanced MRI, which can assess renal blood flow and filtration fraction as well as GFR. However, the agreement between measured GFR assessed by MRI and plasma clearance of iohexol was only moderate.[41] More study is required before MRI technology can be used for GFR measurement in clinical practice.[40-42]

Exogenous Filtration Markers

Inulin was used as the filtration marker in the classic studies by Homer Smith and remains the gold standard for exogenous filtration marker. There are now a wide variety of exogenous isotopic and nonisotopic filtration markers that are more available and simpler to use than inulin.[38] The properties of inulin and these alternative filtration markers are described later (Table 2.1).

1. *Inulin.* Inulin, a 5200-dalton, inert, uncharged polymer of fructose, meets all of the criteria for an ideal filtration marker.[2] It is administered as a continuous intravenous infusion with a long interval for equilibration throughout extracellular fluid because of its large molecular radius. However, inulin is difficult to dissolve in aqueous solutions, difficult to measure, and in short supply. Because of these disadvantages, inulin is unsuitable for clinical assessment of GFR; other filtration markers are required.
2. *Iothalamate.* Iothalamate is commonly administered labeled with radioactive iodine for ease of assay, but it can also be administered in its nonradioactive form and measured using high-performance liquid chromatography (HPLC) or mass spectroscopy methods. The filtration properties are not affected by the radiolabeling. ^{125}I-iothalamate, widely available in a pure, stable form (half-life of ^{125}I is 60 days), is bound to protein to a minor degree. Most, but not all, studies comparing urinary clearance of iothalamate with inulin show a small positive bias (overestimation of inulin clearance), likely due to tubular secretion of iothalamate.[41] Iothalamate is generally administered as a bolus subcutaneous injection in urinary clearance procedures, but it can also be administered as bolus intravenous infusion for plasma or urinary clearance or a continuous subcutaneous infusion for urinary clearance.[43]
3. *Iohexol.* Iohexol is a nonionic radiographic contrast agent that is administered using bolus intravenous injection and can be used for both plasma and urinary clearance. Recently there has been much interest in iohexol as it provides several theoretical advantages over iothalamate.[34] It appears to exhibit neither protein binding nor tubular secretion, extrarenal elimination is minimal, it is stable in biological fluids, its adverse reactions are rare given the small dose (5 mL 300 mg/mL iodine when assayed with a sensitive assay, described later), and it does not require radioactive tags. Plasma clearance of iohexol appears to underestimate urinary inulin clearance, and renal tubular reabsorption of iohexol has been suggested.[41, 44] The major disadvantage of iohexol is the complexity and expense of its assay. High-performance liquid chromatography, requiring a skilled technician and expensive equipment, must be used when low doses of iohexol (e.g., 5 mL of 300 mg/mL iodine) are administered. Other methods include x-ray fluorescence, but that necessitates administration of significantly larger doses of iohexol (10 to 90 mL of 300 mg/mL iodine); capillary electrophoresis; and neutron activation analysis.[34]
4. *Ethylene-diaminetetraacetic acid (EDTA).* There is extensive European experience with ^{54}Cr-EDTA in humans.[34,41] This marker is not commercially available in the United States. The urinary clearance of ^{54}Cr-EDTA appears to underestimate urinary inulin clearance by 5% to 15% in most, though not all, studies, suggesting tubular reabsorption or protein binding.
5. *DTPA.* An analog of EDTA, DTPA is usually labeled with ^{99m}Tc and is available in the United States. The advantages of ^{99m}Tc-DTPA include a short half-life (6 hours) that minimizes radiation exposure, the high counting efficiency of ^{99m}Tc, its availability on a daily basis in most nuclear medicine departments, and the convenience of using it to measure GFR at the time of renal imaging studies.[34] DTPA is freely filtered at the glomerulus, with minimal reabsorption by the tubules, but may undergo extrarenal elimination.

TABLE 2.1 **Properties of Exogenous Filtration Markers**

Marker	Molecular Weight (Daltons)	Protein Binding	CLEARANCE METHODS		TUBULAR EFFECTS		Extrarenal Elimination	Assay	Serious Adverse Side Effects
			Administration	Plasma or Urinary	Secretion	Reabsorption			
Inulin	5200	No	IV bolus	Urinary	None	None	Small	Chemical	None
Iothalamate (^{125}I or Nonradioactive)	614	Small	IV or SC bolus	Plasma[a] or urinary	Small (?)	None	None	Gamma counter. T½ 60 d/HPLC/ mass spectroscopy	Oral KI required to protect the thyroid from ^{125}I Anaphylatic reaction and contrast nephropathy at higher doses
Iohexol	821	No (?)	IV or SC bolus	Plasma* or urinary	None	Small	Small	HPLC MS	Anaphylatic reaction and contrast nephropathy at higher doses
^{51}Cr-EDTA[b]	292	Small	IV or SC bolus	Plasma* or urinary	None	Small	None	Gamma counter T½ 28 d	
^{99m}Tc-DTPA[c]	393	Small	IV or SC bolus	Plasma* or urinary	?	Small	None	Gamma counter T½ 6 h	None
Gadolinium	157	Small	IV or SC bolus	Plasma* or urinary	?	?		RIA	Nephrogenic systemic fibrosis at low GFR

[a]Plasma clearances can be calculated only when marker is administered using intravenous route.
[b]Ethylenediaminetetraacetic acid.
[c]Diethylenetriaminepentaacetic acid.

One disadvantage is dissociation of ^{99m}Tc from the DTPA and protein binding of ^{99m}Tc, leading to underestimation of GFR. Rigorous quality control is necessary to minimize this error, making it more difficult to standardize across centers. The MRI contrast agent gadolinium (Gd)-DTPA has recently been discussed as a novel exogenous filtration marker.[34] There is a highly sensitive novel immunoassay technique for serum and urine Gd. However, there is some concern about the risk of systemic nephrogenic fibrosis due to toxicity of Gd, even at the low levels administered for GFR measurement. The safety of Gd-DTPA and its accuracy and precision have not been thoroughly tested compared with other exogenous filtration markers.

ESTIMATION OF GLOMERULAR FILTRATION RATE

Clearance measurements are difficult to perform in clinical practice. Instead, the level of GFR is usually estimated from the plasma or serum level of an endogenous filtration marker. In this section, we review the relationship of GFR to plasma solute concentrations, and then we focus on specific markers, including creatinine, cystatin C, and urea (Table 2.2).

Relationship of Glomerular Filtration Rate to Plasma Solute Concentrations

The plasma concentration of solute x reflects the balance of its rate of generation in body fluids (either from endogenous production or exogenous intake) and its rate of elimination from body fluids (either from excretion or metabolism) (Fig. 2.3). In the steady state, the rates of generation and elimination from body fluids are equal and the plasma concentration of solute x is constant, thus the following equation applies.

$$Gx = Ux \times V + Ex \qquad \textbf{(Eq. 9)}$$

where Gx is the rate of generation of x, and Ex is the extrarenal elimination of x.

For solutes excreted only in the urine (no extrarenal elimination), an important corollary is that, in the steady state, the rate of generation can be assessed from the urinary excretion rate.

TABLE 2.2 Properties of Endogenous Filtration Markers

Marker	Molecular Weight (daltons)	Generation	TUBULAR EFFECTS: Secretion	TUBULAR EFFECTS: Reabsorption	Extrarenal Elimination[a]
Metabolites					
Creatinine	113	Muscle, diet	++	None	Gut flora with advanced CKD
Urea	60	Liver, dietary protein	+	+++	Not described
Low Molecular Weight Proteins					
Cystatin C	~13,300	Nucleated cells	Not described	Catabolized	Not described
β-2 microglobulin	~11,818	Nucleated cells	Not described	Catabolized	Not described
β-trace protein	23,000–29,000	Choroid plexus, testes, ovaries	Not described	Catabolized	Not described

[a]Magnitude of effect.

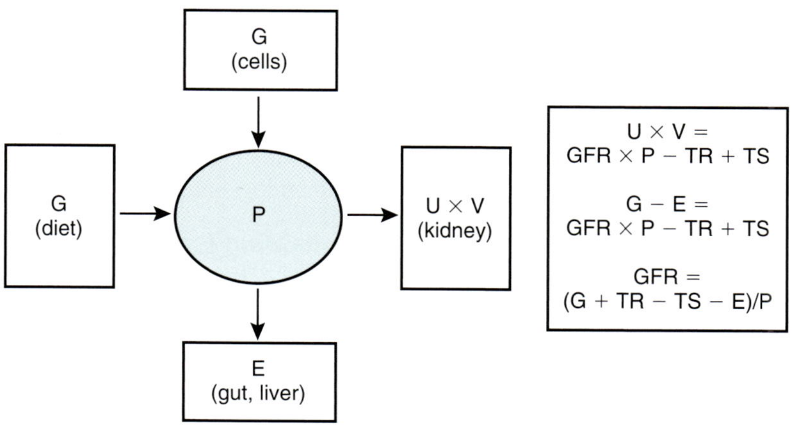

FIG. 2.3 Determinants of the serum level of endogenous filtration markers. The plasma level (*P*) of an endogenous filtration marker is determined by its generation (*G*) from cells and diet, extrarenal elimination (*E*) by gut and liver, and urinary excretion (U × V) by the kidney. Urinary excretion is the sum of filtered load (GFR × P), tubular secretion (*TS*), and reabsorption (*TR*). In the steady state, urinary excretion equals generation (plus) and extrarenal elimination (minus). By substitution and rearrangement, GFR can be expressed as the ratio of the non-GFR determinants (G, TS, TR, and E) to the plasma level.[34] (From Stevens LA, Levey AS. Measured GFR as a confirmatory test for estimated GFR. *J Am Soc Nephrol.* 2009;20:2305–2313.)

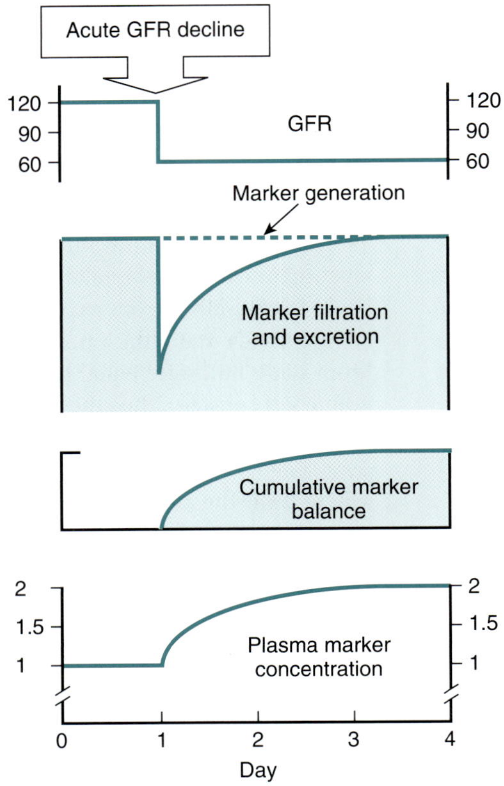

Day	P_{marker}	eGFR
1	1	120
1.5	1.6	79
2	1.8	69
2.5	1.9	65
3	2	60

FIG. 2.4 Effect of an acute GFR decline on generation, filtration, excretion, balance, and serum level of endogenous filtration markers. After an acute GFR decline, generation of the marker is unchanged, but filtration and excretion are reduced, resulting in retention of the marker (a rising positive balance) and a rising plasma level (nonsteady state). During this time, estimated GFR (eGFR) is lower than measured GFR (mGFR). Although GFR remains reduced, the rise in plasma level leads to an increase in filtered load (the product of GFR times the plasma level) until filtration equals generation. At that time, cumulative balance and the plasma level plateau at a new steady state. In the new steady state, eGFR approximates mGFR. GFR expressed in units of mL/min/1.73 m^2. Tubular secretion and reabsorption and extrarenal elimination are assumed to be zero.[34,46] (Modified and reproduced with permission from Kassirer JP. Clinical evaluation of kidney function-glomerular function. *N Engl J Med.* 1971;285:385-389; Used with permission from Stevens LA, Levey AS. Measured GFR as a confirmatory test for estimated GFR. *J Am Soc Nephrol.* 2009;20:2305–2313.)

By substitution of eq. 9 and rearrangement, the plasma level can be related to the level of GFR and its non-GFR determinants (Gx, TRx, TSx, and Ex).

$$Px = (Gx + TRx - TSx - Ex)/GFR \quad \textbf{(Eq. 10)}$$

Fig. 2.4 shows hypothetical changes in generation, excretion, balance, and plasma level of solute x after a 50% decrement in GFR, assuming TR, TS, and E are zero. In the steady state, changes in the plasma level would reflect reciprocal changes in GFR. For example, a decline in GFR to two-thirds, one-half, or one-third of the baseline level would be reflected by a rise in the plasma level to 1.5, 2.0, and 3.0 times the baseline level, respectively. Expression of the change in plasma level as its reciprocal (1/Px) would more clearly reflect the magnitude of changes over time in GFR in an individual.

Further rearrangement of eq. 10 provides the conceptual framework for estimating GFR from plasma solute levels of endogenous filtration markers.

$$GFR = (Gx + TRx - TSx - Ex)/Px \quad \textbf{(Eq. 11)}$$

In practice, the non-GFR determinants of plasma solute levels are not measured. However, if the rates of these physiological processes were similar among all individuals and constant over time, then the level of GFR could be estimated directly from the inverse of the plasma concentration. Unfortunately, this is not the case for any of the currently used endogenous filtration markers.

Estimating Equations for Glomerular Filtration Rate

GFR estimating equations are equations that permit more accurate estimation of measured GFR from plasma levels of endogenous filtration markers and clinical and demographic variables than from the plasma level alone. GFR estimating equations are derived from regression analysis in which the level of measured GFR is related to the plasma solute concentration and observed clinical and demographic variables that serve as surrogates for the non-GFR determinants of plasma levels.

$$GFR = (b \times X + c \times Y + d \times Z)/a \times Px + \varepsilon \quad \textbf{(Eq. 12)}$$

where
X, Y, and Z = numerical values for clinical and demographic variables
a, b, c, and d = coefficients relating Px and other variables to measured GFR
ε = the error based on uncertainty due to measurement, biological variability, and statistical techniques used to derive the coefficients

Estimating equations for GFR are often developed on the logarithmic scale, then exponentiated to report estimated GFR (eGFR) on the linear scale, and therefore have the appearance of:

$$eGFR = (Px)^{-a} \times X^b \times Y^c \times Z^d \times \varepsilon \qquad \textbf{(Eq. 13)}$$

where eGFR is estimated GFR, and the negative sign for the coefficient a reflects the inverse relationship of plasma level of solute x to GFR. If the coefficient a is −1.0 and the variables b, c, and d are 0, then a rise in Px to 1.5, 2, and 3 times the baseline level would be reflected in a decline in eGFR to two-thirds, one-half, or one-third of the baseline level, respectively.

In principle, use of multiple endogenous filtration markers with differing non-GFR determinants can improve the accuracy of GFR estimation. In multiple marker equations, the magnitude of the coefficient for each filtration would be closer to zero and the coefficients for clinical and demographic variables would be closer to 1.0, thereby lessening the dependence of eGFR on each filtration marker and factors associated with its non-GFR determinants.

Clinical use of GFR estimating equations would be facilitated if clinical laboratories reported eGFR when plasma concentrations of endogenous filtration markers were measured, and a single equation were used for each filtration marker or combination of markers. Here, we use the notation eGFRx to refer to estimated GFR based on plasma concentration of solute x. For endogenous filtration markers in current use, plasma and serum concentrations are generally equivalent.

Interpretation of Glomerular Filtration Rate Estimates

Development of accurate and generalizable estimating equations for widespread clinical use requires strict adherence to epidemiological and statistical principles.[45] In general, it is recommended that equations be developed in a large study population (>500 subjects), including a variety of racial and ethnic groups for international comparisons, using high-quality GFR measurements; validated to have adequate precision and low bias against a gold standard measure of GFR in an independent study population; and practical to implement, taking into consideration cost, required data elements, assay considerations, and generalizability. Accuracy of GFR estimates in the validation population reflects bias, defined as average difference between the estimated and measured value for each subject, and precision, inversely related to the distribution of the differences between estimated and measured value for each subject. Table 2.3 lists some of the metrics that can be used for the assessment of bias, precision, and accuracy, as well as the causes for bias and imprecision.[44] In general, knowledge of the sources of bias and imprecision can assist in interpretation of plasma levels of endogenous filtration markers and GFR estimates based on these levels. In this section, general principles are discussed; interpretation

TABLE 2.3 Metrics for Evaluation of GFR Estimating Equations and Causes of Bias and Imprecision

Criteria	Metric	Definition	Causes[a]
Bias	Median difference	Measured GFR-Estimated GFR[b]	Systematic difference between development and validation population in GFR measurement error (clearance method or exogenous filtration marker) Assays for endogenous filtration markers Non-GFR determinants of endogenous filtration marker (selection criteria) Mean level of measured GFR
	Median percent difference	(Measured GFR-Estimated GFR)/Measured GFR	
Precision	SD difference	Standard deviation of the differences	Larger random variation in the validation than the development population True GFR (biological variation) GFR measurement error (clearance method or exogenous filtration marker) Non-GFR determinants of endogenous filtration markers
	IQR difference[c]	Interquartile range of (Measured GFR–Estimated GFR)	
	IQR 96 difference[c]	Interquartile range of ((Measured GFR–Estimated GFR)/Measured GFR)[a] 100	
Accuracy	Median absolute difference	Median of the absolute value of eGFR–mGFR	All of the above
	P30	Percent of estimates within 30% of measured GFR	
	RMSE	Square root of mean (log Measured GFR–log Estimated GFR)^2	

Accuracy measures precision when bias is 0 (development data set).
[a]Differences between development and validation population.
[b]May also be expressed as Estimated GFR–Measured GFR.
[c]IQR is the width of the 25th to 75th percentile.

of GFR estimates from specific endogenous filtration markers are discussed separately later.

The coefficients for the clinical and demographic variables reflect average values for the relationship of the observed variables to the unmeasured surrogates in the development population. Systematic differences in these relationships between the development and validation populations is reflected as bias and generally reflects differences in selection between the development and validation populations. Random differences among individual patients are reflected as imprecision. In principle, use of multiple endogenous filtration markers with differing non-GFR determinants would cancel errors due to systematic bias in each filtration marker and improve precision.

There can be substantial variation among clinical laboratories in assays for endogenous filtration markers, leading to bias in GFR estimates between the development population and the validation population. This source of bias can be overcome by calibration of the clinical laboratory to the laboratory in which the equation was developed. In practice, this is best accomplished by standardization of clinical laboratories and reexpression of the GFR estimating equation for use with standardized values.

Measurement error in GFR in the development population is another source of inaccuracy in GFR estimates. This is a special case, however, because the difference is between measured and true GFR rather than between estimated and measured GFR. Systematic error in GFR measurement, due to the clearance method or the exogenous filtration marker, introduces a bias in GFR estimates compared with true GFR, which can lead to a bias in comparing GFR estimates to measured GFR in the validation population. Random error in GFR measurement leads to lower precision of GFR estimates compared with measured GFR than compared with true GFR in both the development and the validation populations.

A property of the statistical technique of regression is to "shrink" estimates to the mean of the development population. In the development population, the mean eGFR is unbiased, but higher values for measured GFR are systematically underestimated and lower values for measured GFR are systematically overestimated. In a validation population with a substantially different mean measured GFR, the estimates may be systematically biased due to "regression to the mean" of the development population. Because most GFR estimating equations are derived in a population with a wide range of GFR, this would lead to an underestimation of measured GFR in a validation population drawn from the general population, in which most subjects would be expected to have normal measured GFR, and an overestimation of measured GFR in a validation population with low GFR.

All of these factors tend to cause larger errors in GFR estimation at higher values, in large part because estimating equations are usually developed in study populations with a large number of patients with reduced GFR and because development on the logarithmic scale leads to larger errors at the higher levels when estimates are reexpressed on the linear scale. Thus eGFR is likely to be more accurate at lower values, as encountered in patients with kidney disease, and less accurate at higher values, as encountered in the general population.

Finally, it is difficult to estimate GFR in the nonsteady state because the change in the endogenous filtration marker lags behind the change in GFR (see Fig. 2.4). This limitation applies both to plasma levels of endogenous filtration markers and to GFR estimates based on plasma levels. Nonetheless, a change in the plasma levels and eGFR based on plasma levels in the nonsteady state can be a useful indication of the magnitude and direction of the change in kidney function. If the plasma level is rising due to declining kidney function, then the decline in eGFR would be less than the decline in measured GFR. Conversely, if the plasma level is falling due to rising kidney function, then the rise in eGFR would be greater than the rise in measured GFR. The more rapid the change in the filtration marker or in eGFR, the larger the change in measured GFR. As kidney function stabilizes, the endogenous filtration marker reaches a new steady state, and eGFR more accurately reflects measured GFR.

ENDOGENOUS FILTRATION MARKERS

Creatinine

Creatinine is the most commonly used endogenous filtration marker for estimation of GFR. Understanding basic concepts of metabolism, renal physiology, and analytical chemistry related to creatinine is essential to the interpretation of GFR estimates based on serum creatinine (Table 2.4).[45,47]

1. Structure and Function

Creatinine is a 113-dalton amino acid derivative that serves as a nitrogenous waste. It is distributed throughout total body water and has no known toxicity.

2. Plasma Levels

The normal level of GFR is sufficient to maintain a low concentration of creatinine in serum, approximately 0.64 to 1.36 mg/dL.

3. Generation

Creatinine is generated in muscle from the nonenzymatic conversion of creatine and phosphocreatine. Creatine is synthesized from arginine and glycine in the liver and actively concentrated in muscle. Thus creatinine generation reflects the size of the creatine pool, which is proportional to muscle mass. In the steady state, creatinine generation can be estimated by creatinine excretion, and related to age, gender, and body size.[48]

$$Ucr \times V = 28.2 - 0.172 \times age \text{ (men)} \qquad \textbf{(Eq. 14)}$$

$$Ucr \times V = 21.9 - 0.115 \times age \text{ (women)} \qquad \textbf{(Eq. 15)}$$

where creatinine excretion is expressed in mg/kg/d and age is expressed in years.

These equations do not take into account racial and ethnic differences in muscle mass. African American (black) males and females have higher muscle mass and consequently higher creatinine excretion than their Caucasian (white) counterparts. Asians have lower muscle mass and

TABLE 2.4 **Clinical Conditions Affecting Interpretation of GFR Estimates**

	Creatinine	Cystatin C	Urea
	OVERESTIMATION OF GFR (LOWER SERUM LEVELS)		
Generation	Reduction in muscle mass; vegetarian diet	Hypothyroidism, female sex, older age	Severe malnutrition and liver disease
Renal handling	Proximal tubular injury; e.g., sickle cell disease	Not described	Decreased tubular reabsorption in absence of ADH
Extrarenal elimination	Increase with severe reduction in GFR (gut)	Increased with severe reduction in GFR (spleen, diaphragm, heart, liver, and lungs)	Not described
Assay	Not described	Not described	Not described
	UNDERESTIMATION OF GFR (HIGHER SERUM LEVELS)		
Generation	Higher muscle mass and ingestion of cooked meats and creatinine supplements	Corticosteroids, inflammation, hyperthyroidism, male sex, younger age, obesity, transplant recipients	Dietary protein intake, corticosteroids, diuretics, or tetracyclines; absorption of blood from the gut, infection, acute kidney injury, trauma, congestive heart failure, and sodium depletion
Renal handling	Decreased secretion with drugs such as cimetidine, trimethoprim, possibly fenofibrate	Not described	Increased tubular reabsorption in presence of ADH
Extrarenal elimination	Decrease with antibiotic use	Not described	Not described
Assay	Keto acids, some cephalosporins may interfere with alkaline picrate; flucytosine may interfere with enzymatic by as much as 60%	At high levels of bilirubin interference with the PETIA assay	Ammonium in reagents or use of ammonium heparin; drugs such as chloral hydrate, chlorbutanol, and guanethidine

lower creatinine excretion rate than their Caucasian counterparts.[49,50] Other equations to estimate creatinine excretion have been proposed, but precision is limited; approximately 20% of estimates deviate by more than 30% of measured creatinine excretion rate.[51]

Creatinine generation is affected by diet and disorders of skeletal muscle. Muscle wasting is associated with a decreased creatine pool, leading to decreased creatinine generation and excretion. Reduction in dietary protein causes a decrease in the creatine pool by 5% to 15%, probably by reducing the availability of creatine precursors. Of greater importance is the effect of creatine in the diet. Creatine is contained largely in meat; elimination of creatine from the diet decreases urinary creatinine excretion by as much as 30%. Conversely, ingesting a creatine supplement increases the size of the creatine pool and increases creatinine excretion. Meat intake also affects creatinine generation and excretion independent of its effect on the creatine pool. During cooking, a variable amount of the creatine in meat is converted to creatinine, which is absorbed from the gastrointestinal tract. After ingestion of cooked meat, there is a sudden transient increase in the serum creatinine concentration and urinary creatinine excretion.

4. Renal Handling

a. *Glomerular filtration.* The small molecular diameter of 0.3 nm and the lack of binding to plasma proteins assures the free passage of creatinine through the glomerular capillary wall into the Bowman space (sieving coefficient of 1.0).

b. *Tubular secretion.* Creatinine is actively secreted by the tubules, probably by the same pathway used for other organic cations in the proximal tubule; hence creatinine clearance exceeds GFR.

$$\mathrm{Ucr} \times \mathrm{V} = \mathrm{GFR} \times \mathrm{Pcr} + \mathrm{TScr} \qquad \textbf{(Eq. 16)}$$

where TScr is the rate of tubular secretion. The relationship between creatinine clearance and GFR is as follows:

$$\mathrm{Ccr} = \mathrm{GFR} + \mathrm{TScr}/\mathrm{Pcr} \qquad \textbf{(Eq. 17)}$$

where TScr/Pcr represents creatinine clearance due to secretion (CTScr). Thus Ccr exceeds GFR, but the magnitude of the difference is not well established. Using older assays for serum creatinine, which overestimated the level of serum creatinine in the low range, as described later, creatinine secretion in normal individuals was observed to account for 5% to 10% of excreted creatinine, on average; hence creatinine clearance exceeded GFR by approximately 10 mL/min/1.73 m^2, and creatinine clearance was considered an accurate index of measured GFR. However, with the newer assays, creatinine clearance can exceed measured GFR by much larger amounts, suggesting higher rates of creatinine excretion.[55] Some studies find the level of measured GFR, type of kidney disease, and quantity of dietary protein intake to be determinants of creatinine secretion.[56] Several commonly used medications, including cimetidine and trimethoprim, competitively inhibit creatinine secretion, thereby reducing creatinine clearance and raising the serum creatinine concentration, despite having no effect on measured GFR. Clinically, it can be difficult to distinguish a rise in serum creatinine due to drug-induced inhibition of creatinine secretion from a decline in GFR.

A clue to inhibition of creatinine secretion is that the concentration of other endogenous filtration markers, such as cystatin C and urea, remains unchanged.

c. *Tubular reabsorption.* To a limited extent, creatinine may also be reabsorbed by the tubules, possibly due to its passive back-diffusion from the lumen to blood because of the high tubular creatinine concentration that occurs during low urine flow. Based on the clearance ratios observed in these studies, the maximum effect of creatinine reabsorption probably would be a 5% to 10% decrease in creatinine clearance.

5. Extrarenal Elimination

Extrarenal loss of creatinine is not detectable in normal individuals but may account for a larger proportion of daily creatinine generation in patients with severe decrease in GFR. Thus in patients with kidney disease, creatinine excretion underestimates creatinine generation:

$$\mathrm{Ucr} \times \mathrm{V} = \mathrm{Gcr} - \mathrm{Ecr} \qquad \textbf{(Eq. 18)}$$

where Ecr is the rate of elimination of creatinine by extrarenal routes. One likely, but still not established, mechanism is degradation of creatinine within the intestinal lumen by microorganisms due to induction of the enzyme creatininase. Possibly, elimination of intestinal bacteria by broad-spectrum antibiotics could reduce extrarenal elimination of creatinine, thus causing a rise in serum creatinine without an effect on GFR. In practice, it would be difficult to distinguish a rise in serum creatinine due to drug-induced reduction in extrarenal creatinine elimination from a decline in GFR. As discussed previously for drug-induced reduction in creatinine secretion, a clue to inhibition of extrarenal elimination would be that urea clearance and blood urea nitrogen concentration remain unchanged.

6. Assay

Creatinine can be measured easily in serum, plasma, and urine by a variety of methods.[51-53] No systematic differences between serum and plasma have been noted. The gold standard method for creatinine assay is isotope dilution mass spectrometry (IDMS) using either gas or liquid chromatography. Various methods are in use in clinical laboratories to assay serum and urine creatinine. Calibration of autoanalyzers differs among clinical laboratories, irrespective of the method for measurement of serum creatinine. The National Kidney Disease Education Program (NKDEP) and the International Federation of Clinical Chemistry and Laboratory Medicine (IFCC) have standardized serum creatinine assays to methods traceable to IDMS to minimize differences in across clinical laboratories. However, standardization does not eliminate patient-specific factors that interfere with creatinine measurement, as discussed below.

a. *Alkaline-picrate methods.* The classic method used the Jaffe reaction, in which creatinine reacts directly with picrate ion under alkaline conditions to form a red-orange complex that is easily detected and quantified. In normal subjects, up to 20% of the color reaction in serum or plasma is due to solutes other than creatinine, resulting in an apparent creatinine value that is 20% higher than the true value. Noncreatinine chromogens are not present in sufficient concentration in urine to interfere with creatinine measurement. In patients with kidney disease, noncreatinine chromogens are not retained to the same degree as creatinine; consequently, the overestimation of serum creatinine is reduced, as is the underestimation of creatinine clearance at lower GFR. The kinetic alkaline-picrate method takes advantage of the differential rate of color development for noncreatinine chromogens compared with creatinine. It significantly reduces but does not eliminate the positive interferences described previously. As discussed earlier, with standardization of creatinine assays, the discrepancy between creatinine clearance and GFR in normal individuals became apparent.

b. *Enzymatic methods.* To circumvent interferences in the alkaline picrate reaction, a variety of enzymatic methods have been developed. Two are in use in clinical laboratories: the creatinine iminohydrolase method and the creatininase, creatinase, and sarcosine oxidase method. Both methods have been reported to have fewer interferences than the alkaline-picrate methods.

c. *HPLC.* HPLC is a fairly sensitive and analytically specific method for measuring serum creatinine. Many of the protocols include deproteinization to obviate the effects from interfering compounds. All of the commonly used methods are imprecise in the lower range of serum creatinine. The imprecision makes it difficult to interpret changes in serum creatinine within the normal range, as one cannot readily distinguish between differences in serum creatinine levels due to errors in the assay or due to biological variability in GFR.

7. Creatinine as a Filtration Marker

Based on the previous considerations, the relationship of GFR to serum creatinine is expressed as follows:

$$\mathrm{GFR} = (\mathrm{Gcr} - \mathrm{TScr} - \mathrm{Ecr}) / \mathrm{Scr} \qquad \textbf{(Eq. 19)}$$

The use of serum creatinine as an index of GFR rests on the assumption that generation, tubular secretion, and extrarenal elimination of creatinine are similar among individuals and constant over time. As described previously, none of these assumptions is strictly correct, and it is difficult to estimate the level of GFR from serum creatinine alone (see Table 2.4). The rate of creatinine generation is lower in people with reduced muscle mass (women, children, the elderly, and malnourished individuals) and those with restricted meat intake.

Estimating equations overcome some of these limitations of using serum creatinine alone to estimate GFR by incorporating known demographic and clinical variables as observed surrogates for creatinine generation. Over the years, a large number of equations have been developed to estimate creatinine clearance and GFR in adults (eCcr and eGFRcr, respectively).[57] However, fewer equations have been expressed for use with standardized creatinine.

One of the first widely used estimating equations was the Cockcroft-Gault formula.[58]

$$\mathrm{eCcr} = [(140 - \mathrm{Age} \times \text{body weight}) \times 0.85 \ (\text{if female})] / [(\mathrm{Scr} \times 72)] \qquad \textbf{(Eq. 20)}$$

where eCcr is estimated creatinine clearance in mL/min, Scr is expressed in mg/dL, age is expressed in years, and body weight is expressed in kg. The Cockcroft-Gault formula was derived in 249 Caucasian men with a mean mCcr of 73 mL/min. The formula for women was based on the assumption that creatinine generation is 15% less in women than in men. Comparison to normal values for creatinine clearance requires computation of BSA and adjustment to 1.73 m^2. The Cockcroft-Gault formula has several limitations. First, it is not precise, in particular in the GFR range above 60 mL/min/1.73 m^2. Second, it estimates Ccr rather than GFR and thus is expected to overestimate GFR. Third, the formula was derived by older assay methods for serum creatinine, which cannot be calibrated to newer assay methods and would be expected to lead to a systematic bias in estimating creatinine clearance. Fourth, it systematically overestimates Ccr in edematous or obese patients. Fifth, the large age term means that all older adults will have lower levels of estimated GFR. Sixth, because it was derived in Caucasians, it may underestimate creatinine clearance in African Americans.

The most commonly used equation to estimate GFRcr has been the four-variable Modification of Diet in Renal Disease (MDRD) Study equation using standardized creatinine.[59]

$$eGFRcr = 175 \text{ standardized } Scr^{-1.154} \times Age^{-0.203} \times 0.742 \text{ (if female)} \times 1.21 \text{ (if African American)} \quad \textbf{(Eq. 21)}$$

where eGFRcr is expressed in mL/min/1.73 m^2, Scr is expressed in mg/dL, and age is expressed in years. The MDRD Study equation was developed in a study population of 1628 patients with chronic kidney disease (mean mGFR 40 mL/min/1.73 m^2) who were predominantly Caucasian and had predominantly nondiabetic kidney disease. GFR was measured using urinary clearance of ^{125}I-iothalamate, and serum creatinine was measured using a kinetic alkaline-picrate assay, which was subsequently calibrated to standardized creatinine. It includes a variable for race (African American vs. other). As shown by the Scr coefficient of less than −1, the relationship of eGFR to Scr is more steep than in the hypothetical relationship in which there are no non-GFR determinants of the filtration markers. A rise in the serum creatinine level to 1.5, 2, and 3 times the baseline value is associated with a decline in eGFRcr to 73%, 45%, or 28% of the baseline value, respectively, if all other factors are constant. The MDRD Study equation is more accurate than the Cockcroft-Gault equation and has been validated extensively. It is unbiased in individuals with eGFRcr less than 60 mL/min/1.73 m^2, but it underestimates measured GFR at higher levels of eGFRcr, and it is relatively imprecise.[69] The main limitations of the MDRD Study equation are (1) because it systematically underestimates mGFR at higher eGFRcr, numeric values cannot be reported for eGFRcr levels greater than 60 mL/min/1.73 m^2, and (2) because the race variable includes coefficients only for African Americans vs. other, it may be more biased in populations of other races and ethnicities.

The Chronic Kidney Disease Epidemiology Collaboration (CKD-EPI) equation has been developed to overcome some of the limitations of the MDRD Study equation.[64]

$$eGFRcr = 141 \times [\min(Scr/\kappa), 1)^{\alpha} \times [\max(Scr/\kappa), 1]^{-1.209} \times 0.993^{Age} \times 1.018 \text{ (if female)} \times 1.159 \text{ (if African American)} \quad \textbf{(Eq. 22)}$$

where eGFRcr is expressed in mL/min/1.73 m^2, Scr is standardized serum creatinine expressed in mg/dL, age is expressed in years, κ is 0.7 for females and 0.9 for males, α is −0.329 for females and −0.411 for males, min indicates the minimum of Scr /κ or 1, and max indicates the maximum of Scr/κ or 1.

The CKD-EPI creatinine equation was developed in a study population of 5504 individuals, derived from 10 studies, with a mean measured GFR of 68 mL/min/1.73 m^2 and a wide range of age, and included men and women, whites and blacks, and subjects with and without kidney disease, diabetes, and kidney transplants. GFR was measured as urinary clearance of ^{125}I-iothalamate. The equation was validated in a separate population of 3859 individuals from 16 studies. The CKD-EPI creatinine equation is based on the same variables as the MDRD Study equation; additional terms to characterize individuals according to presence or absence of diabetes, history of organ transplantation, or weight did not improve accuracy. The CKD-EPI creatinine equation differs from the MDRD Study equation principally by having a two-slope relationship between eGFRcr and Scr and a steeper relationship between eGFRcr and age. Fig. 2.5 compares the performance of the two equations in the validation population. The CKD-EPI creatinine equation has a lower bias than the MDRD Study equation, especially at higher GFR. Precision is improved, but it is still suboptimal. As with the MDRD Study equation, the CKD-EPI creatinine equation does not include terms for racial or ethnic groups other than blacks or whites.

GFR estimating equations based on creatinine have been implemented in laboratory information systems for automated reporting of eGFR when serum creatinine is measured.[68] A systematic review comparing the CKD-EPI creatinine and MDRD Study equations confirmed the greater accuracy of the CKD-EPI creatinine at higher eGFRcr and recommended it for use in general populations.[69] Current guidelines by the international group Kidney Disease Improving Global Outcomes (KDIGO) recommend using eGFRcr as the "first test" for evaluation of kidney function in routine general practice.[3] The guidelines recommend reporting eGFRcr by clinical laboratories whenever serum creatinine is measured, and using the CKD-EPI creatinine equation in North America, Europe, and Australia, and other equations elsewhere if they are more accurate than the CKD-EPI equation. For example, a Japanese creatinine equation is more accurate in Japanese populations than the CKD-EPI creatinine equation and is in widespread use there.[67] Since the KDIGO guidelines were developed, other GFR estimating equations for use with standardized creatinine assays have been reported, including the Lund-Malmo revised equation, Berlin Initiative Study (BIS) creatinine equation, and Full Age Spectrum (FAS) creatinine

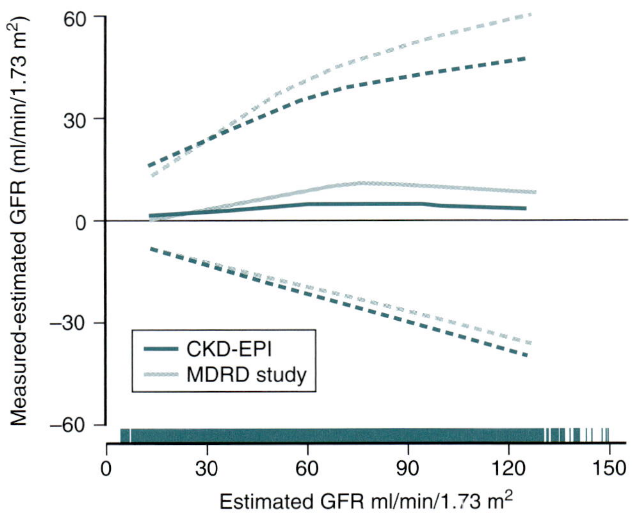

FIG. 2.5 Comparison of performance of MDRD Study and CKD-EPI equations by estimated GFR shown are lowest smooth line (*solid curve*) and 95% CI using quantile regression (*dashed lines*), for the CKD-EPI validation data set excluding lowest and highest 2.5% of estimated GFR values. The CKD-EPI equation is in darker color, and the MDRD Study equation is in gray. The CKD-EPI equation has improved performance compared with the MDRD Study equation with a decrease in median difference (IQR) from 2.7 (14.7) to 0.4 (16.4), and P30 from 83% to 86%.[58] (Reproduced with permission from Levey AS, Stevens LA, Schmid CH, et al. A new equation to estimate glomerular filtration rate. *Ann Intern Med.* 2009;150(9):604–612.)

equation.[62-65] These equations are not more accurate than the CKD-EPI creatinine equation in the overall adult population but may perform better in some subgroups.[69,67]

There are limitations to the use of all estimating equations based on serum creatinine. Age, sex, and race serve as surrogates of creatinine generation but do not account for differences in creatinine generation due to effects of diet, nutritional status, and chronic illness on muscle mass. This is especially important in acute and chronic kidney diseases that may lead to reduced creatinine generation due to reduction in protein intake (especially meat), malnutrition, and muscle wasting, and may enhance creatinine secretion and extrarenal elimination. These factors tend to blunt the rise in serum creatinine as GFR declines, and they may cause serious overestimation of the level of GFR from serum creatinine.

Even among patients without kidney disease, differences in race and ethnicity are likely to be confounded with differences in creatinine generation, thus requiring development and validation of multiple terms for use throughout the world.[68] Malnutrition and chronic illness are likely to be more common in the elderly. Accurate GFR estimates are especially important in the elderly due to the high prevalence of chronic kidney disease. It is not likely that variation in other non-GFR determinants of serum creatinine, such as drug-induced inhibition of secretion or extrarenal elimination, will be captured by routinely used equations. Standardized assays have overcome limitations due to variation in creatinine calibration, but even standardized assays are less precise at low values; therefore errors in GFR estimates may be greater in normal adults, in whom serum creatinine is low because of normal GFR, and in children, in whom serum creatinine is low because of lower muscle mass. Finally, GFR estimates are less accurate in the nonsteady state than in the steady state. Table 2.4 lists clinical situations in which estimating equations for GFR may not be accurate and confirmatory tests for evaluation of kidney function may be indicated.

Cystatin C

Cystatin C has been proposed as an endogenous filtration marker to be used as an alternative or in addition to creatinine. A summary of issues related to its structure, generation, renal handling, metabolism, measurement, and use as an index of GFR is presented below.

1. Structure and Function

Cystatin C is a 13,343-dalton protein consisting of 120 amino acid residues in a single polypeptide chain.[69] Cystatin C regulates the activities of cysteine proteases to prevent uncontrolled proteolysis and tissue damage.[70,71]

2. Plasma Levels

The reference range for serum cystatin C is listed as 0.52 to 0.98 mg/L. However, the true "normal level" is not well known because, as with other filtration markers, it depends on the level of GFR. In a sample of noninstitutionalized US population, the third National Health and Nutrition Examination Survey (NHANES III), the median plasma cystatin C level was 0.85 mg/L, with 1.12 mg/L as the upper 99th percentile for young people 20 to 39 years of age who did not have hypertension and diabetes.[72] The level of cystatin C was related to age, sex, and ethnicity, with the median serum level estimated at 8% lower in women than men, and it increased steeply with age and was greater in non-Hispanic whites. Prevalence of increased serum cystatin C levels (>1.12 mg/L) were 1%,

41%, and greater than 50% in people younger than 20 years, 60 years and older, and 80 years and older, respectively. In a multivariable analysis, older age; non-Hispanic white ethnicity; hypertension; current smoking; lower levels of education; lower high-density lipoprotein; and higher body mass index, C-reactive protein, and triglyceride values are associated with increased serum cystatin C levels.[72]

3. Generation

Cystatin C is thought to be produced by all human nucleated cells at a stable rate.[70,71] As described later, in contrast to creatinine and urea, cystatin C is not excreted in the urine; therefore studies of its generation in humans have evaluated the association of demographic and clinical factors with variation in plasma levels after taking into account the level of measured Ccr or GFR. These studies show that cystatin C is less dependent on muscle mass and diet than creatinine, and consequently is less strongly related to age and sex than creatinine and not related to race. Higher BMI, C-reactive protein, and smoking are among the most consistent factors associated with higher cystatin C.[73,74-77]

4. Renal Handling

Cystatin C is thought to be completely filtered at the glomerulus, taken up by the proximal tubular cells, and then catabolized, such that only small amounts of cystatin C are lost in the urine under normal conditions.

a. *Glomerular filtration.* The molecular diameter of cystatin C (3 nm) suggests that it can be freely filtered by the glomerulus.
b. *Tubular reabsorption and secretion.* Cystatin C is degraded by proximal tubular cells after its passage through the glomerular membrane.[78] In kidney disease, loss of cystatin C in the urine increases due to failure of reabsorption due to tubular damage.[79-81] There is no suggestion of tubular secretion.

5. Extrarenal Elimination

Extrarenal elimination of cystatin C was observed to occur in the spleen, diaphragm, heart, liver, and lungs in nephrectomized rats and was estimated at approximately 15% of the total cystatin C elimination.[82,83]

6. Assay

There are two primary methods by which commercially available autoanalyzers assay cystatin C: particle-enhanced turbidimetric immunoassay (PETIA)[84] and particle-enhanced nephelometric immunoassay (PENIA).[85] With the PENIA method, no interference is noted with common interfering factors such as bilirubin, rheumatoid factor, hemoglobin, or triglycerides. The PETIA method also shows minimal interference with these substances, but bilirubin levels of 150 to 300 μmol/L (8.8 to 17.5 mg/dL) raise cystatin C levels by less than 10%.[84] An International Federation of Clinical Chemistry and Laboratory Medicine (IFCC) Working Group on Standardization of Cystatin C has produced and characterized both a primary and a secondary reference preparation for cystatin C, but international standardization of the assay is still in process, and important differences remain.[86-88]

7. Cystatin C as a Filtration Marker

Based on the previous considerations, the relationship of GFR to plasma cystatin C concentration is expressed as follows:

$$\text{GFR}\ (\text{Gcys} + \text{TRcys} - \text{Ecys})/\text{Scys} \qquad \textbf{(Eq. 23)}$$

The first GFR estimating equations for use with standardized cystatin C in general populations were the CKD-EPI 2012 cystatin C and creatinine-cystatin C equations.[89]

$$\begin{aligned}\text{eGFRcys} = {} & 133 \times \min(\text{Scys}/0.8,\ 1)^{-0.499} \\ & \times \max(\text{Scys}/0.8,\ 1)^{-1.328} \times 0.996^{\text{Age}} \\ & \times 0.932\ [\text{if female}]\end{aligned} \qquad \textbf{(Eq. 24)}$$

where eGFRcys is expressed in mL/min/1.73 m^2, Scys is serum cystatin C expressed in mg/L, age is expressed in years, min indicates the minimum of Scys or 1, and max indicates the maximum of Scys or 1.

$$\begin{aligned}\text{eGFRcr} - \text{cys} = {} & 135 \times \min(\text{Scr}/\kappa,\ 1)\ \alpha \\ & \times \max(\text{Scr}/0.8, 1)^{-0.601} \\ & \times \min(\text{Scys}/0.8,\ 1)^{-0.375} \\ & \times \max(\text{Scys}/0.8,\ 1)^{-0.711} \\ & \times 0.995^{\text{Age}} \times 0.969\ [\text{if female}] \\ & \times 1.08\ [\text{if African American}]\end{aligned} \qquad \textbf{(Eq. 25)}$$

where eGFRcr-cys is expressed in mL/min/1.73 m^2, Scr is serum creatinine expressed in mg/dL, Scys is serum cystatin C expressed in mg/L, κ is 0.7 for females and 0.9 for males, α is −0.248 for females and −0.207 for males, min indicates the minimum of Scr/κ or 1, and max indicates the maximum of Scr/κ or 1.

The CKD-EPI 2012 cystatin C and creatinine-cystatin C equations were developed in a diverse study population of 5352 individuals from 13 studies with a mean GFR of 68 mL/min/1.73 m^2.[89] The equation was validated in a separate population of 1119 individuals from 5 studies. Although serum cystatin C levels correlated more strongly with measured GFR than serum creatinine levels, eGFRcys is not more accurate than eGFRcr. In contrast, eGFRcr-cys is more accurate than either eGFRcr or eGFRcys, but requires age, sex, and race (Fig. 2.6).[89] As discussed earlier, the likely explanation for the increased accuracy of eGFRcr-cys is that the non-GFR determinants of each marker (creatinine and cystatin C) contribute less when both markers are included than the non-GFR determinants of either marker when only one marker is included.

Of interest, the risks of cardiovascular disease and mortality, but not kidney failure, are more strongly related to decreased eGFRcys than eGFRcr, presumably due to differential risk associations of non-GFR determinants of cystatin C and creatinine.[90] For example, increased risk for cardiovascular disease and mortality is associated with factors that are associated with decreased eGFRcys, such as inflammation, obesity, and smoking, but with increased eGFRcr, such as malnutrition and chronic illness.

The KDIGO guidelines recommend eGFRcys and eGFRcr-cys as confirmatory tests for the evaluation of kidney function.[3] In general, eGFRcys is a useful confirmatory test in patients in whom eGFRcr is suspected to be inaccurate. In other patients, eGFRcr-cys is the more accurate confirmatory test. The KDIGO guidelines recommend reporting eGFRcys or eGFRcr-cys whenever serum cystatin C is measured and using the CKD-EPI cystatin C equation or creatinine-cystatin C equations in North America, Europe, and Australia, and other equations elsewhere, if they are more accurate than the CKD-EPI equations. Of interest, the Japanese creatinine-cystatin C equation, but not the Japanese cystatin C equation, is more accurate than the CKD-EPI equations in Japan.[91] Other recently reported equations, including BIS creatinine-cystatin C equation, the Caucasian and Asian Pediatric and Adult (CAPA) cystatin C equation, and the FAS cystatin C equation, are not more accurate than the CKD-EPI equations in adults.[65,64-67] As with eGFRcr, the accuracy of eGFRcys is limited by factors associated with the non-GFR determinants of serum cystatin C, nonstandardized assays, and the nonsteady state (see Table 2.4).

One common application for eGFRcys or eGFRcr-cys is for confirmation of the diagnosis of CKD in patients with eGFRcr below the threshold for diagnosis (60 mL/min/1.73 m^2), but without markers of kidney damage. In such patients, if eGFRcys or eGFRcr-cys is <60 mL/min/1.73 m^2, the likelihood of measured GFR <60 mL/min/1.73 m^2 and the risks of cardiovascular disease and mortality are greater than in patients with eGFRcys or eGFRcr-cys ≥60 mL/min/1.73 m^2, and the diagnosis of CKD can be considered confirmed.

Urea

A relationship between plasma urea and kidney function was recognized long before the development of the concept of clearance or of techniques to assess GFR.[92] The factors influencing both the generation of urea and its excretion by the kidneys are considerably more complex and variable than those for creatinine and cystatin C (see Table 2.4).[93] As a result, serum urea nitrogen concentration (SUN, for historical reasons, often referred to as the blood urea nitrogen or BUN) has been replaced largely by the serum creatinine and cystatin C concentrations as an endogenous filtration marker in routine clinical practice. Nonetheless, measurement of the SUN remains useful in some clinical circumstances. A brief summary of the properties of urea is presented hereafter.

1. Structure and Function

Urea is a 60-dalton molecular weight compound derived from deamination of amino acids. It is a nitrogenous waste product, accounting for more than 75% of nonprotein nitrogen excreted by the body. Urea is freely distributed in total body water. At high BUN levels (greater than 100 mg/dL), urea has neurotoxicity.

2. Plasma Levels

Plasma urea is affected by numerous factors in addition to GFR; thus BUN levels in normal individuals vary over a wider range than creatinine, from approximately 8 to 22 mg/dL.

3. Generation

The metabolism of urea, its relationship to dietary protein intake, and the effect of kidney disease on protein metabolism are discussed in detail in Chapter 13. Briefly, urea is the product of protein catabolism and is synthesized primarily by the liver. Approximately one-quarter of synthesized urea is metabolized in the intestine to carbon dioxide and ammonia, and the ammonia thus generated returns to the liver and is reconverted to urea.

Dietary protein intake is the principal determinant of urea generation and may be estimated as follows:

$$EPI = 6.25 \times GUN \quad \textbf{(Eq. 26)}$$

where EPI is estimated protein intake, GUN is urea generation, and both are measured in g/d.[93]

Usual protein intake in the United States is approximately 100 g/d, corresponding to a usual value for urea nitrogen generation of approximately 15 g/d.

In the steady state, urea generation can be estimated from measurements of urea excretion, as shown here:

$$GUN = UUN \times V + 0.031 \times weight \quad \textbf{(Eq. 27)}$$

where GUN and UUN × V are measured in g/d, weight is measured in kg, and 0.031 g/kg/d is a predicted value for nitrogen losses other than urine urea nitrogen.[94]

For a 70-kg individual with a dietary protein intake of 100 g/d, urea excretion and other nitrogen losses would be approximately 13 g/d and 2 g/d, respectively.

Urea generation is also influenced by factors other than protein intake (see Table 2.4). An increase is observed after administration of corticosteroids, diuretics, or tetracyclines; after absorption of blood from the gut; and in infection, acute kidney injury, trauma, congestive heart failure, and sodium depletion. Decreases in urea generation may occur in severe malnutrition and liver disease.

4. Renal Handling of Urea

Urea (molecular diameter 0.36 nm) is uncharged, not bound to plasma proteins, and freely filtered by the glomerulus and reabsorbed in both the proximal and distal nephron. Hence urea excretion (UUN × V) is determined by both the filtered load and tubular reabsorption (TRUN):

$$UUN \times V = GFR \times SUN - TRUN \quad \textbf{(Eq. 28)}$$

where TRUN is tubular reabsorption of urea.

Consequently, clearance of urea (or urea nitrogen, CUN) is less than GFR:

$$CUN = GFR - TRUN/SUN \quad \textbf{(Eq. 29)}$$

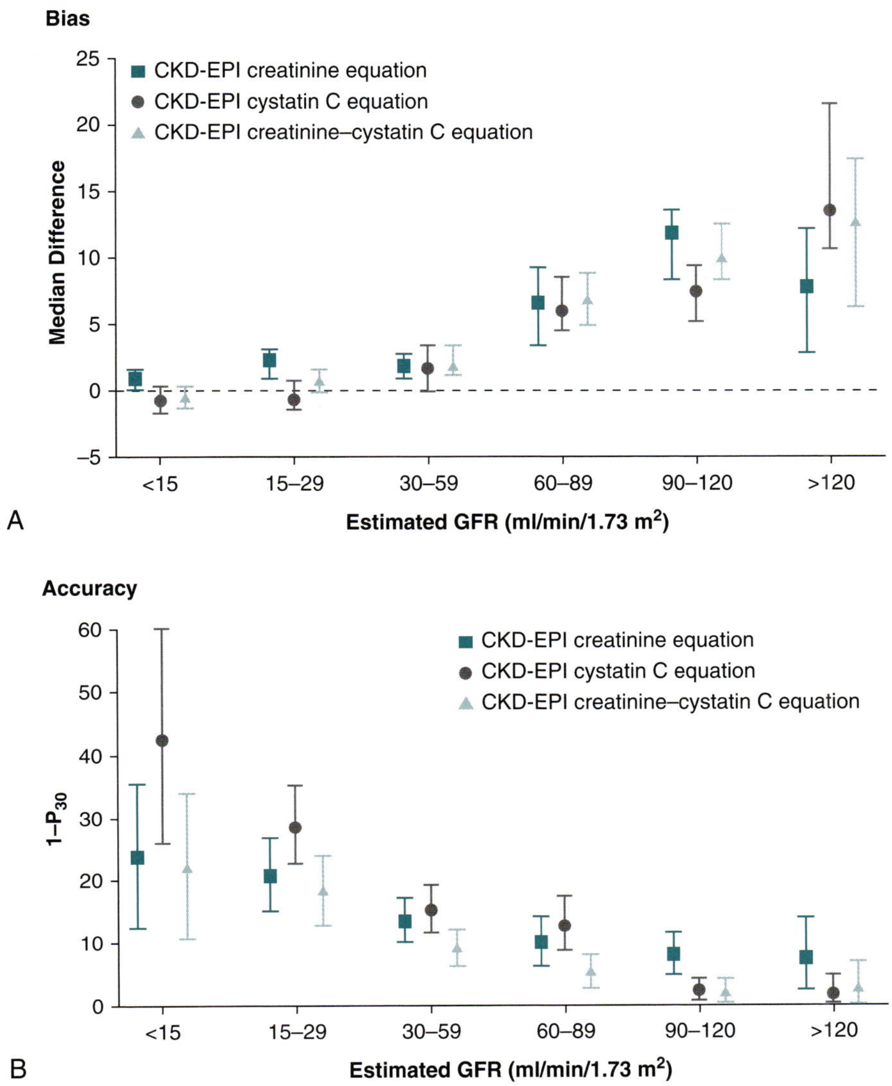

FIG. 2.6 Comparison of performance of CKD-EPI equations for creatinine, cystatin C, and the combination by estimated GFR. Panel A shows the median difference between measured and estimated GFR. The bias is similar with the equation using creatinine alone, the equation using cystatin C alone, and the combined creatinine–cystatin C equation. Panel B shows the accuracy of the three equations with respect to the percentage of estimates that were greater than 30% of the measured GFR (1 – P30). Mean values for the study population for 1-P30 were 12.8% for eGFRcr, 14.1% for eGFRcys, and 8.5% for eGFRcr-cys. I bars indicate 95% confidence intervals.[89] (Reproduced with permission from Inker LA, Schmid CH, Tighiouart H, et al. Estimating glomerular filtration rate from serum creatinine and cystatin C. *N Engl J Med.* 2012;367(1):20–29.)

where TRUN/SUN is clearance of UN by tubular reabsorption.

In the proximal convoluted tubule, a large fraction of the filtered load of urea is reabsorbed regardless of the state of diuresis. In the medullary collecting duct, urea reabsorption is closely linked to water reabsorption. In the absence of antidiuretic hormone (diuresis), the medullary collecting duct is relatively impermeable to urea; thus urea reabsorption is minimal. Conversely, in the presence of antidiuretic hormone (antidiuresis), permeability rises and urea reabsorption increases. In normal individuals, the urea clearance ranges from as high as 65% of GFR during diuresis to as low as 35% of GFR during antidiuresis.

In patients with GFR less than 20 mL/min/1.73 m^2, the urea clearance ranges from 70% to 90% of GFR and is not influenced greatly by the state of diuresis. Thus urea clearance is approximately 5 mL/min less than GFR. By coincidence, at this level of GFR, the difference between the values of GFR and urea clearance is similar to the difference between the values of creatinine clearance and GFR, providing a relatively simple method to assess GFR in patients with severely decreased GFR.[95,96] This method has also been used to assess the level of residual kidney function in patients with chronic kidney failure undergoing maintenance dialysis.[100]

$$GFR = (Ccr + CUN)/2 \quad \textbf{(Eq. 30)}$$

However, the kidney handling of urea and creatinine is influenced by different physiological and pathological processes and may vary independently, causing deviations from this approximation. In addition, kidney functions other than GFR may contribute importantly to residual kidney function.[97]

5. Extrarenal Elimination

More than 90% of urea is excreted by the kidneys, with losses through the gastrointestinal tract and skin accounting for most of the remaining fraction.

6. Assay

The urease method assays the release of ammonia in serum or urine after reaction with the enzyme urease.[53] A variety of systems for detection of ammonium are available, all with good precision and specificity. The presence of ammonium in reagents or use of ammonium heparin as an anticoagulant may falsely elevate the SUN. Urea is also subject to degradation by bacterial urease. Bacterial growth in urine samples can be inhibited by refrigerating the sample until measurement or by adding an acid to the collection container to maintain urine pH below 4.0.

7. Urea as a Filtration Marker

In the steady state, the SUN level reflects the levels of urea clearance and generation.

$$GFR = (GUN + TRUN)/SUN \quad \textbf{(Eq. 31)}$$

Consequently, many factors influence the level of SUN (see Table 2.4); thus estimating equations based on SUN (eGFRUN) would not be generally useful. Nonetheless, SUN can be a useful tool in some clinical circumstances.

As mentioned earlier, the state of diuresis has a large effect on urea reabsorption and a small effect on GFR, but it does not affect creatinine secretion. Hence the state of diuresis affects urea clearance more than creatinine clearance and is reflected in the ratio of SUN to Scr. The normal ratio of SUN to Scr is approximately 10:1. In principle, a reduction in GFR without a change in the state of diuresis would not alter the ratio. However, conditions causing antidiuresis (dehydration or reduced kidney perfusion) would decrease GFR and increase urea reabsorption, thus raising the SUN-to-Scr ratio. Consequently, the SUN-to-Scr ratio may be a useful aid in the differential diagnosis of acute kidney injury (AKI). Conversely, overhydration or increased kidney perfusion would raise GFR and decrease urea reabsorption, thus lowering the serum creatinine and the SUN-to-Scr ratio. However, conditions affecting urea generation may also affect the SUN and the SUN-to-Scr ratio when GFR is decreased, limiting the use of this ratio as a guide to the status of hydration and kidney perfusion in patients.

Also important is the well-recognized relationship of the level of kidney function, the SUN level, and clinical features of uremia. A traditional rule of thumb is that a SUN level greater than 100 mg/dL is associated with a higher risk of complications in both acute and chronic kidney failure and may indicate the need to initiate dialysis, although SUN may exceed this level without apparent clinical effects in many clinical circumstances.[98-100] The role of high concentrations of urea versus other retained nitrogenous wastes in causing symptoms of uremia is not well known, despite decades of investigation. In both acute and chronic kidney disease, restriction of dietary protein intake to 40 to 50 g/d would reduce urea nitrogen excretion to approximately 4.5 g/d. Consequently, the SUN level might rise to only 40 to 60 mg/dL, despite severe reduction in GFR. Although protein restriction may temporarily ameliorate some of the uremic symptoms, severe reduction in GFR is associated with development of uremic symptoms, despite only moderate elevation in SUN.

Another application of SUN measurement is to estimate the adequacy of hemodialysis treatment. A large body of evidence relates the urea reduction ratio (URR) to urea clearance (expressed as Kt/Vurea) during hemodialysis and clinical outcomes.

$$URR = (\text{Predialysis SUN} - \text{Postdialysis SUN})/\text{Predialysis SUN} \quad \textbf{(Eq. 32)}$$

$$Kt/Vurea = -\ln(R - 0.03) + [(4 - 3.5 \times R) \times (UF/W)] \quad \textbf{(Eq. 33)}$$

where K is the dialyzer clearance of urea in mL/min, t is dialysis session time in minutes, V is the volume of distribution of urea in mL, R is the ratio of the postdialysis to predialysis SUN, UF is the ultrafiltration volume in liters, and W is the postdialysis weight in kg.[101,102]

For a hypothetical patient with postdialysis weight of 70 kg and UF of 2 L, a URR of 65% would correspond to a Kt/V of approximately 1.2 per dialysis session. If the volume of urea distribution is 42,000 mL and dialysis session time is 240 minutes, 3 sessions per week would correspond to an average dialyzer urea clearance of approximately 15 mL/min throughout the week, or approximately 12% of normal GFR. A detailed description of urea kinetic modeling and hemodialysis adequacy is given in Chapter 24.

Novel Markers

There are several alternative novel endogenous markers under investigation as potential filtration markers that could be used in addition or in combination with creatinine or cystatin C. For optimal clinical use, it will be important to understand their non-GFR determinants and factors associated with deviations in these determinants, as discussed previously. Because of the large number of low-molecular-weight serum proteins and metabolites correlated with measured GFR, development of a panel eGFR may be practical. An important consideration for the introduction of novel filtration markers is the availability of assays that can be easily implemented and standardized across all clinical laboratories.

It is beyond the scope of this chapter to discuss novel markers in detail. β2-microglobulin (β2M) and β-trace protein (βTP) are low-molecular-weight serum proteins (see Table 2.2). As with cystatin C, β2M and βTP are freely filtered by the glomerulus and extensively reabsorbed and degraded by the proximal tubule, with only small amounts lost in the urine under normal conditions. Like cystatin

C, serum levels of β2M and βTP are more strongly correlated with measured GFR than serum creatinine and are less influenced by age, sex, and race than creatinine.[76,103] However, GFR estimating equations using β2M and βTP these markers derived in CKD populations are not more accurate than equations using creatinine and cystatin C.[104] Whether they provide an advantage in diverse populations is under study.

Metabolites associated with eGFR other than creatinine and urea have been discovered using metabolomic techniques in large populations. Serum levels of pseudouridine (a nucleic acid metabolite) and acetylthreonine (an amino acid metabolite) are more strongly correlated with mGFR than creatinine and urea and may have promise for GFR estimation.[105]

ACKNOWLEDGMENTS

The authors are grateful to Sara Couture, BS, for assistance with manuscript preparation.

A full list of references is available at www.expertconsult.com.

3

Diabetic Kidney Disease

Radica Z. Alicic, MD, FHM, FACP, Emily J. Johnson, PhD, and Katherine R. Tuttle, MD, FACP, FASN, FNKF

OUTLINE

INTRODUCTION

Diabetic kidney disease (DKD) is the leading cause of chronic kidney disease (CKD) worldwide and one of the most serious complications of diabetes.[1,2] It is a major, yet underrecognized contributor to the global burden of chronic diseases.[3] Despite many improvements in diabetes care over the past two decades, DKD still develops in approximately 30% of individuals with type 1 diabetes and nearly 50% of those with type 2 diabetes.[1,4,5] Although the incidence of end-stage renal disease (ESRD) has in fact stabilized over the past decade, the increasing prevalence of diabetes due to obesity, aging, and reduction in cardiovascular disease–related deaths has greatly expanded the number of people living with diabetes.[3] In 2015 there were an estimated 415 million cases of diabetes throughout the world; by 2040, this number is projected to increase to 642 million cases, of which 90% to 95% will be type 2 diabetes.[6] These data clearly show that prevalence of DKD is growing at an unprecedented pace.[7-9]

Development of DKD in people with diabetes amplifies the risk of cardiovascular diseases, infections, and cancers, as well as cardiovascular-related and all-cause mortality.[3,10] Indeed, recent studies indicate that excess mortality associated with diabetes is mainly noted in those who developed kidney disease.[11,12] Compared with the nondiabetic population, individuals with diabetes alone have a twofold higher risk of cardiovascular mortality, whereas individuals with both diabetes and kidney disease exhibit a threefold to twelvefold higher mortality risk.[12-14]

Due to the frequent occurrence of death, only a minority of individuals with DKD survive to ESRD.[15] Moreover, those with diabetes who survive to ESRD exhibit a 10- to 100-fold higher mortality risk than age-matched controls with normal kidney function.[3] Due to the impact of DKD on diabetes-related complications and deaths, as well as the rising prevalence of diabetes, the global number of deaths attributed to DKD rose by 94% between 1990 and 2012.[16] As the burden of DKD and diabetes-attributable ESRD grows, limited accessibility to renal replacement therapy (RRT) presents an increasingly emergent global healthcare challenge.[17]

DIAGNOSIS AND CLASSIFICATION OF DIABETIC KIDNEY DISEASE

DKD is diagnosed by macroalbuminuria (albumin-to-creatinine ratio [ACR] >300 mg/g) or microalbuminuria (ACR 30 to 300 mg/g) associated with retinopathy (type 1 diabetes or type 2 diabetes), and in type 1 diabetes, more than 10 years' duration of diabetes.[18] Because a high glomerular filtration rate (GFR), or hyperfiltration, often occurs early after a diagnosis of diabetes, GFR <90 mL/min/1.73 m^2 may represent substantial loss of kidney function in DKD[18] (Table 3.1).

The preferred test for albuminuria is the urinary albumin-to-creatinine ratio (UACR) measured in a spot urine sample, preferably in the morning.[19,20] Because UACR results are characterized by substantial day-to-day variability (up to 40%), abnormal results must be confirmed by at least two specimens collected over a 3- to 6-month period.[20] In clinical practice, estimated GFR (eGFR) is usually calculated from serum creatinine concentration. Although the Modification of Diet in Renal Disease (MDRD) equation is commonly reported by clinical laboratories, the Chronic Kidney Disease-Epidemiologic Prognosis Initiative (CKD-EPI) equation is more accurate, particularly at eGFR levels in the normal or near-normal range.[20]

Screening for DKD should be performed annually, starting 5 years after diagnosis of type 1 diabetes or at the time of type 2 diabetes diagnosis.[20,21] The following features should prompt evaluation for non-DKD causes of kidney disease: absence of diabetic retinopathy, sudden onset of low eGFR, or rapidly decreasing eGFR; abrupt increase in albuminuria; development of nephrotic syndrome; presence of active urinary sediment; refractory hypertension; signs or symptoms

TABLE 3.1 Likelihood of Diabetic Kidney Disease Staged According to Glomerular Filtration Rate and Level of Albuminuria

		ALBUMINURIA		
GFR (mL/min)	**CKD Stage**	**Normoalbuminuria**	**Microalbuminuria**	**Macroalbuminuria**
>60	1 + 2	At risk	Possible DKD	DKD
30–60	3	Possible DKD	Possible DKD	DKD
<30	4 + 5	Unlikely DKD	Unlikely DKD	DKD

Normoalbuminuria (<30 mg/g urinary creatinine in spot sample or 24-hour collection), microalbuminuria (30–300 mg/g urinary creatinine in spot sample or 24-hour collection), macroalbuminuria (>300 mg/g urinary creatinine in spot sample or 24-hour collection).
CKD, Chronic kidney disease; *DKD*, diabetic kidney disease; *GFR*, glomerular filtration rate.
(Adapted from Liyanage T, Ninomiya T, Jha V, et al. Worldwide access to treatment for end-stage kidney disease: a systematic review. *Lancet.* 2015; 385(9981): 1975-1982.)

of another systemic disease; and/or >30% decline in eGFR within 2 to 3 months of initiating treatment with a renin-angiotensin system (RAS) inhibitor.[18]

Novel Biomarkers in Development

Current diagnostic methods are imprecise and lack adequate sensitivity for identifying patients with DKD. For example, many diabetic patients remain normoalbuminuric despite kidney structural damage that is severely advanced by the time eGFR declines.[22,23] Testing for albuminuria and serum creatinine as primary diagnostic indicators also carries a number of limitations such as high biological and assay variability, lack of standardization, and low specificity.[24] A number of new candidate biomarkers representing various molecular processes and disease pathways are under investigation for applications, including DKD diagnosis, risk stratification, monitoring, and prognosis (Box 3.1). However, none are currently validated for clinical use.

BOX 3.1 Potential Biomarkers Under Study for Diabetic Kidney Disease Classified by Mechanism and Source

Inflammation
Tumor necrosis factor alpha (TNF-α) – blood
Tumor necrosis factor receptor-1 (TNFR-1) – blood
Tumor necrosis factor receptor-2 (TNFR-2) – blood
Serum amyloid A (SAA) – blood and urine
Macrophage chemotactic protein-1 (MCP-1) – urine

Fibrosis
Connective tissue growth factor (CTGF) – urine
Transforming growth factor-β (TGF-β) – urine
Type IV collagen – urine

Angiogenesis
Vascular endothelial growth factor-A (VEGF-A) – blood

Endothelial Dysfunction
Amino terminal pro C-type natriuretic peptide (NT-proCNP) – blood

Mineral Metabolism
Fibroblast growth factor 23 (FGF-23) – blood

Tubular Injury
Neutrophil gelatinase associated lipocalin (NGAL) – urine
Kidney injury marker (KIM-1) – urine
Epidermal growth factor (EGF) – urine

RISK FACTORS

Demographic Factors

Several studies indicate that older age is an important predictor of progressive albuminuria and kidney dysfunction in diabetes.[25,26] Male sex is a risk factor for kidney function decline in type 2 diabetes.[25,27,29] Certain ethnicities also appear to exhibit greater susceptibility to, and/or a worse prognosis for, DKD.[5,30] For instance, people of South Asian, African, American Indian, and Pacific Islander ancestry or Hispanic ethnicity are at higher risk of kidney function decline compared with people of European descent.[30-33]

Alterations of Developmental Programming

Exposure to maternal diabetes during gestation increases the risk of DKD and high birth weight (≥4500 grams).[31] Both low (<2500 grams) and high (≥4500 grams) birth weight are associated with an elevated risk of albuminuria in the offspring.[34] For low-birth-weight infants, the proposed mechanism underlying increased risk of DKD is growth retardation, resulting in low nephron number and alterations of developmental programming that may predispose these infants to development of kidney disease later in life.[34]

Hereditary Risk Factors

The fact that recognized risk factors fail to account for the variability of incident DKD suggests a genetic component underlying risk. Evidence for such inherited susceptibility to DKD comes from family studies that have shown increased risk of kidney disease in family groupings.[35,36] The diabetic offspring of parents with diabetes and DKD have a cumulative risk of developing kidney disease of >70% and a threefold to fourfold increased incidence of kidney disease compared with children of diabetic parents without kidney disease.[35,37,38] It appears that any inherited predisposition for developing DKD does not follow simple Mendelian rules.[39] Genes that may be associated with DKD risk include those with functional networks related to the RAS, lipid metabolism, polyol pathways, fibrinogenesis, and kidney development; however, to date, no specific gene or gene combination has been definitively implicated in DKD risk.[40]

Hyperglycemia

A relationship between elevated blood glucose and diabetic complications was observed as early as the 1930s, but five decades elapsed before an association between glycemic control and development of DKD was recognized.[41,42] It is currently accepted that poor glycemic control independently predicts progression to development of albuminuria and ESRD in patients with type 1 diabetes and normoalbuminuria.[43] Similarly, higher hemoglobin A1C (HbA1C) levels are among the strongest determinants of DKD progression independent of albuminuria in patients with type 2 diabetes.[26,44-47]

Two landmark trials conducted in patients with either early-stage type 1 diabetes or type 2 diabetes found that early, intensive glycemic control reduced the long-term risk of DKD onset.[48,49] The Diabetes Control and Complications Trial (DCCT) enrolled individuals with early, uncomplicated type 1 diabetes and compared effects of intensive versus conventional glycemic control. Time-averaged HbA1C during the 6-year study was 7.3% in the intensive therapy group and 9.1% in the conventional therapy group.[50] The original DCCT participants were followed for another two decades in the Epidemiology of Diabetes Interventions and Complications (EDIC) study. Although the original differences in glucose control dissipated during the EDIC study, with HbA1C approximating 8% in both groups, an interim analysis including 9 years of EDIC data clearly showed that the intensive glycemic control group exhibited a 34% and 56% lower risk of developing microalbuminuria and macroalbuminuria, respectively.[51] Pooled data from 22 years of follow-up showed that intensive glucose control was associated with about 50% lower risk of developing eGFR <60 mL/min/1.73 m^2 and ESRD, but the incidence of ESRD was small ($n = 8$ participants in intensive care group, $n = 16$ participants in standard therapy group). The average rate of eGFR loss was significantly reduced from 1.56 mL/min/1.73 m^2 per year in the standard therapy group to 1.27 mL/min/1.73 m^2 per year in the intensive therapy group ($P < 0.001$).[52]

The United Kingdom Prospective Diabetes Study (UKPDS) enrolled individuals with newly diagnosed type 2 diabetes and compared the effect of conventional therapy to intensive therapy with either sulfonylurea or insulin or, in overweight patients, metformin.[53,54] Between-group differences in glycemic control were lost 1 year into posttrial monitoring. Nevertheless, 10 years of posttrial follow-up data showed a 24% reduction in development of microvascular complications, including DKD, in the intensive therapy group compared with the conventional therapy group ($P = 0.001$).[55] After 12 years of posttrial follow-up, the intensive therapy group exhibited a 33% reduction in the risk of development of microalbuminuria or "clinical grade" proteinuria (macroalbuminuria) and a significant reduction in the proportion of patients with a doubling of blood creatinine level, relative to the conventional therapy group (0.9% vs. 3.5%, $P = 0.0028$).[55,56]

In the wake of these studies, it was hypothesized that the observed beneficial effect of early strict glycemic control, termed the *legacy effect* or *metabolic memory*, could be explained by prevention of metabolism-driven epigenetic modifications.[57] The mechanistic role of epigenetic alterations in DKD is supported by the observation that periods of uncontrolled hyperglycemia are associated with an elevated risk of developing DKD that does not reflect real-time HbA1C levels.[58,59] Indeed, recent studies have indicated that greater glycemic variability, rather than real-time HbA1C levels, may better reflect the risk of DKD.[58-60] The "legacy effect" may, at least in part, explain discrepant results from different observational studies evaluating the predictive value of HbA1C for DKD.

Hypertension

In patients with newly diagnosed type 2 diabetes followed for a median of 15 years, treatment to a target blood pressure of <150/85 mmHg compared with treatment to a target blood pressure <180/105 mmHg resulted in a significant reduction in overall risk of microvascular complications (37%, $P = 0.009$). Each 10 mmHg increase in mean systolic blood pressure was associated with a 13% ($P < 0.0001$) increase in hazard ratio (HR) for development of both microalbuminuria and macroalbuminuria and impaired kidney function, defined as eGFR <60 mL/min/1.73 m^2, or doubling of the blood creatinine level.[61] A baseline systolic blood pressure >140 mmHg in patients with type 2 diabetes has also been shown to increase the risk for ESRD and death.[62,63] In contrast to the legacy effects observed with intensive glycemic control, benefits of blood pressure control are transient and are lost if blood pressure rises again.[56]

Obesity

The presence of obesity often precedes the diagnosis of diabetes by years or decades and exerts a continuously additive effect on the risk of DKD.[64,65] The Verona Diabetes Study reported that obese participants with type 2 diabetes and preserved kidney function (baseline eGFR ≥60 mL/min/1.73 m^2) exhibited significantly faster age-adjusted annual eGFR decline during 10 years of follow-up (-1.2 ± 0.1 mL/min/1.73 m^2/year) compared with normal-weight individuals.[47] Although the specific mechanisms for obesity-induced kidney damage remain to be fully elucidated, a major insult appears to arise from glomerular hyperfiltration with resultant endothelial injury and activation of inflammatory pathways.[66] For example, inflammatory adipokines and abnormalities of fatty acid metabolism may contribute to structural changes in the glomerulus leading to albuminuria.[67,68] Obesity also exerts indirect effects by exacerbating other DKD risk factors, including hypertension, hyperglycemia, and insulin resistance.[40]

Acute Kidney Injury

Several prospective and retrospective studies have identified a strong relationship between diabetes and incidence of acute kidney injury (AKI).[69-72] This association is not age limited: a

TABLE 3.2 **Risk Factors for Diabetic Kidney Disease**

Risk Factor	Susceptibility	Initiation	Progression
Demographics			
Older age	+		
Sex (male)	+		
Race/ethnicity (African American, American Indian, Hispanic, Asian/Pacific Islanders)	+		+
Development			
Low birth weight/high birth weight	+		+
Exposure to maternal diabetes	+		+
Heredity			
Family history of diabetic kidney disease	+		
Systemic Conditions			
Hyperglycemia	+	+	+
Hypertension	+		+
Obesity	+	+	+
Kidney Injuries			
Acute kidney injury		+	+
Smoking	+		+
Dietary Factors			
High protein intake	+		+

high proportion of children hospitalized with diabetic ketoacidosis developed AKI.[73] Among 4000 diabetic patients followed from the years 1999 to 2008, a single episode of AKI was associated with over threefold increased risk for developing eGFR <30 mL/min/1.73 m^2, independent of other major risk factors for DKD. This effect was dose dependent, such that each episode of AKI increased the risk of progression to advanced CKD stages.[74]

Protein Intake

An elevation in circulating amino acids is an established inducer of hyperfiltration; consequently, the relationship of dietary protein intake to DKD prevention and progression has been under study for many years.[75] Research in this area is limited by inherent difficulties associated with the conduct of nutritional studies, such as variability of diet composition and adherence to study diets. However, data from experimental studies suggest that long-term consumption of a lower-protein diet may reduce DKD progression via suppression of glomerular hyperfiltration, albuminuria, and inflammation.[76]

In patients with type 2 diabetes, high protein intake is associated with development of albuminuria.[77] Likewise, in patients with type 1 diabetes, reduced protein intake (0.89 g/kg/day) versus usual protein intake (1.02 g/kg/day) is associated with fewer cases of ESRD or death (10% in the reduced-protein diet group vs. 27% of patients on the usual-protein diet group, $P = 0.042$).[78] However, presumably due to differences in diet composition, adherence, and study duration, other studies and metaanalyses have not consistently reported positive results.[79,80].

Risk factors contributing to the susceptibility, initiation, or progression of DKD are detailed in Table 3.2.

NATURAL HISTORY

Progressive albuminuria followed by decline in GFR is the classical paradigm of DKD presentation.[81] However, accumulating knowledge challenges this concept.

The UKPDS offered a unique opportunity to observe the natural history of DKD in patients with type 2 diabetes from early in the course of the disease. Approximately 2% of study participants per year progressed from normoalbuminuria to microalbuminuria and from microalbuminuria to macroalbuminuria. At a median of 15 years after diagnosis, 40% of UKPDS participants developed albuminuria and 30% developed either an eGFR <60 mL/min/1.73 m^2 or a doubling of the blood creatinine level.[27,82] These data raised awareness that albuminuria and declining eGFR do not always coincide: 60% of individuals developing kidney functional impairment did not have preceding albuminuria, and 40% of study participants never developed albuminuria.[27]

The Developing Education on Microalbuminuria for Awareness of Renal and Cardiovascular Risk in Diabetes (DEMAND) study confirmed that albuminuria and declining kidney function do not co-occur in a significant number of patients. Overall, 21% of individuals with normoalbuminuria, 31% of individuals with microalbuminuria, and 35% of individuals with macroalbuminuria developed a creatinine clearance of <60 mL/min.[22] In a different study, about 20% of individuals with type 2 diabetes had eGFR <60 mL/min/1.73 m^2 and about 50% had albuminuria, with presentation varying across different races and ethnicities.[83]

The classical paradigm of DKD is further complicated by recent data indicating that albuminuria is a dynamic, fluctuating condition rather than a linearly progressive

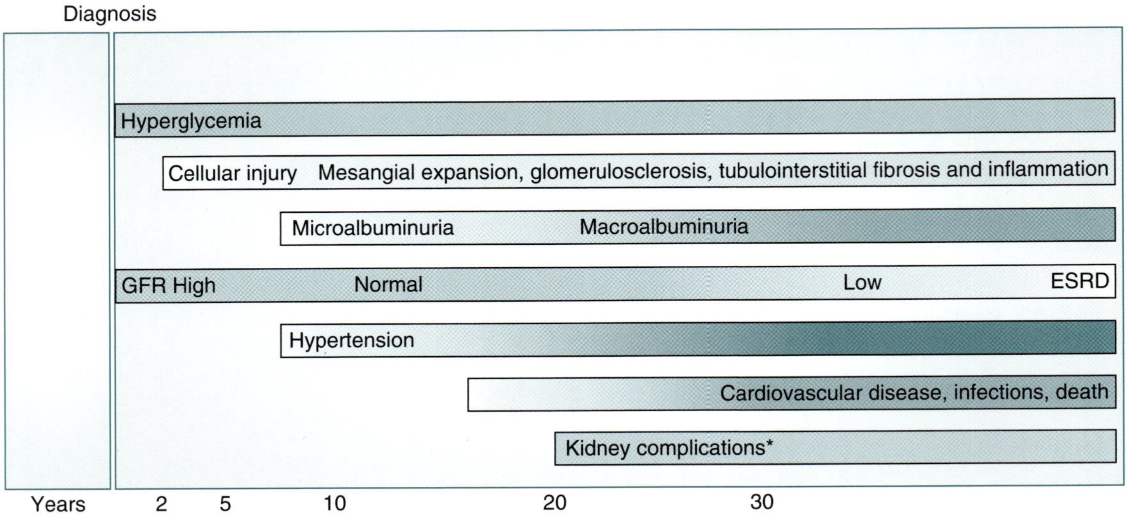

FIG. 3.1 Conceptual model of the natural history of diabetic kidney disease. Duration of diabetes in years is presented on the horizontal axis. Timeline is well characterized for type 1 diabetes mellitus; for type 2 diabetes mellitus, timeline may depart from the illustration due to the variable timing of the onset of hyperglycemia. *Diabetic kidney disease (DKD)–related complications: anemia, bone and mineral metabolism (From Alicic RZ, Rooney MT, Tuttle KR: Diabetic kidney disease: challenges, progress, and possibilit es. *Clin J Am Soc Nephrol.* 2017; 7:12(12):2032-2045.)

process. For example, during nearly 8 years of follow-up in the Multifactorial Intervention for Patients with Type 2 Diabetes Study (Steno-2), 31% of participants with microalbuminuria progressed to macroalbuminuria, whereas 31% regressed to normoalbuminuria. Another 38% remained microalbuminuric during this period.[84]

Over time, the clinical presentation of DKD has changed. In a representative US population, the prevalence of albuminuria alone as a clinical presentation decreased from 21% (1988 to 1994) to 16% (2009 to 2014). Across the same time span, the prevalence of low eGFR (<60 mL/min/1.73 m^2) increased from 9% to 14%, and severely reduced GFR (<30 mL/min/1.73 m^2) increased from 1% to 3%.[85] Data from large clinical trial databases have also revealed different patterns of clinical DKD presentations associated with type 1 diabetes and type 2 diabetes. In data from over 20,000 patients, those with type 1 diabetes showed a lower frequency of eGFR <60 mL/min/1.73 m^2 and albuminuria compared with type 2 diabetes after a mean of 19 years. Frequencies of low eGFR and albuminuria were 8% and 19% in type 1 diabetes and type 2 diabetes, respectively.[86] Factors underlying different presentations of DKD in type 2 diabetes may include longer exposure to hyperglycemia before diagnosis, older age, a higher burden of comorbidities, and other types of kidney diseases.

The practice of diagnosing DKD based on clinical presentation alone has been challenged by recent reports of kidney histology. Autopsies of diabetic individuals found a considerably higher prevalence of histologically diagnosed DKD compared with that shown by clinical laboratory testing. Of 168 patients with type 1 and type 2 diabetes, 106 (63%) exhibited histopathological changes characteristic of DKD. However, albuminuria and low eGFR were absent in 20% (20/106) of these patients throughout their lifetime. Structural changes were highly variable and encompassed a variety of histopathological classes of DKD.[23]

CKD complications develop relatively early in DKD (Fig. 3.1). There are several possible explanations why anemia and bone and mineral metabolism disorders manifest earlier in DKD than in other types of CKD. Predominant tubulointerstitial fibrosis associated with damage to the peritubular interstitial cells that produce erythropoietin is frequently seen in DKD. As a result, patients with diabetes are prone to erythropoietin deficiency and are nearly twice as likely to have anemia compared with patients with nondiabetic CKD and comparable eGFR.[87] DKD is associated with lower parathyroid hormone levels compared with other types of CKD, probably because insulin is a cofactor for parathyroid hormone release.[88] Lower parathyroid hormone levels may predispose DKD patients to adynamic bone disease.

Deaths due to cardiovascular diseases and infections are highly prevalent and compete with progression to ESRD. The UKPDS study showed that the overall death rate after onset of DKD among patients with blood creatinine levels >2 mg/dL or among those receiving kidney replacement therapy was nearly 20% per year[82]. More recent data show that the annual mortality rate in individuals with DKD was 64.1 per 1000 individuals (95% confidence interval [CI], 60.2 to 68.3) The mortality rate sharply increased with severity of kidney disease and ranged from 37 per 1000 individuals in stage 3A, 58 per 1000 individuals in stage 3B, 98 per 1000 individuals with stage 4, and 199 per 1000 individuals with stage 5 DKD.[89]

KIDNEY STRUCTURAL CHANGES IN DIABETIC KIDNEY DISEASE

Diagnosis of DKD is made based on a constellation of histological findings, with no single histological change being

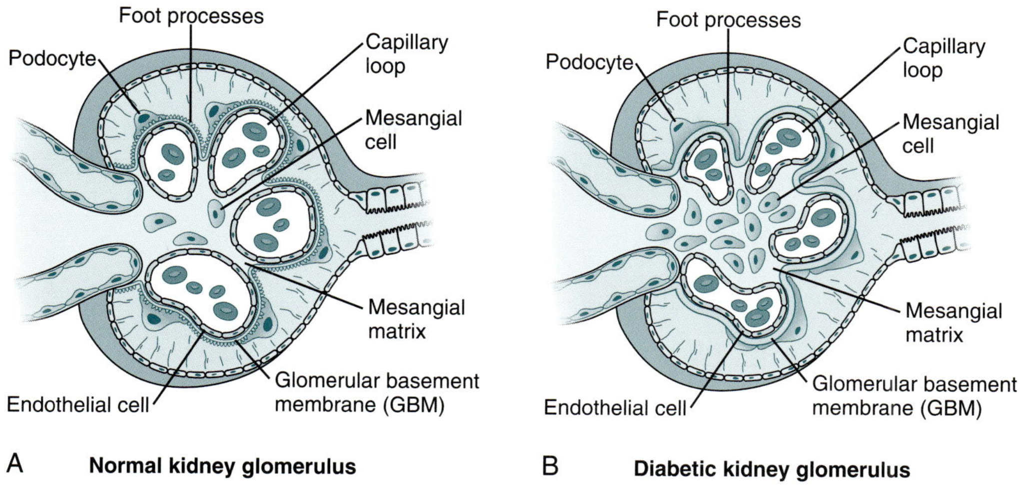

FIG. 3.2 Normal kidney morphology and structural changes in diabetes mellitus. Diabetes induces structural changes, including thickening of the glomerular basement membrane, fusion of foot processes, loss of podocytes with denuding of the glomerular basement membrane, and mesangial matrix expansion. (From Alicic RZ, Rooney MT, Tuttle KR: Diabetic kidney disease: challenges, progress, and possibilities. *Clin J Am Soc Nephrol.* 2017;7:12(12):2032-2045.)

characteristic of DKD (Fig. 3.2). Structural changes in both types of diabetes are similar, but changes in type 2 diabetes are more heterogeneous and less predictably associated with clinical presentations.[90] Knowledge of structural kidney changes in patients with types 1 and 2 diabetes is derived mostly from clinical biopsies, and is therefore limited by selection bias, because most who undergo a biopsy have atypical presentations. Selection bias for kidney biopsy contributes to a high prevalence of nondiabetic kidney disease by histology, especially in type 2 diabetes.[91] However, recent clinical biopsy studies estimate prevalence of nondiabetic kidney disease in patients with diabetes and albuminuria to be about 10%.[92,93]

An early histological finding in DKD is thickening of the glomerular basement membrane, which is typically apparent 1.5 to 2 years after type 1 diabetes diagnosis. It is paralleled by capillary and tubular basement membrane thickening.[43,93,94] Other glomerular changes include loss of endothelial fenestrations, mesangial matrix expansion, and loss of podocytes with effacement of foot processes (Fig. 3.3). Mesangial volume expansion is detectable within 5 to 7 years of type 1 diabetes onset.[43,93,95,96] Later, segmental mesangiolysis with disruption of capillary tufts gives rise to microaneurysms. Classical Kimmelstiel–Wilson nodules and microaneurysms often present together.[97,98]

With progression, efferent arterioles as well as capillary loops become hyalinized. The exudative lesions result from subendothelial deposits of plasma proteins, which form periodic-acid–Schiff-positive and electron-dense deposits and accumulate in small arterial branches, arterioles, and glomerular capillaries, as well as microaneurysms. These deposits result in luminal compromise (e.g., hyaline arteriosclerosis). Similar subepithelial deposits are seen in Bowman capsule ("capsular drop lesion") and proximal renal tubules. In later stages of DKD, there is coalescence into segmental and global sclerosis[99] (Figs. 3.4 and 3.5). An international consensus working group has provided a pathological classification system to address the heterogeneity of DKD presentation (Tables 3.3 and 3.4).[100]

PATHOPHYSIOLOGICAL MECHANISMS IN DKD

Pathophysiology of DKD is a complex and dynamic process. It involves multidirectional and self-perpetuating signaling pathways, with crosstalk between various mediators regulating initiation and progression of the disease.

Glomerular hyperfiltration is an early hemodynamic change in DKD. It occurs in up to 75% of patients with early type 1 diabetes. Among patients with type 2 diabetes, prevalence of glomerular hyperfiltration is approximately 40%.[101] Although mechanisms underlying glomerular hyperfiltration in diabetes are incompletely understood, one plausible mechanism is increased proximal tubular reabsorption of glucose via sodium–glucose cotransporter 2 (SGLT-2), which decreases distal delivery of solutes, particularly sodium chloride, to the macula densa.[101-103] The resulting decrease in tubuloglomerular feedback dilates the afferent arteriole to increase glomerular perfusion, while concurrently, high local production of angiotensin II at the efferent arteriole produces vasoconstriction. These mechanisms operating in tandem produce high intraglomerular pressure and glomerular hyperfiltration.[102,104] In type 2 diabetes, systemic hypertension and obesity also contribute to glomerular hyperfiltration via mechanisms such as high transmitted systemic blood pressure and glomerular enlargement[104] (Fig. 3.6).

The inability of the endothelial cells to downregulate glucose transport in response to hyperglycemia results in excessive intracellular glucose flux, leading to mitochondrial generation of reactive oxygen species (ROS), formation of advanced glycation products (AGE), increased expression of receptors for advanced glycation products (RAGE), and activation of various protein kinase C (PKC) isoforms[105-107] (Fig. 3.7). Recent proteomic studies indicate that activation of inflammatory pathways antedates development of DKD, and inflammatory markers are detected in the urine of patients

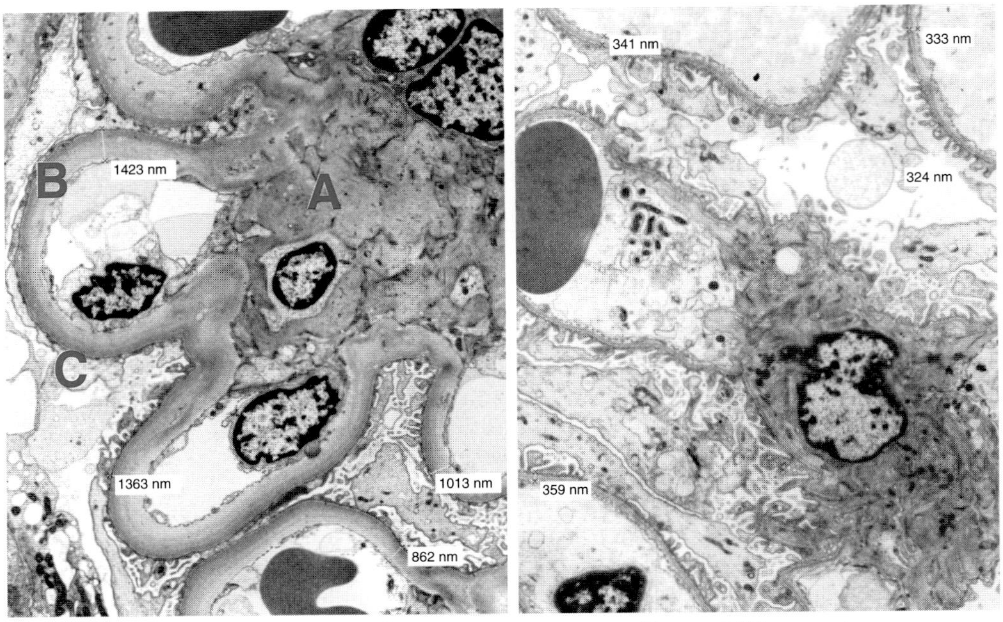

FIG. 3.3 Electron microscope image of structural changes in diabetic kidney disease. Structural changes in diabetic glomerulopathy found with electron microscopy (magnification: 3500×): *A*, Marked expansion of the mesangium. *B*, Marked diffuse thickening of capillary basement membranes (to 3× the normal thickness in this case). *C*, Segmental effacement of the visceral epithelial foot processes. (From Alicic RZ, Rooney MT, Tuttle KR: Diabetic kidney disease: challenges, progress, and possibilities. *Clin J Am Soc Nephrol.* 2017.)

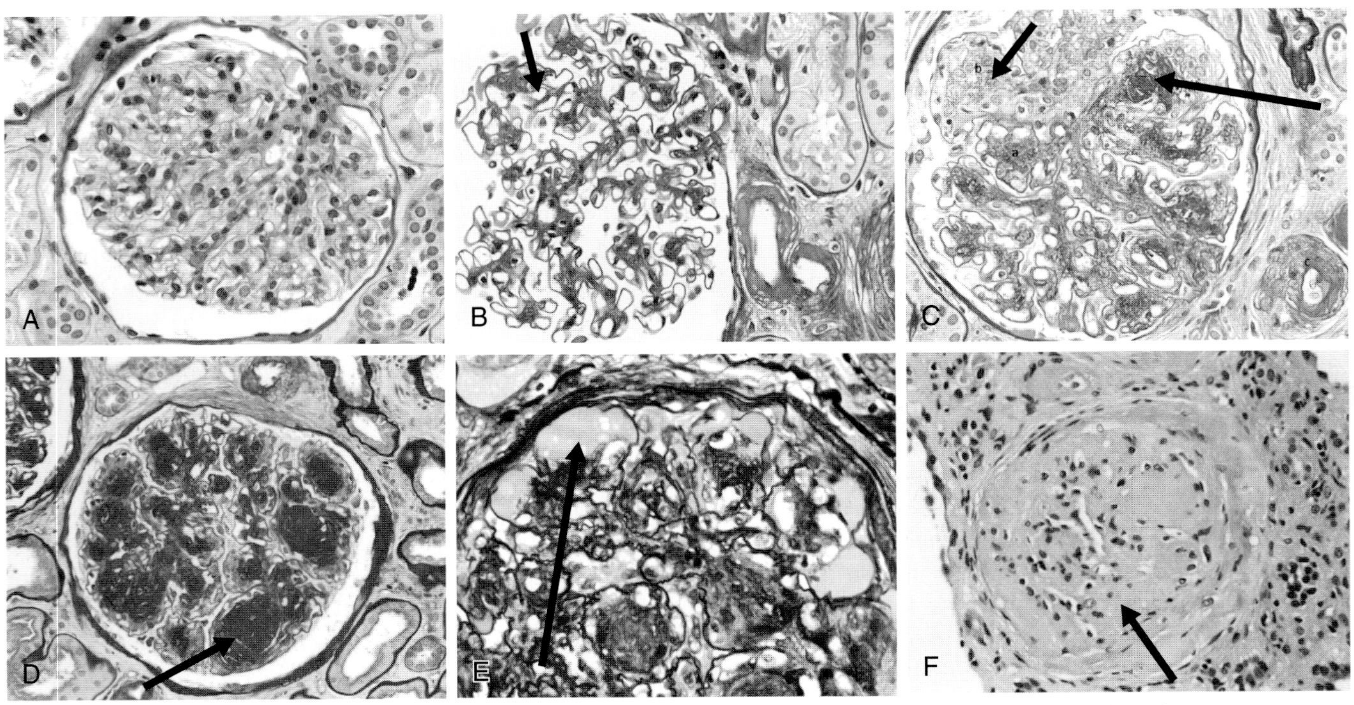

FIG. 3.4 Diabetic glomerulopathy. Changes in glomerular histology in diabetic glomerulopathy (magnification 400×; A–D and F stained with periodic-acid–Schiff stain, E stained with methenamine silver stain): (A) Normal glomerulus. (B) Diffuse mesangial expansion with mesangial cell proliferation. (C) Prominent mesangial expansion with early nodularity and mesangiolysis. (D) Accumulation of mesangial matrix forming Kimmelstiel–Wilson nodules. (E) Dilation of capillaries forming microaneurysms, with subintimal hyaline ("plasmatic insudation"). (F) Obsolescent glomerulus. (From Alicic RZ, Rooney MT, Tuttle KR: Diabetic kidney disease: challenges, progress, and possibilities. *Clin J Am Soc Nephrol.* 2017;7:12(12):2032-2045.)

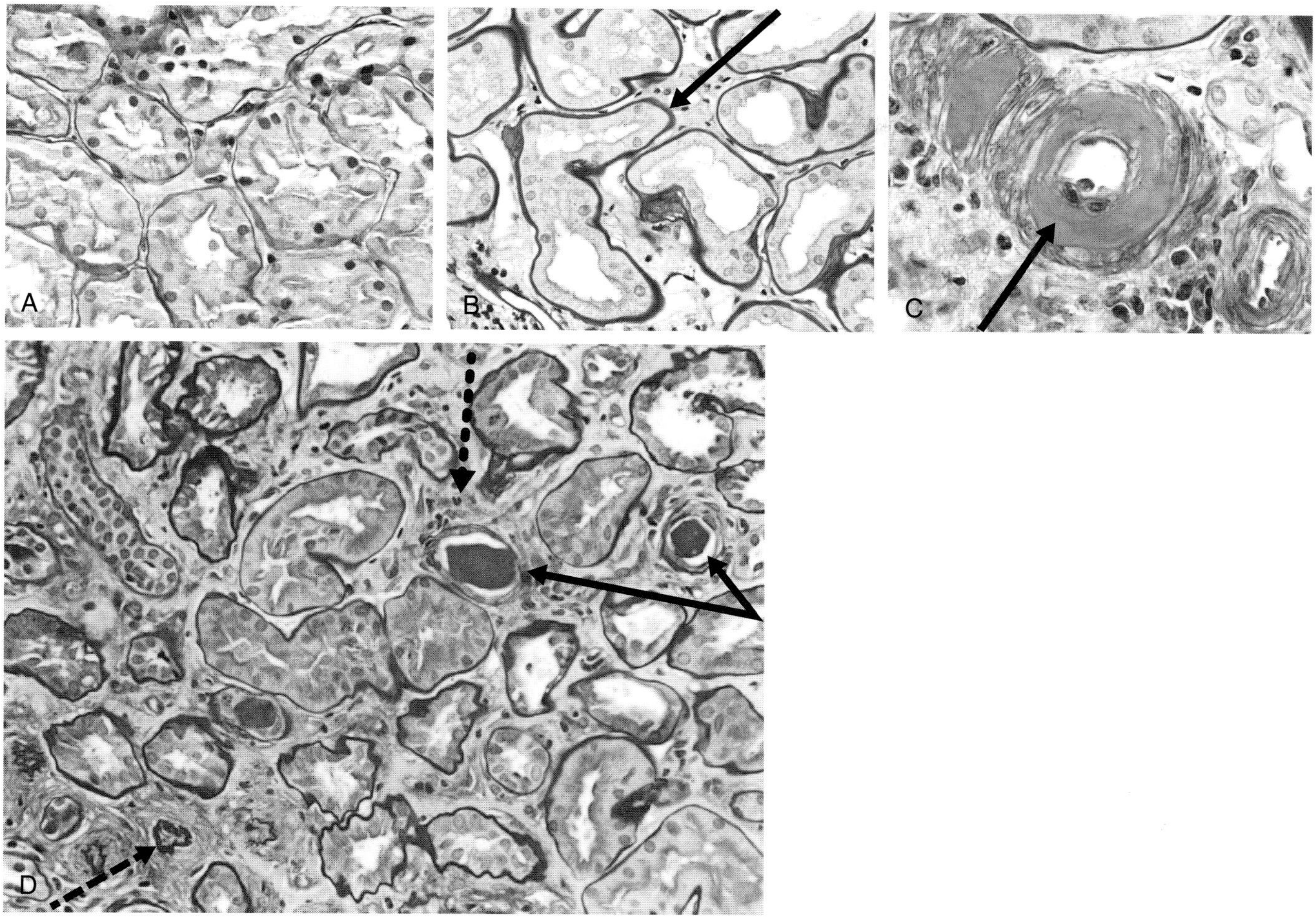

FIG. 3.5 Tubulointerstitial changes and arteriolar hyalinosis in diabetic kidney disease Tubulointerstitial changes in diabetic kidney disease (magnification: 200×, all sections stained with periodic acid–Schiff stain): (A) Normal renal cortex. (B) Thickened tubular basement membranes and interstitial widening. (C) Arteriole with an intimal accumulation of hyaline material with significant luminal compromise. (D) Kidney tubules and interstitium in advancing diabetic kidney disease, with thickening and wrinkled tubular basement membranes (*solid arrows*), atrophic tubules (*dashed arrow*), some containing casts, and interstitial widening with fibrosis and inflammatory cells (*dotted arrow*). (From Alicic RZ, Rooney MT, Tuttle KR: Diabetic kidney disease: challenges, progress, and possibilities. *Clin J Am Soc Nephrol.* 2017;7:12(12):2032-2045.)

TABLE 3.3 International Classification of Interstitial and Vascular Lesions in Diabetic Kidney Disease

Type of Lesion	Criterion	Score
Interstitial fibrosis and tubular atrophy (IFTA)	Absent	0
	<25%	1
	25%–50%	2
	>50%	3
Interstitial inflammation	Absent	0
	Infiltration only in relation to IFTA	1
	Infiltration in areas without IFTA	2
Vascular lesions arteriolar hyalinosis	Absent	0
	At least one area of arteriolar hyalinosis	1
	More than one area of arteriolar hyalinosis	2
Presence of large vessel arteriosclerosis	No intimal thickening	0
	Intimal thickening less than thickness of media	1
	Intimal thickening greater that thickness of media	2

TABLE 3.4 International Pathological Classification of Glomerular Changes in Diabetic Kidney Disease

Class	Description	Inclusion Criteria
I	Mild or nonspecific light microscopy changes and electron microscopy–proven GBM thickening	GBM >395 nm in female and >430 nm in male individuals 9 years of age and older Biopsy does not meet any of the criteria mentioned later for class II, III, or IV
IIa	Mesangial expansion, mild	Mild mesangial expansion in >25% of the observed mesangium Biopsy does not meet criteria for class III or IV
IIb	Mesangial expansion, severe	Severe mesangial expansion in >25% of the observed mesangium Biopsy does not meet criteria for class III or IV
III	Nodular sclerosis (Kimmelstiel–Wilson lesion)	At least one convincing Kimmelstiel–Wilson lesion Biopsy does not meet criteria for class IV
IV	Advanced diabetic glomerulosclerosis	Global glomerular sclerosis in >50% of glomeruli Lesions from classes I through III

GBM, Glomerular basement membrane.
Mild mesangial expansion occupies an area smaller than the area of the capillary lumen; severe mesangial expansion occupies an area greater than the area of the capillary lumen.
(Adapted from Tervaert TW, Mooyaart AL, Amann K, et al. Pathologic classification of diabetic nephropathy. *J Am Soc Nephrol.* 2010; 21(4): 556-563.)

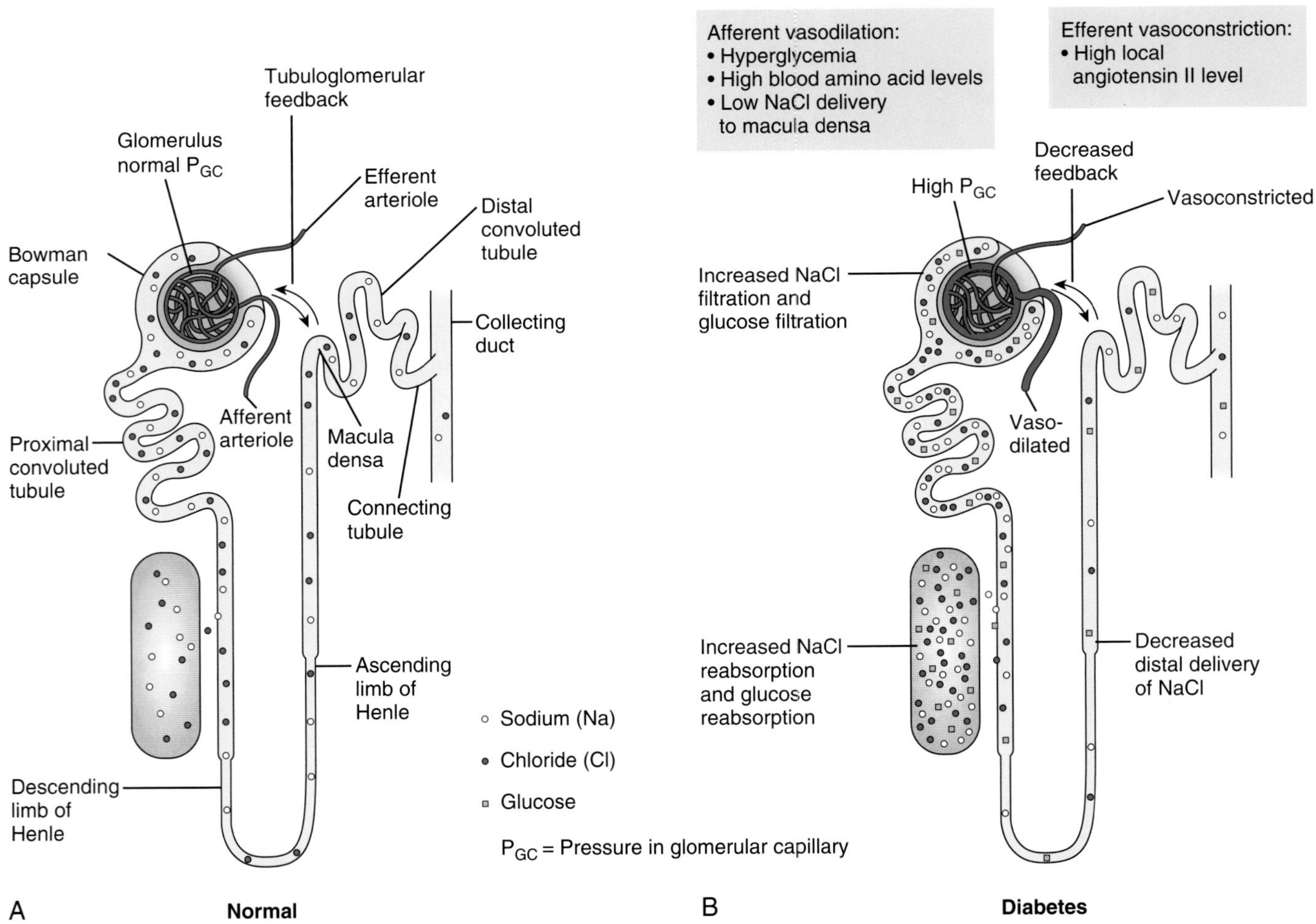

FIG. 3.6 Normal and diabetic nephron with altered renal hemodynamics. In diabetes mellitus the glomerular filtration of glucose is increased in a linear manner with increasing plasma glucose concentrations. As an adaptive response to this increase, there is an amplified expression of sodium–glucose cotransporter 2 (SGLT-2) transporters, resulting in increased glucose and sodium chloride reabsorption. The increased reabsorption leads to decreased distal delivery of sodium chloride to the macula densa with a decrease in the tubuloglomerular feedback. (From Alicic RZ, Rooney MT, Tuttle KR: Diabetic kidney disease: challenges, progress, and possibilities. *Clin J Am Soc Nephrol.* 2017; 7:12(12):2032-2045.)

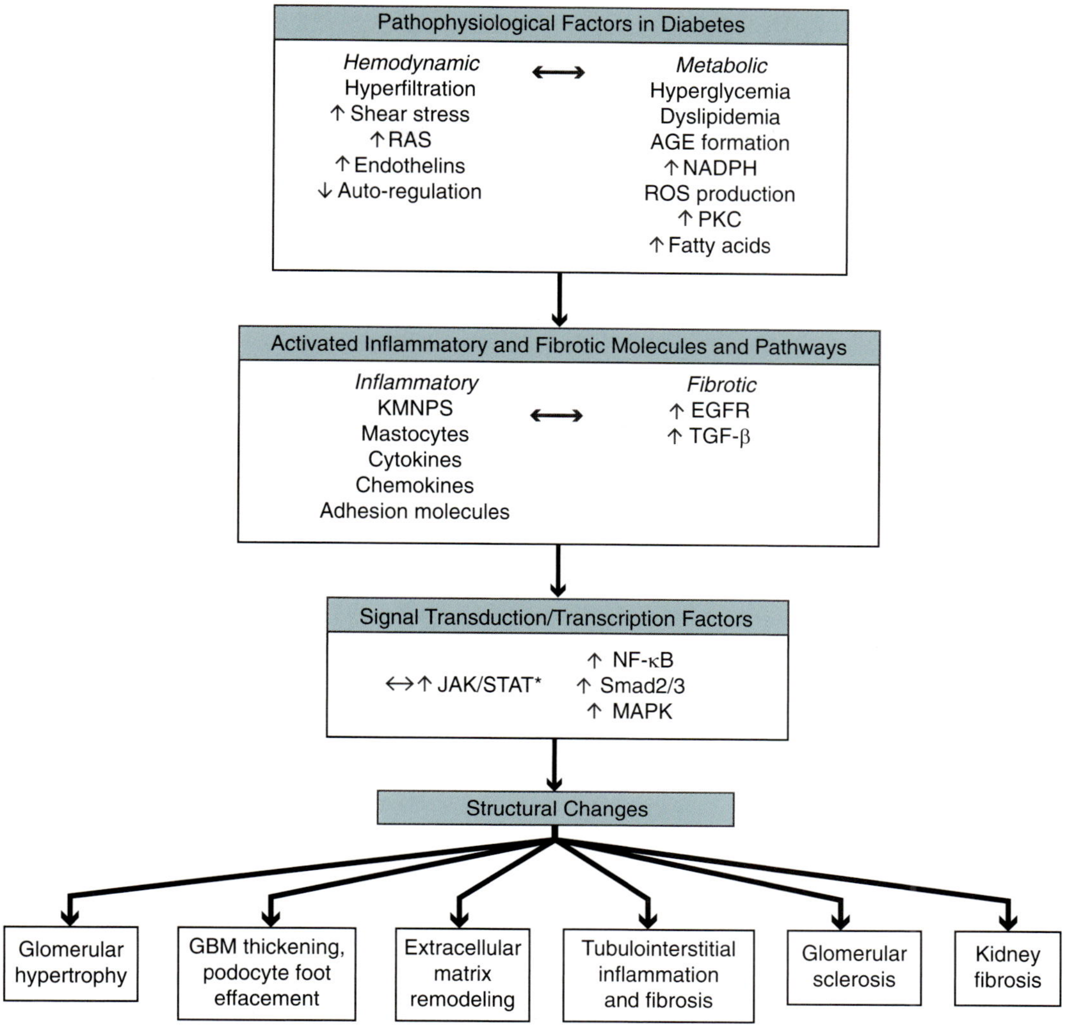

FIG. 3.7 Pathways and networks involved in the initiation and progression of diabetic kidney disease. *AGE,* Advanced glycation end product; *EGFR,* epidermal growth factor receptor pathway; *GBM,* glomerular basement membrane; *JAK-STAT,* Janus kinase/signal transducer and activator of transcription; *KMNPs,* kidney mononuclear phagocytic system; *MAPK,* mitogen-activated protein kinase; *NADPH,* nicotinamide adenine dinucleotide phosphate; *NF-κB,* nuclear factor kappa B; *PKC,* protein kinase C; *RAS,* renin-angiotensin-system; *ROS,* reactive oxygen species; *SMAD,* mothers against decapentaplegic homolog; *TGF-β,* transforming growth factor beta. *JAK/STAT signaling can be unchanged or upregulated in early and later stages of diabetes, respectively. ↑ upregulated; ↔ unchanged.

with early diabetes.[107] It is now believed that ongoing activity of inflammatory and fibrotic molecules and pathways underlies the structural and functional changes observed in DKD (Figs. 3.8 and 3.9).

CURRENT TREATMENT OF DKD

Glycemic Control

A recent metaanalysis of over 27,000 individual participants from four large-scale randomized trials (the UKPDS, Action to Control Cardiovascular Risk in Diabetes [ACCORD] trial, the Action in Diabetes and Vascular Disease: Preterax and Diamicron MR Controlled Evaluation [ADVANCE] trial, and the Veterans Administration Diabetes Trial [VADT]) confirmed the importance of intensive glucose control in the prevention of microvascular complications in adults with type 2 diabetes. Analysis found that an absolute difference in HbA1C of 0.9% (mean HbA1C 7.7% vs. 6.8% in standard and intensive treatment groups, respectively) was associated with 20% relative risk reduction of development of macroalbuminuria, ESRD, renal death, and eGFR <30 mL/min/1.73 m^2 (Fig. 3.10).[108]

In contrast to the role of intensive glucose control in the development of kidney disease, intensive glucose control targeting low HbA1C (6% to 6.9%) after the onset of diabetic complications has a nominal effect on DKD progression and does not improve overall clinical outcomes.[51,53,54,56,109,110] Compared with standard therapy, intensive glucose control incurs greater risk of hypoglycemia and does not reduce the

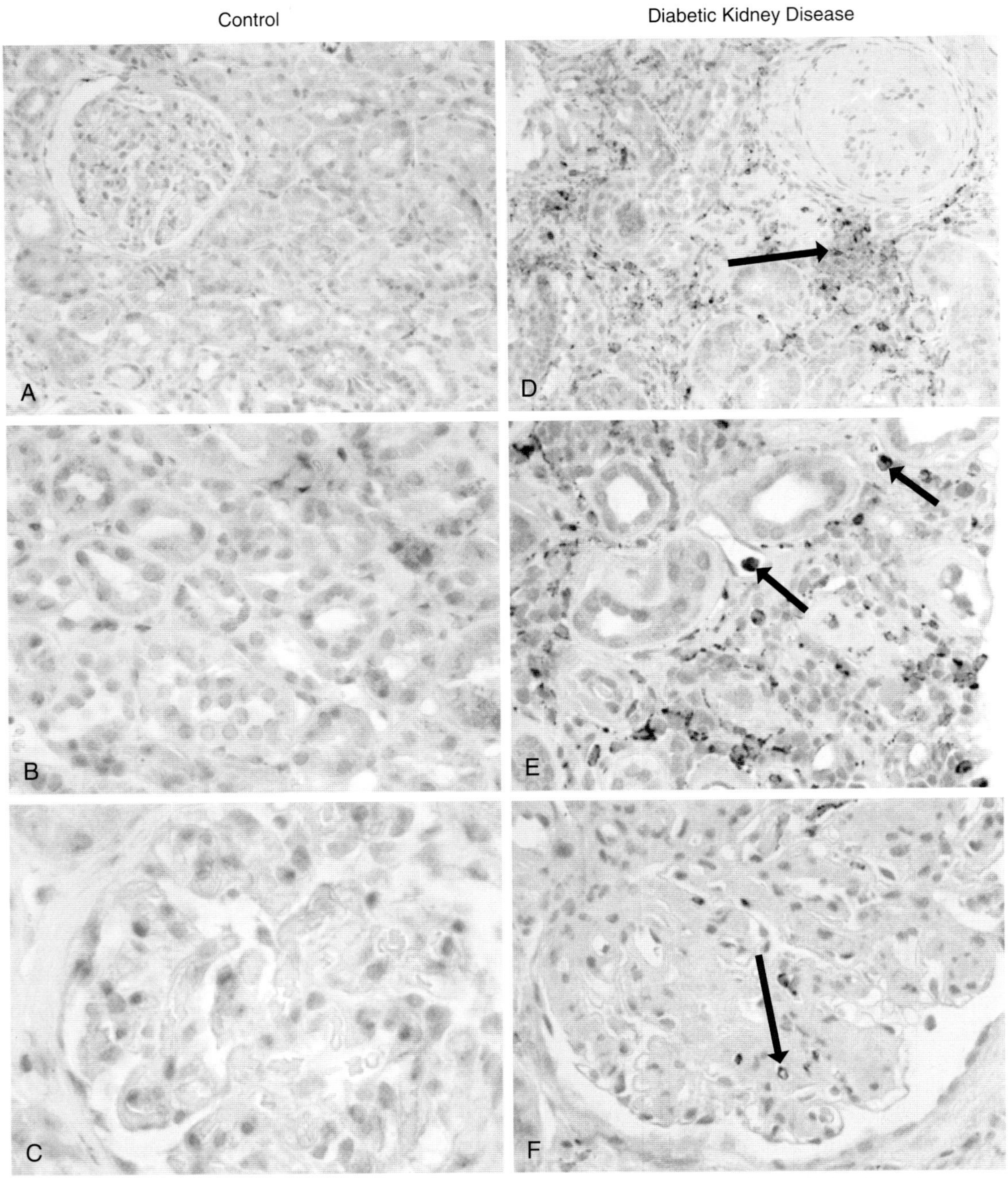

FIG. 3.8 Anti-CD68 (KP-1) immunohistochemistry of kidney biopsies from diabetic patients without and with histological features of diabetic kidney disease. CD68 antibodies highlight the influx of macrophage lineage cells in different kidney structures. Immunohistochemistry with anti-CD68 (KP-1) antibody (Roche Diagnostics, Indianapclis, IN) used at a concentration of 0.4 micrograms/mL. (A–C) Human kidney from diabetic patient without histological features of diabetic kidney disease (control) [magnification: 200× (A), 400× (B), 600× (C)]. (D) Interstitial macrophage lineage cells infiltrates in diabetic kidney disease (magnification: 200×). (E) Macrophage lineage cells in peritubular capillaries (magnification: 4C0×). (F) Macrophage lineage cells in glomerular capillary (magnification: 600×).

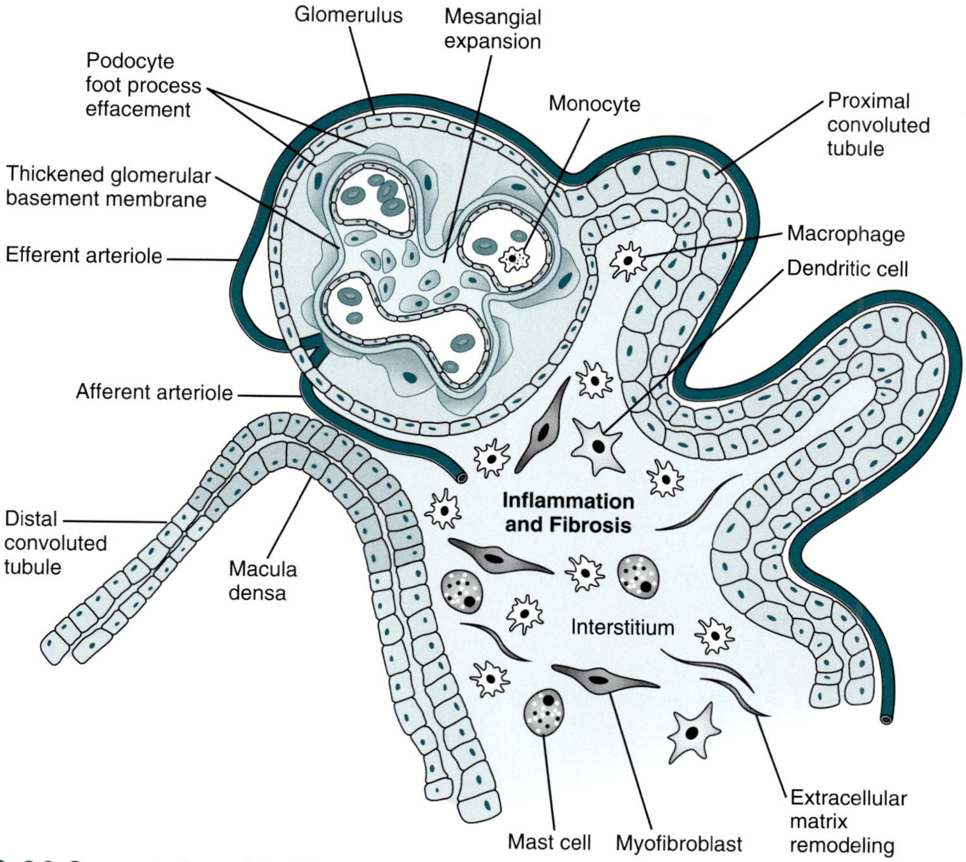

FIG. 3.9 Conceptual model of immunity, inflammation, and fibrosis in diabetic kidney disease. Metabolic and hemodynamic abnormalities induced by diabetes instigate cytokine production and activate resident macrophages, dendritic cells, and mast cells. This leads to recruitment of the additional immune cells and further cytokine release. Biological effects of the inflammatory and fibrotic processes include podocyte foot process effacement, thickening of the glomerular basement membrane, mesangial expansion, extracellular matrix remodeling, and phenotypic transformation of a variety of kidney cells to myofibroblasts (e.g., podocyte to myofibroblasts transformation).

risk of cardiovascular complications.[111-113] Furthermore, an analysis of patients with type 2 diabetes and even early-stage CKD showed 30% and 40% higher risk for all-cause mortality and cardiovascular mortality, respectively, with intensive glycemic control compared with standard therapy.[114] A small benefit of intensive glycemic control on the risk of ESRD was observed, but the absolute number of cases was minute.[115] A stratified analysis demonstrated that the greatest benefit of intensive glycemic control for preventing ESRD was seen in participants without kidney disease at study entry, further supporting intensive glycemic control for DKD prevention during early diabetes.[116]

The American Diabetes Association (ADA) recommends the following goals for blood glucose control: (1) HbA1C <6.5% for patients with a shorter duration of diabetes, younger age, absence of complications, and a longer life expectancy; and (2) HbA1C <8% for patients with long-standing diabetes, older age, microvascular and macrovascular complications, and limited life expectancy. Similarly to the ADA, the National Kidney Foundation-Kidney Disease Outcomes Quality Initiative (NKF-KDOQI) and the Kidney Disease: Improving Global Outcomes (KDIGO) guidelines recommend a target HbA1C of about 7.0% to prevent or delay progression of the microvascular complications of diabetes. However, patients at risk for hypoglycemia, such as those with diabetes and CKD, should not be treated to an HbA1C target of <7.0%.[21]

Antihypertensive Therapy

There is clear evidence that RAS blockade with either an angiotensin-converting enzyme (ACE) inhibitor or an angiotensin receptor blocker (ARB) reduces the progression of established DKD in patients with macroalbuminuria.[117] The Eighth Joint National Committee (JNC-8) recommends initiation of pharmacological treatment at a systolic blood pressure ≥140 mmHg or diastolic blood pressure ≥90 mmHg, irrespective of diabetes status. In the general hypertensive population, the JNC-8 recommends that initial antihypertensive treatment include a thiazide-type diuretic, calcium-channel blocker (CCB), ACE inhibitor, or ARB. In black patients with diabetes, the JNC-8 recommends initial treatment with a thiazide diuretic or CCB.[118] The KDIGO 2012 guidelines recommend treatment with an ACE or ARB to a blood pressure goal ≤130/80 mmHg in all patients with CKD and urine albumin excretion >30 mg per 24 hours, or equivalent, irrespective of diabetes status.[119]

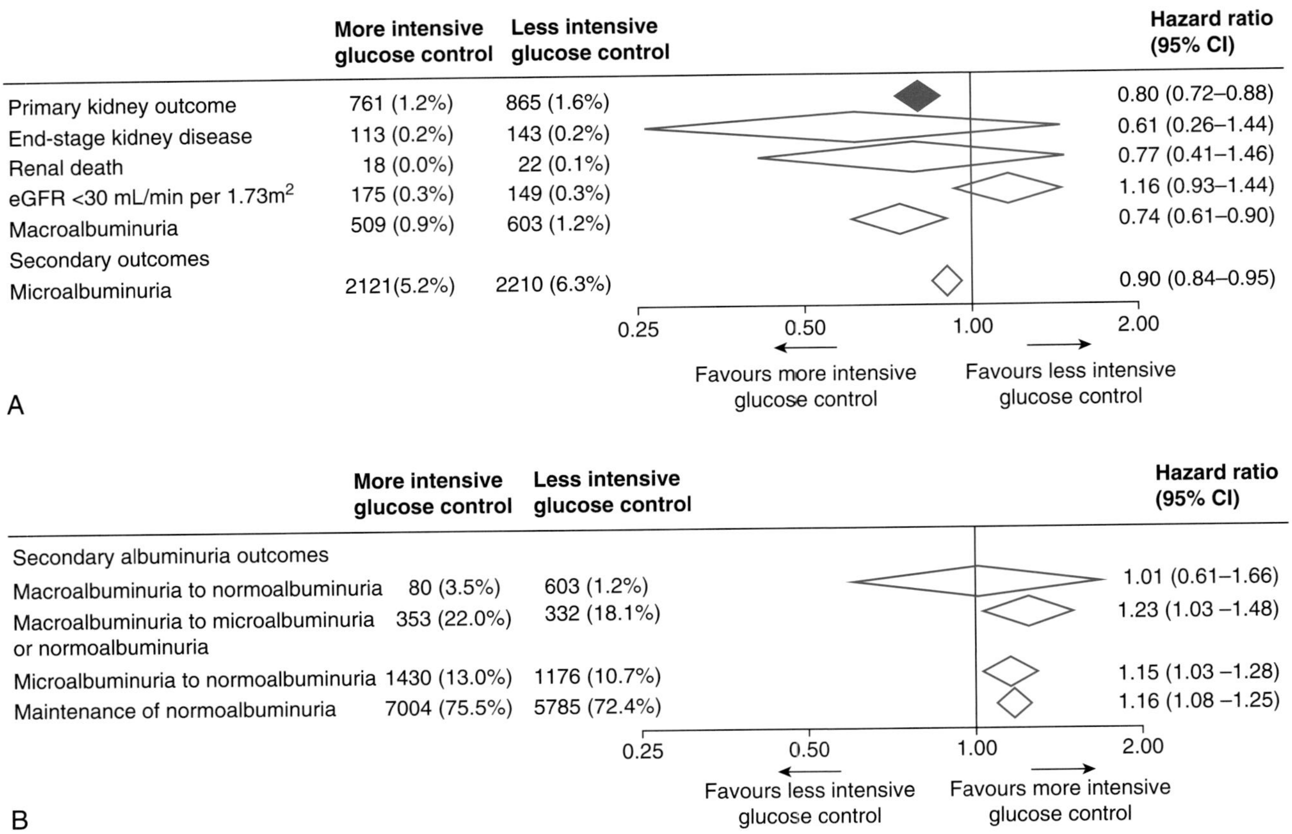

FIG. 3.10 **Kidney outcomes from glycemic control trials (The United Kingdom Prospective Diabetes Trial [UKDPS], Action to Control Cardiovascular Risk in Diabetes [ACCORD], Action in Diabetes and Vascular Disease: Preterax and Diamicron MR Controlled Evaluation [ADVANCE], and the Veterans Administration Diabetes Trial [VADT]).** (A) Effect of more intensive glucose control (mean HbA1C 6.8%) versus less intensive glucose control (mean HbA1C 7.7%) on primary kidney outcomes (end-stage renal disease, renal death, eGFR <30 mL/min/1.73 m^2, macroalbuminuria) and the secondary outcome of microalbuminuria. (B) Regression of albuminuria. Data are events (annual rate), unless specified otherwise. Diamonds represent summary data centered on the pooled estimates, and their width spans the corresponding 95% CIs. *eGFR*, Estimated glomerular filtration rate. (From Zoungas S, Arima H, Gerstein HC, et al.: Effects of intensive glucose control on microvascular outcomes in patients with type 2 diabetes: a meta-analysis of individual participant data from randomised controlled trials. *Lancet Diabetes Endocrinol.* 2017;5(6):431-437.)

A recent ADA position statement on treatment of hypertension recommends that the majority of diabetic patients should be treated to JNC-8 recommended goals of systolic blood pressure <140 mmHg and diastolic blood pressure <90 mmHg. Lower systolic and diastolic goals such as 130/80 mmHg may be appropriate for individuals at high risk of cardiovascular disease, if they can be achieved without undue burden. Use of the maximal tolerated dose of an ACE inhibitor or ARB is recommended as a first-line treatment in patients with diabetes and UACR ≥30 mg/g creatinine, and particularly in those with UACR ≥300 mg/g creatinine. ACE inhibitors and ARBs can be interchanged. While on an ACE inhibitor or ARB, eGFR and serum potassium should be closely monitored.[120] Combination therapy (an ACE inhibitor and an ARB administered together) increases the risk of serious side effects, primarily hyperkalemia and AKI, and offers no apparent clinical benefits.[120-122] The risk of hyperkalemia increases when eGFR <45 mL/min/1.73 m^2 or serum potassium is >4.5 mEq/L.[123]

Following the liberalized JNC-8 recommendations, target blood pressure goals have been challenged by results of the Systolic Blood Pressure Intervention Trial (SPRINT). SPRINT included 9361 nondiabetic participants with hypertension and high cardiovascular risk. Participants randomized to an intensive (<120 mmHg) systolic blood pressure goal experienced reduction in the rates of the primary outcomes (myocardial infarction, acute coronary syndrome, stroke, heart failure, or death from cardiovascular causes) and all-cause mortality by 25% and 27%, respectively, compared with the standard regimen group. These results held across prespecified subgroups defined according to CKD stages, advancing age (>75 years), sex, race, previous cardiovascular disease, and baseline levels of systolic blood pressure.[124,125] In contrast to the SPRINT trial, the ACCORD trial, which included 4733 diabetic patients at high risk for cardiovascular events, showed that achieving the same systolic blood pressure targets (<120 vs. <140 mmHg) did not exert a significant effect on the risk of nonfatal myocardial infarction, nonfatal stroke, death from cardiovascular cause, or death from any causes.[126] One of the possible explanations for this incongruent finding is that ACCORD was underpowered to show between-group differences, because cardiovascular morbidity and mortality occurred at substantially lower rates than predicted. In the SPRINT trial, intensive blood pressure control did not reduce incident ESRD, 50% decline in eGFR, or ≥30% decline in eGFR to a value of <60 mL/min/1.73 m^2 among participants who had CKD at the time of entering the study. Furthermore, hospitalizations or emergency room visits for AKI occurred more frequently in the intensive treatment group than in the standard regimen group (4.4% vs. 2.6%; HR: 1.71)[124,127] ACCORD also detected a possible negative effect of intensive blood pressure control on kidney function. Even among participants who had normal kidney function at baseline, the instances of eGFR ≤30 mL/min/1.73 m^2 were almost doubled in the intensive treatment group.[126] Results from these and other trials examining the effect of blood pressure control on kidney outcomes in diabetic patients are summarized in Table 3.5.

Dietary Management

The optimal diet for patients with DKD is determined by unique metabolic abnormalities characteristic of diabetes and kidney disease (i.e., hyperglycemia, altered glomerular hemodynamics, lipid metabolism abnormalities, alterations in mineral metabolism, metabolic acidosis, anemia, vitamin D deficiency, loss of lean muscle mass), as well as the high burden of hypertension and cardiovascular disease in this population. The relationship between protein intake and DKD development and progression was specifically addressed in the NKF-KDOQI Clinical Practice Guidelines and Clinical Practice Recommendations for Diabetes and Chronic Kidney Disease. A target protein intake of 0.8 g/kg body weight per day (the recommended daily allowance) for nondialysis-dependent DKD is recommended.[24] The KDIGO 2012 guidelines also suggest a dietary protein intake of 0.8 g/kg/body weight per day in adults with diabetes and GFR <30 mL/min/1.73 m^2, as well as appropriate nutritional education.[21,24,128] Both NKF-KDOQI and KDIGO guidelines recommend avoidance of a high-protein diet, defined as more than 20% of kcal from protein or >1.3 g/kg/day of protein for individuals with CKD.[129] Dietary sodium reduction has been shown to reduce blood pressure irrespective of diabetes status.[24] A daily limit <2 g is recommended based on the Dietary Approaches to Stop Hypertension (DASH) and DASH–sodium diet.[129,130] Healthful dietary approaches, such as Mediterranean and DASH-style diets, emphasize intake of whole grains, fruits, vegetables, and plant proteins by nuts, seeds, and beans. These dietary approaches have been associated with improvement in blood pressure, body weight, and cardiovascular risk.[24]

Effect of Multiple Risk Factor Interventions in Diabetes

In the Steno-2 study, participants received step-wise introduction to lifestyle and pharmacological interventions aimed at keeping HbA1C <6.5%, blood pressure <130/80 mmHg, total cholesterol <175 mg/dL, and triglycerides <150 mg/dL in patients with type 2 diabetes and microalbuminuria. The lifestyle component of the intensive intervention included reduction in dietary fat and promotion of regular exercise and smoking cessation. After 7.8 years of follow-up, only 24% of participants in the intensive group had a cardiovascular event compared with 44% of participants in the conventional group—a relative risk reduction of nearly 50%. Relative risk of secondary endpoints (nephropathy, retinopathy, and autonomic neuropathy) was diminished by about 60% in the intensive group compared with the conventional treatment group.[131] After approximately 13 years of follow-up, the intervention led to a 20% absolute risk reduction for all-cause death and a 13% absolute risk reduction for cardiovascular death among participants who received intensive therapy compared with the standard therapy. Only one patient in the multifactorial intervention group progressed to ESRD, compared with six patients in the conventional therapy group.[132]

Population-Based Approaches

Success of population-based strategies has been demonstrated by recently available data from the Centers for Disease Control. A 54% decrease in diabetes-related kidney failure occurred between 1996 and 2013 among American Indians, a group with an historically high prevalence of diabetes and DKD. Interventions associated with this improvement included systematic implementation of guidelines for the treatment of hypertension and diabetes, regular albuminuria testing, use of ACE inhibitors and ARBs, services to support nutrition, physical activity, and diabetes education.[133] These results reinforce the importance of public health initiatives and widespread population-based approaches for prevention of DKD (Fig. 3.11).

NEW THERAPIES FOR DIABETIC KIDNEY DISEASE

Despite current advances in the management of diabetes and hypertension, including the use of ACE inhibitors and ARBs, there is still a large residual risk of DKD progression, ESRD, and death. As a consequence, there is a great need for new therapeutic agents for DKD.

Newer Antihyperglycemic Agents

In 2008 the US Food and Drug Administration (FDA) mandated that new antihyperglycemic therapies seeking approval for the treatment of type 2 diabetes must demonstrate cardiovascular safety. This mandate resulted in a number of cardiovascular outcome (CVO) trials, some of which demonstrated beneficial kidney outcomes.

Glucagon-like Peptide-1 Receptor Agonists

Glucagon-like peptide-1 (GLP-1) receptors are located in glomerular endothelial and mesangial cells, macrophages, and proximal tubular cells.[134] Proposed mechanisms for their antioxidant, antiinflammatory, and antifibrotic effects in the kidneys of diabetic patients include inhibition of renal nicotinamide adenine dinucleotide phosphate (NADPH),

TABLE 3.5 Clinical Trials Examining the Effect of Blood Pressure Control on Kidney Outcomes in Diabetic Patients

Study Name	Study Population	Follow-up	Intervention	Outcomes	Results
UKPDS 38, 1998[165]	*n* = 1148 with DM2 and HTN	8.4 y (median)	Target BP <150/85 mmHg vs. <180/105 mmHg	Microvascular disease (albuminuria, retinopathy)	37% risk reduction in microvascular endpoints
RENAAL, 2001[166]	*n* = 1513 with DM2, HTN, UAE > 300 mg/24 h, and Cr 1.3–3 mg/dL	3.4 y (mean)	Losartan vs. placebo	Primary: composite of doubling of the baseline Cr, ESRD or death Secondary: composite of CV morbidity and mortality, proteinuria, progression of kidney disease	16% risk reduction of primary outcome 28% ESRD reduction 25% reduction of doubling of Cr 35% proteinuria reduction in losartan group
IDNT, 2001[167]	*n* = 1715 with DM2, HTN, albuminuria (>900 mg/24 h), Cr 1.0–3.0 mg/dL	2.6 y (median)	Irbesartan vs. amlodipine vs. placebo	Primary: composite of doubling of Cr, ESRD, or death of any cause	Irbesartan group showed: ↓20% risk of primary composite endpoint ↓30% risk of doubling the creatinine 24% slower Cr concentration increase
IRMA-2, 2001[168]	*n* = 590 with DM2 and HTN, UAE 20–200 μ/min, Cr < 1.5 mg/dL in men and <1.1 mg/dL in women	2 y (median)	Irbesartan vs. placebo	Primary: developing nephropathy defined as UAE ≥200 mg/24 h UAE 30% higher than baseline Secondary: level of albuminuria, changes in CrCl, restoration of UAE <20 μ/min	↓UEA by 24% in 150 mg/24 h group ↓UEA by 38% in 300 mg/24 h group Nonsignificant change in creatinine decline
BENEDICT, 2004[169]	*n* = 1204 with DM2, HTN, UAE 20 μ/min, and Cr ≤1.5 mg/dL	3.6 y (median)	Trandolapril vs. verapamil vs. trandolapril + verapamil vs. placebo	Primary: onset of microalbuminuria Secondary: magnitude of treatment effect	Trandolapril + verapamil delayed albuminuria by factor of 2.6 Trandolapril only delayed albuminuria by factor of 2.1
ADVANCE, 2007[170]	*n* = 11,140 with DM2, HTN, and history of major CV disease or at least one factor for CV disease	4.3 y (mean)	Perindopril-indapamide vs. placebo	Primary: major macrovascular and microvascular events	9% risk reduction in macrovascular and microvascular events
ACCORD BP, 2010[171]	*n* = 4733 with DM2 (34% with previous CV disease)	4.7 y (mean)	SBP <120 mmHg (intensive) vs. SBP <140 mmHg (standard)	Primary: composite of nonfatal MI, nonfatal stroke of CV death	Significant increase of SAE (eGFR, elevations of Cr, GFR <30) in intensive treatment group
ROADMAP, 2011[172]	*n* = 4447 with DM2 mean baseline BP 136.5/80.5 mmHg, 33% with previous CV disease	3.2 y (median)	Olmesartan vs. placebo	Primary: time to onset of microalbuminuria	Delayed onset of microalbuminuria by 23% in olmesartan group
VA NEPHRON, 2013[173]	*n* = 1448 with DM2, UACR ≥300 mg/g, eGFR 30.0–89.9, 23% with CV disease, mean baseline BP 137/72.7 mmHg	2.2 y (median)	Losartan vs. losartan + lisinopril	Primary: first occurrence of change in eGFR, ESRD, or death	Combination therapy: offers no benefit with respect to mortality of CV events Increased risk of hyperkalemia and AKI ($P \leq 0.001$) Trial stopped for safety concerns

ACE inhibitor, Angiotensin converting enzyme inhibitor; *AKI,* acute kidney injury; *BP,* blood pressure; *Cr,* serum creatinine in mg/dL; *CrCl,* creatinine clearance; *CV,* cardiovascular; *DM2,* type 2 diabetes mellitus; *eGFR,* estimated glomerular filtration rate in mL/min/1.73 m^2; *ESRD,* end-stage renal disease; *HTN,* hypertension; *SAE,* serious adverse events; *UACR,* urine albumin-to-creatinine ratio in mg/g; *UAE,* urine albumin excretion in mg/24 h or μg/min; *UAE,* urine albumin excretion; *UKPDS,* United Kingdom Prospective Diabetes Study; *RENAAL,* Reduction of Endpoints in NIDDM with the Angiotensin II Antagonist Losartan; *IDNT,* Irbesartan Diabetic Nephropathy Trial; *IRMA,* Irbesartan in Patients with Type 2 Diabetes and Microalbuminuria; *BENEDICT,* Bergamo Nephrologic Diabetes Complications Trial; *ADVANCE,* Action in Diabetes and Vascular Disease: Preterax and Diamicron MR Controlled Evaluation; *ACCORD,* Action to Control Cardiovascular Risk in Diabetes; *ROADMAP,* Randomized Olmesartan and Diabetes Microalbuminuria Prevention; *VA-NEPHRON-D,* Diabetes in Nephropathy Study.

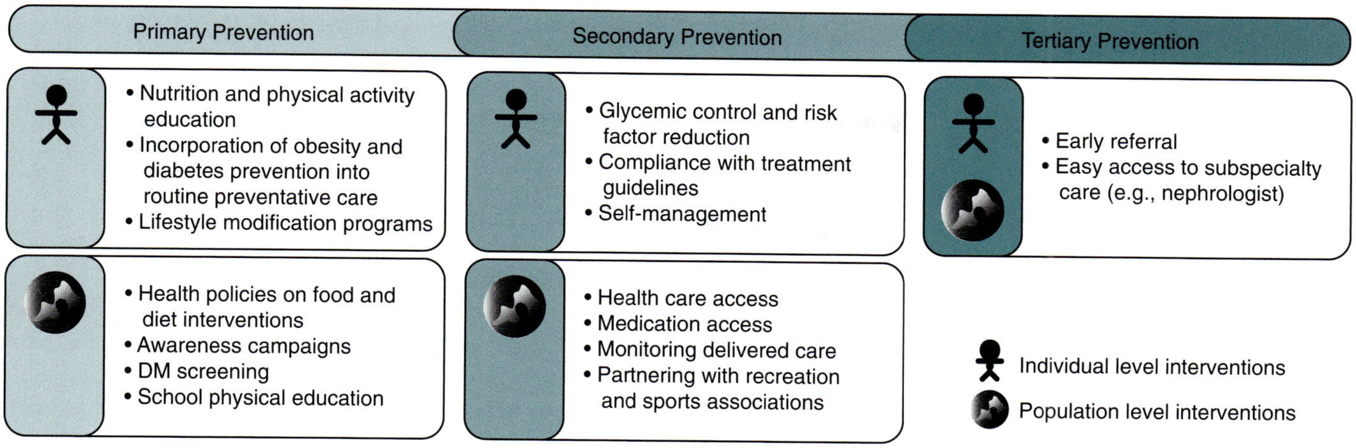

FIG. 3.11 Prevention strategies for mitigating the global burden of diabetic kidney disease.

inhibition or suppression of AGE-induced expression of oxidase monocyte chemoattractant protein-1, inhibition of proinflammatory cytokine production, blockade of angiotensin II action, and inhibition of glucose-mediated expression of transforming growth factor beta (TGF-β).[135-137]

Besides their incretin mimetic effect, GLP-1 receptor agonists reduce the risk of albuminuria and progression of kidney disease.[138] In the Liraglutide Effect and Action in Diabetes: Evaluation of Cardiovascular Outcome Results (LEADER) trial and the Trial to Evaluate Cardiovascular and Other Long-term Outcomes with Semaglutide in Subjects with Type 2 Diabetes (SUSTAIN-6), fewer participants with moderate to severe CKD reached the primary composite cardiovascular endpoint in the liraglutide and semaglutide groups compared with those receiving placebo.[139,140] Initial analysis of the LEADER trial indicated that liraglutide reduced albuminuria in patients with normal kidney function or early-stage CKD.139 This finding was confirmed by the recent report of the prespecified secondary kidney outcome, a composite of new-onset persistent macroalbuminuria, persistent doubling of the serum creatinine level, ESRD, or death due to kidney disease. After a median follow-up of 4 years, the kidney outcomes occurred in fewer participants in the liraglutide group than in the placebo group (268 of 4668 patients vs. 337 of 4672; HR, 0.78; 95% CI, 0.67 to 0.92; $P = 0.003$). This result was driven primarily by the new onset of persistent macroalbuminuria which was 22% lower than in the placebo group.[141] In SUSTAIN-6, new or worsening nephropathy, defined as persistent macroalbuminuria, persistent doubling of serum creatinine, eGFR <45 mL/min/1.73 m^2, or a need for continuous RRT, occurred in 62 patients (3.8%) in the semaglutide group and 100 (6.1%) in the placebo group (HR, 0.64; 95% CI, 0.46 to 0.88; $P = 0.005$). This result was also driven by a reduction in new or persistent macroalbuminuria (HR, 0.54; 95% CI, 0.37 to 0.77; $P = 0.001$).[139,140] A Randomized, Open-Label, Parallel-Arm Study Comparing the Effect of Once-Weekly Dulaglutide with Insulin Glargine on Glycemic Control in Patients with Type 2 Diabetes and Moderate-to-Severe Chronic Kidney Disease (AWARD-7) trial was just completed in 2017, and results will soon be published.[142]

Sodium–Glucose Cotransporter 2 Inhibitors

Another recently introduced class of oral glucose-lowering agents are SGLT-2 inhibitors. These agents may reduce glomerular hyperfiltration and hypertension by reducing tubuloglomerular feedback. In the Empagliflozin Cardiovascular Outcome Event Trial in Type 2 Diabetes Mellitus Patients (EMPA-REG OUTCOME) trial, which enrolled approximately 7000 individuals with an established cardiovascular disease, participants taking the SGLT-2 inhibitor empagliflozin showed significantly lowered rates of death from cardiovascular causes (38% relative risk reduction), hospitalization for heart failure (35% relative risk reduction), and death from any cause (32% relative risk reduction) compared with those taking a placebo.[143,144] Analysis of prespecified secondary outcomes demonstrated that empagliflozin also slowed progression of DKD and lowered rates of clinically relevant kidney outcomes, including ESRD, among patients with CKD stages 2 to 4.[144]

The Canagliflozin Cardiovascular Assessment Study (CANVAS) Program integrated data from two trials that compared effects of another SGLT-2 inhibitor, canagliflozin, versus placebo. These trials enrolled approximately 10,000 individuals with type 2 diabetes who were at high cardiovascular risk. In the canagliflozin group, significantly fewer participants experienced composite outcome of cardiovascular death, nonfatal myocardial infarction, or nonfatal stroke (26.9 vs. 31.5 events per 1000 patient-years; HR 0.86; 95% CI, 0.75 to 0.97; $P < 0.001$). Progression of albuminuria occurred less frequently in the canagliflozin group compared with the placebo group (89.4 vs. 128.7 participants per 1000 patient-years, HR 0.73, 95% CI, 0.67 to 0.79), and a corresponding observation was made for regression of albuminuria (293.4 vs. 187.5 participants per 1000 patient-years, HR 1.70; 95% CI, 1.51 to 1.91, respectively). The composite outcome (40% eGFR reduction, need for RRT, or death from renal causes) occurred less frequently in the canagliflozin group relative to placebo (5.5 vs. 9.0 participants per 1000 patient-years; HR 0.60; 05% CI, 0.47 to 0.77).[145]

New Treatments for Diabetic Kidney Disease Targeting Intrinsic Kidney Mechanisms

Several promising therapies have been evaluated in clinical trials, including ruboxistaurin[146]; atrasentan, a selective endothelin A receptor antagonist[147,148]; finerenone, a selective nonsteroidal mineralocorticoid receptor antagonist[149-151]; and several agents targeting inflammatory pathways[146,152-155] (Table 3.6). However, thus far only finerenone has been evaluated in an ongoing phase III clinical trial, and none of the agents are yet FDA-approved for use in DKD.

The PKC-β inhibitor ruboxistaurin produced significant reduction in albuminuria and preservation of eGFR in a phase II clinical trial of participants with type 2 diabetes and macroalbuminuria on top of receiving standard of care for DKD, including background RAS inhibition. However, drug development was unfortunately halted for business and regulatory reasons.[146]

Pooled data analysis from two similarly designed, parallel, multinational, double-blind clinical trials of a selective endothelin A receptor antagonist, atrasentan, showed >35% reduction in albuminuria in study participants with DKD and no previously observed peripheral edema or heart failure. Participants who had a UACR of 300 to 500 mg/g were managed on the maximum tolerated dose of either an ACE inhibitor or an ARB and had an eGFR of 30 to 75 mL/min/m^2.[147] Atrasentan is currently being evaluated in the Study of Diabetic Nephropathy with Atrasentan trial (SONAR).[147,148]

The highly selective nonsteroidal mineralocorticoid receptor antagonist finerenone was studied in a randomized, double-blind, placebo-controlled clinical trial, Mineralocorticoid Receptor Antagonist Tolerability Study – Diabetic Nephropathy (ARTS-DN). Participants had type 2 diabetes, macroalbuminuria, and eGFR >30 mL/min/1.73 m^2. Forty percent of participants had eGFR <60 mL/min/1.73 m^2. Finerenone produced a dose-dependent reduction in albuminuria when added to a RAS blocker. After 90 days of treatment, finerenone decreased UACR in a dose-dependent manner, from 21% in the lowest to 38% in the highest dose group, compared with placebo. There were no differences between groups in terms of >30% decrease in eGFR or adverse and serious adverse events.[149] Two ongoing phase III trials are evaluating the safety and efficacy of finerenone in DKD patients, as well as its effects on cardiovascular morbidity and mortality in this population (FIGARO-DKD and FIDELIO-DKD).[150,151]

Serum uric acid concentration has been proposed as an independent risk for albuminuria and GFR decline in type 1 diabetes, primarily due to inflammatory and prooxidant properties.[156] An ongoing study, A Pilot Study of Allopurinol to Prevent Kidney Function Loss in Type 1 Diabetes (PERL) is currently evaluating whether allopurinol, a serum uric acid–lowering agent, prevents or delays loss of kidney function.[157]

Effect of Pentoxifylline on Renal Function and Urinary Albumin Excretion in Patients with Diabetic Kidney Disease (PREDIAN) was a randomized, open-label trial evaluating pentoxifylline, a phosphodiesterase inhibitor that exhibits both antiinflammatory and antifibrotic effects. PREDIAN enrolled 169 DKD patients who had macroalbuminuria despite RAS inhibitor treatment. After 24 months, eGFR decreased by 2.1 ± 0.4 mL/min/1.73 m^2 in the treatment group, compared with 6.5 ± 0.4 mL/min/1.73 m^2 in the control group (95% CI, 3.1 to 5.5 mL/min/1.73 m^2; $P < 0.001$). Both the between-group difference in eGFR decrease and the percentage change in albuminuria (5.7 vs. −14.9, $P < 0.001$) were significantly different in the control and treatment groups, respectively. A major limitation of this study was a lack of placebo control in the RAS-only group.[152]

Baricitinib is a Janus kinase-2 (JAK-2) inhibitor that was recently investigated in a phase II clinical trial.[153] Participants had DKD with macroalbuminuria while on RAS inhibitor treatment. Baricitinib reduced UACR in a dose-dependent manner after 3 and 6 months compared with placebo. The highest dose produced approximately a 40% reduction in UACR from baseline and decreased serum levels of inflammatory biomarkers, including tumor necrosis factor receptor 2 (TNFR2) and serum amyloid A (SAA), and urinary levels of monocyte-chemotactic protein-1 (MCP-1)/chemokine C-C motif-ligand 2 (CCL2). Notably, the therapeutic effect on albuminuria and these biomarkers was maintained after completion of the treatment and a 4-week washout period.[153]

Empaticap pegol (NOX-E36) is an antagonist of MCP-1/CCL2, an inflammatory chemokine with an important role in pathogenesis of DKD. NOX-E36 was evaluated in a phase II, placebo-controlled trial that enrolled DKD patients on RAS inhibitor treatment who still exhibited residual macroalbuminuria. After 12 weeks of treatment with empaticap, UACR was reduced 29% compared with baseline ($P < 0.05$). Interestingly, the maximum therapeutic effect of empaticap was delayed and was observed 4 weeks after discontinuation of treatment, as a 40% reduction in UACR compared with baseline ($P < 0.001$). However, this potential therapeutic effect on albuminuria did not reach a significant difference between treatment and the placebo group, and there was no difference between groups in eGFR.[154]

CCX140-B is an inhibitor of the receptor for MCP-1/CC2-chemokine receptor type 2 (CCR2). This agent showed promising results in DKD patients with residual macroalbuminuria who were managed on RAS inhibitors. Treatment with the lower dose resulted in a significant 18% decrease in albuminuria (95% CI, −26% to −8%, $P < 0.001$) in the treatment group compared with the placebo group. The albuminuria-lowering treatment effect persisted throughout the 52 weeks of the study.[155]

CONCLUSIONS

Driven by the escalating prevalence of diabetes across the world, DKD is an expanding global epidemic that incurs enormous human and economic cost. DKD is the most common cause of ESRD worldwide. DKD amplifies the risk of other serious complications such as cardiovascular diseases and death. Many patients with DKD do not follow the classical paradigm of progressive albuminuria followed by declining kidney function. Currently, intensive glycemic control early in the course of types 1 and 2 diabetes produces a long-lasting

Study Name	Intervention	Study Population	Outcomes
Kidney Outcomes in Clinical Trials of New Antihyperglycemic Therapies			
CARMELINA NCT01243424[174]	Linagliptin (DPP-4 inhibitor)	DM2, 6.5% ≥ HbA1C ≤ 10% albuminuria, macrovascular complications, eGFR >15 mL/min/1.73 m^2	In progress, estimated completion in January 2018
LEADER NCT01179048[139]	Liraglutide (GLP-1 receptor agonist)	DM2 HbA1C >7% eGFR <60 mL/min/1.73 m^2 CV coexisting disease	22% reduction of kidney endpoint (new-onset albuminuria, doubling of sCr and CrCl <45 mL/min/1.73 m^2; need for RRT, renal death) (1.5 number of events /100 patient/y vs. 1.9 number events/100 patient/y; $P = 0.003$)
SUSTAIN-6 NCT02054897[139,140]	Semaglutide (GLP-1 receptor agonist)	DM2 HbA1C 7%–10% 83% with CV disease or DKD stage 3 and higher	Reduction of onset of new or worsening of existing nephropathy (ESRD, renal death, eGFR <30 mL/min/1.73 m^2, development of macroalbuminuria) (hazard ratio 0.64, 95% CI, 0.46–0.88, $P = 0.005$)
AWARD-7 NCT01621178[142]	Dulaglutide (GLP-1 receptor agonist)	DM 2 7.5% ≥ HbA1C ≤10.5% 15 ≥ eGFR ≤60 mL/min/1.73 m^2	Estimated completion in July 2018
EMPA-REG OUTCOME NCT01131676[144]	Empagliflozin (SGLT-2 inhibitor)	DM2 eGFR ≥30 mL/min/1.73 m^2 High CV risk	44% relative risk reduction of doubling of SCr (1.5% vs. 2.6%) 38% relative risk reduction of progression to macroalbuminuria (11.2% vs. 16.2%) 55% relative risk reduction of initiation of RRT (0.3% vs. 0.6%) Slowing GFR decline (annual decrease 0.19 ± 0.11 mL/min/1.73 m^2 vs. 1.67 ± 0.13 mL/min/1.73 m^2, $P < 0.001$)
CREDENCE NCT02065791[175]	Canagliflozin (SGLT-2 inhibitor)	DM2 6.5% ≥ HbA1C ≤12% High CV risk 300 mg/g ≥UACR ≤5000 mg/g 30 ≥ eGFR ≤90 mL/min/1.73 m^2	In progress, estimated completion in June 2019
CANVAS and CANVAS R NCT01032629 NCT01989754[145]	Canagliflozin (SGLT-2 inhibitor)	DM2 7 ≥ HbA1C ≤10.5% High CV risk Median UACR 12.3 mg/g Mean eGFR 76.5 mL/min/1.73 m^2	34% ↓progression of albuminuria in UACR >30 mg/g group 36% ↓ progression of albuminuria in UACR >300 mg/g group 40% reduction of composite outcome (40% reduction of eGFR, RRT, or renal death)
Kidney Outcomes in Clinical Trials of Novel Therapies			
RADAR NCT01356849 and RADAR/JAPAN NCT01424319[147]	Atrasentan (ETA)	DM 2 eGFR 30–75 mL/min/1.73 m^2 UACR 300–3500 mg/g On maximal tolerated dose of ACE/ARB	35% reduction of albuminuria
SONAR NCT01858532 [148]	Atrasentan (ETA)	HTN eGFR 15–90 mL/min/1.73 m^2 UACR > 30 < 5000 mg/g On maximal tolerated dose of ACE/ARB	Results pending
PERL NCT01575379[157]	Allopurinol (Xanthine oxidase)	DM 1 eGFR 40–99 mL/min/1.73 m^2 UAE 18–5000 mg/d	Active, not recruiting
ARTS-DN NCT01874431[149]	Finerenone (Steroid mineralocorticoid receptor antagonist)	DM 2 UACR ≥30 mg/g eGFR >30 mL/min/1.73 m^2 On maximal tolerated dose of ACE/ARB	No difference in eGFR 21%–38% albuminuria reduction dose dependent

Continued

TABLE 3.6 **Clinical Trials of New Treatments for Diabetic Kidney Disease—cont'd**

Study Name	Intervention	Study Population	Outcomes
FIGARO-DKD NCT02545049[151]	Finerenone (Steroid mineralocorticoid receptor antagonist)	DM 2 UACR ≥30 but ≤5000 mg/g eGFR ≥25 but ≤75 mL/min/1.73 m^2 Serum K ≤4.8 mmol/l On maximal tolerated dose of ACE/ARB	Actively recruiting
FIDELIO-DKD NCT02540993[150]	Finerenone (Steroid mineralocorticoid receptor antagonist)	DM 2 UACR ≥30 but ≤5000 mg/g eGFR ≥25 but ≤75 mL/min/1.73 m^2 Serum K ≤4.8 mmol/l On maximal tolerated dose of ACE/ARB	Actively recruiting
PREDIAN NCT01858532[176]	Pentoxifylline (antiinflammatory, antifibrotic action)	DM2, eGFR 15–60 mL/min/1.73 m^2 UAE >300 mg/24 h On maximal tolerated dose of ACE/ARB	Pentoxifylline group: eGFR decline 4.3 mL/min/1.73 m^2 less than control group Mean difference in albuminuria of 21%
Tuttle et al., 2005[146]	Ruboxistaurin (PKC inhibitor)	DM2, macroalbuminuria On maximal tolerated dose of ACE/ARB	Decreased albuminuria, stabilized kidney function
Study to Test Safety and Efficacy of Baricitinib in Participants with Diabetic Kidney Disease NCT01683409[153]	Baricitinib (JAK-1/2 inhibitor)	DM2, eGFR 20–75 mL/min/1.73 m^2 macroalbuminuria On maximal tolerated dose of ACE/ARB	Albuminuria reduction by 40% in the highest treatment group No effect on eGFR
Empaticap pegol (NOX-E36) NCT01547897[154]	Empaticap pegol (direct MCP-1 inhibitor)	DM 2 eGFR >25 mL/min/1.73 m^2 ACR >100 mg/g On maximal tolerated dose of ACE/ARB	29% ACR reduction compared with baseline ($P < 0.05$) The maximum effect a 40% reduction of albuminuria from baseline achieved 4 weeks after discontinuation of treatment
CCX140-B, NCT01447147[155]	CCX140-B (CCR2 inhibitor)	DM2 HbA1C 6%–10% eGFR ≥25 mL/min/1.73 m^2 UACR 100–3000 mg/g On maximal tolerated dose of ACE/ARB	5-mg group : 18% reduction of albuminuria , −16% ($P = 0.01$) compared with placebo 10-mg group: nonsignificant reduction of albuminuria

ACE, Angiotensin-converting enzyme inhibitor; *ARB,* angiotensin II receptorblockers; *ARTS-DN,* Safety and Efficacy of Different Oral Doses of BAY94-8862 in Subjects With Type 2 Diabetes Mellitus and the Clinical Diagnosis of Diabetic Nephropathy; *AWARD-7,* A Randomized, Open-Label, Parallel-Arm Study Comparing the Effect of Once-weekly Dulaglutide With Insulin Glargine on Glycemic Control in Patients With Type 2 Diabetes and Moderate or Severe Chronic Kidney Disease; *CARMELINA,* Cardiovascular and Renal Microvascular Outcome Study With Linagliptin in Patients With Type 2 Diabetes Mellitus; *CCR2,* receptor type 2 for MCP-1; *CrCl,* creatinine clearance; *CI,* confidence interval; *CREDENCE,* A Randomized, Double-blind, Event-driven, Placebo-controlled, Multicenter Study of the Effects of Canagliflozin on Renal and Cardiovascular Outcomes in Subjects With Type 2 Diabetes Mellitus and Diabetic Nephropathy; *CV,* cardiovascular; *DM2,* type 2 diabetes mellitus; *DM1,* type 1 diabetes mellitus; *DKD,* diabetic kidney disease; *DPP-4,* dipeptidyl peptidase-4 inhibitor; *eGFR,* estimated glomerular filtration rate in m/1.73 m^2; *EMPA-REG,* A Phase III, Multicentre, International, Randomised, Parallel Group, Double Blind Cardiovascular Safety Study of BI 10773 (10 mg and 25 mg Administered Orally Once Daily) Compared to Usual Care in Type 2 Diabetes Mellitus Patients With Increased Cardiovascular Risk; *FIDELIO-DKD,* Finerenone in Reducing Kidney Failure and Disease Progression in Diabetic Kidney Disease; *FIGARO- DKD,* Finerenone in Reducing Cardiovascular Mortality and Morbidity in Diabetic Kidney Disease; *GLP-1,* glucagon-like peptide-1; *HbA1C,* hemoglobin A1c; *HTN,* hypertension; *JAK 1/2,* Janus kinases 1/2; *LEADER,* A Long-term, Multi-centre, International, Randomised Double-blind, Placebo-controlled Trial to Determine Liraglutide Effects on Cardiovascular Events; *MCP-1,* monocyte chemotactic protein-1; *PCR,* protein-to-creatinine ratio in mg/g; *PERL,* A Multicenter Clinical Trial of Allopurinol to Prevent Kidney Function Loss in Type 1 Diabetes; *PIONEER,* A Phase 3 Randomized, Double-Blind, Placebo-Controlled, Multi-Center Study to Evaluate the Safety and Efficacy of Pyridorin (Pyridoxamine Dihydrochloride) in Subjects With Nephropathy Due to Type 2 Diabetes; *PREDIAN,* Effect of Pentoxifylline on Renal Function and Urinary Albumin Excretion in Patients with Diabetic Kidney Disease; *RADAR,* Evaluate the Efficacy and Safety of Once Daily Administration of Atrasentan Tablets (Low and High) Compared to Placebo in Reducing Residual Albuminuria in Type 2 Diabetic Patients With Nephropathy Who Are Treated With the Maximum Tolerated Labeled Dose of a Renin Angiotensin System Inhibitor; *RRT,* renal replacement therapy; *SAVOR-TIMI,* The Saxagliptin Assessment of Vascular Outcomes Recorded in Patients with Diabetes Mellitus-Thrombolysis in Myocardial Infarction; *SUSTAIN-6,* Trial to Evaluate Cardiovascular and Other Long-term Outcomes with Semaglutide in Subjects with Type 2 Diabetes; *SCr,* serum creatinine in mg/dL; *SGLT-2,* sodium glucose cotransporter 2; *UACR,* urinary albumin-to-creatinine ratio in mg/g; *UAE,* urine albumin excretion in mg/day.

preventive effect on DKD development. However, once DKD is established, intensive glycemic control increases the risk of hypoglycemia and has a nominal effect on DKD progression. Antihypertensive treatment with either an ACE inhibitor or an ARB reduces progression of established DKD to ESRD, but these agents do not prevent DKD onset. New approaches to improve DKD awareness, detection, and intervention are urgently needed to reduce its devastating complications.

ACKNOWLEDGMENTS

The authors would like to acknowledge Michele Rooney, MD, for creating and sharing histology images for Figs. 3.4, 3.5, and 3.8.

A full list of references is available at www.expertconsult.com.

4

Hypertensive Chronic Kidney Disease

Anna C. Porter, MD, Amatur Amarah, MD, Esteban Cedillo-Couvert, MD, and James P. Lash, MD

OUTLINE

INTRODUCTION

Hypertension affects around one-third of the US population[1] and is one of the main preventable risk factors for death and chronic disease progression, including kidney disease.[2] According to the US Renal Data System, hypertension was reported as the second leading cause of incident end-stage renal disease (ESRD) cases.[3] Yet controversy remains over whether hypertension alone initiates chronic kidney disease (CKD) and leads to subsequent ESRD, or if hypertension as a cause of ESRD represents a subset of patients with diverse but uninvestigated or unrecognized etiological reasons for kidney disease.[4] Indeed, hypertension and CKD can be viewed as a bidirectional relationship: CKD causing uncontrolled hypertension, and hypertension causing CKD. However, except for accelerated and malignant hypertension, the evidence supporting a causal relationship between mild to moderate hypertension and CKD is inconsistent and therefore this causality is still debated. On the other hand, it is well accepted that CKD causes and contributes to hypertensive disease. In that regard, we know that the prevalence of hypertension is higher in patients with CKD compared with the general population,[5] and that this prevalence increases further as patients progress to ESRD. Furthermore, the severity of hypertension in CKD increases the risk for ESRD[6]; and lower blood pressure (BP) levels in patients with proteinuric kidney diseases are associated with lower CKD progression rates.[7]

Management of hypertension in the context of CKD remains an evolving field. Recent data from the Systolic Blood Pressure Intervention Trial (SPRINT) have lent important insights regarding BP goals in the management of individuals with hypertensive CKD. Nonpharmacological management strategies, such as dietary changes, also remain a field of active investigation. Here we review clinical manifestations of hypertensive kidney disease; therapeutic strategies, including recent findings about BP goals; antihypertensive agents; and nonpharmacological management strategies.

POTENTIAL MECHANISMS OF RENAL INJURY IN HYPERTENSION

The mechanisms by which chronic mild to moderate hypertension may induce renal injury are less clear than those by which it perpetuates progression and acceleration of CKD. The pathophysiology of hypertension causing CKD in individuals with previous normal kidney function depends both on its chronicity and severity. Clear distinct pathological changes are described for long-term chronic mild to moderate hypertension and malignant/accelerated hypertension.[8]

Pathophysiology of Renal Injury in Hypertensive Nephrosclerosis

The pathophysiology of mild to moderate hypertension causing renal injury is, as discussed before, inconsistent across animal and human clinical studies.[4,9,10] The histological changes associated with this type of hypertension are arteriolar hyalinosis, medial hypertrophy, and intimal fibrosis.[8] Arteriolar hyalinosis is not specific to hypertension and can be found in other conditions such as diabetes and aging. Nevertheless, these changes lead to ischemic glomerulosclerosis demonstrated by the collapse of capillary loops and wrinkling of the capillary basement membrane leading to wall thickening. This ultimately results in glomerular tuft retraction and filling of the Bowman space with collagen.[8] In addition, the tubules may show areas of atrophy and tubular lumen dilatation as well as chronic interstitial inflammatory cells surrounding the areas of tubular atrophy.

Evidence suggests that impaired renal autoregulation results in the transmission of systemic pressure to the renal microvasculature. Most of the evidence for impaired renal autoregulation derives from animal models, but the ideal animal model to elucidate the real contribution of hypertension to renal injury has not been identified.[4,8-10] When the threshold of autoregulation is exceeded, as is seen in malignant hypertension, an acute injury is expected despite a normal autoregulation mechanism. The presence of chronic hypertension tends to increase the limits of renal blood flow autoregulation as a means of adaptation.[11] However, there are situations in which lower degrees of systemic BP can be transmitted to the capillary loop in the presence of additive preglomerular vasodilatory states (e.g., inhibition of prostaglandin production by nonsteroidal antiinflammatory drugs) and/or other causes of impaired renal autoregulation. In addition, local, genetic or acquired factors may also increase the susceptibility and degree of renal injury (e.g., impaired structural integrity of the podocyte in glomerular hypertrophy or blood-pressure independent activation of downstream pathways involving angiotensin II, aldosterone, and other deleterious molecules).[10]

Once kidney disease is established, additional pathophysiological mechanisms interact to perpetuate a hypertensive state that consequently contributes to the progression of CKD. The prevalence of hypertension in CKD is high and increases with the severity of renal function ranging from 75% to 89% in advanced CKD stages.[12-15] Ultimately, the main factors that account for the presence and exacerbation of hypertension in CKD include increased extracellular volume and increased vascular resistance. The main mechanisms that contribute to the presence and exacerbation of these factors are sympathetic nervous system overactivity and activation of the renin-angiotensin-aldosterone system (RAAS), which result in arterial stiffness and impaired renal and water excretion.[16-20]

Increased volume and cardiac output are the first changes that begin even before any change in BP manifests. Once the vascular bed compliance can no longer compensate for the increase in the blood volume, hypertension develops.[16,17] The increased extracellular volume expansion is related to the impaired salt and water excretion that occurs in CKD as a consequence of altered pressure natriuresis in the presence of a decreased glomerular filtration rate (GFR) and the presence of angiotensin II resultant from RAAS activation.[18-20] This is also influenced by high dietary sodium intake. Most of the patients with moderate to advanced CKD face a state of volume expansion, which correlates with higher BP levels and worse clinical outcomes.[21,22] These adverse outcomes are the result of not only hypertension but the direct and independent effects of volume expansion and sodium load.[21,23]

The overactivity of the sympathetic nervous system in CKD contributes both to increased volume expansion and vascular resistance. There have been several stimuli identified for increased sympathetic activity in CKD (i.e., renal ischemia, hyperleptinemia, RAAS, uremic toxins, smoking, obesity, hypercapnia, and decreased nitric oxide availability).[24-26] This overactivity has been documented in individuals with nondiabetic predialysis CKD.[26,27] The consequences of this hyperactive sympathetic system are activation of the RAAS with increased release of renin and angiotensin II,[26,28] vasoconstriction of renal vasculature with arterial smooth muscle and fibroblast proliferation, and salt and water retention. There is also evidence that sympathetic overactivity can result in increased local inflammatory cytokines, which could additionally potentiate the progression of CKD.[29,30]

The components of the RAAS activation also result in both increased extracellular volume and vascular resistance. In the presence of decreased cardiac output, renin release is mediated by the sympathetic nervous system along with a fall in distal convoluted tubular sodium delivery due to increased proximal tubular sodium reabsorption with resultant afferent arteriole dilation by tubuloglomerular feedback.[31] Renin has a bidirectional relationship with the sympathetic nervous system, which stimulates it further and results in the production of angiotensin II.

The effects of angiotensin II lead to several hemodynamic and nonhemodynamic changes that promote inflammation, extracellular matrix accumulation, and direct glomerular injury, which lead to hypertension exacerbation and CKD progression through increased glomerular and tubulointerstitial fibrosis. These effects are mainly mediated by the angiotensin type 1 (AT1) receptor. The main hemodynamic changes are to increase glomerular hypertension, upregulate the sympathetic nervous system, and impair the normal pressure natriuresis.[18,26,32] There are many nonhemodynamic effects of angiotensin II that can also contribute to CKD progression, which are predominantly mediated through activation of the AT1 receptor. These include proteinuria and loss of glomerular size permselectivity, stimulation of mesangial proliferation, tumor growth factor-β (TGF-β) expression, extracellular matrix deposition, endothelial production of plasminogen activator inhibitor-1 (PAI-1), macrophage activation, phagocytosis, and adrenal aldosterone production.[32] Furthermore, the contribution of increased renal tubular sodium reabsorption by aldosterone as a result of RAAS activation in CKD is also important for the increased extracellular volume component of hypertension in this state.

Finally, other factors that influence vascular resistance are endothelin and secondary hyperparathyroidism.[33,34] The role of endothelin is important given its role in promoting vasoconstriction; increasing arterial stiffness; and promoting endothelial dysfunction, inflammation, and atherosclerosis, which exacerbate hypertension and progression of CKD.[14,35] In addition, secondary hyperparathyroidism of CKD influences arterial stiffness through its association with arterial calcification among other cardiovascular (CV) effects.[34]

Genetic Risk Markers

One important finding involves the recent identification of the genetic contribution of the apolipoprotein L1 (*APOL1*) gene in the development of nondiabetic kidney disease in individuals of African ancestry (see Chapter 7: Genetic Causes of Chronic Kidney Disease). *APOL1* is a gene located on chromosome 22 that produces a protein that is a component of circulating high-density lipoprotein.[36] Two alleles, APOL1 G1 and APOL1 G2, which are found with greater frequency in individuals with African ancestry, confer an increased risk of development of nondiabetic kidney disease in an autosomal recessive manner; that is, persons who possess two of these renal-risk alleles in APOL1 have a 10.5-fold greater risk for idiopathic focal segmental glomerulosclerosis (FSGS) and a 7.3-fold greater risk for hypertension-related ESRD compared with those with zero or one allele.[37] It has been postulated that APOL1 G1 and G2 (the so-called "renal-risk alleles") became more common in populations with African ancestry as the gene products of these alleles confer resistance against *Trypanosoma brucei* infection (the causative agent of African sleeping sickness) due to the trypanolytic actions of these proteins.[37] Overall, *APOL1*-associated nephropathy may account for a significant proportion of nondiabetic kidney disease in African Americans, including cases previously identified as hypertensive nephropathy, with estimates of up to 70% of all nondiabetic kidney disease in African Americans being due to *APOL1*-associated nephropathy.[9]

DIAGNOSIS AND CLINICAL MANIFESTATIONS

Clinical Manifestations and Risk Factors

The clinical diagnosis of hypertensive CKD includes a long period of antecedent, poorly controlled hypertension, subnephrotic proteinuria (typically less than 1 g/day), and features suggestive of other end-organ complications of uncontrolled hypertension, such as hypertensive retinopathy or left ventricular hypertrophy, as well as a bland urine sediment. There are no well-defined criteria for clinical diagnosis of hypertensive CKD, and biopsy is typically unnecessary for diagnosis.[38] Historically, the African American race has been recognized as a risk factor[39] for hypertensive CKD, though more recent recognition of APOL1 risk alleles raises the possibility that the diagnosis of hypertensive CKD could represent a distinct clinical entity in people with African ancestry.[40-42] One study that retrospectively compared biopsy specimens of African Americans diagnosed with hypertensive CKD with those of whites with the same diagnosis found that there were morphological differences in the global glomerulosclerosis lesions between the two groups, with African Americans having more of a "solidified" global glomerulosclerosis lesion, and that these differences were independent of BP and degree of proteinuria.[40] A later study examined about 200 kidney biopsy specimens from African Americans diagnosed with hypertensive CKD and the relationship between these morphological differences and presence of APOL1 renal-risk alleles on genotyping.[41] Individuals with two APOL1 renal-risk alleles were more likely to have a solidified global glomerulosclerosis lesion, compared with those with zero such alleles.[41] Taken together, these studies suggest the possibility of different mechanisms of renal injury between individuals having two APOL1 renal-risk alleles and those who do not carry these genotypes.

Role of Kidney Biopsy

As the diagnosis of hypertensive CKD is primarily a clinical one, most patients receiving this diagnosis do not undergo biopsy, unless doubt on the part of the clinician exists as to the etiology of CKD. One study that affirms this approach drew data from the African American Study of Kidney Disease and Hypertension (AASK), in which 39 participants carrying a clinical diagnosis of hypertensive nephrosclerosis underwent renal biopsy, and histopathological examination showed changes consistent with this diagnosis in all but one biopsy specimen.[43] Pathological findings of hypertensive nephrosclerosis include changes in the glomeruli, tubulointerstitium, and vasculature.[8] Glomeruli may be normal or show wrinkling, or later global or segmental sclerosis (Fig. 4.1A). Tubular atrophy and hyaline casts may be present. Fibrous intimal thickening may be present in the arcuate and larger arteries (Fig. 4.1B).[8] As discussed earlier, recent studies have demonstrated that renal biopsy specimens from individuals with two APOL1 renal-risk alleles may show different histopathological findings compared with those from individuals without such alleles.[41] Malignant hypertension results in acute glomerular injury when the limits of autoregulation are exceeded and is characterized by focal fibrinoid necrosis (usually segmental), mesangiolysis, and occlusion of the capillary lumen by endothelial swelling and fibrin and platelet thrombi (Fig. 4.1C).[3] This eventually leads to thickening of capillary walls and subendothelial widening resulting in double contour of the basement membrane. These acute changes may be indistinguishable from those of acute thrombotic microangiopathy (Fig. 4.1D). The chronic glomerular changes of malignant hypertension can involve either similar changes to those seen in benign hypertension; or a collapsed, almost acellular, glomerulus with subendothelial widening.[8]

THERAPEUTICS

In the next section, we will review evidence regarding the optimal BP goal for patients with hypertensive CKD and discuss the use of individual antihypertensive agents. These sections will also include a discussion of the recent major studies regarding BP control in CKD (Table 4.1).

Target Level of BP Control

The 2014 Eighth Joint National Committee guidelines recommend a goal BP for adults with hypertension and CKD of ≤140/90 mmHg.[44] However, this consensus recommendation is not without some controversy given the conflicting findings of recent clinical trials including individuals with and without CKD. One further complication is that these trials have had heterogeneity in ascertained outcomes, depending on the population under study. For example, the Modification of

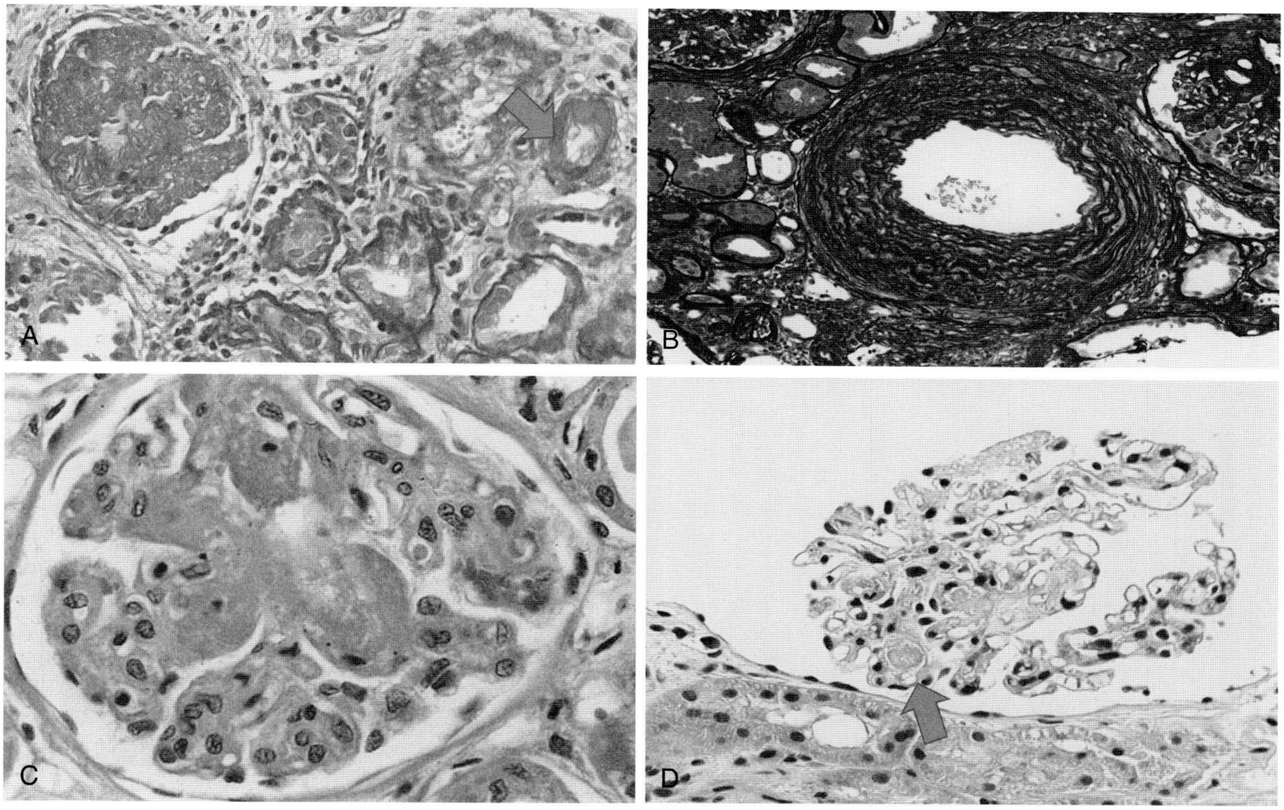

FIG. 4.1 Histopathological changes of hypertension in the kidney. (A) A sclerotic glomerulus with replacement of capillary loops by collagen, adjacent atrophic tubules, and an arteriole with hyaline material deposited in the intima (*arrow*) (PAS, original magnification ×400). (From UIC Pathology Archives, courtesy Dr. Suman Setty.) (B) An interlobular artery with multilayering of the internal elastic lamina (Jones' silver stain, original magnification ×200). (From UIC Pathology Archives, courtesy Dr. Suman Setty.) (C) Hemolytic uremic syndrome (TMA). Some of the glomerular capillary tufts are permeated by eosinophilic acellular material. This change is often described as fibrinoid necrosis. Intraluminal thrombi are also present (original magnification ×400). (From Jennette JC, Heptinstall RH. [Eds.]. *Heptinstall's pathology of the kidney.* [6th ed.]. Philadelphia, PA: Lippincott Williams & Wilkins; 2007.) (D) Change of acute thrombotic microangiopathy with fibrin thrombi (*arrow*) in lumen of glomerular capillary loops (H&E, original magnification ×400). (From UIC Pathology Archives, courtesy Dr. Suman Setty.)

Diet in Renal Disease (MDRD)[45] and AASK[46,47] failed to find benefit of intensive BP control in terms of CKD progression, whereas the SPRINT found benefit of intensive BP control in terms of CV but not renal outcomes (see the following discussion).[48]

SPRINT enrolled more than 9000 hypertensive adults age 50 and older.[49] Although diabetics were excluded, all participants had either an additional CV risk factor or CKD with an estimated GFR (eGFR) at study entry of 20 to 59 mL/min/1.73 m^2 (28% of the study cohort). Individuals with proteinuria of more than 1 g/day were excluded. Participants were randomized to two systolic BP control arms. The standard arm goal was a systolic blood pressure (SBP) goal of ≤140 mmHg and the intensive arm goal was a systolic BP goal of ≤120 mmHg. The study did not focus on a particular antihypertensive medication class, of which any or a combination could be prescribed at the investigators' discretion to achieve the desired level of BP control. The primary endpoint was a composite outcome of myocardial infarction, stroke, acute coronary syndrome not classified as myocardial infarction, stroke, acute decompensated heart failure, or death related to CV cause. For participants with CKD, a renal endpoint was also assessed, defined as a loss of 50% of eGFR from baseline value or development of ESRD requiring long-term maintenance dialysis or transplantation. Participants in the intensive-treatment arm achieved a mean SBP of 121.4 mmHg vs. 136.2 mmHg in the standard-treatment arm within the first year, and the level of BP control was maintained over the course of the study for each group.[48] The study was stopped early (at a median follow-up of 3 years) due to a statistically significant difference in the primary outcome between the BP control arms (1.65% per year in the intensive-treatment arm compared with 2.19% per year in the standard-treatment arm, $P < .001$).[48] There was no difference in renal outcomes among participants with CKD (1.1% per year in both groups) (Fig. 4.2). However, among participants without CKD, the risk of acute kidney injury was higher (4.1% in the intensive-treatment arm compared with 2.5% in the standard-treatment arm, $P < .001$). A more recent subgroup analysis of SPRINT participants with CKD found that intensive BP control resulted in a 19% lower risk of CV

TABLE 4.1 Summary of Clinical Trials in CKD and Hypertension

Study	Population	Study Design	Intervention	Endpoints	Outcome
ACCOMPLISH[147,148]	11,506 people with hypertension at high risk for a cardiovascular event, including 1093 with CKD	Double-blind RCCT	Benazepril-amlodipine vs. benazepril-hydrochlorothiazide combination, follow-up over 2.9 years	CV death and CV event composite	Benazepril-amlodipine superior in preventing CV death/events (19.6% RR reduction). CKD patients also had lower rates of CKD progression
ALLHAT[60]	>33,000 hypertensive adults age 55 and up who had at least one other CV disease risk factor; about 18% had CKD III or IV	Double-blind RCCT	Chlorthalidone vs. amlodipine vs. Lisinopril vs. doxazosin, follow-up 4.9 years	CV death and CV event composite	Chlorthalidone group had better BP control, lower CV events than lisinopril group; No difference in CKD progression rates
AASK[46]	1094 African Americans with hypertensive CKD	3-by-2 factorial design	Ramipril, metoprolol, or amlodipine in intensive (MAP ≤92 mmHg) or standard (MAP 102–107 mmHg) BP control arms, follow-up over 3–6.4 years	Composite of eGFR loss of 50% from baseline, ESRD, or death	No difference between levels of BP control; lower risk of composite outcome with ramipril use
IDNT[149]	1715 hypertensive adults with diabetic nephropathy	Double-blind RCCT	Amlodipine, irbesartan, or placebo, followed over 2.6 years	Composite of doubling of serum creatinine from baseline, ESRD, or death	Irbesartan reduced the risk of the primary outcome by about one-third compared with amlodipine or placebo despite similar achieved blood pressure control
REIN[150]	186 patients with nonnephrotic proteinuria and CKD	Double-blind RCCT	Ramipril vs. placebo + conventional antihypertensive therapy, follow-up over a median of 2.7 years	Change in GFR and time to ESRD	Ramipril reduced the risk of progression to ESRD compared with placebo and also reduced proteinuria
SPRINT[48]	9361 hypertensive adults >50, without diabetes, including 2646 with nonproteinuric CKD (eGFR 20–60 mL/min/1.73 m^2 and urine protein <1 g/d)	RCCT	Two arms: standard BP goal of <140 mmHg SBP or intensive BP goal of <120 mmHg SBP. Different classes of medications could be used at the investigator's discretion to achieve BP control. Follow-up over 3 years	CV events, decrease in GFR by 50% or ESRD, and death	Participants in intensive control arm (including those with CKD) had lower risk of CV events and death. Increased rate of AKI in intensive arm but not CKD progression

AKI, acute kidney injury; *BP*, blood pressure; *CKD*, chronic kidney disease; *CV*, cardiovascular; *eGFR*, estimated glomerular filtration rate; *ESRD*, end-stage renal disease; *GFR*, glomerular filtration rate; *MAP*, mean arterial pressure; *RCCT*, randomized controlled clinical trial; *RR*, relative risk.

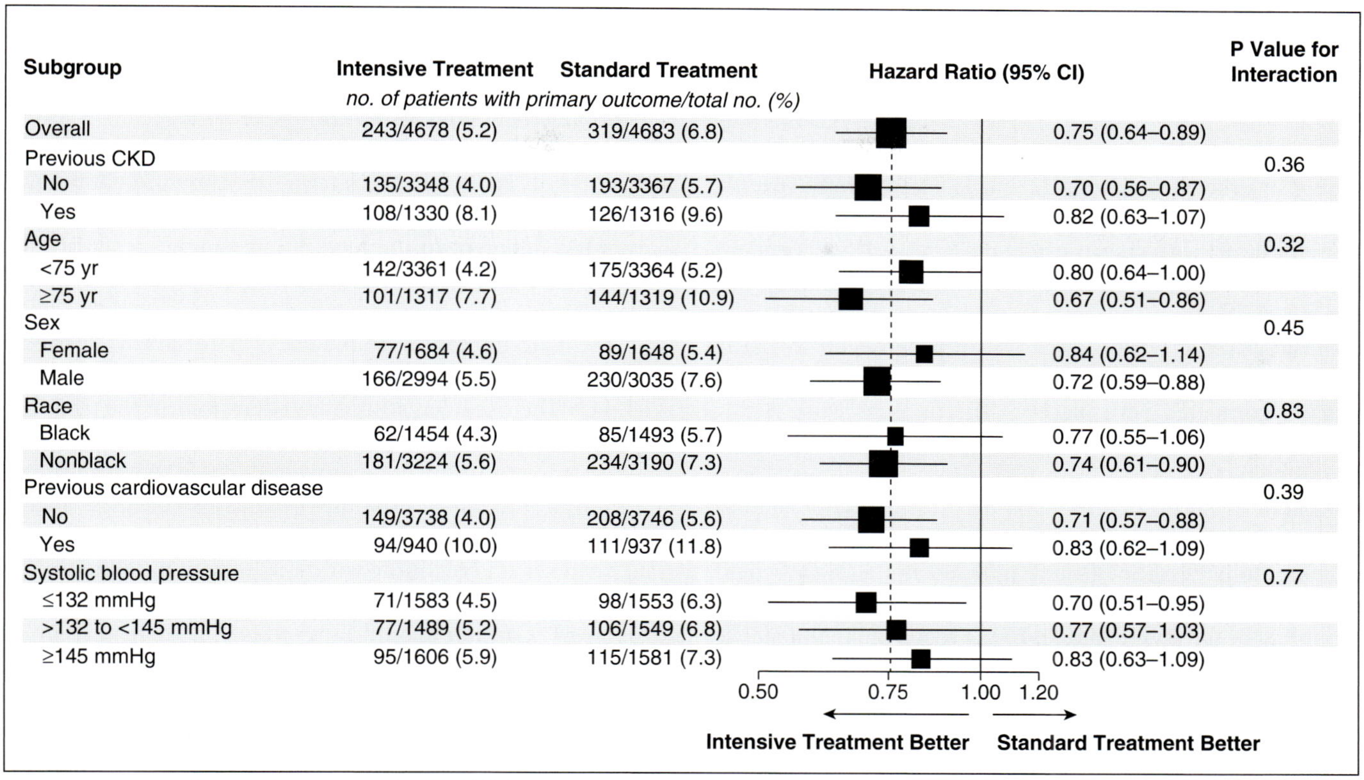

FIG. 4.2 Outcomes in SPRINT according to participant subgroups. (From SPRINT Research Group, Wright JT Jr, Williamson JD, et al. A randomized trial of intensive versus standard blood-pressure control. *N Engl J Med.* 2015;373(22):2103-2116.)

events and a 28% lower risk of all-cause mortality compared with standard BP control but did not have a significant effect on CKD progression rates.[50] It should be noted that SPRINT participants with CKD had a mean eGFR of 47 mL/min/1.73 m^2, and individuals were excluded with proteinuria >1 g/day at baseline. Therefore findings may not be generalizable to all patients with CKD.[51]

In choosing optimal BP, the clinician and the patient need to balance pros and cons and take into consideration comorbid and demographic propensity for the development of CV events, as well as the risk for adverse events from increased BP control. The role of specific agents and lifestyle modification strategies are discussed in the following section.

THERAPEUTIC AGENTS

RAAS Blockade

The RAAS, through the mediation of angiotensin-II, contributes to the progression of CKD in both its hemodynamic and nonhemodynamic effects.[52] The pharmacological blockage of this system results in the lowering of BP in individuals with primary hypertension and CKD.[46,53-55] In addition to this hemodynamic effect, there is considerable evidence from animal models of CKD that RAAS blockade using either angiotensin-converting enzyme inhibitors (ACEIs) or angiotensin receptor blockers (ARBs) results in decreased glomerular pressure and consequently proteinuria, protects against arterial wall thickening, prevents activation of profibrotic and proinflammatory cytokines and macrophage recruitment.[32] Human trials have confirmed the protective effects of these agents in both diabetic and nondiabetic individuals with CKD.[46,55,56] We focus on those with nondiabetic hypertensive CKD in this section.

ANGIOTENSIN CONVERTING ENZIME INHIBITORS

ACEIs inhibit the enzymatic conversion of angiotensin I to angiotensin II and have been shown to attenuate the decline of renal function in nondiabetic CKD populations. Although the first trial showing the benefit of ACEI was in a diabetic population,[57] subsequent trials that have analyzed moderate nondiabetic, mostly hypertensive, CKD populations with eGFR ranging between 39 and 50 mL/min/1.73 m^2 have reported improved renal outcomes in this group.[7,46,55,58] Maschio et al.[58] randomized 583 European individuals with baseline creatinine clearance of 42 mL/min to benazepril or placebo. After 3 years of follow-up, these investigators found greater systolic and diastolic lowering effects in the benazepril group. The placebo group experienced a small increase in both SBP and diastolic blood pressure (DBP). There was a 53% overall risk reduction in the endpoint of doubling of serum creatinine or need for dialysis in the benazepril group compared with placebo. Also, the Ramipril Efficiency in Nephropathy (REIN) study randomized 352 individuals with two different strata of protein excretion (1 to 3 g per 24 h vs. >3 g per

24 h) to receive ramipril or placebo.[55] Mean measured GFR was 40 mL/min/1.73 m^2 for the treatment group and 37 mL/min/1.73 m^2 for the placebo group. This trial saw a decrease in both SBP and DBP compared with baseline, but this was not statistically different between the ramipril and placebo groups in either stratum of proteinuria. However, the investigators observed a slower decline in GFR in the ramipril group from the strata with greater proteinuria that was independent of baseline and follow up BP levels. Although this finding was not seen for the ramipril group in the lower proteinuric strata, they did observe a 56% lower risk of progression to ESRD and 52% lower risk to progress to overt proteinuria in this stratum compared with placebo. The findings from AASK further support the role of ACEI to slow CKD progression. In this trial, 1094 African Americans were randomized to a normal or lower mean arterial blood pressure (MAP) and to one of three antihypertensive agents: ramipril, amlodipine, or metoprolol.[46] Although this trial did not show a benefit of lower MAP in the primary outcome of CKD progression (doubling of serum creatinine, ESRD requiring maintenance dialysis or transplantation, or death), differences were seen with respect to this outcome between the groups treated with different antihypertensive agents: the ramipril group had 22% and 38% lower risk of the composite outcome of GFR decline, ESRD, or death compared with metoprolol and amlodipine, respectively. After the initial trial phase of AASK, participants were invited to enroll in an observational cohort phase and were followed for up to 12 years. An analysis of overall event rates during both the trial and cohort phase found no difference in the primary outcome over the entire period of follow-up between those initially randomized to intensive vs. standard control.[47] However, the effects differed by level of baseline proteinuria ($P = .02$ for interaction). Compared with individuals in the intensive BP control group with a protein–creatinine ratio of ≤0.22, individuals with a ratio >0.22 had a reduced risk for CKD progression (hazard ratio, 0.73; $P = .01$). Of note, follow-up BPs during this trial were similar between these three drug groups. The findings from this and other trials[59] suggest a long-term effect of ACEI independent from its effect on BP. In the metaanalysis by Jafar et al.,[7] the slowing of CKD progression was more effective when antihypertensive regimens included ACEI. Whether this independent effect is driven by additional proteinuria decline from that attributed to BP lowering, or from other influence on the nonhemodynamic effects of RAAS, is still unclear. However, this concept of an independent RAAS blockade effect has been challenged by the results of the Antihypertensive and Lipid Lowering Treatment to Prevent Heart Attack Trial (ALLHAT) in nondiabetic CKD and some animal studies.[58-60] The ALLHAT followed more than 33,000 adults older than 55 years with hypertension and one risk factor for heart disease randomized to receive chlorthalidone, amlodipine, or lisinopril for a combined primary outcome of fatal heart disease or nonfatal myocardial infarction.[60] Approximately 18% of participants had CKD stage 3 or 4 at baseline. After almost 5 years of follow-up, ALLHAT investigators reported a superiority of chlorthalidone in preventing CV disease and no difference on the secondary outcome of reaching ESRD between the chlorthalidone and lisinopril groups.[60] A post hoc analysis of CKD participants found no difference in the incidence of ESRD or a combined endpoint of ESRD and/or 50% decline in eGFR between the lisinopril and chlorthalidone groups. However, these results are difficult to interpret because proteinuria was not reported in this trial, and those in the lisinopril group were less adherent to the medication and had a statistically significant 2 mmHg higher BP level than the chlorthalidone group.[61]

The main limitations to the use of ACEI in CKD patients are its associated increase in serum creatinine and hyperkalemia.[62] The rise in creatinine noted in some of the trials has been attributed to the hemodynamic effect of the hypertensive therapy resulting in an initial fall in GFR within the first 2 months of therapy initiation[58] but has also been associated with subsequent long-term renal protection.[32,63,64] Therefore a rise in serum creatinine within 30% from baseline should not be of concern if stable within the first 2 months of therapy.[65] Caution should be exercised if there is a larger increase in serum creatinine. In terms of hyperkalemia >5.0 mEq/L, the trials by Maschio et al.[58] reported an increase of 0.5 mEq/L per liter in the serum potassium concentration in the ramipril group as opposed to no change in the placebo group. Five patients, three in the ramipril group and two in the placebo group, withdrew from the study due to hyperkalemia. In the REIN trial, only one patient withdrew from the study due to hyperkalemia, as opposed to two in the placebo group.[55] The AASK trial had only three reports of hyperkalemia, but this was not statistically different from the other drug groups compared (amlodipine and metoprolol).[66] Therefore the incidence of hyperkalemia observed in a nondiabetic CKD population treated with RAAS blockade remains low.

ANGIOTENSIN RECEPTOR BLOCKERS

The ARBs have a similar BP lowering effect as the ACEIs in the general population of hypertensive patients.[53] These agents block the AT1 receptor resulting in blockage of angiotensin-II stimulation from any source, and produce elevations in both renin and angiotensin-II due to impaired feedback suppression.[32] This potentially leads to stimulation of angiotensin receptor-2, which could counterbalance some of the effects mediated by AT1. However, the clinical significance of this is still unknown. Moreover, although there is plenty of evidence of similar BP control and proteinuria reduction to ACEI in animal models, the ARBs' clinical effectiveness is based on large trials investigating diabetic kidney disease.[56,57] There is currently no large randomized clinical trial available in a nondiabetic CKD population, and the clinical application of ARBs is based on results from smaller trials, which find similar BP control and reduction in proteinuria compared with ACEI in individuals with nondiabetic CKD.[67-75] A stable, small rise in creatinine resultant from similar hemodynamic effects as ACEI has been observed for ARBs as well.[32]

COMBINATION THERAPY ACEI AND ARBS

There are several animal model and small trials that suggest that RAAS inhibition may be improved with combination therapy using both ACE and ARBs.[76-79] However, a favorable clinical effect has not been shown when tested in large clinical trials. Specifically, the only trial that had reported a favorable effect of combination therapy in nondiabetic CKD has been discredited due to data inconsistencies.[80-83] Therefore the evidence relies on other main trials showing an increased adverse effect of the combination therapy in different populations: those at high risk for vascular disease and those with diabetes.[85] The Ongoing Telmisartan Alone and in Combination with Ramipril Global Endpoint Trial (ONTARGET) randomized more than 25,000 individuals at high risk for vascular disease to receive telmisartan, ramipril, or the combination of both.[85] Despite a lower mean BP in the telmisartan and combination group compared with the ramipril group, there was no difference among the study groups in the composite CV primary outcome. However, the combination group had higher risk for hypotension, syncope, renal dysfunction, and hyperkalemia. A later post hoc analysis confirmed a higher risk for both a renal primary composite (dialysis, doubling serum creatinine, and death) and secondary outcomes (dialysis and doubling serum creatinine) for the combination group compared with the ramipril group.[86] Most of these outcomes were driven by acute dialysis needs in the combination group; and the risk for chronic dialysis was not different among groups. Of note, this population had mild CKD with a baseline mean eGFR of 73 mL/min/1.73 m^2 and mean albuminuria of 82 mg/mmol of creatinine. Similar findings were noted in studies focusing on individuals with type 2 diabetes.[84,87]

DIRECT RENIN INHIBITORS

The newer medication class acting on the RAAS is that of direct renin inhibitors, which act by binding to several active sites of renin. There is evidence of its BP lowering effect as monotherapy in hypertensive patients[88] and similar efficacy to ACEI and ARBs.[54] Additionally, there is evidence for an antiproteinuric effect in both hypertensive diabetic[89] and nondiabetic[90] individuals with early stage CKD (eGFR >60 mL/min/1.73 m^2). Two studies in different Asian populations have examined the effects of aliskiren as an add-on therapy in cohorts that included individuals with both moderate diabetic CKD and moderate nondiabetic CKD (<60 mL/min/1.73 m^2).[91,92] In an open-label trial, Abe et al.[91] added the direct renin inhibitor aliskiren to the medication regimen of 67 Japanese patients with moderate CKD who had suboptimal hypertensive control on their regular regimen. They found a reduction in SBP, DBP, and albuminuria after 24 weeks. These reductions in albuminuria and eGFR did not differ in subgroup analysis by diabetic status. In China, Wu et al.[92] added aliskiren to the medication regimen of 103 individuals with moderate CKD with persistent proteinuria and uncontrolled hypertension despite treatment with ACEI or ARBs. After 6 months, they found that the addition of aliskiren resulted in almost 8 mmHg reduction of mean arterial pressure and 23% reduction in urine protein–creatinine ratio without significant changes in eGFR. Neither of these trials reported a significant change in potassium levels by the end of their respective study. Importantly, neither of these trials had a control group. In Singapore, however, an open-label study by Woo et al.[93] randomized 155 individuals with moderate nondiabetic CKD to therapy with aliskiren, losartan, or a combination of both. After 3 years of follow-up, they reported similar efficacy for three groups in proteinuria reduction and change in eGFR from baseline. They also reported a significantly higher incidence of hyperkalemia in the combination group compared with the aliskiren alone or ARB alone groups. Therefore at this time the evidence in nondiabetic hypertensive CKD, although scattered, does not support an improved efficacy of the combination of a direct renin inhibitor and ACEI or ARB, but does raise concern regarding potential serious side effects.

ALDOSTERONE ANTAGONISTS

As reviewed earlier, the RAAS has an important role in the perpetuation of hypertension in CKD and ultimately contributes to its progression. However, this construct was not confirmed in the CKD population of the prospective observational Chronic Renal Insufficiency Cohort (CRIC) Study in which aldosterone levels were not found to be an independent risk factor for all-cause mortality, ESRD, nor atherosclerotic events.[94] Nonetheless, the authors found that high aldosterone levels were a risk factor for heart failure, especially in men. Beside the BP reduction in patients with resistant hypertension and normal renal function,[36,37,95] some experimental animal studies and pilot human trials suggest their influence in reducing proteinuria and slowing CKD progression independent of BP control.[96,97]

A recent systematic review of 27 studies (including 1549 individuals with CKD) found that aldosterone antagonists combined with ACEI, ARB, or both had a significant effect in reduction of BP and proteinuria at the expense of increased risk of hyperkalemia and gynecomastia.[98] The effect on proteinuria was similar for individuals with both diabetic and nondiabetic CKD in those studies comparing spironolactone plus ACEI or ARB (or both) to ACEI or ARB (or both). The findings on proteinuria and BP are consistent with a prior review by Bomback et al.,[99] which shared 8 of the 15 studies with the review by Bolignano et al.[98] It is important to note that most of the studies analyzed by both reviews lacked data on the relevant clinical outcomes including CKD progression and CV events. However, there is some evidence from two prespecified subgroup analyses in two major trials testing mineralocorticoid receptor antagonists in patients with heart failure that confirm a reduced risk for death and reduced risk of combined endpoints that included hospital admission and hospital stay for heart failure in individuals with eGFR between 30 and 60 mL/min/1.73 m^2.[100,101] Similarly, another post hoc analysis found that in individuals with severe heart failure and severe renal dysfunction (creatinine clearance [CrCl] <30 mL/min) that the use of RAAS antagonists, including mineralocorticoid receptor antagonists, was associated with reduced all-cause mortality.[102] At present, there is little evidence suggesting that aldosterone antagonists have a renoprotective effect. Well-designed trials in patients with CKD are needed to evaluate this question.

Diuretics

Diuretics are a critical component of therapy in hypertensive CKD and help address the sodium retention and concomitant volume expansion that perpetuate hypertension in CKD. By doing so, they also enhance the BP reduction and antiproteinuric effects of RAS blockade.[103-105] Additionally, these agents may be helpful in the management of hyperkalemia and acidosis, which become more common in severe CKD. Thiazides have been the most studied antihypertensive agent and have been found to reduce the risk of major CV outcomes.[106] This was confirmed in ALLHAT, which was a large randomized study in which chlorthalidone efficacy was similar to amlodipine and lisinopril for the primary CV outcome of fatal coronary heart disease or nonfatal myocardial infarction.[60] A post hoc analysis stratified by renal function showed that in those with eGFR less than 60 mL/min/1.73 m^2, chlorthalidone was not inferior either to amlodipine or lisinopril for the outcomes of CV events, mortality, eGFR reduction, and ESRD.[61,107] The question frequently arises regarding the comparable benefit of chlorthalidone versus hydrochlorothiazide. Compared with hydrochlorothiazide, chlorthalidone has been more widely studied, has a longer duration of action, and has approximately 1.5 to 2 times more potency. Whether both drugs have similar effects in CV event reduction is questionable.[106,108] The use of thiazides has been usually recommended for individuals with eGFRs more than 30 mL/min/1.73 m^2 due to their presumed poor efficacy in more severe CKD.[109] However, the combination of a thiazide in addition to a loop diuretic in advanced CKD has been advocated in patients with resistant edema. Metolazone is another thiazide diuretic with erratic absorption that has been found to have a better diuretic response in advanced CKD when given in combination with a loop diuretic.[110] Loop diuretics have a good diuretic response and a BP lowering effect; however, their duration of action is shorter than thiazides.[111]

CALCIUM CHANNEL BLOCKERS

Calcium channel blockers are very effective agents for lowering BP in hypertensive individuals. The two main subclasses are dihydropyridines (amlodipine, nifedipine, felodipine) and non-dihydropyridines (verapamil and diltiazem). Their effects differ in terms of renal hemodynamics and seem to depend on their differential blockade of the T-channel receptors and L-channel receptors within the glomerular vasculature. This difference renders the dihydropyridine agents, which exert their effect mainly on the L-channel receptors in the afferent arteriole, more likely to interfere with renal autoregulation, transmitting the systemic hypertension to the glomerular vasculature and potentially influencing albumin excretion.[112] This probably translates to the different effects on proteinuria observed in individuals with CKD. In AASK, amlodipine was shown to be inferior to ACEI in terms of CKD progression in individuals with protein–creatinine ratio >0.22.[46] However, the effect of amlodipine was equivalent to ACEI in individuals with a protein–creatinine ratio ≤0.22. Therefore in patients with nonproteinuric CKD, any calcium channel blocker can be used for BP control. However, a nondihydropyridine is preferred in CKD patients with proteinuria. If a dihydropyridine is used, it is recommended to be used in combination with an ACEI or ARB.[113]

ADRENERGIC BLOCKERS

As discussed earlier, the activation of the sympathetic nervous system is increased in CKD, and it plays a significant role in the perpetuation of hypertension as well as conferring increased CV risk. Therapy with beta blockers has been shown to increase survival in individuals with heart disease.[114] With CV death being the most common cause of mortality in individuals with CKD, there is a role for the use of beta blockers in this population. Evidence suggests a survival benefit from beta-adrenergic blockade in hemodialysis patients.[115,116] However, in nondiabetic hypertensive CKD, although beta blockers compare with ACEI in BP reduction, these agents are inferior to ACEI in terms of proteinuria reduction and renal function preservation.[46,59,117] Carvedilol is the better-studied vasodilating beta and alpha blocker that has shown favorable renal hemodynamic outcomes in individuals who are hypertensive.[118,119]

Nebivolol is a newer β1 blocker with vasodilatory properties mediated through nitric oxide with favorable renal hemodynamics in experimental animal models.[120] The main clinical evidence in CKD comes from the Study of the Effects of Nebivolol Intervention on Outcomes and Rehospitalization in Seniors with Heart Failure (SENIORS) Trial that studied adults older than 70 years with heart failure in which, compared with placebo, nebivolol showed a reduced composite primary endpoint of all-cause mortality or CV hospitalizations.[121] In a post hoc analysis, upon stratification by renal function tertiles, similar trends were detected for all GFR tertiles, although these did not reach statistical significance.[122] Both diabetic and nondiabetic patients were included in this analysis.

The main evidence for peripheral alpha blockers comes from ALLHAT in which the group assigned to doxazosin had to be terminated early because of a significantly increased incidence of CV events, especially stroke and heart failure, compared with chlorthalidone.[60] Although the ESRD events did not differ between doxazosin and chlorthalidone in this population, with a well-preserved mean baseline eGFR of 78 mL/min/1.73 m^2, it is unclear whether these effects are different in CKD patients.[61,107,123]

Surgical Management

Renal artery denervation has been proposed for the management of refractory hypertension. The SYMPLICITY HTN-3 trial,[124] motivated by previous positive results in unblinded studies of catheter-based renal artery denervation,[125-127] enrolled 535 patients with refractory hypertension (defined as a SBP of ≥140 mmHg despite use of a medication regimen of three antihypertensive agents, including a diuretic) into a single-blind, randomized trial in which participants either underwent the denervation procedure or a sham procedure. Though participants with eGFR less than 45 mL/min/1.73 m^2 were excluded from the study,[128] about 10% of the participants had CKD. However, there was no significant difference in mean SBP assessed by 24-hour ambulatory BP 6 months after the procedure, and the effects of this procedure on long-term renal outcomes is not known.[124]

Lifestyle Modification

Recommended strategies in treatment of hypertension in individuals without CKD include weight loss if overweight, smoking cessation, regular moderate physical activity, and adherence to a sodium-restricted healthy diet.[113] Studies of lifestyle modification and its effects on outcomes in individuals with hypertensive CKD have been mixed in their results.

Smoking is associated with an increased risk of incident ESRD, as demonstrated in a 25-year follow-up of participants in the Multiple Risk Factor Intervention Trial.[129] In an analysis of data from the CRIC Study, which included individuals with and without diabetes, participants who were nonsmokers were found to have a lower risk of CKD progression compared with smokers over a follow-up period of 4 years (Fig. 4.3). In the Study of Heart and Renal Protection (SHARP),[130] involving more than 6000 persons with CKD not on dialysis, smoking was associated with vascular events but not with CKD progression.[131] Additionally, data from CRIC and the Cardiovascular Health Study demonstrated that nonsmokers with CKD have a lower risk of CV events compared with smokers with CKD (see Fig. 4.3).[132]

A sodium-restricted diet (<2 g/day of dietary intake) has been shown to improve hypertensive control in individuals with CKD.[133] There is emerging evidence suggesting that there may be a link between healthy dietary patterns and CKD. A recent analysis of participants in the Atherosclerosis Risk in Communities Study (ARIC) found that consuming a healthy diet rich in fruits and vegetables and low in sodium and fat was associated with a lower risk for the development of kidney disease.[134] Furthermore, a recently published

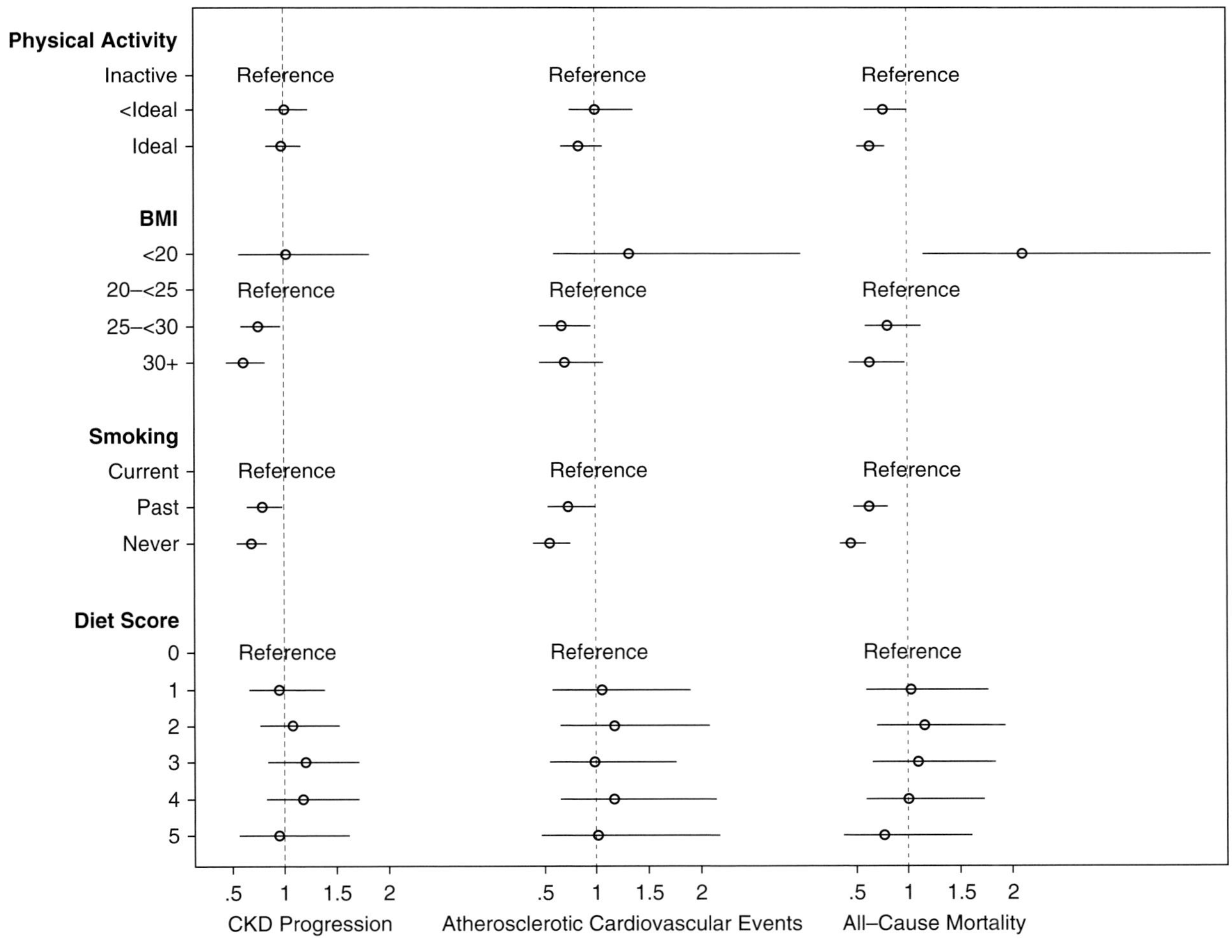

FIG. 4.3 Impact of lifestyle choices in CRIC participants on CKD progression, cardiovascular events, and all-cause mortality. (From Ricardo AC, Anderson CA, Yang W, et al. Healthy lifestyle and risk of kidney disease progression, atherosclerotic events, and death in CKD: findings from the Chronic Renal Insufficiency Cohort (CRIC) Study. *Am J Kidney Dis Off J Natl Kidney Found*. 2015;65(3):412-424.)

systematic review, which included over 15,000 individuals with CKD, found that healthy dietary patterns were associated with lower mortality but not incident ESRD.[135] However, the study did not evaluate the outcome of incident CKD. In another study that also used data from ARIC, Rebholz et al.[136] found that consumption of a Dietary Approaches to Stop Hypertension (DASH)-style diet was associated with lower risk for incident kidney disease. Using data from the Northern Manhattan Study, Khatri et al.[137] found that adherence to a Mediterranean diet was associated with a reduced incidence of CKD and lower risk for eGFR decline. In summary, these studies suggest that dietary patterns, which have been found to be beneficial in the general population, are also beneficial for CKD patients.

Studies in non-CKD populations have found obesity to be an independent risk factor for the development of CKD and ESRD.[2,138] However, in the CRIC study, overweight status as assessed by body mass index ≥25 kg/m^2 was associated with better outcomes compared with being at a normal weight: notably, lower risk of CKD progression and risk of all-cause mortality (see Fig. 4.3).[139] This paradoxical association has been observed in other CKD populations.[140,141] Reasons for the paradox are not understood, but some have hypothesized that it is related to protein-energy malnutrition and inflammation in underweight patients.

With the growth of bariatric surgery as a treatment for increasing rates of obesity in the United States, there is an interest in evaluating its effects on renal outcomes. In one study, bariatric surgery patients showed a lower risk of 50% decline in eGFR or ESRD compared with a matched cohort of obese individuals. However, the number of CKD patients in this study was relatively low.[142] In a recent retrospective study, individuals with CKD who underwent bariatric surgery had a higher eGFR at 3 years of follow-up compared with propensity score-matched controls with CKD and obesity.[143] However, the accuracy of GFR estimating equations in the setting of large changes in body weight is not known.

CRIC participants who reported recommended levels of physical activity had a lower risk of all-cause mortality over the period of follow-up, but did not have a reduced risk of CKD progression compared with sedentary participants (see Fig. 4.3).[139] In individuals with CKD, there is evidence of a reduction in all-cause mortality conferred by regular physical activity.[139,144] Aerobic exercise has been shown to improve BP control in individuals without CKD.[145] However, exercise interventions in CKD aimed at slowing CKD progression have not definitively shown benefit.[146]

CONCLUSION

Hypertension remains a primary driver of CV morbidity and mortality in individuals with and without CKD, and the diagnosis of hypertensive nephrosclerosis remains a leading cause of CKD and incident ESRD in the United States. New insights into genetic risk variants in African Americans may explain a significant proportion of increased risk for nondiabetic kidney disease in African Americans. Though a significant body of research has identified RAAS blockade along with appropriate diuretic management as a mainstay of antihypertensive therapy in hypertensive CKD, important questions remain as to the appropriate BP targets of antihypertensive therapy and the role of lifestyle modification in improving patient outcomes.

A full list of references is available at www.expertconsult.com.

5

Chronic Kidney Disease in the Elderly

Jessica W. Weiss, MD, MCR, and Tyler B. Woodell, MD

OUTLINE

INTRODUCTION

This chapter will review core questions and concepts of chronic kidney disease (CKD) in older adults including physiologic changes associated with aging, identification and epidemiology of CKD in older populations, and differences in manifestations and management that directly affect the care of older individuals with abnormal kidney function.

KIDNEY STRUCTURAL AND PHYSIOLOGIC CHANGES ASSOCIATED WITH AGING

As in all body systems, the kidneys experience significant structural and consequent physiologic changes with advancing age. These changes affect all parts of the kidney, including the glomerulus, tubules, and vasculature with resultant changes in renal function including decreased filtration, decreased vascular responsiveness, and changes in water and sodium balance. Understanding usual, age-related changes in the kidneys can help delineate the difference between usual effects of age versus non–age-related pathology and can support age-appropriate individualization of patient care.

Changes in the Glomerulus

It is long established that prevalence of glomerulosclerosis increases with age, affecting approximately 5% to 10% of nephrons in the fourth decade of life and increasing thereafter.[1,2] In 1975 Kaplan et al.[1] examined autopsy-obtained renal tissue from people aged <1 to 90 years who died of nonrenal causes (primarily trauma, overdose, and alcohol in younger subjects compared with cancer, liver disease, and pneumonia in older subjects). They observed less than 10% glomerulosclerosis in subjects who died before age 40, compared with an increased but variable rate of sclerosis more than 10% in adults older than age 40 (most marked in adults over age 50). Although the degree of glomerulosclerosis varied over a 10-year age range examined, a linear increase in glomerulosclerosis was generally noted as age increased.[1] Similarly, Rule et al. noted linear increases in the percentage of glomerulosclerosis indicated on biopsy samples from live kidney donors, with as little as 3% in adults under age 30 to as much as 70% in adults over age 70.[2]

The etiology behind increasing glomerulosclerosis in older age is likely multifactorial. Rat models have demonstrated decreased pressure in the afferent arteriole with advancing age, which may result in increased transmission of hydrostatic pressure to the glomerular capsule.[3,4] Hyalinosis of the afferent arterioles has also been demonstrated in humans. Hill et al. noted that, in kidneys removed due to malignancy, hyalinosis of afferent arterioles not only correlated with increased luminal size but also was strongly associated with hypertrophy and glomerulosclerosis.[5] With progressive loss of functioning glomeruli, compensatory hypertrophy may also occur. Studies have identified a clear relationship between glomerular hypertrophy and the development of glomerulosclerosis.[6,7]

Concurrent with a decline in glomerular filtration rate (GFR), kidney morphology also changes with increasing age. Like GFR, overall renal mass peaks in the fourth decade of life; at its greatest, renal mass is around 400 grams and declines by up to 25%, or as low as 300 grams in the ninth decade of life.[8] This decline in renal mass is thought to correlate with the overall change in body surface area that occurs with aging and is primarily attributed to a loss of cortical tissue. Overall change in glomerular shape has also been observed in older adults, specifically a more lobular appearance than the spherical glomeruli of younger adults. These increased lobulations may potentially result in less filtration area, contributing to an overall decline in GFR with age.

Changes in Renal Vasculature and Renal Tubules

Significant changes in renal vasculature occur with increasing age, which may not only predispose to increased glomerular pressure but also diminish the ability of glomeruli to autoregulate and adjust renal blood flow during acute events. In addition to afferent arteriolar dilation due to hyalinosis, described previously, anastomoses can form between glomerular capillary loops, and the glomerular basement membrane may show increased folding and thickening with eventual hyalinosis and collapse.[9,10] Juxtamedullary glomeruli have been shown to develop channels between the afferent and efferent arterioles, leading to glomerular ischemia and eventual aglomerular vasculature.[10] These combined changes to the typical and appropriate vasodilatory and vasoconstrictive capacities of the renal vasculature hinder the ability of the kidneys to autoregulate blood flow. This may lead to an inappropriate or exaggerated decline in GFR, for example in lower blood flow states (intravascular depletion, poor cardiac output), or an inappropriate transmission of higher pressures to the glomerulus (sustained systolic hypertension), fostering and exacerbating glomerular hypertrophy and injury. Renal tubules also experience changes with advancing age, including decreased tubule mass, thickening of basement membranes, and increased atrophy and fibrosis.[11,12]

Age-Related Changes in Renal-Active Hormones and Vasodilators

In addition to changes within the vasculature, hormonal influences on the vasculature also change with age. Both renin and aldosterone levels decline with advancing age, which is thought to primarily occur due to decreased renin production and release in older versus younger adults.[13] It has been found that older adults have relatively higher basal rates of atrial natriuretic peptide (ANP), which can suppress renin release.[14] Decreases in renin and aldosterone levels compromise the ability of the kidneys to autoregulate via efferent vasoconstriction and appropriate sodium conservation in states of decreased renal blood flow.

Changes in nitric oxide may also contribute to differences in vasodilatory capacity of the vasculature in older adults. Nitric oxide is known to decrease with advancing age, particularly in the renal cortex.[15] Animal models suggest that this may be related to increased oxidative stress with age, leaving fewer cofactors for nitric oxide generation, as well as a decline in L-arginine with age, which is a key for nitric oxide production.[16] Decreased asymmetrical dimethyl arginine (ADMA) also occurs with increasing age and may lead to a decline in nitric oxide synthase, directly affecting the body's ability to produce nitric oxide.[17] Lower levels of nitric oxide may lead to increased renal vasoconstriction, as well as increased matrix production and mesangial fibrosis.

$$Kf(P_{GC} - P_{BS}) - (\pi_{GC} - \pi_{BS})$$

P_{GC} – hydrostatic pressure in the glomerular capillary
P_{BS} – hydrostatic pressure in Bowman space
π_{GC} – oncotic pressure in glomerular capillary
π_{BS} – oncotic pressure in Bowman space

FIG. 5.1 Formula components of GFR.

Changes in Glomerular Filtration Rate

GFR is known to decline with age, and many factors that determine GFR can be impacted by age-associated changes (Fig. 5.1). Davies and Shock first described the decline in GFR with age in 1950 in their hallmark study of 70 men between the ages of 24 and 89 years; using directly measured GFR, they described a decline in GFR by 8 mL/min/1.73 m^2 per decade after age 20.[18] Population-level studies have described peak GFR, which occurs around the fourth decade of life, as being 140 mL/min/1.73 m^2 in men and 120 mL/min/1.73m^2 in women, with a decline thereafter to mean levels around 80 mL/min/1.73 m^2 in the ninth decade of life and 60 mL/min/1.73 m^2 in the eighth decade of life for men and women, respectively.[19] Hoang et al. noted decreases in GFR, renal plasma flow, and the filtration coefficient (*Kf*) in older versus younger adults.[20] GFR declined by 22% and renal plasma flow declined by up to 28% in adults over age 55 compared with adults ages 40 and younger. They also observed a decrease in both two-kidney and single-kidney *Kf*, which was thought to be most likely related to a decrease in filtration surface as well as an observed decline in permeability.

Proteinuria

Loss of functioning glomeruli is associated with increased rates of albuminuria. Early animal studies noted an increase in proteinuria related to increased permeability of the glomerular basement membrane.[21] More recent animal models suggest that increased glomerular size is not necessarily accompanied by increases in podocyte size. Increased markers of podocyte stress occur with prolonged hypertrophy followed by eventual widening of foot processes and consequent increases in proteinuria.[22]

Electrolyte Management

Both sodium and potassium homeostasis have been observed to change with age. Much of this change is hypothesized to stem from differences in the decreased production of and reduced sensitivity to renin and aldosterone in older adults. Overall sodium homeostasis is less reliable in older adults. Epstein described excess sodium excretion when conservation would be appropriate, such as during a state of volume depletion.[13] Conversely, the rate of sodium excretion after a large sodium load may also be slowed, increasing the risk of volume overload. This observation is thought to result from a decreased responsiveness to aldosterone, as well as decreased overall GFR in the setting of fewer functioning nephrons. Potassium excretion is also relatively decreased in older versus younger adults and, like sodium, is hypothesized to stem from a decreased aldosterone response to a potassium load.[14]

Clinical Implications of Age-Associated Physiological Changes

Despite significant changes in renal structure and function, clinically meaningful changes in renal function are not uniform or consistent across older adults. The documented loss of 8 mL/min/m^2 per decade noted by Davies and Shock, starting from GFR of ~140 mL/min/1.73 m^2, would still result in a GFR greater than 90 mL/min/1.73 m^2 by the ninth decade, well above the threshold for the current CKD definition.[18,23] Population studies of GFR over time do show significant decline between the fourth and ninth decades, but the mean GFR even in the oldest age group is ≥60 mL/min/1.73 m^2 (with stage 3 CKD beginning at ≤59 mL/min/1.73 m^2).[19] Fliser and colleagues notably described intact renal reserve (defined as increased GFR in response to an amino acid load), even among the adults as old as 90 years, in both those who were healthy and those who were chronically ill.[18,24] Moreover, in otherwise healthy older adults, hemoglobin and erythropoietin levels typically remain normal, whereas lower erythropoietin levels are a hallmark of CKD in younger adults with abnormal kidney function.[25] Perhaps most striking, in patients included in the study by Rule and colleagues, which demonstrated as much as 73% prevalence of nephrosclerosis in adults aged 70 to 77 years (the oldest age group examined), all had eGFR >60 mL/min/1.73 m^2 because all participants were active kidney donors at the time of this study.[2] The mean eGFR in the oldest age group was 70 ± 7 mL/min/1.73 m^2. This does not negate the described and documented changes in kidney structure and function with age, but it does place perspective on the clinical ramifications of these changes, particularly in comparison to more severe decrements in GFR that may satisfy the formal definition of CKD.

IDENTIFICATION OF CKD IN OLDER ADULTS

The definition of CKD is age neutral, with the same criteria applied to both older and younger adults. The Kidney Disease Improving Global Outcomes (KDIGO) work group defines CKD as decreased GFR (<60 mL/min/1.73 m^2) or other markers of kidney damage (albuminuria >30 mg/day, history of kidney transplantation, urine findings associated with renal disease including glomerular hematuria, or abnormalities on renal imaging studies or pathology); any one criterion present for >3 months establishes the diagnosis of CKD.[23]

The prevalence of CKD is notably high among older adults and increases with age when using the current KDIGO definition of CKD. Twenty-five to thirty percent of adults aged 65 to 79 years meet the criteria for CKD diagnosis, and this increases to as much as 40% to 50% in the oldest age group (adults over age 80).[26,27] It should be noted that although there was an increase in the reported prevalence of CKD between the late 1980s and the early 2000s, these data come from population level studies often using diagnostic codes. As such, this trend could represent greater CKD recognition rather than a true change in disease frequency, because the time period over which this increase in CKD prevalence occurred coincides with the development of the first GFR estimating equation and institution of automated eGFR reporting by laboratories.[28]

A point of some debate related to CKD prevalence is the severity of identified CKD. The majority all adults over age 18 with CKD have modest reductions in GFR,[27] a pattern that holds true for both older and younger adults. In older individuals, however, the diagnosis of CKD is more likely to be established based on eGFR alone rather than alternative or additional criteria, including albuminuria. In a population of veterans aged 18 years and older, 72% of adults aged 65 years and younger meeting the definition of CKD did so with some contribution from albuminuria, compared with just under one-third of adults over age 65.[29] In that same cohort, 44% of adults over age 60 met CKD criteria by GFR alone, versus less than 25% of adults younger than age 60. Even when present, proteinuria in older adults is less likely to be found in larger amounts (200 mg/g) compared with their younger counterparts. In the National Health and Nutrition Examination Survey (NHANES) cohort, the rate of albuminuria >200 mg/g declined with advancing age, from 38% in adults aged 20 to 54 years, 18% in adults aged 55 to 70, and only 12.9% in adults older than age 70.[30] The relatively lower incidence of proteinuria and comparatively larger role of GFR in identifying CKD among older adults highlights the importance that estimating GFR plays in determining CKD incidence and prevalence for older adults.

The two most commonly utilized GFR estimating equations are the Modification of Diet in Renal Disease (MDRD) study equation and the Chronic Kidney Disease Epidemiology (CKD-EPI) equation. Both equations include an age variable to model the decline in creatinine generation that accompanies normal aging (associated with decreased muscle mass), but the cohorts from which these equations were validated had relatively few individuals >65 years.[31]

Multiple studies have compared the performance of the MDRD and CKD-EPI equations at estimating GFR in older adults, and the CKD-EPI equation generally produces more accurate estimates, including at correctly estimating CKD stage compared with the gold standard of measuring GFR (Table 5.1).[32-38] The improved diagnostic accuracy of the CKD-EPI equation has important clinical implications; the CKD-EPI equation better predicts mortality and end-stage renal disease (ESRD) compared with MDRD and other equations in adult populations, and subgroup analysis indicates this is true for adults <65 and ≥65 years alike.[39,40]

One concern raised by creatinine-based estimating equations of particular relevance to older adults is the dependence of creatinine on muscle mass.[41] Because there is a predictable

TABLE 5.1 **Comparison of Equations' Performance at Estimating GFR Among Older Adults**

Study	Population	Age (years)	Gold Standard	Outcome of Interest	Result
Kilbride et al., 2013[32]	394 community-dwelling older adults in England; all of European ancestry; median measured GFR 53.4 mL/min	Median age 80 (range 74–97)	Iohexol clearance	Accuracy of estimating equation (defined as estimate within 30% of measured GFR)	Accuracy for MDRD, CKD-EPI(cr), CKD-EPI(cys), and CKD-EPI(cr-cys) was 81%, 83%, 86%, and 86%, respectively (MDRD inferior to CKD-EPI[cr] with P =.004)
David-Neto et al., 2016[33]	70 older adults with a functioning kidney transplant in Brazil; mean measured GFR 47 mL/min	Mean age 65 ± 4	Creatinine EDTA clearance	Bias and accuracy (defined as estimate within 30% and, separately, 10% of measured GFR)	CKD-EPI(cr) had the best 30% and 10% accuracy at 74% and 34%, respectively (P < .04 compared with MDRD, BIS, and CG)
Lopes et al., 2013[34]	95 community-dwelling older adults in Brazil; mean measured GFR 55 mL/min	Mean age 85 (range 80–97)	Iohexol clearance	Accuracy of estimating equation (defined as estimate within 30% of measured GFR)	Compared with MDRD, CKD-EPI(cr-cys) had greater accuracy at 85.3% vs. 70.5% (P < .01)
Liu et al., 2013[35]	431 older adults in China; mean measured GFR 53.4 mL/min	Mean age 69.9 ± 6.8	^{99m}Tc-DTPA	Median absolute difference between estimating equation and measured GFR	CKD-EPI(cr-cys) had best accuracy with median absolute difference of 10.5 mL/min (P < .05 compared with CG and MDRD); 30% accuracy not statistically significant between equations
Bevc et al., 2011[36]	317 Caucasian older adults; mean measured GFR 34.5 mL/min	Mean age 72.7 ± 5.1	Creatinine EDTA clearance	Diagnostic accuracy as defined by area under the ROC curve	No statistically significant difference in diagnostic accuracy between MDRD and CKD-EPI at measured GFR ≤60 mL/min; CKD-EPI (cr-cys) performed better than MDRD or CKD-EPI(cr) at measured GFR ≤45 mL/min (P < .013)
Stevens et al., 2010[37]	Pooled dataset of 3896 people across 16 studies; mean measured GFR 68 mL/min	Mean age 50 ± 15; 15% of sample >65 (n =568)	A variety of exogenous filtration markers	Bias (reported as measured GFR – eGFR)	Though bias was significantly improved for the whole population, subgroup analysis for participations >65 years demonstrated no significant improvement in bias using CKD-EPI(cr) compared with MDRD; cystatin C was not examined
Fan et al., 2015[38]	805 older adults enrolled in the community-based Age, Gene/Environment Susceptibility (AGES)-Reykjavik Study; mean measured GFR 64 mL/min	Mean age 80.3 ± 4.0	Iohexol clearance	24 comparisons of measured bias, precision and accuracy between three CKD-EPI equations, BIS equation, and CAPA equation	CKD-EPI equations performed better than other equations in 9 metrics, similar in 13 and worse in 2; among CKD-EPI equations, the combined CKD-EPI equation performed better than $eGFR_{cr}$ in all 4 metrics examined, better than $eGFR_{cys}$ in 2 and similar to $eGFR_{cys}$ in 2

^{99m}Tc-DTPA, Technetium-99m diethylenetriamine pentaacetic acid.

decline in muscle mass with age, and because older adults are more likely to have comorbid conditions that contribute to decreased muscle mass, the generation of creatinine can be quite heterogeneous across individuals and demographic characteristics. Cystatin C is an alternative endogenous biomarker filtered freely at the glomerulus that is thought to be less dependent on muscle mass and demographic characteristics, thus providing an opportunity for improved GFR estimation.[42] Indeed, compared with creatinine, cystatin C is a stronger predictor of risk of death and cardiovascular events in older adults.[43] Modifications of the original CKD-EPI equation that use cystatin C alone or in combination with creatinine have been developed for clinical practice and have been shown to provide more accurate estimates of renal function.[38,44] Fan and colleagues examined the performance of the three CKD-EPI equations (creatinine alone, cystatin C alone, or the two in combination) in comparison to measured GFR using plasma clearance of iohexol among 805 older adults with a mean age of 80.3 years.[38] The combined CKD-EPI equation performed better than the creatinine-based CKD-EPI equation in all four metrics examined; better than the cystatin C-based CKD-EPI equation in two metrics; and similar to the cystatin C-based CKD-EPI equation in two metrics. Given the wide clinical use of creatinine, it remains the recommended tool for estimating GFR, but KDIGO suggests the addition of cystatin C to creatinine when there is uncertainty about the diagnosis and need for confirmation of CKD.[23]

Recently the Berlin Initiative Study (BIS) developed two novel equations utilizing creatinine (BIS-1) or the combination of creatinine and cystatin C (BIS-2) for estimating GFR that, in contrast to other equations, were specifically derived from a cohort of older adults ($n = 610$, mean age 78.5 years).[45] Despite internal validation that performed well compared with measured GFR and resulted in less CKD-stage misclassification than the CKD-EPI equation, the BIS equations demonstrated increased bias at age <80 years and higher GFR when externally validated in two cohorts.[46,47] Currently, KDIGO only recognizes the MDRD and CKD-EPI equations as recommended tools for estimating GFR, though it must be noted that the BIS equations were derived after the most recent KDIGO Practice Guideline on this topic. The Cockcroft-Gault formula has not been validated for use with standardized creatinine assays and, as for all adults, its use in estimating GFR is not recommended for older adults.[23]

CHARACTERISTICS OF OLDER ADULTS WITH CKD

Older adults with CKD are likely to experience a high burden of additional comorbid diseases.[48] Approximately 75% of older adults with CKD have two or more comorbid conditions; in one study, 74% of older adults with CKD had four or more comorbidities.[49] Hypertension is the most common condition associated with CKD in older adults (prevalence ~90%), followed by dyslipidemia (39% to 50%), diabetes mellitus (21% to 45%) and coronary artery disease (21% to 27%). The prevalence of coronary artery disease is almost three times higher in CKD patients ≥75 years versus those ≤45 years, consistent with the linear relationship observed between aging and cardiovascular disease.[50] Frailty, a state of non–disease-specific decline characterized by the presence of any three of five measures (weight loss, self-reported exhaustion, poor grip strength, slow walking speed, and low physical activity), is three times as likely among older adults with CKD as it is among those with normal renal function.[51,52] This association remains significant even after adjusting for other comorbidities and demographic factors. The prevalence of anemia is increased in community-dwelling older adults with severe CKD (eGFR <30 mL/min/1.73 m^2) compared with older adults with normal renal function, and associates with decreased quality of life.[53,54] CKD is also associated with cognitive impairment as determined by performance on the Mini-Mental State Examination in older adults.[55] Taken together, these findings underscore the importance of recognizing the presence of CKD in older adults and, when appropriate and in line with goals of care, comprehensively evaluating for and managing associated conditions.

OUTCOMES ASSOCIATED WITH CKD IN OLDER ADULTS

The relatively modest reductions in estimated eGFR as well as less frequent proteinuria have stirred debate about the accuracy and clinical relevance of the current standard for CKD definition among older individuals. Differences in outcomes associated with abnormal renal function in older versus younger adults have further stirred that controversy.

Older adults with CKD have significantly increased risk of morbidity and mortality. In a community-based prospective cohort study of 4893 adults ≥65 years, Manjunath and colleagues identified an inverse linear relationship between eGFR and incident cardiovascular disease (myocardial infarction, coronary angioplasty, coronary artery bypass graft, angina pectoris, heart failure, cardiac death, peripheral vascular disease, stroke, and transient ischemic attack); for every 10 mL/min/m^2 reduction in eGFR the risk of cardiovascular disease increased 5%.[56] Risk of hospitalization is also increased among older adults with severe CKD (eGFR <30 mL/min/m^2); older individuals with CKD are 60% more likely than those with normal renal function to be hospitalized at least twice over a 2-year period, even after adjusting for additional cardiovascular disease risk factors.[57] Although the risk of AKI is increased among those with CKD compared with those without CKD, this risk does not appear to be different for older versus younger adults.[58]

Older adults represent nearly 40% of all prevalent ESRD patients in the United States and nearly half of all new ESRD cases each year.[59] This presumably stems from the profound prevalence of CKD in older adults. However, older adults with abnormal renal function actually experience a decreased risk of progression to ESRD than do their younger counterparts with comparable levels of eGFR. Data suggest this difference may stem more from an age-dependent increase in mortality, compared with a true difference in CKD pathology in older versus younger adults. For instance, the Cardiovascular Health Study (CHS) determined that, in a cohort of community-dwelling adults ages 65 years and older, participants were 13 times more likely to die of any cause than progress to ESRD and six times more likely to die of cardiovascular causes than progress to ESRD over almost 10 years of follow up.[60] The importance of these competing risks in older adults highlights the need to explore patient goals and preferences to individualize CKD-related care in the context of each patient's preferences and expectations.

Older adults experience an increased risk of death compared with their age-matched peers with normal renal function. Data from the United States Renal Data System (USRDS) indicate that the risk of death is more than twice as high among older adults with CKD than those without CKD after adjusting for age, sex, and race (111.2 deaths compared with 45.2 deaths per 1000 patient-years at risk among older adults with and without CKD, respectively).[59] The risk of death associated with CKD varies, however, by severity of renal dysfunction. In particular, the risk of death is attenuated among those older adults with moderate reductions in GFR (eGFR 45 to 59 mL/min/1.73 m^2).[27] In older individuals, the risk of death with moderate reductions in GFR is only slightly greater than that in their age-matched counterparts with GFR >60 mL/min/1.73 m^2.[61] The risk of death associated with CKD also varies by CKD trajectory (the rate of renal function decline); older adults with a steeper decline in renal function (more rapidly progressive CKD) experience an increased risk of death compared with their peers with more stable (less progressive) renal disease. The trajectory of renal function decline can help identify older adults who may benefit from more frequent follow up and discussion regarding goals of care.[62]

MANAGEMENT OF SPECIFIC COMORBIDITIES AND CHARACTERISTICS IN OLDER ADULTS WITH CKD

Hypertension Management

Ever since publication of the landmark Veterans Affairs health studies in the 1960s, evidence from randomized controlled trials has highlighted the effect that treating high blood pressure has on reducing the risk of cardiovascular complications and death.[63,64] Although these data have been reliably replicated across more diverse populations, this cornerstone concept of hypertension management was not immediately applied to the care of older adults because the populations examined in these early trials were not elderly (mean ages ranged 50 to 52).[65,66] Moreover, long established dogma held to the notion that higher blood pressures, particularly systolic blood pressures (SBPs), were acceptable and perhaps even preferable for perfusion of older organs. As a result, customary practice was to adopt the tenet that SBP values up to "100 + age"—that is, 100 mmHg plus 1 mmHg per year alive—were clinically acceptable. This premise was disproven, however, by the end of the 20th century when randomized trials demonstrated that a reduction in both systolic and diastolic blood pressure decreased the risk of cardiovascular disease and stroke even in adults over the age of 60.[67-69] Further, in 2008, investigators from the Hypertension in the Very Elderly Trial (HYVET) demonstrated that treatment of blood pressure, compared with no treatment, led to lower risk of cardiovascular disease, stroke, and death even among the oldest age group (veterans aged 80 and older).[70]

Available hypertension guidelines through the seventh issue of The Joint National Committee (JNC-7) recommended an age-neutral blood pressure target of less than 140/90 mmHg, with a lower target for those patients who also experienced diabetes or kidney disease (<130/80 mmHg). The generalizability of these lower targets to older adults, however, remains unclear. Studies involving adults over age 60 who demonstrated reduced rates of stroke and major cardiovascular events in the treatment arm generally achieved SBPs greater than 140 mmHg and less than 160 mmHg (compared with higher values in the usual care or higher SBP goal arms).[67,69-72] In contrast, studies of older adults who achieved SBPs less than 140 mmHg compared with higher values reported more mixed results without consistent across-study reduction in stroke or major cardiovascular events.[68,73-81] Historically, data from trials of younger adults were extrapolated to older individuals, and hypertension management guidelines remained age-neutral. The JNC's eighth guideline was the first to recommend a higher blood pressure target (<150/90 mmHg) for adults over age 60, and a lower target (<140/90 mmHg) for younger adults, based on available trial data specific to adults over age 60.[82] These recommendations were echoed in subsequent recommendations by the American College of Physicians and American Academy of Family Physicians, which were based on a large evidence review and metaanalysis of data in older adults.[83,84]

The applicability of these guidelines to older adults with CKD remains unclear. The vast majority of trials of hypertension management in older adults have explicitly excluded individuals with moderate to severe kidney disease. Importantly, most trials used creatinine rather than eGFR to identify CKD and exclude study participants. Because relatively "normal" creatinine values (correlating to eGFR closer to or >60 mL/min/1.73 m^2) are more likely to correlate with mildly abnormal eGFR in older adults with lower muscle mass, adults with mild CKD (stage 3, eGFR 45 to 59 mL/min/1.73 m^2) were less often explicitly excluded. Adults with eGFR less than 45 mL/min/1.73 m^2, however, and certainly less than 30 mL/min/1.73 m^2 in men and less than 25 mL/min/1.73 m^2 in women, were not included in most hallmark trials of hypertension management in older adults.[70-72,74,78,81,85] For this reason, hypertension targets for older adults with CKD have been generalized from trials of younger CKD populations. Studies by Shulman et al. and Walker et al. in 1989 and 1992, respectively, were akin to the early Veterans Affairs Cooperative trials in that these studies demonstrated that compared with no control, "some" blood pressure control could slow renal function decline (Table 5.2).[86,87] Subsequent studies evaluating lower blood pressure targets (SBP ≤130

TABLE 5.2 **Trials That Examined the Effect of Blood Pressure Control on Renal Disease Progression**

Trial	Population	Age (years)	BP Target by Treatment Group (mmHg)	Medications Used	Achieved BP (mmHg)	CKD	Outcomes
Shulman et al., 1989[36]	10,940 patients with hypertension	Range 30–69 Mean 50.8	Stepped vs. referred care Goal: DBP <90 or 10 below baseline (if 90 at baseline)	Diuretics Antiadrenergics CCBs	Not reported	Subgroup: patients with creatinine >1.5 and >1.7 mg/dL (~200 patients)	**More rapid decline in renal function for those with higher vs. lower BPs**
Walker et al., 1992[87] (MRFIT)	5524 men with DBP >90 mmHg at baseline	Range 35–57 Mean 46.5	Usual BP care vs. "special" care (stepped approach)	Diuretic Antiadrenergics β-Blockers Hydralazine Guanethidine	<140 mmHg in special care Remainder 150–159 mmHg and >160 mmHg	Unclear: excluded if creatinine >2	**More rapid decline in renal function for those with higher vs. lower BPs**
Klahr et al., 1994[90] (MDRD)	840 pts total; 585 patients with elevated creatinine in BP arm	Range 18–70 Mean 52	Low BP (<125/75) vs. usual care (<140/90)	Any allowed. Encouraged ACE inhibitor as first line, CCB as second line	MAP 92 low BP group vs. ~98 usual care	All had CKD • Mean creatinine clearance 49–51 mL/min • Mean eGFR 37–38 mL/min/1.73 m^2	**Lower blood pressure significantly slowed GFR decline ONLY in subgroup of those with proteinuria >1 g/d**
Wright et al., 2002[88] (AASK)	African Americans with DBP ≥95, GFR 20–65	Range 18–70 Mean 54	BP usual care (MAP 102–107) vs. low BP (MAP ≤92)	Metoprolol Ramipril Amlodipine	BP 128/78 mean low BP group vs. 141/85 usual BP group	All had CKD	No significant difference GFR slope or composite of GFR decline/ESRD/death
Ruggenenti 2005 (REIN-2)	Men and women with nondiabetic nephropathy and persistent proteinuria	Range 37–69 Mean 53–54	<130/80 vs. diastolic <90	Ramipril Felodipine	130/80 vs. 134/82	All had CKD (nondiabetic nephropathy with proteinuria)	No significant difference in ESR or change in eGFR

AASK, African American study of kidney disease trial; *MDRD*, modified diet in renal disease trial; *MRFIT*, multiple risk factor intervention trial; *REIN-2*, Ramipril efficacy in nephropathy trial 2.

mmHg) compared with higher targets (SBP >130 mmHg) did not show a consistent benefit of more intensive blood pressure control in slowing kidney disease progression.[88-90] One exception to these findings was the subgroup of patients in the MDRD study who had more than 1 gram of proteinuria per day, among whom blood pressure less than 130/80 mmHg slowed eGFR decline.[90] The mean age across all of these studies, however, was 46 to 54 years, and no patients over age 70 were included.

Observational data of older adults with CKD have consistently demonstrated a U-shaped association between SBP and mortality, with risk of death increased at very low (SBP <120 mmHg) and very high (SBP >160 mmHg) thresholds.[91,92] The risk of residual confounding persists in these studies, particularly as relates to impact of other diseases, which both lower blood pressure and increase risk of death (e.g., heart failure, cirrhosis, severe malnutrition), and causation cannot be established from this work. More recently, the Systolic Blood Pressure Intervention Trial (SPRINT) has added to these data. SPRINT evaluated the effect of very low (SBP <120 mmHg) versus more moderate (SBP 140 mmHg) blood pressure control on risk of cardiovascular events, stroke, and mortality.[73] SPRINT was terminated early when participants in the SBP less than 120 mmHg arm were found to have a 25% reduction in all-cause mortality and 30% reduction in cardiovascular events compared with participants in the higher blood pressure arm. SPRINT oversampled for both older adults and adults with CKD, and found no difference in the reduction in mortality or cardiovascular events for their CKD subgroup or adults over age 75. Individuals in the more intensive treatment arm did experience an increased risk of adverse events and severe adverse events, including hypotension, syncope, and electrolyte abnormalities (categorized as severe when emergency care was needed). The overall population of SPRINT notably did not reach required numbers to power for statistical significance due to the earlier than anticipated stop date, and subgroup analyses were not of sufficient size for powered analyses. The population included in SPRINT was also specific to adults with increased cardiovascular risk (defined by age >75, presence of clinical or subclinical cardiovascular disease, presence of CKD, or Framingham score 10-year risk of cardiovascular disease of at least 15%).[93] Overall, these data add to our understanding of the effect of low versus moderate blood pressure targets in this population, and suggest that lower blood pressure targets even in older adults with CKD may result in benefit in terms of reduced cardiovascular disease and death, with the potential countering cost of increased adverse effects.

Perhaps the greatest challenge in examining available trial data on hypertension management in older adults is how to apply those data to individuals who would have been excluded from those trials. Adults with certain comorbid conditions are often excluded from clinical trials due to the concern that those additional comorbidities may cofound interpretation of the efficacy of the therapy or management strategy being evaluated. Older adults with dementia, poor functional status, and those who reside in skilled nursing facilities are explicitly excluded from many studies of hypertension management in older adults, presumably due to the concern that these conditions would directly interfere with an individual's ability to adhere to trial regimens and trial-related appointments (Table 5.3).[67,70,71,94-98] The end result is the absence of trial data specific to those older adults with CKD and hypertension who providers may see as most vulnerable, or the most likely to have competing risks associated with more aggressive blood pressure control. Moreover, for patients who experience multiple comorbidities and potentially significant symptom burden from multiple comorbidities, outcomes including quality of life, independence, and functional status may hold greater import than traditional outcomes in trials of hypertension management such as mortality and composite cardiovascular events. These less traditional and less disease-specific outcomes have not been the primary focus of major hypertension studies in older adults (Fig. 5.2).[67-72,76,77,81,94,95,97-103] For those older adults with CKD who would not have qualified for inclusion in clinical trials based on frailty, poor functional status, or other markers of fragility, providers must incorporate and interpret available trial data in concert with specific patient characteristics and goals to provide a more tailored and individualized approach to blood pressure management.

TABLE 5.3 Heart Failure Typically New York Heart Class III or IV but Sometimes Less Specific*

Patient Characteristic	Trials of Hypertension Management in Older Adults Which Excluded Patients Based on This Characteristic
Dementia	HYVET, SCOPE, SHEP, SPRINT, Syst-Eur
Living in skilled nursing facility	ACCORD, HYVET, SPRINT
Poor functional status (explicit/implicit)	EWPHE, HYVET, PROGRESS, Syst-Eur, TRANSCEND

*Exclusion for implicit or explicit poor functional status included exclusion based on inability to sit or stand and exclusion for significant disability thought likely to preclude regular follow up or attendance at study appointments.

ACCORD, Action to Control Cardiovascular Risk in Diabetes; *EWPHE*, European Working Party on High Blood Pressure in the Elderly; *HYVET*, Hypertension in the Very Elderly Trial; *PROGRESS*, Perindopril Protection Against Recurrent Stroke Study; *SCOPE*, Study on Cognition and Prognosis in the Elderly; *SHEP*, Systolic Hypertension in the Elderly Program; *SPRINT*, Systolic Blood Pressure Intervention Trial; *Syst-Eur*, Systolic Hypertension in Europe; *TRANSCEND*, Telmisartan Randomized Assessment Study in ACE Intolerant Subjects With Cardiovascular Disease.

Proteinuria

Multiple studies have demonstrated the ability of renin angiotensin system blockade (particularly angiotensin-converting enzyme inhibitors [ACEIs] and angiotensin receptor blockers [ARBs]) to reduce the risk of progression to ESRD, cardiovascular events, and death among patients with proteinuria.[89,104-107] The generalizability of these data

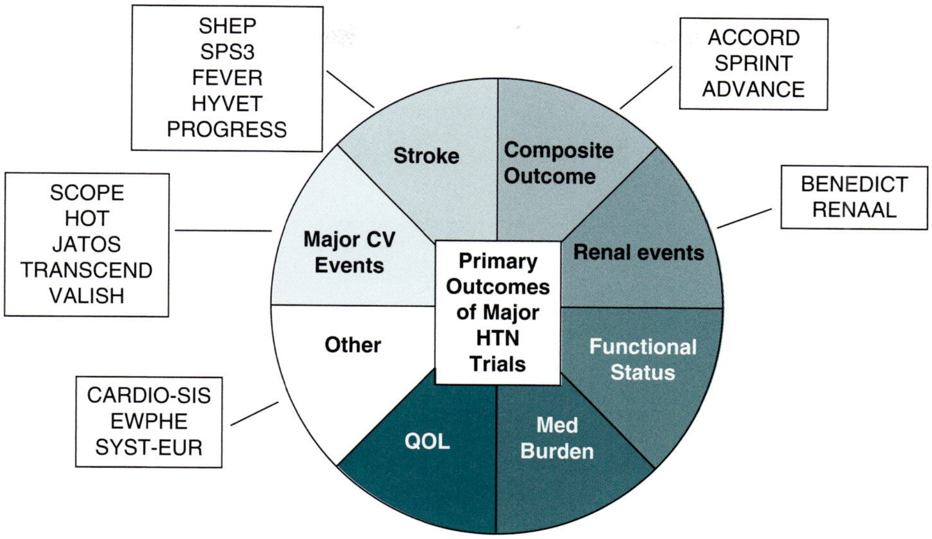

FIG. 5.2 Primary outcomes examined in hypertension trials of older adults.

to older populations, however, and particularly to the oldest age group (adults aged >80 years), is unclear. Studies demonstrating the benefit of antiproteinuric therapy in decreasing risk of adverse events among adults with CKD routinely excluded patients over the age of 70; the mean age of these studies ranged from 48 to 58. It remains unknown whether age affects the relationship between reduction in proteinuria and risk of outcomes such as ESRD and death. Moreover, previously described changes in renal vasculature associated with aging may affect usual autoregulation mechanisms in the kidneys of older adults. Compounding those age-related changes with loss of efferent vasoconstriction associated with use of ACEI and ARB may lead to an increased risk of acute kidney injury events in older adults who use these medications. Extrapolation of the benefits of ACEI and ARB therapy to older patients should be considered on a case by case basis, with consideration given to both the potential risks and benefits associated with antiproteinuric therapy, in particular ACEI and ARB use, among older patients.

MULTIMORBIDITY AND COMPLEXITY IN OLDER ADULTS WITH CHRONIC KIDNEY DISEASE

The number of medical diagnoses experienced by a patient is known to increase with both advancing age and decreasing eGFR.[48] Review of Medicare data found that almost 50% of older adults with CKD carried diagnoses of five or more comorbidities; a study of the oldest age group with severe CKD (stages 4/5), noted that up to 75% of these patients may experience multiple medical problems.[108,109] Understanding the role that CKD plays in patients' overall approach to healthcare is essential in optimizing management and individualizing care for older adults with CKD who experience multimorbidity.

The dominant paradigm for medical practice in the United States is a disease-specific model of care.[110] Within this model, practitioners rely on evidence-based clinical practice guidelines to inform decisions about management strategies for each individual disease state. Available data from clinical trials, however, frequently exclude adults with CKD and complex comorbid conditions such that the generalizability of these data to frail, medically complex patients remains unclear.[111,112] In older adults, hypertension is almost always found alongside at least one additional comorbid condition, but even trials of hypertension management routinely excluded adults with dementia, frailty, and poor functional status in addition to those with significant CKD.[84,113] Importantly, disease-specific guidelines rarely consider the interaction between two diseases, or between a disease and its proposed treatment. Strict adherence to multiple, separate, disease-specific guideline recommendations may result in a cumbersome burden of therapy and an increased risk of undesirable, competing outcomes.[114,115] Moreover, older adults with multiple chronic conditions may be more likely to experience geriatric syndromes; constellations of symptoms such as delirium and urinary incontinence, which may arise from a combination of different comorbidities and that are unlikely to be addressed by recommendations pertinent to a single disease state.[116,117]

The risk of frailty and declining functional status increase as renal function declines, and these changes can occur independent of comorbidity burden.[51,118] Changes in frailty and functional status can negatively affect a patient's ability to understand and enact complicated healthcare regimens. How well patients practice self-care and adhere to complicated healthcare regimens is also influenced significantly by social and systems-based resources, including degree of social support, quality of health insurance coverage, and the ability to afford medications.[119] The interplay of a patient's medical and social characteristics, in combination with the characteristics of the healthcare system in which he or she exists, all contribute to the complexity of

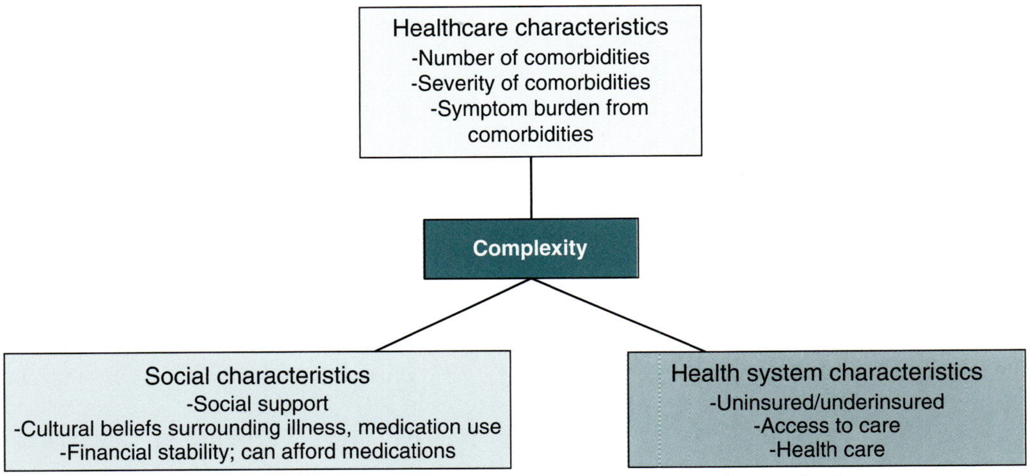

FIG. 5.3 Pictorial representation of components of complexity.

that individual.[120-122] Older adults with CKD may experience a high degree of care complexity, which can adversely affect their ability to self-manage their CKD, particularly in the context of multiple other chronic conditions[123] (Fig. 5.3).

Understanding the effect that a diagnosis of CKD may have on a given individual can help guide how to appropriately implement CKD-specific care that is consistent with his or her larger healthcare picture. Often, patients may experience a dominant comorbidity—a disease that has such significant effect on a patient's quality or quantity of life—whose management supersedes that of other concurrent illnesses.[124] Not all patients have a dominant comorbidity or the same dominant comorbidity over time, but recognition of where CKD falls in the hierarchy of a patient's medical problems and symptoms is critical. Older adults with CKD are less likely than their younger counterparts with kidney dysfunction to experience progression to require dialysis during their lifetime, and may experience highly varied trajectories of renal function.[125,126] This variability in disease course, in combination with the frequent lack of symptoms associated with CKD before advanced-stage disease, can influence a patient's perception of the importance of CKD and CKD self-care.[123]

The multimorbidity and overall complexity of care for older adults with CKD may be best addressed by an individualization of care based on a patient's personal preferences and healthcare priorities.[127] Guidelines on management of multiple chronic conditions in older adults support integration of patient concerns and priorities with information on prognosis and potential benefits and burdens of therapy when considering treatment regimens for older patients.[128] Use of patient goals and preferences to guide care across disease states may lead to a more integrated treatment plan that is better equipped to address symptoms related to geriatric syndromes and which may be less likely to result in conflicting or competing outcomes. The ability of nephrologists to understand how CKD fits into the overall context of care for older adults with multiple medical problems is the cornerstone to provision of comprehensive, individualized, and patient-centric care.

MANAGEMENT OPTIONS IN ADVANCED RENAL DISEASE IN OLDER ADULTS

The decision to initiate dialysis for older adults can be challenging, and available data suggest this decision is often influenced by factors other than patient preference or made without having conversations with patients.[129-132] When discussing the potential for dialysis with older adults, it is imperative to learn what their expectations are regarding dialysis and to educate them about how dialysis may affect their lives differently than younger adults. An appropriate alternative to dialysis is conservative care, whereby medical management is provided with the express purpose to minimize symptoms of kidney failure with a focus on patient comfort and quality of life.[133] Whenever possible, an interdisciplinary approach that involves the patient, nephrology, primary care and, if appropriate, family members and palliative care, is an effective way to understand the patient's goals and reach a joint decision that reflects and respects those goals.

Dialysis Initiation in Older Adults

Adults over age 75 are one of the most rapidly increasing groups of incident dialysis patients in the United States.[59] The decision for older adults to initiate dialysis, however, is not always straightforward, as they typically carry with them a greater burden of illness and complex treatment regimens. As such, what an older adult may gain from dialysis initiation in terms of both quality and quantity of life may be different from what would be experienced by a younger individual.

Dialysis is, at its core, a form of life support and is typically considered a therapy specifically initiated to extend life. The risk of death among older adults who initiate dialysis, however, is high and is considerably worse than for younger adults. In the United States, mortality among adults aged 65 to 74 years who initiate dialysis is twice that of younger adults; and adults over age 75 who are on dialysis experience a threefold increased risk of mortality compared with younger adults on dialysis.[59] Although age intuitively plays an important role in this mortality difference, older adults receiving dialysis also experience an increased risk of death compared with their age-matched counterparts who have alternative serious chronic conditions including heart failure, stroke, myocardial infarction, and even cancer.

Whether an older person who initiates dialysis will experience prolonged life due to dialysis therapy depends on particular patient characteristics. Evaluation of the ability of dialysis to prolong life is complex, as randomized controlled trials cannot ethically assign patients to receive or not receive dialysis therapy. The majority of data comparing longevity among older adults who do versus do not receive dialysis are derived from observational data comparing older adults who elect to receive dialysis and those who pursue conservative care, with a set level of estimated GFR to represent the time point of dialysis initiation. These observational data suggest that, although life is generally longer for older adults who choose dialysis compared with those who do not choose dialysis, the amount of time gained is influenced by a combination of age and the burden of comorbidity of a given individual (Table 5.4).[134-140] In particular, adults over age 80 who have coronary artery disease and a high burden of comorbid illness (defined by scales such as Charlson Comorbidity Index) may experience little to no life extension via dialysis initiation compared with their peers who choose to not initiate dialysis. The generalizability of these data is unclear, as most of the data related to life extension after dialysis initiation are derived from single-center studies of predominantly Caucasian populations in the United Kingdom and other European countries. Nevertheless, a better understanding of how much (or how little) dialysis may be expected to extend life in an older individual can be a critical addition to the decision-making process surrounding dialysis initiation in older adults.

Another important factor when considering dialysis initiation in older adults, beyond amount of time gained, is the type or quality of time that older adults may anticipate having after starting dialysis. Older patients considering dialysis should be counseled on the logistical aspects of such therapy, including the considerable time commitment required and the potential limitations such therapy may impose on activities. One study reported that adults ages 70 and older on hemodialysis spent an average of 173 days per year in the hospital or at dialysis, compared with an average of 16 days per year in the hospital for patients who chose conservative care.[140] Studies have specifically described reductions in both physical and mental components of quality of life among older adults who chose to receive dialysis that have not been observed in older adults who pursue conservative care.[50,137] These objectively measured reductions in quality of life do not appear to recover to predialysis levels over the study period examined, highlighting the need to set realistic expectations with older adults about how dialysis may affect both quantity and quality of life.[141] For some, the trade-off between quantity of life gained compared with quality of life lived after dialysis initiation may not be acceptable or reasonable.

Older adults on dialysis also frequently experience loss of independence. In one study of over 3700 nursing home residents with a mean age of 73.4 years, Kurella and colleagues identified an independent association between the initiation of dialysis and decreased functional status that was maintained after adjusting for age, sex, multiple medical conditions, and trajectory of functional decline before dialysis initiation.[142] Similar findings have been observed in community-dwelling older adults; among 76 adults ages 80 and older who were living independently at time of dialysis initiation, just 14% continued to live independently without assistance 2 years after dialysis initiation.[108]

Research shows that the majority of older adults, including those >85 years, received or were preparing to receive dialysis.[131] Importantly, these population level data will not apply to each unique individual in the same way, but do provide general trends about the amount and type of life that an older adult can expect after dialysis initiation. Further, they provide an important framework for discussion with older adults as they consider dialysis initiation in the context of their own patterns of comorbidity and functional status. Studies have found that older adults value and want to have discussions about dialysis initiation, particularly with their nephrologists.[143] Resources exist to support providers in having these sometimes challenging and important conversations with their patients.[144]

Resources to Inform Productive Discussion

Multiple resources are available to facilitate a productive dialogue with patients who have advanced kidney disease and may be considering dialysis or other treatment options.[145-147] The Renal Physicians Association (RPA) released its second edition of a Clinical Practice Guideline on *Shared Decision-Making in the Appropriate Initiation of and Withdrawal from Dialysis* in 2010, which serves as a useful starting point.[148] The Guideline provides 10 specific recommendations on how to frame the discussion with patients about dialysis planning, it and begins by acknowledging that shared decision-making is the preferred model for medical decision-making.

One important aspect of the shared decision-making model is to fully inform patients about their prognosis, including time estimates that are specific to an individual patient's condition. Although the ability to precisely predict an individual's prognosis is limited, validated prediction tools have been developed to guide the nephrologist or other healthcare provider.[149-154] Risk equations exist for progression from CKD to ESRD, CKD to mortality, and ESRD to mortality, some of which are available for use through electronic applications (e.g., http://www.qxmd.com/calculate-online/nephrology). Some of these tools utilize the surprise question *("Would you be surprised if this patient died in the next 12 months?")*, which is reliably associated with mortality among older adults with advanced CKD.[155]

Tangri and colleagues developed four risk equations to predict progression from CKD to ESRD over 2 and 5 years utilizing demographic and laboratory data of 3449 patients with CKD in Canada, of which the four-variable and eight-variable equations performed best.[150] Recently, these equations were validated in 31 multinational cohorts, involving 721,357 patients with CKD in >30 countries over four continents.[156]

TABLE 5.4 Survival Comparison Among Older Adults Choosing Dialysis versus Conservative Treatment

Study	Population	Study Period	Outcome of Interest	Findings	Comments
Martinez Echevers et al., 2016[134]	314 patients ≥70 years at single center in Spain, of whom 162 had or reached stage 5 CKD	2007–2013	Survival in stage 5 subgroup receiving dialysis vs. conservative treatment	Among patients ≥80 years, survival was not statistically different between those on dialysis (n = 15) vs. conservative treatment (n = 40; P = .2)	
Hussain et al., 2013[135]	441 patients ≥70 years in a predialysis clinic in the UK; 172 chose conservative treatment and 269 chose dialysis	2006–2011	Survival (primary); hospital admission (secondary)	Survival not statistically different among patients ≥80 years, or among patients with a World Health Organization performance score of ≥3 Relative risk of hospitalization among patients receiving dialysis compared with conservative treatment was 1.6 (1.1–2.1, P < .05)	Analysis performed from time of eGFR <20 mL/min; <15 mL/min; and <12 mL/min, all with the same results for the comparisons of interest
Verberne et al., 2016[136]	311 patients ≥70 years at single center in the Netherlands who were diagnosed with ESRD and elected to either pursue (n = 204) or withhold (n = 107) dialysis	2004–2014	Survival from 4 starting points (treatment decision; and eGFR <20, 15, or 10 mL/min) comparing those choosing dialysis to those choosing conservative treatment	No survival difference among patients ≥80 years, regardless of starting point	Though survival difference remained statistically significant, the magnitude of difference was greatly reduced in the presence of cardiovascular disease (CVD) for the entire cohort (survival 7.3 vs. 1.9 years (P < .001) without CVD; 2.3 vs. 1.5 years (P = .003] with CVD, dialysis vs. conservative treatment)
Brown et al., 2015[137]	467 older adults at single center in Australia who received conservative therapy (n = 122, mean age 82 years) or either planned for or started dialysis (n = 273, mean age 67 years)	2009–2013	Survival, symptom burden and quality of life (QOL)	No survival difference when restricted to patients >75 years of age with heart disease and at least one other comorbidity	No difference in change in symptoms and QOL over time between those choosing conservative treatment vs. dialysis
Murtagh et al., 2007[138]	129 adults >75 years with stage 5 CKD at four predialysis clinics in the UK who either chose dialysis (n = 52) or conservative treatment (n = 77)	2003–2005	Survival from the date eGFR was first <15 mL/min	No survival difference between dialysis (n = 10) and conservative treatment (n = 15) among those with Davies comorbidity score of 2 No survival difference between dialysis (n = 17) and conservative treatment (n = 30) among those with ischemic heart disease	

Da Silva-Gane et al., 2012[139]	170 patients attending predialysis clinics in the UK who chose dialysis (n = 122) conservative treatment (n = 30) or were undecided (n = 16) Not restricted to older adults (mean age for HD patients, PD patients and conservative treatment patients 60.6, 48.0, and 77.5 years, respectively)	2005–2010 (minimum follow-up of 30 months)	Median survival from recruitment date; QOL assessment	After adjusting for comorbidity, Karnofsky performance score, age, physical health score, and propensity score, median survival was 13 months shorter in the conservative treatment group than in HD patients, though not statistically significant (P = .08)	Patients choosing conservative treatment maintained QOL; patients choosing dialysis had reduced global satisfaction with life (P = .01) compared with predialysis that did not improve over the study period
Carson et al., 2009[140]	202 patients ≥70 years with ESRD in the UK choosing dialysis (n = 173) or conservative treatment (n = 29)	1997–2005	Median survival; hospitalization rate; location of death	Median survival 37.8 months for dialysis patients vs. 13.9 months for conservative treatment patients (no subgroup analysis performed) Dialysis patients hospitalized an average of 6.9% of days alive, compared with 4.3 % among conservative treatment patients (P < .05) Patients choosing conservative treatment four times as likely to die at home or in hospice than dialysis patients (OR 4.15, 95% CI 1.67–10.25)	Dialysis patients spent an average of 173 days per year in the hospital or at dialysis; conservative treatment patients spent an average of 16 days per year in the hospital

Older adults were well represented in these cohorts, and the ability to differentiate those who developed kidney failure from those who did not among older adults was very good (*C* statistic 0.874 to 0.905 depending on using 2-year or 5-year prediction and four-variable or eight-variable equation for patients ≥65 years). It is important to note that these equations are based on population level data and also overestimate risk in some non–North American cohorts.

Despite these resources and support from nephrology and other care providers, the decision of whether or not to initiate dialysis is a great challenge to most older adults. Uncertainty often remains even after circumstances develop that would otherwise prompt initiation of therapy (e.g., uremia, volume overload, etc.). In these types of circumstances, where undecided individuals may be at risk of adverse outcomes related to not starting dialysis but are not committed to conservative care, the RPA recommends that a time-limited trial of dialysis be offered.[148] If the decision is made to proceed with a time-limited trial of dialysis, the patient and provider should jointly define a time period over which the trial will tentatively occur (typically this is 1 to 3 months), the interval(s) at which the patient and provider will convene to discuss the progress of the trial and specific factors (e.g., physical status, quality of life, etc.) that will be considered during the trial to help determine the appropriate course of action (i.e., continuation vs. withdrawal of dialysis) upon completion of the trial.[157,158] As with all older adults who choose to initiate dialysis, patients receiving a time-limited trial should have the opportunity to routinely reevaluate how dialysis complements, or contradicts, their personal values in light of changes in physical status, quality of life, or other factors.

Palliative Support as an Alternative or Adjunct to Dialysis Preparation

There is increasing recognition in the nephrology community that additional expertise is needed in palliative management to support older adults who have or are progressing to ESRD.[159,160] Studies describing symptom burden in older adults with CKD stage 5 who have chosen conservative care identify an average of at least seven prevalent symptoms, which become more severe in the month before death.[161,162] Common symptoms experienced include weakness/decreased energy, poor appetite, sleep disturbances, dyspnea, and pain. Nephrologists and other members of the healthcare team must be prepared to identify and address these symptoms. Although clinical standards do not exist to guide the delivery of palliative care to patients with CKD, in 2013 KDIGO held the first consensus conference to define palliative care in the context of CKD and create a framework for how to ultimately develop international guidelines to improve quality of life and standard of care for patients with advanced CKD.[163] Although consistent with the World Health Organization's definition of palliative care, the term *kidney supportive care* has been proposed in response to the misconception that palliative and terminal care are synonymous among patients and providers alike.[159] The overarching goals of palliative care are to improve CKD patients' quality of life, deliver optimal care, and help patients reach clinical decisions driven by their personal values. It should be emphasized that palliative care is not restricted to older adults who elect not to pursue dialysis; palliative care can complement dialysis in any individual. Indeed, the implementation of palliative care among hemodialysis patients greatly improves documentation of patients' goals of care and recognition of code status.[164]

Although resources exist to facilitate the integration of palliative care concepts into the care of older adults with CKD, knowledge gaps remain as to how best to translate these concepts into improved patient outcomes or standards of care.[133,159,165] A prospective, multicenter study is currently under way in Europe to longitudinally measure quality of life and other factors such as cognition, frailty, and healthcare costs among patients choosing conservative care and palliative treatment.[166] Discussions to better inform older adults about the risks and benefits of, as well as alternatives to, dialysis initiation can foster a more comprehensive and individualized approach to decisions regarding dialysis initiation for this complex and growing patient population.

A full list of references is available at www.expertconsult.com.

6

The Pediatric Patient With Chronic Kidney Disease

Michelle C. Starr, MD, MPH, and Sangeeta R. Hingorani, MD, MPH

OUTLINE

Although less common in children than in adults, pediatric chronic kidney disease (CKD) is a significant health problem with the potential for serious long-term consequences. As in adults, CKD is as a state of irreversible damage to the kidneys with reduction of kidney function, representing a continuum of disease from mild kidney abnormalities with normal metabolic function and solute clearance to end-stage kidney disease (ESKD). Although similarities are seen between adult and pediatric populations, childhood CKD has many unique features and issues not present in adults. For example, growth and cognitive development issues are prominent because infants and children are in the formative phase of physical and neurodevelopmental growth, both of which can be adversely affected by CKD. Because physical growth and cognitive development are two of the essential components of childhood, these issues are particularly pertinent; a substantial percentage of pediatric CKD populations develop their disease early in life as the result of inherited or congenital disorders. Other CKD-associated complications, such as metabolic bone disease, anemia, nutrition, and cardiovascular disease (CVD), also pose unique challenges in pediatric patients. Despite these challenges, opportunities exist to decrease CKD-related morbidity and mortality and slow the loss of kidney function with early recognition and intervention. This chapter will focus on the identification and treatment of clinical issues that develop in children with CKD, as defined by a creatinine clearance <75 mL/min/1.73 m^2, irrespective of the primary kidney disorder.

EPIDEMIOLOGY OF PEDIATRIC CHRONIC KIDNEY DISEASE

Information on the incidence and prevalence of pediatric CKD is limited and imprecise; early CKD is often asymptomatic, so estimates of CKD in children often represent those with moderate or severe CKD or ESKD. Epidemiological information is often limited, and caution must be used when extrapolating data from small reference populations in the few well-designed studies. This study bias is important to recognize, as earlier stages of CKD are often more amenable to therapeutic interventions that can slow the rate of progression.[1]

Small, international studies provide the most comprehensive data regarding incidence and prevalence of pediatric CKD. The ItalKid project, a prospective population-based registry that includes 20 years of Italian pediatric cases of CKD, as defined by a glomerular filtration rate (GFR) <75 mL/min/1.73 m^2, reported a yearly incidence and prevalence of CKD of 12.1 and 74.7 cases per million children and adolescents per year.[2] Studies that have focused on severe CKD (e.g., GFR <30 mL/min/1.73 m^2) in Sweden and Chile also report similar rates but are limited by small reference population size.[3,4]

In contrast to adult CKD, where hypertension and diabetes are the most common etiologies, the majority of CKD in pediatric patients is due to congenital renal disorders, including dysplasia, hypoplasia, and aplasia as well as obstructive uropathy. In the United States the North American Pediatric Renal Trials and Collaborative Studies (NAPRTCS) registry has collected data on children with CKD since 1994[5]; however, it does not provide information on incidence and prevalence rates.[6] Of the 11,186 patients represented in the 2014 NAPRTCS data, almost half of the cases are due to congenital anomalies of the kidney and urinary tract (CAKUT), with aplasia/hypoplasia/dysplasia (15.8%), obstructive uropathy (15.3%), and reflux nephropathy (5%).[6] Although CAKUT represents the majority of causes of CKD in younger children, glomerular diseases resulting in CKD increase in those older than 12 years of age with focal segmental glomerulosclerosis (FSGS), the third most common diagnosis (11.7%) and the most prevalent acquired renal disease. Other glomerulonephritis (e.g., immunoglobulin [Ig]A nephritis, membranoproliferative glomerulonephritis) make up less than 10% of the causes of pediatric CKD. Similar trends are reported in the Chronic Kidney Disease in Children (CKiD) study, an ongoing prospective study of children with CKD. In their initial cohort of 587 children, nonglomerular disease was the underlying cause of the majority of CKD (78%), with obstructive uropathy being the most common diagnosis. Of those children with glomerular disease as the cause of their CKD, FSGS was the most common diagnosis (7%).[7] For reasons that remain incompletely understood but may partially be due to genetic polymorphisms, FSGS is more than three times more common in blacks (22.6%) than in whites (9.0%) and is especially prevalent among black adolescents (35%).[6]

Due to a lack of data from low- and middle-income countries, it is difficult to estimate the causes of pediatric CKD, although more registry-based data has been published in recent years.[8,9] A similar distribution for the etiology of CKD has been reported in Europe by the Italian and Belgian registries. The slightly higher proportions of hereditary nephropathy (15% to 19%) may be due to differences in cohorts racial or ethnic distribution.[2] However, there are significant geographic and cultural differences in epidemiological trends of pediatric CKD due to genetic, environmental, and racial factors. For example, heritable causes of CKD (e.g., cystinosis, Alport syndrome, congenital nephrotic syndrome) are more common in areas of the world where consanguinity is more frequent, such as in Iran[10] and Jordan.[11] In Japan, a high percentage of pediatric CKD is due to glomerulonephritis, such as FSGS and IgA nephropathy.[12] In less-developed areas of the world, glomerulonephritis continues to represent a significant percentage of kidney disease, suggesting the ongoing burden of infectious causes of CKD, including hepatitis, malaria, schistosomiasis, tuberculosis, and HIV.[8]

DEFINING CHRONIC KIDNEY DISEASE

The effort to standardize the definitions of CKD has led to the Kidney Disease: Improving Global Outcomes (KDIGO) 2012 Clinical Practice Guideline (CPG) for Evaluation and Management of Chronic Kidney Disease, which includes kidney function based on GFR and the presence of urinary albumin and excretion rate.[13] There are five stages of CKD, with lower stages (e.g., stage 1) representing higher GFR (Table 6.1). The diagnosis of CKD in pediatric patients requires fulfilling one of the criteria:

TABLE 6.1 GFR Category

GFR Category	Glomerular Filtration Rate
G1	90 mL/min/1.73 m^2
G2	60–89 mL/min/1.73 m^2
G3a	45–59 mL/min/1.73 m^2
G3b	30–44 mL/min/1.73 m^2
G4	15–29 mL/min/1.73 m^2
G5	<15 mL/min/1.73 m^2

(Adapted from Kidney International Supplements. KDIGO 2012 Clinical Practice Guideline for the Evaluation and Management of Chronic Kidney Disease. Chapter 1: Definition and classification of CKD. *Kidney Int.* Suppl. 2013; 3:19.)

TABLE 6.2 GFR Change With Age

Age (Sex)	Mean GFR ± SD
1 wk (males and females)	41 ± 15 mL/min/1.73 m^2
2–8 wk (males and females)	66 ± 25 mL/min/1.73 m^2
>8 wk (males and females)	96 ± 22ml/min/1.73 m^2
2–12 y (males and females)	133 ± 27 mL/min/1.73 m^2
13–21 y (males)	140 ± 30ml/min/1.73 m^2
13–21 y (females)	126 ± 22 mL/min/1.73 m^2

Wk, Weeks; *y*, years.
(Adapted from National Kidney Foundation's Kidney Disease Outcomes Quality Initiative Clinical Practice Guidelines for Chronic Kidney Disease in Children and Adolescents: Evaluation, Classification, and Stratification. *Pediatrics* 111 (2003) 1416–1421.)

1. GFR of less than 60 mL/min/1.73 m^2 for greater than 3 months regardless of whether other CKD markers are present
2. GFR greater than 60 mL/min/1.73 m^2 accompanied by markers of functional kidney abnormalities such as proteinuria, albuminuria, renal tubular disorders, or pathological abnormalities, or evidence of structural damage based on imaging or history

This classification has been widely adopted since its introduction; however, it does have significant limitations in pediatric patients. Although GFR is the primary criteria used to define and stage CKD, its use is challenging in younger children. In pediatric populations, the normal level of GFR varies depending on body size, age, and gender. Although normal GFR in adolescents and adults is approximately 120 mL/min/1.73 m^2, the norms are much lower in early childhood, even when adjusted for body surface area. GFR slowly increases to adult levels over the first year or two of life before reaching normal levels[14] (Table 6.2).

A gold standard measurement of GFR can be estimated from clearance of a filtration marker, either inulin or iohexol, in serum or blood at set time points after infusion.[15] These studies can be challenging to perform for routine clinical use in children.[16] Creatinine clearance can also be determined by 24-hour urine collection; however, this can often be compromised by incomplete collection and tends to overestimate GFR in advancing CKD due to enhanced renal tubular creatinine secretion.[13] There has been growing evidence that cystatin C may be a more accurate marker of kidney function[17] because it has less intrapatient variability and, in patients over 2 years old, levels are inversely associated with kidney function independent of body composition, age, gender, and height.[18,19]

Given these limitations, GFR is often estimated by equations based on endogenous markers. The Schwartz formula, used since the 1980s, is based on serum creatinine as determined by the Jaffe technique.[20] The Schwartz formula is the most widely used formula in pediatric practice, with GFR calculated as:

$$\text{CrCl (mL/min per } 1.73\text{m}^2 = 0.55 \times \text{Height (cm)} / \text{S Cr (mg/dL)} \quad \textbf{Eq. 1}$$

Of note, the constant is 0.45 for infants <1 year and 0.7 for adolescent boys. Despite its simplicity, with the introduction of enzymatic creatinine measurement the equation has become imprecise. Investigators have developed more accurate GFR-estimating equations using enzymatically determined creatinine, which can be used for children with CKD and which have been validated for children with an estimated GFR between 15 and 75 mL/min/1.73 m^2.[21]

$$\text{CrCl (mL/min per } 1.73\text{m}^2 = 0.413 \times \text{Height (cm)} / \text{S Cr (mg/dL)} \quad \textbf{Eq. 2}$$

NATURAL HISTORY AND PROGRESSION OF CHRONIC KIDNEY DISEASE

The progression of CKD to ESKD results in many of the health consequences of this disease; however, the natural history and the rate of progression are both highly variable and unpredictable. Pediatric data suggest that there is a slower progression of disease in those with congenital renal disorders compared with those with glomerular etiologies of their CKD.[22] Studies have demonstrated that the progression of CKD can be influenced by multiple factors, many of which are not modifiable (e.g., underlying renal pathology, genetics, race, age, and gender).[23] However, some risk factors can be modified, such as obesity, hypertension, and proteinuria.[24] There is evidence in both adult and pediatric studies that hypertension and proteinuria are the most significant risk factors for CKD progression; minimizing proteinuria and maximizing blood pressure control can slow progression of CKD.[25,26]

It is postulated that proteinuria contributes to CKD progression due to tubular damage resulting in interstitial inflammation, fibrosis, and subsequent apoptosis of proximal tubular cells.[27] In adult studies, both microalbuminuria and overt proteinuria are independent risk factors for CKD progression.[28,29] Results from several pediatric cohort studies demonstrate similar trends, with an analysis of 202 patients in the CKiD cohort finding that those with proteinuria had mean eGFR that was 16 mL/min/1.73 m^2 lower than those without proteinuria.[30] In children with CKD stage 3 and 4 in the European Study Group for Nutritional Treatment of Chronic Renal Failure in Childhood, both proteinuria and hypertension were major independent risk factors for progression of CKD.[31] Finally, a secondary analysis from the Evaluation Study of Congestive Heart Failure and Pulmonary Artery Catheterization Effectiveness (ESCAPE) trial found that residual urinary protein excretion during ACE inhibition therapy was associated with CKD progression.[32]

Although proteinuria is a well-established biomarker in the progression of CKD, it does appear to have some limitations and some investigators suggest that urinary tubular proteins, such as β 2-microglobulin, may better predict the clinical course and progression of CKD. Other biomarkers, previously used in acute kidney injury, such as neutrophil gelatinase-associated lipocalin (NGAL), also show promise in pediatric CKD.[33] Children with kidney disease resulting in a high load of tubular protein excretion are not commonly associated with renal insufficiency or rapid progression of CKD.

There is clear and consistent evidence from large trials that hypertension is a modifiable risk factor for CKD progression. Although data was primarily from adult populations, within the last 10 years several large studies have provided consistent evidence that, among children with CKD, uncontrolled hypertension is associated with significantly faster declines in GFR.[31,34,35] Results from the ESCAPE trial show that intensified blood pressure control, defined as 24-hour mean arterial pressure below the 50th percentile for age, in children aged 3 to 18 with CKD (GFR between 15 and 80 mL/min/1.73 m^2) was beneficial.[36] Primary analysis showed that fewer patients in the intensified blood pressure control group reached the primary end point of 50% decline in GFR or progression to ESKD (29.9% vs. 41.7%).

Other factors contribute to the progression of pediatric CKD. Obesity and metabolic syndrome are associated with dyslipidemia, hypertension, and albuminuria, all of which may influence the progression of kidney disease.[37] Although the mechanisms by which obesity potentiates and exacerbates CKD are largely speculative, studies suggest that a combination of lipotoxicity, a proinflammatory state, glomerular hyperfiltration, and resultant hemodynamic disturbances may all play a role.[38] Race and genetics are two nonmodifiable risk factors for CKD progression. There is strong concordance of kidney disease in African American families, and African Americans have a faster rate of progression compared with all other populations after controlling for other factors.[39] In the CKiD cohort, among 419 children with CKD, Caucasian children had significantly less proteinuria than other ethnicities at any GFR, regardless of underlying renal disease.[25] The clustering of CKD in families suggests genetic and/or familial predisposition in some cases. In addition, several studies demonstrate links between CKD and various polymorphisms in genes encoding mediators of CKD (such as the renin-angiotensin system [RAS]) and an increased susceptibility to progression in disease such as IgA nephropathy.[40,41]

Low birth weight (LBW) is another nonmodifiable factor associated with a reduction in the number of nephrons and a subsequent predisposition to CKD and hypertension in later life.[42] In a cross-sectional analysis of the fourth National Health and Nutritional Examination cohort, adolescents (aged 12 to 15) who were born at LBW (<2500 g) were more likely to have a decreased GFR (OR = 1.49, $P = 0.02$) than those in the normal weight cohort.[43] Using a cross-sectional national survey linked to birth records in Japan, investigators found that the risk ratio for CKD was significantly higher in the LBW group and those born prematurely.[44] Finally, regardless of the degree of CKD, puberty appears to be associated with a steep decline in kidney function.[45] This progression pattern may be due to an adolescent-specific pathophysiological mechanism: either the result of an imbalance between rapidly growing body size and residual nephron mass or related to sex hormones. Data pertaining to a variety of risk factors potentially associated with the progression of CKD, including those discussed in this section, are currently being collected by the CKiD study.

PREVENTION OF PROGRESSION

Although many of the risk factors that potentiate progression of pediatric CKD are nonmodifiable, several antiproteinuric and antihypertensive therapies have demonstrated promising results in slowing the progression of CKD. Three large adult studies—the Appropriate Blood Pressure Control in Diabetes (ABCD) study, the African American Study of Kidney Disease and Hypertension (AASK), and the Modification of Diet in Renal Disease (MDRD) study—found that blood pressure control also decreases proteinuria.[28,46,47] Although large pediatric studies are limited, results from the ESCAPE trial and CKiD cohort suggest that antiproteinuric treatment is protective in pediatric CKD patients. The goal of antiproteinuric treatment is to reduce proteinuria to <300 mg/m^2/day, a value that appears to be associated with the maximal renoprotective effect in adult studies.

Treatment with either angiotensin-converting enzyme inhibitors (ACEIs) or angiotensin II type I receptor blockers (ARBs) has been shown to be more effective for both blood pressure control and reduction in proteinuria compared with other agents currently available.[48] By decreasing either angiotensin II tone (ACEI) or action (ARB), these agents reduce pressure within the glomerulus and decrease proteinuria, downregulate activation of inflammatory pathways, and attenuate local release of cytokines and chemokines. These changes appear to attenuate glomerular hypertrophy and sclerosis, tubulointerstitial inflammation, and fibrosis.[49]

Well-matched studies assessing the efficacy of RAS antagonists for renoprotection in children with CKD are limited. Small uncontrolled studies in children with CKD provide evidence of stable kidney function and proteinuria in those treated with losartan for 2.5 years.[50] A recent randomized controlled trial of ARB therapy in pediatric CKD patients found that ARB therapy significantly reduced proteinuria (35.8%) compared with the amlodipine/placebo (1.4%) group independent of blood pressure control.[51] Similarly, in the CKiD cohort, Wong et al. observed an antiproteinuric effect of renin-angiotensin-aldosterone system blockade in those with glomerular diseases as a cause of their CKD.[24,25] In the ESCAPE study, treatment with ACE inhibition lead to a 50% reduction in proteinuria in hypertensive children and a 2.2 mmHg decrease in mean arterial blood pressure (BP) in children with CKD, with similar efficacy in patients with hypo/dysplastic kidneys and glomerular disease.[36]

Intensive blood pressure control, in addition to proteinuria, is also associated with significant risk reduction. The recently concluded ESCAPE trial found that fewer patients in the intensified-control group (blood pressure target below the 50th age-related percentile of 24-hour mean arterial pressure) than in the conventional-control group (target of 50th to 95th percentile) reached the composite primary end point of doubling serum creatinine, GFR deterioration to less than 10 mL/min/1.73 m^2, or need for renal replacement therapy (29.9% vs. 41.7%; hazard ratio, 0.65; 95% confidence interval [CI], 0.44 to 0.94; $P = 0.02$).[36] This corresponds to a risk reduction of 35% and suggests that controlling blood pressure to reach a target of less than the 50th percentile may improve outcomes.

Finally, existing studies do not support the use of a low-protein diet to protect from CKD progression. One of the largest trials in adults, the MDRD trial, did not show an effect of a low-protein diet on CKD progression in patients with nondiabetic kidney disease.[52] In children, data do not show a clear benefit, either. In a 2-year prospective, randomized multicenter study of 191 children with CKD, the use of a low-protein diet (0.8 to 1.1 g/kg) failed to affect the decline in creatinine clearance.[31] Furthermore, a low-protein diet with intake below the Dietary Reference Intake (DRI) may have an adverse effect on growth. The current consensus is to provide children with CKD the age-appropriate recommended daily allowance for protein.[53]

GROWTH FAILURE

Growth impairment is one of the most visible complications for children with CKD and is associated with significant morbidity and mortality. Pediatric CKD patients often fail to reach an adult height equivalent to either their genetic potential or population norms.[54] Growth impairment is common in children with CKD, with data from NAPRTCS showing more than 35% of children had impaired growth with height less than third percentile (standard deviation score [SDS] of −1.88).[55] On average, patients with CKD are 1.44 SD below sex- and age-specific norms for height, with the youngest patients (those under 1 year) having the most severe growth failure with a mean SDS of −2.34.[56] Because one-third of postnatal stature is obtained in the first 2 years of life, this may have a profound effect on adult height.[57] There is an increased risk for poor growth with decreasing renal function; however, growth failure is seen at all stages of CKD. Approximately one-fifth of patients in the 2008 NAPRTCS registry with an estimated CrCl <60 mL/min/1.73 m^2 had an SDS of −1.85.[56] The CKiD study estimates that for each decline of 10 mL/min/1.73 m^2 in GFR, there is a corresponding decrease in height SDS by 0.12 to 0.16.[58] Additionally, as puberty is both delayed and shortened in CKD, the height growth during puberty in children with CKD is only half that in children with normal kidney function.[54]

Poor growth is also associated with an increased risk of both morbidity and mortality, with each SDS decrease in height associated with a 14% increased risk of death.[59] Analysis of data from the United States Renal Data System (USRDS) found that children with ESKD on dialysis with growth failure had a threefold increased risk of death. Results from the NAPRTCS cohort also demonstrate that children with growth failure (height SDS <−2.5 at time of dialysis initiation) had a significantly higher risk of hospitalization and twice the risk of death compared with children with normal growth.[60] In addition, severe growth impairment is associated with more complex clinical courses and with more hospitalizations, both of which affect health-related quality of life for these children and families.[61] Short stature is associated with poor physical functioning and may affect the psychological development of patients.[62,63] Short children are often treated as younger than their chronological age and may have lower expectations set for them compared with their average height peers.[64]

Growth failure in children with CKD is multifactorial, but disturbances in growth hormone (GH) and insulin-like growth factor-1 (IGF-1) appear to be the primary contributing factors. Other risk factors for poor growth in children with CKD include secondary hyperparathyroidism, metabolic acidosis, inadequate nutrition, anemia, and disturbances of water and electrolyte balance. In normal growth, GH is released by the anterior pituitary in a pulsatile manner under the stimulation of growth hormone–releasing hormone (GHRH) and is then bound by GH receptors in the liver, resulting in the production of insulin growth factor (IGF)-1.[65] A majority of IGF-1 is bound to insulin growth factor–binding protein 3 (IGFBP-3), and the remaining free (unbound) IGF-1 stimulates growth by acting on cartilaginous receptors in bone.[66] In CKD, levels of GH are increased due to a decrease in metabolic clearance and IGF-1 feedback is attenuated, leading to amplified pulsatile release of GH.[67] However, despite these increases in GH concentrations, there is a downregulation of IGF-1 synthesis in the liver as well as decreased bioavailability.[68] In some patients with CKD, GH secretion is decreased as metabolic acidosis inhibits GH action on peripheral tissue and steroid therapy reduces GH pulsatility.[69]

In pediatric CKD patients with persistent growth impairment, recombinant human GH (rhGH) is the standard therapy to correct and prevent the growth failure associated with CKD and ESKD.[70] Recommendations of the 2008 KDOQI Clinical Practice Guideline suggest considering rhGH therapy for pediatric CKD stages 2 through 5 with short stature (defined as height SDS less than −1.88) and linear growth potential after metabolic abnormalities have been corrected and nutritional issues addressed.[71] The treatment dose of rhGH is 0.05 mg/kg daily given via subcutaneous injection.[72] Of note, the amount of rhGH given to pediatric CKD patients is higher than those with GH deficiency because CKD causes GH insensitivity and pharmacologic rather than replacement dosing is required in this population. rhGH is beneficial for children with CKD throughout the continuum of disease from mild CKD to ESKD to post–renal transplantation. Studies have demonstrated that improved clinical response to GH treatment is seen in patients with initiation in younger children (prepubertal), the degree of bone age delay, extent of height SDS gain within first year of treatment, and renal dysplasia as the primary renal disease.[57,73,74] Cumulative height gain is predicted based on the height deficit at therapy initiation and the duration of treatment, suggesting that rhGH may help "unlock" growth potential. The largest response to rhGH treatment is seen within the first year of therapy, with less effect after 1 year; however, sustained use may allow achievement of a final adult height within the normal range.[75]

Before the initiation of rhGH therapy, evaluation should include assessment of concomitant metabolic bone disease, including a serum parathyroid hormone (PTH) level as well as baseline hip x-rays due to the theoretical increased risk of femoral head avascular necrosis and slipped capital femoral epiphysis (SCFE).[76] Evidence is mixed on obtaining bone age with x-ray imaging; however, many providers do obtain a bone age in older children and adolescents before initiation of rhGH.[77] Despite initial concern that it may contribute to advancing CKD via induction of glomerular hyperfiltration, there is no evidence that rhGH accelerates progression of CKD.[78] Ongoing monitoring is required to adjust treatment dose for changes in weight, to detect adverse effects, and to evaluate the response to rhGH, with an adequate response defined as a growth velocity greater than 2 cm/year.[13] Adverse effects are rare in children undergoing rhGH treatment, but there may be a slightly higher risk of developing idiopathic intracranial hypertension, SCFE, or worsening of existing scoliosis.[72,79] Treatment with rhGH should be stopped when epiphyses are closed, the patient has achieved target height, and/or when adverse events occur. Studies suggest that discontinuation of therapy at the time of kidney transplant did not adversely affect growth velocity.[80] A simple approach to the use of rhGH is provided in Fig. 6.1.

There is good evidence that the adult height of pediatric patients with CKD has improved significantly over the last several decades and, though multifactorial, rhGH had a primary role in this change.[58,81] Long-term follow-up of a cohort of German children showed that patients with CKD who received rhGH grew significantly better than patients who did not, without differences in the duration of the pubertal growth spurt.[82] Despite these findings, however, a significant percentage of pediatric CKD patients do not receive treatment. In the 2008 NAPRTCS report, only 11.1% of pediatric patients with CKD received rhGH at baseline and only 22.1% by the end of their first year.[6] Although multiple factors appear to contribute, psychosocial concerns (including family refusal and/or noncompliance) were the ascribed cause in 30% of patients not receiving rhGH therapy, and waiting for insurance company approval delayed initiation of treatment in 18% of children.[83] Additionally, there is substantial variation in nephrologist utilization of rhGH.[77] These findings suggest an opportunity for improvement in our care of children with CKD.

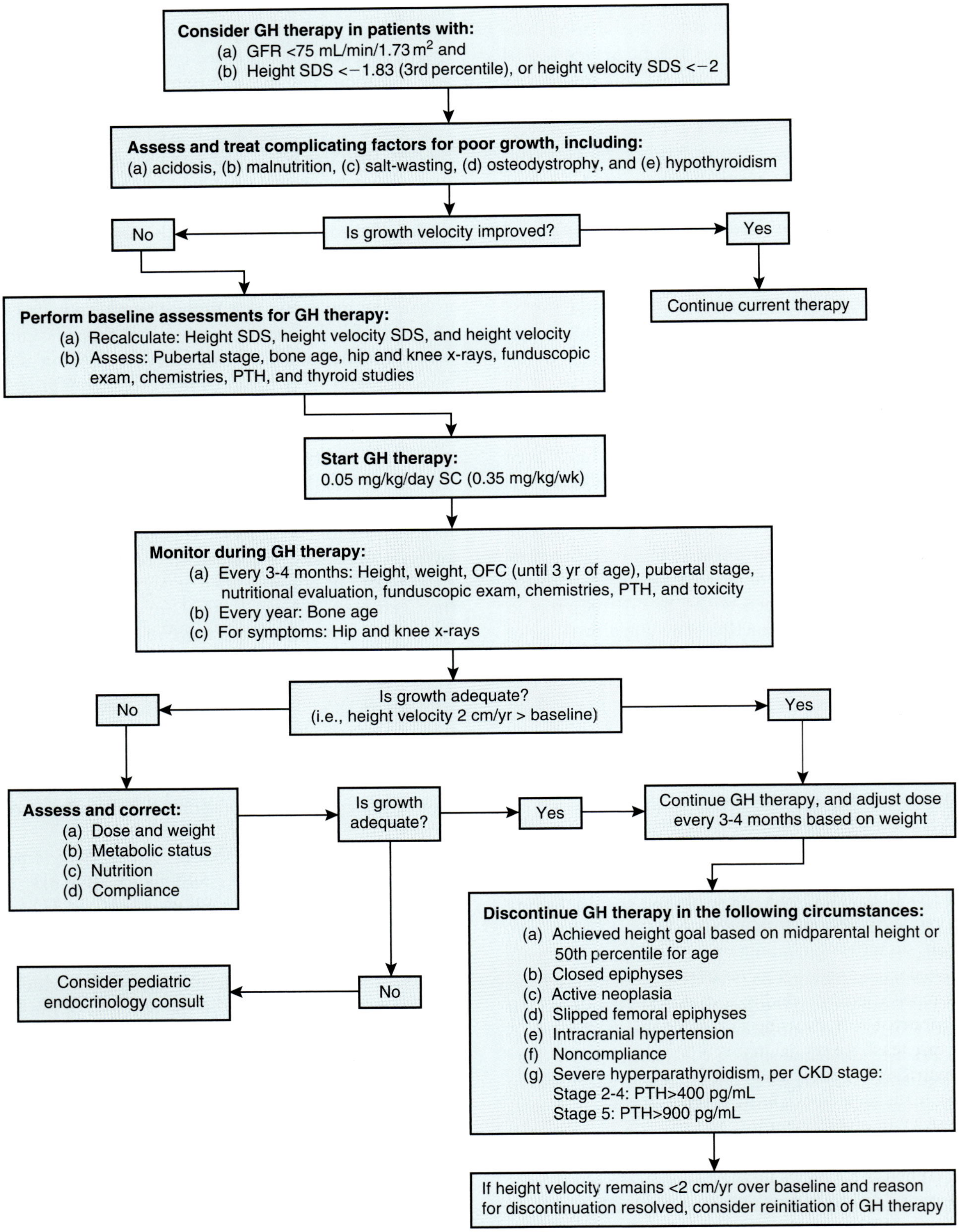

FIG. 6.1 Management of GH therapy.

BOX 6.1 Causes of Protein Energy Malnutrition (PEM) in Children With Chronic Kidney Disease

Inadequate food intake due to:
Altered taste sensation
Prescribed diets
Anorexia
Nausea/vomiting/impaired gastric motility
Illness
Food insecurity
Chronic inflammatory stage
Catabolic state due to chronic illness
Uremic toxins and ingestion of exogenous toxins
Removal of nutrition with dialysis

Endocrinologic causes:
Insulin and IGF-1 resistance
Hyperparathyroidism

(Adapted from National Kidney Foundation, KDOQI clinical practice guideline for nutrition in children with CKD: 2008 update, *Am. J. Kidney Dis.* 53 (Suppl. 2) (2009) S1–S124.)

NUTRITIONAL ISSUES AND METABOLIC CONCERNS

In children with CKD, protein energy malnutrition (PEM) is a common and important complication. PEM has a significant effect on linear growth and neurocognitive development and is particularly important in infants and young children, where deficits in linear growth and neurocognitive development may not be fully correctable. Although PEM is a well-known complication of CKD, the published prevalence rates range from 6% to 65%. The wide range is due to use of varying diagnostic criteria for PEM among studies.[84,85] Given the obesity epidemic, it is important to balance concerns for PEM with avoidance of excessive nutrition, given its role in potentiating GFR decline in patients with CKD. Recent data from the CKiD cohort found that children with CKD consumed more sodium, protein, and calories than recommended by guidelines and that this intake was heavily driven by consumption of milk and fast food.[86] In childhood CKD, the focus of nutritional care should be on maintenance of optimal nutritional status, avoidance of metabolic abnormalities, and reduction in the risk of associated morbidity and mortality in adulthood. A collaborative effort involving all members of the multidisciplinary care team is essential in nutritional management.

Malnutrition in children with CKD is often multifactorial; however, inadequate intake is often a major contributing factor (Box 6.1). In infants, vomiting and delayed gastric emptying are common and may be worsened by gastroesophageal reflux.[87] When these issues limit nutritional intake, medical management (e.g., antireflux measures with proton pump inhibition or H2-blockers) or surgical intervention (e.g., gastrostomy tube placement) may be required.[88] Adolescents and older children may be at increased risk of malnutrition due to poor dietary habits, as well as alterations in smell and taste, which can have an effect on food intake.[89]

BOX 6.2 Recommended Nutritional Assessment for Chronic Kidney Disease

Dietary intake
Height or length-for-age percentile or SDS
Height or length velocity-for-age percentiles or SDS
Estimated dry weight and weight-for-age percentiles or SDS
BMI-for-height/age percentile or SDS
Head circumference-for-age or SDS (for children <3 year)
nPRC (for adolescents maintained on hemodialysis)

BMI, Body mass index; *nPCR*, normalized protein catabolic rate; *SDS*, standard deviation score.
(Adapted from National Kidney Foundation, KDOQI clinical practice guideline for nutrition in children with CKD: 2008 update, *Am. J. Kidney Dis.* 53 (Suppl. 2) (2009) S1–S124.)

Nutritional assessment requires a comprehensive approach, including dietary evaluation, anthropometric measurements, and physical markers, in addition to laboratory monitoring. The most recent KDOQI pediatric nutrition guidelines recommend using dietary intake plus a combination of measurements to assess nutritional status more completely (Box 6.2).[71] Evaluation of anthropometric parameters, though an important part of this evaluation because they have been closely associated with mortality, must be interpreted carefully.[59,60] Some of the challenges in identifying children with PEM include finding comparable reference population differences between growth charts offered by the CDC and the World Health Organization, and that the severe growth failure common in CKD requires normalization by height rather than by chronological age.[71] Additionally, abnormalities in body composition in children with CKD may confound evaluation because alterations in total body water and fat mass make assessment more challenging. A recent study evaluating pediatric CKD patients found a dramatically discordant body composition characterized by relatively high fat mass, which was not accurately assessed by calculated body mass index (BMI).[90]

Various biochemical parameters are used as markers of nutritional status, the most commonly cited being serum albumin. Despite the historical use of albumin as a marker of nutritional status, recent studies have demonstrated that nutritional interventions do not have an effect on serum albumin levels in pediatric CKD. In a trial of intradialytic parenteral nutrition therapy in adolescents on hemodialysis, no change in serum albumin was noted. In a separate cohort of 44 patients on hemodialysis, there was no correlation between albumin and weight loss.[91,92] Although serum albumin may be a poor marker of nutrition, it does appear to be a useful marker of increased risk of mortality In the CKiD cohort, investigators found that for each 1 g/dL decrease in serum albumin 45 days before the start of dialysis, there was a 54% higher risk of death.[93] Given the challenges of assessment of PEM in children with CKD, recent work has focused on creating pediatric specific criteria using alternative definitions of PEM to allow for better risk discrimination through inclusion of criteria based on growth.[94]

Energy

As CKD advances and renal function deteriorates, children with CKD often experience a decrease in spontaneous energy intake.[95] Despite this decline, energy requirements of children with CKD appear to remain the same as other pediatric populations. Guidelines suggest that energy requirements for children with CKD should be 100% of the estimated energy requirement for age as adjusted for physical activity level and BMI.[71] Infants often have inadequate energy intake; however, in older children energy intake is often relatively normal.[87] Studies have demonstrated that optimizing energy intake in infants with CKD improves height velocity.[96] Similar findings have also been described outside the infant population. In a group of 35 children younger than 5 years with CKD stages 4 to 5, weight gain and accelerated linear growth were demonstrated in those starting enteral feeding at <2 years of age, with both improved weight gain and maintenance of growth velocity in those starting enteral feeds at age 2 to 5 years.[97]

Supplementary nutritional support should be considered in every child with CKD, particularly when the usual intake of the child fails to meet energy requirements or the patient is not achieving the expected rate of weight gain or linear growth for age. Infants with CKD often require fluid restriction and greater caloric density of nutritional feeds, and poor appetite or vomiting often precludes adequate oral intake. Conversely, in pediatric patients with polyuric CKD, fluid requirements may require supplementary support, as well. The institution of tube feeding should be considered in patients unable to take adequate oral intake. Nasogastric tubes, gastrostomy tubes, and gastrojejunostomy tubes can all be used to provide enteral feeding in children with CKD, and each has its own benefits and drawbacks.[88] More detailed recommendations regarding tube feeds are available in the 2008 update of KDOQI Clinical Practice Guideline for Nutrition in Children with CKD.[71]

Irrespective of the administration route or caloric density, nutritional therapy should provide a balance of calories from carbohydrate and unsaturated fat within the ranges recommended as the Acceptable Macronutrient Distribution Range (AMDR) in the DRI. The recommended AMDR for children older than 4 years is 45% to 65% from carbohydrate, 25% to 35% from fat, and 10% to 30% from protein, with children younger than 3 years needing a somewhat greater proportion of fat (30% to 40%) in their diets to meet energy needs.

Protein

Nitrogenous waste products and inorganic ions potentiate many of the metabolic disturbances and clinical manifestations of uremia; therefore low-protein diets reduce the generation of these products. Studies have demonstrated that protein intake is linearly matched to phosphorus intake, resulting in the association between high phosphorus levels and a high-protein diet.[98] Not surprisingly, low-protein diets decrease the development of electrolyte disorders, including hyperphosphatemia, hyperkalemia, and metabolic acidosis.[99] A large number of trials and studies have examined the effect of dietary protein restriction on the rate of progression to ESKD in adults.[100,101] In the large MDRD trial, there was no significant beneficial effect of decreasing Dietary Protein Intake (DPI) from 1.3 to either 0.58 or 0.3 g/kg/day, although subtle signs of a suboptimal nutritional status were noted with these restrictive diets.[52,102]

TABLE 6.3 Recommended Dietary Protein Intake in Children With CKD Stages 3 to 5

Age	DRI (g/kg/d)	Recommended for CKD Stage 3 100%–140% DRI	Recommended for CKD Stages 4 to 5 100%–120% DRI
0–6 mo	1.5	1.5–2.1	1.5–1.8
7–12 mo	1.2	1.2–1.7	1.2–1.5
1–3 y	1.05	1.05–1.5	1.05–1.25
4–13 y	0.95	0.95–1.35	0.95–1.15
14–18 y	0.85	0.85–1.2	0.85–1.05

DRI, Daily recommended intake; *mo*, months; *y*, years.
(Adapted from National Kidney Foundation, KDOQI clinical practice guideline for nutrition in children with CKD: 2008 update, *Am. J. Kidney Dis.* 53 (Suppl. 2) (2009) S1–S124.)

In children, there is concern that dietary protein restriction may have effects on the growth and neurocognitive development in infants and young children with CKD. Studies in experimental animal models showed that dietary protein restriction may slow renal function deterioration but adversely affects growth.[103] Few clinical studies of dietary protein restriction have been conducted in children due to these concerns. In a 2-year prospective, stratified, and randomized multicenter study of 191 children with CKD stages 3 to 4, the use of a low-protein diet (0.8 to 1.1 g/kg) did not adversely affect growth or serum albumin. Neither did protein restriction affect the rate of renal function decline as indicated by creatinine clearance.[31] Although there is no evidence of a protective effect of dietary protein restriction on kidney function, protein intake can be restricted safely to 0.8 to 1.1 g/kg/day in children with CKD.

Current KDOQI pediatric nutrition guidelines recommend dietary protein intake at 100% to 140% of the DRI for ideal body weight in children with CKD stage 3 and at 100% to 120% of the DRI in children with CKD stages 4 to 5 (Table 6.3).[71] Interestingly, although dietary protein intake is reduced in children with CKD similar to the reduction in energy intake, the energy intake tends to be critically low (<85% of RDA), whereas the DPI is typically far in excess of the average requirements, ranging from 150% to 200% of the RDA.[31,102] Recommendations are that at least 50% of the total protein intake be from high biological value protein such as milk, eggs, meat, fish, and poultry.[104] Additionally, protein requirements may be increased in patients with proteinuria and during intercurrent illness, and may be adjusted to height age instead of chronological age if evidence of protein deficiency exists.[71]

Acid-Base and Electrolytes

Fluid and electrolyte requirements of children with CKD vary dramatically based on primary kidney disease as well as the degree of residual renal function. This is particularly true when it comes to sodium balance and intravascular volume; children who have CKD due to renal dysplasia or obstructive uropathy often have poor urinary concentrating capacity and are polyuric with substantial urinary sodium losses, even with advanced degrees of CKD. The growth of children with polyuric CKD may be severely limited if ongoing sodium and water losses are not corrected.[105] In contrast, children with primary glomerular CKD, as well as those who have oliguria or anuria, often require both sodium and fluid restriction to minimize fluid gain, edema, and hypertension. According to the most recent dietary guidelines, the sodium intake for children 4 to 8 years of age should be restricted to 1.2 g/day, and to 1.5g/day for those older than 8 years. The sodium intake for those younger than 2 years is 1 to 2 mmol/kg/day.[106] As the majority of sodium (75%) in pediatric diets comes from salt added during food processing, children with CKD should be encouraged to avoid processed food as much as possible.[86] Families should be taught to monitor nutritional sodium intake carefully, and the sodium content of medications may need to be monitored, as well.

Because children have a relatively larger endogenous hydrogen ion load (2 to 3 mEq/kg) compared with adults (1 mEq/kg), metabolic acidosis is a common manifestation of CKD in children and is characteristically present when the estimated GFR falls below 30 mL/min/1.73 m^2 (CKD stage 4). Persistent metabolic acidosis confers worse nutritional outcomes and is associated with increased protein degradation, oxidative damage, and decreased albumin synthesis.[107] Additionally, chronic metabolic acidosis is associated with impaired bone health and abnormal hydroxyapatite integration into bone because the body uses hydroxyapatite as a buffer to bind excess circulating hydrogen ions. Current guidelines recommend that the serum bicarbonate level should be maintained at or above 22 mEq/L by supplementation with oral bicarbonate therapy.[71]

Potassium handling in children with CKD is usually preserved until the GFR falls to less than 10% of normal. However, in children with severe reflux nephropathy, renal dysplasia, postobstructive kidney damage, or interstitial nephritis, renal tubular resistance to aldosterone is often present and may be exacerbated by volume contraction, resulting in hyperkalemia, even when GFR is relatively well preserved. In patients with persistent hyperkalemia, dietary potassium intake should be limited. Because potassium content is challenging for families to identify, assistance from a trained renal dietician may be required to recognize foods with high potassium content. Moderate to severe hyperkalemia may necessitate treatment with potassium binders (e.g., sodium polystyrene sulfonate), and in infants being fed formula, the potassium content of the formula can be reduced by pretreatment with a potassium binder.[108] New agents with improved efficacy and decreased side effect profile are entering the market but are not yet approved for use in pediatric patients.[109] Commonly used medications, such as potassium-sparing diuretics, ACEIs, and calcineurin inhibitors that may cause or exacerbate hyperkalemia, should be monitored.

Vitamins and Micronutrients

Children with CKD are prone to deficiencies of vitamins and micronutrients due to dietary restrictions, poor appetite, and chronic illness; however, they are also at risk of developing toxic levels as GFR declines. Vitamins and minerals are essential for normal growth and development, and either deficiency or excess can be harmful. Unfortunately, the vitamin and mineral needs of pediatric patients with CKD are not clearly defined.

The current KDOQI pediatric nutrition guidelines recommend a dietary intake of at least 100% of the DRI for thiamine (B_1), riboflavin (B_2), niacin (B_3), pantothenic acid (B_5), pyridoxine (B_6), biotin (B_8), cobalamin (B_{12}), ascorbic acid (C), retinol (A), α-tocopherol (E), vitamin K, folic acid, copper, and zinc for children with CKD stages 2 to 5. If dietary intake does not meet DRI, supplementation is recommended.[71] Most infant milk formulas, including Similac PM 60/40, are fortified with both water-soluble and fat-soluble vitamins; therefore the majority of infants with CKD receive the DRI for all vitamins by dietary intake alone and do not require vitamin supplementation. In children with low levels of GFR (stage 5 CKD), the lack of renal clearance of vitamins places children at risk for hypervitaminosis A, and children should receive vitamin A supplementation only if documented to have low levels.[110]

Carnitine

Carnitine is an essential component in the formation of adenosine triphosphate as well as oxidative processing of fatty acids, and the kidney serves as the major site for synthesis in humans.[111] Carnitine deficiency can result in the development of cardiomyopathy, anemia, and muscle weakness. Although there is evidence of carnitine deficiency in both adult and pediatric patients undergoing hemodialysis, there is little information on the carnitine status of children with CKD. Studies in pediatric dialysis patients demonstrated increases in plasma carnitine level after supplementation; however, there was no associated change in symptoms.[112] Currently, there is insufficient evidence to support the routine use of carnitine in either the pediatric CKD or the dialysis patient population.

NEUROCOGNITIVE DEVELOPMENT AND SCHOOL PERFORMANCE

The effect of CKD on cognition and neurological development is an area of growing focus. Historically, a high prevalence of intellectual disability, seizures, and severe impairment was noted in children with CKD. However, with recognition of the effect of malnutrition and aluminum exposure, more favorable outcomes are seen with aggressive nutritional management and minimizing the use of aluminum-containing compounds and binders.[113-115] Although uremia has long been associated with alterations in cognition and may affect neurodevelopmental achievement in children, only recently have studies attempted to discriminate between neurocognitive effects of those with early-stage CKD compared with

ESKD. A broad range of neurological findings are associated with CKD, from seizures and significant intellectual disability to more subtle deficits with poor school performance and academic achievement.

There is growing evidence that children with CKD have an increased risk of neurodevelopmental delays, which appear more frequently in children with younger onset of kidney disease, longer duration of disease, and more severe CKD.[116] Recent data from the CKiD cohort found that although most children with mild to moderate CKD had no major neurocognitive deficits, a substantial percentage (21% to 40%) scored lower on measures of intelligence quotient (IQ), academic achievement, executive functioning, or attention regulation.[117] Subsequent evaluation of this cohort correlates duration of disease with abnormalities in attention regulation and inhibitory control.[118] In a case-control study of 92 subjects between 8 and 25 years of age with CKD stages 2 to 5, children with CKD had lower performance in all neurocognitive domains, with statistically significant differences in attention, memory, and inhibitory control compared with a control population of either siblings or individuals similar in age, gender, and insurance status.[119] Although cognitive function does appear to be affected by uremia (studies show lower IQ among children with CKD compared with their sibling controls),[120] the severity of CKD may influence developmental outcomes, with some studies showing higher scores on neurocognitive testing for toddlers with CKD compared with those with ESKD.[121]

Neurodevelopmental impairment can be minimized by optimizing nutrition, dialysis, and anemia management. Warady and colleagues found that in a group of 19 children with severe CKD requiring peritoneal dialysis (PD) as infants, of those undergoing neurocognitive testing as children (mean age 6.6 ±1.3 years), 79% (15/19) had normal IQ and 94% (15/16) were attending school full-time in age-appropriate classrooms.[115] More recently, Icard and colleagues found significant cognitive improvement in a cohort of children with CKD after transplantation compared with children with CKD without transplantation.[122]

Studies that assess specific aspects of development and neurocognitive function in children with CKD have found impairments in both memory skills and verbal performance, which lead to impairment in academic functioning. Gipson and colleagues evaluated children and adolescents with CKD and found that, compared with controls, children with CKD had significantly lower memory abilities, decreased new learning capacity, and impairments in short-term visual and verbal memory, and were deficient in both initiation and sustaining behaviors within the executive function domain, even after controlling for IQ and age.[123] Because impaired cognition has effects on academic performance, children with CKD are at high risk for difficulties in school. These are likely exacerbated by issues related to quality of life, school absenteeism, depression, and behavioral concerns.[63,124]

Monitoring for developmental delays merits close follow-up. In young children, frequent monitoring of developmental parameters, including head circumference and age-appropriate developmental evaluations, is necessary. A more formal neurodevelopmental assessment should be considered in older children, especially if they have poor school performance. When necessary, educational support systems should be utilized by timely referral to early intervention programs for young children and individualized learning programs for older children.

ANEMIA

Anemia is a near-universal complication of advanced pediatric CKD, with lower levels of GFR associated with lower levels of hemoglobin. Anemia in CKD results in a number of physiological abnormalities, including decreased tissue oxygen delivery, increased cardiac output, ventricular hypertrophy, and congestive heart failure, and appears to result in decreased cognition, abnormal immune responsiveness, and poor quality of life.[125] Although many factors, such as shortened lifespan of red blood cells, inflammation, and iron deficiency, contribute to CKD-associated anemia, the primary etiology is progressive loss of peritubular fibroblast–like interstitial cells that produce erythropoietin.[126] Anemia in both pediatric and adult CKD patients appears to be an important marker of morbidity and mortality,[127] with data from the NAPRTCS study demonstrating that anemia (defined as a hematocrit <33%) 1 month after dialysis initiation was associated with an increased risk of prolonged hospitalization and an estimated 52% greater risk of death.[128] Using the same database, an analysis of more than 2500 children with predialysis CKD (stages 2 through 5a), anemic children (defined as hematocrit <33%) were 55% more likely to be hospitalized compared with nonanemic children (OR = 1.55, 95% CI, 1.23 to 1.94).[129]

Recent evidence suggests that anemia may be an independent risk factor for CKD progression. Proposed mechanisms include kidney tissue hypoxia and cytokine-induced fibrosis. Although most data are in adults, a study among adolescents with predialysis CKD found anemia was associated with an accelerated decline in GFR compared with those with normal hemoglobin levels.[130] Data from NAPRTCS have shown that anemia is an independent risk factor for CKD progression.[129] Erythropoietin trials in adults suggest that improvement in anemia may decrease the risk of CKD progression.[130]

Anemia due to reduced renal erythropoietin production typically develops when GFR declines below 30 mL/min/1.73 m^2. Data from the CKiD study suggest that hemoglobin begins to decline significantly below a GFR of 43 mL/min/1.73 m^2 as measured by iohexol clearance (which is equivalent to a GFR of 58 mL/min/1.73 m^2 when estimated by the Schwartz formula), with a 0.3 g/dL hemoglobin decrease for every 5 mL/min/1.73 m^2 decline in GFR.[131] In that analysis, the prevalence of anemia increased from 18.5% in CKD stage 2 to more than 93% in CKD stage 5.[129,132] Of note, there is a sizable prevalence of anemia even in early-stage CKD, emphasizing that all patients with CKD, regardless of the underlying cause or disease stage, should have their hemoglobin (Hb) checked at least annually.

Defining anemia in children with CKD is complex and requires a nuanced clinical and laboratory evaluation. In adult CKD patients, fixed values (Hb <11 g/dL) have been used to define anemia.[13] Current standards include monitoring by Hb level over hematocrit, because Hb is a stable analyte that is measured directly and is not influenced by differences in measurement or volume status. Although previous versions of the KDOQI pediatric guidelines have applied this adult cut-off to children, this substantially underestimated the prevalence of anemia.[133] In North America, the most recent KDOQI Clinical Practice Guideline and Clinical Practice Recommendations for Anemia in Chronic Kidney Disease changed the threshold for anemia from less than fifth percentile for age and sex to standardized age-based Hb thresholds: 6 months to 5 years <11 g/dL, 5 to 15 years <11.5 g/dL, 12 to 15 years <12 g/dL, and >15 years <13 g/dL (males) and <12 g/dL (females).[13]

Iron deficiency in pediatric CKD is multifactorial and complex. It may be due to absolute iron deficiency from poor dietary intake, increased losses from the gastrointestinal track, or frequent phlebotomy required for disease monitoring. In addition, there is an element of functional iron deficiency due to inadequate iron for erythropoiesis and impaired iron trafficking due to inflammation. Iron status should be assessed by use of serum ferritin and transferrin saturation (TSAT), which is calculated as serum iron × 100 divided by total iron-binding capacity (TIBC) and reflects adequacy of available iron for erythropoiesis. KQODI guidelines suggest that serum ferritin levels >100 ng/mL and TSAT >20% reflect adequate iron stores.[13] However, despite adequate iron stores, children with CKD often have "functional" iron deficiency, which is characterized by the presence of adequate iron stores by conventional criteria but inability to mobilize this iron to support erythropoiesis. Hepcidin, an iron-regulating antimicrobial peptide, appears to play an important role between inflammatory response and the handling of iron for erythropoiesis. Studies have demonstrated that this is mediated through the downregulation of ferroportin, the major transmembrane iron transporter present on the surface of iron-storing cells, leading to degradation and effectively trapping iron in enterocytes and macrophages and making iron unavailable for erythropoiesis.[134,135] As hepcidin is freely filtered at the glomerulus, decreased hepcidin excretion with declining GFR likely contributes to anemia. In a study of 48 children with CKD (stages 2 through 4) and 26 children on dialysis, serum hepcidin levels were significantly higher than levels in healthy controls.[135]

Annual evaluation for anemia in all children with CKD should be performed, regardless of the cause or stage. Once anemia is detected, evaluation should focus on eliminating causes of anemia other than CKD and determining the iron status of the patient. The initial workup should include red blood cell indices (MCV, MCHC, MCH), reticulocyte count, iron parameters to assess stores such as serum iron, TIBC, TSAT, and serum ferritin.[13]

Treatment of CKD-associated anemia was revolutionized in 1986 with the introduction of recombinant human erythropoietin (rHuEPO) therapy.[136] Management of anemia in children with CKD often includes iron supplementation and administration of an erythropoiesis-stimulating agent (ESA). rHuEPO (such as epoetin alpha) may be administered either subcutaneously or intravenously, and it effectively treats anemia in children with predialysis CKD and those on maintenance dialysis.[137] It is important to note that dosing requirements may differ dramatically between children and adults; the recommended starting dose of 150 units/kg/week is based on adult clinical trial data, and data from NAPRTCS demonstrate that young children may need higher doses (ranging from 275 to 350 units/kg/week for infants to 200 to 250 units/kg/week for adolescents).[138,139] This higher dose requirement in the youngest age group may be due to increased clearance of rHuEPO in these patients, which has been speculated to be caused by the presence of nonhematopoietic binding sites for the erythropoietin molecule. Unlike most drug dosing in pediatrics, rHuEPO dose should be based on target hemoglobin level independent of weight, with dose based on hemoglobin deficit.[140] Epoetin alpha is often administered by subcutaneous injection, and although patients on hemodialysis often use intravenous dosing, erythropoietin-alfa is more cost-effective when administered subcutaneously.[141] However, the psychological effect of painful subcutaneous injections is an important consideration when determining the dosing route, and patient reports show that epoetin alpha injections from a multidose vial are less painful than those from preloaded syringes because multidose vials contain benzyl alcohol, which acts as an anesthetic.[142] The 2011 NAPRTCS annual report revealed that 95% of children on PD were administered an ESA by the subcutaneous route as opposed to only 15% of the hemodialysis (HD) population.[143]

Darbepoetin alpha, an erythropoietin analog with a longer half-life than rHuEPO, is an effective alternative with less frequent administration.[144-146] The usual starting dose of darbepoetin is 0.45 ug/kg/week in ESA naïve patients; for those converting from rHuEPO, a conversion dose of 0.25 to 0.75 ug/kg/week for each 200 U of rHuEPO is recommended.[137] A potential limiting factor in the use is reported discomfort associated with administration, which appears to be more than with rHuEPO, which may be due to the buffer used in the dilution.[142]

The second element of anemia management in patients with CKD is iron therapy. It is recommended that iron studies (serum ferritin and TIBC), Hb level, and ESA dose be collectively evaluated to guide iron therapy.[147] Several pediatric studies have shown that the iron supplementation in pediatric CKD patients on ESA therapy allows for a reduction in the ESA dose.[148] Many children with CKD stages 2 to 4 benefit from oral iron therapy, and oral iron is readily available and inexpensive. However, because iron often has limited efficacy due to issues of compliance and poor gastrointestinal absorption, only 28% of children with CKD in the NAPRTCS registry were receiving oral iron therapy.[143] The recommended doses of oral elemental iron range from 2 to 3 mg/kg/day up to 6 mg/kg/day (maximum 300 mg) in 2 to 3 divided doses. Iron administration can be complex for families because it

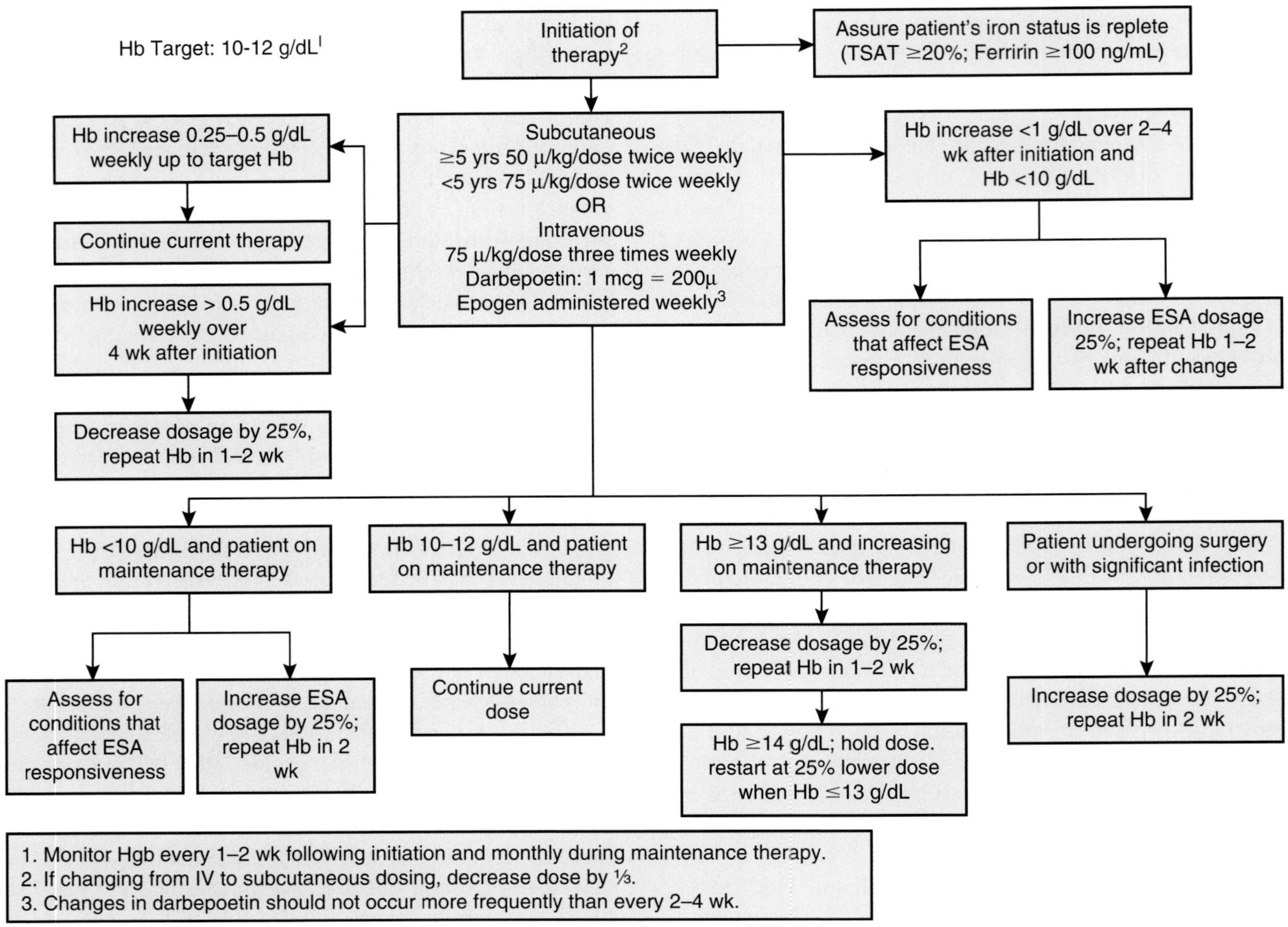

FIG. 6.2 Management of ESA therapy.

must be administered 2 hours before or 1 hour after phosphate binders containing calcium and food to maximize absorption. Despite proper administration, some patients may not tolerate or may fail to respond to oral iron therapy and require intravenous iron. In the setting of functional iron deficiency, children may have levels within target range of both TSAT and ferritin but still benefit from intravenous (IV) iron; therefore occasionally a "trial" of IV iron in an iron-replete anemic patient may be indicated. Monitoring iron status in patients with CKD should be done monthly during initial ESA adjustment and then at every 3 months after a stable ESA treatment regimen has been reached.[148]

With rHuEPO treatment initiation or with changes to dosage, Hb level should be monitored every 1 to 2 weeks, and monitoring intervals changed to monthly when the patient has reached a target Hb level and is on a stable dose of ESA (Fig. 6.2). The goal for the rate of increase in Hb level should be an increase of 1 to 2 g/dL per month.[137] The question of the appropriate hemoglobin target in pediatric CKD remains up for debate, but current recommendations target hemoglobin levels of 10 to 12 g/dL. Many pediatric nephrologists argue that growth, cognitive development, and avoidance of CVD are reasons to target normal hemoglobin levels in children. Decreased response to ESAs is a common issue in children with CKD; more than 20% of children with CKD stage 4 have persistently low hemoglobin despite appropriate ESA treatment. Poor response to ESA therapy can be associated with chronic inflammation, nutritional deficits, inadequate dialysis, chronic blood loss, and hyperparathyroidism.[138] Treatment for decreased ESA responsiveness often involves escalation in ESA dose. However, adult experience over the last 10 years has led to caution in aggressive use of ESA agents. Recent studies in adults (CHOIR and CREATE trials) demonstrated that ongoing ESA escalation to meet a therapeutic Hb target was associated with an increased risk of cardiovascular events and death without improvement in quality of life. In pediatric patients, however, recent studies have shown higher levels of Hb appear to be safe.[149] At this time target Hb levels ≥13 g/dL in children are not recommended due to the uncertain but potentially devastating risk of myocardial infarction or stroke.[141,150]

MINERAL AND BONE DISORDERS

Mineral metabolism abnormalities and bone disease are almost universal complications of CKD. Dysregulation of mineral metabolism leads to complications similar to those in adults (e.g., bone pain, pathological fractures) as well as those unique to children (e.g., growth failure and skeletal deformities).[151] Recent guidelines by KDIGO have called this collection of complications CKD-mineral and bone disorder (CKD-MBD) to define the broad clinical syndrome that develops as a systemic disorder of mineral, skeletal, and vascular abnormalities associated with CKD.[152,153] Changes in homeostatic mechanisms—including disturbances in calcium and phosphate handling, reduced synthesis of active vitamin D, and altered regulation of PTH—lead to the development of CKD-MBD and renal osteodystrophy.[13] Additionally, the accumulation of fibroblast growth factor (FGF-23), secreted by bone-forming osteoblasts, contributes to CKD-BMD through phosphaturic actions that are PTH-independent and inhibition of renal 1α-hydroxylase activity. Abnormalities in FGF-23 appear to be one of the earliest detectable markers in children with CKD. FGF-23 may help maintain normal serum phosphate levels but at the cost of suppressing calcitriol levels and worsening secondary hyperparathyroidism (SHPT). CKD-MBD becomes more significant with advancing CKD. Children with early CKD (stage 2) usually have no symptoms of bone abnormalities; however, laboratory testing may show decreased serum calcitriol (1,25-dihydroxyvitamin D) and elevated PTH.[154] Clinical signs may develop when the GFR falls below 50% (stage 3 CKD), starting with high serum phosphorus levels. Physical findings, including weakness, muscle pain, and long bone abnormalities, are often seen. In a study of children with predialysis CKD, defective mineralization was seen in 29% of children with CKD stage 2 and in 79% of those with CKD stages 4 and 5; abnormal bone turnover was observed in 13% with CKD stage 3 and in 29% of those with CKD stages 4 and 5.[154] Among pediatric patients on dialysis, studies have shown abnormal bone histology in over two-thirds of patients, with low bone turnover states most commonly found.[155]

Renal osteodystrophy is a broad term for bone abnormalities due to CKD. It includes osteitis fibrosa cystica, adynamic bone disease, mixed osteodystrophy, and osteomalacia. These manifestations appear to worsen with the advancement of CKD.[156] Low bone turnover states (adynamic bone disease, osteomalacia) are characterized by low osteoblastic activity and bone formation rates, and they are the most common lesion in children with ESKD on dialysis due to excessive parathyroid gland suppression. Adynamic bone disease increases the risk of fractures and metastatic calcification and should be managed by decreasing or discontinuing calcium-containing therapy and vitamin D supplementation. Osteomalacia is due to increased undermineralized bone due to decreased number of osteoblast and osteoclast cells.

Soft tissue calcification (calcinosis) is a complication that can lead to significant long-term morbidity. Although calcinosis can result in ocular, periarticular, and visceral calcifications, vascular calcifications are the most well studied in regard to the effect on children with CKD. Vascular calcification is increased with both low and high bone turnover states. In low bone turnover, vascular calcification is due to the inability of bone to buffer changes in calcium and phosphate; in high turnover, it is a result of high PTH levels that mobilize calcium and phosphate from bone, increase tubular reabsorption of calcium, and promote gut absorption of calcium and

TABLE 6.4 Target Range of Serum PTH by Stage of CKD

CKD Stage	GFR Range (mL/min/1.73 m^2)	Target Serum PTH (pg/mL)
3	30–59	35–70
4	15–29	70–110
5	<15	200–300

(Adapted from National Kidney Foundation, KDOQI Clinical practice guidelines for bone metabolism and disease in children with chronic kidney disease, *Am. J. Kidney Dis.* 46 (Suppl. 1) (2005) S1–S122.)

phosphate by hydroxylation of 25(OH) Vitamin D_3. Although underlying pathophysiological mechanisms responsible for the vascular calcification that results from CKD-MBD have not yet been fully elucidated, studies have demonstrated a direct correlation between the presence and severity of calcification and the levels of serum phosphorus, PTH, FGF-23, dosages of calcium containing phosphorus binders and calcitriol, and the duration of dialysis.[157] Vascular calcification in CKD is mainly localized in the medial layer of blood vessels (measured by carotid intima-media thickness or CIMT) and appears to be an active cell-mediated process.[158] Recent studies have shown that serum 1,25-dihydroxyvitamin D levels had a U-shaped distribution for vascular calcifications with children with both low and high levels at increased risk for elevated CIMT, as well as an increased risk of increased CIMT in those with PTH levels at twice the upper limit of normal.[159] With the recognition of early-onset coronary artery calcification and increased cardiovascular morbidity in patients with CKD, there has been a shift in the recommended management of mineral and bone disorders.

Current management of CKD-MBD hinges on the concept of achieving an optimum serum PTH for each CKD stage to promote normal bone turnover without increasing the risk for calcification.[13] Although bone biopsy is the gold standard to establish the type of renal osteodystrophy, PTH level is often used as a more accessible marker of bone turnover. The optimum range of PTH in CKD likely changes with the progression of disease due to increasing skeletal resistance to PTH, with higher PTH levels necessary to maintain normal bone turnover (Table 6.4).[160] Only a handful of small studies in children have attempted to identify the range of PTH levels that correlate with normal bone histology, with most of the data generated in the ESKD and not the CKD population.[161] One study of children on peritoneal dialysis found that a PTH of >200 pg/dL and serum calcium <10 mg/dL identified patients with high turnover bone disease with 85% sensitivity and 100% specificity.[162] Both KDOQI and KDIGO provide guidelines on when to consider bone biopsy to assess for high- versus low-turnover bone disease, to determine the type of renal osteodystrophy and to guide therapy.[151,160] Serum levels of calcium, phosphorus, and PTH should be measured routinely in all children with CKD, as early detection helps ensure that therapeutic interventions can be initiated and CKD-MBD effects minimized. The most recent guidelines recommend monitoring of serum calcium and phosphorus levels at least yearly for those with mild CKD and monthly measurements for those with ESKD. Irrespective of the target, PTH level can be manipulated by the control of dietary calcium and phosphate, use of phosphate binders, and judicious utilization of vitamin D and analogs as detailed in the most recent guidelines.[153,160]

Calcium

Achieving a positive calcium balance and ensuring adequate dietary calcium intake in periods of high growth during childhood is essential for appropriate skeletal development and optimization of bone mass, with a goal calcium intake of 100% of the DRI recommendations for pediatric CKD patients.[163] For infants and young children, this can usually be met with breast milk or formula; in older children dairy products serve as one of the largest sources of dietary calcium. However, these foods are also rich in phosphorus, and phosphorus restriction substantially decreases calcium intake. Often, calcium supplementation or calcium-fortified products are required to meet DRI. Calcium can also be supplemented in as calcium-containing medication such as carbonate or acetate salts commonly used as phosphate binders. High calcium intake coupled with excessive activated vitamin D analogs can lead to systemic hypercalcemia, adynamic bone disease, and vascular calcification. Accordingly, the most recent guidelines recommend that the elemental calcium intake from both nutritional sources and phosphate binders not exceed two times the DRI for age, except for ages 9 to 18 years, where two times the DRI (2600 mg) exceeds the tolerable upper intake level (UL) of 2500 mg.[163] Serum calcium and phosphorus product should be kept below 55 mg/dL in adolescents over 12 years and <65 mg/dL in younger children, and total corrected calcium should be maintained within normal range (8.8–9.5 mg/dL), preferably toward the lower end and ideally not more than 10.2 mg/dL.[151]

Phosphorus

Serum phosphorus should be maintained in the normal range in patients with CKD to control associated bone disease because phosphorus is a key component of bone matrix. Phosphorus retention begins early in the course of CKD and is a primary driver in the development of SHPT: first by reduced production of calcitriol and, in more advanced CKD, due to direct effect on parathyroid glands.[98] Even in early CKD with normal serum phosphorus levels, phosphorus dietary intake affects the severity of SHPT. Of note, avoiding deficiencies in phosphorus is equally important, especially in infants and young children, where higher physiological phosphorus concentrations are required for rapidly growing bones and to avoid rickets (Table 6.5).[160] Although studies of children with CKD do not suggest an association between restricted phosphorus intake and poor growth, hypophosphatemia should be avoided due to potential effect on linear growth.[31] The most recently published guidelines suggest that, in children with CKD when serum PTH concentration exceeds the target range and serum phosphorus concentration remains normal, the dietary phosphorus intake should be restricted to 100% of the DRI, and when the serum phosphorus concentration is above the normal range, dietary intake should be restricted to 80% of the DRI.[71] After dietary phosphorus restriction, the serum phosphorus concentration should be monitored every 3 months in children with CKD stages 3 to 4 and monthly for those with CKD stage 5.

TABLE 6.5 Normal Ranges of Calcium and Phosphorus for Age

Age	Total Calcium (mg/dL)	Ionized Calcium (mmol/L)	Phosphorus (mg/dL)
0–5 mo	8.7–11.3	1.22–1.4	5.2–8.4
6–12 mo	8.7–11	1.2–1.4	5.0–7.8
1–5 y	9.4–10.8	1.22–1.32	4.5–6.5
6–12 y	9.4–10.3	1.15–1.32	3.6–5.8
13–20 y	8.8–10.2	1.12–1.3	2.3–4.5

mo, Months, *y*, years.
(Adapted from National Kidney Foundation, KDOQI clinical practice guidelines for bone metabolism and disease in children with chronic kidney disease, *Am. J. Kidney Dis.* 46 (Suppl. 1) (2005) S1–S122.)

Although dietary phosphorus restriction is important, overly strict restriction below the levels may be impractical and can inadvertently lead to poor dietary protein intake.[98] Infants may be managed by a low-phosphorus-containing milk formula such as Similac PM 60/40 (Ross Laboratories, OH); whereas most older CKD patients require oral phosphate binders to control hyperphosphatemia. Notably, for vegetarians phosphorus restriction is especially difficult because phosphorus content is greater in protein derived from vegetable sources (average 20 mg of phosphorus per gram of protein) than animal protein (average 11 mg of phosphorus per gram of protein).[160] Calcium-based phosphate binders are safe and effective in lowering serum phosphate and PTH levels and are recommended as the initial therapeutic choice. Phosphorus binders should be taken 10 to 15 minutes before or during meals; the effect is diminished when taken between meals because phosphorus has already been absorbed. Phosphorus binders have a limited binding capacity and will be effective in lowering levels only if restriction is continued: 1 g of calcium carbonate binds 39 mg of phosphate, 1 g of calcium acetate binds 45 mg of phosphate, and 400 mg of sevelamer binds 32 mg of phosphate.[164] The choice of calcium binder is made based on patient tolerance and clinician preference; there does not seem to be an advantage of one over another. However, the total dose of elemental calcium should not exceed twice the DRI, and calcium citrate should not be used because it increases intestinal aluminum absorption.[160]

Given growing concern that calcium-based binders may contribute to vascular and soft tissue calcification, sevelamer hydrochloride (RenaGel) and sevelamer carbonate (Renvela) are more frequently used as initial therapy.[165] A randomized, open-labeled, crossover study demonstrated that sevelamer was as effective as calcium acetate in reducing serum phosphorus and was associated with a reduction in cholesterol, low-density lipoprotein (LDL) cholesterol, and

TABLE 6.6 Supplementation for Vitamin D Deficiency in Children With CKD

Category	Serum 25-hydroxyvitamin D level	Ergocalciferol or Cholecalciferol dosing	Duration
Severe vitamin D deficiency	<5	8000 International Units (IU) daily enterally x 4 weeks (50,000 IU/week x 4 weeks), then 4000 IU daily (or 50,000 IU every other week) x 2 months	3 mo
Mild vitamin D deficiency	5–15	4000 IU daily enterally x 12 weeks (50,000 IU every other week)	3 mo
Vitamin D insufficiency	16–30	2000 IU daily (50,000 IU every month)	3 mo

(Adapted from National Kidney Foundation, KDOQI clinical practice guidelines for bone metabolism and disease in children with chronic kidney disease, *Am. J. Kidney Dis.* 46 (Suppl. 1) (2005) S1–S122.)

the frequency and severity of hypercalcemia.[164,166] Although aluminum hydroxide and aluminum carbonate were once widely used as phosphate binders, their use has been abandoned (other than on rare occasions for restricted periods of time, and with a closely monitored low dose [<30 mg/kg/day] until more definitive therapy is instituted and effective) because they were found to be associated with severe toxicity in adults and children with renal insufficiency. Pretreatment of breast milk, infant formula, and cow's milk with sevelamer has been shown to effectively reduce the phosphorus content in the supernatant by 80% to 90%. Lanthanum carbonate (Fosrenol), a calcium- and aluminum-free binder with high affinity for phosphorus and minimal intestinal absorption, is also effective in controlling serum phosphorus without inducing hypercalcemia, adynamic bone disease, or osteomalacia; however, it is a heavy metal and accumulates in tissue, so more studies are required before it is recommended for pediatric patients.[167]

Vitamin D

In children with CKD, production of 1, 25-dihydroxyvitamin D (calcitriol) is disrupted due to phosphate retention, low serum 25-hydroxyvitamin D, and increased FGF-23. There is a high prevalence (80% to 90%) of nutritional vitamin D insufficiency in children with CKD. Ali and colleagues reported 20% to 75% prevalence of vitamin D deficiency (defined as a 25-hydroxyvitamin D <15 ng/mL) in children with CKD stages 1 to 5, with higher prevalence rates in Hispanics and African Americans, likely due to increased melanin skin content.[168] Data from the CKiD cohort found that nearly 30% of patients had vitamin D deficiency, with increased prevalence in those with lower daily milk intake, more advanced CKD, nonwhite race, and higher body mass index.[169] Vitamin D appears to have a renoprotective effect, with a post hoc analysis of the ESCAPE trial finding that, in children with renal impairment (mean GFR 51 mL/min/1.73 m^2), serum 25-hydroxyvitamin D levels above 50 nmol/L were associated with greater preservation of GFR than those with levels below 50 nmol/L.[170] Systematic reviews have found that vitamin D therapy improves bone disease and PTH levels regardless of formulation or administration route.[171]

The most recent KDOQI pediatric nutrition guidelines suggest monitoring serum 25-hydroxyvitamin D levels once per year in children with CKD stages 2 to 5. If the serum level of 25-hydroxyvitamin D is <30 ng/mL, supplementation with vitamin D_2 (ergocalciferol) or vitamin D_3 (cholecalciferol) is suggested, with the specific dosing regimen dependent on the severity of the deficiency (Table 6.6). During the treatment phase, laboratory monitoring, including measurement of serum levels of calcium and phosphorus, should be performed 1 month after the initiation or a change in the dose of vitamin D and at least every 3 months thereafter. Once patients are replete, supplemental vitamin D should be continued and levels checked yearly. Recent studies have suggested that cholecalciferol may be more potent than ergocalciferol; however, responsiveness to treatment appears to decline with advancing CKD.[172]

For pediatric CKD patients with normal vitamin D levels (>30 ng/mL) and PTH levels exceeding the target range for the CKD stage, therapy with an active vitamin D agent (calcitriol) or dihydrotachysterol (requires only hepatic activation) is recommended, as long as the serum level of corrected total calcium is <10 mg/dL and the serum level of phosphorus is within normal range.[13] Calcitriol usage increases intestinal phosphorus absorption by 50% and thus may worsen hyperphosphatemia. Calcitriol can be administered either orally or intravenously, with initial doses ranging from 5 to 10 ng/kg/day,[151] and it may be administered daily or intermittently with equivalent efficacy in controlling SHPT.[173] The use of calcitriol in patients with elevated calcium or phosphorus may lead to soft tissue calcification due to increased calcium phosphorus product. Given the concerns about side effects, several newer, noncalcemic vitamin D analogs, such as paricalcitol, alfacalcidol, and doxercalciferol, have been developed to reduce the risk of hypercalcemia and hyperphosphatemia by selectively suppressing the parathyroid gland with a lower incidence of hypercalcemia compared with current agents. These agents have been used successfully in children.[174] In adults, calcimimetic agents such as cinacalcet can be used to suppress PTH secretion and decrease the risk of hypercalcemia associated with calcitriol, by increasing the sensitivity of the calcium-sensing receptor in the parathyroid gland to ionized calcium; these agents can also be used to treat hyperparathyroidism. Although anecdotal experience in children does exist, cinacalcet has not been approved for use in children. We anticipate more evidence should be forthcoming, given that a recent open-label study of its dosing in pediatric ESKD patients showed it was effective and well tolerated without any significant adverse effects.[175]

CARDIOVASCULAR DISEASE

Historically, atherosclerotic disease and CVD were thought to be complications isolated to adults with CKD, where rates of mortality and morbidity greatly exceed the general population.[176,177] However, growing evidence shows that not only do atherogenic deposits begin to form in childhood, but that children with CKD likely have years of accelerated atherosclerosis during their childhood and young adult years.[178] Although overall mortality rates in pediatric patients with ESKD have improved dramatically, the mortality rates are still 30 times higher than the general pediatric population and CVD is the most common cause of death.[179] Children with CKD have an extremely high prevalence of both traditional (e.g., hypertension and hyperlipidemia) and CKD-related (e.g., anemia, malnutrition, chronic inflammation, and hyperparathyroidism) cardiovascular risk factors, and the combination of risk factors initiates and accelerates CVD in the pediatric CKD patients.

The pathophysiology of CVD in CKD is characterized by two separate processes: vascular injury and cardiac remodeling. Vascular injury, including atherosclerosis, begins with lipid-containing foam cells (macrophages) entering the vascular intima, followed by the accumulation of smooth muscle cells and collagen fibers and formation of plaques or atheromas, which then result in local stenosis and occlusion.[180] Arteriosclerosis, on the other hand, results in arterial stiffening involving the entire arterial tree, especially elastic arteries, and leads to both intimal and medial thickening, leading to increased vascular-wall thickness and lumen enlargement.[181] CVD in children with CKD develops early in the course of CKD and becomes more severe as CKD progresses; surrogate markers of CVD include measurements of carotid intima media thickness (IMT) and endothelial dysfunction.[182] This results in increased systolic blood pressure and pulse pressure. There appears to be a direct correlation between the severity of vascular calcification and markers of CKD-MBD, including phosphorus, calcium-phosphorus product, and PTH, as well as the duration of dialysis.[157]

Cardiac remodeling involves both concentric and eccentric left ventricular hypertrophy (LVH), with concentric changes due to increased resistance from hypertension, and eccentric changes from volume overload and anemia. LVH is defined as a left ventricular mass (LVM) index greater than the 95th percentile for age, and can be assessed with echocardiography. Approximately one-third of children with mild to moderate CKD have an increased LVM index. LVH develops early during mild to moderate CKD and progresses with worsening kidney function. In a longitudinal study of 31 pediatric subjects with CKD stages 2 to 4, Mitsnefes and colleagues showed that a substantial proportion (19%) of children had a significant increase in the LVM index, and 32% of the patients who initially had a normal LVM index developed LVH over the study period.[183] Similar to adults, pediatric CKD studies have demonstrated a significant association between low hemoglobin levels and an increased LVM index.[184] Elevation of PTH levels has been associated with the progression of LVH in children with CKD, which may be due to direct effect of PTH on cardiomyocytes and/or indirect effect through elevated BP.[178] Although in adults systolic dysfunction is frequently associated with early cardiac failure and mortality, in children with CKD systolic function is often preserved, whereas diastolic dysfunction is often the initial abnormality; the clinical significance of this is unclear.[185]

In addition to these unique CKD-associated risk factors, the severity of CVD in children with CKD appears to be influenced by conventional CVD risk factors such as hypertension and dyslipidemia; in children receiving dialysis, hyperparathyroidism, hyperphosphatemia, and treatment with calcium-containing phosphate binders are major determinants.[181]

Hypertension

The National High Blood Pressure Education Program Working Group (NHBPEP) defines hypertension as either systolic and/or diastolic blood pressure greater than or equal to the 95th percentile measured on three or more occasions. Hypertension is highly prevalent in children with CKD, even in early stages of the disease, and increases with incremental decline in GFR. Data from CKiD report a prevalence rate for hypertension of 47% in children with GFR between 30 and 90 mL/min/1.73 m^2, with only a third of patients receiving antihypertensive therapy.[35] In that cohort, hypertension was more common in African American children, even after adjustment for age, cause, and duration of CKD, and antihypertensive use. In another study using CKiD data, 38% of children with CKD had masked hypertension (defined as normal office blood pressure but elevated ambulatory blood pressure) and 18% had confirmed hypertension.[186] Among children with ESKD, hypertension was observed in two-thirds of a cohort of patients 6 months after initiation of dialysis, despite the use of antihypertensive agents.[187] These studies suggest that underdiagnoses and inadequate treatment of blood pressure in children with CKD is quite common.

Recommendations for the evaluation and treatment of risk factors in children with CKD have primarily been derived from adult data and expert opinion, and they focus on addressing traditional risk factors such as hypertension and dyslipidemia. Several studies suggest that ambulatory blood pressure monitoring (ABPM) may serve as a better means of predicting end-organ injury than office blood pressure measurement in children with CKD.[188] ABPM may be a helpful adjuvant tool to evaluate blood pressure in children with CKD when consistent blood pressure data are difficult to obtain, or to evaluate the efficacy of antihypertensive therapy in difficult to control hypertension. Findings from two recent studies in pediatric CKD cohorts suggest that ABPM may provide important data. In a report from the CKiD study, ABPM data resulted in normal blood pressure categorization for 42%, masked hypertension in 35%, ambulatory hypertension in 14%, and white-coat hypertension in 4%.[189]

Additionally, children with CKD appear to have higher systolic and diastolic blood pressure variability and lower heart rate variability, which is thought to be a precursor for cardiovascular morbidity in adults.[190] Given these data, the most recent guidelines suggest the use of ABPM to assess blood pressure and monitor treatment in children with CKD.[191]

In children with CKD, recommendations from both NHBPEP and KDOQI for target blood pressure are below the 90th percentile based on age, gender, and height of the patient or <120/80 mmHg, whichever is lower.[137,192] Recent data from the ESCAPE trial suggest that more aggressive blood pressure control (defined as blood pressures below the 50th percentile) slows the progression of CKD; children in the intensified blood pressure control group were less likely to develop ESKD compared with those in the conventional blood pressure control group.[36] Similar data from the CKiD study also found that elevated office blood pressures may predict quicker decline in GFR.[22] Based on the ESCAPE trial findings, KDIGO guidelines target blood pressure goals of less than or equal to the 50th percentile for age, sex, and height. New guidelines published in 2017 endorse stricter blood pressure goals, targeting a 24-hour mean arterial pressure (MAP) of less than the 50th percentile based on ABPM.[13,191]

Therapy for hypertension in CKD includes both nonpharmacologic and pharmacologic interventions. Conservative measures such as aerobic exercise, weight reduction, and dietary restriction should be the first step in treatment, with KDIGO guidelines recommending hypertensive children with CKD be restricted to the age-based dietary sodium intake (1.2 g/day for children 4 to 8 years and 1.5 g/day for older children).[13,192] ACEIs and ARBs, which act to interrupt the RAS, are recommended as first-line agents for the management of hypertension in CKD.[193] RAS antagonists appear to offer better preservation of kidney function than other antihypertensive agents, especially in those with proteinuria. Several large studies, including the ESCAPE trial, demonstrated slower progression of CKD in patients on treatment,[36] and secondary analysis of CKiD study data showed that there was an association between ACE inhibition and improved blood pressure control.[35]

Other classes of antihypertensive therapy such as calcium-channel blockers (CCBs) and diuretic therapy can be used in pediatric CKD. CCBs are safe and effective antihypertensive agents in patients with CKD; however, CCBs of the dihydropyridine type (e.g., amlodipine, nifedipine) have been shown to increase proteinuria and have been associated with poorer outcomes in large adult trials compared with RAS antagonists.[193] Diuretic therapy may be indicated in children with early stages of CKD to address the sodium and fluid overload that may be present. Thiazide diuretics may be used in patients with earlier stages of CKD, but they become less effective monotherapy as GFR declines to less than 30 mL/min/1.73 m^2.[193] Other classes of antihypertensive therapy, such as beta blockers, α-adrenergic, and direct vasodilators, may also be considered depending on their efficacy and side effect profile in the individual patient.

Lipids

The prevalence of dyslipidemias in children with CKD is high (39% to 65%) and varies based on the etiology of CKD (more common in glomerular disease), degree of proteinuria, and duration of CKD.[7,194] In children with CKD, the most common dyslipidemia is hypertriglyceridemia, with an inverse relationship between renal function and serum triglycerides and total cholesterol levels.[7] Dyslipidemia becomes more frequent with more severe stages of CKD; hypercholesterolemia and hypertriglyceridemia have been reported in 69% and 90% of children with CKD stage 3 and stage 5, respectively. The pattern of dyslipidemia seen in CKD has been labeled "atherogenic," and the potential effect of dyslipidemia is profound, because elevated lipid levels are an independent risk factor for CVD. The Pathobiological Determinants of Atherosclerosis in Youth (PDAY) study demonstrated that children can develop fatty streaks during adolescence that may quickly progress to atheromatous plaques during early adulthood.[178,195]

Although data regarding CVD risk in pediatric CKD populations remain lacking, multiple large adult studies demonstrate that the mortality rate due to CVD in adults with ESKD is 10- to 20-fold higher than the general population. In adult patients with CKD, statins have been shown to reduce both serum lipid levels and the incidence of CVD.[196] The American Heart Association (AHA) classifies children with CKD as a high-risk pediatric patient population due to their high risk of CVD.[181]

Despite the strong association between dyslipidemia and CVD, the optimal management in children with CKD remains unclear. The American Academy of Pediatrics (AAP), AHA, KDIGO, and an expert panel sponsored by the National Heart, Lung, and Blood Institute (NHLBI) all published guidelines with recommendations for dyslipidemia management in CKD. Although most of the guidelines focus on adult patients, several pediatric recommendations were made by all groups.[197] All guidelines recommend that children with CKD be screened for dyslipidemia, with the 2013 KDIGO clinical practice guidelines suggesting that children with CKD have a fasting lipid profile obtained annually, because growth and development may influence lipid levels.[198] In all children with CKD, measures to prevent and manage dyslipidemia include diet and daily exercise (therapeutic lifestyle changes or TLC), with more restricted dietary modifications suggested for those with ESKD or severe hypertriglyceridemia. Studies suggest that in children with CKD, correction of metabolic acidosis, vitamin D therapy, and treatment of anemia with erythropoietin each have a normalizing effect on dyslipidemia.[199,200] Additionally, fish oil has been shown to reduce hypertriglyceridemia in two small studies of children with ESKD and renal transplantation, and there are limited reports of statin usage in children with nephrotic syndrome.[201,202]

Although the 2013 KDIGO guidelines do not recommend statin treatment in children with CKD under age 10 years, the group does note that statin initiation may be considered on a case-by-case basis for boys older than 10 years and postmenarchal girls with severe LDL elevation.[198] The use of lipid-lowering drugs such as statins should be considered in selected patients, such as in adolescents with stage 5 CKD if LDL cholesterol is ≥160 mg/dL, as well as those whose LDL cholesterol remains above 130 mg/dL after a trial of TLC. Although the efficacy and safety of statins have been demonstrated in short-term studies, long-term data are required before statins can be recommended for use in all children. An adolescent who begins stain therapy will receive a higher total dose over their lifetime than most adults; the effect of this cumulative dose is unclear.[203] Although clinical trials in adolescents have not demonstrated adverse effects of statin therapy on growth, pubertal development, myopathy, or rhabdomyolysis, they may have been too short in duration and underpowered to detect such effects. Additionally, because statins are potent teratogens, adolescents prescribed statin therapy must be educated about effective birth control. Despite their frequent usage in adults, there is insufficient evidence to support the regular, long-term usage of the standard lipid-lowering therapies such as statins in children of all ages.

QUALITY OF LIFE AND TRANSITIONS TO ADULTHOOD

Like any pediatric chronic disease, CKD affects the quality of life for children and their families.[204] A survey of families with children with mild to moderate CKD (mean GFR of 42.5 mL/min/1.73 m^2) found an overall low health-related quality of life and lower scores compared with healthy peers in all four measured domains: physical, emotional, social, and school.[62] Social stressors and psychological difficulties are common in children with CKD. The normal progression from childhood to independence is impeded, and achievement of normal childhood and adolescent developmental milestones is often delayed or impaired, both in those with early-stage CKD and in those with ESKD.[205] Depression and poor self-esteem are more common in children with CKD than their age-matched peers.[206] In the CKiD cohort, 5% of children had depressive symptoms and another 2% were being treated for depression, and these patients had lower quality-of-life and achievement scores.[207]

The negative effect of chronic disease also extends to parents and siblings.[208] Siblings of children with CKD often have negative emotional consequences; they may feel neglected due to the care required by their sibling while simultaneously feeling conflicting emotions regarding their sibling's disease. Studies have demonstrated that parents of children with CKD and ESKD experience depression and posttraumatic stress disorder at much higher rates than the general population.[206]

These challenges appear to continue into adulthood, where patients with childhood ESKD are more likely than their age-matched peers to be unemployed and to have lower income and lower quality-of-life scores.[206,209] Employment security appears to be a major concern, given ongoing medical issues in this population.[210] Optimal management of these psychosocial stressors should involve a multidisciplinary team, including social workers and mental health specialists, to proactively screen for these psychosocial concerns and address them early.

Transition of care from pediatric to adult care for children with CKD is a challenging task, requiring complex care coordination by a multidisciplinary team as well as increased autonomy and disease self-management by the patient.[211] Transitions of care are a particularly high-risk time for children with chronic disease, with increased risk of complications, nonadherence, and poor outcomes.[212] Although disease-specific interventions have been implemented to aid transitions from pediatric to adult medicine, this area is becoming an important focus to improve the care and long-term outcomes of children with CKD.

A full list of references is available at www.expertconsult.com.

7

Genetic Causes of Chronic Kidney Disease

Gentzon Hall, MD, PhD

OUTLINE

INTRODUCTION

Chronic kidney disease (CKD) is a global public health burden affecting an estimated 10% of the world population. It is a major cause of morbidity and mortality as all stages of CKD are associated with increased risks of death and cardiovascular disease, in addition to end-stage kidney disease (ESKD). CKD can be caused by multiple factors including genetic diseases. This chapter will discuss the genetics of two major causes of CKD and review therapeutic options for the treatment of inherited kidney diseases.

NEPHROTIC SYNDROME

Nephrotic syndrome (NS) is the most common glomerular disease in children and adults.[1] The annual incidence of idiopathic NS is estimated to be 7/100,000 in children and 3/100,000 in adults.[2,3] Clinically, NS is characterized by proteinuria, hypoalbuminemia, peripheral edema, and hyperlipidemia. NS is considered to be a manifestation of multiple pathologic processes affecting the glomerular epithelial cell (i.e., podocyte), slit diaphragm, and glomerular basement membrane.[4] NS can manifest in utero or in the early postnatal period as with congenital NS of the Finnish type (CNF)[5] or later in life with pathologic findings consistent with focal segmental glomerulosclerosis (FSGS).[4] NS is broadly classified as steroid-sensitive (SSNS) or steroid-resistant (SRNS) based on the clinical response to corticosteroid treatment. Classically, 80% to 90% of cases in the pediatric age group are steroid sensitive and are therefore classified as SSNS. The remaining 10% to 20% are called SRNS and it is estimated that nearly 30% of these cases are caused by single-gene (i.e., monogenic) defects.[6] SRNS is more prevalent in adults and most commonly manifests with the pathological lesions of FSGS.[7] SRNS is estimated to account for 15% of CKD cases.[8] For reasons that remain unclear, the incidence of FSGS has increased more than 10-fold over the past three decades, and some believe that up to 18% of FSGS cases are caused by hereditary disorders.[9]

Autosomal Recessive Diseases

Congenital Nephrotic Syndrome

Monogenic causes of NS vary with respect to the timing of disease onset and the response to therapy based on the effects of the genetic mutation and the mode of inheritance.[7] Autosomal recessive glomerular diseases typically manifest early in life, whereas autosomal dominant diseases manifest in the adolescent or adult years. CNF is a rare autosomal recessive glomerular disease with an incidence of 1 in 8000 live births in Finland.[10] CNF can be seen worldwide but occurs less frequently in non-Finnish populations.[11] First described by Ahvenainen et al. in 1956, CNF is characterized by massive proteinuria, edema, hypoalbuminemia, and hyperlipidemia at or shortly after birth.[5] The kidneys of affected children typically exhibit cystic dilation of the proximal tubules and diffuse mesangial sclerosis (DMS), which can be observed by light microscopy and podocyte foot process effacement with loss of the slit diaphragm by electron microscopy.[12] CNF is caused by mutations in Nephrin (*NPHS1*), a critical component of the glomerular slit diaphragm that is expressed by podocytes (Table 7.1).[13] Nephrin is composed of a short intracellular domain, a single-pass transmembrane domain and an extracellular domain containing eight immunoglobulin G–like domains and one fibronectin type III–like module.[14] The intracellular domain has been shown to interact with other key slit diaphragm proteins such as CD2-associated protein (CD2AP) and podocin (NPHS2) to modulate cell-survival signaling and actin cytoskeletal dynamics through the phosphoinositol-3 kinase (PI-3K) and mitogen-activated protein kinase (MAPK) signaling pathways.[15-17] The extracellular domain

TABLE 7.1 **Congenital Nephrotic Syndrome of the Finnish Yype and Autosomal Recessive Steroid-Resistant Nephrotic Syndrome**

Gene	Protein	Affected Podocyte Compartment	Clinical Presentation	Histologic Features	Mechanism of Disease
NPHS1	Nephrin	Slit diaphragm	CNF, resistant to conventional therapy, transplant is the only option	Cystic dilation of proximal tubules and DMS	Disruption of the podocyte slit diaphragm
NPHS2	Podocin	Slit diaphragm	Disease manifests in childhood, variable clinical presentation, resistant to corticosteroids	Ranges from MCN to FSGS	Disruption of the podocyte slit diaphragm
CD2AP	CD2AP	Slit diaphragm	Disease manifests in the first year of life, resistant to corticosteroids	FSGS	Disruption of the podocyte slit diaphragm
CRB2	CRB2	Slit diaphragm	Disease manifests in childhood, resistant to corticosteroids	FSGS	Disruption of the podocyte slit diaphragm
MAGI2	MAGI2	Slit diaphragm	Disease manifests in the early postnatal period, resistant to corticosteroids	CNS and MCN	Disruption of the podocyte slit diaphragm
NUP107	NUP107	Nuclear pore	Disease manifests in childhood, resistant to corticosteroids	FSGS	Impaired nucleocytoplasmic translocation of proteins, RNAs, and ribonuclear particles
NUP93	NUP93	Nuclear pore	Disease manifests in childhood, resistant to corticosteroids	FSGS	Impaired nucleocytoplasmic translocation of proteins, RNAs, and ribonuclear particles; dysregulated SMAD4 signaling
NUP205	NUP205	Nuclear pore	Disease manifests in childhood, resistant to corticosteroids	FSGS	Impaired nucleocytoplasmic translocation of proteins, RNAs, and ribonuclear particles
XP05	Exportin 5	Nuclear pore	Disease manifests in childhood, resistant to corticosteroids	FSGS	Impaired nucleocytoplasmic translocation of proteins, RNAs, and ribonuclear particles; dysregulated SMAD4 signaling
WT1	WT1	Nucleus	Disease manifests in childhood, resistant to corticosteroids	DMS and FSGS	Impaired transactivation of various podocyte-enriched genes
ADCK4	ADCK4	Mitochondria	Disease manifests in the early postnatal period through adulthood, can reverse some symptoms of disease with CoQ10 supplementation	FSGS	Impaired CoQ10 biosynthesis
COQ2	COQ2	Mitochondria	Disease manifests in the early postnatal period, can reverse some symptoms of disease with CoQ10 supplementation	FSGS, collapsing glomerulopathy, crescentic glomerulonephritis	Impaired CoQ10 biosynthesis
Myo1e	Myo1e	Actin cytoskeleton	Disease manifests in childhood, resistant to steroids, partial remission with cyclosporine A in some patients	FSGS	Impaired organization of actin filaments
ARHGDIA	ARHGDI-α	Actin cytoskeleton	Disease onset in the early postnatal period through early childhood, resistant to corticosteroids	DMS	Dysregulated actin cytoskeletal dynamics
KANK4	KANK4	Actin cytoskeleton	Disease onset in the early postnatal period, resistant to corticosteroids	FSGS	Dysregulated actin cytoskeletal dynamics
PLCε1	PLCε1	Actin cytoskeleton	Disease manifests in early childhood; partial remission possible with cyclosporine A in some patients	DMS and FSGS	Dysregulated actin cytoskeletal dynamics
GLEPP1	GLEPP1	Actin cytoskeleton	Disease manifests in childhood through early adolescence; partial remission with immunosuppression and ACE inhibition	MCN and FSGS	Dysregulated actin cytoskeletal dynamics
TTC21B	TTC21B	Microtubules	Disease manifests in the first through the fourth decade of life, resistant to corticosteroids	FSGS or MCN with severe tubulointerstitial lesions	Dysregulated microtubular dynamics
CFH	CFH	Glomerular basement membrane	Disease manifests in childhood through adolescence, resistant to corticosteroids; may be responsive to factor H replacement (i.e., fresh frozen plasma)	MPGN type II (DDD)	Impaired suppression of complement-mediated damage to the glomerular basement membrane

CNF, Congenital nephrotic syndrome of the Finnish type; *CNS*, congenital nephrotic syndrome; *DDD*, dense deposit disease; *DMS*, diffuse mesangial sclerosis; *FSGS*, focal segmental glomeris a critical component of the slit diaphragm, involved in homodimeric interactions between adjacent foot processes and heteromultimeric assemblies with proteins such as Neph 1 and Ephrin-B1.[18-20] The most common mutations in nephrin, Fin-major and Fin-minor, account for 90% to 95% of CNF, but more than 180 other nephrin mutations have been reported.[21] In addition, nephrin mutations have also been shown to cause childhood- and adult-onset SRNS.[22,23] Renal biopsies in these patients can show mesangioproliferative lesions, minimal-change nephropathy (MCN), or FSGS without the characteristic tubular lesions of CNF.[22]

Patients with CNF do not respond to cytotoxic therapy or corticosteroids (see Table 7.1). For patients with the Fin-major mutation, which results in a total absence of nephrin protein expression, nephrectomy may be considered to manage overwhelming daily urinary protein losses.[24] For less severe nephrin mutations, some reports suggest that dual therapy with angiotensin-converting enzyme (ACE) inhibitors and nonsteroidal antiinflammatory drugs (NSAIDs) alone or in combination with unilateral nephrectomy may be of benefit in controlling proteinuria.[25,26] Ultimately, renal transplantation is the only curative therapy for CNF; however, disease recurrence has been reported in nephrin-naïve patients (i.e., homozygous Fin-major genotype) who have developed antinephrin antibodies.[27-29]

Corticosteroid-Resistant Nephrotic Syndrome

The slit diaphragm. Over the past three decades, more than 50 genetic causes of SRNS have been identified.[7] Because these disease-causing mutations have been identified predominantly in genes expressed by podocytes, these terminally differentiated epithelial cells of the glomerular filtration barrier have emerged as central to disease pathogenesis. Podocytes synthesize various components of the slit diaphragm.[30] Pathogenic mutations in *NPHS2,* the gene that encodes the slit diaphragm protein Podocin, have been found in 40% of familial (i.e., autosomal recessive) and 6% to 17% of sporadic SRNS.[31,32] Affected individuals typically manifest with nephrotic-range proteinuria and rapid progression to ESKD. Histologic findings vary on the spectrum of MCN to FSGS (see Table 7.1).[31] Podocin is a hairpin-shaped transmembrane protein that is expressed by podocytes.[33] Podocin is a lipid raft-associated protein that localizes to podocyte foot processes and participates in various intracellular signaling processes through recruitment of other slit diaphragm proteins such as nephrin and CD2AP.[33] Disease-causing podocin mutations most commonly manifest in children between 3 months and 5 years of age but can also manifest later in life.[34-37] The age of disease onset can vary with the specific podocin mutation. Patients who are homozygous for the *R138Q* mutation or who have a heterozygous truncating mutation manifest disease at ~2 years of age, whereas patients with two missense podocin mutations will manifest disease at ~5 years of age.[36] In addition, adult-onset FSGS has been reported in patients who are compound heterozygotes for the *R229Q* podocin mutation and a second mutant NPHS2 allele.[35,37]

CD2-associated protein (CD2AP) is a multifunctional scaffolding protein that links membrane proteins to the cytoskeleton.[38] CD2AP is an essential component of the glomerular slit diaphragm that participates in the regulation of actin cytoskeletal dynamics[39,40] and is involved in various aspects of podocyte motility and survival signaling through interactions with proteins such as nephrin, podocin, anillin, and the p85 subunit of PI-3K.[15,41,42] Disease-causing mutations in CD2AP can cause both autosomal dominant and autosomal recessive SRNS but are exceedingly rare (see Table 7.1).[43-45] Pathogenic *CD2AP* mutations have also been associated with sporadic FSGS.[46] Individuals with autosomal recessive SRNS manifest disease within the first year of life and show FSGS on renal biopsy.[45] In mice, targeted deletion of *cd2ap* induced congenital nephrotic syndrome (CNS).[47]

Mutations in crumbs homolog 2 (CRB2) have also been found to cause SRNS.[48] CRB2 is a conserved regulator of epithelial cell polarity that is highly expressed in podocytes.[49] CRB2 is a transmembrane protein that is involved in podocyte foot process arborization, slit diaphragm formation, and nephrin trafficking.[50] Individuals with pathogenic *CRB2* mutations manifest disease between 3 and 9 years of age and show histology consistent with FSGS (see Table 7.1).[48] Targeted deletion of *crb2b* in zebrafish induced edema, foot process effacement, irregular podocyte morphology, and impaired apical basal patterning in podocytes.[48]

Mutations in membrane-associated guanylate kinase, WW, and PDZ domain-containing 2 (MAGI2) have also been reported to cause familial and sporadic CNS.[51] Patients with pathogenic *MAGI2* mutations manifest disease in the first few months of life and show the histologic lesions of late-stage CNS and MCN on renal biopsy (see Table 7.1).[51] MAGI2 is a multifunctional adaptor protein that is highly expressed in podocytes.[52] MAGI2 interacts with nephrin in a heteromultimeric protein complex at the slit diaphragm and participates in the regulation of intracellular signaling and actin cytoskeletal dynamics.[52,53] Patients with disease-causing *MAGI2* mutations showed reduced and irregular glomerular nephrin and MAGI2 staining.[51]

The nuclear compartment. Mutations in a variety of genes encoding nuclear pore proteins (NUPs) and karyopherins cause autosomal recessive SRNS.[54,55] NUPs are a diverse group of almost 30 structural proteins that assemble within the bileaflet nuclear membrane to form channels known as *nuclear pore complexes* (NPCs).[56] In humans, each NPC has a molecular mass of 120 to 125 MDa and is composed of 500 to 1000 NUPs.[56] These complex macromolecular assemblies negotiate a broad array of functions including nucleocytoplasmic transport, chromatin organization, regulation of gene expression, and DNA repair.[56] Karyopherins, also known as *importins* or *exportins,* are a superfamily of nuclear transport receptors that facilitate the translocation of proteins, RNAs, and ribonuclear particles across the NPC in a Ran GTP hydrolase-dependent process.[57] In 2015 pathogenic mutations in *NUP107* were reported to cause early-onset SRNS.[55] Affected individuals ranged in age from 2 to 11 years at disease onset and all show findings consistent with FSGS on renal biopsy (see Table 7.1).[55] In vivo, the targeted knockdown of *NUP107* in zebrafish induced glomerular hypoplasia and irregular podocyte foot process architecture.[55] In vitro, the heterozygous D831A mutation, which was common to all the affected individuals in a small Korean cohort, impaired NUP107 binding to NUP133 and disrupted the localization of NUP107 to the NPC.[55] Subsequently, the frequency of biallelic *NUP107* mutations in a small cohort of Korean children with SRNS was determined to be 44.4% in familial cases and 4.3% in sporadic cases.[58]

Further evidence for the role of NUPs in the pathobiology of SRNS was provided in 2016 with the identification of novel disease-causing mutations in *NUP93*, *NUP205*, and *exportin 5* (*XP05*).[54] Affected individuals manifest disease between 1 and 6 years of age and the predominant histologic finding on renal biopsy was FSGS (see Table 7.1).[54] *NUP93* knockdown attenuated basal podocyte motility and proliferation, increased podocyte apoptosis and impaired NUP205 recruitment to the NPC.[54] Reciprocally, the pathogenic NUP205 mutation abrogated NUP93 binding.[54] Disease-causing NUP93 mutations impaired the assembly of intact NPCs, disrupted the interaction of NUP93 and *XP05* with the transcriptional regulator SMAD4 and attenuated SMAD4 transcriptional activity.[54] Disruptions in podocyte SMAD signaling are proposed as a potential mechanism of disease in these patients (see Table 7.1).

Wilms' tumor 1 (WT1) is widely recognized for its multifaceted role in the pathobiology of renal disease.[59] WT1 is a zinc-finger transcription factor that regulates the expression of a variety of genes that regulate podocyte function, viability, and differentiation.[60,61] Mutations in *WT1* can occur de novo or be inherited in an autosomal dominant or autosomal recessive fashion.[59] Pathogenic mutations cause syndromic and nonsyndromic disease.[59] Mutations associated with isolated SRNS most commonly occur in exons 8 and 9, which encode zinc-finger domains 2 and 3, respectively.[62] Affected individuals with isolated autosomal recessive SRNS mutation manifest disease in early in childhood and the predominant histologic finding was DMS; however, FSGS can also be seen (see Table 7.1).[62-64]

The mitochondria. Mutations in genes involved in the coenzyme Q10 (CoQ10) biosynthetic pathway cause syndromic and nonsyndromic forms of autosomal recessive SRNS.[65-68] CoQ10 is an essential lipophilic antioxidant required for proper functioning of the mitochondrial electron transport chain. CoQ10 deficiency has been demonstrated to cause mitochondrial depolarization and increased apoptosis in podocytes.[66] Pathogenic mutations in the aarF domain-containing kinase 4 (*ADCK4*), an enzyme involved in CoQ10 biosynthesis, cause nonsyndromic autosomal recessive SRNS.[69] Affected individuals manifest disease between <1 and 21 years of age and FSGS was the predominant histologic lesion on renal biopsy (see Table 7.1).[69] ADCK4 is expressed in podocytes and localizes to mitochondria and foot processes.[69] ADCK4 was found to interact with other enzymes of the CoQ10 biosynthetic pathway and individuals with disease-causing mutations were found to have reduced serum levels of CoQ10.[69] Knockdown of *adck4* caused nephrosis and podocyte foot process effacement in zebrafish.[69] Further, *ADCK4* knockdown in podocytes reduced podocyte motility; however, this effect was reversible with administration of CoQ10.[69]

Pathogenic mutations in the Coenzyme Q2 *COQ2* gene have also been identified as causes of syndromic and nonsyndromic SRNS.[65,67,70] COQ2 is an enzyme in the CoQ10 biosynthetic pathway that catalyzes prenylation of parahydroxybenzoate, the second step in the final reaction sequence of CoQ biosynthesis.[71] Affected individuals manifest disease in the first few months of life and renal histology can show features of classical FSGS, collapsing glomerulopathy, or crescentic glomerulonephritis (see Table 7.1).[67] Electron microscopy can show a "wrinkled and folded" glomerular basement membrane and hyperplastic podocytes populated with numerous dysmorphic mitochondria.[67]

Corticosteroid-resistant nephrotic syndrome is the hallmark renal injury of primary CoQ10 deficiency.[72] It is often the initial manifestation of disease and can present as isolated kidney involvement or in association with other conditions such as encephalopathy, hypertrophic cardiomyopathy, retinopathy, optic atrophy, or sensorineural hearing loss.[72] The genetic diagnosis of primary CoQ10 deficiency is made with identification of biallelic pathogenic variants in one of the nine genes encoding proteins directly involved in the synthesis of coenzyme Q10 (i.e., *COQ2*, *COQ4*, *COQ6*, *COQ7*, *COQ8A*, *COQ8B [ADCK4]*, *COQ9*, *PDSS1*, and *PDSS2*).[72] Early diagnosis and treatment with high-dose oral CoQ10 supplementation (ranging from 5 to 50 mg/kg/day) have been shown to limit disease progression and reverse some manifestations; however, established severe kidney and/or neurologic damage cannot be reversed by CoQ10 supplementation.[72] ACE inhibitors may be used in combination with CoQ10 supplementation in persons with proteinuria and kidney transplantation is an option for those with ESKD.[72]

The actin cytoskeleton. The actin cytoskeleton plays a critical role in the regulation of podocyte size, shape, and adhesion.[73] Monogenic causes of SRNS that effect actin-associated proteins or regulators of actin cytoskeletal dynamics are well described and have greatly informed our understanding of the essential role of the actin cytoskeleton in podocyte function. Myosin 1e (*Myo1e*) is a long-tail, class I (nonmuscle) myosin that participates in the organization of actin filaments at lamellipodia and filopodia to facilitate cell motility.[74] Disease-causing mutations in *Myo1e* cause autosomal recessive SRNS.[75] Affected individuals present in childhood with nephrotic-range proteinuria, microscopic hematuria, and FSGS on kidney biopsy (see Table 7.1).[35] Partial remission can be achieved in some patients with cyclosporine treatment; however, some will progress to ESKD.[75] Targeted deletion of *Myo1e* in mice induces proteinuria, podocyte injury, and CKD.[76] Disease-causing mutations of *Myo1e* and transient gene knockdown cause mislocalization of the protein from plasma membrane puncta and impair podocyte motility in podocytes.[75]

Members of the Rho family of small guanine nucleotide triphosphate hydrolases (GTPases) are widely recognized as critical regulators of actin cytoskeletal dynamics.[77] In humans, the six known subfamilies of Rho GTP hydrolases (GTPases) are composed of more than 25 proteins encoded by multiple alternatively spliced gene transcripts.[77] Dysregulated activity of the Rho GTPase family members RhoA, Cdc42, and Rac1 is implicated in the pathogenesis of both hereditary and idiopathic forms of NS.[78] Rho GDP dissociation inhibitors (ARHGDIs) are a family of three evolutionarily conserved Rho GTPase interacting proteins that negatively regulate Rho GTPase activity by preventing the transition from the inactive GDP-bound state to the active GTP-bound state.[79] Pathogenic mutations in ARHGDI-α (*ARHGDIA*) cause autosomal recessive CNS and SRNS.[80] Affected individuals manifest disease between 14 days and 2.4 years of age and show DMS on kidney biopsy (see Table 7.1).[80] Disease-causing *ARHGDIA* mutations abrogated interactions with Rho GTPases, increased active GTP-bound RAC1 and CDC42 and enhanced migration of cultured human podocytes.[80] In vivo, knockdown of *arhgdia* reproduced the nephrotic phenotype.

Kidney ankyrin repeat-containing proteins (KANKs) are another class of Rho GTPase regulatory proteins that have been linked to the pathobiology of SRNS.[81] The KANK family is composed of four evolutionarily conserved proteins (KANK1–4) that are all expressed in the kidney.[82] KANKs negatively regulate the formation of actin stress fibers and cell migration through the inhibition of RhoA activity.[82,83] Disease-causing mutations in KANK4 cause autosomal recessive SRNS.[81] Affected individuals manifest disease at 2 months of age and show FSGS on kidney biopsy (see Table 7.1).[81]

Phospholipase Cε1 (*PLCε1*) is a ubiquitously expressed enzyme that catalyzes the hydrolytic cleavage of phosphoinositide 4,5 bisphosphate into diacylglycerol (DAG) and inositol triphosphate (IP3).[84] Both DAG and IP3 regulate a diversity of intracellular processes, in part, through the activation of Ca^{2+}-dependent signaling.[84] Disease-causing mutations of *PLCε1* cause autosomal recessive SRNS.[85,86] Affected individuals manifest disease before 4 years of age and DMS is the predominant histologic finding on kidney biopsy; however, FSGS was also observed (see Table 7.1).[85,86] Treatment with corticosteroids or cyclosporine A, an inhibitor of Ca^{2+}-induced calcineurin/nuclear factor of activated T-cell (Cn/NFAT) signaling, stabilized disease in some cases but most progress to ESKD.[85] PLCε1 colocalizes with the IQ motif-containing Rho GTPase activating protein (IQGAP) and they were shown to physically interact by coimmunoprecipitation.[85] This interaction may be integral to the pathobiology of some *PLCε1* mutations, because IQGAP has been shown to interact with slit diaphragm and cytoskeletal proteins, it is an activator of Rho GTPase actin cytoskeletal signaling, and it is negatively regulated by its association with calmodulin, a Ca^{2+}-binding modulatory protein.[87] In vivo, targeted knockdown of *plce1* produced nephrosis in zebrafish but *plce1* deletion in mice did not induce a kidney disease phenotype.[85]

Glomerular epithelial protein 1 (GLEPP1), also known as *Protein Tyrosine Phosphatase Receptor type O* (PTPRO), is a receptor membrane protein tyrosine phosphatase located on the apical membrane of podocyte foot processes.[88,89] Though the molecular functions of GLEPP1 in podocytes are not fully understood, it seems that GLEPP1 may play a role in the regulation of podocyte foot process architecture consistent with its known involvement in actin cytoskeletal and cell motility signaling.[88,90] Disease-causing mutations in *GLEPP1* cause autosomal SRNS.[91] Affected individuals manifest disease between 7 and 14 years of age and kidney histology can show lesions consistent with FSGS or MCN (see Table 7.1).[91] Partial remission was achieved with treatment regimens that included immunosuppression and renin-angiotensin system blockade, but some progressed to ESKD.[91] In *glepp1*-deficient mice, electron microscopy revealed blunting and widening of podocyte foot processes in association with altered distribution of the podocyte intermediate cytoskeletal protein vimentin by electron microscopy.[87] In association with these structural changes, these mice also had a reduced filtration surface area, which was confirmed by the finding of reduced glomerular nephrin content and reduced glomerular filtration rate.[87]

The microtubular network. Tetratricopeptide repeat domain 21B (*TTC21B*) gene encodes an intraflagellar transport component-A, IFT139, which localizes to the base of the primary cilium in developing and undifferentiated cultured podocytes and along the extended microtubular network in mature podocytes.[92] Disease-causing mutations in *TTC21B* cause autosomal recessive SRNS.[92] Affected individuals manifest disease in the first through the fourth decades of life and can show FSGS or MCN with severe tubulointerstitial lesions on kidney biopsy (see Table 7.1).[92] Targeted *TTC21B* knockdown induced ciliary structural defects, actin cytoskeletal abnormalities, and decreased motility in cultured podocytes.[92] Expression of the disease-causing mutation partially rescued the phenotype suggesting a hypomorphic effect of the mutation.[92]

The glomerular basement membrane. Pathogenic mutations in the complement factor H (*CFH*) gene cause membranoproliferative glomerulonephritis type II, also known as *dense deposit disease*.[93] Deletion of a single amino acid (lysine 224) within the complement regulatory domain of CFH impaired its ability to bind and inactivate the complement component C3b resulting in complement-mediated destruction of the glomerular basement membrane.[93] Affected individuals manifest disease in childhood through adolescence and about half will progress to ESKD within 10 years of symptom onset.[94] Replacement of functional factor H by administration of fresh frozen plasma has been shown to be of benefit.[93]

Corticosteroid-Sensitive Nephrotic Syndrome

The slit diaphragm. In contrast to SRNS, there are fewer known genetic causes of SSNS.[95] Although disease-causing mutations in nephrin are most commonly associated with CNF and SRNS, pathogenic nephrin mutations have been shown to cause childhood-onset SSNS with histologic lesions of DMS and MCN (Table 7.2).[96,97]

The actin cytoskeleton. As previously noted, some individuals with NS caused by pathogenic *PLCε1* mutations received therapeutic benefit from corticosteroid therapy (see Table 7.1).[85,86] In addition, pathogenic mutations in KANKs 1 and 2 cause SSNS (see Table 7.1).[81]

Membrane trafficking. Pathogenic mutations of epithelial membrane protein 2 (*EMP2*) have been identified as causes of SSNS.[98] EMP2 is a member of the tetraspanin family of membrane scaffolding proteins that regulate a variety of cellular processes including cell morphology, motility, invasion, membrane fusion, membrane trafficking, and cell signaling.[99] Tetraspanins alter the biologic and functional properties of their membrane protein partners by functioning as organizers of multimolecular membrane complexes.[99] Disease-causing *EMP2* mutations caused childhood-onset SSNS by 2.5 years of age.[98] Notably, one case of SRNS was observed in a 3-year-old patient with MCN on kidney biopsy (see Table 7.1).[98] In podocytes, EMP2 localized to the cell body and foot processes but did not colocalize with podocyte proteins such as synaptopodin.[98] In addition, targeted knockdown of *EMP2* attenuated podocyte proliferation and induced an increase in caveolin-1 expression consistent with the known roles of EMP2 in membrane trafficking and as a negative regulator of caveolin-1 transcription.[98,100] Expression of caveolin-1 was also increased in podocytes expressing the disease-causing truncating *EMP2* mutation. In vivo, *emp2* knockdown recapitulated the nephrosis phenotype.[93]

Disorders of lipid metabolism. Lecithin-cholesterol acyltransferase (*LCAT*) deficiency is an autosomal recessive disease characterized by anemia, corneal opacities, low serum HDL, proteinuria, and often NS with progressive kidney failure.[101] Affected individuals often present in adulthood and show irregular thickening of the glomerular capillaries with vacuolization of the capillary basement membrane due to lipid droplet deposition.[101] Electron-dense lamellar aggregates in the mesangium and basement membrane are characteristic diagnostic features of the disease (Table 7.3).[101] Currently, there is no specific therapy for familial LCAT deficiency.[101]

Pathogenic mutations of apolipoprotein E (*APOE*) are associated with lipoprotein glomerulopathy, a disease characterized by type III hyperlipidemia and proteinuria often with a rapid progression to ESKD.[102] Lipoprotein glomerulopathy is generally considered to be a hereditary disease largely because of the early studies of the disease in a number of Japanese kindreds.[102] Affected individuals usually present in adulthood and show characteristic deposition of laminated lipid droplets containing apolipoproteins A, B, and E in the

TABLE 7.2 Autosomal Recessive Steroid-Sensitive Nephrotic Syndrome

Gene	Protein	Affected Podocyte Compartment or Function	Clinical Presentation	Histologic Features	Mechanism of Disease
NPHS1	Nephrin	Slit diaphragm	Disease manifests in childhood, variable clinical presentation, responsive to corticosteroids	DMS and MCN	Disruption of the podocyte slit diaphragm
PLCε1	PLCε1	Actin cytoskeleton	Disease manifests in early childhood; partial remission possible with cyclosporine A in some patients	DMS and FSGS	Dysregulated actin cytoskeletal dynamics
KANK1 and *KANK2*	KANK1 and KANK2	Actin cytoskeleton	Disease manifests in the early postnatal period, responsive to corticosteroids	MCN	Dysregulated actin cytoskeletal dynamics
EMP2	EMP2	Membrane trafficking	Childhood onset of disease, responsive to corticosteroids	MCN	Dysregulated membrane trafficking

DMS, Diffuse mesangial sclerosis; *FSGS*, focal segmental glomerulosclerosis; *MCN*, minimal-change nephropathy.

TABLE 7.3 Autosomal Recessive Disorders of Lipid Metabolism

Gene	Protein	Affected Podocyte Compartment	Clinical Presentation	Histologic Features	Mechanism of Disease
LCAT	LCAT	Glomerular basement membrane	Disease manifests in adulthood	Electron-dense lamellar aggregates in the mesangium and glomerular basement membrane	Lipid deposition in the mesangium and glomerular basement membrane
APOE	APOE	Actin cytoskeleton	Disease manifests in adulthood, responsive to lipid lowering therapy	Deposition of laminated lipid droplets containing apolipoproteins	Lipid deposition in the mesangium and glomerular basement membrane

glomerular capillaries.[102] Intensive lipid-lowering therapy has been shown to be effective in reversing glomerular lipid deposition and reducing proteinuria (see Table 7.3).[103]

Two independent sequence variants in the apolipoprotein L1 (*APOL1*) gene have been associated with an increased risk for the development of FSGS and hypertension-attributed ESKD in people of African descent.[104] APOL1 is a serum factor that lyses trypanosomes and the two sequence variants enhance the trypanolytic activity of APOL1 in vitro.[104] Although APOL1 has not been established as a cause of FSGS, investigations into potential pathogenic mechanisms are ongoing.

Autosomal Dominant Diseases

The slit diaphragm. As previously noted, pathogenic mutations in *CD2AP* can cause autosomal dominant SRNS.[44] Affected individuals manifest disease in adulthood and show histologic lesions of FSGS (Table 7.4).[44] Pathogenic mutations in anillin (*ANLN*), a critical binding partner of CD2AP at the slit diaphragm, have also been shown to cause autosomal dominant FSGS.[42] Anillin is a ubiquitously expressed nucleocytoplasmic scaffolding protein that regulates various intracellular functions including cytokinesis, cell proliferation, cell motility, F-actin bundling, and cell-survival signaling.[105] Anillin derives its name from the Spanish word for ring, *anillo*, given its prominent role in the formation of the cytokinetic contractile ring; however, its nonmitotic functions are highly dependent on interactions with a diversity of cytoskeletal proteins and signaling intermediates.[106,107] In podocytes, anillin localizes to the slit diaphragm where it binds CD2AP at a conserved N-terminal conserved Px(P/A)xxR motif.[108] Anillin was shown to colocalize with CD2AP to peripheral membrane blebs in migratory podocytes and disease-causing mutations in anillin disrupted the anillin–CD2AP interaction.[42] Affected individuals typically manifest disease in the second and third decades of life and show FSGS on kidney biopsy (see Table 7.4).[42] Anillin expression is upregulated in the podocytes of patients with collapsing FSGS and in experimental models of HIV-associated nephropathy.[42] In addition, overexpression of anillin induced hypermotility in podocytes.[42] In vivo, targeted knockdown of *anln* induced nephrosis and irregular foot process architecture in zebrafish.[36,42]

Disease-causing mutations in the transient receptor potential cation channel, subfamily C, isotype 6 (*TRPC6*) were first recognized to cause autosomal dominant FSGS in 2005, and since then, more than 20 other pathogenic mutations have been reported.[109,110] TRPC6 is a receptor operated, nonselective cation channel with a high affinity for Ca^{2+}.[111,112] TRPC6 is directly activated by DAG and induces its own gene expression through the activation of Ca^{2+}-induced Cn/NFAT signaling.[113,114] TRPC6 localizes to podocyte foot processes where it interacts with proteins such as podocin and nephrin in multimolecular complexes at the slit diaphragm.[115] Dysregulated TRPC6-mediated Ca^{2+} conductance is thought to induce podocyte injury through alterations in actin cytoskeletal dynamics and derangement of foot process architecture.[116] Most of the disease-causing *TRPC6* mutations exert "gain-of-function" effects, inducing an increase in Ca^{2+} conductance through the channel; however, "loss-of-function" mutations have also been reported.[101,110] Affected

TABLE 7.4 Autosomal Dominant Steroid-Resistant Nephrotic Syndrome

Gene	Protein	Affected Podocyte Compartment	Clinical Presentation	Histologic Features	Mechanism of Disease
CD2AP	CD2AP	Slit diaphragm	Disease manifests in adulthood	FSGS	Disruption of the podocyte slit diaphragm
ANLN	ANLN	Slit diaphragm	Disease manifests in the second and third decades of life	FSGS	Disruption of the podocyte slit diaphragm and actin cytoskeletal dynamics
TRPC6	TRPC6	Actin cytoskeleton	Disease manifests in the third and fourth decades of life, some instances of childhood SRNS have been reported	FSGS	Disruption of Ca^{2+}-dependent actin cytoskeletal dynamics
WT1	WT1	Nucleus	Disease manifests in adolescence through adulthood	FSGS	Impaired transactivation of various podocyte-enriched genes
LMX1β	LMX1β	Nucleus	Disease manifests in adolescence through adulthood	Variable	Impaired transactivation of various podocyte-enriched genes
PAX2	PAX2	Nucleus	Disease manifests in adolescence through adulthood	FSGS	Impaired transactivation of various podocyte-enriched genes
ACTN4	α-Actinin-4	Actin cytoskeleton	Disease manifests in adolescence	FSGS	Enhanced cytoskeletal rigidity
INF2	INF2	Actin cytoskeleton	Disease manifests in adolescence through adulthood	FSGS	Dysregulation of actin cytoskeletal dynamics
ARHGAP24	ARHGAP24	Actin cytoskeleton	Disease manifests in the second and third decade of life	FSGS	Dysregulation of actin cytoskeletal dynamics
PODXL	Podocalyxin	glycocalyx	Disease manifests in adolescence through adulthood	FSGS	Impaired glycocalyx formation

FSGS, Focal segmental glomerulosclerosis.

individuals usually manifest in the third and fourth decades of life although some cases of early-onset childhood SRNS have been documented.[117] It is estimated that as many as 60% of affected individuals will progress to ESKD within 10 years of disease onset (see Table 7.4).[118]

In addition to its role in familial FSGS, TRPC6 has been implicated in the pathobiology of other forms of acquired proteinuric kidney disease such as MCN, membranous nephropathy, and diabetic kidney disease.[119,120] Podocyte injury in these diseases is thought to result, in part, from an inappropriate upregulation of TRPC6 expression and activity.[108,121] Although there are no selective TRPC6 inhibitors currently in clinical use, these findings suggest that therapies targeting reduced TRPC6 expression may be of therapeutic value. This hypothesis is supported by a growing number of animal studies that show amelioration of TRPC6-induced glomerular injury with pharmacologic or molecular genetic inhibition of TRPC6 expression.[121,122]

The nuclear compartment. In addition to its role in autosomal recessive and sporadic forms of SRNS, pathogenic mutations in *WT1* have been found to cause nonsyndromic autosomal dominant FSGS.[123] Affected individuals manifest disease in adolescence through adulthood, and it is thought that the mechanism of disease involves podocyte injury through downregulation of essential slit diaphragm and actin cytoskeletal proteins and increased apoptosis (see Table 7.4).[123]

Similar to WT1, Lin-11, Isi-1, and Mec3 (LIM)-homeobox-1β (LMX1β) is another nuclear transcription factor that regulates many facets of kidney development and differentiation.[124] In podocytes, LMX1β plays an essential role in the formation of the actin cytoskeleton, slit diaphragm, and glomerular basement membrane through the transcriptional regulation of genes such as *NPHS1, NPHS2, CD2AP, GLEPP1*, collagen IV α3 (*COL4A3*), and collagen IV α4(*COL4A4*).[125-128] In addition, LMX1β differentially regulates the transcription of *WT1* isoforms to selectively modulate WT1-mediated gene regulation.[127] Pathogenic mutations in LMX1β can cause syndromic kidney disease (i.e., Nail Patella syndrome [NPS]) or isolated FSGS without extrarenal manifestations (i.e., Nail Patella–Like Renal disease [NPLRD]).[129] Pathogenical mutations of the LIM homeodomain cause NPLRD.[127,130,131] Affected individuals manifest disease in adolescence through adulthood and the kidney histology can vary widely (see Table 7.4).[116,118,119]

The Paired Box family of nuclear transcription factors is composed of the principal regulators of cellular lineage determination through the maintenance and specification of progenitor cells during embryonic development.[132] PAX2 is essential for the development of the kidney epithelial cells and pathogenic mutations in *PAX2* cause kidney coloboma syndrome in childhood.[133] In adults, pathogenic mutations in *PAX2* have been found to be associated with isolated autosomal dominant FSGS.[134] Affected individuals manifest disease from late adolescence through adulthood and show histologic lesions consistent with FSGS on kidney biopsy (see Table 7.4).[134] Functional analysis of FSGS-associated variants revealed that *PAX2* variants perturbed protein function by disrupting its DNA binding and transactivation functions or by altering the interaction of PAX2 with repressor proteins, resulting in enhanced repressor activity.[134]

The actin cytoskeleton. α-Actinin-4 (*ACTN4*) is one member of a family of four actin-bundling proteins (ACTN1–4) that plays an essential role in podocyte foot process architecture and adhesion.[135,136] α-Actinin-4 is a Ca^{2+}-responsive, nonmuscle myosin that localizes to F-actin bundles with synaptopodin and MAGI1.[137,138] Mutations in *ACTN4* cause autosomal dominant and sporadic SRNS by a mechanism that involves impaired relaxation of F-actin–ACTN4 cross-bridges, which results in dysregulation of podocyte foot process architecture and function.[139] Interestingly, this cytoskeletal rigidity only manifests in podocyte dysfunction and glomerular sclerosis despite the broad tissue expression of ACTN4.[139] This highlights the essential role of the actin cytoskeletal network for proper podocyte function.[139] Affected individuals manifest disease in adolescence, and some progress to ESKD.[139] Kidney histology shows areas of podocyte foot process effacement and lesions consistent with FSGS (see Table 7.4).[139] Similarly, mice expressing a disease-causing *ACTN4* mutation developed proteinuria and exhibited histologic features consistent with human FSGS including segmental sclerosis, tuft adhesion, tubular dilation, mesangial matrix expansion, podocyte vacuolization, and foot process fusion.[140]

Inverted formin 2 (*INF2*), also known as *WH-domain containing formin 1* (WHIF1), is an actin-associated protein that binds to actin monomers to accelerate polymerization or depolymerization of F-actin filaments.[141] In podocytes, *INF2* negatively regulates lamellipodial actin dynamics and the trafficking of slit diaphragm proteins by opposing Rho/mDia-mediated actin polymerization.[142,143] Pathogenic mutations in *INF2* have been identified as causes of autosomal dominant FSGS.[144] Notably, pathogenic *INF2* mutations account for 9% to 16% of familial FSGS making it the most common genetic cause of the disease.[145,146] Affected individuals can manifest disease in adolescence through adulthood (see Table 7.4).[144] Interestingly, mice expressing a disease-causing mutation in *INF2* showed no significant kidney pathology or proteinuria at baseline despite diminished INF2 protein levels.[147] However, *INF2* mutant podocytes showed impaired reversal of protamine sulfate-induced foot process effacement by heparin sulfate perfusion.[147]

Rho GTPase-activating proteins (ARHGAPs) negatively regulate Rho GTPases by accelerating the hydrolytic conversion of GTP to GDP.[148] Disease-causing mutations in *ARHGAP24* cause autosomal dominant FSGS.[149] Affected individuals manifest disease in the second and third decades of life and show FSGS on kidney biopsy (see Table 7.4).[149] *ARHGAP24* knockdown in podocytes increased Rac1 and CDC42 activity, podocyte motility, and membrane ruffling[149] Similarly, a disease-causing *ARHGAP24* mutation demonstrated diminished Rac1-GAP activity in HEK 293 cells.[149]

The glycocalyx. Mature and healthy podocytes are covered by a polyanionic mucinous coating of sulfated molecules and sialated glycoproteins referred to as the *glycocalyx*.[150] The components of this protective coating are synthesized and secreted by podocytes and are thought to act as an antiadhesin, which maintains the patency of the filtration slits between adjacent podocytes through electrostatic repulsion.[151-154] Podocalyxin (*PODXL*) is the major sialoglycoprotein of the glycocalyx and disease-causing variants in *PODXL* are associated with autosomal dominant FSGS.[155,156] Affected individuals presented in early adolescence though adulthood with proteinuria and FSGS on kidney biopsy (see Table 7.4).[143] Notably, an FSGS-associated *PODXL* variant induced podocalyxin dimerization but did not alter protein stability, extracellular domain glycosylation, cell-surface expression, global subcellular localization, or interaction with its intracellular binding partner, ezrin.[143]

Syndromic Proteinuric Kidney Disease

Autosomal Recessive Diseases

The nuclear compartment. The SWI/SNF-related, matrix-associated, actin-dependent regulator of chromatin, subfamily a like 1 (*SMARCAL1*) is an ATP-dependent annealing helicase that assists in the repair of damaged DNA replication forks to promote genome stability during replicative stress.[157,158] SMARCAL1 is ubiquitously expressed and localizes to the nuclei of glomerular podocytes, tubular cells, and endothelial cells.[159] Pathogenic mutations in *SMARCAL1* cause Schimke immuno-osseous dysplasia (SIOD). SIOD is a rare autosomal recessive multisystem disorder characterized by disproportionate growth failure, impaired T-cell function, and SRNS.[160] Affected individuals manifest in childhood and adolescence and the predominant histologic finding is FSGS (Table 7.5).[160] Although the mechanisms of disease remain unclear, increased DNA fragmentation and dysregulated gene expression have been observed in human tissue and experimental models of *SMARCAL1* deficiency.[160,161]

Pathogenic mutations in the *WT1* gene cause Denys–Drash syndrome (DDS) and Frasier syndrome.[162] Both are rare diseases characterized by congenital NS, male pseudohermaphroditism, and development of urogenital tumors.[162] The glomerular lesion of DDS is DMS and patients typically progress to ESKD within 3 years (see Table 7.5).[162] Alternatively, the glomerular lesion of Frasier syndrome is FSGS, which usually manifests slowly over the course of a decade. Individuals with Frasier syndrome progress to ESKD in the second or third decade of life.[162]

The actin cytoskeleton. Loss-of-function mutations in diacylglycerol kinase ε (*DGKE*) have been identified as causes of familial atypical hemolytic uremic syndrome (aHUS) with

TABLE 7.5 Syndromic Proteinuric Kidney Diseases (Autosomal Recessive)

Gene	Protein	Affected Podocyte Compartment or Function	Clinical Presentation	Histologic Features	Mechanism of Disease
SMARCAL1	SMARCAL1	Nucleus	Schimke immuno-osseous dysplasia (SIOD), disease manifests in childhood through adolescence, disproportionate growth failure, impaired T-cell function, SRNS	FSGS	Chromatin instability and dysregulated gene expression
WT1	WT1	Nucleus	DDS and Frasier syndromes, congenital nephrotic syndrome, DDS typically progresses to ESKD within 3 years, Frasier syndrome manifests slowly over a decade.	DMS with DDS, FSGS with Frasier syndrome	Impaired transactivation of various developmental genes of the kidney and urogenital tract
DGKE	DGKε	Actin cytoskeleton	aHUS, SRNS	Foot process effacement (rare)	Dysregulated Ca^{2+}-dependent actin cytoskeletal dynamics
SGLP1	SGLP1	Actin cytoskeleton	Adrenal insufficiency, congenital nephrotic syndrome, SRNS, disease manifests in the early postnatal period	FSGS	Dysregulated actin cytoskeletal dynamics
WDR73	WDR73	Microtubules	Galloway–Mowat syndrome, disease manifests in childhood	FSGS	Dysregulated microtubular dynamics
FAT1	FAT1	Slit diaphragm	SRNS with tubular ectasia, hematuria, and facultative neurologic involvement, disease manifests in early childhood through late adolescence	Glomerulotubular nephropathy	Disruption of the podocyte slit diaphragm

Continued

TABLE 7.5 Syndromic Proteinuric Kidney Diseases (Autosomal Recessive)—cont'd

Gene	Protein	Affected Podocyte Compartment or Function	Clinical Presentation	Histologic Features	Mechanism of Disease
EXT1	Exostosin-1	Glomerular basement membrane	Glomerular sclerosis with multiple exostoses, disease manifests in childhood through adulthood	Glomerular sclerosis with abundant fibrillary collagen deposits	Disruption of glomerular basement membrane composition and function
ITGA3 and *ITGB4*	ITGα3 and ITGβ4	Adhesion to the glomerular basement membrane	Disease manifests in the first year of life	FSGS	Impaired adhesion to the glomerular basement membrane
CD151	CD151	Glomerular basement membrane	Disease manifests in adulthood	Classical changes of Alport syndrome without COL4A5 mutations	Impaired formation of the glomerular and tubular basement membranes
LAMB2	LAMB2	Glomerular basement membrane	Pierson syndrome, disease manifests in the early postnatal period	Glomerular sclerosis, DMS	Impaired formation of the glomerular basement membrane
ZMPSTE24	ZMPSTE24	Glomerular basement membrane	Disease manifests in adulthood	FSGS	Impaired formation of the glomerular basement membranes
COQ6	COQ6	Mitochondria	Disease manifests in first decade of life, SRNS and sensorineural hearing loss; responsive to CoQ10 supplementation	FSGS	Impaired CoQ10 biosynthesis
PDSS2	PDSS2	Mitochondria	Disease manifests in the early postnatal period, Leigh syndrome and SRNS	Renal tubulopathy or diffuse glomerulocystic kidney damage	Impaired CoQ10 biosynthesis
MTTL1	MTTL1	Mitochondria	Disease manifests in childhood through adulthood, MELAS syndrome with nephropathy, A3243G mutat on particularly associated with adult-onset FSGS	FSGS	Impaired mitochondrial function
SCARB2	SCARB2	Membrane trafficking	Disease manifests in the second decade of life, action myoclonus-renal failure syndrome, substrate removal therapy targeting reduction of glucocerebrosidase accumulation found to be effective in one patient	C1q nephropathy	Impaired lysosomal formation and function
CUBN	CUBN	Membrane trafficking	Disease manifest in the first decade of life; intermittent proteinuria and megaloblastic anemia secondary to vitamin B_{12} deficiency	Unknown	Impaired protein reuptake from glomerular filtrate
ALG1	ALG1	Glycosylation	Disease manifests in the early postnatal period, congenital nephrotic syndrome with congenital disorder of glycosylation	FSGS	Impaired N-glycosylation and targeting of slit diaphragm proteins
PMM2	PMM2	Glycosylation	Disease manifests in the early postnatal period, Jaeken syndrome with congenital nephrotic syndrome	DMS with focal tubular dilation	Impaired N-glycosylation and targeting of slit diaphragm proteins

DDS, Denys–Drash syndrome; *DMS*, diffuse mesangial sclerosis; *FSGS*, focal segmental glomerulosclerosis; *MCN*, minimal-change nephropathy; *SRNS*, steroid-resistant nephrotic syndrome.

SRNS.[163] DGKE is a critical negative regulator of Ca^{2+}-dependent signaling through the phosphorylation and inactivation of arachidonic acid diacylglycerol (AADAG).[164,165] DGKE is expressed in podocytes and it is proposed that DGKE deficiency may cause podocyte injury through dysregulated Ca^{2+} signaling, derangement of actin cytoskeletal dynamics, and perturbation of the slit diaphragm complex.[166] Although proteinuria is a rare feature of aHUS, podocyte foot process effacement has been observed in the kidney biopsies of affected patients (see Table 7.5).[163]

Homozygous truncating mutations in the sphingosine-1-phosphate lyase (*SGPL1*) gene catalyzes the irreversible degradation of endogenous and dietary sphingosine-1-phosphate, the final step of sphingolipid catabolism, and of other phosphorylated long-chain bases.[167] Sphingosine-1-phosphate is a bioactive phospholipid that signals through G-protein–coupled receptors to influence a variety of cellular processes including cell growth and survival, angiogenesis, cell motility and migration, and lymphocyte trafficking.[168] Homozygous truncating mutations in *SGPL1* cause autosomal recessive syndromes characterized by adrenal insufficiency with associated CNS or SRNS.[167,169] Affected individuals manifest disease in the early postnatal period and show histologic lesions consistent with FSGS on kidney biopsy (see Table 7.5).[162,164]

The microtubular network. WD repeat domain 73 (*WDR73*) is a microtubule-associated protein that interacts with microtubules to regulate cell-cycle progression, proliferation, and survival in the brain and kidney.[170] Pathogenic mutations of *WDR73* cause Galloway–Mowat syndrome, a rare autosomal recessive disorder characterized by the combination of NS and various CNS abnormalities.[171] Affected individuals manifest disease in childhood and show histologic lesions consistent with FSGS on kidney biopsy (see Table 7.5).[171] WDR73 localizes diffusely in the cytoplasm during interphase but is relocalized to spindle poles and astral microtubules during mitosis.[171] Fibroblasts from one affected child and WDR73-depleted podocytes displayed abnormal nuclear morphology, diminished cell viability, and alterations of the microtubule network.[171]

The slit diaphragm. Adherens junctions are dynamic, multimolecular complexes that bridge the plasma membranes of adjacent cells.[172] The slit diaphragm is considered to be a "modified" adherens junction given that it functions as a region of cell–cell contact and is partially composed of typical adherens junction proteins such as catenins, p-cadherins, and FAT proteins.[173] FAT1 is an atypical cadherin that localizes to the slit diaphragm complex in podocytes.[174] FAT cadherins play a role in the regulation of cell migration, lamellipodia formation, cell polarity, and cell–cell adhesion.[175] Disease-causing mutations in FAT1 have been identified as causes of autosomal recessive SRNS with tubular ectasia, hematuria, and facultative neurologic involvement.[176] Affected individuals manifest disease in early childhood though late adolescence with histologic lesions of a glomerulotubular nephropathy (see Table 7.5)[176] Mice with podocyte-specific deletion of *FAT1* display abnormal glomerular filtration barrier development, proteinuria, foot process effacement, and FSGS.[176] In addition, *FAT1* knockdown in podocytes induced decreased cell adhesion and migration, which was partially reversed by an activator of the Rac1/CDC42 Rho GTPase.[176] Similarly, *FAT1* knockdown in tubular cells decreased migration, attenuated Rac1 activation, and impaired luminal formation in spheroids demonstrating a role for FAT1 in the modulation of Rho GTPase-dependent signaling.[176,177]

The glomerular basement membrane. The exostosin-1 gene (*EXT1*) encodes a glycosyltransferase required for the synthesis of heparan sulfate glycosaminoglycans, which are critical components of the glomerular basement membrane.[178] Pathogenic mutations in *EXT1* cause autosomal dominant SRNS with multiple exotoses.[179] Affected individuals manifest disease in childhood through adulthood and show glomerular sclerosis and abundant fibrillar collagen deposits on kidney biopsy (see Table 7.5).[179] The mechanism of disease is thought to be due to impaired glomerular basement membrane composition and function.[179]

Integrins are a family of ubiquitously expressed, divalent cation-dependent transmembrane receptors that mediate cell adhesion dynamics and mechanotransduction.[180] Pathogenic mutations in integrin-α 3 (*ITGA3*) and integrin-β 4 (*ITGB4*) have been found to cause syndromic forms of autosomal recessive SRNS.[181,182] Affected individuals manifest disease in the first year of life and show FSGS on kidney biopsy (see Table 7.5).[167,168] The mechanism of disease is thought to involve impaired podocyte adhesion and defective transmission of extracellular signals to the intracellular compartment.[167,168]

Cluster of differentiation 151 (*CD151*) is a tetraspanin that is essential for the proper assembly of the glomerular and tubular basement membranes in the kidney and skin.[183] Tetraspanin CD151 forms laminin-binding complexes with integrins-α3β1 and -α6β1 in kidney and -α3β1 and -α6β4 in the skin.[183] Disease-causing mutations *CD151* cause syndromic autosomal recessive SRNS.[183] Affected individuals manifest disease in adulthood with classic changes of Alport syndrome on kidney biopsy without collagen IV-α 5 mutations (see Table 7.5).[183]

Laminin subunit β 2 (*LAMB2*) is a multidomain, trimeric glomerular basement membrane protein that regulates cell adhesion and migration through its interaction with integrin-α3β1 and other glomerular basement membrane components.[184] Disease-causing mutations in *LAMB2* cause Pierson syndrome, a rare genetic disease that is characterized by a combination of developmental defects affecting the kidney and eyes.[185,186] Affected individuals present in the early postnatal period with hypoplasia of the ciliary body, microcoria, massive proteinuria, and rapid progression to ESKD (see Table 7.5).[171]

Zinc metallopeptidase STE24 (*ZMPSTE24*) is a membrane-bound endoprotease involved in posttranslational proteolytic cleavage of carboxy terminal residues of prelamin A to form mature lamin A.[187] Disease-causing mutations in

ZMPSTE24 cause mandibuloacral dysplasia with autosomal recessive SRNS.[187,188] Affected individuals manifest with disease in adulthood and show histologic lesions consistent with FSGS on kidney biopsy (see Table 7.5).[173,174]

The mitochondria. Coenzyme Q10 biosynthesis monooxygenase 6 (*COQ6*) is an essential component of the Q10 biosynthetic pathway. Pathogenic mutations in COQ6 cause autosomal recessive SRNS with sensorineural deafness.[66] Affected individuals manifest disease within the first decade of life and the predominant histologic finding on kidney biopsy was FSGS (see Table 7.5).[66] Partial remission was achieved in some cases with cyclosporine A.[66] CoQ10 supplementation decreased proteinuria in all cases, whereas sensorineural deafness only improved in some patients.[66]

Decaprenyl diphosphate synthase subunit 2 (*PDSS2*) is another critical enzyme in the CoQ10 biosynthetic pathway that has been linked to the pathogenesis of autosomal recessive SRNS.[189] Disease-causing mutations in *PDSS2* cause Leigh syndrome with SRNS and CoQ10 deficiency.[68] Affected individuals present in the early postnatal period with massive proteinuria, hypoalbuminemia, and reduced kidney function (see Table 7.5).[68]

Pathogenic mutations in mitochondrially encoded TRNA leucine 1 (UUA/G) (*MTTL1*) cause mitochondrial myopathy, encephalopathy, lactic acidosis, and stroke (MELAS) syndrome, a multisystem disorder that can present with cerebral vascular accidents, seizures, hearing loss, cardiomyopathy, diabetes, and nephropathy.[190,191] Affected individuals can manifest disease in childhood through adulthood and can show FSGS on kidney biopsy (see Table 7.5).[192] Notably, the *A3243G MTTL1* point mutation is particularly associated with the development of adult-onset FSGS and should be considered in patients with maternally inherited diabetes or hearing loss presenting with FSGS.[192]

Membrane trafficking. Scavenger receptor class B member 2 (*SCARB2*) is a lysosomal membrane protein that is required for the normal biogenesis and maintenance of lysosomes and endosomes.[193] SCARB2 participates in lysosomal/endosomal membrane trafficking and has been identified as the principle receptor for the glycosphingolipid hydrolase glucocerebrosidase.[194] Disease-causing mutations in *SCARB2* cause action myoclonus-renal failure syndrome.[195] Affected individuals presented in the second decade of life and had evidence of C1q nephropathy on kidney biopsy (see Table 7.5).[195] Notably, substrate removal therapy, to correct the possible accumulation of glucocerebrosidase in cells, ameliorated disease in one patient.[194]

Cubilin (*CUBN*) is an endocytic membrane trafficking protein that is highly expressed in the kidney tubular epithelium.[196] Cubilin is thought to be responsible for the reuptake of proteins filtered through the glomeruli.[196] Pathogenic mutations in the *CUBN* gene cause intermittent nephrotic range proteinuria.[196] Affected individuals manifest disease in the first decade of life (see Table 7.5).[196] Mice deficient in cubilin demonstrate decreased albumin uptake and proteinuria.[197]

Disorders of glycosylation. Asparagine-linked glycosylation 1 (*ALG1*) is a ubiquitously expressed mannosyltransferase that participates in the formation of the lipid-linked precursor oligosaccharide for N-glycosylation of membrane proteins.[198] N-glycosylation is essential for the proper membrane localization of the slit diaphragm and glomerular basement membrane proteins such as nephrin and α-dystroglycan.[199,200] Disease-causing mutations of *ALG1* cause congenital NS with congenital disorder of glycosylation (CGD).[201] Affected individuals present in the early postnatal period and collapsing FSGS with marked foot process effacement and microvillous transformation can be seen on kidney biopsy (see Table 7.5).[201]

Pathogenic mutations in the N-glycosylase phosphomannomutase-2 (*PMM2*) gene cause the most common subtype of CGD known as CGD-1a or Jaeken syndrome.[202] CGD-1a is a rare cause of congenital NS and the mortality rate is nearly 20% within the first year of life.[203] Affected individuals manifest disease in the early postnatal period and DMS with focal tubular dilation can be seen on kidney biopsy (see Table 7.5).[202]

X-Linked Diseases

The nuclear compartment. Nuclear RNA export factor 5 (*NXF5*) is an RNA-binding protein that may function as a nucleocytoplasmic RNA export protein.[204] Disease-causing mutations in *NXF5* cause X-linked recessive SRNS with heart block[204] Affected individuals manifest disease in adulthood and show FSGS on kidney biopsy (Table 7.6).[204]

Immune dysregulation, polyendocrinopathy, enteropathy, X-linked (IPEX) syndrome is a rare familial disorder of the immune regulatory system caused by mutations in the transcriptional regulator, Forkhead box P3 (*FOXP3*).[205] The Forkhead family of nuclear transcription factors regulates the expression of genes involved in cell proliferation, differentiation, growth, and longevity.[205] FOXP3 plays an essential role in the regulation of T cells with regulatory properties.[205] Individuals with pathogenic mutations in *FOXP3* manifest disease in childhood and kidney histology can show a variety of glomerular injury patterns including MCN and membranous nephropathy (see Table 7.6).[206]

Membrane trafficking. Inositol polyphosphate-phosphatase or the Oculocerebrorenal Syndrome of Lowe (*OCRL*) protein is a phospholipid phosphatase that regulates cellular levels of phosphatidylinositol 4,5-bisphosphate.[207] OCRL is heavily expressed in the proximal tubule where it participates in a variety of functions including endocytic membrane trafficking, cell migration and polarity, phagocytosis, intracellular signaling, and ciliogenesis.[207] Disease-causing mutations in *OCRL* cause both Dent disease and Lowe syndrome; proximal tubulopathies are characterized, in part, by low molecular weight proteinuria and hypercalcemia.[208] Affected individuals manifest disease in the first decade of life with Dent disease and in the fourth and fifth decades of life with Lowe syndrome. Interestingly, focal global sclerosis, mild segmental foot process effacement, interstitial

TABLE 7.6 **Syndromic Proteinuric Kidney Diseases (X-Linked)**

Gene	Protein	Affected Podocyte Compartment or Function	Clinical Presentation	Histologic Features	Mechanism of Disease
NXF5	NXF5	Nucleus	Disease manifests in adulthood, SRNS with heart block	FSGS	Impaired nucleocytoplasmic transport of RNAs
FOXP3	FOXP3	Nucleus	Disease manifests in childhood, IPEX syndrome with nephrotic syndrome	MCN and membranous nephropathy	Impaired transactivation of various genes of the kidney and immune system
OCRL	OCRL	Membrane trafficking	Dent disease and Lowe syndrome, disease manifests in the first decade of life with Lowe syndrome and the fourth or fifth decades with Dent disease	Focal global glomerulosclerosis, mild segmental foot process effacement, interstitial lymphocytic infiltration, and tubular damage	Impaired endocytic trafficking
COL4A5	COL4A5	Glomerular basement membrane	Alport syndrome, 95% of patients have X-linked form of the disease, which manifests in adolescence through adulthood	Diffuse thickening and splitting ("tram-tracking") of the glomerular basement membrane	Impaired assembly of the glomerular basement membrane

FSGS, Focal segmental glomerulosclerosis; *MCN*, minimal-change nephropathy; *SRNS*, steroid-resistant nephrotic syndrome.

lymphocytic infiltration, and tubular damage has been observed in kidney biopsies of patients with Dent disease but glomerular injury is not commonly associated with Lowe syndrome (see Table 7.6).[209]

The glomerular basement membrane. Alport syndrome is a hereditary, progressive, hematuric nephropathy characterized by glomerular basement membrane abnormalities with frequent hearing defects and ocular anomalies.[210] Pathogenic mutations in collagen IV α3, α4, and α5 genes (i.e., *COL4A3*, *COL4A4*, and *COL4A5*) have long been recognized as causes of Alport syndrome and SRNS.[211] Collagen IV α3, α4, and α5 are principle components of the glomerular basement membrane and are synthesized by mature podocytes.[212] It is estimated that 95% of Alport syndrome cases are due to X-linked mutations in *COL4A5*. Affected individuals can manifest disease in adolescence though adulthood and show a typical histologic lesion characterized by diffuse thickening and splitting (i.e., tram-tracking) of the glomerular basement membrane on kidney biopsy (see Table 7.6).[210]

Autosomal Dominant Diseases

The nuclear compartment. The nuclear lamina is a dense fibrillar network of structural proteins that lines the inner nuclear membrane of eukaryotic cells.[215] Lamin A (*LMNA*) is a principle component of the nuclear lamina that functions as a scaffolding molecule to assist in the organization of chromatin.[215] Pathogenic mutations in *LMNA* have been identified as causes of familial partial lipodystrophy (FPLD) with kidney disease, a syndrome characterized by partial lipodystrophy, proteinuric nephropathy, cardiomyopathy, and atypical myopathy.[215] Affected individuals manifest disease in adolescence through adulthood, and kidney histology can show glomerular sclerosis and mesangial proliferation (Table 7.7).[215] Although the mechanisms of disease are not fully understood, lamin A participates in a variety of cellular processes that may be dysregulated including cell-cycle regulation, chromatin organization, DNA replication, cell differentiation, and apoptosis.[215]

The actin cytoskeleton. Pathogenic mutations in *INF2* have previously been discussed as causes of nonsyndromic, autosomal dominant FSGS. Disease-causing mutations in *INF2* have also been shown to cause FSGS associated with Charcot–Marie–Tooth neuropathy.[216] Affected individuals manifest in adolescence through adulthood and show FSGS on renal biopsy (see Table 7.7).[216] The mechanism of disease is suspected to involve dysregulation of actin cytoskeletal dynamics in podocytes and Schwann cells.[216]

The glomerular basement membrane. Heterozygous mutations in *COL4A3* and *COL4A4* can cause autosomal dominant Alport syndrome. It is estimated that 5% of individuals with Alport syndrome have the autosomal dominant form of the disease.[213] Affected individuals have a decreased risk of developing ocular or hearing manifestations of the disease but are at a higher risk of developing adult-onset kidney failure.[213] Notably, thin basement membrane nephropathy can also be observed in individuals with pathogenic *COL4A3* and *COL4A4* mutations.[214] In these individuals, kidney histology may show lesions consistent with FSGS and potentially lead to a misclassification of the disease (see Table 7.7).[214] In these cases, complimentary molecular genetic screening may be required in addition to histologic analysis for accurate diagnosis.[214]

TABLE 7.7 Syndromic Proteinuric Kidney Diseases (Autosomal Dominant)

Gene	Protein	Affected Podocyte Compartment or Function	Clinical Presentation	Histologic Features	Mechanism of Disease
LMNA	LMNA	Nucleus	Familial partial lipodystrophy, disease manifests in adolescence through adulthood	Glomerular sclerosis and mesangial proliferation	Dysregulated chromatin organization
INF2	INF2	Actin cytoskeleton	Charcot–Marie–Tooth neuropathy with FSGS, disease manifests in the second and third decades of life	FSGS	Dysregulated actin cytoskeletal dynamics in podocytes and Schwann cells
COL4A3 and *COL4A4*	COL4A3 and COL4A4	Glomerular basement membrane	Alport syndrome, 5% of patients have autosomal dominant form of the disease, which manifests in adulthood	FSGS	Impaired assembly of the glomerular basement membrane
MYH9	MYH9	Glomerular basement membrane	Epstein–Fechtner syndromes, manifest in infancy with proteinuria ± hematuria and rapid progression to ESKD, MYH9 R702 mutations cause progressive nephritis	FSGS	Impaired assembly of the glomerular basement membrane

FSGS, Focal segmental glomerulosclerosis.

TABLE 7.8 Sporadic Proteinuric Kidney Diseases

Gene	Protein	Affected Podocyte Compartment or Function	Clinical Presentation	Histologic Features	Mechanism of Disease
E2F3	E2F3	Nucleus	Sporadic FSGS, disease manifests in childhood	FSGS	Glomerular injury resulting from inappropriate VEGF expression
ACTN4 and *SYNPO*	ACTN4 and SYNPO	Actin cytoskeleton	Sporadic FSGS, disease manifests in adulthood	FSGS	Dysregulation of actin cytoskeletal dynamics

FSGS, Focal segmental glomerulosclerosis.

Pathogenic mutations in myosin heavy chain 9 (*MYH9*) cause Epstein–Fechtner syndromes; diseases characterized by thrombocytopenia, giant platelets, granulocyte inclusion bodies, progressive hearing loss, and nephritis.[217] In particular, *MYH9 R702* mutations have been identified as causes of proteinuric kidney disease in infancy, which rapidly progresses to ESKD in adolescence.[217] Affected individuals show findings consistent with FSGS on kidney biopsy; however, ACE inhibitor therapy has been shown to significantly reduce proteinuria in some patients (see Table 7.7).[217] Notably, *MYH9* has also been established as a major-effect risk gene for the development idiopathic FSGS or ESKD in African Americans, further highlighting the significance of this molecule in the pathobiology of FSGS.[218]

Sporadic Disease

Pathogenic mutations in the E2F transcription factor 3 (*E2F3*) cause sporadic FSGS with cognitive impairment.[219] The E2F family of transcription factors controls the cell cycle-dependent expression of genes that are essential for cellular proliferation and differentiation.[220] In particular, E2F3 is a rate-limiting transcriptional regulator of the G_1/S-phase transition that has been shown to attenuate cellular proliferation during vascular development through inhibition of vascular endothelial growth factor (*VEGF*) gene expression.[219-221] Individuals with disease-causing *E2F3* mutations manifest disease in childhood and the mechanism of glomerular injury is thought to involve inappropriate upregulation of *VEGF* expression in the absence of E2F3-mediated *VEGF* gene repression (Table 7.8).[219]

Pathogenic mutations in the promoter regions of the *ACTN4* and synaptopodin (*SYNPO*) genes have been identified in individuals with sporadic FSGS.[222] Both of these genes encode actin-associated proteins that are essential for the maintenance of podocyte cytoskeletal architecture.[223] Pathogenic promoter mutations in the *ACTN4* and *SYNPO* genes reduced gene transactivation in vitro and protein expression in the kidneys of affected individuals (see Table 7.8).[222]

POLYCYSTIC KIDNEY DISEASE

Polycystic kidney disease (PKD) is a complex disorder characterized by the development of fluid-filled cysts in the kidney.[224] It is a progressive disease and many affected individuals develop decreased kidney function in the fifth and sixth decades of life.[224] PKD is the fourth leading cause of ESKD and accounts for approximately 5% of all ESKD.[224] PKD can be inherited or acquired and cystogenesis is thought to arise from the dysregulated proliferation of a monoclonal population of kidney tubular epithelial cells.[225] The cysts originate from the epithelia of only 1% to 5% of nephrons and are bordered by a single layer of tubular cells that proliferates more rapidly and are less differentiated than normal.[226]

Autosomal dominant polycystic kidney disease (ADPKD) is the most common form of inherited kidney disease worldwide. Prevalence estimates for ADPKD vary from approximately 1/1000 in the United States to just over 1/4000 in Japan. ADPKD is caused by mutations in the *PKD1* or *PKD2* genes that encode polycystin-1 (PC1) and polycystin-2 (PC2) respectively.[227] An estimated 85% of ADPKD is attributable to mutations in PC1; the remaining 15% is due to mutations in PC2.[226] PC1 is a large, 11-transmembrane protein that localizes to the base of primary cilia where it interacts with PC2, a Ca^{2+}-permeable TRP channel.[228] The complex is thought to function as a mechanosensor of fluid dynamics, which influences various cellular processes including cell proliferation, differentiation and apoptosis.[229,230] The mechanisms of cystogenesis are not completely understood but it is clear that mutations in *PKD1* or *PKD2* lead to a reduction in intracellular calcium, an increase in cyclic adenosine monophosphate (cAMP), activation of protein kinase A, and an increase in sensitivity of collecting duct principal cells to the constant tonic effect of vasopressin.[226] This results in the activation downstream signaling pathways responsible for impaired tubulogenesis, cell proliferation, increased fluid secretion, and interstitial inflammation.[226] ADPKD cysts increase in size and number over the space of decades, displacing and destroying adjacent parenchyma, leading ultimately to ESKD in ~50% of cases.[227] The prominent role of vasopressin signaling in the pathobiology of ADPKD has provided a rationale for the use of vasopressin receptor antagonists (VRAs) in the treatment of this hereditary disease.[231] VRAs block vasopressin-induced fluid influx into cysts. Although not currently approved for clinical use in ADPKD, VRAs have shown promising results in clinical trials, reducing total kidney volume and eGFR decline.[232,233] In addition to VRAs, statins have been shown to be of benefit in the treatment of ADPKD.[234] Although the mechanism of action remains unclear, statins were shown to slow progression of structural kidney disease in children and young adults with ADPKD.[234]

Autosomal recessive PKD (ARPKD) is caused by mutations in the *PKHD1* gene, which encodes a large multidomain integral membrane protein known as fibrocystin/polyductin (FPC).[235] FPC is a membrane-associated receptor-like protein that colocalizes with PC2 in the primary cilia of tubular epithelial cells.[236] It has been shown to regulate both the expression and function of PC2.[236] ARPKD has an annual incidence of 1:20,000 to 1:40,000.[237] In contrast to ADPKD, ARPKD is a disease of the very young. The majority of affected individuals present in the neonatal period with enlarged echogenic kidneys.[237] Kidney disease is characterized by nephromegaly, hypertension, and varying degrees of kidney dysfunction. More than 50% of affected individuals progress to ESKD within the first decade of life.[237] All ARPKD patients are invariably afflicted with congenital hepatic fibrosis of varying degrees of severity.[237] The suspicion of a diagnosis of ARPKD is based on clinical findings in an affected patient and the absence of kidney disease in their biological parents.[237] Identification of pathogenic homozygous mutations in *PKHD1* in the affected individual establishes the diagnosis ARPKD.[237]

Recently a pathogenic mutation in the promoter region of the *PMM2* gene was identified as a cause of PKD with hyperinsulinemic hypoglycemia (HIPKD).[238] As previously noted, mutations in *PMM2* cause CGD-1a; a rare syndromic disorder that can be associated with congenital NS.[203] The disease-causing *PMM2* promoter mutation (c.167G>T) was identified in a small European cohort as either a homozygous mutation or as a heterozygous mutation combined with another pathogenic *PMM2* mutation.[238] The mutation impaired binding of the transcription factor ZNF143 to the *PMM2* promoter and reduced *PMM2* gene expression in vitro.[238] Affected individuals presented in the early postnatal period through adulthood and none showed any of the classic features of CDG-1a.[238] The promoter mutation is thought to cause disease through the tissue-specific distortion of chromatin loop formation and impaired *PMM2* gene expression.[238]

Treatment of Genetic Disease

With the advent of next-generation sequencing technologies, the pace of gene discovery in CKD has accelerated tremendously. With each new discovery, new facets of previously illusive mechanisms of disease are revealed exposing novel therapeutic opportunities or common molecular targets that underlie the pathogenesis of multiple disease processes. In this regard, the aggressive genetic characterization of inherited kidney diseases is justified by the wealth of mechanistic information derived from the efforts. The previously held notion that "genetic diseases are untreatable" is belied by examples of treatable genetic disease such as the inherited CoQ10 deficiency-associated nephropathies.[239] Similarly, advances in our understanding of the mechanisms of ADPKD have led to promising rational clinical trials of a class of therapeutic agents, VRAs (i.e., vaptans), which have been repurposed to target a well-characterized signaling pathway that is common to ADPKD and several other disease processes.[240] These advances were made possible by decades of rigorous, multidisciplinary scientific investigation. To extend this progress, it will be necessary to pair advanced genomics with high-throughput biochemical and physiological characterizations of disease mechanisms for the design or repurposing of patient-specific therapies.

A full list of references is available at www.expertconsult.com.

SECTION II

Complications and Management of Chronic Kidney Disease

8

The Role of the Chronic Kidney Disease Clinic and Multidisciplinary Team Care

Melissa Nataatmadja, MBBS, MPH&TM, FRACP, Judi M. Graham, MBBChBAO, Monica C. Beaulieu, MD, FRCPC, MHA, Nadia Zalunardo, MD, SM, FRCPC, and Adeera Levin, MD, FRCPC

OUTLINE

INTRODUCTION

Chronic kidney disease (CKD) is defined by the Kidney Disease Improving Global Outcomes (KDIGO) as an abnormality of kidney structure or function that is present for greater than 3 months and has implications for health[1]. CKD affects 10% of the global population.[2,3] The numbers of people affected are growing exponentially, and certain populations from low-income backgrounds and geographical areas such as Asia and Africa are disproportionately affected.[2,4,5] CKD is an increasingly common cause of morbidity and mortality, climbing from the 27th greatest contributor to global deaths in 1990 to the 18th greatest in 2010.[5,6] United States Renal Data System (USRDS) data suggest that mortality in patients with CKD is greater than double that of patients without CKD, at 111.2 per 1000 patient years (after adjusting for age, sex, and race) in 2014.[7] Likewise, hospitalization rates are much higher among patients with CKD compared with those without, with the 2014 USRDS data showing it to be two to three times higher.[7] In the United States, the crude incidence rate of end-stage kidney disease (ESKD) was 370 per million per year in 2014, and the number of dialysis and transplant patients rose by 3.5% from 2013.[7] Caring for patients with CKD and ESKD is costly, with 2014 estimates of cost per person per year in the United States equaling $32,586 for transplant patients, $73,612 for peritoneal dialysis patients, and $87,638 for hemodialysis patients.[7]

Both awareness and adoption of CKD guidelines are generally considered to be suboptimal among nonnephrologist physicians.[2] International CKD guidelines may only be accessible in around 50% of cases,[8] and the availability of renal registries may be extremely low in developing countries.[8]

Historically, the focus of CKD care was to coordinate placement of vascular access, to attend to uremic symptoms and complications, and to provide dialysis. However, it is increasingly recognized that conditions associated with CKD, such as anemia and malnutrition, and comorbidities such as diabetes and hypertension, may result in significant morbidity, even if the patient does not progress to ESKD. Thus the goals of therapy are to (1) delay progression of CKD; (2) delay and treat known cardiovascular disease (CVD) comorbidities; (3) manage uremic symptoms (such as fatigue, pruritis, anorexia) and complications (such as anemia, CKD-mineral bone disease [CKD-MBD], malnutrition, and hypertension); (4) educate and engage patients and families in modality choice; (5) initiate

TABLE 8.1 Glomerular Filtration Rate (GFR) Categories in Chronic Kidney Disease

GFR category	GFR (mL/min/1.73 m^2)	Terms
G1	≥90	Normal or high
G2	60–89	Mildly decreased, compared with young adult level
G3a	45–59	Mildly to moderately decreased
G3b	30–44	Moderately to severely decreased
G4	15–29	Severely decreased
G5	<15	End-stage kidney failure

(Adapted from Kidney Disease: Improving Global Outcomes (KDIGO) CKD Work Group, KDIGO 2012 Clinical Practice Guideline for the Evaluation and Management of Chronic Kidney Disease, *Kidney Int. Suppl.* 3 (2013) 1-150.)

TABLE 8.2 Albuminuria Categories in Chronic Kidney Disease

Category	Albumin/creatinine ratio (ACR) (mg/mmol)	ACR (mg/g)	Terms
A1	<3	<30	Normal to mildly increased
A2	3–30	30–300	Moderately increased, compared with young adult level
A3	>30	>300	Severely increased, compared with young adult level

(From Kidney Disease: Improving Global Outcomes (KDIGO) CKD Work Group, KDIGO 2012 Clinical Practice Guideline for the Evaluation and Management of Chronic Kidney Disease, *Kidney Int. Suppl.* 3 (2013) 1-150.)

timely kidney replacement therapy, including timely placement of access or transplant workup (including preemptive transplantation where feasible); and (6) facilitate goals of care discussions and patient autonomy in decision making and support a conservative approach to CKD management where this is in line with patient wishes. Each of these goals requires education and effective communication between patients and caregivers and comanagement by different health professionals, including nursing and allied health. With the main aim to maintain health, it is essential that the structure of the clinic reflect all goals and the demand for communication and investigation to ensure success.

This chapter describes the principles of chronic disease management and a model of integrated multidisciplinary team-based care structured on these goals. The structure and function of a clinic-based approach for the comprehensive care of patients with CKD are outlined, and the potential uses of such a clinic are also discussed. The described structure and function may serve as a template for the development of such clinics. To ensure a context for such a clinic, we also review the evidence and rationale supporting this concept.

STAGING AND TERMINOLOGY FOR CHRONIC KIDNEY DISEASE AND EFFECT ON NEED FOR COORDINATED CARE

The 2012 KDIGO guideline suggested a classification of CKD based on cause, glomerular filtration rate (GFR) category and albuminuria category. After determining the etiology of the kidney disease, patients can be assigned to six different GFR categories (Table 8.1), and three different albuminuria categories (Table 8.2), to assess in two dimensions: severity and prognosis. The aim of this classification system was to recognize the importance of other markers of CKD, such as albuminuria or structural kidney abnormalities, which can occur even when GFR is preserved. Recognition of CKD as a spectrum of disease, and these abnormalities as points along this spectrum, may permit the earlier identification and intervention of CKD in individuals, thereby providing the greatest opportunity to reduce morbidity and mortality.

The adoption of a universal language and terminology, initially through the 2002 National Kidney Foundation–sponsored Kidney Disease Outcomes Quality Initiative (K/DOQI) guidelines,[9] and more recently through the aforementioned KDIGO guidelines, has helped facilitate knowledge acquisition by the medical community, patients, and public bodies and has improved research clarity and applicability. The KDIGO staging system has helped clarify the previously used terms (*predialysis, progressive renal disease, progressive renal insufficiency*), which were often confusing and sometimes misleading.

The estimates of populations with CKD generated from the new CKD classification system and the accompanying public awareness campaign around the world have helped identify the large burden of CKD that exists. The focus on earlier identification has identified a large number of patients whose CKD would have remained undetected much longer based on creatinine levels alone, and thus there is the need to create appropriately structured care delivery systems as described herein, including the education of other healthcare providers in CKD care. Furthermore, evidence has accumulated regarding the need for more proactive care and for the early institution of strategies to delay CKD progression, as well as CVD risk reduction, which is the most common cause of death among the CKD population.[7] As a result, CKD screening and prevention strategies should be employed alongside management strategies in high-risk populations, such as people with diabetes. Kidney health promotion campaigns and education have already been shown to be effective in reducing rates of ESKD in Taiwan, Uruguay, and Chile.[5,10]

OVERVIEW OF CHRONIC KIDNEY DISEASE CLINIC

Philosophical Basis

In contrast to the case of diabetes or heart failure, the role of a multidisciplinary clinic in facilitating the care of patients with CKD has not been clearly defined. Thus data to support the concept and implementation are often drawn from experience with other chronic diseases. Clinics for the care of CKD should be based on the fundamental principle of ensuring the delivery of longitudinal, complex care to a large, diverse group of individuals. This requires that the structure of the clinic and services offered optimize communication within and between individuals, including the patient and other physicians and allied health teams. One of the key roles of the care should be to integrate medical, psychological, and social aspects of chronic disease to optimize patient outcomes.

Health literacy is defined by the Institute of Medicine as "the degree to which individuals can obtain, process and understand the basic health information and services they need to make appropriate health decisions."[11] It represents a complex set of skills that allow an individual to optimize their healthcare interactions, which encompasses not only their numeracy, reading, and writing (print literacy) and listening and speaking (oral literacy) but also their cultural and conceptual knowledge as applied to health information,[12,13] and their personal skills and confidence, which allow individuals to take action on healthcare issues.[14]

It is clear that patients who have poor health literacy and a poor understanding of their health conditions and management have worse outcomes, including lower likelihood of receiving kidney transplantation[15,16] and increased mortality.[15,17] Limited health literacy is common, and prevalence can range between 12% and 20% among patients with CKD and ESKD.[15-18] Certain groups of patients may be particularly at risk of poor outcomes due to poor health literacy, as limited health literacy has been demonstrated to have an independent association with low socioeconomic status,[15-19] nonwhite ethnicity,[19] poor English fluency,[16] and comorbidities[16] in patients with kidney disease. Kidney transplant recipients are less likely to have poor health literacy,[19] particularly those who have received preemptive transplantation and live-donor transplantation.[16] This may suggest that the intensive education process typically performed pretransplant could improve health literacy and lead to better clinical outcomes. Causality cannot be established, however, as it is possible that health literacy directly affects access to transplantation,[19] where patients with higher health literacy at baseline are better equipped to seek live kidney donors and have regular medical follow-up to allow preemptive transplantation. In any case, improving health literacy among patients with CKD is likely to result in better clinical outcomes.

Adult learning operates five assumptions: (1) adults are independent and self-directing; (2) adults have accumulated a great deal of experience, which is a rich resource for learning; (3) adults value learning that integrates with the demands of their everyday life; (4) adults are more interested in immediate, problem-centered approaches than subject-centered ones; and (5) adults are more motivated to learn by internal drives than by external ones.[20] Knowles and colleagues suggested seven principles of adult learning based on these, including (1) establishing a safe and effective learning environment, (2) involving learners in mutual planning of methods and learning content, (3) involving learners in identifying their own needs, (4) facilitating learners to define their own learning objectives, (5) encouraging learners to identify and use resources appropriately to achieve their objectives, (6) supporting learners to carry out their own learning plans, and (7) allowing learners to critically reflect on and evaluate their own learning.[20,21] The importance of the application of these principles in the development and application of tools for use in multidisciplinary clinics should be emphasized.

BOX 8.1 Current KDIGO Recommendations Regarding Referral to a Nephrologist

- Acute kidney injury (AKI) or abrupt sustained fall in glomerular filtration rate (GFR);
- GFR <30 mL/min/1.73 m^2;
- a consistent finding of significant albuminuria (albumin/creatinine ration [ACR] >300 mg/g;
- progression of chronic kidney disease (CKD) (irrespective of GFR);
- urinary red cell casts, red blood cell >20 per high-power field sustained and not readily explained;
- CKD and hypertension refractory to treatment with four or more antihypertensive agents;
- persistent abnormalities of serum potassium;
- recurrent or extensive nephrolithiasis; or
- hereditary kidney disease.

(From Kidney Disease: Improving Global Outcomes (KDIGO) CKD Work Group, KDIGO 2012 Clinical Practice Guideline for the Evaluation and Management of Chronic Kidney Disease, *Kidney Int. Suppl.* 3 (2013) 1-150.)

Role of Multidisciplinary Clinics

Early referral to a nephrologist is associated with a lower chance of needing to commence dialysis by temporary vascular access, increased uptake of independent therapies such as peritoneal dialysis, reduced hospitalization rates, and reduced mortality compared with late nephrology referral.[1,22-27] Moreover, multidisciplinary nephrology clinics have been shown to be cost-effective compared with general nephrology clinics, especially when patients were referred early, leading to increased life-years free of dialysis and fewer days spent in hospital.[23] KDIGO provides recommendations for criteria for referral to a nephrologist (Box 8.1); however, the decision to refer must be considered on a case-by-case basis.

Given the multiplicity of goals of CKD care, the complexity of treatment options, wide disparities in patient health literacy, and patient educational needs, it is clear that a team of individuals is required to achieve optimal management. Treatment targets, such as blood pressure, may be reached by involving expert nurses, pharmacists, or other members of the team in conjunction with the physician. Thus a team approach with well-defined roles, responsibilities, and objectives appears to be both logical and practical. Improved patient care and outcomes due to a multidisciplinary team clinic have been demonstrated in disciplines such as endocrinology,[28-30] cardiology,[31-36] rheumatology,[37-38] and oncology.[39] Similarly, compared with standard care by a nephrologist alone, there is evidence that a multidisciplinary care team approach is beneficial for both children[40,41] and adults with CKD.[42-50]

Structure and Definition of Multidisciplinary Clinics

Formal Multidisciplinary Team

A multidisciplinary team is defined as nurses, nurse educators, dietitians, pharmacists, social workers, and physicians who are allied in a formal relationship and who interact with the patient and each other. Although it is recognized that there are a number of different configurations due to funding and local healthcare system issues, for the purpose of definition, this team is readily identifiable as dedicated (part time or full time) to CKD care.

Informal Multidisciplinary Resources

Nurses, social workers, dietitians, pharmacists, and physicians associated with the kidney team to whom patients are referred may constitute informal resources, because there is no defined team or expectation of standardization of team interactions with each other or the patient. In such an arrangement, patient access is dependent on individual patient needs, and the group of individuals may or may not interact as a team or necessarily be involved with longitudinal follow-up of patients. Each team member is able to interact with the patient on a regular basis as necessary, but coordination with other team members is not necessary to its structure.

No Multidisciplinary Team

Nurses, social workers, pharmacists, and dietitians may or may not be available to the patient. There is an absence of team structure or function.

KEY GOALS OF CHRONIC KIDNEY DISEASE CARE

This section describes the key goals of comprehensive CKD care, including diagnosis, education, delay of progression, identification and treatment of comorbidities associated with CKD, and complications of CKD. The institution of primary prevention strategies, including vaccination programs and the preparation of patients for kidney replacement therapy as appropriate, is also discussed. The goals described are comprehensive and complex, thus the need for a structured delivery system with protocols, such as delivery in formal longitudinal clinic care.

Diagnosis

The first goal of the nephrology clinic team should be to attempt to establish or confirm a diagnosis and to determine the rate of progression of kidney disease. A review of current medications is necessary to ensure the absence of nephrotoxic medications. Past medical and family history should be investigated, with effort to elucidate the presence of systemic disease including diabetes, vascular disease, connective tissue disorders, infections, and malignancy. Kidney disease may be multifactorial in nature, and consideration should be given to the possibility of several contributory factors.

The nephrologist should ensure that appropriate tests have been undertaken to establish a diagnosis. In early visits, reversible causes of kidney disease should be sought, even if a chronic etiology is suspected, especially if there has been a rapid decline in kidney function. For example, noninvasive imaging may be helpful to rule out potentially reversible obstructive causes.[51] Invasive tests, such as kidney biopsy, may be performed when needed to establish diagnosis or guide treatment.[1]

BOX 8.2 Components of Chronic Kidney Disease (CKD) Education

- Explanation of normal kidney function, blood pressure, and laboratory test results and their significance
- Explanation of specific disease conditions, symptoms, and complications of CKD
- Dietary teaching
- Diabetes education, if appropriate
- Facilitating medication knowledge and adherence
- Discussions about vein preservation in preparation for future vascular access (avoiding blood taking and intravenous cannulae on selected side)
- Anemia management education, including risks and benefits of iron and erythrocyte-stimulating agents (ESAs), teaching of self-administration, and provision of educational materials to the primary care provider
- Discussions about self-management, values, and decision-making considerations.
- Discussion of choices for treating end-stage kidney disease, including conservative therapy, hemodialysis, peritoneal dialysis, and discussion of the benefits of home-based modalities, if appropriate
- Discussion about option of kidney transplantation (live or deceased donor), if appropriate

Education

CKD education covers a broad range of topics and skills (Box 8.2). Patient education and awareness are integral components of the clinic. Education is important from a decision-making perspective and to alleviate fear and psychological suffering. In addition, people who have received disease and management education are more likely to take an active part in their care, with better outcomes noted in other chronic health conditions,[52-53] especially for those previously failing to meet treatment goals.[54] Ongoing feedback to increase patient knowledge regarding interventions and their outcomes has been demonstrated to improve effectiveness of treatment in the case of dyslipidemia.[55] Patients receiving comprehensive education programs in the predialysis period are more likely to opt for independent dialysis therapies, including peritoneal dialysis and home hemodialysis.[56] In the present and emerging technological era, promising new opportunities for education exist, such as computer-based, online, mobile phone applications, and virtual environment training.[57-59]

Ideally, education should also involve family members or support-network individuals. Education should commence in early stages of CKD, to allow patients a better understanding of their disease and to equip them with knowledge and skills so they can best preserve kidney function and avoid complications

TABLE 8.3 **Prevention of Chronic Kidney Disease (CKD) Progression in Adults**

	Treatment Target	Treatment Options
Blood pressure and renin-angiotensin-aldosterone system (RAAS) interruption	If urine ACR <3 mg/mmol: ≤140 mmHg systolic and ≤90 mmHg diastolic If urine ACR >3 mg/mmol: ≤130 mmHg systolic and ≤ 80mmHg diastolic Minimizing proteinuria in people with diabetes and urine ACR 3 to 30 mg/g, and in all individuals with AER >30 mg/g	Antihypertensive medications ACE inhibitor or ARB in people with diabetes and urine ACR 30 to 300 mg/g, and in all individuals with ACR >300 mg/g Fluid status management with dialysis
Reducing risk of AKI	Avoiding AKI	Careful consideration when performing investigations or procedures which may increase risk of AKI Careful management of patients with intercurrent illnesses that may increase risk of AKI Provision of educational material for patients regarding AKI risks
Protein intake	If GFR <30 mL/min/1.73 m^2: ≤0.8 g/kg/d If at risk of CKD progression: <1.3 g/kg/d	Dietary protein limitation, avoid excess while providing sufficient intake for adequate nutrition
Glycemic control	HbA_{1c} <7% for prevention of diabetic kidney disease HbA_{1c} 7%–8% with established CKD	Dietary modification Oral Various hypoglycemic agents Injectable Insulin Glucagon-like peptide -1 receptor agonists
Salt intake	<90 mmol (<2 g) per day	Dietary salt restriction
Lifestyle	Physical activity compatible with cardiovascular health and tolerance ≥30 min, 5 times per wk BMI 20–25 kg/m^2 (according to country specific demographics) Nonsmoker	Physical activity Dietary modification Bariatric surgery (in appropriate patients) Smoking cessation
Additional dietary advice	Dependent on individual	Individualized dietary advice regarding phosphate and potassium intake when indicated

ACE, Angiotensin-converting enzyme; *ACR*, albumin/creatinine ratio; *AER*, albumin excretion rate; *AKI*, acute kidney injury; *ARB*, angiotensin receptor blocker; *BMI*, body mass index; *GFR*, glomerular filtration rate; *HbA_{1c}*, hemoglobin A1c.
(From Kidney Disease: Improving Global Outcomes (KDIGO) CKD Work Group, KDIGO 2012 Clinical Practice Guideline for the Evaluation and Management of Chronic Kidney Disease, *Kidney Int. Suppl.* 3 (2013)1-150. ADA, Standards of Medical Care in Diabetes, *Diabetes Care* 40 (2017) S50.)

of CKD for as long as possible. As CKD progresses, education must expand and intensify to include more complex management concepts, such as preparations for dialysis.

Delay of Kidney Disease Progression

The cornerstone of CKD care is to delay progression of kidney disease and thereby to reduce complications related to kidney failure, including death and ESKD. This involves treatment of the primary kidney disease, if possible, as well as optimizing factors and systemic disease that may otherwise contribute to CKD progression. Lastly, management also involves the avoidance of future kidney insults where possible, such as hypotension, hypovolemia, and nephrotoxic medications. Although guidelines exist regarding management targets for intervention, treatment goals and methods must be individualized, with consideration of risks versus benefits for each patient (Table 8.3).

Management of Comorbidities

These topics are covered in-depth in other, dedicated chapters. This section will identify how multidisciplinary clinics can help facilitate optimal care.

Cardiovascular Disease

Patients with CKD are more likely to have cardiovascular risk factors, including smoking, obesity, hypertension, dyslipidemia, hyperuricemia, anemia, elevated glycosylated hemoglobin, chronic inflammation with elevated C-reactive protein (CRP), and albuminuria.[60] Patients with CKD are at an increased risk of cardiovascular events and death,[61-63] and this risk increases with declining GFR.[64-65] In fact, CVD is the most common cause of death in the CKD population, accounting for close to 50% of deaths,[66] and mortality due to CVD may be 10 to 30 times higher in dialysis patients compared with the general population.[67] Furthermore, not only is declining GFR a predictor for CVD, but albuminuria is also an independent predictor for CVD-related death, even at low levels.[61,68,69] Again, the risk of major cardiovascular events has been shown to increase with increasing levels of proteinuria.[70]

Patients with CKD therefore require assessment and therapy for vascular disease and associated risk factors. It should be noted that many risk factors for CVD are also associated with the risk of progression of CKD.[71] Traditional risk factors, such as hypertension, smoking, obesity, and diabetes, are common in the CKD population; thus risk factor reduction strategies used to prevent CVD in the general population can be applied to patients with CKD and may have the added effect of slowing the progression of kidney disease.[72] However, these risk factors fail to adequately explain the increased cardiovascular risk among patients with CKD, and management strategies used in the general population, such as aspirin and statins, do not always result in similar benefits in the CKD population.[73] Other nontraditional risk factors, such as calcific vascular disease,[74] volume overload, and uremic toxins, may help account for the disproportionately increased risk among patients with CKD.

Multidisciplinary clinics may help facilitate cardiovascular risk reduction by enhancing the adherence to a healthy lifestyle and medication use and by complementing other cardiovascular risk reduction strategies that patients may receive in other circumstances (i.e., from primary care or other specialists).

Anemia

Anemia in CKD patients is due to reduced erythropoietin production by the kidneys, reduced red cell life span, functional iron deficiency, and chronic inflammation.[75] Anemia is an important predictor of morbidity and mortality in the dialysis population and has been associated with ischemic heart disease,[72] left ventricular hypertrophy,[76-78] congestive heart failure,[76,78] reduced quality of life,[79,80] and increased mortality.[76,81]

Erythrocyte-stimulating agents (ESAs) are currently recommended in patients with CKD who are iron replete to achieve partial correction of anemia. There have been several studies investigating the optimal target hemoglobin for patients with CKD who are treated with ESAs. Several large randomized controlled trials have evaluated clinical outcomes with ESA use to achieve normal versus near-normal hemoglobin targets, including the Correction of Hemoglobin and Outcomes in REnal Insufficiency (CHOIR),[82] Cardiovascular Risk Reduction by Early Anemia Treatment with Epoetin Beta (CREATE),[83] and Trial to Reduce Cardiovascular Events with Aranesp Therapy (TREAT)[84] studies. Overall, the evidence has suggested that targeting normal hemoglobin levels with ESA use does not result in a significant difference in mortality, cardiovascular events, or progression to ESKD, but may be associated with a higher risk of hypertension and vascular complications, including stroke and vascular access thrombosis.[85] As a result, KDIGO recommends that ESAs generally should not be used to target a hemoglobin of greater than 11.5 g/dL, and should not be used to intentionally increase the hemoglobin to greater than 13.0 g/dL.[86]

To maintain hemoglobin in the target range, regular blood tests are required. Pharmacists and doctors can then review blood work results and make adjustments to doses if needed. Nursing staff are also vital to this process, first to educate patients in how to self-administer ESAs, decreasing the number of clinic visits required, and to facilitate administration of ESAs for those patients who are unable to self-administer due to dexterity, cognitive issues, or other concerns. In addition, nurses are an important bridge to communicate and reinforce changes in dose or administration to patients.

CKD-MBD

Hyperphosphatemia, hypercalcemia, and hyperparathyroidism observed in ESKD have been independently associated with increased mortality.[87] It is likely that disordered calcium/phosphate metabolism contributes to the excessively high incidence of CVD in patients with CKD. Vessel wall calcification, as well as atherosclerotic plaque with high calcium component, has been demonstrated in patients with CKD.[74]

Phosphate-binding treatments have been the mainstay of managing calcium/phosphate abnormalities in the past, with calcium-based binders generally being used as a first line due to their low cost and availability. More recently, however, evidence has suggested that calcium-based phosphate binders may contribute to vascular calcification and to increased cardiovascular events and mortality.[88] The use of noncalcium-based binders is becoming more common, and newer products are also being developed, including sevelamer, lanthanum, and iron-based binders. However, limited is known about the long-term effects and complications of these medications. Moreover, phosphate-lowering therapy, though effective at normalizing biochemical CKD-MBD parameters, has not demonstrated a mortality benefit thus far.[89] As such, the most recent, updated KDIGO guidelines on CKD-MBD management suggest aiming for normal phosphate levels, avoiding hypercalcemia, and restricting both the use of calcium-based phosphate binders and dietary phosphate intake.[90,91]

The input of dieticians and nurse educators is vital to ensure that patients have adequate knowledge about their dietary goals and to assist them with strategies to reduce excessive phosphate intake, thereby reducing the need for calcium-based binders and patients' pill burden.

Nutrition

Malnutrition is common in patients in later stages of CKD. There is a strong association between decreased albumin and worse nutritional status, with adverse outcomes including increased mortality.[92-96] Unfortunately, albumin is a late indicator of malnutrition and is a negative acute phase reactant. Acidosis also contributes to protein breakdown and mineral metabolism aberrations. Thus assessment of nutritional status cannot be adequately performed by only using biochemical markers, but also requires the expertise of a dietitian.

Reduced protein diets have been extensively studied as a means to slow the progression of kidney disease, with mixed results. Metaanalyses and a large, randomized trial suggest that the effect may be slight and there is a potential for protein malnutrition, which would result in adverse outcomes.[97-99] The optimal level of dietary protein restriction to derive maximal benefits and avoid harm is not clear,[99] and protein restriction to slow CKD progression is controversial, especially in advanced CKD. A reasonable approach is to limit protein with a goal to avoid excess while providing sufficient intake for adequate nutrition. Thus the KDIGO guidelines currently suggest protein intake of 0.8 g/kg/day in adults with a GFR <30 mL/min/1.73 m^2, when accompanied with appropriate education, and that adults at risk of CKD progression should avoid high protein intake of >1.3 g/kg/day.[1]

Formulation of a dietary plan that optimizes nutritional state, individually caters to a patient's nutritional needs (whether that be weight loss or weight gain), and avoids excessive loads of nutritional elements that may add to complications in patients with CKD (such as phosphate, potassium, and salt) is challenging and requires dietetics expertise. Furthermore, ensuring adherence to a prescribed diet is difficult and requires frequent, continuous input from dietitians and nurse educators. This becomes only more important as the patient approaches ESKD, because worsening malnutrition may become the principal indication to initiate dialysis.

Primary Prevention

The main content for the topics in this section is covered in-depth by other dedicated chapters. This section will identify how multidisciplinary clinics can help facilitate optimal care.

Primary prevention strategies are also important in the management of patients with CKD and may sometimes be overlooked due to the time-intensive management of conditions associated with uremia and its complications. Vaccinations, lipid-lowering agents and other CVD primary prevention strategies, diabetes control, smoking cessation, and lifestyle modification are important. This section briefly reviews these strategies in CKD patients.

Vaccinations

Infection is the second leading cause of death among patients on dialysis.[1] As a result, patients with CKD may benefit from immunization against communicable diseases, including pneumococcal infections and influenza, which are common sources of morbidity and mortality in hospitalized patients and those with chronic illnesses. Vaccination programs have been less successful among CKD patients compared with the general population, both in terms of implementation and response to vaccine. Reasons for poor response include malnutrition, uremia, and the generally immunosuppressed state of patients with CKD.

Variations in vaccination dose and dosing schedule to increase response rates in dialysis patients have been tried with reasonable success, which could be implemented among patients at all stages of CKD. In the case of hepatitis B, KDIGO recommends that patients with a GFR <30 mL/min/1.73 m^2 and risk of CKD progression should be vaccinated. Intradermal hepatitis B vaccination may be able to achieve higher rates of seroconversion and higher peak antibody titers and thus should be considered for patients who do not respond to intramuscular vaccination, especially those in high-risk populations.[100-103] In general, patients with higher GFR levels are more likely to seroconvert after hepatitis B vaccination[104]; thus it is clear that early identification of CKD and provision of comprehensive care is invaluable.

Aspirin

The use of low-dose aspirin to prevent cardiovascular events is widespread in the general population; however, results in the literature are inconsistent as to whether aspirin therapy results in a clinically significant effect on either cardiovascular or all-cause mortality in patients with CKD.[105-107] In addition, aspirin therapy may increase the risk of bleeding.[106-108] As a result, it remains unclear whether aspirin therapy is beneficial in patients with CKD, and this therapy is currently recommended only for secondary prevention in patients with known coronary artery disease, not as primary prevention in patients with CKD.[1]

Dyslipidemia

Like aspirin, statin use for correcting dyslipidemia and reducing cardiovascular risk has become extremely common in the general population. Studies including the Prospective Pravastatin Pooling (PPP) project,[109] the Deutsche Diabetes Dialyse (4D) study,[110] and A Study to Evaluate the Use of Rosuvastatin in Subjects on Regular Hemodialysis: An Assessment of Survival and Cardiovascular Events (AURORA)[111] have evaluated the use of statins in patients with CKD and found that statins are effective in lowering cholesterol levels; however, these studies did not show convincing reductions in cardiovascular events or mortality. More recently (2011) the Study of Heart and Renal Protection (SHARP) trial evaluated combined statin and ezetimibe use in patients with CKD in the largest, prospective, double-blind, placebo-controlled trial to date, and found a significant reduction in major atherosclerotic events and stroke in the treatment group.[112] However, this trial did exclude patients with a history of cardiovascular events, limiting its applicability to many CKD patients. Although the study demonstrated effectiveness of the lipid-lowering strategy in CKD patients, that effect was proportional to the reduction in cholesterol (as in other populations). In those patients who were on dialysis, the proportional reduction was lower and the benefit smaller. As a result, the most recent KDIGO guidelines recommend initiation of statin use for primary prevention of cardiovascular events only in non–dialysis-dependent CKD patients and also recommend the continuation, but not initiation, of statins for patients with CKD on dialysis or kidney transplant, in those who have not had a previous CVD event.[113] In addition, the guidelines recommend that statin dose should not be titrated up to achieve a target low-density lipoprotein (LDL) due to the lack of benefit with higher doses, and therefore that monitoring follow-up LDL levels is not necessary.[113]

Diabetes Control

Optimal diabetes management should be encouraged and facilitated with referral to a diabetes program if possible. Intensive glucose control in both type 1 and type 2 diabetes may prevent or stabilize the early stages of microvascular complications, including CKD,[114,115] and the benefits from early intensive glucose control appear to be sustained even years later, in a so-called "legacy effect."[116] However, despite reductions in progression of albuminuria and microvascular disease, tight glycemic control is not associated with a reduced risk of kidney failure, major cardiovascular events, or death in the CKD population.[117]

Sodium-glucose cotransporter 2 (SGLT2) inhibitors have gained recent attention through the EMPA-REG OUTCOME trials, a large, randomized, double-blind, placebo-controlled trial, where empagliflozin was associated reduced cardiovascular events and death in patients with diabetes,[118] and was also associated with slower progression of CKD in diabetic patients.[119] The canagliflozin cardiovascular assessment study (CANVAS) confirmed these results with canagliflozin, another SGLT2 inhibitor.[120] These agents represent a new therapeutic direction for prevention, and possibly treatment, of CKD in diabetes. These agents appear to produce beneficial effects beyond glycemic control to reduce risk of CVD and CKD progression.

Lifestyle Modification and Rehabilitation

Smoking cessation is recommended for reducing cardiovascular and malignancy risk, but also because cigarette smoking is associated with CKD progression.[121-123] Obesity, poor diet, and sedentary lifestyle contribute to diabetes, hypertension, and vascular disease. Patients with CKD should be encouraged to maintain a healthy weight, and those who are able should be encouraged to increase physical activity because this has been demonstrated to result in improved aerobic capacity, cardiovascular function, and health-related quality of life.[124,125]

Multidisciplinary clinics therefore offer another opportunity to assist patients with lifestyle interventions through facilitating and encouraging healthy diet, smoking cessation, and individual appropriate exercise interventions.

PREPARATION FOR KIDNEY REPLACEMENT THERAPY

Individuals with progressive CKD require timely preparation for either kidney replacement therapy (dialysis or transplantation) or conservative care. Creating and implementing these care plans is an iterative process that takes time and requires a multidisciplinary team approach. The different modalities should be seen as complementary, and individuals may transition through several modalities. Home-based therapies that foster independent care are encouraged. The optimal timing of dialysis initiation remains unknown but is usually influenced by a combination of low estimated GFR (eGFR), patient symptoms, and careful clinical evaluation. Close follow-up of patients at the later stages of CKD, with objective assessment of global functioning, permits appropriate timing of dialysis initiation.

Modality Selection

Predialysis counseling programs provided through the CKD clinic may help patients chose a dialysis modality, confront the prospect of dialysis, and prepare themselves for life on dialysis. Education and knowledge influence both readiness to decide and decision making itself. A multidisciplinary team should identify possible barriers to various modalities, including physical, visual, cognitive, psychological, and social problems, and help overcome such barriers where possible by adequate care, education, and psychological counseling. Predialysis nurses have an important role in supporting patients who must make decisions when kidney replacement therapy is needed. Dialysis modalities include hemodialysis, either in-center or at home, peritoneal dialysis (peritoneal dialysis), including continuous ambulatory peritoneal dialysis (CAPD), and automated peritoneal dialysis (APD). The selection of dialysis modality is influenced by a number of factors, including availability and accessibility, patient comorbidities, socioeconomic circumstances, the patient's living situation, and the method of clinician financial reimbursement.[126-129]

Suboptimal preparation for kidney replacement therapy can result in a high rate of hospitalizations in patients with advanced CKD, low uptake of home dialysis or preemptive transplantation, urgent hospitalization to initiate dialysis, and decreased likelihood of commencing dialysis with an arteriovenous fistula (AVF). A number of factors may contribute, including fragmented treatment, poorly delivered patient education, healthcare infrastructure, inadequate communication among healthcare providers, and delayed decision making.[130] Both time and healthcare support are necessary for patients to process their dialysis options. In one study, around 25% of patients were undecided about modality choice, despite receiving predialysis education.[131] Stage of behavioral change has been shown to influence patients' ability to make medical treatment-related decisions and act on the basis of those decisions.[132] As a result, there is a need for structured dialysis decision-making education tools that facilitate patient behavioral change and support the multidisciplinary team in addressing the diverse lifestyle barriers and learning requirements of patients.

The availability of a comprehensive predialysis education program has been shown to facilitate increased uptake of home-based therapies among CKD patients, particularly in centers with established home dialysis programs.[56] Home-based dialysis (home hemodialysis and peritoneal dialysis) has been associated with improved quality of life and cost-effectiveness compared with in-center hemodialysis.[133] Despite this, the overall uptake remains low, with 90% of patients with ESKD in the United States undertaking in-center dialysis, compared with less than 10% on home dialysis. Reasons for this are multifactorial and include patient comorbidities, late referral to a nephrologist, inadequate dialysis modality education, and unfavorable social circumstances.[134-136] Furthermore, it has been reported that CKD patients who select home dialysis (especially peritoneal dialysis) as their initial modality of choice may still end up initiating dialysis in-center and are more likely to start with a central venous catheter (CVC) as opposed to an AVF.[131] Thus there is a need to develop and test the effectiveness of comprehensive and standardized education programs to address this issue. Through the CKD clinic, there should be ongoing evaluation of patients' expectations, reinforcement of modality choice, and ongoing education of patients regarding benefits and timing to improve preparedness for home dialysis.

In terms of dialysis therapies, observed survival is generally highest in patients treated with home hemodialysis.[137] There is currently no compelling evidence to show a difference in survival between in-center hemodialysis and peritoneal dialysis. Studies attempting to compare survival outcomes between these two modalities have been mainly observational in nature and yielded variable results due to selection bias, flawed study design, variances in mortality effects with time from initiation of dialysis, differences in patient comorbidities, and other factors. Although several studies have found an early survival benefit associated with peritoneal dialysis, this has been largely attributed to higher baseline residual kidney function and less comorbidity.[138]

Transplantation is the optimal treatment for kidney replacement therapy and is associated with improved cost effectiveness, patient survival, and quality of life.[139,140] Living versus deceased kidney donation affords an increased survival benefit to both recipient and graft,[141] in addition to facilitating earlier transplantation.[142] At any given time, approximately 50% to 60% of patients receiving dialysis are eligible for transplantation, but estimates are not available for those with earlier stages of CKD. A significant proportion of patients may be ineligible for transplantation, such as those with extensive vascular calcification or severe CVD. Preemptive transplantation, that is, before the need for dialysis, is only generally an option for patients with an available living donor. In the United States approximately 30% of transplants are from living donors, with one-fifth of these being unrelated to the recipient.[143]

It is generally preferred that patients commence dialysis either on peritoneal dialysis, or hemodialysis using an AVF rather than a CVC. This is especially relevant in today's reimbursement environment, where patients with optimal starts can lead to healthcare savings of tens of thousands of dollars per year. For this reason, modality selection should be explored with the patient in a timely manner, with early identification of contraindications to a particular modality. A perspective on the relative amount of time required to prepare for each of the options, including transplantation, should be provided. The option of conservative care should also be discussed with patients, particularly those who wish to focus on quality of life rather than extending life expectancy.

Vascular Access Creation

For most patients considering hemodialysis, the preferred vascular access option is an AVF, due to longer patency, lower infectious complications, improved quality of life, improved cost effectiveness, and lower all-cause mortality compared with AVGs and CVCs.[144-147] Timely referral is recommended to ensure sufficient time for creation and maturation, particularly as more than one procedure may be required to establish functionality. If creation of an AVF is delayed, it may not mature in time for dialysis initiation and subsequently a CVC may be required. The patient should be reassured that the presence of a functioning AVF does not signify that dialysis must be initiated; rather, it reduces the chance that additional procedures, such as placement of a temporary dialysis catheter, might be needed at the actual time of dialysis initiation. Creating an AVF too early has been associated with a small increase in complications and potential utilization of the limited lifespan before hemodialysis is needed. The process for access creation begins with timely referral to the CKD clinic and patient education, followed by appropriate investigations and interventions in preparation for the desired access, including venous mapping and surgical referral where appropriate. After access creation, the multidisciplinary team should coordinate surveillance of the dialysis access.

Although traditionally a fistula-first approach has been adopted, recent studies suggest that not all patients may benefit from AVF compared with AVGs and CVCs. When considering options for vascular access, clinicians should consider the patient's risk of death before reaching ESKD, their anticipated life expectancy after initiating dialysis, expected duration of therapy, and risk of complications with each type of access. Elderly patients are more likely to have limited life expectancy and lower likelihood of AVF maturation, necessitating multiple procedures, which may mitigate the relative benefits of AVFs over AVGs and CVCs.[148] Furthermore, recent data suggest that for patients with an estimated life expectancy of 2 years, AVFs are no more cost effective than AVGs, and neither form of vascular access is more cost effective than CVCs for patients with a life expectancy of 6 months.[149] Therefore AVG placement and, in some cases, continued CVC use after dialysis initiation may be reasonable vascular access options for older adults with reduced life expectancy. For patients requiring a temporary period of hemodialysis, either as a bridge to living donor kidney transplantation or while awaiting transition to peritoneal dialysis, a CVC may also be acceptable vascular access option due to the anticipated short duration of therapy.

Planning for vascular access creation should begin at least 6 months in advance of the anticipated need to start. According to most published guidelines, vascular access should be created when the eGFR is approximately 15 to 20 mL/min/1.73 m^2 in those who are anticipated to progress and who do not have a reasonable chance for a preemptive transplant.[150] The timing of AVF creation in any individual patient should also take into account the rate of CKD progression. Reasons for lack of permanent access at the start of dialysis may include patient factors such as denial of inevitable dialysis, being too unwell to undergo permanent access procedures, failure of AVF maturation, acute deterioration of kidney function in a previously stable patient, or late decision to undertake chronic dialysis. However, this may also reflect the multidisciplinary team's inability to predict the start of dialysis, lack of resources, or poor planning. Late recognition of CKD and late referral to nephrology contribute to the problem. In consultation with the patients and the clinic team, optimal timing around education, decision making, and access creation should be undertaken.

Timely Initiation

When to initiate dialysis is a complex decision that involves the consideration of many variables. Although there are some easily identified absolute indications for initiation,[151] debate exists with respect to "timely" dialysis when these indicators are not so apparent. Indeed, since the 1970s some have advocated for initiation of dialysis before clinically significant markers of uremia appear.[151-153] These studies suggested a positive association between residual kidney function at dialysis initiation and clinical outcomes. Unfortunately, lead-time bias, patient selection, or referral bias may favor outcomes in the population of patients starting "timely" dialysis.

According to USRDS data, there has been a trend toward early dialysis initiation in the United States since 1996,[154] with the fraction of patients transitioning to dialysis with eGFR of 10 to 14 mL/min/m^2 rising from 20% to 52% and from 4% to 17% for patients with eGFR of ≥15 mL/min/m^2.[155] The appropriate timing for initiating hemodialysis in patients with advanced CKD in terms of optimal patient outcomes and cost effectiveness remains unclear. Recent randomized controlled trial data, together with large registry-based studies corrected for confounding, show no survival advantage to early-start dialysis. The Initiating Dialysis Early and Late (IDEAL) study examined whether early initiation of dialysis influenced survival among 828 patients with progressive CKD.[156] They found no difference in survival or clinical outcomes (cardiovascular events, infectious events, and complications of dialysis) between early (MDRD eGFR 9 mL/min/1.73 m^2 versus late eGFR 7.2 mL/min/1.73 m^2) start dialysis. Furthermore, several recent studies have reported reduced comorbidity-adjusted survival rates for early-start hemodialysis,[157] raising the possibility that dialysis may be incurring more harm than benefit. A further observational study found that planned early initiation of dialysis has also been shown to be more costly and was not associated with an improvement in quality of life.[158] The failure to find benefit of early hemodialysis by the IDEAL study and the potential harm of early initiation of hemodialysis reported in recent studies raises questions relating to the trend to early start of hemodialysis.

Given the risks and benefits of kidney replacement therapy, the decision to start dialysis should be individualized and based on symptoms rather than relying solely on a laboratory estimate of kidney function, which is subject to imprecision unless this measure is accompanied by definitive ESKD-related indications for dialysis. The 2012 KDIGO guidelines recommend considering initiation of dialysis for the treatment of progressive CKD if one or more of the following are present: symptoms or signs attributable to kidney failure (serositis, acid base or electrolyte abnormalities, pruritus); inability to control volume status or blood pressure; a progressive deterioration in nutritional status refractory to dietary intervention; or cognitive impairment.[1] Invariably, most patients will experience these with eGFR 5 to 10 mL/min/1.73 m^2. Earlier initiation may be required in patients with certain complications of CKD.

The decision should be individualized with a careful assessment of the benefits and risks each patient may incur with each therapy option. Overall, the key factor is to avoid commencing dialysis when the patient is so ill that education opportunities and the chances for maintaining independence are missed.

Independent Therapies

Home Hemodialysis

Time taken for home hemodialysis training can vary widely according to patient characteristics, vascular access, machine selection, and delivery method of the training program. CKD patients electing for home hemodialysis normally require initial hemodialysis sessions in-center to assess for early complications, such as a dialyzer reaction, before transitioning to home hemodialysis training. The role of the CKD clinic is to ensure that patients are referred in a timely manner for assessment for home hemodialysis and vascular access creation. Coordination between the clinic and dialysis unit is vital to ensure smooth transition for the patient through these various initiation steps.

Peritoneal Dialysis

Patients should be oriented to the peritoneal dialysis unit and staff. The role of the CKD clinic in organizing peritoneal dialysis catheter placement will vary according to the center. However, the timing, placement, and preliminary education should be done in concert with the peritoneal dialysis team. As in hemodialysis, specific orders and transfer summaries should be sent to the peritoneal dialysis unit and the training/initiating schedule coordinated with appropriate team members, family members, and other health professionals.

In-Center Hemodialysis

The goal is a smooth transition to hemodialysis care, and the CKD clinic staff should ensure the appropriate commencement of dialysis with a functional vascular access. Patients should be oriented to the hemodialysis unit in advance and schedules coordinated with appropriate team members in the hemodialysis unit, family members, and other medical professionals. The CKD clinic should send initial dialysis orders and transfer summaries to the hemodialysis unit.

Transplant

As part of the educational process early in the course of CKD, the concepts of transplantation, including living donation, should be explored with patients and families. Conversations with individuals about RRT and transplantation are individualized, but given that most centers require a 3 to 12 month period for living transplantation processes, education should likely commence in potentially living donor–eligible patients, when GFR trajectory is steep, or at GFR values around 25 mL/min with evidence of progression over time. The 2012 KDIGO guidelines suggest that preemptive transplantation should be considered when the GFR is less than 20 mL/min/1.73 m^2 along with evidence of irreversible progression of their CKD over the previous 6 to 12 months.[1] However, education and discussions regarding transplantation should ideally take place earlier in the patients' CKD course, given potential complex barriers to transplantation.[159] The CKD clinic, working closely with the transplant assessment team, can help determine eligibility for a kidney transplant and assist with the identification of living donors, which may facilitate preemptive transplantation.

Maximum Conservative Management

Maximum conservative management (MCM) has been proposed as an alternative care pathway for some patients with progressive CKD for whom dialysis is unlikely to confer improved survival or quality of life.[160] Elderly patients with advanced CKD often have a higher burden of comorbidity and frailty that may influence their treatment choices and outcomes. Furthermore, advancing age, increased comorbidities, and higher level of dependency at initiation of dialysis have been associated with adverse survival.[161] Clinical tools such as the Charlson Comorbidity Index (CCI) and Clinical Frailty Scale (CFS) have been shown to be independent predictors of mortality in patients with CKD[162] and may serve as useful adjuncts to identify patients appropriate for a conservative pathway.

Observational data have shown that dialysis may extend survival of patients with ESKD and comorbidities by up to 2 years compared with MCM; however, patients choosing MCM may achieve a similar number of hospital-free days and are more likely to die at home or in a hospice.[163] When discussing treatment options with patients, establishing patient-centered goals of care are important to ascertain what is important to the patient. Often patients are willing to accept shorter life expectancy in return for improved quality of life.

Patients considering conservative management often have many anxieties related to life expectancy, anticipated symptoms, and family expectations. If appropriate, consultation with psychiatric practitioner may be warranted to ensure the patient has the capacity to make a decision regarding their care. A conservative care pathway for patients choosing not to undergo dialysis should focus on symptom control, management of anemia and other complications, social support, and palliative care. Patients may require varying levels of specialist palliative care support, with the option to intensify services in the event of clinical deterioration.

Once the decision to decline kidney replacement therapy is made, end-of-life wishes should be formalized, in particular resuscitation status, with appropriate consent and documentation. The patient should have referrals for home care and for palliative care when appropriate.

Advanced Care Planning

Advance care planning (ACP) for patients with CKD helps identify life goals and can be a useful guide for discussions among patients, their families, and their healthcare providers. ACP should be a dynamic process with the ability to adapt to the changing healthcare needs of the patient with CKD and allow for intervention as necessary. Early initiation of ACP provides time for thoughtful and deliberate consideration of the options available for kidney replacement therapy, their potential effect on a patient's day-to-day life, and time to contemplate and discuss the choices and preferences that best reflect a patient's values and life goals.[164] The results of such discussions are typically recorded as an advance care directive.

Patients often enter dialysis programs unaware that ESKD confers such a poor prognosis, with patients considerably overestimating even their 2-year survival rates.[165] The CKD clinic should facilitate timely, consistent, and detailed discussions regarding ACP for all CKD patients as part of a patient-centered approach to nephrology care, including guidance on relevant and timely prognostic data.

Planning ahead for care is preparatory to making decisions about kidney replacement therapy and can facilitate a smooth transition to dialysis as well as optimize the chance that dialysis is not initiated solely because symptoms prompt an urgent decision. To emphasize the role of ACP and prognosis sharing with CKD and ESKD patients and their families, the Renal Physicians Association issued guidelines in 2010. They encourage nephrology practitioners to address ACP within the first 90 days of providing care and to review these care plans at least annually or more frequently if a change in patient status arises.[166]

CLINIC LOGISTICS

Services

CKD clinics presumably exist within a healthcare system and society in which the common goal is promoting health of the patients. Comprehensive care delivered in a sole location is presumed to be beneficial. The frequency with which any individual patient accesses care is determined by several factors, including the infrastructure of the specific healthcare system, other primary physicians involved in the patient's care, additional patient comorbidities, and the specific stage of disease. The clinic should provide a wide range of services for patients with kidney disease and their physicians, with the overall goals of:

1. Ensuring patient and family understanding of kidney disease.
2. Ensuring understanding of healthcare or hospital systems and services available to patients with CKD.
3. Identifying potential issues related to long-term patient management.
4. Facilitating longitudinal and parallel care of patients with CKD.

Key Components of the Clinic

Ideally, the CKD clinic should operate consistently from the same outpatient facility to facilitate continuity of care and improved accessibility for patients. Locations in close proximity to hospitals and dialysis units can promote familiarity with the services and hospital logistics. If the patient does not speak the primary language of the clinic, translation by a medical interpreter should be provided by the healthcare facility to ensure unbiased translation. If this is unavailable, friends or family members who speak the primary language of the clinic should be encouraged to accompany the patient.

Patients should be given an information pack with an introduction to how the clinic operates, along with various educational materials and information regarding peer support groups. Patients and families should also be introduced to each member of the multidisciplinary team, with a clear explanation of their roles and responsibilities. In addition to continuous assessment of the patient by the team through regular clinic visits, weekly multidisciplinary rounds should be organized to facilitate communication among team members and to allow development of a care plan. This enables comprehensive follow-up by nurses, clerical staff, and others and will facilitate:

- Scheduling for tests (ultrasound, computerized tomography, etc.) and referrals to other specialists
- Medication changes, tolerance, and side effects
- Reminders for appointments and laboratory tests
- Follow-up of test results
- Liaison with laboratories and pharmacies
- Liaison with primary care providers and other consultants, including palliative care team
- Education about kidney or kidney-pancreas transplant and screening for potential donors and referrals as appropriate
- Timely referral for dialysis access creation

Individual Roles

To ensure effective and cohesive teamwork among CKD team members, definition and clarification of individuals' roles is important. This section lists key roles and responsibilities for each of the key staff involved in the delivery of CKD care. The specifics may vary depending on local policies, but the principal roles need to be clearly defined.

Nurse

The CKD nurse functions as a case manager and educator and facilitates care of patients, both directly and through the physician and team member liaison. Nursing support should be available by telephone or in person to triage medical concerns, answer questions, and provide education or emotional support and referral to other team members or community resources. This should allow for ongoing collaboration and reevaluation with the patient and should enable adaptions in the care plan with input from team members. A regular review of symptoms, medications, and monitoring of laboratory work results should occur, with response to important values by notifying physician, pharmacist, patient, and dietitian as necessary. The nurse should be able to liaise with family physicians and other primary care providers, consultants, and other chronic health condition clinics (e.g., diabetes clinic, heart health clinic).

Nurses should be able to implement protocols such as hepatitis screening and vaccination programs. Similarly, they should be able to arrange and coordinate treatments such as intravenous iron and arrange dialysis access referrals as necessary.

If a patient progresses to kidney failure, the nurse should ensure coordination of initiation of dialysis or referral for transplantation and transfer of relevant data to the prospective dialysis or transplant facility. Finally, the nurse should coordinate services in remote settings for patient convenience.

Dietitian

Dieticians should evaluate the nutritional status and diet history of each patient to ensure proper nutrition for optimal kidney function. The dietitian should develop an individualized nutrition care plan with each patient and provide education on dietary self-management. Ongoing periodic dietary review with incorporation of blood work results is encouraged to help reach goals and optimize kidney function. Dieticians should also be equipped to address the needs of patients who have specific nutrition issues, such as cachexia, metabolic abnormalities, obesity, fluid management, and CKD-related bone disease.

Social Worker

Social workers provide a wide range of support services, including emotional and practical assistance for patients and their families to help them adjust to life with CKD. They serve as patient advocates to ensure patients receive maximum allowable benefit from available resources such as home support, financial and insurance assistance, employment, and housing. Often, they play a key role in ACP and transition to kidney replacement therapies by facilitating communication of the patient's needs to the rest of the CKD team.

Pharmacist

Pharmacists, in collaboration with physicians, play an important role in educating patients about medications for managing CKD. They also address medication costs, pill burden, and possible drug interactions. The pharmacist should be available to perform a medication review with patients at their initial clinic visit and continue to follow-up at subsequent visits to assess for any alterations. In addition, the pharmacist should help optimize medication administration for each patient with CKD and address any potential side effects. Electronic medication records are encouraged to facilitate uniform care across the spectrum of CKD.

Clerical or Administrative Support

Clinics should have a dedicated unit coordinator or clerical support worker. This person's main role is to ensure that patient data and health records are maintained accurately. A paper or electronic chart should be established with complete information available and maintained with ongoing follow-up data, including laboratory test results, medications, and cumulative comorbidities. The coordinator is essential for scheduling and coordinating appointments with other clinics, consultants, and diagnostics. In addition, the coordinator is integral for information and chart transfer to programs within the kidney programs, such as dialysis or transplant clinic. They may also triage patient concerns with the team and organize appointment reminders for patients. Finally, they should identify interpreter requests and book interpreters as needed.

Chronic Kidney Disease Clinic Role in Longitudinal Care: Different Stages of Chronic Kidney Disease

Given the current estimates of CKD prevalence in the population (between 40 and 50 million in the United States[7]), it is unlikely that the optimal resources described in this chapter are available to all patients with CKD. It is still debated whether a nephrologist must see all patients with early CKD, because it is not clear who will and who will not progress. Although there is consensus that nephrologists and teams need to see the patients at least 6 months, and ideally 12 months, before dialysis starts for access, there remains some skepticism regarding the intensity and need of nephrology input before that time. However, because it is not so easy to identify those who will and will not progress or the timing or duration of that progression, developing referrals based on these criteria does not seem practical.

An inclusive approach is recommended, with individualization of intensity of follow-up based on demographics, rates of progression, and intercurrent events as a practical solution. Although much has been learned about the care of patients close to initiating dialysis, it is not known how to care optimally for patients in early CKD (frequency of visits and laboratory testing, when to initiate drug therapies, etc.). It seems reasonable that a phased approach is applicable. As outlined, the focus of the clinic must be adjustable from early CKD detection and risk factor modification to preparing for kidney replacement therapy. Communication and education are key at all CKD stages, among patients, health caregivers, and allied care teams.

One end of the spectrum is an early referral (CKD stages 1 to 2) and a broad plan outlined to another caregiver about goals of treatment to follow. Patients could be familiarized with the clinic and kidney disease at this initial period and seen infrequently (annually or every 6 months), with increasing frequency if, or as, kidney function deteriorates for further education and refinement of management plan. In this scenario, both the patient and the other caregivers and health professionals are informed that the CKD clinic is available for consultative purposes as needed, and none of these parties will presume to comanage the patient. With worsening kidney function, the CKD team may assume more of the care planning and execution, surrounding issues pertaining to kidney disease and related issues such as diabetes management. Appropriate discussion of comanagement expectations with other specialists and primary care physicians is necessary and can be helpful in minimizing visits, medication changes, and confusing messages for patients. The frequency of testing and visits should be somewhat standardized, but individualization is needed depending on circumstances. To date there are no studies that have systematically evaluated the effect of different methods of care at earlier stages of CKD; thus there is a paucity of data to inform health system design to optimize outcomes for patients with CKD.

Chronic Kidney Disease Clinic Role in Parallel Care: Integrating With Other Caregivers

The clinic should be viewed as a resource for both patients and their health caregivers, such as family physicians and other primary care providers, thereby integrating care with other caregivers. It is vital for such a clinic to communicate information about patient status, medications, plans, and so forth, not only to the patient but to all other caregivers involved (e.g., family physicians, diabetes clinics, and hospital systems).

When patients access different healthcare systems, due to the complex nature of their disease or due to practical issues such as locale, it is not always clear how to determine the responsibility of each individual medical practitioner. For example, should the CKD clinic assume the angiotensin-converting enzyme (ACE) inhibitor is being managed by the cardiovascular clinic? Or does the CKD clinic assume the diabetes clinic is managing glycemic control or counseling about smoking cessation? At what stage of CKD does the CKD clinic take a more active role? These are not questions that will be answered in clinical trials, so practical solutions to the issue of responsibility for care implementation will need to be developed.

Coordination of clinical care is complicated by the variety of caregivers involved and the variation in levels of responsibility among them. Members of the clinical team need to state clearly their individual roles and responsibilities among themselves, as well as to the patient. Doctors bear ultimate responsibility for clinical care and must play the central, coordinating role, although members of the team who have closer or more frequent contact with the patient may be appropriate channels of information.

Patients with serious, life-limiting illness often face challenging treatment choices. A shared decision-making model is particularly important for these patients to reach an informed decision regarding treatment based on their individual values. Shared decision making is the process whereby the clinical and patient jointly participate in a healthcare decision after a discussion on the options, benefits, and risks, and considering the patient's values, preferences, and circumstances. This enhances the patient-clinician interaction and is central to good clinical care. When the evidence of benefit and harm is similar or uncertain, a patient's values and preferences are vitally important to inform medical decisions.[167,168]

Other Benefits of the Chronic Kidney Disease Clinic and Organized Protocol-Based Care

The key to the care of patients with chronic health conditions is acknowledgment of the complexity of the condition(s) and the need for longitudinal follow-up by a well-trained and prepared team. As in other areas of medicine, the care of patients with CKD requires adoption of protocols for evaluation, therapy, and follow-up. Through this approach, sensible strategies can be based on data, and management of selected conditions will be uniformly undertaken, and aim to reduce resource use and to enhance patient adherence.

The additional advantages to the clinic models for the care of CKD include the ability to optimize holistic aspects of care by using each team member's expertise appropriately and to manage follow-up and monitoring of large groups of patients in one area. Furthermore, a clinic-based approach allows database development and evaluation of outcomes in large cohorts of patients, the ability to enroll patients in clinical trials, and importantly, the adoption of newly proven therapies that may be facilitated more readily by the CKD clinic setting than in individual physicians' offices.

The clinic structure may also ensure that patients have access to appropriate, up-to-date information and materials that may not be available in individual physicians' offices. Also, it will permit coordination of care plans and execution of those plans within health system structures.

Barriers to care or implementation of strategies are more likely to be identified within a clinic setting, where social workers, pharmacists, and others may more readily identify issues not solely identified by physicians. The importance of an asymptomatic condition can be reinforced in clinic settings where the patient-team interaction is far longer than the usual patient-doctor visit.[49]

RECENT AND FUTURE STUDIES

There are few large studies describing best care models for CKD in different healthcare systems. We list some here that have attempted to describe some of what is known.

The CAN-CARE (Canadian Care Prior to Dialysis) study was a prospective multicenter cohort study of incident CKD patients referred to nephrologists across Canada between the years 2000 and 2004.[169] The study demonstrated that in 2000, referral to nephrology remained relatively late, with the mean referral eGFR of approximately 23 mL/min/1.73 m^2. Outcomes of those referred to nephrologists appeared to be different from those described in population-based studies, in that there was a greater likelihood of commencing dialysis than of dying. In a large cohort of patients in British Columbia (BC), Canada,[170] followed in more standardized multidisciplinary clinics, the probability of commencing dialysis also was higher than that of dying. In the BC observational cohort study, factors that lead to more rapid CKD progression of a referred population include younger age, male gender, proteinuria, lower hemoglobin levels, and higher serum phosphate levels. Some of these factors remain amenable to interventions, but none has been rigorously studied in randomized control trials within the context of healthcare system delivery models to determine the most cost-effective approaches to management.

The CANN-NET (Canadian Kidney Knowledge Translation & Generation Network) was developed in partnership with the Canadian Society of Nephrology, focused on systematic identification of shortcomings in CKD care and development of an evidence base on which to inform changes. In the year 2012, the CANN-NET developed a questionnaire that was used to survey the CKD clinic structure and models of care in 71 of 84 multidisciplinary adult CKD clinics across Canada. Again, almost a decade after the CAN-CARE study, there is a large variation in clinic structure and function, with particular emphasis on staffing ratios (nephrologist, dieticians, pharmacists, and nurses to patients), and even in referral criteria. They also noted that dialysis initiation decisions were usually made by nephrologists. The majority of clinics (57%) had a consistent model of care (the same nephrologist and nurse per patient), whereas others had a different nephrologist and nurse seeing patients at sequential visits.[171]

The Canadian Prevention of Renal and Cardiovascular Endpoints Trial (CanPREVENT) was a Canada-wide, multicenter clinical trial that compared care coordinated by a general practitioner (controls) with care provided by a nurse-coordinated team including a nephrologist (intervention) for patients with CKD identified through community-based clinical laboratories. Over a median follow-up period of 24 months, the study found that the overall risk of progression to ESKD in this largely unreferred population was low; however, there was a substantial risk of cardiovascular events despite optimization of traditional risk factors.[172] The study also concluded that although it was more cost effective, the nurse-coordinated model did not affect rate of GFR decline or control of most risk factors compared with usual care. Of note, the laboratory case finding strategy employed in this study resulted in a substantial number of patients being enrolled with relatively well-preserved kidney function.

Two ongoing prospective, observational studies evaluated clinical characteristics of CKD patients at baseline and continue to follow patients to predict a variety of outcomes, including ESKD. These include the Study of Treatment for Renal Insufficiency: Data and Evaluation (STRIDE) registry,[173] which will study data on prevalent CKD patients in nephrology practices in the United States, and the Chronic Renal Insufficiency Cohort (CRIC) study, which will examine risk factors for progression of CKD and the incidence of CVD among patients with CKD.[174-176] The CRIC study enrolled a total of 3612 patients with mild to moderate CKD between the years 2003 and 2007. This cohort included a racially and ethnically diverse group of patients, approximately half of whom had diabetes. Lower eGFR was associated with lower socioeconomic and educational level, cigarette smoking, and self-reported CVD.[175] Longitudinal follow-up of CRIC participants will enable a more precise assessment of these newly recognized, but less studied, risk factors on CVD and CKD outcomes. Multiple publications describing the association of novel biomarkers, including cystatin C–based GFR,[177] KIM-1/Cr,[178] interleukin-6,[179] c-reactive protein,[179] and FGF-23,[179] with cardiovascular, kidney, and mortality outcomes have been forthcoming from this study over the last decade.

The Kidney Early Evaluation Program (KEEP) is a United States–based free health screening program run by the National Kidney Foundation to increase awareness of kidney disease among those at highest risk and, subsequently, to improve outcomes through early detection and referral for care. Participation in this kidney disease screening and education program has been associated with improved preparation for ESKD with significantly higher rates of pre-ESKD nephrologist care, peritoneal dialysis, preemptive kidney transplant listing, and transplantation.[180]

The Canadian Study of Prediction of Death, Dialysis and Interim Cardiovascular Events (CanPREDDICT) is a large, prospective, Canada-wide cohort study established in the year 2008 with the primary aim of describing the associations between traditional and novel biomarkers in the prediction of kidney and cardiovascular events in patients with CKD managed by nephrologists.[181] Early data from this cohort suggests that elevated trimethylamine N-oxide (TMAO) levels may represent a new potentially modifiable cardiovascular risk factor for CKD patients[182] and that in patients with different causes of CKD, at the same level of eGFR, different biomarker profiles are associated with adverse outcomes.[183]

The Palliative Care in Chronic Kidney Disease (PACKS) study is a prospective, multicenter, longitudinal study conducted in the United Kingdom to assess quality of life, symptoms, cognition, frailty, performance decision making, costs, and effect on caregivers in people with advanced CKD managed conservatively without dialysis.[184] It aims to explore interactions and experiences leading to clinical care decisions and the effect these have on caregivers, with the intention of improving clinical outcomes of patients and experiences for their caregivers.

Currently, more well-designed studies are needed to better understand the effect of various therapeutic regimens on patient perceptions of health and wellness. Furthermore, it is imperative that we better understand the effect of various aspects of the professional care delivered (e.g., time spent, education provided) and assess the association of these with outcomes. The use of specific interventions, alone or in combination, also needs to be better understood in various stages of CKD or subpopulations.

CONCLUSION

Kidney disease involves complex physical, mental, and social aspects of health, mandating an understanding and rational use of available resources. Opportunities exist to improve early identification and follow-up of patients with CKD and to ensure better outcomes overall, regardless of whether patients ultimately require dialysis. To focus on these complex aspects of care, a multidisciplinary team approach, with protocol-based goals and systematic approaches to longitudinal follow-up, is required. It is hoped that the information supplied herein will help develop templates and deliveries of care models for further evaluation, so that, ultimately, the outcomes of patients with CKD at all stages are improved.

A full list of references is available at www.expertconsult.com.

9

Anemia in Chronic Kidney Disease

Jeffrey S. Berns, MD, Tiffany C. Wong, MD, and Solomon Dawson, MD

OUTLINE

Anemia, a reduction in blood hemoglobin (Hgb) concentration or hematocrit (Hct), is common among patients with chronic kidney disease (CKD), stemming primarily from a reduction in endogenous erythropoietin production by the diseased kidneys. There is an incremental and monotonic increase in the prevalence of anemia with reduced glomerular filtration rate (GFR).[1] Using the World Health Organization (WHO) definition of anemia as a Hgb concentration less than 13.0 g/dL for adult males and postmenopausal women, and an Hgb less than 12.0 g/dL for premenopausal women,[2] as many as 90% of patients with CKD and a GFR less than 30 mL/min have anemia, and many have Hgb levels less than 10 g/dL.[3] The prevalence of anemia in any population sample with CKD varies depending on the level of GFR and definition of anemia. In general population studies, the prevalence of anemia defined as an Hgb level less than 11.0 g/dL was approximately 1.3%, 5.2%, and 44.1% among patients with estimated GFRs of 60 to 89, 30 to 59, and 15 to 29 mL/min/1.73 m^2, respectively.[4]

The low Hgb concentration in individuals with anemia reduces the oxygen carrying capacity of blood and in turn reduces tissue oxygenation delivery, which may adversely affect health and quality of life and predispose individuals to excess morbidity and mortality. There has been a proliferation of research and clinical practice guidelines seeking to define the effects of anemia and its treatments in patients with CKD, including those on dialysis, and to identify therapeutic goals that maximize health outcomes. Limitations of treatments for CKD-associated anemia and the potential risks of such therapies have also been more clearly delineated.

In this chapter, we discuss the pathogenesis of anemia in CKD, the clinical consequences of anemia, current therapies, and recommended therapeutic goals for patients with CKD.

PATHOGENESIS

Anemia in CKD is characterized by a normochromic normocytic appearance of circulating red blood cells without the expected increase in bone marrow erythroid progenitor cells and circulating reticulocytes expected with an observed low Hgb concentration. The anemia associated with CKD derives principally from inadequate production of the hormone erythropoietin by the kidneys, with reduced red cell life span and other factors contributing.[5] Identification and purification of erythropoietin and cloning of the erythropoietin gene led to the production of a recombinant erythropoietin hormone[6,7]; therapeutic administration of this agent confirmed the primacy of erythropoietin in the pathogenesis of the anemia from CKD.[8,9] Impairment of the erythropoietic response to endogenous or exogenous erythropoietin due to the "uremic milieu" may also contribute to the anemia of CKD, with various polyamines, parathyroid hormone, and inflammatory cytokines being other potential inhibitors of erythropoiesis.[10] Interestingly, recent evidence has demonstrated the capacity to pharmacologically stimulate erythropoietin synthesis by the kidneys even in individuals with very advanced kidney disease and anemia.[11]

Erythropoietin is a circulating glycoprotein of 165 amino acids with three N-linked and one O-linked carbohydrate chains. Before birth, the hormone is produced in the liver, whereas postnatally it is synthesized primarily by peritubular interstitial cells in the kidneys.[12] Erythropoietin is normally present in the circulation in low concentrations (0.01 to 0.03 U/mL) under basal conditions, but the concentration increases 100-fold to 1000-fold in response to hypoxia and anemia,[13] in a process regulated by hypoxia-inducible factor-1 (HIF-1). HIF-1 is a transcription factor that binds to a hypoxia response element in the erythropoietin gene and other hypoxia-responsive genes, increasing their transcription; expression of the HIF-1α subunit of the HIF-1 complex increases rapidly in response to hypoxia, whereas in the presence of oxygen, HIF-1α rapidly undergoes proteosomal degradation after ubiquitination by the von Hippel–Lindau protein complex.[14,15]

Erythropoietin receptors are present on erythroid precursors, with the greatest expression on colony forming unit-erythroid cells; stimulation by erythropoietin induces their proliferation and maturation into mature erythrocytes. Erythropoietin receptors are not found on mature red blood cells. The erythropoietin receptor is a preformed dimer. Binding of erythropoietin to the receptor changes its conformation, leading to activation of the intracellular mediator kinase Janus kinase-2 (JAK-2) via transphosphorylation, subsequent phosphorylation of other intracellular tyrosine kinases, and stimulation of a complex signal transduction cascade that eventuates in erythrocyte production.[16,17]

Erythropoietin deficiency and the anemia of CKD may be preceded or exacerbated by states of absolute or functional iron deficiency; these will be discussed in detail later in this chapter. In addition, patients with CKD may have anemia on the basis of other conditions, such as vitamin B_{12} or folate deficiency, bleeding, hemolysis, infection/inflammation, bone marrow infiltration, inherited hemoglobinopathies, and medications. Among patients on chronic hemodialysis (HD), other factors include blood loss during the dialysis treatment, subclinical infection, or inflammation related to HD catheters or thrombosed synthetic bridge grafts, severe secondary hyperparathyroidism, and grossly inadequate dialytic solute clearance.

CLINICAL CONSEQUENCES OF ANEMIA AND EFFECTS OF CORRECTION

Health-Related Quality of Life (HRQoL)

The symptoms of anemia are nonspecific and can overlap with those of advanced kidney failure and uremia. They include fatigue, shortness of breath and dyspnea on exertion, impaired exercise tolerance, difficulty concentrating, headaches, lightheadedness, impaired sexual function, and diminished sense of well-being. Before the availability of recombinant human erythropoietin and other similar agents, many patients on dialysis had Hgb levels in the range of 5 to 7 g/dL.[8,18] Once it became possible to improve Hgb levels with recombinant human erythropoietin in both dialysis patients and patients with CKD not on dialysis, it became clear that various measures of health-related quality of life (HRQoL) improved in association with partial correction from very severe to more moderate degrees of anemia.[19-22]

There has been a renewed interest in this area, particularly as the potential benefits and risks of using erythropoiesis-stimulating agents (ESAs; a general term that will be used in this chapter to refer to the recombinant human erythropoietin, darbepoetin, and other similar or related pharmacological preparations) to raise Hgb levels from moderate to more normal Hgb levels have been examined. With this intervention, improvement in various HRQoL parameters, such as physical function, energy, and fatigue, school performance in children, and vitality, as well as reduction in hospitalization rates have been documented in some randomized controlled trials and observational cohort studies, whereas other studies have found minimal or no benefit.[23-31] A recent metaanalysis of 17 randomized controlled trials concluded that use of ESAs to raise Hgb levels did not significantly improve overall HRQoL in patients with CKD, including those on dialysis.[32] Heterogeneity among the patient populations studied and the short duration of most studies is a limitation of assessments of HRQoL in this population, and the long-term persistence of HRQoL benefit occurring in response to anemia in CKD patients remains unknown. Depending on the instrument used for assessment and the population studied, some HRQoL domains, such as fatigue and vitality, may show more improvement than others such as social and emotional functioning, mental health, and pain. In addition, some domains not measured by some of the more commonly used instruments such as sleep, cognitive functioning, and sexual functioning may improve with ESA treatment.[33] In the absence of definitive evidence in this regard, the US Food and Drug Administration (FDA) revised ESA product labeling to remove claims that ESAs improve patients' quality of life, symptoms of anemia, fatigue, or general well-being. Nonetheless, it is still recommended that ESA therapy be individualized, particularly in younger patients, a group that has not been well studied, and in those with fewer comorbidities.[34-37]

Cognitive Function

Decreased oxygen delivery to the central nervous system is expected to result in impairment in cognitive function, an effect that should be amenable through anemia correction. A number of randomized trials have demonstrated a favorable effect of anemia treatment on cognitive function in dialysis patients. In this population, full[38] and partial[39] anemia correction have been demonstrated to improve performance on neuropsychiatric testing and electrophysiological markers of cognitive function. Additional evidence suggests that complete normalization of Hgb is superior to partial correction in this regard,[40] an effect that must be weighed against potential detrimental effects on survival (discussed in the next section). Partial anemia correction has also been associated with improvement in intelligence quotient, concentration, memory, and speed of information processing,[41] as well as improvements in sleep quality and wakefulness.[42]

To date, little work has been done to examine the cognitive effects of anemia correction among patients with earlier stages of CKD who are not on dialysis. One study demonstrated that anemia correction results in improvement in electrophysiological markers of cognitive function,[43] but none have examined clinical outcomes such as neuropsychiatric testing. Given the lesser severity of anemia in the milder stages of CKD, it is unclear whether extrapolation of data from dialysis patients is warranted. In fact, in a recent prospective observational study, anemia (using the WHO definition) was not associated with either baseline cognitive impairment or change in cognitive function over time.[44] Thus for CKD patients who are not on dialysis, provision of anemia therapy with the intent of improving cognitive function is probably not warranted at this time.

Cardiovascular Disease and Mortality

As Hgb concentration falls, there is a commensurate reduction in blood-oxygen carrying capacity. To maintain constant tissue oxygen delivery, cardiac output is increased via augmentation of heart rate and stroke volume in conjunction with peripheral vasodilatation. As part of the compensatory process, left ventricular geometry is altered, with increases in left ventricular end-diastolic volume and wall thickness. Thus left ventricular hypertrophy (LVH) is common among patients with CKD,[45] and its prevalence is strongly associated with the degree of anemia.[46] In this population, LVH is a potent marker for cardiovascular morbidity and mortality,[47] with observational data demonstrating a clear association between greater degrees of anemia and increased risk of myocardial infarction, stroke, cardiovascular events, and all-cause mortality among patients with CKD.[48] These observations led some to hypothesize that anemia correction would result in both an improvement in left ventricular geometry with reduction in LVH (e.g., decreased hypertrophy) and better cardiovascular outcomes.

Studies have demonstrated a beneficial effect of partial correction of severe anemia on cardiac structural markers among patients with CKD not on dialysis.[49-51] Anemia therapy has been shown to induce regression of LVH and echocardiographic evidence of favorable left ventricular remodeling. Evidence suggests that complete correction of anemia to normal Hgb levels does not provide benefit beyond partial correction in this regard.[24,52,53] Similarly, studies generally have failed to demonstrate a beneficial effect of normalization or near-normalization of anemia therapy on clinical cardiovascular outcomes among HD patients and patients with CKD not on dialysis.[24,53-55] In the only large randomized placebo-controlled trial of ESA therapy (darbepoetin) in diabetic patients with CKD not on dialysis, treatment did not reduce death or occurrence of adverse cardiovascular events, but was associated with an increased stroke risk.[29,56,57]

Among patients with CKD who are not on dialysis, observational studies suggested that higher Hgb levels were associated with improved survival,[48,58] and that anemia therapy was associated with improved longevity among patients going on to require dialysis.[59,60] Observational studies examining the association between higher Hgb levels and mortality among patients on hemodialysis have yielded mixed findings, with some demonstrating a benefit,[61-65] and others not.[26,66,67] However, Hgb levels are likely to reflect underlying health status, suggesting that these findings may be confounded. Several large randomized trials, including the placebo-controlled study noted previously, have not demonstrated a mortality benefit of ESA treatment aimed at restoring normal or near-normal Hgb levels.[24,54,55,57,68] Recent systematic reviews and updated clinical practice guidelines have cautioned against the normalization of Hgb levels with ESA treatment in dialysis and nondialysis CKD patients.[35,69-71]

THERAPIES FOR CHRONIC KIDNEY DISEASE–RELATED ANEMIA

Erythropoiesis-Stimulating Agents

Since the first descriptions of the use of recombinant human erythropoietin in hemodialysis patients in the late 1980s,[8,18] ESAs have been the mainstay of anemia therapy for anemia in adults and children with CKD including those not on dialysis, on HD and peritoneal dialysis, and after renal transplantation. Many studies have demonstrated the efficacy of ESAs in raising blood Hgb concentration. Erythropoietin alpha was the first ESA approved for use and was demonstrated to be superior to placebo in this regard among patients with CKD.[8,18,72,73]

Currently available ESAs are a class of recombinant preparations of human erythropoietin or its structural analogs, although other types of agents are undergoing clinical trials. In the United States, this includes epoetin alpha, darbepoetin alfa, and methoxy polyethylene glycol-epoetin beta (Table 9.1). A variety of other similar agents are available in other countries. Recombinant human erythropoietin (epoetin) has an identical amino acid backbone as the native hormone and has biochemical and immunological properties that are virtually indistinguishable from human erythropoietin. Darbepoetin alfa is a hyperglycosylated structural analog of recombinant human erythropoietin with a five amino acid substitution and five N-linked carbohydrate chains, two more

TABLE 9.1 Erythropoiesis Stimulating Agents Approved for Use in the United States

Preparation	Approved Starting Dosage[a]	Comments[b]
Epoetin alpha	50–100 U/kg 3 times per wk	IV recommended in HD patients Weekly or every 2 wk SC dosing typically used in patients with CKD not on dialysis US dosage forms: 2000; 3000; 4000; 10,000; 20,000; 40,000 U/mL
Darbepoetin alpha	0.45 mcg/kg IV or SC weekly or 0.75 mcg/kg every 2 weeks	IV recommended in HD patients Weekly to monthly dosing typically used US dosage forms: 10, 25, 40, 60, 100, 150, 200, 300, 500 mcg/0.4–1.0 mL
Methoxy polyethylene glycol-epoetin beta	0.6 mcg/kg every 2 weeks	IV or SC administration Every 2 wk to monthly dosing typically used US dosage forms: 30, 50, 75, 100, 200 mcg/0.3 mL

[a]All require subsequent dose titration depending on goal Hgb level.
[b]Dialysis facilities typically use specific dosing protocols. In many patients with CKD not on dialysis and on home dialysis, unit-based dosing rather than weight-based dosing will be used.
CKD, Chronic kidney disease; *HD*, hemodialysis; *Hgb*, hemoglobin; *IV*, intravenous; *SC*, subcutaneous.

than erythropoietin, which increases the potential maximum number of sialic acid residues from 14 to 22, increases its in vivo potency, and extends its serum half-life approximately twofold to threefold.[74] Methoxy polyethylene glycol-epoetin beta is a chemically synthesized substituted analog of erythropoietin with receptor-binding kinetics that are different from other ESAs and a very low plasma clearance. The biological half-life is approximately 6 times greater than darbepoetin and 20 times greater than epoetin alpha.[75-77]

"Biosimilar" erythropoietic agents (also termed *follow-on biologicals*)[78] have been approved for use in the European Union and elsewhere but are not yet approved in the United States. These agents are similar to already approved biological medicines such as recombinant human erythropoietin. Due to inherent heterogeneity of biological agents, including biosimilar ESAs, different regulations are required compared with other generic medications. As such, specific regulatory approval pathways have been established in the United States, Europe, and elsewhere that allow for approval of these products as being similar but not necessarily identical to the original product.[79] Although it is difficult to directly compare two versions of a biopharmaceutical agent and prove equivalent efficacy and safety, studies to date suggest that most of these agents are generally equivalent to ESAs previously in use, although further analysis is needed to confirm that the side-effect profile is also similar.[80-82]

Currently available ESAs can be given in patients with CKD not on dialysis and in patients who are on dialysis by either intravenous (IV) or subcutaneous (SC) administration. Although the clinical efficacy of darbepoetin and methoxy polyethylene glycol-epoetin beta appear to be similar regardless of whether they are administered IV or SC, studies have found that the shorter-acting epoetin is more effective by approximately 50% when administered subcutaneously.[83] Each of these may be administered by IV or SC injection. SC administration is generally preferred for those patients with CKD who are not on dialysis or who are on home hemodialysis or peritoneal dialysis, whereas the approved prescribing information for those treated by maintenance HD in the United States recommends IV administration of epoetin and darbepoetin with either IV or SC administration of methoxy polyethylene glycol-epoetin beta.

Unlike currently available ESAs, which require parenteral (IV or SC) administration, a new class of orally available agents is undergoing testing in clinical trials and may be available in the near future. Hypoxia-inducible factor (HIF) prolyl hydroxylase inhibitors stimulate endogenous synthesis of erythropoietin and also enhance iron utilization.[84-88] If approved, these agents have the potential to markedly change anemia management in patients with CKD, including those on dialysis, due to their oral administration, avoidance of high peak levels of ESAs, and beneficial effects on iron utilization and balance.[89]

SC administration of one particular formulation of erythropoietin alpha has been associated with an unusually high risk of developing neutralizing antierythropoietin antibody-mediated pure red cell aplasia (PRCA)[90]; fortunately, with product reformulation, PRCA related to its use appears to have largely disappeared.[91] Isolated instances of antibody-mediated PRCA related to other ESAs have been rarely reported.[91,92]

Recommendations vary regarding the initial ESA dosing regimen and the specific Hgb level at which initiation of ESA therapy should be considered. Depending on individual circumstances, an Hgb level <10 g/dL is often considered an appropriate level in many patients to start an ESA, provided that iron deficiency and other causes of anemia have been excluded or treated (Table 9.2).[71] Once started, usage should be tailored to individual clinical circumstances, patient comorbidities, pretreatment Hgb levels, and quality-of-life expectations. In addition, after initiation of ESA therapy, care should be taken to titrate dosing to maintain Hgb levels in the desired range (generally in the range of 10 to 11.5 g/dL), avoid targeting and maintaining Hgb levels greater than 13 g/dL (discussed in the next section), and to ensure adequate provision of iron necessary for adequate erythropoiesis.[35,71,93] The short-acting epoetin is typically administered three times weekly to maintenance HD patients and once every 1 to 2 weeks in patients with CKD who are not on dialysis.[94,95] Darbepoetin and methoxy polyethylene glycol epoetin beta, with their longer biological half-lives, can often be effectively administered once or twice monthly.[96-99]

Besides induction of iron deficiency, the primary adverse effects of ESAs are exacerbation of hypertension and hemodialysis access thrombosis.[100] As discussed elsewhere in this chapter, in several large prospective, randomized controlled trials, however, hemodialysis patients and patients with CKD not on dialysis targeted to achieve normal or near-normal Hgb levels tended to have poorer outcomes, leading to an ongoing discussion of whether the high ESA doses (needed to achieve higher Hgb levels) are directly toxic in some way.[24,53-55] A secondary analysis of one of the recent large trials in patients with CKD suggested that high ESA doses appeared to independently explain the poorer outcome in patients assigned to the higher Hgb target group.[101] Others have also found that requiring or receiving higher ESA doses was independently associated with higher mortality.[63] This has led some to speculate that particularly high doses of ESAs may have adverse effects on survival not mediated by changes in Hgb concentration,[101-103] although the mechanism for this effect, if real, remains obscure. Nonetheless, this has led to increasing caution about the use of very high ESA doses.

Two other concerns with ESA therapy relate to use in patients with a history of stroke or malignancy. The TREAT study found an increased risk of stroke among patients with CKD receiving darbepoetin, particularly in those with a prior stroke, and also noted an increased risk of cancer-related death in those with a history of cancer.[30] An increased stroke risk with ESAs was also seen in an older study among dialysis patients[104] and a more recent study among US veterans with CKD[105] but not others.[106,107] Nonetheless, caution is advised about ESA use in patients with a history of stroke or malignancy.[35,71]

TABLE 9.2 **Kidney Disease: Improving Global Outcomes Guidelines for Anemia Management (2012)**[71]

Use of iron agents	Balance the potential benefits of avoiding or minimizing blood transfusions, ESA therapy, and anemia-related symptoms against the risk of harm in individual patients Suggest a trial of IV iron (or in CKD ND patients alternatively a 1–3 mo trial of oral iron therapy) if an increase in Hgb concentration, avoidance of an ESA or an ESA dose reduction is desired, if TSAT is <30% and ferritin is <500 ng/mL
Iron monitoring	Evaluate iron status (TSAT and ferritin) at least every 3 mo during ESA therapy; more frequently when initiating or increasing ESA dose, with blood loss, after a course of iron
Cautions regarding IV iron	Monitor for 60 min after infusion with iron dextran (recommended) and other irons (suggested) Avoid administering IV iron to patients with active systemic infections
Initiating use of ESAs	Suggest ESA therapy not be initiated for CKD ND patients with Hgb ≥10 g/dL Individualize decision to initiate ESA therapy in CKD ND patients with Hgb <10 g/dL Suggest ESA therapy be used in CKD 5D patients to avoid having Hgb <9.0 g/dL by initiating ESA when Hgb is 9.0–10.9 g/dL
ESA maintenance therapy	Suggest ESAs not be used to maintain Hgb >11.5 g/dL Individualize therapy as some patients may have improvement quality of life with Hgb <11.5 g/dL and be willing to accept the risks
Cautions regarding ESA use	Use ESA therapy with great caution, if at all, in CKD patients with active malignancy, history of stroke, or history of malignancy Recommend that ESAs not be used to intentionally increase Hgb >13.0 g/dL In patients with ESA hyporesponsiveness, suggest avoiding repeated dose escalations beyond doubling the initial weight-based dose

CKD, Chronic kidney disease; *CKD ND,* CKD not on dialysis; *CKD 5D,* patients on dialysis; *ESA,* erythropoiesis-stimulating agent; Hgb, hemoglobin; *IV,* intravenous; *TSAT,* transferrin saturation.

Iron

Adequate iron stores are essential for erythropoiesis, whether in response to endogenous erythropoietin or ESA therapy. Because erythropoiesis itself consumes iron, assessment of the adequacy of available iron before and during ESA administration is a routine part of anemia management in patients with CKD, including those on dialysis. Inadequacy of iron can take one of two forms: absolute iron deficiency and functional iron deficiency. Absolute iron deficiency is defined by a lack of bone marrow iron and is common among hemodialysis patients, in particular, due to loss of iron via the dialytic circuit, access surgery, and frequent phlebotomy, but is also common among CKD patients who are not on dialysis. Although the diagnosis of absolute iron deficiency in this population has been suggested by transferrin saturation (TSAT) <20% or serum ferritin level <100 ng/mL for patients with CKD not on dialysis or on peritoneal dialysis and <200 ng/mL for hemodialysis patients,[108] these tests are of rather low sensitivity and specificity.[109-112] In fact, little or no bone marrow iron may be present in patients with CKD despite serum ferritin and TSAT levels that would not have predicted such severe iron deficiency.[112,113] As such, simply supplementing iron and observing whether there is an increase in Hgb and/or a reduction in required ESA dose for a goal Hgb level is often undertaken in practice. Other markers of iron status and availability are also used, primarily outside the United States, which may have better operational characteristics compared with serum ferritin and TSAT.[110,111,114]

Functional iron deficiency is defined by normal bone marrow reticuloendothelial iron stores, but inability to mobilize iron for erythropoiesis, usually stemming from systemic inflammation and/or malnutrition.[115,116] Complexities of iron handling in the body and the impact of inflammation on the hepcidin–ferroportin axis have become increasingly elucidated.[117] The presence of functional iron deficiency is suggested when serum ferritin levels are >200 ng/dL with TSAT levels <30%. Although total body iron stores are not reduced in this setting, and some experts and clinical practice guidelines recommend against administration of additional IV iron to most patients with serum ferritin levels greater than 500 to 800 ng/mL,[71] evidence nonetheless suggests that a course of iron repletion in such patients may raise Hgb levels[118] and lower ESA requirements.[119] A recent meta-analysis of 34 studies of supplemental iron in hemodialysis patients with functional iron deficiency found that IV iron significantly increased Hgb levels, serum ferritin, and TSAT without increased risk of adverse events, although increases in some markers of oxidative stress of uncertain clinical relevance were noted.[120]

A full evaluation of a patient's anemia, including complete blood count, reticulocyte count, tests for iron stores, and vitamin B_{12} and folate levels should be assessed when Hgb levels fall below normal,[121] and certainly before the initiation of ESA therapy. Patients with absolute iron deficiency should receive iron supplementation, either as oral or intravenous iron, and have their Hgb levels remeasured when iron stores have normalized before initiation of ESA therapy. This is particularly important because intravenous iron supplementation alone will significantly increase Hgb levels in patients with iron deficiency, with many patients achieving Hgb levels of 10 to 12 g/dL without ESA treatment. Adequacy of iron stores should be reassessed 1 to 2 months after initiation of

TABLE 9.3 **Parenteral Iron Preparations**

Iron Preparation	Dosage (single dose)[a] (as elemental iron)	Test Dose Requirement? Special Precautions
Low MW iron dextran	100 to >1000 mg	Yes (25 mg); FDA black box warning regarding risk of anaphylaxis
Iron sucrose	200–300 mg	No[b]
Ferric gluconate	125 mg/250 mg	No[b]
Ferumoxytol	510 mg/1020 mg	No[b]; FDA black box warning regarding risk of hypersensitivity/ anaphylaxis reactions Only limited experience with >510 mg dosing; should not administer faster than 510 mg/15 min
Ferric carboxymaltose	750 mg to 20 mg/kg body weight	No[b]
Iron isomaltoside (not available in United States)	500 mg to 20 mg/kg body weight	No[b]
Ferric pyrophosphate citrate (via dialysate)	Provides 5–7 mg per dialysis treatment	No[b]

[a]Includes off-label use with higher single dose than approved.
[b]Slow infusion for all intravenous products initially with observation for infusion reactions is recommended.
FDA, US Food and Drug Administration; *MW*, molecular weight.

ESA therapy and periodically thereafter, as treatment will often deplete iron stores. By virtue of repeated blood loss nearly all hemodialysis patients will require maintenance therapy to maintain adequate iron stores.[122] Patients demonstrating continued (or new) iron insufficiency with an Hgb level less than desired and levels of TSAT <30% and ferritin <500 ng/mL (see Table 9.2) should receive another course of iron repletion. Consideration should be given in such patients to maintenance iron therapy to avoid ongoing iron insufficiency.[123-125] Once Hgb has reached a steady state and a stable ESA dose has been reached, measurement of iron stores can be made every 3 months.

Supplemental iron can be given orally, intravenously, or via dialysate (hemodialysis). Most oral iron preparations are inexpensive, available without a prescription, and of relatively similar efficacy. Use of oral iron avoids bypassing the normal gastrointestinal (GI) tract regulation of iron balance but use of one of the most commonly used oral iron preparations, ferrous sulfate, in particular is limited by GI side effects. Metaanalyses and systematic reviews have consistently shown superiority of IV compared with oral iron for treatment of anemia in patients with CKD, on dialysis and not.[126-128] Intravenous preparations including iron dextran, iron sucrose, ferric gluconate in sucrose complex, ferumoxytol, and ferric carboxymaltose are available in the United States (Table 9.3). A high-molecular-weight formulation of iron dextran is no longer readily available and is not recommended for use due to a higher risk of serious allergic/anaphylactic reactions compared with a low-molecular-weight formulation and other parenteral iron products.[129-131] Iron isomaltoside is available in some countries outside the United States. The choice among intravenous agents is often governed by formulary considerations in dialysis units, hospitals, and clinics; there is little evidence to suggest superior efficacy of any one agent over another. Iron sucrose is the most commonly used preparation among HD patients in the United States. Iron dextran requires a test dose before initial administration to assess for allergic reactions although some recommend cautious administration with the initial dose of other IV irons as well. Ferumoxytol and ferric carboxymaltose can be given in higher doses per administration than the others, reducing the number of needed infusions. Iron dextran and ferumoxytol have "black box" warnings in the United States regarding risk of severe hypersensitivity reactions and anaphylaxis; other side effects with these products seem to be similar to other iron preparations.[132-134] Ferric carboxymaltose has been associated with development of hypophosphatemia caused by renal phosphate wasting in patients with CKD not on dialysis[135-137] but otherwise appears to be generally well tolerated.[138]

Ferric pyrophosphate citrate is available in the United States for delivery of iron via dialysate during hemodialysis by adding it to the liquid bicarbonate concentrate and appears to be helpful in maintaining iron stores and reducing need for supplemental IV iron.[139-141] Oral ferric citrate is approved for use as a phosphate binder but has also been shown to be a potential source of supplemental iron in both dialysis patients and patients with CKD not on dialysis, increasing Hgb levels and iron stores while reducing the need for IV iron.[139,142-145]

Oral iron repletion should be accomplished using a total daily dose of 200 mg of elemental iron. This is often given in divided doses to minimize GI side effects such as constipation. Individual iron preparations vary in their content of elemental iron; none has been shown to be clearly superior in terms of efficacy or tolerability. One small study suggested that an oral heme iron preparation may be effective and well-tolerated in HD patients[146]; this preparation was not effective in patients on peritoneal dialysis[147] but may be of benefit in patients with CKD who are not on dialysis.[148]

In hemodialysis patients, IV iron is the preferred route for iron supplementation.[35,71] For patients with CKD who are not on dialysis and peritoneal dialysis patients who do not respond to or tolerate a 1 to 3 month course of oral iron, intravenous iron repletion should be administered. Typically, iron repletion for iron deficiency is accomplished via administration of approximately 1000 mg of iron with subsequent assessment of iron stores, Hgb level, and ESA responsiveness. The Kidney Disease: Improving Global Outcomes (KDIGO) recommendations suggest limiting iron replacement to patients with TSAT <30% and serum ferritin <500 ng/mL (see Table 9.2). There continues to be a debate about the need to limit additional iron in patients with high serum ferritin levels, particularly when TSAT levels are not elevated.[35,118,149-152]

The use of IV iron has increased among HD patients, in particular.[153,154] This has come with concern about the long-term safety of large cumulative doses of parenteral iron. Iron sequestration is one means by which the body protects itself against invading pathogens. Thus some have speculated that administration of intravenous iron may promote infection as well as increase cardiovascular disease and mortality. Some early observational studies indicated an association between increased rates of bacterial infection and colonization and intravenous iron administration in hemodialysis patients.[155,156] However, others have concluded that there is not a significant risk of infection or mortality with IV iron administration in HD patients,[157-160] although one recent study suggested the possibility of infection-related mortality, but not all-cause or cardiovascular mortality, with high cumulative doses.[161] Two recent prospective trials of IV iron supplementation in patients with CKD provided discordant results, with one indicating an increased risk of infection,[162] whereas another found no evidence of this concern.[138] Nonetheless, many clinicians avoid supplemental iron administration in the presence of an active infection due to the theoretical risk and likelihood of poor response to supplemental iron in this setting.[35]

Other Therapies

Whereas ESAs and iron repletion are the primary therapeutic modalities for anemia management in CKD, other agents have been investigated for potential roles in augmenting the effect of ESA treatment, although none are of proven efficacy or clinical value and none have been shown to enhance patient outcomes.[35,71,163-165] Vitamin C (ascorbic acid), administered intravenously at each hemodialysis session, has been shown in several small short-term studies to improve ESA responsiveness, particularly in hemodialysis patients with high serum ferritin levels and functional iron deficiency.[166-170] This effect is thought to be through antioxidant effects, mobilization of iron stores for erythropoiesis, and enhancement of iron utilization. Long-term safety has not been proven and the affect on important clinical outcomes is unknown.

Other adjuvants to ESA therapy that have been used in the past or proposed for clinical use include L-carnitine,[171,172] androgens,[173-175] pentoxifylline,[176-178] and statins.[179,180] Due to limitations previously mentioned, most notably absence of convincing evidence that these agents improve patient outcomes, their use is generally not recommended.

TARGET HEMOGLOBIN LEVELS FOR ERYTHROPOIESIS-STIMULATING AGENT–TREATED PATIENTS

Ideally, the Hgb level achieved in each ESA-treated patient with CKD would be individually tailored depending on such factors as functional capacity and limitations, other comorbidities such as coronary artery disease and heart failure, and life expectancy. Historically, target Hgb levels have generally instead been influenced more by regulation by the FDA and healthcare payers, quality assurance programs in dialysis units, and clinical practice guideline recommendations. Whereas many observational cohort studies in the past indicated an association between Hgb levels greater than 12 to 13 g/dL in both dialysis patients and patients with CKD not on dialysis, more recent evidence, including that from prospective randomized trials, indicates that there is little benefit, and even potential risk to targeting or maintaining Hgb levels of 13 g/dL or higher in many CKD patients.[24,30,53-55,69,100]

Data From Clinical Trials

There are now at least four large prospective randomized controlled trials evaluating target Hgb levels in patients with CKD. The "Normal Hematocrit Trial," in hemodialysis patients with cardiac disease, was terminated early when it was determined that the group targeted to normal values had a higher mortality that was approaching, but had not yet attained, statistical significance. Mortality rates were 7% higher in the normal Hct group than in the low Hct group.[54,68]

The CHOIR trial (Correction of Anemia with Epoetin Alfa in Chronic Kidney Disease) randomly assigned CKD patients with anemia to achieve a target Hgb of either 13.5 or 11.3 g/day, with the primary study endpoint being a composite of death, myocardial infarction, stroke, and hospitalization for heart failure without renal replacement therapy.[55] The study was stopped early when it was determined that is was unlikely to show any benefit of the higher Hgb level and there was a significantly higher number of events in the higher Hgb group. There was no improvement in quality of life with higher Hgb levels. In the CREATE trial (Cardiovascular Risk Reduction in Early Anemia Treatment with Epoetin Beta), patients with CKD and anemia were randomly assigned to a normal (13 to 15 g/dL) or subnormal (10.5 to 11.5 g/dL) Hgb level.[24] The primary endpoint was a composite of eight cardiovascular events, including sudden death, myocardial infarction, acute heart failure, stroke, transient ischemic attack, hospitalization for angina pectoris or arrhythmia, or complications of peripheral vascular disease. At 3 years, there was a similar risk of experiencing the primary endpoint in both groups, although there was a nonsignificant trend toward more events in the higher Hgb group.

In the TREAT trial (Trial to Reduce Cardiovascular Events with Aranesp Therapy), patients with CKD and diabetes were randomly assigned to receive darbepoetin alfa to achieve an Hgb level of approximately 13 g/dL or placebo, with darbepoetin given only as "rescue" therapy if the Hgb was <9.0 g/dL.[30] The primary endpoints were the composite of death or a cardiovascular event and death or end-stage renal disease (ESRD). At 48 months, there was not a significant difference between groups for either composite endpoint but there was a significant increase in the risk of fatal and nonfatal stroke in the darbepoetin group.[56] Of note is that this is the only large placebo-controlled trial assessing outcomes associated with ESA use in patients with CKD.

A systematic review of 27 studies including over 10,000 subjects found that using ESAs to target a higher Hgb level of 12 to 15 g/dL compared with a lower Hgb level of 9.5 to 11.5 g/dL was associated with an increased risk of stroke, hypertension, and vascular access thrombosis but did not find a higher risk for mortality, serious cardiovascular events, or progression of CKD to ESRD.[181]

US Regulatory and Fiscal Policy

The use of ESAs in dialysis patients in the United States has been governed by various regulatory policies since recombinant human erythropoietin was approved by the FDA in 1989, including policies governing reimbursement for ESAs to dialysis and other healthcare providers. The target Hct range for EPO therapy approved by the FDA when the drug was initially introduced was 30% to 33%. The ESA label in the United States now warns of a greater risk of death, serious adverse cardiovascular events, and stroke when ESAs are used to target Hgb levels >11 g/dL and recommends initiation of treatment with an ESA only when the Hgb is <10 g/dL. The package insert also notes that no Hgb level, ESA dose, or ESA dosing strategies have been identified that reduce these risks and recommends use of the lowest possible ESA dose sufficient to reduce the need for red blood cell transfusions. A specific Hgb target or minimum Hgb level is not recommended.[93,182]

In 2011 the Centers for Medicare & Medicaid Services (CMS) in the United States introduced a new prospective payment system for dialysis treatment reimbursements that included the costs of certain medications, including ESAs (often referred to as *bundling*), creating a disincentive for high ESA dose use. This was followed by a decline in ESA use and Hgb levels, an increase in intravenous iron use, rising serum ferritin levels, and a small increase in blood transfusion rates, without an increase in mortality or other major cardiovascular events.[153,183,184]

Clinical Practice Guidelines for Erythropoiesis-Stimulating Agents and Iron Therapy

Several national and international organizations and societies have developed clinical practice guidelines and recommendations for anemia management in patients with CKD including specific target Hgb and iron levels; these are generally similar, although differences in some of the specifics, such as upper and lower Hgb level limits, do exist.[35,71,110,185,186] All have concluded that partial correction of anemia to an Hgb level of approximately 10 to 11 g/dL is reasonable in many patients with ESRD and CKD who are not on dialysis but that higher Hgb targets should generally be avoided.

Major recommendations of the most recent anemia guideline regarding Hgb target levels and iron tests from the KDIGO are summarized here.[35,71] These international guidelines, last updated in 2012, recommend that ESA therapy not be initiated in patients with CKD who are not on dialysis if the Hgb is ≥10.0 g/dL and if <10.0 g/dL that ESA therapy be individualized based on the rate at which the Hgb is falling, response to iron replacement, estimated transfusion risk, symptoms, and potential risks of ESA treatment. For patients on dialysis, it is recommended that ESA therapy be used to avoid having the Hgb concentration fall to <9.0 g/dL by initiating treatment when the Hgb is in the 9.0 to 10.0 g/dL range, although it was noted that some individual patients might benefit from starting an ESA even with a Hgb >10.0 g/dL. These guidelines recommend that ESAs not be used to maintain Hgb concentrations >11.5 g/dL in most patients, noting that a somewhat higher level may be appropriate in some patients (who understand and are willing to accept the risks). Others have suggested that a target Hgb <11.0 g/dL is more appropriate given the available evidence and FDA statement.[35] A strong recommendation was also made to avoid intentionally increasing the Hgb to >13.0 g/dL with ESAs.

Erythropoiesis-Stimulating Agent Hyporesponsiveness

Not all patients have a brisk or fully desired therapeutic response to standard ESA doses and are thus considered to have ESA hyporesponsiveness or resistance. Hyporesponsiveness to ESA therapy is clearly associated with poorer outcomes than is responsiveness to lower ESA doses.[187-191] Although there is no widely accepted and scientifically validated definition, a reasonable definition of ESA hyporesponsiveness is a weekly epoetin requirement of more than 450 U/kg IV or 300 U/kg SC in a hemodialysis patient.[115,192] ESA hyporesponsiveness has been even less well defined in patients with CKD not on dialysis and those on peritoneal dialysis. Another approach to defining hyporesponsiveness, from the KDIGO guidelines, is the lack of an increase in Hgb after the first month of appropriate weight-based dosing and/or a need for two increases in ESA dose up to 50% beyond the dose as which the patient was previously stable.[71] This recommendation stems in part from a report from the TREAT study in patients with CKD who were not on dialysis[188] and may not be relevant or applicable to a dialysis-treated population.[35]

The most common cause of ESA hyporesponsiveness is iron deficiency.[115] Provided that adequate monitoring and repletion of iron stores is undertaken, this cause should be apparent and treatable with oral or intravenous iron administration. Among iron-replete patients, inflammation and infection are important causes of ESA hyporesponsiveness.[193] The proposed mechanism is thought to be disruption of erythropoiesis in the bone marrow by proinflammatory cytokines such as interleukin-1, tumor necrosis factor-α, and interferon-γ.[193,194] In cases where systemic inflammation is suspected as a cause of ESA hyporesponsiveness but no source is identified, consideration should be given to the possibility of occult infection of thrombosed arteriovenous access grafts.[195] Hospitalized patients have lesser degrees of ESA responsiveness than their nonhospitalized counterparts.[196] Likely, this relates to the higher prevalence of inflammation, infection, and malnutrition—and frequent phlebotomy—in this population. Other potential causes or contributors to ESA hyporesponsiveness include inadequate dialytic clearance, secondary hyperparathyroidism, aluminum overload, and deficiency in vitamin B_{12} and folic acid. Administration of angiotensin-converting enzyme inhibitors (ACE) inhibitors and angiotensin receptor blockers (ARBs) has also been suggested to inhibit the response to ESAs. The underlying mechanisms may relate to reduction in erythroid burst forming units in the bone marrow due to decreased angiotensin II synthesis or decreased degradation of an inhibitor of erythropoiesis by ACE inhibitors or ARBs by direct inhibition of the erythropoietic stimulating effect of angiotensin II.[197,198] Although the clinical impact of this effect is small in most patients, adjustment of the renin angiotensin system inhibition can be considered as an approach that may improve Hgb levels or responsiveness to ESA. Severe secondary hyperparathyroidism may also be associated with impaired erythropoiesis, presumably due to disruption of the bone marrow architecture although toxic effects of parathyroid hormone on erythropoietin synthesis, erythropoiesis, and red blood cell survival have also been postulated.[199,200] As noted previously, PRCA should also be considered in assessing patients with ESA hyporesponsiveness, particularly if they were previously responsive.

A full list of references is available at www.expertconsult.com.

10

Mineral Bone Disorders in Chronic Kidney Disease

Jessica Kendrick, MD, MPH, Anna Jovanovich, MD, and Sharon Moe, MD

OUTLINE

INTRODUCTION

Chronic kidney disease (CKD) is associated with an increased risk of death and cardiovascular disease. Disorders of bone mineral metabolism and regulatory hormones seen in CKD are thought to play a key role in the excess morbidity and mortality. In people with healthy kidneys, normal serum levels of phosphorus and calcium are maintained through the interaction of three hormones: parathyroid hormone (PTH), $1,25(OH)_2D$ (calcitriol, the active metabolite of vitamin D), and fibroblast growth factor 23 (FGF-23). These hormones act on three primary target organs: bone, kidney, and intestine. The kidneys play a critical role in the regulation of normal serum calcium and phosphorus concentrations, convert vitamin D into calcitriol, and respond to PTH and FGF-23. Thus derangements are common in patients with CKD. Abnormalities in mineral metabolism occur early in the course of CKD, even as early as stage 2, and progress as kidney function worsens. The progression of kidney disease is eventually associated with (1) altered serum levels of calcium, phosphorus, PTH, FGF-23 and vitamin D; (2) disturbances in bone modeling or remodeling with the development of fractures or impaired linear growth in children; and (3) extraskeletal calcification in soft tissues and arteries. Collectively, these abnormalities are called *chronic kidney disease-mineral bone disorder* (CKD-MBD) (Box 10.1).[1] In this chapter, the physiology and clinical consequences of CKD-MBD will be discussed, followed by treatment recommendations.

Phosphorus

Normal Physiology

Phosphorus is critical for numerous physiological functions, including skeletal development, mineral metabolism, cell membrane phospholipid content and function, cell signaling, platelet aggregation, and energy transfer through mitochondrial metabolism. Because of its importance, normal homeostasis maintains serum phosphorous concentrations between 2.5 and 4.5 mg/dL (0.81 to 1.45 mmol/L). The serum phosphorus concentration is maintained under the direction of hormonal regulators including FGF-23, PTH, and calcitriol. In an average diet, approximately 1 gram of phosphorus is ingested daily. Of this, 300 mg is excreted in the stool and 700 mg is absorbed. Eighty-five percent of phosphorus is contained in bone in the form of hydroxyapatite. Of the remainder, 14% is intracellular, and only 1% is extracellular. Of this extracellular phosphorus, 70% is organic (phosphate) and contained within phospholipids, and 30% is inorganic. The inorganic fraction is 15% protein bound, and the remaining 85% is either complexed with cations or circulates as the free monohydrogen or dihydrogen forms. Thus serum measurements only reflect a minor fraction of total body phosphorus and therefore do not accurately reflect total body stores in the setting of the abnormal homeostasis that occurs in CKD. The terms *phosphorus* and *phosphate* are often used interchangeably, but the term *phosphorus* means the sum of the two physiologically occurring inorganic ions in serum, hydrogen phosphate (HPO_4^{2-}), and dihydrogen phosphate ($H_2PO_4^-$).

Most of the phosphorus (60% to 70%) is absorbed in the duodenum and jejunum with minimal absorption occurring in the ileum. Phosphorus absorption is dependent on both passive transport, related to the concentration in the intestinal lumen, and active transport stimulated by calcitriol, the active metabolite of vitamin D. The passive absorption is dependent on luminal phosphate concentration and occurs via the epithelial brush border sodium-phosphorus cotransporter (Npt2b).[2] Calcitriol can upregulate the sodium-phosphate cotransporter and therefore actively increase phosphate absorption; however, there is near normal intestinal absorption of phosphorus in the absence of vitamin D. Medications or foods that bind intestinal phosphorus (antacids, phosphate binders, and calcium) can decrease the net amount of phosphorus absorbed by decreasing the free phosphate for absorption.

Most inorganic phosphate is freely filtered by the glomerulus. Approximately 70% to 80% of the filtered load is reabsorbed in the proximal tubule, which serves as the primary regulated site of the kidney. The remaining 20% to 30% is reabsorbed in

BOX 10.1 Kidney Disease Improving Global Outcomes (KDIGO) Classification of CKD-MBD and Renal Osteodystrophy

Definition of CKD-MBD

A systemic disorder of mineral and bone metabolism due to CKD manifested by either one or a combination of the following:

- Abnormalities of calcium, phosphorus, PTH, or vitamin D metabolism
- Abnormalities in bone turnover, mineralization, volume, linear growth, or strength
- Vascular or other soft tissue calcification

Definition of Renal Osteodystrophy

- An alteration of bone morphology in patients with CKD
- One measure of the skeletal component of the systemic disorder of CKD-MBD that is quantifiable by histomorphometry of bone biopsy

(From Moe S, Drueke T, Cunningham J, et al. Definition, evaluation, and classification of renal osteodystrophy: a position statement from Kidney Disease: Improving Global Outcomes (KDIGO). *Kidney Int.* 2006;69:1945–1953.)

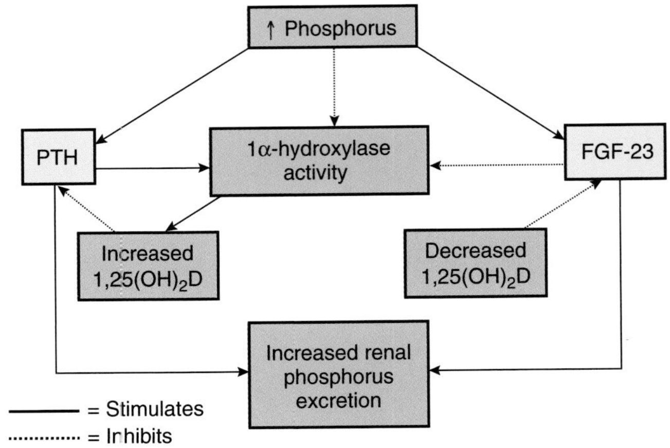

FIG. 10.1 Regulation of serum phosphorus levels. As phosphorus levels increase (or there is a chronic phosphorus load), both PTH and FGF-23 are increased. Both the elevated PTH and FGF-23 increase urinary phosphorus excretion. The two hormones differ in respect to their effects on the vitamin D axis. PTH stimulates 1α-hydroxylase activity, thereby increasing the production of $1,25(OH)_2D$, which in turn negatively feeds back on the parathyroid gland to decrease PTH secretion. In contrast, FGF-23 inhibits 1α-hydroxylase activity, thereby decreasing the production of $1,25(OH)_2D$ feeding back to stimulate further secretion of FGF-23. *Solid line*, stimulates; *dashed line*, inhibits.

the distal tubule. Factors that increase phosphorus excretion are primarily increased plasma phosphate concentration, PTH, and FGF-23. Conversely, acute or chronic phosphorus depletion will decrease excretion. Renal phosphorus excretion is also increased, although to a lesser extent, by volume expansion, metabolic acidosis, glucocorticoids, calcitonin, growth hormone, and thyroid hormone. The majority of this regulation occurs in the proximal tubule via sodium-phosphorus cotransporters. Similar to the intestine, the sodium-phosphorus cotransporters can be acutely moved to the brush border in the presence of acute or chronic phosphorus depletion. Alternatively, after a phosphorus load or in the presence of PTH, the exchanger is removed from the brush border and catabolized.[3]

Renal phosphorus excretion is exquisitely sensitive to changes in the serum phosphorus level due to hormones that regulate phosphate excretion including PTH and FGF-23 (both are discussed in detail later). The normal homeostatic response to increased phosphorus levels is increased PTH and FGF-23. Both PTH and FGF-23 increase phosphorus excretion, but FGF-23 is the principle phosphaturic hormone. FGF-23 is predominately produced from bone cells (osteocytes and bone-lining cells) during active bone remodeling, but messenger RNA is also found in heart, liver, thyroid/parathyroid, intestine, and skeletal muscle.[4] FGF-23 requires the coreceptor klotho for binding to its receptor[5,6] as inactivating klotho in FGF-23 overexpressing mice reverses biochemical and skeletal abnormalities.[7] Klotho is found in the distal tubule and is downregulated in aging and CKD.[6] Once active, FGF-23 regulates Npt2a independently of PTH and affects the conversion of 25 hydroxyvitamin D to calcitriol ($1,25[OH]_2D$) by inhibition of the 1α-hydroxylase enzyme in the renal tubules,[8] leading to hypophosphatemia and inappropriately normal or low calcitriol levels. FGF-23 also stimulates PTH.[9] Mice with targeted ablation of FGF-23 confirm these physiological effects of FGF-23: hyperphosphatemia, inappropriately low PTH, increased calcitriol, and bone loss.[10] Overexpression of FGF-23 in mice leads to the progressive development of secondary hyperparathyroidism.[11] FGF-23 gene expression in bone is regulated by both phosphorus and calcitriol, even in uremic animals.[12] In contrast, PTH stimulates 1α-hydroxylase activity, thereby increasing the production of $1,25(OH)_2D$, which in turn negatively feeds back on the parathyroid gland to decrease PTH secretion. Because PTH is also stimulated in response to hypocalcemia, this proposed homeostatic loop implies that the effects of PTH would predominate in the setting of high phosphorus and low calcium, whereas FGF-23 would predominate in the setting of high phosphorus and normal or high calcium.[13]

Abnormal Physiology in Chronic Kidney Disease

The ability of the kidneys to control phosphate becomes impaired at glomerular filtration rates (GFRs) of approximately 50 to 60 mL/min/1.73 m^2. Frank hyperphosphatemia is not observed in most subjects until the GFR is less than 25 to 30 mL/min/1.73 m^2. Although phosphorus levels are maintained in the "normal" range in patients with CKD stages 3 and 4 (GFR 30 to 60 mL/min/1.73 m^2 and 15 to 29 mL/min/1.73 m^2, respectively), there is a gradual increase in the serum level[14,15] with progressive CKD. Phosphate retention plays a pivotal role in the development of CKD-MBD (Fig. 10.1). With the initial fall in GFR there is a decrease in the amount of filtered phosphate and subsequently excreted phosphate. The remaining nephrons increase single-nephron phosphate excretion due to rises in FGF-23 and PTH. FGF-23 rises very early in CKD, before changes in the serum calcium phosphorus or PTH levels. The

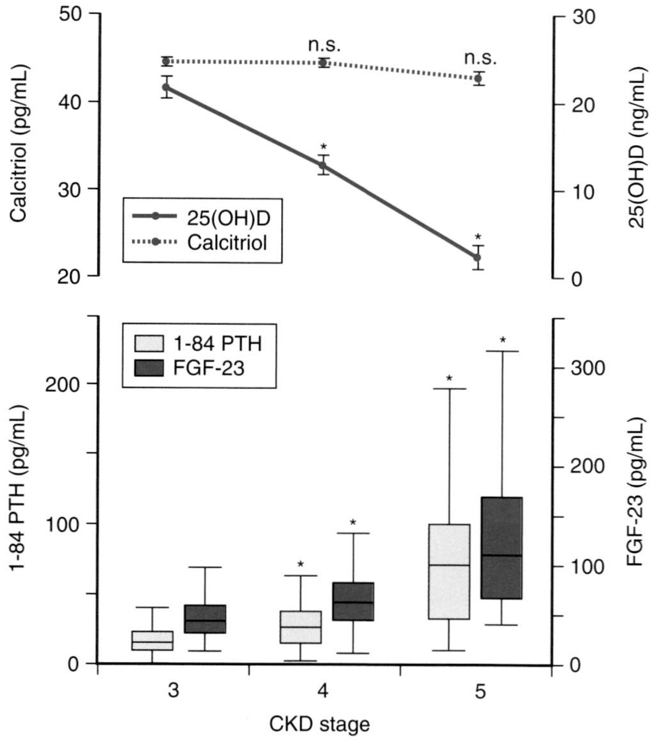

FIG. 10.2 Hormone changes with progression of CKD. As GFR declines, there is a progressive decline in calcitriol levels, a rise in parathyroid hormone and FGF-23 levels, and persistent vitamin D deficiency. Data are presented as mean ± SEM for upper figure, and median with 25th and 75th percentiles for lower figure. (From Tomida K, Hamano T, Mikami S, et al. Serum 25-hydroxyvitamin D as an independent determinant of 1-84 PTH and bone mineral density in nondiabetic predialysis CKD patients. *Bone*. 2009;44:678-683.)

rise in FGF-23 leads to a decrease in calcitriol levels inhibiting intestinal phosphate absorption but also decreasing serum calcium levels and subsequently leads to a rise in serum PTH (Fig. 10.2). The rise in serum PTH and FGF-23 at the expense of maintaining normal serum phosphorus is often referred to as the *trade off hypothesis*.[16] Phosphorus loading increases FGF-23 and PTH, and conversely, phosphorus restriction inhibits the rise in PTH.[17] Additional studies in isolated parathyroid glands or cells confirm a direct role of phosphorus on the regulation of PTH synthesis through multiple mechanisms.[18-21] Hyperphosphatemia also indirectly increases PTH by inhibiting the activity of 1α-hydroxylase, thereby reducing the conversion of 25(OH)D to 1,25(OH)$_2$D. In the skeleton, phosphorus stimulates FGF-23 secretion from osteocytes.[22]

Clinical Consequences of Abnormal Phosphate

Higher serum phosphate levels consistently associate with clinical and subclinical cardiovascular disease among patients with and without kidney disease. Adverse effects occur both from consequences of hyperphosphatemia and elevations in hormones designed to maintain phosphate balance. Hyperphosphatemia is associated with increased vascular stiffening, arterial calcification, calciphylaxis, and valvular calcification.[23] Epidemiological data suggest that serum phosphorus levels above the normal range are associated with increased morbidity and mortality in patients with CKD. These studies differ in their sample size, analyses, and their chosen reference range. The inflection point or range at which phosphorus becomes significantly associated with increased all-cause mortality in dialysis patients varies between studies being 5.0 to 5.5 mg/dL (1.6 to 1.8 mmol/L), greater than 5.5 mg/dL (>1.8 mmol/L), 6.0 to 7.0 mg/dL (1.9 to 2.3 mmol/L), and greater than 6.5 mg/dL (>2.1 mmol/L).[24-26] A Dialysis Outcomes and Practice Patterns Study (DOPPS) analysis demonstrates that the relationship between elevations in serum phosphorus and mortality is consistent across all countries analyzed and that if a facility had 10% more patients with phosphorus levels between 6.1 to 7.0 mg/dL and greater than 7.0 mg/dL (1.97 to 2.26 mmol/L and greater than 2.26 mmol/L), mortality risk was 5.3% and 4.3% higher, respectively.[26] Even in the nondialysis population, higher levels of serum phosphorus, even within the normal range, have been associated with increased risk of all-cause or cardiovascular mortality in patients with normal renal function who were free of cardiovascular disease,[27] in patients with coronary artery disease and normal renal function,[28] and in patients with CKD stages 3 through 5.[29] In addition, hyperphosphatemia is a risk factor for more rapid progression of CKD.[30] Increases in FGF-23 resulting from disordered phosphate metabolism may be a greater risk factor for cardiovascular disease and death than serum phosphorus. Higher FGF-23 levels are associated with increased mortality, cardiovascular disease, left ventricular hypertrophy, vascular calcification, and progression of kidney disease.[31,32] Thus there is clear epidemiological data to support that patients with lower levels of phosphorus do better. Unfortunately, no study has demonstrated that lowering the serum phosphorus to a specific value leads to improved outcomes.

Management of Elevated Phosphate in Chronic Kidney Disease

Normalizing serum phosphorus is an important therapeutic goal for CKD-MBD. Unfortunately, it remains challenging and requires a combination of dietary restriction, phosphate binders, and enhanced dialytic removal. It should be noted that treatment of CKD-MBD should be based on serial assessments of phosphate, calcium, and PTH levels. There is great interdependency of these parameters and therapies aimed at only one often has unintentional effects on another parameter. Thus phosphate, calcium, and PTH levels should be considered together when making management decisions. The Kidney Disease: Improving Global Outcomes (KDIGO) guidelines recommend focusing treatment on patients with hyperphosphatemia.[33]

Diet. Phosphorus is contained in almost all foods. Unfortunately, foods high in phosphate are generally also high in protein, making it challenging to balance dietary phosphorus restriction against the need for adequate protein intake in patients with CKD. Indeed, most well-nourished dialysis patients are in positive phosphorus balance. Roughly 60% to

70% of consumed phosphorus is absorbed, so about 4000 to 5000 mg of phosphate per week enters the extracellular fluid. Phosphate is often added to processed foods, and the amount of phosphate from these sources is significant but difficult to quantify as manufacturers are not required to list the amount of phosphate in foods. Prescription medications, over the counter medications, and dietary supplements have been found to be hidden sources of phosphate.[34] Data regarding the amount of phosphate contained in the medications is limited but data does suggest that they contribute significantly to the phosphate load due to the large number of medications that CKD patients take.[34] The KDIGO 2017 guidelines recommend limiting dietary phosphate intake in patients with CKD stages 3 to 5D. The source of phosphorus (organic vs. inorganic) also needs to be taken into consideration as the bioavailability of phosphorus is different. Organic phosphate is found in animal- and plant-based foods whereas phosphate additives contain inorganic phosphate. Forty percent to 80% of animal-based phosphate and 20% to 50% of plant-based phosphate is absorbed, whereas greater than 90% of phosphate in additives is absorbed.[35] Educating patients on how to read food labels is helpful in reducing phosphate intake.[36] Nutrition education should focus on how to help patients make the best choices as restricting phosphate must not compromise adequate protein intake. Dietary phosphate restriction alone, although an important component of effective phosphorus management, is usually not sufficient to control serum phosphate levels in most dialysis patients.

Phosphate binders. Phosphate binders are the mainstay of treatment of hyperphosphatemia in dialysis patients. Nearly all dialysis patients are prescribed binders. In the nondialysis population there is lack of data demonstrating efficacy of phosphate binders for lowering serum phosphate. A recent trial comparing placebo to active phosphate binder therapy in patients with CKD stages 3B to 4 found a minimal decline in serum phosphate from 4.2 mg/dL at baseline to 3.9 mg/dL after 9 months.[37] Active binder therapy also resulted in a significant increase in coronary artery and abdominal aorta calcification. Although the data suggest that this observed increase in calcification was due to calcium-based binders, those treated with noncalcium-based binders had no advantage over placebo in regard to calcification. Thus the updated recommendations by KDIGO are to focus treatment on CKD stage 3 to 4 patients with hyperphosphatemia, and decisions about treatment should be based on progressive or persistently elevated serum phosphate.

The current phosphate binders available work by binding phosphate in the gastrointestinal (GI) tract and excreting phosphate in feces. Current binders are based on metals (aluminum, lanthanum), calcium, magnesium, polymers, and iron. Advantages and disadvantages of the currently available binders are shown in Table 10.1.

The use of aluminum as a phosphorus binder was popular throughout the 1970s and 1980s. But as evidence emerged implicating aluminum's role in osteomalacia and dialysis encephalopathy, the therapeutic trend shifted to the use of calcium carbonate. In the decade that followed, it was noted that calcium acetate would reduce the elemental load of calcium while controlling the serum phosphorus level compared with calcium carbonate, although there was no difference in the incidence of hypercalcemia.[38] Subsequent studies demonstrated that the calcium-containing phosphate binders were associated with increased burden of vascular calcification in some, but not all studies.[39,40] This and the increased risk of hypercalcemia with the concomitant use of vitamin D led to a need for noncalcium-containing, nonaluminum-containing phosphate binders. In 1998 sevelamer hydrochloride (HCl) was introduced and was shown to be as effective as calcium acetate in maintaining the serum phosphorus without hypercalcemia in crossover trials.[41,42]

It is now recommended to restrict the dose of calcium-based phosphate binders in adult patients with CKD due to data suggesting that excess exposure to calcium (either through diet or medications) may be harmful in patients with CKD regardless of GFR. Two recent randomized controlled trials (RCTs) in predialysis and dialysis patients found a significant survival benefit in patients treated with sevelamer versus calcium-containing binders over a 3-year period.[43,44] Dialysis patients treated with sevelamer had a 10-fold reduction in the risk of experiencing a lethal cardiac arrhythmia and all-cause cardiovascular death compared with patients treated with calcium-based binders.[44] However, one of the largest studies to date, the Dialysis Clinical Outcomes Revisited (DCOR) trial, in which 2103 dialysis patients were randomized to either sevelamer or a calcium-based binder did not find a difference in all-cause or cause-specific mortality rates between the two groups.[45] The study did find a decrease in all-cause hospitalizations with sevelamer. The very high dropout rate (47% in the sevelamer arm and 51% in the calcium-based arm) made the study underpowered; thus it should not be considered a negative study, but rather an inadequate study.

Studies have also found that calcium-based binders may worsen vascular calcification. In a nonblinded study called the *Treat-to-Goal* study, patients were randomized to either a calcium-based binder or sevelamer HCl for 1 year. Despite equivalent phosphorus control, patients taking a calcium binder had progression in coronary and aorta calcification, whereas patients treated with sevelamer HCl did not progress.[46] In an open-label extension of this study in Europe for a second year, calcification scores continued to rise significantly in patients treated with a calcium-based binder, but not in the sevelamer HCl group.[47] The Renagel in New Dialysis Patients (RIND) study[48] found that approximately 65% of patients new to dialysis have coronary artery calcification. In this 18-month trial, 60 incident hemodialysis patients were randomized to calcium-based binders and 54 to sevelamer HCl. Similar to the Treat-to-Goal study, patients had equivalent control of serum phosphorus levels, yet patients treated with calcium-based binders had progressive calcification and those treated with sevelamer HCl did not.[48] In a study of 90 binder-naive patients with CKD stages 3 to 5 who were not receiving dialysis, Russo and colleagues randomized patients (30 per group) to either a low-phosphate diet alone, a low-phosphate diet in combination

Binder	Advantages	Disadvantages	Forms	Dosage (mg)
Calcium Carbonate	• Effective • Inexpensive • Readily Available (over the counter) • Long-term experience	• Potential hypercalcemia • Potential for progression of vascular calcification • GI side effects • Low-turnover bone disease	• Tablet, chewable • Capsule • Liquid • Gum	• Contains 40% elemental calcium (200 mg elemental calcium per 500 mg) • Total dose of elemental calcium should not exceed 2000–2500 mg/d
Calcium Acetate	• Effective • Inexpensive • Readily Available • Long-term experience • Potentially less calcium absorption than calcium carbonate	• Potential hypercalcemia • Potential for progression of vascular calcification • GI side effects • Low-turnover bone disease	• Tablet • Capsule	• Contains 25% elemental calcium (160 mg elemental calcium per 667 mg capsule) • Total dose of elemental calcium should not exceed 2000–2500 mg/d
Magnesium Carbonate/ Calcium Acetate	• Effective • Inexpensive • Decreased calcium load compared with calcium-based binders	• Potential hypermagnesemia • Potential hypercalcemia • GI side effects • No long-term experience	• Tablet	• 235 mg/435 mg • Maximum dose is 3–6 pills/day
Aluminum hydroxide	• Very effective • Inexpensive	• Potential for aluminum toxicity • GI side effects • Altered bone mineralization • Anemia	• Tablet • Capsule • Liquid	• 300–600 mg 3 times per day • Aluminum content varies from 100 to >200 mg per tablet • Limit use to no more than 4 wk
Lanthanum Carbonate	• Effective • Calcium free	• Expensive • Potential for lanthanum accumulation in bone and tissue • GI side effects • No long-term data	• Tablet, Chewable • Powder	• 500–1000 mg (3–6 chewable tablets) 3 times per day
Sevelamer hydrochloride	• Effective • Calcium free • Pleiotropic effects • Potentially decreased vascular calcification	• Expensive • GI side effects • Metabolic acidosis • Potentially interferes with vitamin D and vitamin K absorption	• Tablet	• 800–1600 mg 3 times per day • Maximum dose studied 13 g/d
Sevelamer Carbonate	• Effective • Calcium free • Pleiotropic effects • No metabolic acidosis • Potentially decreased vascular calcification	• Expensive • GI side effects • Potentially interferes with vitamin D and vitamin K absorption	• Tablet • Powder	• 800–1600 mg 3 times per day • Maximum dose studied 14 g/d
Sucroferric Oxyhydroxide	• Effective • Calcium free • Less pill burden than sevelamer • Potential to raise transferrin, iron and hemoglobin levels	• Expensive • GI side effects • Cannot be prescribed with oral levothyroxine • Long-term side effects unknown • Unknown if iron accumulation long-term	• Tablets, chewable	• 500 mg (1 tablet) 3 times per day • Maximum dose studied is 3000 mg/d
Ferric Citrate	• Effective • Calcium free • Less pill burden than sevelamer • Potential to raise transferrin, iron and hemoglobin levels • Potential to decrease iron and ESA usage	• Expensive • GI side effects • Long-term side effects unknown • Unknown if iron accumulation long-term	• Tablets	• Each tablet contains 210 mg ferric iron • Starting dose: 2 tablets 3 times per day • Maximum dose is 12 tablets per day

ESA, Erythropoietin stimulation agents; *GI*, gastrointestinal.

with fixed doses of calcium carbonate (2 g/day), or a low-phosphate diet in combination with sevelamer HCl (1600 mg/day), and they followed these individuals for 2 years.[49] The primary endpoint of the study was progression of coronary artery calcification, assessed as the total calcium score using multislice spiral computed tomography (CT). Among the 84 patients who completed the study, final coronary artery calcification scores were greater than initial scores in those receiving diet alone ($P < 0.001$) or diet in combination with calcium carbonate ($P < 0.001$), whereas there was no progression of calcification in the group treated with diet plus sevelamer HCl.[49] Thus three studies found less calcification with the use of sevelamer HCl compared with calcium-based binders. Two studies have failed to find differences in coronary artery calcification with sevelamer HCl compared with calcium-based binders. In the CARE 2 study, chronic hemodialysis patients from the United States were randomized to receive either calcium acetate or sevelamer HCl.[50] The study was designed to assess noninferiority, evaluating coronary artery calcification by electron beam computed tomography (EBCT) at 6 and 12 months after randomization. There was no difference in the progression of arterial calcification between groups. It should be noted though that before 1 year, 30% of patients in the sevelamer HCl arm and 43% in the calcium acetate arm dropped out, leaving the final sample size less than the power needed to determine noninferiority. The second study was the Brazilian Renagel and Calcium (BRIC) study that compared calcium acetate versus sevelamer on coronary artery calcification and bone histomorphometry in hemodialysis patients.[51] The annual rates of progression of coronary calcification scores were not statistically different. However, this study was hampered by several significant confounders: differences in baseline coronary artery calcification scores between the two study arms; the use of high dialysate calcium concentrations in most patients; and multiple interventions during the course of the study allowed by the caring physicians based on bone biopsy results.

Another noncalcium binder, lanthanum carbonate, was introduced in 2005. Lanthanum carbonate effectively binds intestinal phosphorus without sequestering bile acids and is poorly absorbed. The tablets are chewable and well tolerated. Randomized prospective studies have demonstrated that lanthanum carbonate controls serum phosphorus as well as other binders, but with less hypercalcemia.[52-54] Although there has been concern of toxicities similar to aluminum, the clearance of lanthanum is primarily by the liver as opposed to renal clearance for aluminum. Although animal studies are controversial, in human studies no liver toxicity, suppression of erythropoiesis, or change in the mental status examination have been observed.[54] In addition, no direct bone toxicity has been demonstrated. In a randomized, open-label, multicenter study where bone biopsies were performed, lanthanum did not induce osteomalacia, whereas treatment with calcium carbonate increased the incidence of adynamic bone disease.[55-56] To date, there are no human studies demonstrating that lanthanum carbonate can prevent vascular calcification.

There are now two available iron-based phosphate binders in the United States: sucroferric oxyhydroxide and ferric citrate. An open-label, phase III, randomized, active-controlled, parallel-group, multicenter study was performed in 1059 dialysis patients (n = 968 hemodialysis patients, n = 86 peritoneal dialysis patients) over 24 weeks examining sucroferric oxyhydroxide compared with sevelamer.[57] The study demonstrated that sucroferric oxyhydroxide was noninferior to sevelamer for control of serum phosphate. In addition, treatment effect was achieved with 62% fewer sucroferric oxyhydroxide tablets than sevelamer. Transferrin saturation increased significantly in the sucroferric oxyhydroxide group. There was a trend toward increased ferritin levels in the sucroferric oxyhydroxide group but it did not reach statistical significance. Adverse events were more common in the sucroferric oxyhydroxide group than the sevelamer group (83.2% vs. 76.1%). The most frequent adverse events with sucroferric oxyhydroxide were diarrhea, discolored stools, and hyperphosphatemia. The long-term effects of sucroferric oxyhydroxide were examined in a 28-week extension study of the phase III study.[58] Six hundred and forty-four patients participated in the extension study and were continued on the same treatment and dose of phosphate binder that they were receiving at the end of the initial study. Serum phosphate remained within the Kidney Disease Outcomes Quality Initiative (KDOQI) target range for both treatment groups throughout the study. The number of daily tablets was lower in the sucroferric oxyhydroxide group (mean ± SD, 4.0 ± 1.5 tablets/day) compared with sevelamer (mean ± SD, 10.1 ± 6.6 tablets/day). There was no evidence of iron accumulation over the 1-year period of treatment. There were no significant changes in transferrin saturation, ferritin, iron, or hemoglobin concentrations between the two groups. Adverse events were more common with sucroferric oxyhydroxide compared with sevelamer (14.6% vs. 9.0%) and the most common events reported were hypophosphatemia and hyperphosphatemia. Overall, sucroferric oxyhydroxide appears to be an effective and well-tolerated phosphate binder. One disadvantage is that it inhibits GI absorption of levothyroxine, so it cannot be prescribed with levothyroxine.

Ferric citrate is another iron-based binder approved for use in dialysis patients in the United States. In a large, phase III study of >400 dialysis patients randomized to ferric citrate or active control for 56 weeks, ferric citrate was as effective as sevelamer and calcium acetate in controlling serum phosphate levels.[59] Ferric citrate had a lower average pill burden compared with sevelamer (8 tablets/day vs. 9 tablets/day, P = 0.01) but did not have lower pill burden than calcium acetate (8 tablets/day vs. 7.7 tablets/day, P = 0.28). More patients in the ferric citrate group discontinued the study drug compared with the active control in the first weeks of the study (21% vs. 15%). The most common reason for discontinuation of the study drug was nonserious GI side effects. Thirty-nine percent of patients in the ferric citrate group experienced a serious adverse event compared with 49% in the active control group. There was a significant increase in serum ferritin and transferrin saturation in the ferric citrate group. In addition, ferric citrate reduced both intravenous iron and erythropoietin stimulation agent (ESA) usage at 52 weeks. Hemoglobin levels remained stable throughout the study period and were slightly higher in the ferric citrate group. There was no evidence of iron accumulation throughout the study period but the study did not perform radionuclide-tagged balance studies to confirm.

Overall, the iron-based binders appear to be effective with minimal side effects and less pill burden than calcium-based or polymer-based binders. The long-term effects of these medications beyond 1 year have not been determined and there are no studies examining patient outcomes with these binders.

A new agent for the management of hyperphosphatemia has been developed. Tenapanor is a small molecule inhibitor of the sodium/hydrogen exchanger isoform 3 that specifically targets the transepithelial transport of intestinal phosphate. It reduces the absorption of sodium and phosphate in the gut.[60] In a randomized trial of 162 hemodialysis patients randomized to tenapanor versus placebo, tenapanor resulted in a dose-dependent reduction in serum phosphate from baseline (least-squares mean change: tenapanor = 0.47 to 1.98 mg/dL; placebo = 0.54 mg/dL; $P = 0.01$).[60] Diarrhea was the most common adverse event. A phase III trial is currently underway in dialysis patients. Tenapanor is not currently approved for the treatment of hyperphosphatemia in the United States.

The KDIGO guidelines for CKD-MBD now recommend restricting the dose of calcium-based phosphate binders in patients with CKD regardless of whether other markers of risk such as arterial calcification, hypercalcemia, low PTH levels, or adynamic bone disease are also present.[33] It should be noted that none of the studies provide dose-threshold information nor do they give information on moderately dosed calcium-based binders in combination therapies, so there is no current guideline about a maximum dose. In clinical practice, economic factors, patient preference, and GI distress limit adherence to a rigorous diet and binder schedule. The choice of binder should be individualized for each patient because in the end, the best phosphate binder is what works for an individual patient. Ultimately, there are no studies that demonstrate that lowering the phosphorus to a specific level improves mortality or reduces cardiovascular risk in patients with CKD.

Dialysis. Dialysis is an important part of phosphate management in patients on dialysis. Conventional dialysis removes 1000 mg of phosphorus per dialysis, but because 1000 mg is absorbed on a daily basis, the net positive balance may be 4000 mg per week.[38] Patients who undergo nightly dialysis have weekly removal of phosphate that is twice as high. In a study of 10 patients dialyzing 8 to 10 hours, 6 to 7 days per week at blood flows of 100 mL/min/1.73 m^2, it became possible to discontinue binder therapy and increase dietary phosphate (and protein) intake.[61] One prospective RCT has reported the impact of alternative dialysis therapies using biochemical markers of CKD-MBD as a secondary endpoint.[62] In this study, 26 patients receiving nocturnal, prolonged-duration, hemodialysis six times weekly were compared with 25 patients receiving standard hemodialysis given three times weekly for 4 hours each session in a parallel design. The authors found significant decreases in serum phosphorus and intact PTH, but no difference in calcium in the patients allocated to frequent nocturnal hemodialysis. Importantly, the phosphate-binder dose was also reduced. These data suggest that frequent nocturnal hemodialysis can lead to an improvement in mineral metabolism. Thus optimized control of serum phosphorus may require the use of alternative dialytic regimens in addition to diet and phosphate binders in some patients.

Calcium

Normal Physiology

Maintenance of calcium levels within a narrow physiological range is essential to life. Calcium homeostasis is complex and tightly regulated and depends on regulation of calcium fluxes within the intestine, kidney, and bones. The serum calcium level is a poor reflection of overall total body calcium, as serum levels are less than 1% of total body calcium; the remainder is stored in bone. Ionized calcium, generally 40% of total serum calcium levels, is physiologically active, whereas the nonionized calcium is bound to albumin or anions such as citrate, bicarbonate, and phosphate. In the presence of hypoalbuminemia, there is an increase in the ionized calcium relative to the total calcium, thus total serum calcium may underestimate the physiologically active (ionized) serum calcium. A commonly used formula for estimating the ionized calcium from total calcium is to add 0.8 mg/dL for every 1 mg decrease in serum albumin less than 4 mg/dL. However, data in CKD patients has demonstrated that this formula offers no superiority over total calcium alone and is less specific than ionized calcium measurements.[63] In addition, the assay used for albumin may affect the corrected calcium measurement.[64] Thus ionized calcium should be measured if more precise assessment of serum calcium levels is needed.

GI absorption of calcium is a highly selective process as only 20% to 25% of total dietary calcium is absorbed. Calcium absorption across the intestinal epithelium occurs via a vitamin D–dependent, saturable (transcellular) TRPV5 and TRPV6 transporters (animal homologues ECaC2 and CaT1)[65] and independent, nonsaturable (paracellular) pathways. The intracellular calcium then associates with calbindin 9k to be "ferried" to the basolateral membrane where calcium is removed from the enterocytes via the calcium-ATPase. TRPV6 is the main transporter responsible for intestinal calcitriol-dependent calcium absorption, with compensation by TRPV5 when needed.[65] Many factors regulate intestinal calcium absorption. Age, vitamin D and calcium intake, serum levels of calcitriol, and PTH all regulate calcium absorption. Calcitriol is the most important hormonal regulatory factor because it induces calcium channels, calbindin (which binds calcium and removes calcium from the microvilli region), and increases the Ca^{2+}-ATPase.[66]

The kidneys play a key role in calcium regulation. Ninety-eight percent to 99% of the filtered load of calcium is reabsorbed by the renal tubules.[66] The majority (60% to 70%) of calcium is reabsorbed passively in the proximal tubule driven by a transepithelial electrochemical gradient that is generated by sodium and water reabsorption. In the thick ascending limb, another 20% of calcium is reabsorbed via paracellular transport. Only 5% to 10% of the filtered calcium load is reabsorbed in the distal nephron, but the distal nephron is the major site for regulation of calcium excretion.[67] Although the majority of total renal calcium reabsorption is paracellular, the regulation of reabsorption is via transcellular pathways that occur in the distal convoluted tubule, the connecting tubule, and the initial portion of the cortical collecting duct. The calcium enters these cells via TRPV5 and TRPV6 calcium channels down electrochemical gradients, binds with calbindin 28k, and is transported to the basolateral membrane where calcium is actively reabsorbed by the Na^{2+}/Ca^{2+} exchanger (NCX1) and/or the Ca^{2+}-ATPase (PMCA1b).[65] Both TRPV5 and TRPV6 are localized to these distal nephron segments, with upregulation by calcium, PTH, vitamin D, and estrogen. TRPV5 is the most critical, with compensation by TRPV6, which is the opposite from compensation in the intestine.[65]

PTH is the most important regulator of serum calcium. Small reductions in serum ionized calcium lead to the rapid release of PTH due to the existence of a calcium sensor in the parathyroid glands. The calcium-sensing receptor (CaR) belongs to a super family of G-protein–coupled receptors. Activation of the CaR stimulates phospholipase C, leading to increased inositol increased inositol 1,4,5-triphosphate (IP3), which mobilizes intracellular calcium and decreases PTH secretion. In contrast, inactivation reduces intracellular calcium and increases PTH secretion.[68] The CaR is expressed in organs controlling calcium homeostasis, such as parathyroid gland, thyroid C cells, intestine, kidney,[68] and likely bone.[69] In the kidney, the CaR is expressed in mesangial cells and throughout the tubules. The CaR is found not only on the apical membrane of the proximal tubule and the inner medullary collecting duct but also on the basolateral membrane of the medullary and cortical thick ascending limb and distal convoluted tubule. Activation of CaR on the thick ascending limb leads to increased intracellular free Ca^{2+}, which decreases paracellular calcium reabsorption.[70] This CaR also responds to increases in intraluminal calcium concentration by reducing antidiuretic hormone-stimulated water absorption.[71] In theory, this may provide a mechanism by which the urine can stay dilute in the face of hypercalcemia and hypercalciuria to avoid dangerous calcium precipitation, and it may explain the polyuria observed in patients with hypercalciuria. The expression of the CaR is regulated by calcitriol in parathyroid, thyroid, and kidney cells, but the renal effects of CaR are both dependent and independent of PTH. In uremic animals, the expression of CaR in the parathyroid gland is downregulated by high phosphorus diet and occurs after the onset of parathyroid hyperplasia. Once downregulated, the expression can be rescued by a low phosphorus diet.[21]

Calcitriol is another key factor controlling calcium absorption. Cholesterol is synthesized to 7-dehydrocholesterol, which in turn is metabolized in the skin to vitamin D_3. In addition, there are dietary sources of vitamin D_2 (ergocalciferol) and vitamin D_3 (cholecalciferol). Once in the blood, vitamin D_2 and D_3 bind with vitamin D–binding protein (DBP) and are carried to the liver where they are hydroxylated by *CYP27A1* in an essentially unregulated manner to yield 25(OH)D, often called *calcidiol* and measured as "vitamin D." Calcidiol is then converted in the kidney to calcitriol by the action of 1α-hydroxylase (*CYP27B1*). The 1α-hydroxylase enzyme in the kidney is also the site of regulation of calcitriol synthesis by numerous other factors, including low calcium, low phosphorus, estrogen, prolactin, growth hormone, calcitriol itself,[72] and FGF-23.[73] Calcitriol mediates its cellular function via both nongenomic and genomic mechanisms. Calcitriol facilitates the uptake of calcium in intestinal and renal epithelium by increasing the activity of the voltage-dependent calcium channels TRPV5 and TRPV6, upregulating the calcium transport protein calbindins and the basolateral calcium-ATPase.[65] It also is essential for normal bone remodeling.[74]

Abnormal Physiology in CKD

Normal calcium homeostasis is interrupted early in the course of CKD. An increase in FGF-23 levels is the earliest abnormality. Rising FGF-23 levels inhibit production of calcitriol through inhibition of 1α-hydroxylase resulting in decreased calcium reabsorption. In response, PTH levels increase to maintain serum calcium levels. Thus serum calcium levels are maintained in the normal range, at the expense of hyperparathyroidism, throughout the course of CKD until the GFR is less than 30 mL/min/1.73 m^2. Late in the course of CKD, calcitriol levels are inadequate to increase intestinal calcium absorption.[75] In addition, most patients with CKD stages 3 and 4 have very low levels or urinary calcium excretion,[76] suggesting maximum tubular reabsorption.

The inability to maintain normal calcium homeostasis in CKD may lead to inappropriate calcium balance. In CKD, the bone appears less able to take up calcium, at least in low-turnover states that can be present in up to 50% of patients with CKD.[77] This has led to the concept of "calcium loading" when patients are also given a calcium-based binder, because, even with normal serum levels, excess calcium intake can lead to a positive calcium balance. A study of eight patients with CKD (mean estimated GFR [eGFR] 36 mL/min/1.73 m^2) found that patients were in neutral calcium balance while consuming a 957 mg calcium diet, but they went into markedly positive calcium balance of 500 mg per day when treated with calcium carbonate.[78] These data support findings from another study in patients with CKD stages 3 and 4 showing positive calcium balance while consuming a diet of 2000 mg/day calcium.[79] Without net urinary excretion or bone uptake, a positive calcium balance may predispose the person to extraskeletal calcification.[80] In CKD patients, approximately 18% to 20% of calcium is absorbed from the intestine. If patients are taking 2000 mg/day in total elemental calcium intake (1500 mg from binder and 500 mg from diet), and 20% is absorbed, then the net intake is 400 mg per day. On hemodialysis days, this figure is slightly greater because approximately 50 mg of calcium is infused with a 4-hour dialysis treatment using 2.5 mEq/L dialysate calcium concentration. In patients on peritoneal dialysis, there is a slight efflux of calcium using a 2.5 mEq/L dialysate in four daily exchanges. Thus the absorbed intake of elemental calcium from a 2000 mg elemental calcium diet (plus binders) and 2.5 mEq/L calcium dialysate would be 350 to 450 mg/day. In patients taking most forms of vitamin D, net intestinal absorption would be enhanced, thereby increasing the net intake further. In an anuric patient, this positive balance of calcium load has only two "compartments" to go to: bone and extraskeletal locations. If the bone is normally remodeling, then the calcium should be deposited there; however, normal bone is not common in dialysis patients (discussed later). If no calcium-containing phosphate binder is taken, then the patients should be in a neutral or slightly negative balance depending on stool and sweat output. The fraction of the excess calcium that is deposited into bone or into soft tissues (which could promote calcification) is difficult to determine. The KDIGO 2017 guidelines recommend restricting the dose of calcium-based phosphate binders in patients with CKD regardless of whether other markers of risk such as arterial calcification, hypercalcemia, low PTH levels, or adynamic bone disease are also present.[33]

Clinical Consequences of Abnormal Calcium Homeostasis

Both hypocalcemia and hypercalcemia are associated with increased mortality in patients with CKD. Higher serum calcium levels are associated with increased mortality and cardiovascular events in patients with CKD.[81-83] Hypercalcemia can also lead to arrhythmias. As discussed previously, positive calcium balance may lead to vascular calcification, which is associated with an increased risk of cardiovascular disease and mortality in CKD patients. Hypocalcemia contributes to secondary hyperparathyroidism (SHPT) and renal osteodystrophy. High-turnover bone disease is observed in patients with SHPT. In addition, SHPT is associated with an increased risk for cardiovascular events and death. It is unclear at what level of low serum calcium there is an increased risk. It is also important to realize that none of these studies evaluated patients receiving cinacalcet, which lowers calcium by its effects on the CaR, with an expected decrease in the total serum calcium concentration. Thus we do not know whether patients with low serum calcium levels due to cinacalcet have a similar risk to those with similar serum calcium levels who are not on the drug.

Management of Calcium in Chronic Kidney Disease

The KDIGO guidelines do not suggest limits for dietary calcium intake, but they do recommend restricting the dose of calcium-based binders for all patients with CKD stages 3 to 5D. The balance studies discussed previously are consistent in showing that 2000 mg/day of calcium intake is too high for patients with CKD stages 3 to 5D. A more moderate target for dietary calcium intake of 800 to 1000 mg/day may be more appropriate in patients with CKD. The updated KDIGO guidelines do not recommend correction of hypocalcemia in all patients. An individualized approach to the treatment of hypocalcemia should be used because those patients with symptomatic or severe hypocalcemia may benefit from correction. The choice of whether or not to supplement with calcium may also depend on the dietary calcium intake of the individual patient. For those patients with high calcium intakes (>1000 mg/day), calcium supplementation should probably be avoided.

The use of calcium-based phosphate binders also should be restricted in patients with CKD stages 3 to 5D. Several RCTs have shown significant survival benefits for patients treated with sevelamer versus calcium-containing binders.[43,44] It is important to note that none of the available studies provide dose-threshold information about calcium exposure, so a maximum dose of calcium-based binders is unknown. Further research is needed to determine the optimal calcium intake for patients with CKD.

Parathyroid Hormone

Normal Physiology

PTH is cleaved to an 84-amino acid protein in the parathyroid gland, where it is stored with fragments in secretory granules for release. Once released, the circulating 1 to 84 amino acid protein has a half-life of 2 to 4 minutes. It is then cleaved into N-terminal, C-terminal, and midregion fragments of PTH, which are metabolized in the liver and kidney. In addition, fragments are also directly released from the gland. The primary function of PTH is to maintain calcium homeostasis by: (1) increasing bone mineral dissolution, thus releasing calcium and phosphorus; (2) increasing renal reabsorption of calcium and excretion of phosphorus; (3) increasing the activity of the renal 1α-hydroxylase; and (4) enhancing the GI absorption of both calcium and phosphorus indirectly through its effects on the synthesis of calcitriol. PTH is released in response to hypocalcemia, hyperphosphatemia, and low calcitriol levels. The extracellular concentration of ionized calcium is the most important determinant of minute-to-minute secretion of PTH. The secretion of PTH in response to low levels of ionized calcium is a sigmoidal relationship, frequently referred to as the *calcium–PTH curve.*

PTH binds to the PTH1 receptor, which is a member of the G-protein–linked 7-membrane spanning receptor family. PTHrp shares homology with the first few amino acids of PTH and also binds the PTH1 receptor. In general the effects of PTH are systemic, and those of PTHrp is as an autocrine factor. In the kidney, PTHR1 is widely expressed. As detailed earlier, PTH upregulates TRPV5, TRPV6, calbindin$_{28K}$, NCX1, and PMCA1b in these distal tubule segments to facilitate calcium reabsorption.[65] PTH also facilitates phosphorus wasting by inducing the catabolism of the brush border sodium-phosphate cotransporter Npt2b.[2] In bone, PTH receptors are located on osteoblasts with a time-dependent effect. PTH administered chronically inhibits osteoblast differentiation and nodule formation, but administration of PTH in a pulse rather than a continuous manner stimulates osteoblast proliferation and mineralization.[84]

Abnormal Physiology in Chronic Kidney Disease

PTH excess in CKD is a systemic disease with many extraskeletal manifestations. These include encephalopathy, anemia, extraskeletal calcification, peripheral neuropathy, cardiac dysfunction, hyperlipidemia, and impotence. The pathogenesis of SHPT is complex and is driven by hypocalcemia, low levels of calcitriol, decreased phosphate excretion, and skeletal resistance to the actions of PTH. There are also intrinsic abnormalities in parathyroid gland function as parathyroid hyperplasia is an early finding in CKD. There is decreased expression and synthesis of the calcium receptor in SHPT leading to altered calcium-regulated PTH secretion.[85] PTH levels increase when the GFR falls below 60 mL/min/1.73 m^2,[86] and the incidence and severity increases as kidney function declines. High-turnover bone disease is the classic skeletal complication observed in patients with SHPT. Bone disease is discussed later in more detail. Most series demonstrate that at least 50% of patients on dialysis have secondary hyperparathyroidism, and in many series the prevalence is far greater.[26] In addition to increased secretion of PTH, there is altered degradation and resistance to its skeletal effects. As a result, levels of PTH are uniformly increased compared with the general population, and yet levels two to five times the upper limit for the general population may be associated with decreased bone turnover in CKD patients. Although PTH affects multiple organ systems, the focus over the last 20 years has been on bone, and PTH had become a surrogate marker for bone turnover.

Measurement of Parathyroid Hormone

Reliable measurements of the concentration of PTH in serum or plasma are essential for the clinical management of patients with CKD. PTH circulates not only in the form of the intact 84-amino acid peptide but also as multiple fragments of the hormone, particularly from the middle and carboxyl C-terminal regions of the PTH molecule. These PTH fragments arise from direct secretion from the parathyroid gland as well as from metabolism of PTH (1 to -84) by peripheral organs, especially liver and kidney. For these reasons, assays for PTH that were directed toward different parts of the PTH molecule yielded different results. The development of a second generation of PTH assays, the two-site immunoradiometric antibody test (commonly called *intact* assay) improved the detection of entire length of (active) PTH molecules. In this assay, a capture antibody binds within the amino terminus and a second antibody binds within the carboxy terminus. Unfortunately, this "intact" PTH assay also detects accumulated large C-terminal fragments, commonly referred to as *7-84 fragments*, which is a mixture of multiple PTH fragments that include, and are similar in size to, 7-84 PTH.[87] In parathyroidectomized rats, the injection of a truly whole 1-84 amino acid PTH was able to induce bone resorption, whereas the 7-84 amino acid fragment was antagonistic, which explains why patients with CKD may have high levels of "intact" PTH but relative hypoparathyroidism at the bone tissue level.[88]

More recently, a third generation of assays has become available that truly detect only the 1-84 amino acid full-length molecule or "whole" or "bioactive" PTH assays. Early reports suggested that levels of 1-84 PTH or the 1-84 PTH/large C-PTH fragment ratio may be a better predictor of bone histology in end-stage renal disease (ESRD) than standard "intact" PTH values.[89] However, other studies have not confirmed the ability of the whole PTH or the ratio to predict the diagnosis of the underlying bone disease.[90-91] A study demonstrated that although both 1-84 and non–1-84 fragments are secreted from the PTH gland in response to serum calcium levels, the secretory responses are not proportional,[92] perhaps leading to the discrepancy of these reports.

These data highlight that the use of tight PTH ranges as a biomarker for bone turnover is no longer valid. In addition, different available assays measure different quantities of both 7-84 and 1-84 (when added to uremic serum).[93] There are also differences in PTH results when the samples are measured in plasma, serum, or citrate, and depending on whether the samples are on ice or allowed to sit at room temperature.[94] Thus these problems with sample collection and assay variability raise significant concerns with the validity of absolute levels of PTH, and the inability of specific values to predict underlying bone histology limits the clinical use as a bone biomarker at specific values. For these reasons, the KDIGO guidelines recommended that extremes of risk for PTH, which are less than two or greater than nine times the upper limit for a given assay. Values within this range should be evaluated on trends.[33]

Management of Secondary Hyperparathyroidism

The target PTH in the KDOQI guidelines for CKD stage 5D was based on the ability of PTH to predict low and high turnover bone disease.[95] Other studies have demonstrated that intact PTH levels within a range of 150 to 300 pg/mL are not predictive of underlying bone histology.[96] In addition, there are significant problems with assay variation. This raises concerns about the use of PTH as a biomarker of bone turnover, which has been done in clinical practice for years. However, hyperparathyroidism is a systemic disease, with multiple nonbone effects.[97] Thus KDIGO, in establishing optimal PTH ranges, evaluated additional evidence in the form of observational data determining associations between PTH and patient level endpoints (mortality, cardiovascular death, fractures). The inflection point or range at which PTH becomes significantly associated with increased all-cause mortality varies between studies and ranges from >400[98] to >480 pg/mL,[24] to >500[27] to >511 pg/mL,[99] and to >600 pg/mL.[100] Unfortunately, most of these analyses either do not indicate the assay type, or the data comes from PTH measured with multiple assays. Another confounding factor for these analyses is that many studies feature single-baseline PTH values or infrequent (quarterly or less) measurements. Based on these observational data, the KDIGO guidelines considered that levels of intact PTH less than two and greater than nine times the upper limit of normal for the PTH assay (<130 and >585 pg/mL for most kits that have an upper normal limit of 65 pg/mL) represented extreme ranges of risk that should be avoided. Values within that range should be interpreted by evaluating trends, with interventions if the trends are consistently going up or down. However, it is important to recognize that there are no randomized clinical trials that demonstrate that treatment to achieve a specific PTH level results in improved outcomes.

Treatment of elevated parathyroid hormone in patients with chronic kidney disease stages 3 to 5, not on dialysis. In CKD stages 3 to 5, not on dialysis, the ideal PTH level is unknown. The KDIGO guidelines recommend treating hypocalcemia, hyperphosphatemia, high phosphate intake, and vitamin D deficiency in patients with levels of intact PTH that are progressively rising or persistently above the upper limit of normal.[33] As with phosphate and calcium, treatment of an elevated PTH should not be based on a single elevated value. Three RCTs have examined the effect of phosphate binders on PTH levels in the nondialysis population. Two RCTs compared sevelamer with placebo. The first was performed in 109 nondiabetic patients with CKD stage 3 over 36 weeks.[101] The second was performed in 117 CKD patients with a mean GFR of 36 ± 17 mL/min/1.73 m^2 over 24 months.[102] Neither study found significant differences in PTH levels between the two groups. Another RCT of 148 patients with CKD stage 4 compared placebo with three different phosphate binders (calcium-based, lanthanum, and sevelamer) over a 9-month period. This study found that PTH levels increased in the placebo group but remained stable in those on active therapy ($P = .002$).[37]

The use of nutritional vitamin D (ergocalciferol or cholecalciferol) has also only received limited research. A post hoc analysis of the Vitamin D, Calcium, Lyon Study II (DECALYOS II) was conducted by Kooienga and coworkers.[103] This study assessed the impact of treatment with cholecalciferol 800 IU plus calcium 1200 mg daily versus placebo on biochemical parameters in 610 elderly French women, of whom 322 had eGFR values less than 60 mL/min/1.73 m^2 using the MDRD formula. The treatment with vitamin D raised serum levels and lowered PTH in the study, and there was a similar response in individuals with eGFR less than 45 mL/min/1.73 m^2, less than 60 mL/min/1.73 m^2, and greater than 60 mL/min/1.73 m^2 compared with placebo ($P < .001$ for all). However, this study was unable to distinguish between effects of calcium and vitamin D because these treatments were given in combination.[103] A recent RCT in 87 patients with CKD stages 2 to 4 of high-dose cholecalciferol supplementation (20,000 IU/week) versus low dose (5000 IU/week) found that PTH levels decreased significantly in both groups, but PTH levels did not differ significantly between groups at the end of the study.[104]

The use of calcitriol and active vitamin D analogs in patients with CKD not on dialysis should not be routinely used. Several RCTs have shown that calcitriol and active vitamin D analogs reduce PTH compared with placebo.[76,105-107] Two RCTs comparing calcitriol with paricalcitol found that the decrease in PTH was comparable in the two arms and the incidence of hypercalcemia was very low in both groups.[106,107] Despite these findings, the use of calcitriol and active vitamin D analogs should be reserved for patients with severe and progressive hyperparathyroidism. This recommendation is based on two RCTs that found no beneficial effects of paricalcitol compared with placebo on surrogate cardiac endpoints and found a significant increased risk of hypercalcemia.[108,109] Recent metaanalyses confirmed these findings and supported the hypercalcemia risk associated with calcitriol and active vitamin D analogs.[110,111]

A novel vitamin D prohormone, extended-release calcifediol, has been shown in an RCT of 429 patients with CKD stages 3 to 4 to effectively raise 25(OH)D levels and reduce PTH by at least 10% over 12 months.[112] This medication had no significant impact on phosphate, calcium, or FGF-23 levels. Currently, there are no patient-level outcomes reported with this medication and further studies are needed. There is one study using calcimimetics to treat hyperparathyroidism in patients with CKD stages 3 and 4. In this trial, the calcimimetics lowered the PTH effectively compared with placebo, but they also lowered the calcium and raised the phosphorus.[113] Given the concerns over hyperphosphatemia, unless patient-level outcome studies are performed, this agent should be reserved for patients on dialysis. Thus much research is needed in this population.

Treatment of elevated parathyroid hormone in chronic kidney disease stage 5D: Calcitriol and vitamin D analogs. The use of calcitriol has been the key to the management of hyperparathyroidism for nearly 30 years; however, a common side effect has always been hypercalcemia. Initially, the higher level of serum calcium was thought to be a therapeutic advantage, providing additional PTH-suppressive effects independent of vitamin D. However, as hypercalcemia became a concern, new vitamin D analogs were designed to maximize PTH suppression yet minimize intestinal absorption of calcium and phosphate. Two "less calcemic" analogs are commercially available in the United States: 19-nor-1,25(OH)2D2 (paricalcitol) and 1α(OH)D2 (doxercalciferol), and others are available outside the United States.[114] All of these analogs appear effective in suppressing hyperparathyroidism in patients on dialysis.[115-118] A secondary analysis of a trial comparing paricalcitol and calcitriol has been published. This study found that although there was no difference between paricalcitol and calcitriol in the number of subjects who had a single episode of hypercalcemia, paricalcitol led to less sustained hypercalcemia.[119] There are no published direct comparative trials of doxercalciferol to paricalcitol, or doxercalciferol to calcitriol. In addition, there are no prospective studies evaluating patient-level endpoints, and only limited bone studies.[120] The lack of comparative trials makes blanket endorsement of preferential use of any of these analogs over calcitriol premature, and the KDIGO guidelines could not recommend one agent over another.[33] More recent attention has focused on the potential positive effects of these analogs on survival in dialysis patients, apparently independent of their effects on calcium, phosphorus, and PTH. Retrospective analyses demonstrate a survival advantage in patients receiving any form of vitamin D compared with no vitamin D, with paricalcitol and doxercalciferol having superior survival advantage over calcitriol.[98,100,121,122] However, these results must be confirmed in prospective trials as one cannot completely control for the bias of the decision to use vitamin D in a given patient.

Treatment of elevated parathyroid hormone in chronic kidney disease stage 5D: Calcimimetics. Calcimimetics are a group of drugs that are allosteric activators of the CaR, thereby enhancing signaling and decreasing PTH release independent of vitamin D.[123] The only calcimimetic commercially available is cinacalcet HCl. Cinacalcet is effective in suppressing PTH but with some hypocalcemia.[124,125] Composite data from all phase III studies in >1100 patients around the world demonstrated that the use of this agent can lead to suppression of PTH with a lowering of the calcium × phosphorus product,[126] allowing achievement of the current KDIGO guidelines in many more patients that current regimens. Long-term studies have demonstrated continued efficacy.[127] The PARADIGM trial compared cinacalcet to active vitamin D therapy as monotherapy in secondary hyperparathyroidism in 312 dialysis patients and found similar PTH reductions in both groups.[128] A large RCT, the EVOLVE study examined cinacalcet versus placebo on patient-level outcomes in 3883 hemodialysis patients.[129] The primary endpoint was a composite of all-cause mortality, nonfatal myocardial infarction, congestive heart failure, hospitalization for unstable angina, and peripheral vascular events. The trial did not find a reduction in the primary endpoint with cinacalcet (hazard ratio 0.93, $P = 0.112$). However, after adjustment for baseline characteristics that were not similar between the two groups, there was a significant reduction in the primary endpoint (hazard ratio 0.88, $P = 0.008$). In addition, the Evaluation of Cinacalcet Hydrochloride Therapy to Lower Cardiovascular Events (EVOLVE) trial found that cinacalcet significantly reduced the risk of severe unremitting SHPT and parathyroidectomy regardless of baseline PTH.[130] Thus even though EVOLVE did not meet its primary endpoint, the results of secondary analyses suggest that cinacalcet may be beneficial in hemodialysis patients or in a subset of these patients.

Two trials have evaluated the combination use of cinacalcet with active vitamin D versus standard therapy. The trial by Urena-Torres et al.[131] found improved PTH-lowering in subjects treated with both cinacalcet and active vitamin D. Raggi et al.[132] found that cinacalcet plus vitamin D reduced the progression of coronary artery calcium accumulation. No trials have examined the benefits of combination therapy on hard clinical outcomes such as mortality.

At this point, the KDIGO guidelines recommend that calcitriol, vitamin D analogs, calcimimetics, or a combination of calcimimetics with calcitriol or vitamin D analogs can be used in CKD stage 5D to lower PTH.

Treatment of elevated parathyroid hormone: Parathyroidectomy. The need for parathyroidectomy to control secondary hyperparathyroidism should decrease as newer medications offer more flexibility with PTH control. However, patients with serum PTH levels greater than 1000 pg/mL that have been refractory to medical therapy have traditionally been considered candidates. This includes patients who cannot receive vitamin D sterols due to an elevated calcium level and those who do not tolerate cinacalcet secondary to GI disturbances. A study found decreased mortality and lower risk of hip fractures in patients who underwent parathyroidectomy compared with those who did not from the United States Renal Data System database.[133,134] Although this type of data is biased by patient selection for parathyroidectomy, it raises a question about whether the procedure is delayed too long in some patients. Unfortunately, with PTH assays being so problematic, there is no specific level of PTH at which parathyroidectomy is currently recommended.

Fibroblast Growth Factor 23

Normal Fibroblast Growth Factor 23 Physiology

FGF-23 is 251-amino acid protein synthesized by osteocytes and osteoblasts and is a major regulator of phosphate homeostasis. FGF-23 acts as an endocrine hormone by interacting with its coreceptor α-klotho. Elevated FGF-23 levels are responsible for phosphate-wasting syndromes including autosomal recessive hypophosphatemic rickets, X-linked hypophosphatemic rickets, and fibrous dysplasia. FGF-23 downregulates the phosphate transporters Napt2a and 2c, resulting in decreased phosphate reabsorption.[8] It also downregulates 1α-hydroxylase, which decreases the production of calcitriol resulting in decreased intestinal phosphate and calcium reabsorption. FGF-23 also is a regulator of PTH. FGF-23 inhibits parathyroid function and increases the parathyroid expression of the CaSR and vitamin D receptor making the gland more sensitive to the inhibitory actions of calcium and calcitriol.

Whether FGF-23 is regulated by dietary phosphate is unclear. Small, short-term studies have failed to show changes in FGF-23 levels based on changes in dietary phosphate. However, longer studies show that dietary phosphate does modulate FGF-23 levels. A study of phosphate loading found early dose-dependent increases in PTH and FGF-23.[135] It is also unclear whether FGF-23 is regulated by PTH, because studies have found conflicting results. In healthy adults, Burnett-Bowie et al.[136] found that PTH infusion increased FGF-23 over 18 hours, whereas Gutierrez et al.[137] found that PTH infusion over 6 hours lowered FGF-23. FGF-23 is also regulated by calcitriol. Increases in calcitriol levels result in increases in FGF-23. The mechanism by which calcitriol regulates FGF-23 is presumed to be via the vitamin D receptor.

FGF-23 in Chronic Kidney Disease

In CKD, plasma FGF-23 concentrations rise very early before phosphate and PTH. It is not known whether this early increase is in response to phosphate retention, changes in bone or is directly related to CKD progression. In patients with CKD stage 2, bone biopsy samples show increased FGF-23 expression in osteocytes even though serum mineral metabolism parameters are normal.[138] It has been suggested that kidney damage even with preserved GFR sends a signal to bone stimulating FGF-23 secretion. This is based on studies in patients with polycystic kidney disease and preserved GFR as well as in healthy kidney donors after donation showing an increase in plasma FGF-23 levels.[139,140] Interestingly, many patients with CKD may be in negative phosphate balance early in the course of kidney disease due to dietary insufficiency and elevated FGF-23. Epidemiological data show that plasma phosphate concentrations fall in the early stages of CKD (eGFR 60 to 69 mL/min/1.73 m^2) when the plasma FGF-23 levels are high.[141] Increased FGF-23 levels also contribute significantly to the development of secondary hyperparathyroidism through suppression of calcitriol synthesis (see Fig. 10.1) FGF-23 increases progressively as renal function declines to stabilize serum phosphate levels. In patients on dialysis, FGF-23 levels can be up to 1000-fold above the normal range.[142]

Clinical Consequences of Elevated FGF-23

Numerous epidemiological studies have shown an association between higher FGF-23 levels and adverse outcomes in CKD patients. Elevated FGF-23 levels are independently associated with death, cardiovascular disease, and kidney disease progression in both dialysis and predialysis CKD patients.[143-145] Higher FGF-23 levels have also been associated with increased graft loss after kidney transplant.[146] FGF-23 was initially thought of as a risk marker of disordered mineral metabolism, but it is now known that FGF-23 has direct toxicity. Faul and colleagues showed that very high levels of FGF-23 directly induce left ventricular hypertrophy in mice.[147] There is also some evidence that the FGF/α-klotho pathways are protective to the vasculature by inhibiting calcification. However, the association of FGF-23 with vascular calcification is not consistent and seems phosphate dependent, because recent data suggest that FGF-23 has no independent effect on phosphate-driven vascular calcification.[148]

Treatment of Elevated FGF-23

Currently there are several experimental strategies for reducing elevated FGF-23 levels. These include dietary phosphate restriction, use of phosphate binders, use of calcimimetics, and antagonism of FGF receptor signaling or direct neutralization of the FGF-23 protein. Numerous studies have examined the effect of various phosphate binders on circulating FGF-23 levels in CKD patients, and the results are conflicting. A study of 100 CKD stage 4 patients found that sevelamer and not calcium acetate decreased FGF-23 levels.[148] An RCT of 148 patients with CKD stages 3 to 4 randomized to lanthanum, sevelamer calcium acetate, or placebo for 9 months found that none of the phosphate binders had an effect on FGF-23 levels.[37] In dialysis patients, long-term studies have shown that FGF-23 levels are reduced with sevelamer but not with calcium acetate. Given the conflicting findings, further studies are needed to determine whether phosphate binders can lower FGF-23 levels.

Several studies have examined the role of cinacalcet on FGF-23 levels. All of the studies found that cinacalcet reduced FGF-23 levels in dialysis patients.[149-151] Although these studies are suggestive that cinacalcet may reduce FGF-23 levels, it is unclear whether the decrease is due to cinacalcet, to less use of active vitamin D analogs, or to better control of secondary hyperparathyroidism. In addition, it is important to note that in the EVOLVE[129] study there was no improvement in cardiovascular events or mortality in dialysis patients receiving cinacalcet compared with placebo.

Experimental studies have been performed examining the effect of FGF receptor inhibitors and anti–FGF-23 antibodies on various outcomes. FGF-23 neutralization did decrease the progression of SHPT and normalized bone turnover in rats, but it did so at the expense of hyperphosphatemia, increased aortic mineralization, and increased mortality.[152] It is possible that neutralizing FGF-23 or its inhibitor in CKD patients not on dialysis may lead to increases in serum phosphate and increased vascular calcification. Further studies are needed to determine whether there is a role for FGF-23 neutralization.

Currently, there are no data to support that lowering FGF-23 levels results in improved clinical outcomes. Larger, well-powered clinical trials are needed to clarify this situation.

Renal Osteodystrophy

Bone biology. The majority of the total body stores of calcium and phosphorus are located in bone. Trabecular (cancellous) bone is located predominately in the epiphyses of the long bones, and cortical (compact) bone is in the shafts of long bones and is 80% to 90% calcified. Bone consists principally (90%) of highly organized cross-linked fibers of type I collagen; the remainder consists of proteoglycans and noncollagen proteins such as osteopontin, osteocalcin, osteonectin, and alkaline phosphatase. The main bone cells are cartilage cells, which are key to bone development; osteoblasts, which are the bone-forming cells; and osteoclasts, which are the bone resorbing cells. Osteoblasts are derived from progenitor mesenchymal cells located in the bone marrow and become mature osteoblasts. This process is controlled by bone morphogenic proteins, the transcription factor Runx2 early and other hormones and cytokines later. Once bone formation is complete, osteoblasts may undergo apoptosis, or become quiescent cells trapped within the mineralized bone in the form of osteocytes.[153] The osteocytes are interconnected through a series of canaliculi and serve to transmit the initial signaling involved with mechanical loading.[154] Osteoclasts are derived from hematopoietic precursor cells that differentiate and are somehow "signaled" to arrive at a certain place in the bone. Once there, they fuse to form the multinucleated cells known as *osteoclasts* that become highly polarized, reabsorbing bone through the release of degradative enzymes. Once resorption is complete, estrogens, bisphosphonates, and cytokines can induce, and PTH can inhibit, apoptosis.[153] Numerous hormones and cytokines have been evaluated, mostly in vitro, for their role in controlling osteoclast function. The control of bone remodeling is highly complex, but it appears to occur in very distinct phases: (1) osteoclast resorption, (2) reversal, (3) preosteoblast migration and differentiation, (4) osteoblast matrix (osteoid or unmineralized bone) formation, (5) mineralization, and (6) quiescent stage. At any one time, less than 15% to 20% of the bone surface is undergoing remodeling, and this process in a single bone-remodeling unit can take 3 to 6 months.[153] How a certain piece of bone is chosen to undergo a remodeling cycle and how the osteoclasts and osteoblasts signal each other is due to the osteoprotegerin (OPG) and receptor activator of nuclear-factor κB system (RANK). This control system is regulated by nearly every cytokine and hormone thought important in bone remodeling, including PTH, calcitriol, estrogen, glucocorticoids, interleukins, prostaglandins, and members of the transforming growth factor–β superfamily of cytokines.[155] OPG has been successful in preventing bone resorption in animal models of osteoporosis and tumor-induced bone resorption. Not surprisingly, the drug denosumab, a fully human monoclonal antibody that inhibits receptor activator of nuclear-factor κB ligand (RANKL), and is used to treat osteoporosis.[156,157] Abnormalities in the OPG/RANK system have been found in renal failure,[158] although the impact on bone remodeling is not yet clear.

Abnormalities of bone in chronic kidney disease. Disorders of mineral metabolism are also associated with abnormal bone. Bone quality is impaired in CKD, as there is an increased prevalence of hip fracture in dialysis patients compared with the general population in all age groups.[159,160] Dialysis patients in their 40s have a relative risk of hip fracture that is 80-fold higher than that of age- and sex-matched controls.[162] Furthermore, hip fracture in patients on dialysis is associated with a doubling of the mortality rate observed in hip fractures in patients who are not on dialysis.[160,161] In the CKD population, a similar increased risk occurs.

Extremes of bone turnover found in patients with CKD significantly impact fragility and are likely additive to bone abnormalities commonly found in the aging and sedentary general population. These extremes of bone turnover that contribute to abnormal bone quality differentiate renal osteodystrophy from traditional osteoporosis, which is predominately low bone volume. The latter can be determined by bone mineral density (BMD) testing (i.e., with dual energy x-ray absorptiometry (DXA). However, DXA only evaluates how much mineral is present, not how it is arranged. In the case of renal osteodystrophy, the "arrangement" can be so aberrant as to alter quality even at high mineral content. The ability of DXA to predict fractures in patients with CKD has been questioned. However, recent studies have shown that in patients with CKD stages 3 to 5D, DXA does predict fractures.[162-165] In a study of 485 hemodialysis patients, lower baseline femoral neck and total hip BMD predicted a greater risk of fracture.[162] In another study of 131 predialysis CKD patients, low BMD at the hip, lumbar spine, and radius all predicted fracture.[163] Thus DXA is now recommended in patients with CKD stages 3 to 5D to assess fracture risk.[33]

Bone biopsy is the gold standard for the diagnosis and classification of renal osteodystrophy. The patient is given a tetracycline derivative approximately 3 weeks before the bone biopsy and a different tetracycline derivative 3 to 5 days before the biopsy. Tetracycline binds to hydroxyapatite and emits fluorescence, thereby serving as a label of the bone. A core of predominately trabecular bone is taken and embedded in a plastic material and sectioned, requiring special laboratories to process bone biopsy samples. The sections can then be visualized with special stains, and under fluorescent microscopy to determine the amount of bone between the two tetracycline labels, or that formed in the time interval between the two labels. This dynamic parameter assessed on bone biopsy is the basis for assessing bone turnover, which is central to discerning types of renal osteodystrophy. In addition to dynamic indices, bone biopsies can be analyzed by histomorphometry for many static parameters as well. The nomenclature for these assessments has been standardized.[166]

Traditional classification scheme for renal osteodystrophy focused on bone turnover.[167] High-turnover bone disease is due to secondary hyperparathyroidism, with high bone formation rates, increased cell number, and in severe cases, peritrabecular fibrosis (termed *osteitis fibrosa cystica*). Low-turnover bone disease has low bone formation rates with either increased osteoid (unmineralized bone) called *osteomalacia*, or no increased osteoid but decreased cell numbers (adynamic bone disease). In the past, osteomalacia was due to aluminum deposition at the bone mineralization front that prevented appropriate mineralization. Lastly, mixed uremic osteodystrophy is a term used to identify a high-turnover lesion, but with increased osteoid. Unfortunately, the latter diagnosis is not uniformly made throughout the world.

The term renal osteodystrophy is specific to bone pathology found in patients with CKD and is one component of the mineral and bone disorders that occur as a complication of CKD-MBD.[1] In the evaluation of renal osteodystrophy, bone biopsy results are interpreted based on three histological descriptors—bone turnover, mineralization, and volume (TMV system)—with any combination of each of the descriptors possible in a given specimen. The TMV classification scheme provides a clinically relevant description of the underlying bone pathology as assessed by histomorphometry, which in turn helps define the pathophysiology, and thereby guides therapy. Fig. 10.3 shows how the TMV system and the traditional classification terminology intersect. Importantly, by adding the component of volume, one can see that long-standing severe hyperparathyroid bone disease or disease on preexisting conditions of bone volume loss (postmenopausal osteoporosis or corticosteroid use) would be different (and likely more fragile with increased fractures) than newly diagnosed bone disease due to hyperparathyroidism.

Cardiovascular Disease and Vascular Calcification in Chronic Kidney Disease

CKD is associated with significant cardiovascular morbidity and mortality (Fig. 10.4). In fact, nondialysis-dependent CKD patients are more likely to experience a cardiovascular disease event or death than to progress to ESRD.[168] Patients with CKD demonstrate a greater prevalence of traditional cardiovascular risk factors compared with those without CKD[169] in addition to so-called "nontraditional" cardiovascular risk factors. A major contributor to these nontraditional risk factors is CKD-MBD. As discussed previously, patients with CKD develop abnormalities in the serum levels of phosphorus, calcium, PTH, vitamin D, and FGF-23. The bone changes that ensue are associated with these biochemical alterations and other mechanisms. Both the biochemical changes and bone abnormalities contribute to vascular calcification and cardiovascular disease. All three of these processes are closely interrelated and form the rationale for the syndrome CKD-MBD.[1]

Vascular calcification. Extraskeletal calcification can occur in multiple locations in patients with CKD: the cornea,

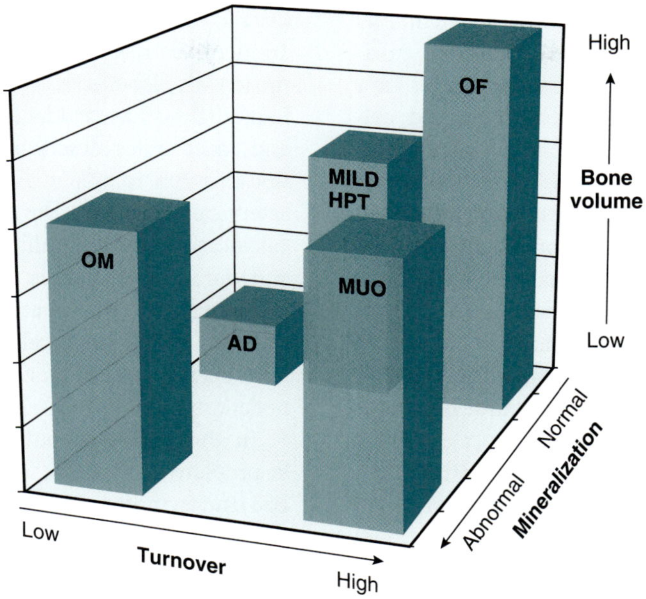

FIG. 10.3 TMV classification system for bone histomorphometry. The figure is a graphical example of how the TMV system provides more information than the present, commonly used classification scheme. Each axis represents one of the descriptors in the TMV classification: turnover (from low to high), mineralization (from normal to abnormal), and bone volume (from low to high). Individual patient parameters could be plotted on the graph, or means and ranges of grouped data could be shown. For example, many patients with renal osteodystrophy cluster in areas shown by the bars. *OM* (osteomalacia) is currently described as low-turnover bone with abnormal mineralization. The bone volume may be low to medium, depending on the severity and duration of the process and other factors that affect bone. *AD* (adynamic bone disease) is currently described as low-turnover bone with normal mineralization, and the bone volume in this example is at the lower end of the spectrum, but other patients with normal mineralization and low turnover will have normal bone volume. *Mild HPT* (mild hyperparathyroid-related bone disease) and *OF* (osteitis fibrosa or advanced HPT bone disease) are currently used distinct categories, but in actuality represent a range of abnormalities along a continuum of medium to high turnover and any bone volume depending on the duration of the disease process. Finally, *MUO* (mixed uremic osteodystrophy) is variably defined internationally. In the present graph, it is depicted as high-turnover, normal bone volume, with abnormal mineralization. In summary, the TMV classification system more precisely describes the range of pathological abnormalities that can occur in patients with CKD. (From Moe S, Drueke T, Cunningham J, et al. Definition, evaluation, and classification of renal osteodystrophy: a position statement from Kidney Disease: Improving Global Outcomes (KDIGO). *Kidney Int.* 2006;69:1945-1953.)

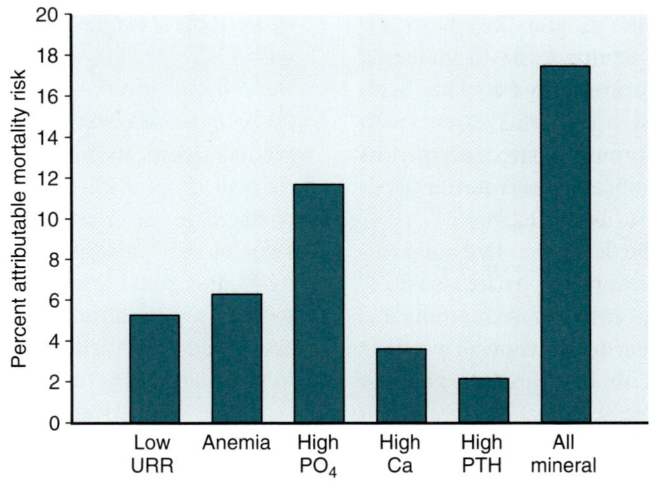

FIG. 10.4 Mortality risk of disturbances in mineral metabolism. A study of 40,538 patients[72] identified the population attributable risk, or the percentage of risk of mortality in ESRD patients attributable to various factors, and demonstrated[72] that hyperphosphatemia conveyed the greatest risk of mortality or even more than anemia and low urea reduction ratio (URR), and that the combination of hyperphosphatemia, hypercalcemia, and elevated PTH accounted for 17.5% of the observed mortality. (From Moe S, Drueke T, Cunningham J, et al. Definition, evaluation, and classification of renal osteodystrophy: a position statement from Kidney Disease: Improving Global Outcomes (KDIGO). *Kidney Int.* 2006;69:1945-1953, using data from Block GA, Klassen PS, Lazarus JM, et al. Mineral metabolism, mortality, and morbidity in maintenance hemodialysis. *J Am Soc Nephrol.* 2004;15:2208-2218.)

areas around joints, pulmonary system, cardiac system, and the vascular system. The high prevalence of vascular calcification in CKD patients is an old observation that is now understood to be a cell-mediated process. Ibels and colleagues (1979)[170] demonstrated that both the renal and internal iliac arteries of patients undergoing a kidney transplant had increased atheromatous/intimal disease and increased calcification compared with transplant donors. In addition, the medial layer was thicker and more calcified in the recipients compared with the donors.[170] When histological changes in coronary arteries from dialysis patients were compared with those of age-matched nondialysis patients who had died from a cardiac event, there was a similar magnitude of atherosclerotic plaque burden and intimal thickness in the dialysis patients compared with controls, but with more calcification. In addition, morphometry of the arteries demonstrated increased medial thickening.[171] When these same authors evaluated more distal segments of the coronary arteries, they found medial calcification adjacent to the internal elastic lamina.[172] Indeed, medial calcification is more specific to CKD and is even found among pediatric patients with CKD.

Biochemical abnormalities of CKD-MBD as well as vascular calcification are noted early in CKD.[173] The pathogenesis of arterial calcification is complex, but it appears that dedifferentiation of vascular smooth muscle cells to osteoblast-like cells is a major initiating factor. Elevated phosphorus, uremic serum, hyperglycemia, oxidative stress, inflammatory cytokines, and other so-called "nontraditional" cardiovascular factors appear to initiate this transformation.[23] Once the vascular smooth muscle cells are osteoblast-like, they appear to mineralize in a manner similar to bone, with the net calcification determined by the balance of promineralizing factors such as elevations in calcium and phosphorus and antimineralizing effects of circulating and local inhibitors such as fetuin-A and matrix gla protein.[23,174] Patients with CKD have elevations of calcium and phosphorus, and they have low levels of the circulating inhibitor fetuin-A due to increased inflammation.[175] Low levels of fetuin-A are associated with vascular calcification and increased mortality in patients with CKD.[176,177] Other bone-derived proteins have emerged as possible mediators of vascular calcification and cardiovascular disease; these are summarized in Table 10.2.[178,179]

EBCT is the gold standard for the detection of vascular calcification; spiral CT and duplex ultrasonography are also used. All of these techniques are thought to be more reproducible than the older method of observing progression of vascular calcification on plain radiographs. EBCT and spiral CT allow rapid imaging of the heart in diastole, such that calcification in the coronary arteries can be easily distinguished and quantified. Hemodialysis patients have twofold to fivefold greater coronary artery calcification than age-matched individuals with normal kidney function that had angiographically proven coronary artery disease.[180] Goodman and colleagues subsequently demonstrated that advanced calcification can also occur in the coronary arteries of children and young adults on hemodialysis and is related to increased doses of calcium-containing phosphate binders, and increased calcium-phosphorus product.[181] Data in patients with CKD not yet on dialysis also demonstrate an increased risk of coronary artery calcification, especially in those with diabetes.[182] Nearly 50% to 60% of patients starting hemodialysis have evidence of coronary artery calcification,[48] and most series describing prevalent hemodialysis patients find that 70% to 80% of all patients have evidence of coronary artery calcification.[39] The only risk factors for coronary artery calcification that are uniform across studies are advanced age and duration of dialysis. Mineral metabolism abnormalities including hyperphosphatemia, elevated calcium-phosphorus product, or excessive calcium load from phosphate binders have been identified as additional risk factors in several, but not all, studies.[40]

In the general population, coronary artery calcification is predictive of future cardiac events in both asymptomatic and symptomatic individuals.[183,184] Likewise, coronary artery calcification is associated with increased morbidity and mortality among those with CKD. Indeed, patients with nondialysis-dependent CKD have an increased risk of all-cause mortality, cardiovascular disease events and mortality, and hospital admission.[185,186] Among both predialysis CKD patients and dialysis-dependent CKD patients, greater coronary artery calcification predicts cardiovascular mortality and events. When coronary artery calcification was measured among 181 predialysis CKD patients using computed tomography, those with an Agatston score greater than 100 units had a threefold higher risk of cardiac events and death.[187] In studies of 114 and 166 dialysis patients, coronary artery calcification scores of more than 400 were associated with a 16-fold increase[188] and greater than eightfold increase[189] in mortality, respectively. Increased valvular calcification in CKD patients is also associated with increased mortality.[190] Interestingly, small studies suggest that nocturnal dialysis[191] and kidney transplantation[192] appear to stabilize the progression of coronary artery calcification.

Peripheral artery calcification is also common in patients with CKD.[193] Dialysis patients with intimal calcification of the femoral artery by plain radiograph had increased all-cause and cardiovascular mortality compared with those with medial calcification, which in turn is significantly greater than in those with no medial calcification.[194] Calcification of the larger arteries is associated with increased pulse wave velocity and pulse pressure.[195] Increased pulse wave velocity[196] and pulse pressure[197] are associated with increased mortality. Alterations in mineral metabolism appear to be associated with increased calcification in peripheral arteries in the majority of studies.[193]

There is an inverse relationship of bone mineralization and vascular calcification. The ability of bone to mineralize appears to peak at ages 25 to 35 years old. Thereafter, bone mineral content decreases gradually, with a 5-year acceleration at the time of menopause in women. These age-related changes appear to be elevated in patients with kidney disease. Interestingly, coronary artery calcification progresses from ages 25 to 35 until death.[23] A cross-sectional study of dialysis patients found a significant inverse correlation between coronary artery calcification by EBCT and BMD by CT.[177] It

TABLE 10.2 Emerging Bone-Derived Proteins That Mediate CKD-MBD

Bone-Derived Protein	Produced By	Function	Role in CKD-MBD
Matrix Gla-protein (MGP)	• Chondrocytes • Vascular smooth muscle cells • Endothelial cells • Fibroblasts	• Prevents ectopic and vascular calcification via numerous suggested mechanisms • Active form (carboxylated and phosphorylated) binds calcium	• Biomarker for vascular disease in CKD • Increased levels of inactive (i.e., under-carboxylated, dephosphorylated) MGP in ESRD • Inactive MGP positively correlated with vascular calcification and mortality in CKD and ESRD
Osteocalcin (OC) aka Bone Gla Protein	• Bone	• Modulates shape and size of hydroxyapatite crystals (bone mineralization) • Modulates osteoblast and osteoclast activity • Active form (carboxylated and phosphorylated) binds calcium	• OC levels positively correlate with bone remodeling in CKD • Link between bone and energy/glucose metabolism, though impact on CKD unknown at this time
Osteoprotegerin (OPG)	• Osteoblasts • Cardiovascular cells • Other cells	• Binds RANKL to prevent RANK/RANKL interaction ○ osteoblast and osteoclast coupling ○ bone remodeling and mass • Inflammatory role along with RANK and RANKL	• In CKD, high OPG levels are strongly associated with vascular stiffness and calcification, as well as cardiovascular mortality possibly mediated by inflammatory role • In CKD, high OPG to RANKL ratio may be associated with high bone turnover
MEPE	• Bone • Kidney	• Modulates bone turnover, mineralization, and vascularization • Modulates renal vascularization	• Bone expression of MEPE increases later in CKD and is inversely related to bone volume
Dentin matrix protein 1 (DMP1)	• Bone	• Modulates bone metabolism	• Inhibits FGF-23 expression • Attenuates extraskeletal calcification • Bone expression of DMP1 increases early in CKD and is inversely related to skeletal mineralization
Sclerostin	• Osteocytes	• Inhibits osteoblast bone formation	• High sclerostin levels in CKD may be associated with adynamic bone disease • Higher sclerostin levels in CKD may be associated with less vascular calcification and better cardiovascular outcomes

CKD, Chronic kidney disease; *ESRD*, end-stage renal disease; *FGF-23*, fibroblast growth factor 23; *MEPE*, matrix extracellular phospho-glycoprotein; *RANKL*, receptor activator of nuclear-factor κB ligand.
Modified from Mazzaferro S, Tartaglione L, Rotondi S, et al. New biomarkers in CKD-MBD. *Semin Nephrol.* 2014;34:598-611; Schiavi SC. Sclerostin and CKD-MBD. *Curr Osteoporos Rep.* 2015;13:159-165.

appears that low-turnover bone disease accounts for the greatest risk of vascular calcification of these patients.[195] Studies of patients who had undergone bone biopsy showed that those with the lowest PTH and lowest bone turnover on biopsy had the greatest arterial calcification by ultrasound[198] and more aortic stiffness.[199] Barreto and colleagues found over a 1-year period that patients with persistent low turnover bone disease were more likely to have progression of their coronary artery calcification.[200] The likely mechanism for these findings is that adynamic bone cannot incorporate an acute calcium load, whereas actively remodeling bone can.[79]

CONCLUSION

CKD-MBD is a systemic disorder of abnormal serum levels of mineral-related biochemistries, abnormal bone, and extraskeletal calcification. The current treatments for CKD-MBD remain focused on only the biochemical abnormalities. Treatment of CKD-MBD should be based on serial assessments of phosphate, calcium, and PTH levels. There is great interdependency of these parameters and therapies aimed at only one often has unintentional effects on another. Thus phosphate, calcium, and PTH levels should be considered together when making management decisions. Further studies are required to determine whether treatment of CKD-MBD results in improvement in hard clinical outcomes including death and cardiovascular events in patients with CKD.

A full list of references is available at www.expertconsult.com.

11

Vitamin D Disorders in Chronic Kidney Disease

Michelle Denburg, MD, MS, and Ian de Boer, MD, MS

OUTLINE

The kidney plays a fundamental role in the metabolism of vitamin D. Humans obtain vitamin D (cholecalciferol and ergocalciferol) from cutaneous synthesis and dietary intake. These forms of vitamin D undergo regulated conversion to compounds with full hormonal activity, most importantly calcitriol. The rate-limiting step in the generation of calcitriol is performed by the enzyme 1-α hydroxylase. This occurs largely in the proximal tubule of the kidney. Thus calcitriol deficiency is a well-recognized consequence of chronic kidney disease (CKD). Also widely recognized are the important effects of calcitriol deficiency on bone and mineral metabolism in CKD. These include hyperparathyroidism, bone disease, and increased risk of fracture (see Chapter 8).

For a number of reasons, interest in vitamin D deficiency has broadened beyond bone and mineral metabolism. First, potential far-reaching pleiotropic effects of vitamin D have been identified. On the basis of these potential pleiotropic effects, vitamin D may help prevent cancer, inflammation, activation of the renin-angiotensin-aldosterone system, cardiovascular disease (CVD), initiation and progression of CKD, and mortality. Second, vitamin D deficiency is highly prevalent among persons with and without CKD. Third, nonrenal synthesis of calcitriol has been described, suggesting that supplementation with cholecalciferol or ergocalciferol, in addition to or instead of calcitriol or its analogs, may have beneficial effects among persons with CKD.

With these concepts in mind, this chapter describes current knowledge of the pathophysiology, epidemiology, consequences, and therapy of vitamin D deficiency in CKD.

PATHOPHYSIOLOGY

Vitamin D

Humans obtain vitamin D as cholecalciferol (vitamin D_3) or ergocalciferol (vitamin D_2) (Fig. 11.1). "Vitamin D" refers jointly to cholecalciferol and ergocalciferol, which differ by their carbon side chains (Fig. 11.2). For healthy individuals, the predominant source of vitamin D is cutaneous synthesis of cholecalciferol.[1-4] Within keratinocytes, ultraviolet light (wavelength 290 to 315 nm, within the UVB range) stimulates the conversion of 7-dehydrocholesterol to previtamin D_3, which is then quickly converted to cholecalciferol. It has been estimated that 5 to 10 minutes exposure of the arms and legs to direct sunlight leads to the production of up to 3000 international units (IU) of cholecalciferol, though this varies by time of day, season, latitude, and skin sensitivity.[2] During winter months at high latitude, particularly higher than 40 degrees north or lower than 40 degrees south, very little light in the 290 to 315 nm range reaches the surface of the earth (Fig. 11.3), and cutaneous synthesis is markedly reduced. Sunlight itself destroys excess cutaneous cholecalciferol so that intense sun exposure does not cause vitamin D intoxication.

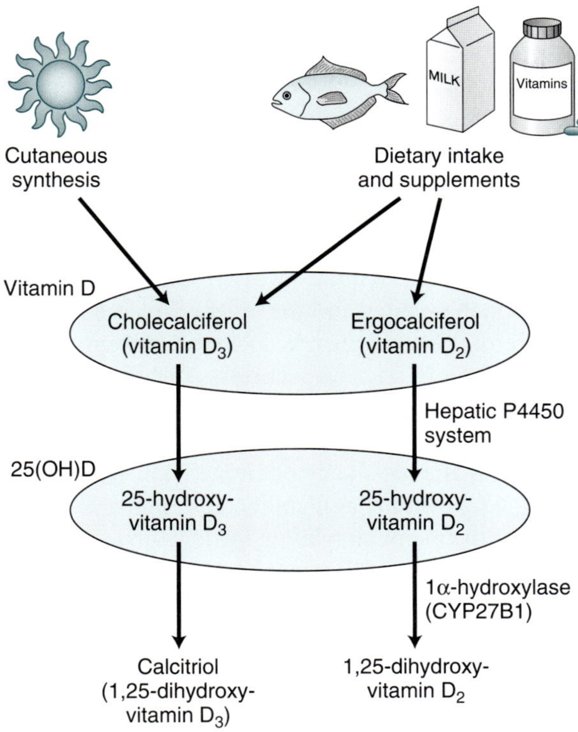

FIG. 11.1 Sources and metabolism of vitamin D. *25(OH)D*, 25-hydroxyvitamin D.

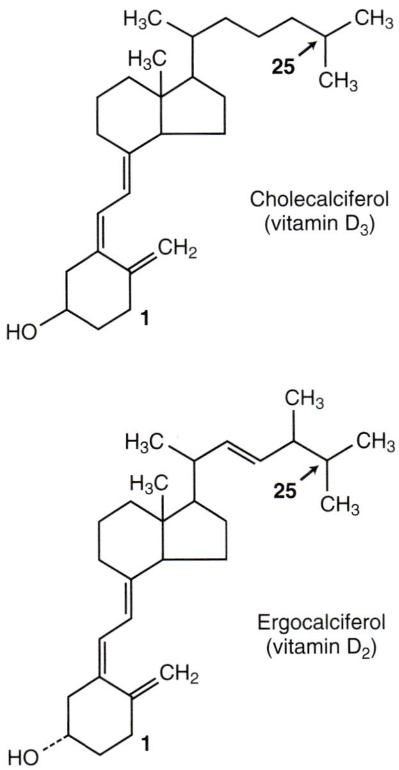

FIG. 11.2 Chemical structures of cholecalciferol (vitamin D_2) and ergocalciferol (vitamin D_3). These two forms of vitamin D differ by their carbon side chain. The 1 and 25 carbons, which are required for hydroxylation for maximum hormonal activity, are labeled.

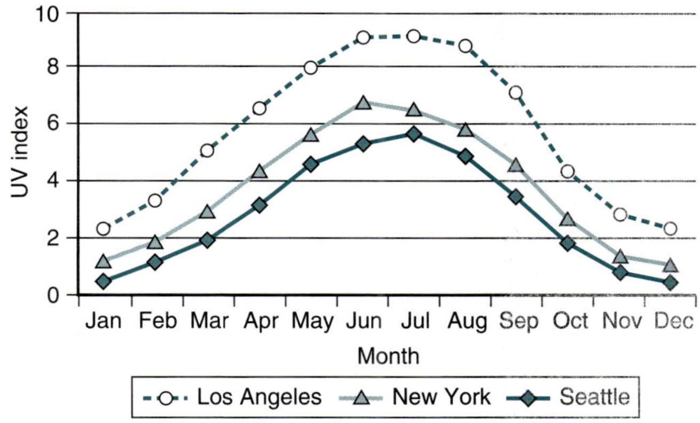

FIG. 11.3 Mean monthly ultraviolet (*UV*) index for Los Angeles, CA (latitude 34 degrees), New York, NY (latitude 41 degrees), and Seattle, WA (latitude 48 degrees). The UV Index is a next-day forecast of the amount of skin-damaging UV radiation expected to reach the earth's surface at the time when the sun is highest in the sky (solar noon). The amount of UV radiation reaching the surface is primarily related to the elevation of the sun in the sky, the amount of ozone in the stratosphere, and the amount of clouds present. To calculate the UV index, irradiances at 290 to 400 nm are weighted so as to reflect the human skin's response to each wavelength; weighting favors the wavelengths also required for cutaneous synthesis of vitamin D. Data presented are means for the calendar years 2000 to 2002, provided by the National Oceanic and Atmospheric Administration/National Weather Service.

Vitamin D is also obtained from the diet and dietary supplements (Table 11.1).[5] Fatty fish provides the largest quantities of cholecalciferol, and milk is fortified with approximately 100 IU of cholecalciferol per cup. Additional foods that sometimes contain supplementary cholecalciferol include other dairy products, orange juice, and breakfast cereals. Mushrooms produce ergocalciferol, and one serving of fresh shiitake mushrooms contains approximately 100 IU. Vitamin D supplements are available over the counter and by prescription. These contain cholecalciferol or ergocalciferol with a wide range of doses. It should be noted that the US Food and Drug Administration does not regulate vitamin D supplements, and in a study of over-the-counter and compounded cholecalciferol preparations, the actual calciferol content was highly variable, with potency ranging from 9% to 146%.[6]

Vitamin D–Binding Protein

Vitamin D is fat soluble. More than 99% of circulating vitamin D is bound to plasma proteins: 85% to 90% to vitamin D–binding protein (DBP) and 10% to 15% to albumin. The binding affinity of DBP for vitamin D metabolites is more than 1000-fold stronger than that of albumin, and therefore the albumin-bound and free fractions together are considered bioavailable.[7-11] DBP, originally named *group-specific component* (Gc-globulin),[12] is a multifunctional 58 kDa circulating glycoprotein that circulates in substantial molar excess to its vitamin D ligands, with less than 5% of vitamin D–binding

TABLE 11.1 Selected Food Sources of Vitamin D

Food	IU per serving
Cod liver oil, 1 tablespoon	1360
Salmon (cooked), 3.5 ounces	360
Mackerel (cooked), 3.5 ounces	345
Tuna fish (canned in oil), 3 ounces	200
Sardines (canned in oil, drained), 1.75 ounces	250
Milk, nonfat, reduced fat, and whole, vitamin D-fortified, 1 cup	98
Margarine, fortified, 1 tablespoon	60
Ready-to-eat cereal, fortified with 10% of the daily value for vitamin D, 0.75–1 cup (more heavily fortified cereals may provide larger quantities)	40
Egg, 1 whole (vitamin D is found in yolk)	20
Liver, beef (cooked), 3.5 ounces	15
Cheese, Swiss, 1 ounce	12

IU, International units.

sites occupied under normal conditions.[13] In addition to transport of vitamin D metabolites, DBP contributes to actin scavenging, fatty acid transport, and chemotaxis.[14-17] Vitamin D absorbed through the gut is also transported on chylomicrons. Storage of vitamin D and its metabolites in adipose tissue is important in intoxication and perhaps in moderation of seasonal fluctuations in cutaneous synthesis. However, the extent, location, and form of vitamin D storage in normal human physiology are not fully understood.

Preclinical studies have established a role for DBP in regulating the availability of 25OHD and 1,25$(OH)_2D_3$ to certain target tissues,[18,19] leading to the hypothesis that free and bioavailable 25OHD concentrations provide superior indices of vitamin D status, compared with the total circulating 25OHD concentration. Assays to measure free and bioavailable vitamin D are not widely available; the concentrations can be estimated using equations that incorporate the 25OHD, DBP, and albumin concentrations and the corresponding binding affinity coefficients. Clinical studies using DBP to estimate concentrations of free/bioavailable 25(OH)D in relation to bone and mineral metabolism in healthy individuals and in children and adults with CKD have yielded conflicting results, with some studies showing bioavailable 25(OH)D to be more tightly correlated with measures of mineral metabolism and bone mineral density[7,20,21] and others not.[22-24] In both healthy and CKD cohorts, prior studies using the monoclonal ELISA to measure DBP have yielded conflicting results regarding whether free and bioavailable 25OHD provide better indices of vitamin D–related bone health as assessed by parathyroid hormone (PTH) concentrations and bone mineral density.

Further complicating the issue of vitamin D binding and bioavailability is that DBP is highly polymorphic. Combinations of two single-nucleotide polymorphisms (SNPs), rs4588 and rs7041, produce three major polymorphic forms (Gc1f, Gc1s, and Gc2) with six resultant allelic combinations that differ in their affinities for vitamin D metabolites, circulating concentrations, and geographical and racial distribution.[25-29] The genetic variation of DBP presents challenges to its accurate measurement, and several recent studies have demonstrated differential performance of the widely used monoclonal DBP ELISA according to genotype and therefore race.[30-33]

Calcitriol

Cholecalciferol and ergocalciferol have little inherent biological activity and require two hydroxylation steps for full hormonal potency. In the liver, cholecalciferol and ergocalciferol are converted to 25-hydroxyvitamin D_3 and 25-hydroxyvitamin D_2, respectively. Together, these are referred to as 25-hydroxyvitamin D, or 25(OH)D (see Fig. 11.1). With normal levels of vitamin D intake, 25(OH)D production by the hepatic cytochrome P450 system is proportional to substrate availability and not rate-limiting. 25(OH)D is the major circulating form of vitamin D.

25-hydroxyvitamin D_3 must be converted to calcitriol (1,25-dihydroxyvitamin D_3) for maximal hormonal function. This is performed by the cytochrome P450 enzyme CYP27B1, or 1-α hydroxylase. The major site of 1-α hydroxylase activity is the proximal tubule of the kidney. 25-hydroxyvitamin D_3 bound to DBP is filtered at the glomerulus, reabsorbed in the proximal tubule in a process facilitated by the luminal receptors megalin and cubilin, freed from DBP within lysosomes, and shuttled across the cytoplasm to mitochondria.[34] Here, conversion of 25-hydroxyvitamin D_3 to calcitriol is tightly regulated by factors including serum phosphorous, PTH, and fibroblast growth factor 23 (FGF-23).[35-37] 25-hydroxyvitamin D_2 is converted to 1,25-dihydroxyvitamin D_2 through parallel steps.

Most known actions of calcitriol require binding to the cytosolic vitamin D receptor. This receptor is similar in many ways to other nuclear receptors for steroid hormones.[38] Once ligand binding occurs in the cytoplasm, the calcitriol-vitamin D receptor complex must translocate to the nucleus, heterodimerize with the retinoid X receptor, bind to vitamin D response elements in the promoter regions of susceptible genes, and recruit coregulatory proteins to the site of binding. The result is upregulation or downregulation of the transcription of specific genes.

Vitamin D Clearance

The main pathway for calcitriol inactivation involves additional hydroxylation at carbon 23 or 24. These hydroxylation steps are catalyzed by specific enzymes that are present in virtually all target cells. CYP24A1 is the key enzyme involved in the catabolism of 25(OH)D and 1,25$(OH)_2D$. Like CYP27B1, CYP24A1 is expressed in most tissues and regulated by 1,25$(OH)_2D$.[39-41] In the kidney, 24-hydroxylase is regulated in a reciprocal manner to 1-α hydroxylase. In vitro and animal studies have shown that renal CYP24A1 is suppressed by PTH[42-44] and induced by FGF-23.[45-47] Once hydroxylation occurs at carbon 23 or 24, further side-chain cleavage leads to inactivation. Additional fates of calcitriol include hydroxylation at carbon 4, formation of lactones, epimerization at the 3-α position, and hepatic conjugation.[38,48-52] 25(OH)D may be inactivated through the same pathways without conversion to calcitriol.

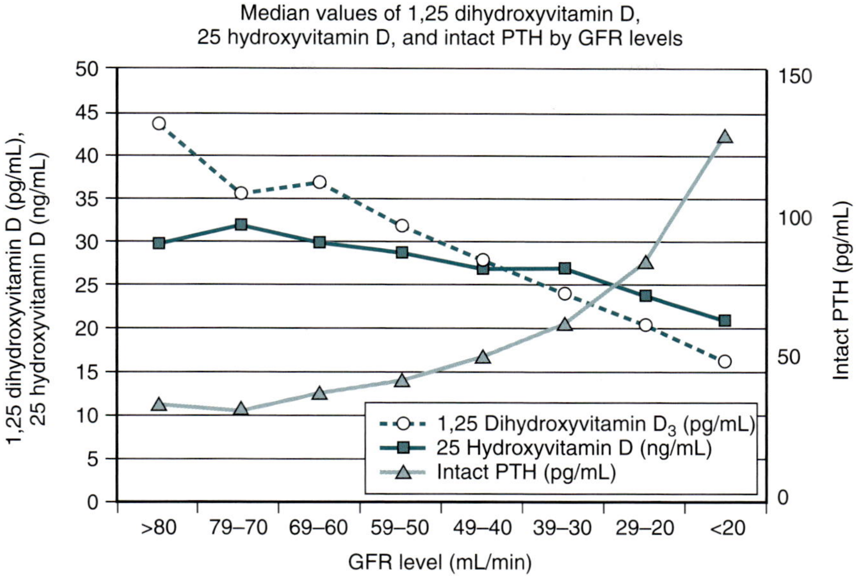

FIG. 11.4 Median concentrations of serum 25-hydroxyvitamin D, calcitriol, and intact parathyroid hormone by estimated GFR. (Reproduced with permission Levin A, Bakris GL, Molitch M, et al. Prevalence of abnormal serum vitamin D, PTH, calcium, and phosphorus in patients with chronic kidney disease: results of the study to evaluate early kidney disease. *Kidney Int.* 2007;71:31-38.)

In adults with CKD, lower glomerular filtration rate (GFR) is strongly associated with lower serum $24,25(OH)_2D$ concentrations, and $24,25(OH)_2D$ is more strongly associated with PTH than 25(OH)D or $1,25(OH)_2D$.[53,54] A pediatric study similarly demonstrated that greater CKD severity is associated with lower $24,25(OH)_2D$ concentrations. Downregulation of CYP24A1 may represent an appropriate response to tissue-concentration deficiency of $1,25(OH)_2D$ [39] in CKD, and it has been suggested that higher $24,25(OH)_2D$ concentrations may provide a more accurate measure of functional vitamin D status.[55]

Disturbances in Chronic Kidney Disease

Vitamin D metabolism is profoundly disordered in CKD. Abnormalities begin during early CKD stages (i.e., before stage 3) and progress as renal function declines.[55,56] The central feature of this process is a decline in circulating calcitriol, which occurs early and is due to diminished 1-α hydroxylase substrate, mass, and activity (Fig. 11.4, Box 11.1).[56-58] 25(OH) D and calcitriol concentrations are directly correlated in CKD, in contrast to persons with normal kidney function, suggesting that calcitriol synthesis may be more substrate-dependent in the setting of CKD.[59-62] Still, diminished 1-α hydroxylase activity is probably the most important cause of declining calcitriol levels in CKD. Hyperphosphatemia, hyperuricemia, metabolic acidosis, and diabetes are associated with decreased 1-α hydroxylase activity.[35,56,58,63,64] Elevated levels of FGF-23, which act to maintain serum phosphorous concentration as GFR falls, potently suppress 1-α hydroxylase activity.[36,37] This is part of a negative feedback loop, whereby calcitriol stimulates FGF-23 release from osteocytes and osteoblasts, and FGF-23 downregulates further calcitriol production. Hyperparathyroidism secondary to calcitriol deficiency is a common complication of CKD (see Fig. 11.4, see Chapter 8).[65]

BOX 11.1 Causes of Calcitriol Deficiency in Chronic Kidney Disease

Reduced vitamin D substrate
Decreased cutaneous synthesis
Older age
Non-Caucasian race/ethnicity
Decreased sun exposure
Inefficient synthesis (uremia)
Decreased dietary consumption
Decreased intake of fatty fish
Decreased intake of fortified dairy products
Obesity
Urinary losses (proteinuria)

Reduced 1-α hydroxylase mass
Loss of nephrons

Reduced 1-α hydroxylase activity
High FGF-23
Hyperphosphatemia
Diabetes
Metabolic acidosis
Elevated uric acid

EPIDEMIOLOGY

Assessment of Vitamin D Deficiency

Measurement of serum 25(OH)D is the cornerstone of evaluation for vitamin D deficiency. Serum 25(OH)D concentration is widely believed to be a valid gauge of vitamin D status because its concentration reliably increases in a dose-dependent fashion with either cutaneous or oral vitamin D intake (Fig. 11.5).[1-3,66-70] Also, the half-life of circulating 25(OH)D is

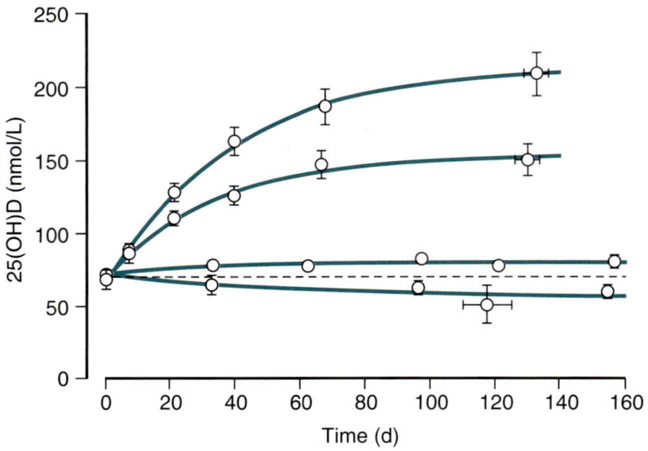

FIG. 11.5 Changes in serum 25-hydroxyvitamin D concentration in response to graded oral dosing of cholecalciferol during winter months among 67 men living in Omaha, Nebraska. The curves, from the lowest upward, are for 0, 25, 125, and 250 µg cholecalciferol per day. (To convert nmol/L to ng/mL, divide by 2.496; to convert µg to IU, multiply by 40.) Points are mean values, and error bars represent 1 SEM. (Reproduced with permission Heaney RP, Davies KM, Chen TC, et al. Human serum 25-hydroxycholecalciferol response to extended oral dosing with cholecalciferol. *Am J Clin Nutr.* 2003;77:204-210.)

10 to 21 days, so that a single measurement plausibly reflects intake over the last 2 to 3 months.

25(OH)D circulates at a reasonably high concentration (ng/mL), and a number of assays are available to accurately measure its concentration in serum.[71] Common methodologies include radioimmunoassay and mass spectrometry. Most assays in wide use today detect both 25-hydroxyvitamin D_3 and 25-hydroxyvitamin D_2. 25-hydroxyvitamin D_3 constitutes most or all of the measureable circulating 25(OH)D in the majority of people. Nonetheless, measurement of both forms (total 25[OH]D) is important, particularly in the setting of ergocalciferol supplementation. When laboratories report 25-hydroxyvitamin D_3 and 25-hydroxyvitamin D_2 concentrations separately, the total 25(OH)D concentration, not its individual components, is most clinically relevant.

Although serum 25(OH)D concentration is a common and useful laboratory assay, two caveats deserve mention. First, there are now two vitamin D quality assurance programs in place, the National Institute of Standards and Technology (NIST) and the international Vitamin D External Quality Assessment Scheme (DEQAS). It is best to use a performance laboratory that utilizes the NIST standard for comparison and has a certificate of proficiency from DEQAS.

Second, although 25(OH)D concentration reliably rises within individuals with vitamin D intake, there are other factors that influence variation in 25(OH)D concentration between individuals (which may include genetic polymorphism in enzymes involved in vitamin D metabolism and DBP, liver disease, nephrotic-range proteinuria, or other host factors).

Definition of Vitamin D Deficiency

Low 25(OH)D concentrations are commonly used to evaluate vitamin D status, but thresholds defining vitamin D deficiency are controversial and have changed over time.[72] Older thresholds (<10 ng/mL, <12 ng/mL) were based on the statistical distribution of 25(OH)D concentration in the general population. However, defining deficiency by a 2.5th or 5th percentile is arbitrary, and it is now realized that many more people may have inadequate vitamin D. Thus newer thresholds based on biological response have been sought.

Several studies have assessed cross-sectional correlations of 25(OH)D concentration with surrogate outcomes thought to respond directly to vitamin D. These outcomes consist of circulating PTH concentration, bone mineral density, and intestinal calcium absorption. In Caucasian populations, serum 25(OH)D and PTH concentrations are inversely correlated below a of 25(OH)D threshold of approximately 30 ng/mL (Fig. 11.6).[73-75] A similar relationship is seen correlating 25(OH)D concentration with bone mineral density.[76,77] Similarly, intestinal calcium absorption was more efficient among participants with a mean 25(OHD) of 35 ng/mL, compared with 20 ng/mL.[78] These relationships have been used to define vitamin D insufficiency as a 25(OHD) concentration less than 30 ng/mL and to advocate for interventions maintaining 25(OHD) concentrations above this threshold.[2,72]

One intervention study assessed the question of 25(OH)D threshold.[79] Change in PTH concentration was examined in response to ergocalciferol supplementation, stratified by baseline 25(OH)D concentration. PTH concentration decreased with therapy when baseline 25(OH)D was <20 ng/mL, but not when baseline 25(OH)D was >20 ng/mL, suggesting that 20 ng/mL was a threshold concentration needed to maximize this outcome.

The 2011 Institute of Medicine Report concluded that a 25(OH)D level of 20 ng/mL meets the requirements of ≥97.5% of the population.[80,81] However, the report explicitly stated that this definition is based solely on the classical skeletal actions of vitamin D and stressed that further research is needed to define the requirements for other facets of health.

Circulating 25(OH)D concentrations vary substantially by race/ethnicity, due to differences in cutaneous synthesis attributable to skin pigmentation, and by season, due to sunlight exposure (see Fig. 11.3). Unfortunately, adequate data have not currently been published to determine whether separate thresholds of 25(OH)D should be used to define vitamin D deficiency by race/ethnicity or season.

Prevalence of Vitamin D Deficiency

Vitamin D deficiency is highly prevalent in the general population when it is defined using any common 25(OH)D threshold (Fig. 11.7). United States prevalence estimates were generated from data collected as part of the National Health and Nutrition Examination Survey.[82] These estimates vary by age, gender, and race/ethnicity.

Race/ethnicity strongly affects vitamin D metabolism. 25-hydroxyvitamin D concentration varies strongly by race/ethnicity due to differences in skin pigmentation and cutaneous

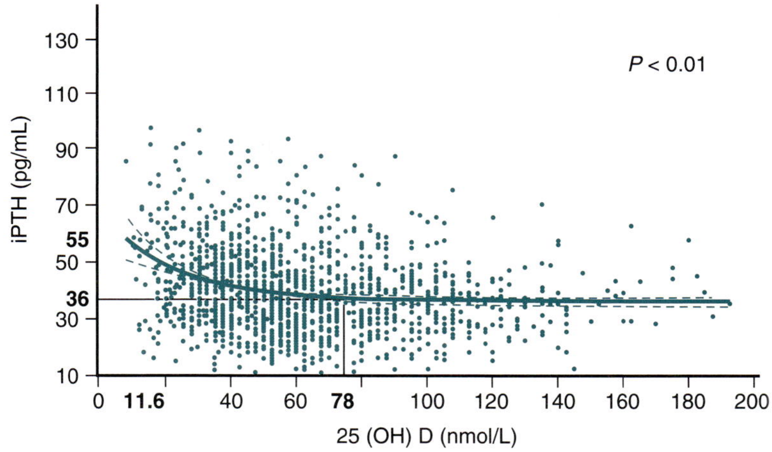

FIG. 11.6 Cross-sectional association of 25-hydroxyvitamin D and intact parathyroid hormone concentrations among French men and women. The curved dark line represents a smoothed mean parathyroid hormone concentration, which begins to rise with a 25-hydroxyvitamin D concentration approximately less than 78 nmol/L. To convert nmol/L to ng/mL, divide by 2.496. (Reproduced with permission Chapuy MC, Preziosi P, Maamer M, et al. Prevalence of vitamin D insufficiency in an adult normal population. *Osteoporos Int.* 1997;7:439-443.)

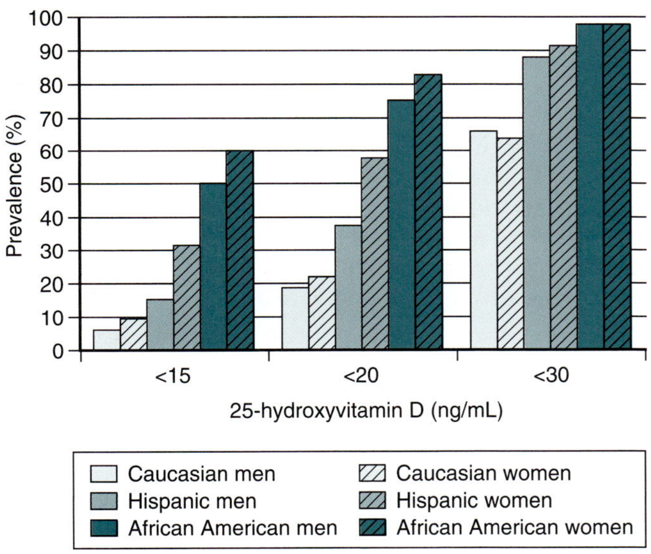

FIG. 11.7 Prevalence of vitamin D deficiency in the US population, ages 20 to 49 years, by threshold 25-hydroxyvitamin concentration, gender, and race/ethnicity. (Data from the National Health and Nutrition Examination Survey (2000 to 2004) are adapted with permission from Looker AC, Pfeiffer CM, Lacher DA, et al. Serum 25-hydroxyvitamin D status of the US population: 1988-1994 compared with 2000-2004. *Am J Clin Nutr.* 2008;88:1519-1527.)

cholecalciferol synthesis, being highest in Caucasian populations, intermediate in Hispanic populations, and lowest in African American populations.[82-84] As would be expected given differences in 25-hydroxyvitamin D, PTH concentrations are highest among African Americans.[85] However, 1,25-dihydroxyvitamin D concentrations are not lower when comparing groups of African American versus Caucasian race, suggesting that racial/ethnic differences in vitamin D metabolism are complex and involve differential regulation of key vitamin D–processing enzymes.[86]

In addition, disease-based and lifestyle risk factors for 25(OH)D deficiency are well described (Box 11.2). The prevalence of 25(OH)D deficiency in the general population appears to be increasing over time, attributable largely to increasing obesity and sunscreen use and decreased intake of fortified dairy products.[82]

The prevalence of 25(OH)D deficiency in persons with CKD has not been studied using rigorous population-based sampling methods. Nonetheless, most studies suggest that the prevalence of 25(OH)D deficiency/insufficiency is quite high in adults[56,61,87-95] and children[62,96-101] with CKD, with the majority (60% to 90%) having 25(OH)D levels <30 ng/mL. Contributing factors may include decreased cutaneous synthesis (due to older age, race/ethnicity, comorbidities, and decreased physical activity); decreased dietary intake of fortified dairy products; obesity; and renal 25(OH)D losses, which are most severe with heavy proteinuria. Many of these risk factors (e.g., age, non-Caucasian race/ethnicity, see Box 11.2) are not unique to CKD but are more prevalent in this population, whereas other risk factors (e.g., proteinuria) are specific to patients with CKD.

Many small studies have documented very low total 25(OH)D levels in nephrotic syndrome (NS),[102-114] attributed to the urinary loss of its DBP and albumin. In a 2015 multicenter study of 61 children with incident idiopathic NS, the prevalence of vitamin D deficiency, defined as a 25(OH)D concentration <20 ng/mL, was 100% at diagnosis and 53% at 2 to 4 months of follow-up.[115] Even in remission, children with steroid-sensitive NS were shown to have lower 25(OH) D concentrations than healthy controls.[116,117] Furthermore, among 182 children and adolescents with CKD and end-stage kidney disease (ESKD), glomerular disease, particularly focal segmental glomerulosclerosis (FSGS), was an independent risk factor for lower 25(OH)D concentrations, adjusted for age, race, season, CKD severity, and hypoalbuminemia.[118] This finding was subsequently corroborated by an analysis in

BOX 11.2 Risk Factors for 25-Hydroxyvitamin D Deficiency

Reduced sun exposure
Residence in northern latitudes
Indoor occupation
Little outdoor leisure-time physical activity

Reduced rate of cutaneous synthesis
Older age
Non-Caucasian race
Use of sun protective clothing
Use of sunscreen

Reduced dietary intake
Low intake of fatty fish
Low intake of fortified dairy products
Inflammatory bowel disease
Gastric/enteric surgery
Other causes of malabsorption

Increased volume of distribution
Obesity

Renal losses
Nephrotic syndrome

the CKiD cohort demonstrating nephrotic-range proteinuria to be a significant risk factor for vitamin D deficiency with an odds ratio (OR) of 8.09, adjusted for age, sex, race, season, body mass index (BMI), milk intake, vitamin D supplementation, and GFR.[119]

Calcitriol Deficiency

As the most potent metabolite of vitamin D, calcitriol is a central molecule in mineral metabolism pathophysiology. Nevertheless, measurement of serum calcitriol has limited application in the clinical evaluation of vitamin D deficiency. This is largely because calcitriol has two unfavorable characteristics as a laboratory assay. First, it is present in blood at very low concentrations (pg/mL), and due to difficult isolation and purification, existing assays may also detect other vitamin D metabolites.[120] Second, the half-life of circulating calcitriol is short (approximately 6 hours), so that single measurements may poorly reflect long-term concentrations. Thus the main clinical use of the serum calcitriol assay is to diagnose cases of hypercalcemia caused by excessive nonrenal calcitriol production (e.g., granulomatous diseases).

Because direct measurement of calcitriol deficiency is difficult, clinical care frequently relies on markers of downstream biological response indicating functional insufficiency of calcitriol. Elevated circulating PTH concentration is the main such marker. Calcitriol and its precursors downregulate PTH by preventing parathyroid hyperplasia and by reducing PTH production and secretion (see Chapter 8).[2,38,121,122] Thus, although elevated serum PTH concentration has a number of implications and consequences, it may in part reflect functional deficiency of vitamin D, and vitamin D therapy is often prescribed in this setting (see Therapy section; see Chapter 8).

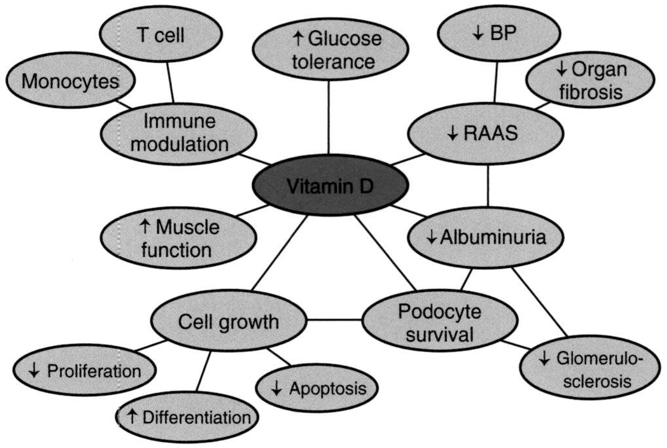

FIG. 11.8 Potential pleiotropic actions of vitamin D. *BP*, Blood pressure; *RAAS*, renin-angiotensin-aldosterone system.

CONSEQUENCES

Pleiotropy

Vitamin D is long recognized as a key factor maintaining calcium, phosphorous, and bone homeostasis (see Chapter 8).[2,121-123] However, vitamin D receptors are present throughout the body in nearly all tissues, and hundreds of human genes contain vitamin D response elements.[38,124] Thus pleiotropic actions have been postulated for vitamin D, beyond those traditionally described for maintenance of calcium homeostasis and bone health (Fig. 11.8). These are described in detail in the following sections.

Autocrine and Paracrine Effects

The enzyme 1-α hydroxylase is also expressed outside of the kidney and nearly ubiquitous, like the vitamin D receptor.[38,124] This observation has led to the suggestion that tissue-specific production of calcitriol may have important autocrine and/or paracrine effects. For example, calcitriol production was demonstrated to be a key autocrine mechanism through which tissue macrophages combat tuberculosis.[125] Binding of tuberculosis antigen to the macrophage cell-surface toll-like receptor leads to upregulated expression of the 1-α hydroxylase and vitamin D receptor genes. Calcitriol then induces a cascade of intracellular signaling pathways that culminate in macrophage synthesis of the antimicrobial peptide cathelicidin and killing of intracellular mycobacteria. Sera from African American individuals with low circulating 25-hydroxyvitamin D concentrations were inefficient in supporting cathelicidin messenger RNA induction, offering a potential explanation for the increased susceptibility to tuberculosis observed in African Americans. Intriguingly, the dependence of macrophage activity on 25(OH)D may have led to improved tuberculosis outcomes when patients were historically moved to tuberculosis sanitaria in sunny locations.

It is important to note that nonrenal 1-α hydroxylase activity is likely to be regulated differently than renal 1-α hydroxylase activity. In addition, the relative contribution of calcitriol produced at the systemic level (kidney) versus tissue level (local) remains to be determined for most potential pleiotropic effects of vitamin D.

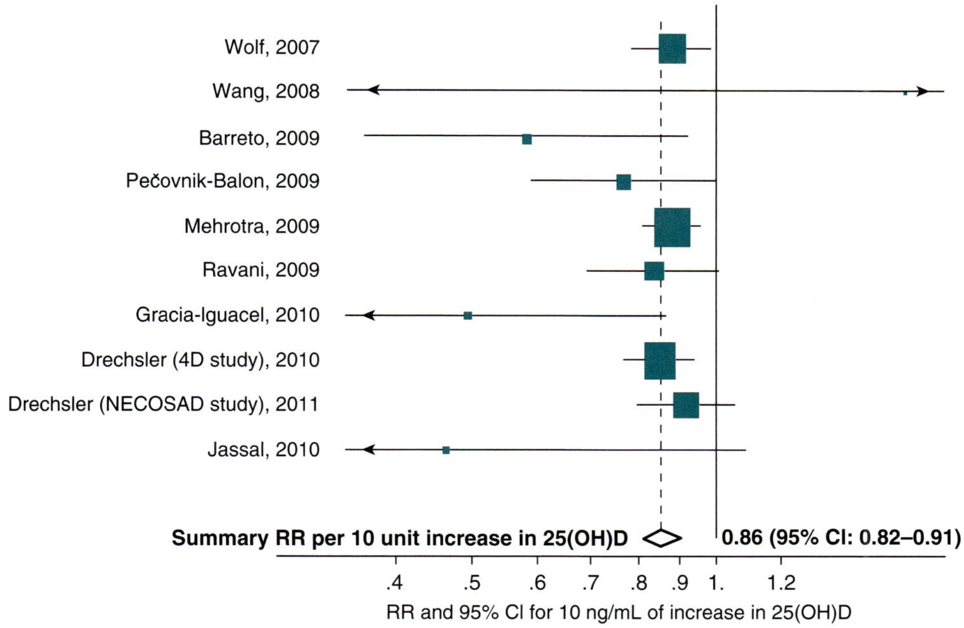

FIG. 11.9 Forest plot and summary relative risk (*RR*) for the association of 25(OH)D level and mortality in patients with CKD. The size of the box is proportional to the weight of the study (1/variance of the estimate). *4D*, Die Deutsche Diabetes Dialyse Studie; *NECOSAD*, Netherlands Cooperative Study on the Adequacy of Dialysis. (Reproduced with permission from Pilz S, Iodice S, Zittermann A, et al. Vitamin D status and mortality risk in CKD: a meta-analysis of prospective studies. *Am J Kidney Dis.* 2011;58:374-382.)

Mortality

Patients with CKD have a markedly increased mortality rate, due in large part to increased risk for CVD.[126,127] Vitamin D deficiency may contribute to poor clinical outcomes. Many observational studies and randomized controlled trials have studied associations between circulating 25(OH)D concentration and a variety of health outcomes. A 2014 umbrella review evaluated the evidence from 107 systematic literature reviews and 74 metaanalyses of observational studies of vitamin D concentrations and 87 metaanalyses of randomized controlled trials of vitamin D supplementation with respect to 137 different clinical outcomes in the general population as well as CKD.[128] Ten of these 137 clinical outcomes, including mortality in patients with CKD and all-cause mortality, were evaluated by both metaanalyses of observational studies and randomized controlled trials. The results of this analysis underscored the discordance between observational studies and randomized controlled trials of vitamin D supplementation. In observational studies, low circulating 25(OH)D and calcitriol concentrations have been associated with increased risks of mortality among incident hemodialysis patients and patients with stages 2 to 5 CKD.[61,88,129] Indeed, a systematic review and metaanalysis of 10 prospective observational studies including a total of 6853 patients with CKD found the relative risk of mortality per 10 ng/mL higher in 25(OH)D concentration to be 0.86 (95% confidence interval [CI], 0.82 to 0.91), with no indication of publication bias or significant heterogeneity (Fig. 11.9).[130]

A number of observational cohort studies have reported that treatment with calcitriol or an activated vitamin D analog is associated with decreased risk for mortality and/or CVD events in CKD.[131-137] A metaanalysis of 14 observational studies (total of 194,932 patients) of calcitriol or synthetic analogs in predominantly hemodialysis cohorts found the relative risk of all-cause mortality to be 0.73 (95% CI, 0.65 to 0.82) and 0.63 (95% CI, 0.44 to 0.92) for cardiovascular mortality (Fig. 11.10).[138] However, observational studies of medications have an important limitation: the potential for confounding by indication.[139] Metaanalyses of randomized clinical trials of vitamin D compounds in patients with CKD and ESKD have failed to confirm a beneficial effect on survival in CKD,[140,141] although the individual trials were inadequately powered to detect an effect on this outcome.

Cell Growth and Differentiation

Vitamin D is known to affect cell proliferation, differentiation, and survival. In general, vitamin D promotes cell differentiation, reduces cell proliferation, and has complex actions to modulate apoptosis.[142-146] These actions are mediated in part through regulation of cell-cycle progression, with effects on the cyclins, cyclin-dependent kinases, and cyclin kinase inhibitors that govern cell-cycle transitions. Due to these and other observations, it has been hypothesized that vitamin D helps prevent a number of cancers, particularly prostate, breast, and colon.[147-150] Data regarding the anticancer effects of vitamin D are not conclusive at this time. Vitamin D may also have important effects on the growth and differentiation of nonmalignant cells (see the following sections: Immune Cell Function; Glucose Metabolism; Cardiovascular Disease; and Chronic Kidney Disease).

CKD stage	Study	Risk ratio	Lower limit	Upper limit	*P* value	Adjusted risk ratio	Relative weight, %
HD	Taniguchi, 2010 [36]	0.54	0.51	0.57	<0.001	Yes	11.8
HD	Naves-Diaz, 2008 [32]	0.55	0.49	0.62	<0.001	Yes	11.0
HD	Wolf, 2008 [40]	0.66	0.50	0.86	0.002	Yes	8.0
HD	Shoji, 2004 [34]	0.70	0.44	1.14	0.15	No	4.7
HD	Melamed, 2006 [31]	0.74	0.56	0.98	0.03	Yes	7.9
HD	Kalantar-Zadeh, 2006 [27, 28]	0.75	0.71	0.79	<0.001	Yes	11.8
HD	Teng, 2005 [37]	0.80	0.76	0.84	<0.001	Yes	11.8
HD	Tentori, 2006 [38]	0.83	0.76	0.91	<0.001	Yes	11.4
HD	Jean, 2011 [26]	0.89	0.74	1.07	0.22	Yes	9.8
HD	Tentori, 2009 [39]	0.89	0.84	0.94	<0.001	Yes	11.8
HD	**Overall** (I^2 = 94%)	**0.73**	**0.64**	**0.83**	**<0.001**		
preHD	Kovesdy, 2008 [29]	0.69	0.55	0.86	0.001	No	43.8
preHD	Shoben, 2008 [33]	0.76	0.58	1.00	0.05	Yes	39.4
preHD	Sugiura, 2010 [35]	0.80	0.44	1.46	0.46	Yes	16.8
preHD	**Overall** (I^2 = 0%)	**0.73**	**0.55**	**0.98**	**0.04**		
Overall (I^2 = 97%)		**0.73**	**0.65**	**0.82**	**<0.001**		

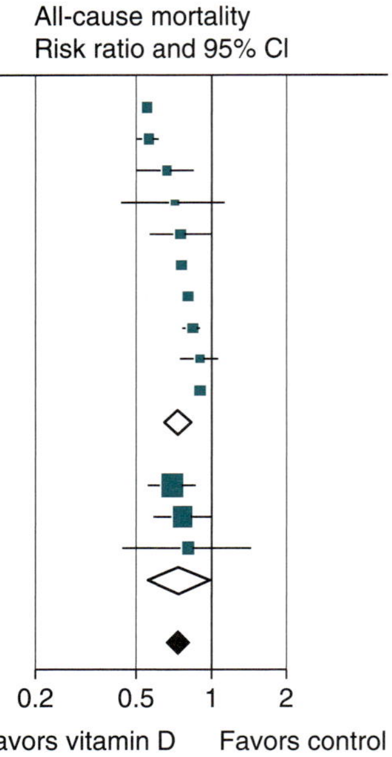

FIG. 11.10 Forest plots and summary estimates of all-cause mortality RRs depending on vitamin D treatment in hemodialysis patients (*HD*) or patients with CKD not requiring dialysis (*preHD*). (Reproduced with permission from Duranton F, Rodriguez-Crtiz ME, Duny Y, et al. Vitamin D treatment and mortality in chronic kidney disease: a systematic review and meta-analysis. *Am J Nephrol.* 2013;37:239-248.)

Immune Cell Function

In vitro cell culture studies and in vivo animal-experimental models demonstrate potent immunomodulatory functions of vitamin D metabolites.[151] In general, vitamin D tends to enhance innate immunity and suppress cellular immunity. Effects on innate immunity include enhanced activity of tissue macrophages, as previously described for tuberculosis (see Autocrine and Paracrine Effects). Regarding cellular immunity, both antigen-presenting cells and T cells are affected. In antigen-presenting cells, including monocytes, calcitriol alters cytokine expression (decreased interleukin (IL)-1, IL-6, IL-8, IL-12, and tumor necrosis factor-α; increased IL-10) and regulates cell growth and cell–cell interaction. These effects decrease cell differentiation, maturation, major histocompatibility complex-II expression, costimulatory molecule expression, and interferon-γ expression, and increase apoptosis.[152-155] Downstream development and activation of T cells is suppressed. Vitamin D also has direct effects on T cells, including inhibition of autocrine IL-2 production. Thus the net result of vitamin D on cellular immunity includes inhibition of antigen presentation, decreased T-cell proliferation, and a shift in the composition of T-cell subpopulations.

Given these effects of vitamin D on immune cell function, vitamin D deficiency has been hypothesized to contribute to a number of autoimmune diseases. Specifically, existing evidence suggests that vitamin D insufficiency may contribute to the pathogenesis of multiple sclerosis, type 1 diabetes, and Crohn disease.[156-158] Vitamin D deficiency may play a role in the systemic inflammation observed in CKD, and vitamin D may have relevant effects on immune tolerance and rejection after kidney transplantation.

Renin-Angiotensin-Aldosterone System

Li et al. demonstrated that calcitriol is a potent suppressor of renin production in the mouse kidney.[159] Renin messenger RNA and protein levels were markedly elevated in vitamin D receptor null mice, which as a result had elevated levels of circulating angiotensin II and blood pressure. Results were confirmed using wild-type mice induced to dietary vitamin D deficiency, whose elevated renin levels were rescued by calcitriol therapy. Cell culture models showed that that calcitriol reduced renin transcription via promoter downregulation. Subsequently, renal production of renin, as well as other components of the renin-angiotensin-aldosterone system (RAAS), was observed to be reduced in a variety of animal models. In humans, circulating calcitriol concentrations are inversely correlated with blood pressure, and lower 25(OH)D concentrations are associated with increased risk of developing hypertension.[160-163]

Glucose Metabolism

Glucose metabolism is frequently impaired in CKD.[164,165] In end-stage renal disease (ESRD), the most profound disturbance is insulin resistance due to a postreceptor defect in skeletal muscle.[166,167] Insulin resistance appears to be common in earlier stages of CKD, as well.[87,168,169] Vitamin D may improve glucose metabolism by stimulating insulin secretion from pancreatic beta cells and by improving peripheral insulin sensitivity.[170-174]

Intervention studies showed benefits of calcitriol therapy on glucose metabolism in the setting of maintenance hemodialysis.[175-183] However, these studies were small and often of suboptimal design, and paricalcitol did not improve glucose metabolism in a randomized trial of people with predialysis

CKD.[184] Studies assessing the effects of vitamin D supplements on glucose metabolism in people without CKD have also been null, although the largest such study is still under way (www.d2dstudy.org).

Cardiovascular Disease

CVD is the most common cause of death among people with CKD.[185] Thus, if vitamin D therapy improves survival in CKD (see Mortality section), it is likely to have a beneficial effect on CVD. There are a number of mechanisms through which vitamin D may help prevent CVD. As one of its effects on immune cell function, vitamin D influences the development of T-cell subsets, promoting the generation of regulatory T-helper type 2 lymphocytes over proatherogenic T-helper type 1 lymphocytes.[186] Through these immunologic effects, as well as the effects on glucose metabolism and the RAAS system discussed previously, vitamin D may help prevent the development of atherosclerosis.

Vitamin D may also have direct effects on vascular smooth muscle cells. Specifically, calcitriol may modulate expression of genes that regulate transformation of vascular smooth muscle cells to an osteoblast-type phenotype.[58,186] In animal models, doses of calcitriol sufficient to suppress PTH reduce vascular calcification, whereas higher doses stimulate vascular calcification, possibly due in part to resultant hyperphosphatemia and hypercalcemia.[187] In humans, low 25(OH)D concentrations have been associated with vascular calcification in cross-sectional analysis and with increased risks of developing coronary artery calcification, and circulating calcitriol concentrations have been reported to correlate inversely with coronary artery calcification.[188-190] The PENNY (Paricalcitol and ENdothelial fuNction in chronic kidneY disease) randomized controlled trial showed that 12 weeks of paricalcitol improved endothelium-dependent vasodilatation in patients with stages 3 to 4 CKD.[191]

In addition, vitamin D may help prevent left ventricular hypertrophy (LVH). Animal models demonstrate that vitamin D deficiency promotes LVH through direct and indirect effects on cardiomyocytes. Rodents with dietary vitamin D deficiency or targeted deletion of the vitamin D receptor or 1-α hydroxylase develop a phenotype of hypertension, cardiomyocyte hypertrophy, and left ventricular enlargement, whereas treatment with 1,25-dihydroxyvitamin D prevents this phenotype.[192-195] In these models, adverse effects of vitamin D deficiency are mediated by activation of the cardiac and systemic RAAS and by direct effects promoting cell growth.[193-196] In humans, LVH leads to coronary ischemia, congestive heart failure, cardiac arrhythmias, and death. In patients with ESRD, low 25(OH)D concentrations have been associated with vascular stiffness.[197] Thus LVH may represent a causal intermediary between vitamin D deficiency and cardiovascular mortality. However, the PRIMO (Paricalcitol Capsule Benefits in Renal Failure–Induced Cardiac Morbidity) randomized controlled trial showed that long-term (48-week) therapy with paricalcitol did not alter left ventricular mass index or improve measures of diastolic dysfunction in patients with CKD, though a post hoc analysis showed reduction in left atrial volume index and attenuation in the rise of brain natriuretic peptide.[198,199] The OPERA randomized controlled trial demonstrated that 52 weeks of treatment with oral paricalcitol significantly improved secondary hyperparathyroidism but did not alter measures of left ventricular structure or function in patients with advanced CKD.[200]

Interestingly, the association of 25(OH)D with cardiovascular outcomes in hemodialysis patients and patients with CKD was found to be more pronounced in the setting of higher FGF-23 concentrations, suggesting that a combination of substrate deficiency and downregulation of CYP27B1 leading to decreased $1,25(OH)_2D$ production may be most detrimental.[201,202]

Chronic Kidney Disease

Vitamin D may help prevent kidney disease through a number of mechanisms. First, suppression of the RAAS may prevent kidney damage by reducing both blood pressure (systemic effect) and transforming growth factor β-mediated fibrosis (local effect).[203] Second, vitamin D has direct effects on podocyte proliferation and differentiation, which appear to prevent apoptosis and cell death. Third, salutary effects on inflammation and metabolism may improve the metabolic milieu of the kidney.

Potent beneficial effects of calcitriol have been observed in animal models of CKD. In five-sixth nephrectomy and streptozotocin models, calcitriol or its analogs reduce local levels of RAAS components, albuminuria, and glomerulosclerosis.[204] These salutary effects appear to be more pronounced with concurrent RAAS inhibitor therapy, which is known to otherwise cause a compensatory increase in renal renin production.[205]

In the US population, low 25(OH)D concentrations are associated with increased risk of albuminuria.[83] Two randomized clinical trials of paricalcitol in stages 3 to 4 CKD have evaluated change in albuminuria as a secondary outcome. Among 118 participants with dipstick albuminuria at baseline, albuminuria regressed in 29 of 57 participants assigned to active treatment for 24 weeks (51%), compared with 25% of participants assigned to placebo ($P = 0.004$).[206] In a 24-person, 1-month trial, albuminuria was reduced by almost 50% among participants assigned to active therapy, compared with an increase of more than 30% for participants assigned to placebo ($P = 0.0005$).[207] Subsequently, the VITAL randomized controlled trial showed that the addition of 2 μg/day of paricalcitol to RAAS inhibition safely reduced residual albuminuria in patients with diabetic kidney disease.[208] A metaanalysis of six trials of active vitamin D analogs (paricalcitol or calcitriol) comprising a total of 688 patients, most of whom were on angiotensin-converting enzyme inhibitor or angiotensin receptor blocker therapy, confirmed a significant reduction in proteinuria (Fig. 11.11).[209] Some observational studies suggest that calcitriol therapy may prevent progression of CKD, though this observation is not consistent.[131,135] No clinical trials of vitamin D, calcitriol, or its analogs have tested whether vitamin D improves long-term renal outcomes.

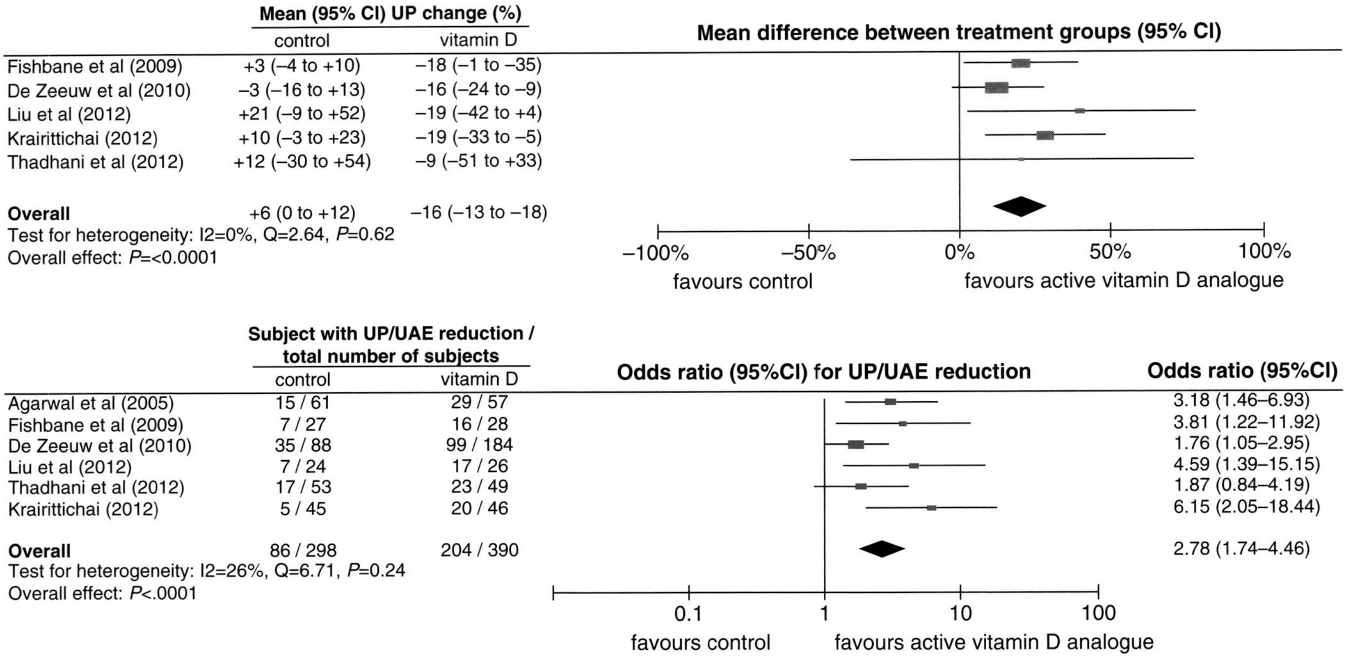

FIG. 11.11 Effect of active vitamin D or control treatment on proteinuria in metaanalysis. (Upper panel) Relative proteinuria change from baseline to last available measurement for all studies with available data. *P* value is for the comparison between the proteinuria change during active vitamin D treatment versus during control treatment. (Lower panel) Odds ratio of a relevant proteinuria reduction for active vitamin D analog versus control treatment. A relevant reduction of proteinuria was defined as a reduction of ≥15% in proteinuria or albuminuria in most studies. *UAE*, Urinary albumin excretion; *UP*, proteinuria. (Reproduced with permission from de Borst MH, Hajhosseiny R, Tamez H, et al. Active vitamin D treatment for reduction of residual proteinuria: a systematic review. *J Am Soc Nephrol.* 2013;24:1863-1871.)

THERAPY

Goals of Therapy

A fundamental challenge in the treatment of vitamin D deficiency is establishing appropriate goals of therapy. As discussed previously, there are many potential pleiotropic actions of vitamin D that may lead to improved patient outcomes. Unfortunately, there are currently no clinical assays available to directly gauge the effect of vitamin D on these pleiotropic pathways. Moreover, several studies suggest that salutary effects of calcitriol therapy do not depend on pretreatment levels of PTH, the traditional measurement used to titrate vitamin D interventions in the setting of CKD. As a result, some experts have suggested that all CKD patients receive vitamin D treatment, regardless of laboratory parameters. More commonly, however, clinicians target vitamin D therapy to one or two laboratory parameters: 25(OH)D and/or PTH. In theory, repletion of 25(OH)D is a relatively safe intervention that maximizes potential autocrine and/or paracrine effects of vitamin D, whereas titration to PTH maximizes bone health and offers a potential "readout" of vitamin D functional status.

Current Practice by Stage of Chronic Kidney Disease

Current approaches to vitamin D therapy vary by the presence and severity of kidney disease. In the general population, renal 1-α hydroxylase activity is generally preserved. "Vitamin D status" is ascertained by 25(OH)D concentration, and forms of vitamin D that require activation by 1-α hydroxylase (cholecalciferol or ergocalciferol) are administered orally. In dialysis patients, 1-α hydroxylase activity is markedly diminished. Vitamin D therapy is usually based on circulating PTH concentration, and therapy is administered as calcitriol or its analogs, often intravenously. In earlier stages of CKD, approaches to evaluation and treatment are heterogeneous. These involve titration to 25(OH)D and/or PTH and use of the full spectrum of vitamin D therapies. After kidney transplantation, bone loss is a major consideration, and calcitriol is commonly prescribed in combination with calcium salts.

Cholecalciferol

Cholecalciferol therapy offers numerous advantages for the treatment of vitamin D deficiency (Table 11.2). It is the best-studied form of vitamin D, and the only form that has been studied for long periods of follow-up in controlled settings. Doses up to 10,000 IU daily have been studied for up to 6 months duration, and doses up to 800 IU daily have been studied for many years duration. In clinical trials, increasing doses of cholecalciferol result in reliable dose-dependent increases in 25(OH)D concentrations (see Fig. 11.2).[70] On average, each 1000 IU/day raises 25(OH)D by 6 to 10 ng/mL (Fig. 11.12).[69,70] Repletion of 25(OH)D should facilitate any autocrine/paracrine actions of vitamin D. Moreover,

TABLE 11.2 Options for Vitamin D Therapy in Chronic Kidney Disease

Therapy	Advantages/Disadvantages
Cholecalciferol	Best-studied form of vitamin D Reliable dose response Proven to prevent fractures* May facilitate autocrine/paracrine effects of vitamin D Can be administered daily or weekly Inexpensive Safety: regulated conversion by 1-α hydroxylase Few short-term adverse effects Hypercalciuria and kidney stones May not adequately increase systemic calcitriol levels May not adequately suppress parathyroid hormone (PTH)
Ergocalciferol	Available in high-dose capsules Can be administered weekly or monthly May facilitate autocrine/paracrine effects of vitamin D Safety: regulated conversion by 1-α hydroxylase May not adequately increase systemic calcitriol levels May not adequately suppress PTH
Calcitriol	Does not require renal activation Known to effectively suppress PTH Associated with improved survival in observational studies Can be administered intravenously with hemodialysis Hypercalcemia and hyperphosphatemia Overtreatment can lead to adynamic bone disease
Other vitamin D receptor agonists	Do not require renal activation Known to effectively suppress PTH Associated with improved survival in observational studies Can be administered intravenously with hemodialysis Less hypercalcemia and hyperphosphatemia than calcitriol Overtreatment can lead to adynamic bone disease

*In the setting of osteoporosis or secondary prevention.

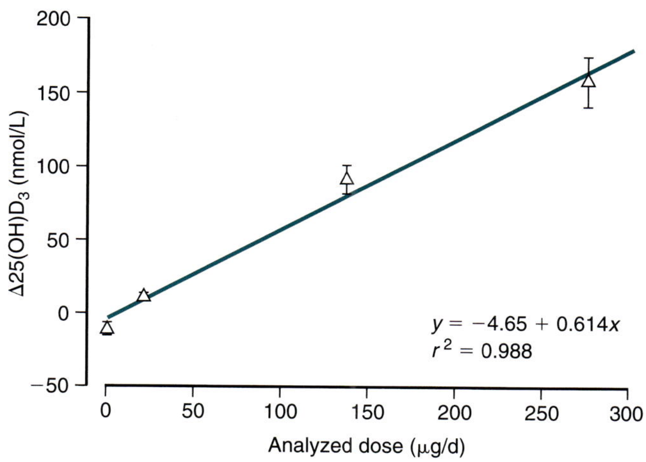

FIG. 11.12 Relationship between oral cholecalciferol dose (*x*-axis) and change in circulating 25-hydroxyvitamin D concentration (*y*-axis) after 5 months of treatment during winter months for 67 men living in Omaha, Nebraska. (To convert nmol/L to ng/mL, divide by 2.496; to convert μg to IU, multiply by 40.) (Reproduced with permission from Heaney RP, Davies KM, Chen TC, et al. Human serum 25-hydroxycholecalciferol response to extended oral dosing with cholecalciferol. *Am J Clin Nutr.* 2003;77:204-210.)

cholecalciferol has been proven in randomized trials to improve some clinical outcomes; when administered with calcium in the setting of osteoporosis, cholecalciferol prevents fractures.[210] Cholecalciferol is also inexpensive. Because of the long half-life of circulating 25(OH)D, cholecalciferol can be administered weekly, and has been evaluated in monthly dosing.

Fewer adverse effects are observed with cholecalciferol therapy, compared with calcitriol therapy, because regulation by 1-α hydroxylase helps prevent excess calcitriol production. Few short-term adverse effects have been reported with cholecalciferol, including administration at very high doses, but long-term therapy does increase the risk of kidney stones when administered with calcium. In the Women's Health Initiative Calcium-Vitamin D trial, administration of calcium plus cholecalciferol (1000 mg plus 400 IU daily, respectively) increased the 7-year cumulative incidence of kidney stones from 2.1% to 2.5% (P <0 .05). This is presumably due to modest chronic increases in dietary calcium absorption with resultant increased urinary calcium excretion.

Among persons with CKD, both before and after the initiation of dialysis, cholecalciferol supplementation has been evaluated in observational studies and clinical trials.[211-214] Over 1 month to 2 years follow-up, cholecalciferol was generally found to effectively raise 25(OH)D concentrations. In pre-ESRD CKD, cholecalciferol tended to reduce PTH concentration by approximately 10%. Few studies evaluated effects on urinary calcium and phosphorous excretion in pre-ESRD CKD, and whether these potentially harmful effects are present or severe is not well defined. The main disadvantage of cholecalciferol therapy in CKD is that it may not restore sufficient circulating calcitriol for important endocrine effects, due to impaired renal 1-α hydroxylase activity. In addition, cholecalciferol alone may not suppress PTH concentrations to recommended targets among persons with established parathyroid hyperplasia. Finally, it is possible that any form of vitamin D therapy may facilitate vascular calcification by increasing dietary calcium absorption. The clinical relevance of this potential adverse effect is not currently clear.

Ergocalciferol

Ergocalciferol therapy offers many of the same potential advantages as cholecalciferol, including facilitation of autocrine/paracrine effects and relative safety (see Table 11.2). Compared with cholecalciferol, ergocalciferol is formulated in capsules of larger dose (50,000 IU). This allows less-frequent administration, which may lower cost and improve patient adherence. However, many experts cite disadvantages of ergocalciferol. Compared with cholecalciferol, ergocalciferol is less effective at raising 25(OH)D concentrations (IU per IU), and its metabolites may be less potent. This may be due to a relatively greater rate of inactivation (including 24-hydroxylation), which is consistent with an observed shorter half-life for 25(OH)D2 compared with 25(OH)D3. In addition, ergocalciferol has not been shown to prevent fractures.

Published evaluation of ergocalciferol in CKD is similar to evaluation of cholecalciferol.[215-217] It does raise 25(OH)D concentration and tends to modestly suppress PTH. Other potential disadvantages, including hypercalciuria, stones, and ineffective conversion to calcitriol, are similar to cholecalciferol. A randomized controlled trial in children with CKD stages 2 to 4 showed that ergocalciferol delayed the onset of secondary hyperparathyroidism.[218] A recent randomized placebo-controlled trial showed that 6 months of supplementation with ergocalciferol raised serum 25(OH)D concentrations in patients on hemodialysis with vitamin D insufficiency or deficiency, but had no effect on epoetin utilization or secondary biochemical and clinical outcomes.

Recently a randomized trial of weekly cholecalciferol versus ergocalciferol for 12 weeks in nondialysis-dependent patients with CKD stages 3 to 5 demonstrated cholecalciferol to be more effective in raising serum 25(OH)D and found no difference in terms of changes in serum PTH or $1,25(OH)_2D$.[219]

Calcifediol

Calcifediol (25-hydroxyvitamin D_3) is another option for treating vitamin D deficiency and is better absorbed in the intestine than ergocalciferol or cholecalciferol. Two randomized, placebo-controlled trials of 429 patients with stages 3 or 4 CKD demonstrated that extended-release calcifediol is safe and effective in treating 25(OH)D insufficiency and secondary hyperparathyroidism in CKD,[220] although it is not clear that this approach offers any clinical benefit compared with more established and less expensive cholecalciferol or ergocalciferol supplementation.

Calcitriol

Calcitriol is commonly prescribed and relatively well studied in the setting of CKD. It does not require renal activation for potent binding to the vitamin D receptor. As a result, it is an established therapy for the treatment of secondary hyperparathyroidism in all stages of CKD and is known to effectively lower serum PTH concentration (see Chapter 8). In addition, calcitriol has been associated with improved survival in observational studies of CKD and ESRD (see the Consequences section). Calcitriol can be administered intravenously with hemodialysis or orally at any stage of CKD. Because calcitriol potently activates the vitamin D receptor, one potential adverse effect is a dynamic bone disease due to oversuppression of PTH (see Chapter 8). In addition, calcitriol carries a risk of hypercalcemia and, less frequently, hyperphosphatemia. Regular monitoring is therefore required. The most recent KDIGO (Kidney Disease Improving Global Outcomes) guideline does not recommend routine use in predialysis CKD.[221]

Other Vitamin D Receptor Agonists

A number of novel vitamin D analogs have been developed. These analogs of calcitriol include paricalcitol and Hectorol, which are available for use in the United States. Vitamin D analogs have differential vitamin D receptor-mediated effects in different tissues and were selected for their ability to reduce circulating PTH concentration while minimizing hypercalcemia, presumably due to a greater ratio of activity in the parathyroid gland versus small bowel. Clinical trials have demonstrated that paricalcitol and Hectorol lower circulating PTH concentrations at least as effectively as calcitriol, with a reduced incidence of hypercalcemia.[222] Relative effects on other tissues, including those that may mediate pleiotropic effects of vitamin D, are not well described. However, one observational study in a large hemodialysis population suggested that paricalcitol use was associated with better survival than calcitriol use.[223]

Recommendations for Therapy

Currently, there is insufficient high-quality evidence from outcomes-oriented randomized clinical trials to confidently define an ideal approach to vitamin D therapy in CKD. Nonetheless, clinicians and patients must make therapeutic decisions based on available data. These decisions should take into account emerging observations that vitamin D therapy may have clinically relevant pleiotropic actions, that some of these actions may be mediated by nonrenal 1-α hydroxylase, and that many patients with CKD are deficient in both 25(OH)D and calcitriol. Therefore one approach is to titrate vitamin D therapy to both 25(OH)D and PTH concentration. With this strategy, 25(OH)D concentrations are routinely measured at any stage of CKD, with low levels repleted using cholecalciferol or ergocalciferol. Simultaneously, intact PTH concentrations are measured as an indicator of functional calcitriol status, with calcitriol and its analogs prescribed to lower PTH when needed. When limited by hypercalcemia, or when no longer effective, calcimimetics and surgical parathyroidectomy can be used to control PTH (see Chapter 8).

UNANSWERED QUESTIONS

There are many unanswered questions in the study of vitamin D deficiency in CKD. Several are especially pressing. In particular, which potential pleiotropic actions of vitamin D are clinically relevant? How do we gauge whether/how much vitamin D is needed to impact relevant targets? In what form or combinations should we provide vitamin D to affect nontraditional actions? These questions require further studies, focusing on intervention studies in CKD with both short-term surrogate outcomes and long-term clinical outcomes.

CONCLUSIONS

Vitamin D deficiency is common in patients with CKD. Low 25(OH)D concentrations reflect inadequate intake of cholecalciferol and ergocalciferol from cutaneous synthesis and dietary intake, and low calcitriol levels reflect decreased metabolism of vitamin D to its active hormonal form. Increasing evidence suggests that vitamin D deficiency may have broad-ranging, clinically relevant effects, beyond those described for calcium and bone homeostasis. Treatment of vitamin D deficiency in CKD is currently guided by measurement of circulating 25(OH)D and PTH concentrations. A number of therapeutic options are available, and there may be benefit to simultaneous treatment with more than one form of vitamin D.

A full list of references is available at www.expertconsult.com.

12

Cardiovascular Disease in Chronic Kidney Disease

Mark J. Sarnak, MD, MS, and Daniel E. Weiner, MD, MS

OUTLINE

EPIDEMIOLOGY

Stage 1 to 2 Chronic Kidney Disease

Even in the absence of reduced estimated glomerular filtration rate (eGFR), kidney damage, which most often is identified through the presence of albumin in the urine, is associated with a higher prevalence of surrogates of cardiovascular disease (CVD), including left ventricular hypertrophy (LVH) in patients with hypertension,[1] arterial intima media thickening in patients with diabetes,[2] and brain white matter hyperintensity volume in the elderly.[3] Albuminuria, even at high normal levels (10 to 29 mg/g) and moderately elevated levels (30 to 299 mg/g), is an independent, graded risk factor for CVD and all-cause death in the general population, identifying a high-risk population even in the absence of reduced kidney function (Fig. 12.1).[4,5] This risk association is present regardless of whether an individual has diabetes.[6]

Stage 3 to 4 Chronic Kidney Disease

Reduced kidney function is defined by a glomerular filtration rate (GFR) below 60 mL/min/1.73 m^2; stage 3a chronic kidney disease (CKD) refers to a GFR of 45 to 59 and CKD stage 3b to GFR of 30 to 44 mL/min/1.73 m^2. CVD is common in all stages of CKD, with the high prevalence of CVD in incident dialysis patients suggesting that CVD develops before the onset of kidney failure. Most observational studies have relied on eGFR to define CKD; accordingly, there has been a proliferation of research in the past two decades, since the 2002 publication of the Kidney Disease Outcomes Quality Initiative (KDOQI) clinical practice guidelines for CKD,[7] on the association between reduced eGFR, typically defined as below 60 mL/min/1.73 m^2, and CVD events.[8] The new paradigm stressed in the KDOQI guideline specifically highlighted people with CKD as a high-risk population for CVD with unique issues and risk factors.[8]

Critically, death from CVD among individuals with CKD is far more common than progression to kidney failure, particularly among individuals with earlier stages of kidney disease and those with relatively low levels of albuminuria, highlighting that targeting CVD risk and risk factor reduction is an essential aspect of care of individuals with CKD.[9] Globally, reduced GFR is associated with 4% of deaths worldwide, and more than half of these deaths attributed to CKD were cardiovascular deaths.[10] Several studies also have shown that manifestations of CVD, including LVH, may be seen relatively early in CKD.[11] The 2016 USRDS Annual Data Report, which used Medicare claims data to explore the associations between CKD and CVD in older US adults, notes a prevalence of CVD of 68.8% among older adults with CKD compared with 34.1% among those without CKD (Fig. 12.2).[12] Those with CKD also fared

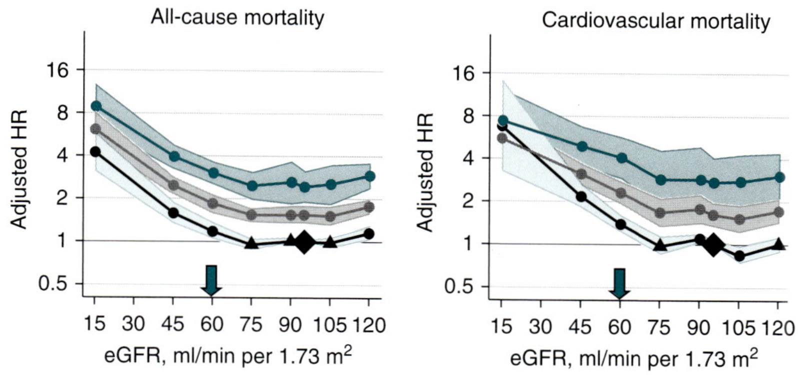

FIG. 12.1 Association of urine albumin-to-creatinine ratio (ACR) and estimated glomerular filtration rate (eGFR) with all-cause and cardiovascular mortality from metaanalysis of population cohorts. The three lines represent urine ACR of <30 mg/g or dipstick negative and trace (black), urine ACR 30 to 299 mg/g or dipstick 1þ positive (gray), and urine ACR 300+ mg/g or dipstick >2 + positive (green). All results are adjusted for covariates and compared with reference point (black diamond) of eGFR of 95 mL/min/1.73 m^2 and ACR of <30 mg/g or dipstick negative. Each point represents the pooled relative risk from a metaanalysis. Solid circles indicate statistical significance compared with the reference point (P<0.05); triangles indicate nonsignificance. Red arrows indicate eGFR of 60 mL/min/1.73 m^2, threshold value of eGFR for the current definition of chronic kidney disease (CKD). *HR*, Hazard ratio. (Reprinted from Levey AS, de Jong PE, Coresh J, et al. The definition, classification, and prognosis of chronic kidney disease: a KDIGO Controversies Conference report. *Kidney Int.* Jul 2011;80(1):17-28.)

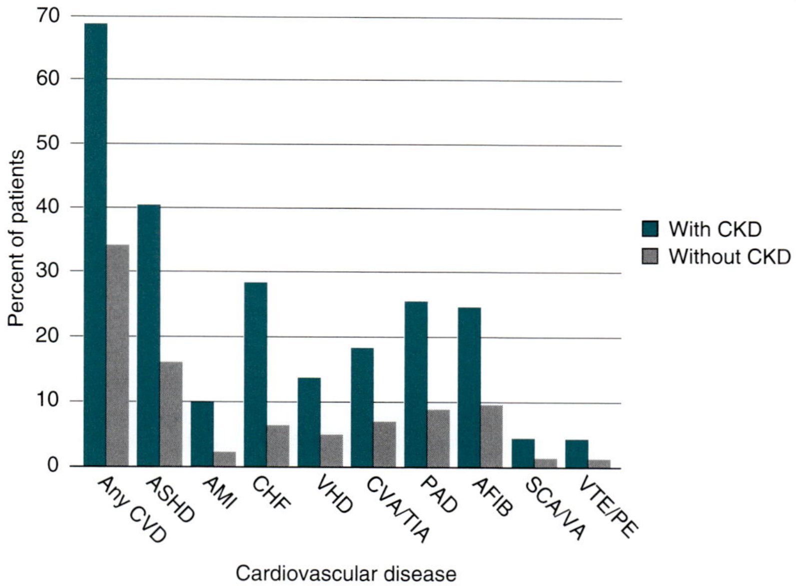

FIG. 12.2 Prevalence of cardiovascular diseases in US adults, age ≥66, with or without CKD. CKD diagnosis is based on administrative codes for CKD stage 3 or worse, and data are derived from the Medicare 5% sample. *AFIB*, Atrial fibrillation; *AMI*, acute myocardial infarction; *ASHD*, atherosclerotic heart disease; *CHF*, congestive heart failure; *CKD*, chronic kidney disease; *CVA/TIA*, cerebrovascular accident/transient ischemic attack; *CVD*, cardiovascular disease; *PAD*, peripheral arterial disease; *SCA/VA*, sudden cardiac arrest and ventricular arrhythmias; *VHD*, valvular heart disease; *VTE/PE*, venous thromboembolism and pulmonary embolism. (Reprinted from the 2016 USRDS Annual Data Report K/DOQI clinical practice guidelines for chronic kidney disease: evaluation, classification, and stratification, *Am J Kidney Dis.* 39 (2 Suppl 1) (2002) S1-266.)

worse when having cardiovascular events. The 2-year survival of patients with acute myocardial infarction (AMI) was 80% among patients without a diagnosis of CKD, compared with 69% for patients with CKD stage 1 to 2, 64% for patients with CKD stage 3, and 53% for patients with CKD stage 4 to 5.[12]

Similarly, among patients with CKD stage 3 to 4 in the Cardiovascular Health Study (CHS, comprising subjects aged 65 years and older), 26% had coronary artery disease, 8% had heart failure, and 55% had hypertension at baseline, whereas among those with eGFR above 60 mL/min/1.73 m^2,

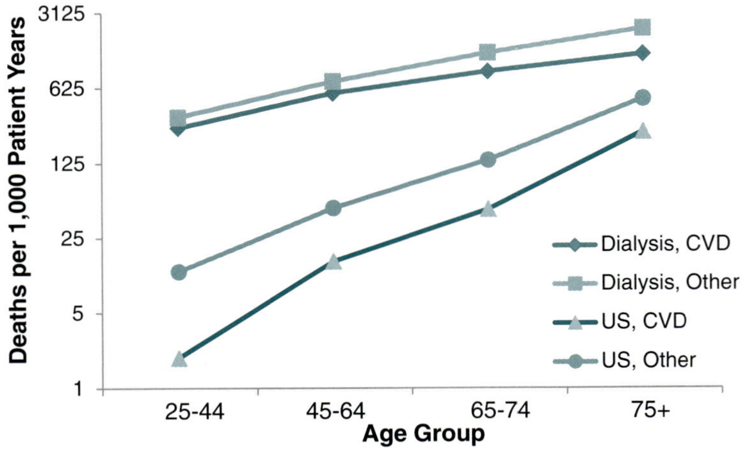

FIG. 12.3 Cardiovascular disease and noncardiovascular disease mortality in the general US population (2014) compared with patients with chronic kidney failure treated by dialysis (2012 to 2014). CVD death in the US population includes "Diseases of the heart" (I00-I09, I11, I13, I20-I51) and "Cerebrovascular diseases" (I60-I69). CVD death in dialysis includes myocardial infarction, pericarditis, atherosclerotic heart disease, cardiomyopathy, arrhythmia, cardiac arrest, valvular heart disease, congestive heart failure, and cerebrovascular disease. The youngest general population group is 22 to 44 years old. Figure created using publicly available data.

13% had coronary artery disease, 3% had heart failure, and 36% had hypertension.[13] Similar findings were noted in the Atherosclerosis Risk in Communities (ARIC) study, a community-based cohort of individuals aged 45 to 64 years, wherein participants with eGFR below 60 mL/min/1.73 m^2 had a baseline prevalence of coronary artery disease, cerebrovascular disease, and diabetes of 11%, 10%, and 24%, respectively, whereas participants with eGFR above 60 mL/min/1.73 m^2 had a baseline prevalence of coronary artery disease, cerebrovascular disease, and diabetes of 4.1%, 4.4%, and 13%, respectively.[14]

Reduced GFR is associated with incident CVD in most cohort studies that have evaluated this relationship.[15-18] The relative strength of this association is similar in high-risk and lower-risk populations, although the absolute risk of CVD events is far greater among those with kidney and CVD risk factors.[19] Of note, risk thresholds for eGFR and albuminuria appear similar regardless of age, sex, or race.[20] Among high-risk populations, the Studies of Left Ventricular Dysfunction (SOLVD) trial included individuals with left ventricular ejection fraction below 35%; participants in SOLVD with CKD had a 40% increased risk of mortality and a 50% to 70% increased risk of death due to heart failure.[21] Similarly, in the Heart Outcomes and Prevention Evaluation (HOPE) trial, patients with CKD had a 40% increased risk of the composite outcome of myocardial infarction (MI), CVD death, and stroke.[22] The largest general population study to date evaluated Kaiser Permanente patients in northern California, who had serum creatinine measured as a part of their clinical care, and noted a strong, graded relationship between eGFR and subsequent CVD outcomes; this was particularly notable below an eGFR of 45 mL/min/1.73 m^2.[23] Accordingly, the presence of reduced GFR identifies a high-risk population.

Dialysis

Among dialysis patients, CVD is the single leading cause of mortality, accounting for approximately 40% of deaths.[12] The majority of cardiovascular events, approximately 30% of all deaths (and 75% of cardiovascular deaths), are classified as either cardiac arrest or arrhythmia.[12] This high burden of CVD mortality is well illustrated by comparing CVD mortality in the dialysis population with the general population; mortality due to CVD is 5 to 37 times higher in dialysis patients who are 45 years old and older and 140 times higher in dialysis patients between the ages of 20 and 45 than in this age group in the general population (Fig. 12.3).

The high CVD mortality rate in dialysis patients likely reflects both a high prevalence of CVD and a high case fatality rate. Based on data obtained from medical claims, at the time of dialysis initiation 73.6% of hemodialysis and 61.3% of peritoneal dialysis patients have CVD, with 46.2%, 43.8%, and 37.9% of incident hemodialysis patients having atherosclerotic heart disease, congestive heart failure, and peripheral artery disease, respectively (Fig. 12.4).[12] Of note, dialysis patients are exceedingly diagnosed with non-ST elevation MI (NSTEMI) rather than ST elevation MI (STEMI), likely reflecting both the pathophysiology of CVD in this population and increased sensitivity of troponin assays.[24]

Dialysis patients with CVD also have a very high case fatality rate. Seminal data from Herzog and colleagues noted a 60% 1-year mortality and 90% 5-year mortality rate after AMI in 34,189 dialysis patients.[25] More recent data evaluating AMI in 2009 to 2011 are essentially unchanged, with 61% 1-year mortality and 74% 2-year mortality for hemodialysis patients and 69% and 80% 1- and 2-year mortality for peritoneal dialysis patients.[26] In-hospital death among dialysis patients hospitalized for AMI is nearly twice that of nondialysis patients (21.3% vs. 11.7%)[27]; risk appears highest in the first several months after dialysis initiation.[28]

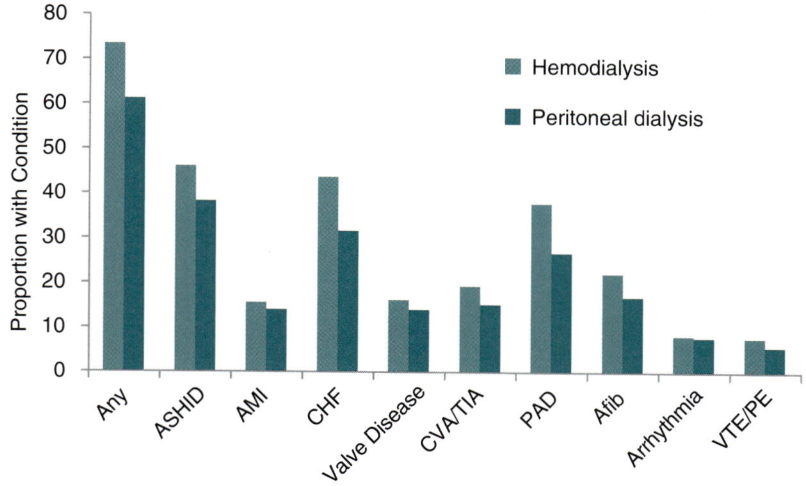

FIG. 12.4 Types of cardiovascular disease in hemodialysis and peritoneal dialysis patients. Plotted from data in the 2016 USRDS Atlas for incident dialysis patients in 2014.[240] Data are derived from Medicare claims. *Afib*, Atrial fibrillation; *ASHD*, atherosclerotic heart disease; *AMI*, acute myocardial infarction; *CHF*, congestive heart failure; *CVA*, cerebrovascular accident; *PAD*, peripheral artery disease; *PE*, pulmonary embolus; *TIA*, transient ischemic attack; *VTE*, venous thromboembolus.

Risk Factors

CVD risk factors are defined as characteristics, both modifiable and nonmodifiable, that increase the risk of developing CVD. Traditional CVD risk factors were identified in the Framingham Heart Study as conferring increased risk of CVD in the general population; these were later incorporated into prediction equations to aid physicians in identifying individuals at higher risk. Traditional risk factors include older age, male sex, hypertension, diabetes, smoking, and family history of coronary disease (Table 12.1).[29] Traditional CVD risk factors are common in individuals with CKD, as suggested by higher coronary risk scores using the Framingham prediction equations in individuals with reduced kidney function (GFR <60 mL/min/1.73 m^2).[30] Nontraditional risk factors include items that were not described in the original Framingham studies; nontraditional risk factors are those risk factors that both increase in prevalence as kidney function declines and have been hypothesized to be CVD risk factors in this population. Nontraditional risk factors may be particular to individuals with kidney disease (such as anemia and abnormalities in mineral metabolism) but also may include factors recognized as important in the general population (such as inflammation and oxidative stress).[31] Of note, the Framingham equations have poor discrimination and calibration in individuals with stage 3 to 4 CKD, perhaps reflecting either greater *severity* of traditional CVD risk factors that are not accounted for in risk equations or the role of nontraditional risk factors.[5,32]

TABLE 12.1 Traditional and Nontraditional Cardiovascular Risk Factors in Individuals With Chronic Kidney Disease

Traditional Risk Factors	Nontraditional Factors
Older age	Lipoprotein (a) and apo (a) isoforms
Male sex	Lipoprotein remnants
Hypertension	Anemia
Higher LDL cholesterol	Mineral and bone disorder
Lower HDL cholesterol	Volume overload
Diabetes	
Smoking	Electrolyte abnormalities
Physical inactivity	Oxidative Stress
Menopause	Inflammation
Family history of cardiovascular disease	Malnutrition
	Thrombogenic factors
Left ventricular hypertrophy	Sleep disturbances
	Sympathetic tone
	Altered nitric oxide/ endothelin balance

HDL, High-density lipoprotein; *LDL*, low-density lipoprotein.
Modified from Sarnak MJ, Levey AS. Cardiovascular disease and chronic renal disease: a new paradigm. *Am J Kidney Dis.* Apr 2000;35(4 Suppl 1):S117-S131.

MECHANISMS OF CARDIOVASCULAR DISEASE RISK IN CHRONIC KIDNEY DISEASE

There are several reasons why reduced GFR may be an independent risk state for CVD outcomes. These include, but are not limited to, residual confounding from traditional risk factors and insufficient adjustment for nontraditional risk factors. In addition, reduced kidney function may be a marker of the severity of either diagnosed or undiagnosed vascular disease. Finally, patients with CKD may not receive sufficient therapy for their disease, including medications such as aspirin, beta blockers, angiotensin-converting enzyme inhibitors (ACEIs), and diagnostic and therapeutic procedures.[33]

Similarly, there are several reasons why albuminuria may be an independent risk factor for CVD outcomes. Albuminuria, even at high normal levels, may represent kidney disease itself, with an associated risk of subsequent CKD progression and

TABLE 12.2 Spectrum of Cardiovascular Disease in Chronic Kidney Disease

Types of CVD	Pathology	Surrogates	Clinical Manifestations of CVD
Arterial vascular disease	Atherosclerosis	Inducible ischemia, carotid IMT, cardiac CT (may be less useful than in the GP for atherosclerosis because of medial rather than intimal calcification), ischemia by ECG	IHD (myocardial infarction, angina, sudden cardiac death), cerebrovascular disease, PAD, heart failure
	Nonatherosclerotic vascular stiffness	Aortic pulse wave velocity, medial vascular calcification, LVH (indirectly), increased pulse pressure	IHD, heart failure
Cardiomyopathy	Concentric LVH as well as LV dilatation with proportional hypertrophy	LVH, systolic dysfunction, and diastolic dysfunction by echocardiogram. LVH by ECG	Heart failure, hypotension, IHD

CAD, coronary disease; *CKD*, chronic kidney disease; *CT*, computed tomography; *CVD*, cardiovascular disease; *ECG*, electrocardiogram; *GP*, general population; *IHD*, ischemic heart disease; *IMT*, intima-media thickness; *LVH*, left ventricular hypertrophy; *PAD*, peripheral vascular disease.

development of elevated and severely elevated albuminuria.[19] Albuminuria likely also represents the kidney manifestation of systemic endothelial disease burden, and it may be associated with systemic inflammatory markers and abnormalities in the coagulation and fibrinolytic systems.[34]

Most CVD risk factors lead to atherosclerosis, nonatherosclerotic vascular stiffness, cardiomyopathy, or any combination of these three conditions (Table 12.2). Both atherosclerosis, defined as an occlusive disease of the vasculature, and nonatherosclerotic vascular stiffness, a function of nonocclusive remodeling of the vasculature, may manifest as ischemic heart disease (IHD) and heart failure. Some risk factors, including dyslipidemia, primarily predispose the patient to development and progression of atherosclerosis, whereas others, including volume overload and elevated calcium-phosphorus product, may predispose the patient to vascular remodeling. Still other risk factors, including anemia and possibly the presence of arteriovenous fistulas, may predispose the patient to cardiac remodeling, LVH, and cardiomyopathy. Essential to the understanding of CVD in CKD is an understanding of the interplay of these various risk factors. A simplified schematic of this interrelationship directed toward individuals with CKD not requiring kidney replacement therapy is displayed in Fig. 12.5.

TRADITIONAL CARDIOVASCULAR DISEASE RISK FACTORS

Hypertension and Blood Pressure

Hypertension is both a cause and a result of kidney disease. About 70% to 80% of patients with stages 1 to 4 CKD have hypertension, and the prevalence of hypertension increases as GFR declines, such that 80% to 90% of patients starting dialysis are hypertensive.[26,35-37]

Chronic Kidney Disease Stage 3 to 4

Blood pressure in stage 3 to 4 CKD has been investigated in more detail than in dialysis patients, although the focus of most studies has been on retarding progression of kidney disease rather than reducing CVD outcomes. Hypertension is highly prevalent in patients with CKD. In adults participating in the National Health and Nutrition Examination Survey (NHANES) from 1999 to 2004, 80% to 90% of individuals with eGFR below 60 mL/min/1.73 m^2 had hypertension, with hypertension more prevalent at lower eGFR levels, compared with approximately 40% of participants with eGFR of 60 to 90 mL/min/1.73 m^2 and 25% of participants with eGFR of 90 mL/min/1.73 m^2 or higher.[38] In the Modification of Diet in Renal Disease (MDRD) study, hypertension was more commonly seen with CKD due to glomerular disease than tubulointerstitial disease.[39]

Elevated systolic blood pressure is an independent risk factor for CVD outcomes in both diabetic and nondiabetic CKD patients. A secondary analysis of the MDRD study, which included a predominantly nondiabetic population, showed a 35% increased risk of hospitalization for CVD for each 10 mmHg increase in systolic blood pressure, and this increased risk remained significant even after adjusting for other traditional risk factors.[40] However, some of the added CVD risk may be driven by an increased rate of kidney disease progression associated with worse blood pressure control; for example, randomization to a lower blood pressure target in the MDRD study reduced the composite outcome of all-cause mortality and kidney failure 7 years after completion of the randomized intervention[41]; this was driven by fewer episodes of kidney failure.

Blood pressure is often insufficiently controlled in individuals with CKD. Fig. 12.6 shows the number of blood pressure medications, on average, to achieve targeted blood pressure thresholds in populations with CKD or diabetes, with achievement of a systolic blood pressure below 140 mmHg often requiring 2 or more medications in a clinical trial setting.[42] In the Chronic Renal Insufficiency Cohort (CRIC), approximately 67% of participants had a systolic blood pressure below 140 mmHg, with the majority of participants using at least three antihypertensive medications.[43] Therapies for hypertension are discussed in detail in Chapter 4, with CKD patients, specifically those with diabetes or albuminuria, prescribed ACEIs and angiotensin receptor blockers (ARBs), often in conjunction with a diuretic.

The Systolic Blood Pressure Intervention Trial (SPRINT) randomized over 9000 individuals without diabetes but with CVD risk factors, including 2646 with eGFR below 60 mL/min/1.73 m^2,

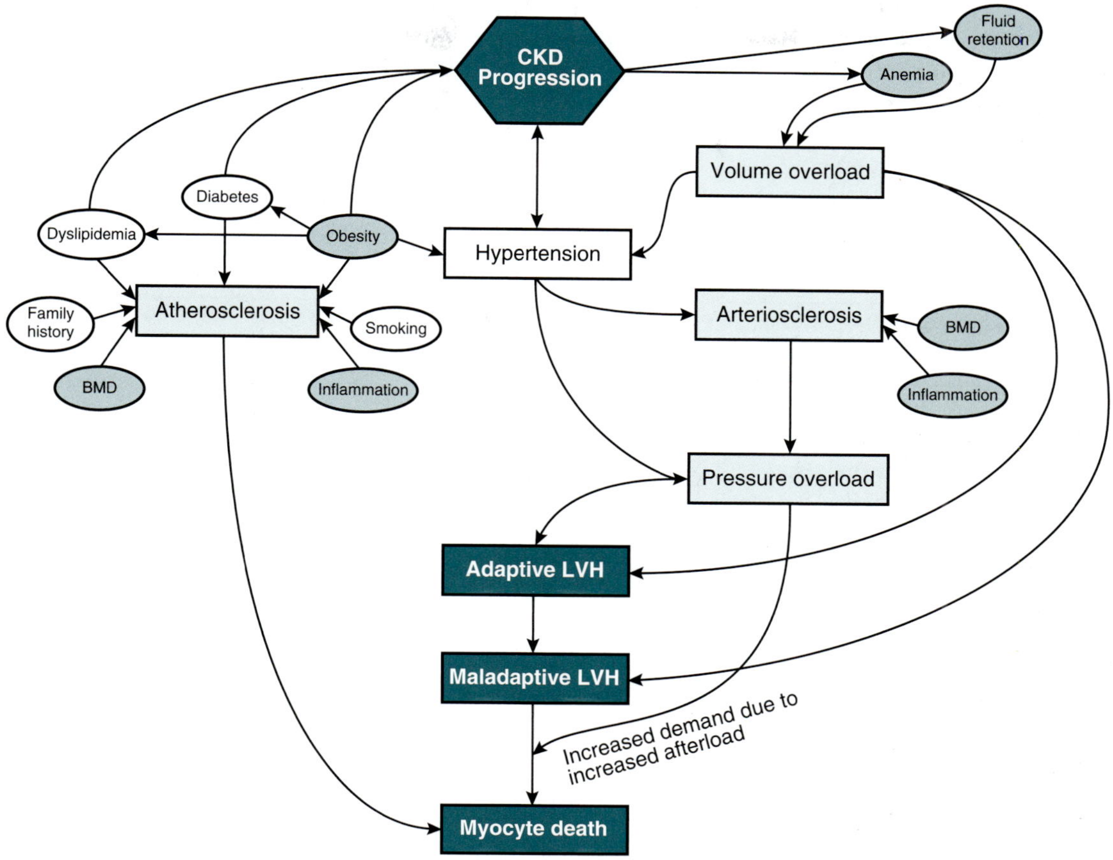

FIG. 12.5 Concept diagram presenting a simplified overview of the relationship among chronic kidney disease, kidney disease risk factors, cardiovascular disease risk factors, and subsequent heart disease. Not all associations presented in this paradigm have been proven causal and, for simplicity, not all potential relationships are included. Selected traditional risk factors are presented in white and nontraditional risk factors are shaded. Outcomes, which themselves may be risk factors, are in black. Hypertension assumes a central role in this paradigm. *BMD*, Bone and mineral disorder of CKD.

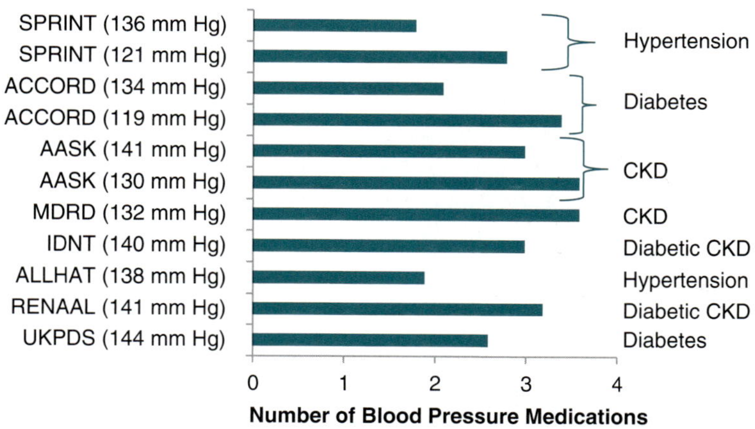

FIG. 12.6 Number of blood pressure medications to achieve a blood pressure target in major hypertension clinical trials, including participants with high-risk hypertension, diabetes, CKD, and diabetic kidney disease. *AASK*, African American Study of Kidney Disease and Hypertension; *ACCORD*, Action to Control Cardiovascular Risk in Diabetes; *ALLHAT*, African American Study of Kidney Disease and Hypertension; *IDNT*, Irbesartan Diabetic Nephropathy Trial; *MDRD*, Modification of Diet in Renal Disease; *RENAAL*, Reduction of Endpoints in NIDDM with the Angiotensin II Antagonist Losartan; *SPRINT*, Systolic Blood Pressure Intervention Trial; *UKPDS*, UK Prospective Diabetes Study Group. *CKD*, Chronic kidney disease.

TABLE 12.3 **Typical Lipid Abnormalities by CKD Subpopulation, Assuming Untreated Status**

	Total Cholesterol	LDL Cholesterol	HDL Cholesterol	Triglycerides	Lp(a)
CKD Stages 1 to 4					
With nephrotic syndrome	↑↑	↑↑	↓	↑↑	↑↑
Without nephrotic syndrome	↑ or ↔	↑ or ↔	↓ or ↔	↑	↑
CKD Stage 5					
Hemodialysis	↓ or ↔	↓	↓	↑ or ↔	↑
Peritoneal dialysis	↑	↑	↓	↑↑	↑↑

CKD, Chronic kidney disease; *HDL*, high-density lipoprotein; *LDL*, low-density lipoprotein; *Lp*, lipoprotein.
Modified and updated from Kwan BC, Kronenberg F, Beddhu S, Cheung AK. Lipoprotein metabolism and lipid management in chronic kidney disease. *J Am Soc Nephrol.* Apr 2007;18(4):1246-1261.

to an intensive systolic blood pressure target of <120 mmHg versus a standard target of <140 mmHg. After median follow-up of 3.3 years, there was a nonstatistically significant lower risk of CVD events and a statistically significant lower risk of death among those randomized to the intensive target without a major difference in serious adverse events between groups.[44] This trial potentially supports a lower blood pressure target for cardiovascular risk reduction in individuals with nondiabetic stage 3 and 4 CKD, although follow-up time was insufficient to draw conclusions regarding kidney disease progression. Blood pressure targets are covered more fully in Chapter 4.

Dialysis

There is a U-shaped relationship between blood pressure and CVD outcomes in the dialysis population, with higher CVD events and mortality rates at both markedly elevated postdialysis systolic blood pressures (>180 mmHg) and lower blood pressures (<110 mmHg) but no apparent increased risk at systolic blood pressure levels that would be consistent with severe hypertension in the general population.[45-49] However, higher blood pressures do not appear entirely benign in dialysis patients, either; hypertension is an independent risk factor for IHD, LVH, heart failure, and cerebral hemorrhage.[50,51] Based on data from the HEMO study, greater visit-to-visit blood pressure variability is associated with a higher risk of all-cause mortality and a trend toward higher risk of cardiovascular mortality, particularly in patients with a lower baseline systolic blood pressure.[52] Similarly, large cohort data suggest that mortality risk is greatest among dialysis patients who have a >30 mmHg drop in systolic blood pressure during the treatment and among those whose blood pressure increases during dialysis.[53]

Intradialytic hypotension is a relatively common occurrence during hemodialysis and may also be an independent marker for CVD outcomes, perhaps representing the inability of the heart or blood vessels to compensate appropriately for reduced blood volume or, alternatively, representing heart failure itself in the absence of overt volume overload.[54] In dialysis patients, where myocardial fibrosis and myocyte-capillary mismatch are common, abrupt decreases in perfusion may further cardiac damage and predispose to arrhythmia or the progression of myocardial fibrosis.[55] Hypotension, both chronic and intradialytic, may also identify high-risk dialysis patients. First, hypotension may be a reflection of the severity of other comorbid conditions, including heart failure, cardiomyopathy, and generalized malnutrition; and, second, low blood pressure may predispose dialysis patients to intradialytic hypotension, which may lead to ischemic events and myocardial stunning.[56-58]

Unfortunately, in the absence of clinical trials delineating blood pressure targets in this population,[59] there is no evidence supporting any blood pressure target or even the best means to achieve a specific blood pressure target, although ultrafiltration to dry weight is generally considered the initial treatment of hypertension.[37] Recent emphasis on volume status and maintaining dialysis patients as close to euvolemia as possible stresses the potential cardiovascular benefits of this approach.[60,61]

Dyslipidemia

Dyslipidemia is common in all stages of CKD (Table 12.3), although the nature of dyslipidemia can be highly variable. As CKD progresses and kidney failure develops, levels of low-density lipoprotein (LDL) cholesterol that previously were high often normalize, perhaps reflecting worse malnutrition, inflammation, and cachexia.[62] Treatment may differ between CKD stage 3 to 4 and dialysis, with studies suggesting cardiovascular benefits of statins in individuals not treated with dialysis.[63]

Chronic Kidney Disease Stage 3 to 4

Earlier stages of CKD are often associated with diabetes, hypertension, CVD, and obesity—conditions that are frequently accompanied by dyslipidemia. In addition, the presence of nephrotic-range proteinuria can also exacerbate dyslipidemia. Among interventions for primary and secondary prevention of CVD in individuals with CKD, lipid-lowering therapies are among the best studied. The Study of Heart and Renal Protection (SHARP), which randomized 9270 individuals with CKD, including 6247 not treated with dialysis, demonstrated a significant benefit associated with simvastatin/ezetimibe use for primary prevention of CVD events in individuals with CKD stage 3b to 5 not receiving dialysis, albeit with no effect on all-cause mortality (Table 12.4).[64] Based on this result, as well as studies conducted in the general population that included individuals with CKD stage 3 and 4,[65-68] the 2013 Kidney Disease

TABLE 12.4 Randomized Controlled Trials of Lipid-Lowering Therapies in Individuals With Chronic Kidney Disease

Study	Intervention	Population	Median Follow-Up	Primary Outcome	Risk of Primary Outcome	Risk of All-Cause Mortality
4D	Atorvastatin 20 mg daily (vs. placebo)	1255 participants Age 18–80 y Type 2 diabetes Hemodialysis for less than 2 y LDL 80–190 mg/dL	4.0 y	Composite of death from cardiac causes,[a] fatal stroke, nonfatal MI, or nonfatal stroke	HR = 0.92 (0.77–1.10)	RR = 0.93 (0.79–1.08)
AURORA	Rosuvastatin 10 mg daily (vs. placebo)	2776 participants Age 50–80 y Hemofiltration or hemodialysis for more than 3 mo	3.8 y	Composite of death from cardiovascular causes, nonfatal MI, or nonfatal stroke	HR = 0.96 (0.84–1.11)	HR = 0.96 (0.86–1.07)
ALERT	Fluvastatin 40 mg daily with dose increase permitted (vs. placebo)	2102 participants Age 30–75 y More than 6 mo from transplant Stable kidney graft function No recent MI Total cholesterol 155–348 mg/dL	5.4 y	Major adverse cardiac event, defined as cardiac death, nonfatal MI, or coronary revascularization procedure	RR = 0.83 (0.64–1.06)	RR = 1.02 (0.81–1.30)
SHARP	Simvastatin 20 mg daily + ezetimibe 10 mg daily (vs. placebo)	9270 participants Age 40+ y No previous MI or coronary revascularization Creatinine more than 1.7 mg/dL (men) or more than 1.5 mg/dL (women)	4.9 y	Composite of coronary death,[b] nonfatal MI, ischemic stroke, or any revascularization procedure	RR = 0.83 (0.74–0.94)	RR = 1.02 (0.94–1.11)
	Subgroups within SHARP[c]	Nondialysis (n = 6247)	Not reported	As above	RR = 0.78 (0.67–0.91)	Not reported
		Hemodialysis (n = 2527)			RR = 0.95 (0.78–1.15)	
		Peritoneal dialysis (*n* = 496)			RR = 0.70 (0.46–1.08)	

[a]In 4D, death from cardiac causes comprised fatal myocardial infarction (death within 28 days after a myocardial infarction), sudden death, death due to congestive heart failure, death due to coronary heart disease during or within 28 days after an intervention, and all other deaths ascribed to coronary heart disease. Patients who died unexpectedly and had hyperkalemia before the start of the three most recent sessions of hemodialysis were considered to have had sudden death from cardiac causes.
[b]In SHARP, the original primary outcome included cardiac death, defined as death due to hypertensive heart disease, coronary heart disease, or other heart disease; the analytic plan was modified before data analysis to focus on death due to coronary heart disease rather than cardiac death.
[c]In SHARP, there was no statistically significant difference in the risk of the primary outcome between dialysis and nondialysis patients ($P = 0.25$) or between hemodialysis and peritoneal dialysis patients ($P = 0.21$).
4D, German Diabetes Dialysis Study; *ALERT,* assessment of Lescol in renal transplantation; *AURORA,* a study to evaluate the use of Rosuvastatin in subjects in regular hemodialysis: an assessment of survival and cardiovascular events; *HR,* hazard ratio; *LDL,* low-density lipoprotein; *MI,* myocardial infarction. *RR,* risk ratio; *SHARP,* Study of Heart and Renal Protection. Data in parentheses represent 95% confidence intervals. HR and RR report the relationship between treatment vs. placebo, with values below 1 favoring treatment and above 1 favoring placebo.

Improving Global Outcomes (KDIGO) Clinical Practice Guideline for Lipid Management in CKD recommended statin or statin/ezetimibe treatment for all adults 50 years old or older with CKD stage 3a to 5 (nondialysis) and for all younger adults with CKD with diabetes, known coronary disease or stroke, or high CVD risk.[69] The KDIGO workgroup stressed a "fire-and-forget" approach to statin use in CKD rather than treating to a specific LDL-cholesterol target. For secondary prevention of CVD, data on treatment of dyslipidemia in individuals with CKD stage 3 to 4 are largely derived from post hoc analyses of clinical trials in the general population and generally show similar benefits to those seen in the general population.[65,67,68] In general, these patients should receive statin therapy.[69]

Dialysis

In hemodialysis patients, high-density lipoprotein (HDL) cholesterol is typically low, whereas triglycerides are highly variable. Other abnormalities include increased levels of lipoprotein (a); a higher proportion of atherogenic, oxidized LDL cholesterol; and abnormal concentrations of apolipoproteins that comprise the major lipoproteins, although LDL and total cholesterol levels are often low or normal (see Table 12.3).[70-72] In peritoneal dialysis patients, the prevalence of hyperlipidemia, defined by elevated LDL cholesterol or triglyceride levels, is approximately 70%. Peritoneal dialysis patients have a somewhat more atherogenic lipid panel than their hemodialysis counterparts, with increased LDL-C, apolipoprotein B, oxidized LDL cholesterol, triglycerides, and lipoprotein (a) and decreased HDL cholesterol. Thus despite total cholesterol levels that may appear relatively normal in many patients, significant dyslipidemia is highly prevalent in the dialysis population.

Observational studies of dialysis patients have noted "reverse epidemiology" between cholesterol levels and risk of death, such that lower cholesterol levels are associated with a higher death rate.[73,74] For example, in an analysis of data from more than 12,000 hemodialysis patients predating widespread use of lipid-lowering medications, individuals with low total cholesterol levels (<100 mg/dL) had a more than fourfold increase in risk of death compared with patients whose cholesterol levels were between 200 and 250 mg/dL.[75] Low cholesterol in these studies may be a surrogate for malnutrition and inflammation, suggesting that higher cholesterol levels may actually be associated with increased cardiovascular risk in dialysis patients with preserved nutritional status (e.g., serum albumin) and low levels of inflammatory markers (e.g., C-reactive protein [CRP]).[74,76]

Clinical trial data have not demonstrated a significant survival benefit with statins in dialysis patients (see Table 12.4). Two large, adequately powered clinical trials, the German Diabetes and Dialysis (4D) study, which tested atorvastatin versus placebo in 1255 hemodialysis patients with diabetes, and AURORA, which tested rosuvastatin versus placebo in nearly 3000 hemodialysis patients, including both individuals with and individuals without diabetes, both show no benefit associated with statins in hemodialysis patients.[77,78] A third trial, SHARP, discussed previously, shows no benefit in the subgroup receiving hemodialysis at trial initiation[64]; peritoneal dialysis patients remain inadequately studied. Based on these results, KDIGO did not recommend routinely initiating statin therapy in hemodialysis patients, although the guideline suggests continuing statins in those who were receiving them predialysis.[79] In patients with longer life expectancies, such as patients expected to receive a kidney transplant, individualized decision making may be most appropriate, with the KDIGO guideline recommending statin therapy in transplant recipients.

Interestingly, data from the United States and from Australia suggest that the rates of CVD death in dialysis patients continue to decrease,[12,80] albeit less markedly than improvements in the general population and for reasons that remain uncertain. Although this improvement temporally relates to the marked increase in statin use in at-risk populations, the failure to demonstrate that specific interventions, including statins, significantly reduce the CVD burden in individuals treated with maintenance dialysis most likely reflects the fact that there are numerous competing causes of death in these patients, and that multiple risk factor adjustment, rather than addressing single risk factors, may result in CVD risk reduction.

Diabetes Mellitus

Diabetes is the leading cause of kidney failure in the United States. The annual incidence of end-stage renal disease (ESRD) in the United States is 370 per million, with the incidence of ESRD due to diabetes at 156 per million—for context, the rate of ESRD due to diabetes exceeds the rate of HIV infection (123 per million) and exceeds the incidence rates of both pancreatic cancer (~127 per million) and leukemia (~139 per million) in the United States.[12,81] Diabetes in CKD is extensively discussed in Chapter 3 and will not be reviewed here except to note that it is a powerful risk factor for CVD and mortality in the general population and in all stages of kidney disease.[6,15,29,32]

In dialysis patients, the presence of diabetes is an independent risk factor for IHD, heart failure, and all-cause mortality.[82,83] Dialysis patients with diabetes also have worse long-term outcomes after coronary interventions than do nondiabetic patients with CKD.[84,85] Notably, similar to other advanced chronic disease populations,[86] the net benefit of rigid diabetes control is uncertain in the dialysis population because microvascular and macrovascular complications already exist and because of a potentially increased risk of hypoglycemia; however, hyperglycemia may still worsen retinopathy, hasten the loss of residual kidney function, cause or worsen peripheral neuropathy, and increase the risk of infection. Several large, observational studies have examined the association between glycosylated hemoglobin level and outcomes in hemodialysis patients. In an analysis of Fresenius data, there was no relationship between glycosylated hemoglobin level and mortality at 1 year[87,88]; similarly, in an analysis of DaVita data, there was no significant increased risk of mortality until glycosylated hemoglobin levels rose above 8%, at which time increased mortality risk was appreciated only after extensive multivariable adjustment for case-mix, nutritional, and inflammatory factors.[89] Notably, this result was driven by cardiovascular mortality and was seen only in individuals with hemoglobin levels stable and 11 g/dL or more. The authors theorized that this relationship was not seen at lower hemoglobin levels due to the effect of atypical red blood cell production and turnover on glycosylated hemoglobin values in hemodialysis patients with variable hemoglobin levels, leading to misclassification of glucose exposure. Reflecting the notable lack of studies in the dialysis population of the relationship between glycemic control and CVD outcomes, currently there are no high-level evidence-based recommendations from KDOQI or KDIGO regarding diabetes management in dialysis patients.[90-93]

Left Ventricular Hypertrophy and Cardiomyopathy

LVH is highly prevalent in both stages 3 and 4 CKD and dialysis patients and represents a physiological adaptation to a

TABLE 12.5 **Causes, Risk Factors, and Manifestations of Left Ventricular Hypertrophy (LVH) in Chronic Kidney Disease**

LVH Risk Factor	Physiology/Etiology	LVH Diagnostic Test	LVH Clinical Sequelae
Pressure overload	Reflects increased afterload due to hypertension, valvular disease (most often the aortic valve), vascular stiffness	Echocardiography Cardiac MRI Electrocardiography	Myocardial infarction Angina Arrhythmia and sudden cardiac death Heart failure
Volume overload	Reflects volume retention due to progressive kidney disease +/- anemia		

MRI, Magnetic resonance imaging.

long-term increase in myocardial work requirements. LVH can be considered both a traditional risk factor, reflecting its inclusion in the original Framingham prediction instrument, and a cardiovascular outcome.

Epidemiology

In the Chronic Renal Insufficiency Cohort (CRIC), the prevalence of LVH assessed by echocardiography was 32% for eGFR above 60 mL/min/1.73 m^2, rising to 48%, 57%, and 75% for eGFR categories, 45 to 59, 30 to 44, and <30 mL/min/1.73 m^2, respectively.[94] These findings contrast with a prevalence of LVH below 20% in older adults in the general population. Prevalence rates may be as high as 70% in incident dialysis patients,[11] likely reflecting the confluence of risk factors predisposing to pressure and volume overload. Among prevalent dialysis patients, LVH is present in 50% to 75% of patients when assessed by echocardiography.[95,96] LVH is even seen in the majority of children requiring hemodialysis, a group typically not subject to IHD.[97] As in the general population, LVH is an independent risk factor for adverse CVD outcomes in patients treated with dialysis[98,99]; this holds true for both concentric LVH and dilated cardiomyopathy.[100]

Pathogenesis

LVH, which may result from either pressure or volume overload, reflects an initially appropriate adaptation by the heart to these forces (Table 12.5, see Fig. 12.5). Higher cardiac workload may be a tenet of CKD, reflecting increased volume retention and blood pressure accompanying deteriorating kidney function. As workload rises over time, increased oxygen demands by the hypertrophied left ventricle may ultimately exceed its perfusion, resulting in ischemia and eventual myocyte death. In individuals with late-stage CKD, including those treated with dialysis, this inability to increase cardiac perfusion is a reflection not only of LVH but also the high prevalence of atherosclerosis, vascular stiffness, and myocyte dropout limiting the ability to upregulate supply to compensate for increased demand.

Pressure overload results from increased cardiac afterload, often due to hypertension, valvular lesions including aortic stenosis, and reduced arterial compliance, at least in part due to medial vascular calcification.[101-103] Volume overload may be related to anemia, as the heart attempts to compensate for decreased peripheral oxygen delivery.[104] Other causes of volume overload include increased extracellular volume seen in CKD and, possibly, the presence of a high-flow arteriovenous fistula or a very high-flow graft.[105-107]

Often LVH is initially concentric, representing a uniform increase in wall thickness secondary to pressure overload, classically reported to be due to hypertension or aortic stenosis. The concentric thickening of the left ventricle wall allows for generation of greater intraventricular pressure, effectively overcoming increased afterload. Volume overload may result in eccentric hypertrophy secondary to the addition of new sarcomeres in series, although hypertension is also associated with eccentric hypertrophy.[108] Eccentric hypertrophy is defined by an increased left ventricle (LV) diameter with a proportional increase in LV wall thickness. The pathophysiology associated with both concentric and eccentric hypertrophy can manifest with heart failure with preserved ejection fraction (HFpEF).[109,110] As left ventricular remodeling progresses, capillary density decreases and subendocardial perfusion is reduced. Myocardial fibrosis may ensue and, with sustained maladaptive forces, myocyte death occurs. In its extremes, the endpoint of this cycle can be dilated cardiomyopathy with eventual reduction in systolic function (see Fig. 12.5).[100]

Diagnosis

LVH is readily diagnosed with echocardiography. Cardiac function is best assessed in the euvolemic state, because significant volume depletion and overload both reduce left ventricular inotropy.[111] Accordingly, in dialysis patients, two-dimensional echocardiogram results may be most meaningful on the interdialytic day, whereas three-dimensional echocardiography may be useful to assess LV structure because it avoids the use of geometrical assumptions of LV shape that are required to estimate LV mass and volume that are used for interpreting two-dimensional echocardiograms.[112] Magnetic resonance (MR) imaging may be more precise for assessing LV structure than echocardiography, but this technique is more costly and time consuming, with many patients having possible contraindications to MR.[113,114] Although screening echocardiography is currently recommended for incident dialysis patients, there is no evidence to date that this results in improvement in clinical outcomes.[115]

Therapy

Given the complexity of its development, LVH and subsequent cardiomyopathy present therapeutic challenges. Potentially modifiable risk factors for LVH (and subsequent heart failure) include hypertension, extracellular volume overload, abnormal mineral metabolism, and possibly anemia and high-flow arteriovenous fistulas. It is notable that in

CKD patients there is a paucity of trial data showing a mortality benefit associated with treating many of these LVH risk factors.

Data from several small observational studies and nonrandomized trials have suggested that regression of LVH can be induced by modification of risk factors, including anemia and systolic blood pressure, and strict management of volume using treatment modalities like daily dialysis.[116-120] This was best described in the Frequent Hemodialysis Network Daily Trial, where frequent in-center hemodialysis was associated with better results in the composite outcome of reduced all-cause mortality and LV mass.[121] In contrast, potentially reflecting effects of erythropoiesis stimulating agents on the vasculature, multiple randomized trials, including studies in both dialysis patients and patients with stage 3 to 4 CKD, have not demonstrated regression of LVH or a decrease in LV mass with near-normalization of hemoglobin.[122-125]

Current treatment for LVH focuses on afterload reduction and volume management; accordingly, ACEIs or ARBs, often in conjunction with diuretics, are a mainstay of treatment in advanced CKD,[126] whereas among dialysis patients the best results may be obtained with volume control. Other therapy at this time is best directed at modifying the multiple risk factors for LVH to prevent its development, particularly in the nondialysis CKD population.

Other Traditional Risk Factors

Other traditional CVD risk factors include advanced age, male sex, and smoking. Of these, only smoking presents an opportunity for intervention.[127,128] Although there have been few studies examining specific effects of smoking in dialysis patients, evaluation of United States Renal Data System (USRDS) data showed that smoking was a strong, independent risk factor for incident heart failure, incident peripheral vascular disease, and all-cause mortality. Importantly, dialysis patients who were former smokers were more similar to nonsmokers than current smokers in risk, demonstrating the potential benefit of smoking cessation efforts in dialysis patients.[129]

NONTRADITIONAL CARDIOVASCULAR DISEASE RISK FACTORS

Oxidative Stress and Inflammation

Oxidative stress and inflammation are proposed as unifying factors linking both traditional and other nontraditional risk factors in CKD.[130] Oxidative stress may be defined as an imbalance between prooxidants and antioxidants (oxidant defenses) that leads to tissue damage.[131] Most oxidation occurs in the mitochondria, although phagocytes also induce production of reactive oxygen species (ROS) in a "respiratory burst" designed to defend the body against infection. ROS can oxidize lipids, proteins, carbohydrates, and nucleic acids, which can then be measured as markers of oxidant burden. This system is balanced by a series of antioxidant defenses, some of which work by enzymatically catalyzing reduction of oxidant species (e.g., superoxide dismutase, catalase), whereas others work nonenzymatically by scavenging for oxidants (e.g., glutathione, vitamin C).[132] There is also a complicated interplay between ROS and advanced glycation end-products (AGEs) in CKD,[133] such that ROS may be both a cause and a consequence of AGE formation in individuals with diabetes and with CKD, and AGE accumulation may result in tissue damage and further oxidative and inflammatory stress.

Numerous factors in CKD patients increase oxidant stress, including inflammation, malnutrition (by reducing antioxidant defenses), uremic toxins, and potentially the dialysis procedure itself. Patients with CKD not only have higher levels of oxidant stress; they also have decreased defenses, particularly plasma protein-associated free thiols such as glutathione.[130] This "double hit" makes CKD patients particularly vulnerable to sequelae of oxidant stress.

The lesions of atherosclerosis may represent a sequence of inflammatory processes affecting the vasculature; elevated and modified LDL cholesterol, genetic factors, infectious microorganisms, free radicals caused by cigarette smoking, hypertension, diabetes mellitus, ischemic injury, and combinations of these all predispose patients to progressive endothelial dysfunction.[134] These factors are all common in individuals with CKD. In the general population, inflammation is a reasonably well-established risk marker for CVD, with leukocytosis and CRP both independently associated with adverse cardiovascular outcomes.[135] In dialysis patients, several studies have demonstrated a strong, independent association between inflammation and the risk of adverse CVD outcomes,[95,136-138] although controversy exists regarding causality.[139] In stage 3 to 4 CKD, inflammatory markers, including CRP, elevated white blood cell count, and fibrinogen, are associated with adverse cardiovascular outcomes.[140,141]

At this time, specific strategies to treat oxidant stress and inflammation in CKD have not been adopted, although potential therapies may be forthcoming. For example, statins are associated with a greater beneficial effect on CVD events and mortality than would be expected by changes in the lipid profile alone in the general population[142]; however, although statins may decrease CRP levels in dialysis patients, there is no evidence of a survival benefit associated with their use.[77,78]

Numerous studies have investigated the use of antioxidants for cardiovascular protection in the general population, including one large trial that demonstrated no benefit of vitamin E supplementation.[143] However, in dialysis patients, a study of 200 patients with prevalent CVD demonstrated a benefit associated with daily use of 800 international units of vitamin E,[144] whereas a separate study showed a benefit with use of 600 mg of acetylcysteine twice daily.[145] Other investigations have used vitamin E–coated dialyzers and noted a decrease in oxidant stress.[146,147] Overall these studies remain preliminary and have not been consistently reproduced. Ongoing studies are examining other inflammatory mechanisms, such as a small study evaluating the interleukin (IL)-1 receptor blocker, anakinra, in hemodialysis.[148]

Nitric Oxide, Asymmetrical Dimethylarginine, and Endothelial Function

Adequate nitric oxide production is critical for local vascular regulation and endothelial function. In individuals with CKD, nitric oxide production is reduced, likely reflecting substrate (L-arginine) limitation and increased levels of circulating endogenous inhibitors of nitric oxide synthase (NOS), most notably asymmetrical dimethylarginine (ADMA). ADMA is a competitive inhibitor of NOS and is chiefly metabolized by dimethylarginine dimethylaminohydrolase (DDAH) to citrulline and dimethylamine. In kidney disease, particularly in states of high oxidative stress, DDAH activity is reduced, resulting in higher plasma and tissue levels of ADMA.[149] Accordingly, the relationship among nitric oxide, endothelial function, and kidney disease may be another example of a vicious circle in this patient population, with chronic NOS inhibition causing systemic and glomerular hypertension, proteinuria, and glomerular and tubular injury, with these ultimately resulting in progressively worse kidney function that leads to further reductions in nitric oxide availability.[149] One cross-sectional study explored these relationships, demonstrating an independent association between higher ADMA levels and lower eGFR, between higher ADMA levels and reduced coronary flow reserve, and between lower eGFR and reduced coronary flow reserve, with the highest ADMA levels seen in individuals with both lower eGFR and reduced coronary flow reserve.[150] A second cross-sectional study showed a significant reduction in nitroglycerin-induced endothelium-independent vasodilation in CKD, suggesting that nitric oxide responsiveness also may be impaired in advanced CKD.[151] These observations require further exploration in longitudinal analyses across a broader range of GFR levels.

Higher ADMA levels occur in individuals with earlier stages of CKD, and ADMA levels continue to rise as GFR declines. Higher ADMA levels are associated with more rapid kidney function decline and all-cause mortality in people with kidney disease.[152,153] Furthermore, ADMA has been independently associated with increased cardiovascular risk in both CKD stage 3 to 4 and dialysis populations. In a post hoc analysis of the MDRD Study, each 0.25 μmol/L higher ADMA was associated with both a 31% higher prevalence of CVD (after adjusting for traditional and nontraditional risk factors) and borderline statistically significant 9% and 19% increases in all-cause mortality and CVD mortality, respectively.[154] Similarly, in a cohort of 225 chronic hemodialysis patients, each 1 μmol/L was associated with a statistically significant 26% increase in all-cause mortality and a 17% increase in incident cardiovascular events.[155] This research has established important groundwork for potentially addressing one aspect of increased cardiovascular risk in CKD. However, there has been no pharmacological intervention to date that reliably reduces ADMA levels in individuals with CKD.[156-158] Accordingly, cardiovascular risk reduction targeting nitric oxide and ADMA remains an active area of research.

Homocysteine

Homocysteine, a metabolite of the essential amino acid methionine, has been implicated in observational studies in the general population as a risk factor for MI and stroke.[159,160] Homocysteine levels increase as GFR declines,[161] and hyperhomocysteinemia is much more common in dialysis patients than in the general population. Further, as elevated levels of homocysteine can often be reduced using pharmacological doses of B vitamins, it is an attractive potential nontraditional risk factor. To date, there have been multiple large, randomized trials of homocysteine-lowering therapies that enrolled patients at high risk of CVD outcomes in the general population and in late-stage CKD, dialysis, and kidney transplant populations, which, despite successfully lowering homocysteine levels, have failed to demonstrate a reduction in cardiovascular events.[162-168] Accordingly, there are no data to suggest a benefit to lowering homocysteine with B vitamins.

Chronic Kidney Disease–Mineral Bone Disorder

Chronic kidney disease–mineral bone disorder (CKD-MBD), discussed more fully in Chapter 10, is an important nontraditional risk factor for CVD in individuals with stage 3 to 5 CKD. The hypothesis that vascular calcification contributes to CVD burden in CKD is supported by several studies in dialysis patients that show independent associations between coronary artery calcification with mortality[169] and between both peripheral artery intimal and medial calcification with mortality.[170]

Arterial calcification, and, specifically, medial calcification, is far more common in individuals with CKD than in the general population,[171,172] likely reflecting a complex interrelationship among hyperphosphatemia, secondary hyperparathyroidism, vitamin D deficiency, and other markers of mineral metabolism that, in conjunction, serve to overwhelm natural defenses against calcification (Table 12.6).[173] A model suggesting that vascular calcification occurs in patients with decreased plasma levels of inhibitory proteins, including fetuin-A, osteoprotegerin, and matrix Gla protein, has been extensively tested, but, to date, these proteins have not been consistent markers of calcification.[174] Additional proteins that may affect this interrelationship include fibroblast growth factor 23 (FGF-23), a phosphatonin that decreases renal phosphate reabsorption, and klotho, a protein facilitating the binding of FGF-23 to its receptor.[175]

As seen with the other nontraditional risk factors, there are extensive observational data implicating vascular calcification and effectors of vascular calcification in the pathogenesis of CVD in individuals with CKD. Providing a physiological basis for the hypotheses that abnormal calcium and phosphorus handling affects vascular calcification, in vitro studies have linked increased vascular calcification to both hyperphosphatemia[176,177] and hyperparathyroidism[178] and have shown that less vascular calcification accompanies low to moderate doses of vitamin D receptor activators.[179]

Multiple longitudinal studies, including an evaluation of DOPPS data, have demonstrated increased cardiovascular and all-cause mortality with higher serum phosphate levels, supporting this hypothesis, with the greatest mortality risks associated with serum calcium levels above 10 mg/dL, phosphorus levels greater than 7.0 mg/dL, and PTH levels greater than 600 pg/mL[180]; other observational data suggest that changes in levels of calcium, phosphate, and PTH to current

TABLE 12.6 Currently Hypothesized Mediators of Arterial Calcification in Chronic Kidney Disease

Factor	Sources and Regulation	Status in CKD	Hypothesized Role in Vascular Calcification
Precipitants			
Phosphorus	Dietary intake Phosphorus binders Vitamin D Dialysis clearance FGF-23/Klotho Parathyroid hormone	↑↑↑	Passive precipitation with calcium Higher intracellular phosphate induces osteogenic behavior of VSMCs
Calcium	Parathyroid hormone Dietary intake Calcium-containing medications Dialysate Vitamin D	↔	Passive precipitation with phosphorus Higher intracellular calcium induces osteogenic behavior of VSMCs
Calcification Inhibitors			
Fetuin A	Negative acute phase reactant	Variable	Inhibits local precipitation of calcium and phosphorus
Osteoprotegerin	Modulates osteoclast activation by indirectly preventing RANKL binding	Likely ↑ (but relative deficiency)	Local inhibition of cartilage and vascular calcification
Matrix Gla protein	Activated by vitamin K-dependent γ-carboxylation (Warfarin reduces active MGP)	Likely ↑ (but relative deficiency)	Local inhibition of cartilage and vascular calcification

FGF-23, Fibroblast growth factor 23; *MGP*, matrix gla protein; *RANKL*, Receptor Activator of NF-kB-ligand; *VSMC*, vascular smooth muscle cell.

clinical target ranges are associated with improved outcomes.[181] Similarly, other large dialysis cohorts have shown worse outcomes in the presence of lower vitamin D levels and benefit associated with vitamin D analog use.[182-184] These data are reviewed in more detail in Chapter 11.

Critically, similar to that seen with the other nontraditional risk factors, there is a paucity of clinical trial data associating management of CKD-MBD with improved cardiovascular and mortality outcomes. Although observational studies suggest that vitamin D analogs, phosphorus binders versus placebo, and noncalcium-containing binders versus calcium-containing phosphorus binders all reduce vascular calcification and CVD in CKD stages 3 to 5,[183,185-187] trial data have not consistently supported a benefit for hard cardiovascular or mortality outcomes for any of these interventions; in particular, the interpretation of studies evaluating phosphate binder selection has been controversial.[169,188,189] The KDIGO MBD guidelines, which were updated in 2016, focused more on CVD than bone disease, reflecting the paradigm that MBD has substantial cardiovascular implications.[190] Citing multiple small studies, mostly in CKD stage 4, that compared calcium carbonate or calcium acetate to noncalcium-containing binders and showed greater vascular calcification with the calcium-containing binders, the CKD-MBD guidelines suggested avoidance of calcium-containing binders.[190] This KDIGO statement, which is based on low-level surrogate data, remains controversial,[191] as does a similar KDIGO statement elevating cinacalcet to a first-line therapy based on the interplay between CKD-MBD and CVD and results from post hoc analyses of the EVOLVE trial.[190-193] Additional research is urgently needed to further evaluate the role of abnormal mineral and bone metabolism in CVD and the effect of MBD management strategies on CVD and mortality outcomes.

Other Nontraditional Risk Factors

Other nontraditional risk factors for CVD include anemia (see Chapter 9), lipoprotein abnormalities, sympathetic tone, malnutrition, and sleep abnormalities.[194] Some of these issues are discussed at length elsewhere in this text, and anemia, in part, is referred to in this chapter's earlier discussion of LVH.

CARDIOVASCULAR DISEASE CLINICAL SYNDROMES

Ischemic Heart Disease

Epidemiology

As discussed earlier, IHD is common in patients with CKD stage 3 to 4 and in dialysis patients. Although there has been considerable improvement in CVD outcomes in the general population, progress in the CKD population, including dialysis, has lagged, with little improvement seen in CVD outcomes, particularly among dialysis patients, relative to improvements in the general population.[80,195-199]

Pathophysiology and Manifestations: Atherosclerosis and Vascular Stiffness

Arterial disease in individuals with CKD can be broadly classified as relating to atherosclerosis, which is a focal process of plaque formation resulting in luminal narrowing, and vascular stiffness, which is a diffuse process resulting in increased systolic blood pressure and pulse pressure and compensatory

LVH in the setting of increased afterload (see Table 10.2). In most cases, it is the interplay between atherosclerosis and vascular stiffness, often accompanied by resultant LVH and cardiomyopathy, that yields clinically apparent ischemic CVD.[200]

Atherosclerosis in CKD, particularly in individuals with advanced CKD, has been dubbed "accelerated" in efforts to explain the high prevalence of CVD (which ironically may not be primarily atherosclerotic in nature). Atherosclerosis in CKD may be a manifestation of increasingly severe risk factors that are prevalent as kidney disease progresses, including a highly atherogenic lipid profile.[201] Importantly, IHD may be present without significant atherosclerosis. In one study, up to 50% of nondiabetic dialysis patients with symptoms of myocardial ischemia did not have significant large-caliber coronary artery disease.[202] The authors of this study hypothesized that the patients may have ischemia secondary to the combined effects of volume overload and LVH causing increased myocardial oxygen demand, and small and larger vessel arterial disease, decreased capillary density, and potentially anemia all causing decreased oxygen supply. This was further explored in a small study of hemodialysis patients where coronary flow reserve, incorporating cardiac microvascular disease, was a strong predictor of mortality.[203] This physiology is likely reflected in chronically elevated troponin levels in some dialysis patients and a high incidence of NSTEMI.[95,204,205]

Arterial stiffness is a state of reduced arterial compliance characterized by diffuse dilatation and hypertrophy of large arteries with loss of arterial elasticity. Commonly occurring in aging, arterial stiffness is far more profound in CKD and is potentially related to the high prevalence of hypertension and disorders of mineral metabolism that promote arterial calcification.[171]Arterial stiffness likely has its onset in the early stages of CKD[41] and is often present at the time of dialysis initiation.[206]

Manifestations of vascular stiffness in CKD patients include LVH and changes in the blood pressure profile. Specifically, with loss of arterial elasticity, increased systolic blood pressure with or without a decrease in diastolic blood pressure is common. This results in an increased pulse pressure, which is an independent risk factor for mortality in dialysis patients.[207,208] Other tests that may be more sensitive for identifying the arteriosclerotic phenotype include measures of aortic pulse wave velocity and augmentation index[209]; abnormal aortic pulse wave velocity and augmentation index both are associated with increased mortality in dialysis patients.[210] Accordingly, the role of CKD and, in particular, the dialysis milieu in promoting arteriosclerosis were nicely demonstrated in a report of 14 children receiving hemodialysis who had markedly increased aortic pulse wave velocity and augmentation index compared with controls.[172]

An additional factor that may be important is the concept of capillary density and cardiomyocyte dropout. In animal models of CKD, a reduction in the number of cardiomyocytes and hypertrophy of the remaining myocytes has been appreciated with lower eGFR,[211] whereas in a small autopsy study, myocardial capillary density was significantly lower in patients with kidney failure receiving dialysis than in patients with essential hypertension and normotensive controls.[212] Taken in sum with recognition of atherosclerotic disease and vascular stiffness in individuals with kidney disease, it is likely that cardiac ischemia in many patients with CKD represents a multifactorial process with synergistic interaction among disease phenotypes.

Diagnosis

Although IHD is extremely common in CKD, routine screening is not currently recommended in the absence of clinical manifestations of CVD. Available diagnostic tools are similar to those used in the general population and include resting echocardiography for evaluation of cardiac structure and function, exercise and pharmacological stress testing for detection of perfusion defects, laboratory tests for assessment of both acute ischemia and chronic cardiac risk, and cardiac catheterization for anatomical description and possible repair of coronary anatomy. There is no single test for identifying IHD in patients with CKD, and each test currently in use has disadvantages specific to CKD that may affect sensitivity and specificity. The best initial option to identify cardiac ischemia is likely a functional assessment of perfusion that includes cardiac imaging (given the high prevalence of baseline electrocardiogram (ECG) abnormalities in CKD patients); readily available options include exercise or pharmacological nuclear stress tests and exercise or pharmacological stress echocardiography. As a single test, stress echocardiography, either exercise or pharmacological if exercise is not feasible, may be particularly useful because echocardiography also provides information on valvular and other structural disease.[213] Although individuals with CKD may represent a higher-risk population for complications of angiography, including bleeding and restenosis with or without stenting, there is no specific contraindication to cardiac catheterization in CKD.[214,215] Although preservation of existing kidney function is an important consideration in all stages of kidney disease, including for those receiving dialysis, many individuals with CKD can avoid significant contrast nephropathy with careful management, preparatory hydration, conservative use of iodinated contrast,[215] and, possibly, periprocedure holding of renin-angiotensin-aldosterone system blocking agents,[216] although further study is required, particularly for this last item.

Several other noninvasive imaging tests may identify coronary disease or increased risk of coronary disease. These include increased intima-media thickness of the carotid wall that is detectable by ultrasound and that may correlate with disease in other arterial beds.[217,218] In addition, electron beam computerized tomography (EBCT) has also emerged as a sensitive method to detect vascular (coronary artery) calcification that correlates with atherosclerosis and predicts development of clinical coronary artery disease in the general population.[219] However, EBCT may not be an ideal method to detect atherosclerosis in CKD because it is unable to distinguish between intimal calcifications of atherosclerosis and medial calcification that is common in CKD,[220] and its utility in clinical practice remains uncertain.[221]

Laboratory evaluation of coronary syndromes in CKD patients also is challenging, as many of the markers used in the general population, including cardiac troponin I and T, N-Terminal pro-B-type natriuretic peptide (NT-proBNP), brain natriuretic peptide (BNP), creatine kinase (CK) and the MB subfraction of creatine kinase (CK-MB), and myoglobin all may be chronically elevated. For example, 20% of asymptomatic hemodialysis patients have cardiac troponin T levels that would be consistent with AMI in the general population (>0.1 μg/L).[222] However, these small elevations in cardiac markers do have prognostic importance. Chronic elevation of troponin T predicts mortality in both stages 3 and 4 CKD and dialysis patients, identifying patients with greater left ventricular dilatation and impaired left ventricular systolic and diastolic function,[95,205,223,224] whereas elevations in NT-proBNP and BNP predict underlying IHD and hypertrophy independent of level of kidney function and are also associated with mortality.[95]

Accordingly, although any elevation in these cardiac markers may identify increased chronic risk, in the absence of a suggestive ECG for AMI, diagnosis of AMI may be best accomplished by monitoring the trend of levels of troponin and other cardiac injury markers, because a sequential rise and fall in levels of these markers is consistent with acute cardiac damage.[225]

Prevention and Treatment

In dialysis patients, to date there are no large randomized clinical trials demonstrating a significant survival benefit with any accepted coronary therapies, leaving current practice decisions dependent on observational data and extrapolations from the non-CKD population. The ongoing ISCHEMIA-CKD Trial (NCT01985360), which is randomizing up to 700 individuals with eGFR below 30 mL/min/1.73 m^2, including dialysis patients, either to a routine invasive strategy with cardiac catheterization followed by revascularization plus optimal medical therapy (OMT) or to a conservative strategy of OMT with catheterization and possible revascularization reserved for those who fail OMT, should be informative for treating patients with advanced CKD.[226]

To date, even risk factor management remains uncertain, reflecting the lack of medical evidence, difficulties of balancing blood pressure control with the risk of hypotension, tempering a healthy diet with the risk of malnutrition in the catabolic dialysis milieu, and the challenge of even adequately assessing risk. With little definitive supporting evidence, opinion-based clinical practice guidelines extrapolating data from the nondialysis population have recommended the targets: (1) predialysis blood pressure goal of >140/90 mmHg while avoiding orthostatic and intradialytic hypotension; (2) statin therapy in nondialysis CKD patients and in dialysis patients who are already using statins; and (3) moderate diabetes control based on frequent glucose assessments, with control tighter for likely transplant candidates and those with longer life expectancy. Blood pressure control may be optimally accomplished by achieving appropriate dry weight followed by pharmacological therapy, with opinion favoring the use of ACEIs or ARBs, potentially reflected in a positive trend among a subgroup of dialysis patients with hypertension randomized to fosinopril versus placebo.[227] Finally, smoking cessation efforts are essential in all stages of CKD.

For primary treatment of IHD in dialysis patients, older observational data largely predating the use of drug-eluting stents suggested a long-term benefit to bypass grafting[84,228,229]; however, there are no trial data demonstrating superiority among any of medical management, bypass grafting, or angioplasty with stenting. Observational data suggest a benefit with drug-eluting stents compared with bare metal stents, but these data also are of limited quality.[229,230] Accordingly, it remains difficult to draw firm treatment conclusions, and most care decisions are extrapolated from general population practices. Perhaps reflecting this lack of trial data, it has been shown that individuals with CKD are less likely to receive revascularization therapies, such as coronary artery bypass grafting and percutaneous angioplasty with stenting, and typically appropriate medications after AMI, including aspirin, beta-blocking agents, ACEIs, and lipid-lowering agents.[33,231]

For individuals with stage 3b or 4 CKD, therapeutic data, particularly data evaluating primary prevention, similarly are lacking, predominantly reflecting the fact that many studies have excluded participants with elevated serum creatinine.[232] Therefore we rely on post hoc subgroup analyses derived from larger clinical trials that often excluded individuals with serum creatinine above 2 or 3 mg/dL. In general, most of these studies demonstrate benefits for stage 3 to 4 CKD patients that are similar to those appreciated in the general population, and treatment strategies for primary prevention of cardiac disease in individuals with CKD mirror those seen in the general population.[66,67] The Systolic Blood Pressure Intervention Trial (SPRINT) was one of the largest trials including patients with CKD stage 3 without diabetes and demonstrated that targeting a lower systolic blood pressure threshold of less than 120 mmHg was associated with a lower risk of CVD events.[233] Notably, there are challenges specific to the CKD population, including more frequent hyperkalemia with blockade of the renin-angiotensin-aldosterone system and an increased risk of rhabdomyolysis seen with statin therapy and, in particular, with dual statin and fibrate therapy (a combination that should be avoided in advanced CKD).

Among individuals with stage 3 to 4 CKD and those receiving dialysis, there are minimal trial data on secondary prevention strategies; however, in the absence of active or chronic gastrointestinal bleeding, there is no specific contraindication to chronic antiplatelet therapy with aspirin or clopidogrel, and SPRINT data again suggest that intensive blood pressure control may be beneficial in those with prior CVD and CKD stage 3.[234] Observational data are extensive, with studies demonstrating that beta blockers, ACEIs, and aspirin are beneficial in patients with stage 3 to 5 CKD and IHD.[235-237]

Heart Failure

Heart failure is generally characterized by volume overload, pulmonary edema, and dyspnea. Heart failure may occur as a result of either left ventricular systolic dysfunction or diastolic dysfunction in which the left ventricle has a normal ejection fraction but impaired filling.

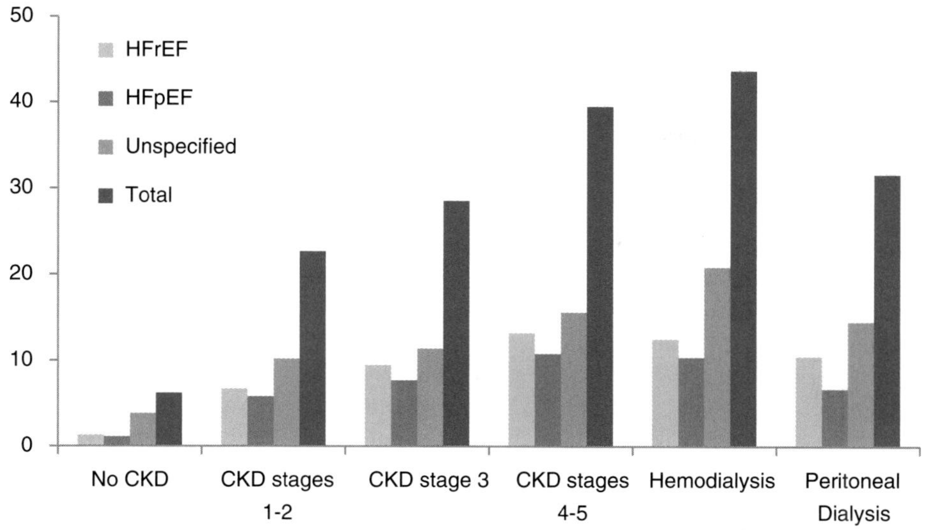

FIG. 12.7 Heart failure prevalence by CKD stage among older US adults in 2014. Data are abstracted from the USRDS 2016 Annual Data Report,[240] which utilized the Medicare 5% sample, limited to patients aged 66 and older, alive, and residing in the United States on 12/31/2014 with fee-for-service coverage for the entire calendar year. Heart failure status is based on diagnosis codes. *CKD*, Chronic kidney disease *HFrEF*, heart failure with reduced ejection fraction; *HFpEF*, heart failure with preserved ejection fraction.

Epidemiology

Both prevalent heart failure and incident heart failure are common in CKD. For incident heart failure, in the ARIC study of individuals aged 45 to 64 years, those with an eGFR less than 60 mL/min/1.73 m^2 at baseline had twice the risk of hospitalization for heart failure and death compared with participants with an eGFR of at least 90 mL/min/1.73 m^2, regardless of the presence of baseline coronary disease.[238] Similarly, in a population of 60,000 insured individuals in northern California with prevalent chronic heart failure, 24% had an eGFR of 45 to 59 mL/min/1.73 m^2, 11% had an eGFR of 30 to 44 mL/min/1.73 m^2, and 4% had an eGFR less than 30 mL/min/1.73 m^2 (not receiving dialysis).[239] Based on claims data, heart failure becomes increasingly common with lower eGFR; among Medicare beneficiaries with CKD stage 4 to 5 (nondialysis), approximately 40% carry a heart failure diagnosis (Fig. 12.7).[240] The high incidence and prevalence of heart failure extends to the dialysis population, where approximately 25% of hemodialysis and 18% of peritoneal dialysis patients in the United States will be diagnosed with heart failure annually, and approximately 55% of prevalent hemodialysis patients are identified as having a history of heart failure.[241] In echocardiography studies in maintenance dialysis patients, prevalence of heart failure is extremely high, likely reflecting long-standing severe hypertension, volume overload, and loss of vascular compliance. In one small study, 57% of stable hemodialysis patients met criteria for HFpEF, whereas only 13% had heart failure with reduced ejection fraction (HFrEF).[242] Similarly, in a study of peritoneal dialysis patients, HFpEF was more common than HFrEF.[243]

Diagnosis

Although heart failure is a clinical diagnosis, echocardiography is a safe, accurate, and readily available tool for assessment of cardiac structure and function. Several factors particular to dialysis patients may affect the accuracy of echocardiography; specifically, as discussed in the section on LVH, assessment of left ventricular mass may be confounded by volume status and timing of dialysis.[244-246] Several biomarkers, notably BNPs, correlate with left ventricular ejection fraction, can be useful for the diagnosis of acute heart failure in stage 3 CKD, and are associated with future CVD events in all CKD stages.[247,248] Although some data suggest that natriuretic peptide levels may be useful to guide therapy in the general population,[249] the GUIDE-IT trial evaluating use of natriuretic peptides to advise diuretic therapy was stopped early for futility.[250] Critically, there are no data addressing this question in patients with advanced CKD.

Treatment

Acute heart failure therapy differs by CKD stage; diuretics are a mainstay of therapy in nondialysis patients, whereas acute fluid overload in dialysis patients is treated with ultrafiltration. Limited data exist regarding CKD-specific chronic treatment of heart failure, but, for earlier stages of CKD, post hoc analyses of clinical trials suggest that most interventions in the general population also apply. For example, two randomized, placebo-controlled trials studying individuals with diabetes and proteinuric stage 3 to 4 CKD have established a role for ARBs in reducing the risk of developing heart failure; however, these studies failed to show a benefit in cardiovascular or all-cause mortality, possibly reflecting insufficient power to evaluate these secondary outcomes.[251,252] Theoretically, further benefits may be associated with aldosterone blockade, although the use of medications such as spironolactone may be limited by hyperkalemia, especially when used in conjunction with ACEIs or ARBs. Newer potassium-binding agents may facilitate more widespread use of renin-angiotensin-aldosterone system blockade in individuals with CKD. Recent data suggest that sodium glucose cotransporter 2 (SGLT2) inhibitors may also have chronic cardiovascular benefits in individuals with CKD stage 3, including a reduction in heart-failure-related hospitalization.[253]

Beta-blocking agents, another mainstay of chronic heart failure therapy in the general population, also appear beneficial in patients with CKD, with evidence supporting carvedilol use to reduce mortality risk in dialysis patients with left ventricular dysfunction.[254] Cardiac glycosides (e.g., digoxin) are frequently used for heart failure in the general population, where they decrease morbidity but not mortality.[255] Although there are no specific studies of cardiac glycosides in CKD, they should be used extremely judiciously, with careful attention to dosage, drug levels, and potassium balance.

STRUCTURAL DISEASE: PERCARDIAL AND VALVULAR CONDITIONS

Pericardial Disease

Pericardial disease in CKD is generally associated with stage 5 CKD. It most commonly manifests as acute uremic or dialysis-associated pericarditis, although chronic constrictive pericarditis may also be seen. Uremic pericarditis describes patients who develop clinical manifestations of pericarditis before or within 8 weeks of initiation of kidney replacement therapy, whereas dialysis-associated pericarditis by definition occurs after a patient is stabilized on dialysis. The precise etiology of uremic pericarditis and dialysis-associated pericarditis is unknown but may be related to inadequate dialysis and volume overload. With high-flux dialysis, uremic pericarditis is exceedingly rare among dialysis patients after initiation.[256]

Pericarditis may be accompanied by nonspecific symptoms including chest pain, fever, chills, malaise, dyspnea, and cough. Physical examination may reveal a pericardial friction rub. When hemodynamically significant, pericardial disease accompanied by an effusion may be characterized by hypotension, particularly during the hemodialysis procedure.[257] Although other expected signs of pericardial effusion may be present, dialysis-related pericarditis often does not manifest with the classic ECG finding of diffuse ST segment elevation because there may be only minimal inflammation of the epicardium.[258] Echocardiography is helpful to diagnose pericarditis in dialysis patients; however, effusions may be absent in patients who have adhesive, noneffusive pericarditis.

Treatment is dependent on symptoms and effusion size. Small, asymptomatic pericardial effusions are fairly common in dialysis patients and require no acute intervention, whereas larger effusions present a risk for tamponade. Initiation of dialysis is the treatment of choice for uremic pericarditis, whereas intensification of hemodialysis is the mainstay of therapy for dialysis-associated pericarditis but is only effective approximately 50% of the time.[256] Traditionally, heparin has been avoided during dialysis out of concern for hemorrhagic tamponade, although this has not been rigorously studied. Adjuvant medical therapies, including oral and intravenous glucocorticoids and nonsteroidal antiinflammatory medications, have generally not been effective. For patients with hemodynamic instability, treatment consists of emergent drainage of the pericardial effusion. This is generally accomplished by pericardiocentesis or pericardiotomy with or without pericardiostomy for the instillation of long-acting, nonabsorbable glucocorticoids.[259]

Endocarditis

Infective endocarditis is a relatively common complication of hemodialysis,[260-263] which reflects the relatively high incidence of bacteremia, chronic use of dialysis catheters, and the high prevalence of preexisting valvular abnormalities.[264-266] The majority of endocarditis in hemodialysis patients is secondary to gram-positive organisms, with *Staphylococcus aureus* predominating.[263,267-269] Dialysis patients with endocarditis usually have fever; murmurs, leukocytosis, and septic emboli may also be common. The mitral and aortic valves are most often affected.[263] Diagnosis is chiefly dependent on positive blood cultures and clinical suspicion; clinical suspicion should be high in settings where bacteremia is persistent and in individuals with prior history of endocarditis. Transthoracic and transesophageal echocardiography are important in establishing the diagnosis.

Treatment of endocarditis begins with appropriate antibiotic therapy; even with appropriate therapy, however, survival is often poor, with case series showing 30% mortality during the initial hospitalization and 1-year mortality over 50%.[261,263] Surgical intervention may also be appropriate, and indications for surgery are the same as in the general population: progressive valvular destruction, progressive heart failure, recurrent systemic emboli, and failure to respond to appropriate antibiotic therapy. Factors associated with mortality include hypoalbuminemia, involvement of multiple valves, and severe valvular insufficiency. In one study, 30-day survival among patients who had surgery was 80%, whereas it was only 47% among those managed medically.[268] Although current data are observational, an important inference to be made is that hemodialysis patients with endocarditis should be considered surgical candidates if they have indications.

Mitral Annular Calcification

Mitral annular calcification may occur in 30% to 50% of patients on dialysis and is also common in patients during the earlier stages of CKD.[270,271] It is recognized on echocardiography as a uniform, echodense, rigid band located near the base of the posterior mitral leaflet and may progressively involve the posterior leaflet. The pathogenesis of mitral calcification may be linked to altered mineral metabolism.[271,272] Serious complications of mitral annular calcification include conduction abnormalities, embolic phenomena, mitral valve disease, and an increased risk of endocarditis.[273]

Aortic Calcification and Stenosis

Aortic valve calcification is common in dialysis patients, occurring in 28% to 55% of patients. Although the overall prevalence is similar to that seen in the general population, dialysis patients experience aortic valve calcification 10 to 20 years earlier than the general population.[274] Age is the most significant risk factor for aortic valve calcification,[273] and abnormal mineral metabolism may also play a role.[275]

The most significant hazard associated with aortic valve calcification is the potential for the development of progressive immobilization of the aortic leaflets, which eventually restricts flow. Aortic stenosis occurs when the valve leaflets thicken to the extent that commissural fusion can no longer occur and a pressure gradient develops across the aortic valve. In one study of dialysis patients the estimated incidence of symptomatic aortic stenosis was 3.3% per year.[275] Progression of aortic valve calcification to aortic stenosis in dialysis patients appears more rapid than in the general population.[276] Very little evidence exists in the nondialysis CKD population as to the prevalence and progression of valvular abnormalities. Angina, heart failure, and syncope are the cardinal symptoms of critical aortic stenosis. Clinical evidence of aortic stenosis may be more readily evident in dialysis patients as they may have more frequent episodes of intradialytic hypotension, particularly as ultrafiltration can rapidly reduce preload.

Treatment of aortic stenosis is multifaceted, encompassing prevention of progression, eventual repair of the valve, and prevention of complications, including endocarditis consistent with general population guidelines for those with prior infective endocarditis or prosthetic valves.[277] Management of mineral metabolism abnormalities could theoretically slow progression of aortic stenosis, although this has not been proven. Valve replacement is the therapy of choice for critical aortic stenosis, and the timing of surgery is dependent on individual patient characteristics with the caveat that surgery should be performed before left ventricular contractility becomes diminished. Currently there is no consensus about a benefit of prosthetic versus bioprosthetic valves in dialysis patients.[278]

Dialysis patients undergoing valve replacement have a high mortality rate: 17% operative mortality for aortic valve replacement in dialysis patients, 23% for mitral valve replacement, 25% for aortic valve replacement and CABG, and 37% for mitral valve replacement and CABG.[279] However, in most cases the prognosis is worse if clinically indicated surgery is not performed or if emergent, rather than elective, surgery is performed.[270] Transcatheter aortic valve replacement (TAVR), increasingly being used in advanced CKD and dialysis patients, likely has lower risks than surgery, although one series did report 1-year mortality of 30% after TAVR in a dialysis population, whereas other studies reported 1-year mortality of 24% to 35% in CKD stage 4. Of note, evaluation for TAVR requires intravenous contrast administration.[280-282]

ARRHYTHMIA AND SUDDEN CARDIAC DEATH

Patients with CKD are at high risk for arrhythmia due to a high prevalence of structural heart disease (including cardiomyopathy, mitral annular calcification, and other valvular disease), heart failure, and coronary disease. Hemodialysis patients are also exposed to rapid shifts in pH and ions, including potassium, calcium, and magnesium.

Atrial Fibrillation

Both atrial and ventricular arrhythmias are common in dialysis patients. Mirroring the general population, atrial fibrillation is the most common of these arrhythmias, with an annual incidence of over 10%.[283] In the USRDS Dialysis Morbidity and Mortality Study (DMMS) Wave 2 cohort, 123 out of 3374 patients (3.6%) were hospitalized with a primary diagnosis of atrial fibrillation (12.5 hospitalizations per 1000 person years),[284] whereas in a contemporary Austrian cohort, 27% of prevalent dialysis patients had either paroxysmal, persistent, or permanent atrial fibrillation.[285]

The major complications of atrial fibrillation include loss of the "atrial kick" and cardiac synchronicity, leading to diminished cardiac function and occurrence of thromboembolic phenomena. Very little data exist as to how common thromboembolism is in dialysis patients with atrial fibrillation. Optimal management involves rate control with or without restoration of sinus rhythm, although patients with symptoms may benefit from a return to sinus rhythm.[286-288] Beta blockers and calcium channel blockers are useful for rate control, whereas amiodarone is useful both for slowing the rate and for chemical cardioversion. Anticoagulation with warfarin has not been prospectively studied in clinical trials in dialysis patients and may be associated with greater risk of vascular calcification and calciphylaxis, making the balance of benefits and risks uncertain.[284,289] At this time, the benefits and risks of anticoagulation in dialysis patients should be considered on an individual patient basis, whereas it is likely that most patients with nondialysis CKD can be treated according to general population recommendations[290,291]; notably, however, the safety of newer oral anticoagulants remains uncertain in advanced CKD.[289] More data are eagerly awaited evaluating the safety and efficacy of both warfarin and newer oral anticoagulants when used for primary stroke prevention in dialysis patients with atrial fibrillation.[289]

Ventricular Arrhythmias and Sudden Death

Ventricular arrhythmias and ectopy are also common in CKD. There are currently no data indicating that cardiac management of patients prone to arrhythmia should be any different than in the general population. Identified arrhythmias and cardiac arrest of unknown cause account for approximately 25% to 30% of all deaths in dialysis patients.[240,292,293] During the first year of dialysis, the rate of cardiac arrest is 93 events per 1000 patient years. Thirty-day survival after cardiac arrest is only 32%, and 1-year survival is 15%. When cardiopulmonary arrest occurs in-hospital in dialysis patients, only 22% survive to hospital discharge, and of these survivors, median life expectancy is only 5 months.[294]

Potential strategies to reduce the risk of fatal cardiac arrhythmias include careful attention to fluid and electrolyte shifts, as well as conscientious use of medications that may be arrhythmogenic or affect the metabolism of potentially arrhythmogenic medications. Hemodialysis units may benefit from the presence of and training in the use of automated external defibrillators. Other potential interventions may include routine use of beta blockers, although this has not been investigated. Finally, studies of the appropriate use of implantable defibrillators in dialysis patients are needed, with subcutaneous implantable defibrillators an attractive option given the lack of transvenous wires.[295]

A full list of references is available at www.expertconsult.com.

13

Nutrient Metabolism and Protein-Energy Wasting in Chronic Kidney Disease

Helen MacLaughlin, BSc, PhD, Hong Xu, MD, Nicola Marsh, BSc, MSc, Derk C.F. Klatte, MD, and Juan J. Carrero, PhD, MBA

OUTLINE

THE ROLE OF THE KIDNEY IN NUTRIENT HOMEOSTASIS

The kidneys regulate dietary sodium, potassium, and phosphate levels in the body.[1,2] As kidney function declines, there are alterations in maintaining nutrient homeostasis. As kidney disease progresses, there is a reduction in the excretion of solutes, resulting in their accumulation in body fluids. The body is therefore less able to adapt to changes in dietary intake. Table 13.1 summarizes the role of the kidney in maintaining nutrient homeostasis and nutritional implications in chronic kidney disease (CKD).

RATIONALE AND NUTRITIONAL REQUIREMENTS FOR PATIENTS WITH CHRONIC KIDNEY DISEASE

Rationale

CKD is a global health problem, and appropriate nutritional intervention strategies are an essential component in the management of CKD across the spectrum of disease.[3] Adopting a healthy diet, addressing obesity, and achieving optimal diabetes control might slow the decline in glomerular filtration rate and reduce the rates of reaching end-stage renal disease (ESRD). Limiting the intake of certain foods or nutrients may reduce the accumulation of metabolic products and prevent hypertension, proteinuria, and other cardiovascular and bone abnormalities.[4] Nutritional management must consider the failing principle functions of the kidney, such as excretion and homeostatic and hormonal regulation (Fig. 13.1). A large body of research has been focused mainly on individual dietary characteristics (single nutrients). More recently, however, there has been a shift toward the evaluation of whole dietary patterns in understanding the role of diet in the development and progression of CKD.[5]

Energy Requirements

Understanding energy needs in the CKD population is important to enable adequate provision of nutrition to avoid protein-energy wasting (PEW) and conversely to limit overweight and obesity given their contribution to the progression of cardiovascular and renal damage. CKD-specific energy intake guidelines suggest that patients with CKD require 30 to 35 kcal/kg/day,[6] which is greater than individuals without CKD because of their increased resting energy expenditure (REE). Inflammation and comorbidities associated with CKD and ESRD may all contribute to an increased REE. Adequate energy intake is usually required to maintain neutral or positive nitrogen balance[7,8]; however, assessment should be made on an individual basis.

Both protein and energy requirements should be adjusted to attain a healthy body weight (express as per ideal body weight [IBW]) and be adjusted for age because of the higher protein needs of the elderly population.[9] A patient's daily energy expenditure should be considered too, because it has been suggested that current energy recommendations (30 to 35 kcal/kg/day) may overestimate a patient's needs. Lean body mass is the primary determinant of energy expenditure, and a low lean body mass is common within the CKD population, offering a possible explanation for their lower than anticipated energy requirements.[10] Furthermore, although reduced food intake is often seen in patients with CKD,[11] a degree of underreporting in energy intake cannot be excluded. As a whole, some authors propose that energy requirements for patients with CKD (30 to 35 kcal/kg/day) should be revised or individualized, especially for those who are sedentary.[12]

TABLE 13.1 Kidney Functions in Nutrient Homeostasis

Kidney Functions in Nutrient Homeostasis	Nutritional Disorders That Appear in CKD
Regulation of sodium and potassium via tight control of body fluid osmolality	Dietary sodium, potassium, and fluid modification
Peptide and amino acid balance via the synthesis, degradation, filtration, and reabsorption of amino acids and the elimination of urea, uric acid, and creatinine	Reduced appetite, nausea, vomiting, and anorexia and thus increased risk for suboptimal energy and nutrient intake
Glucose homeostasis via hormone degradation, excretion, and reabsorption	Altered glucose regulation
Clearance of low-molecular-weight proteins, including insulin, growth hormone, and leptin	Altered appetite signaling
Acid–base balance—the regulation of pH by removing excess hydrogen ions	Acidosis; may consider dietary acid load
Vitamin D_3 activation via hydroxylation of calcidiol to calcitriol for the regulation of calcium, phosphorous, and parathyroid hormone	Altered renal bone metabolism May require modification of dietary phosphorous

CKD, Chronic kidney disease.

A final consideration for determining energy requirements is glucose-based exchanges that take place within peritoneal dialysis (PD). These provide in the region of 300 kcal per exchange, contributing up to 30% of the total daily energy intake of patients undergoing PD.[13] This should be taken into consideration when assessing energy intake in these patients.

Protein Requirements

For stable patients with CKD not requiring dialysis, the recommended protein intake is 0.6 to 0.8 g/kg/day, of which more than two-thirds should be of high biological value.[6] Habitual protein intakes in the general population are usually higher; hence, this level of protein intake is often called *low* or *reduced* protein intake. Reducing protein intake (compared with usual intake in the general population) may result in a reduction in uremic symptoms and slower progression of kidney failure.[7] Lower protein diets may also improve hyperkalemia and hyperphosphatemia.[14] Furthermore, in patients with established CKD, a lower protein intake, compared with an unrestricted intake, has been associated with a 32% lower occurrence of renal death.[9,15]

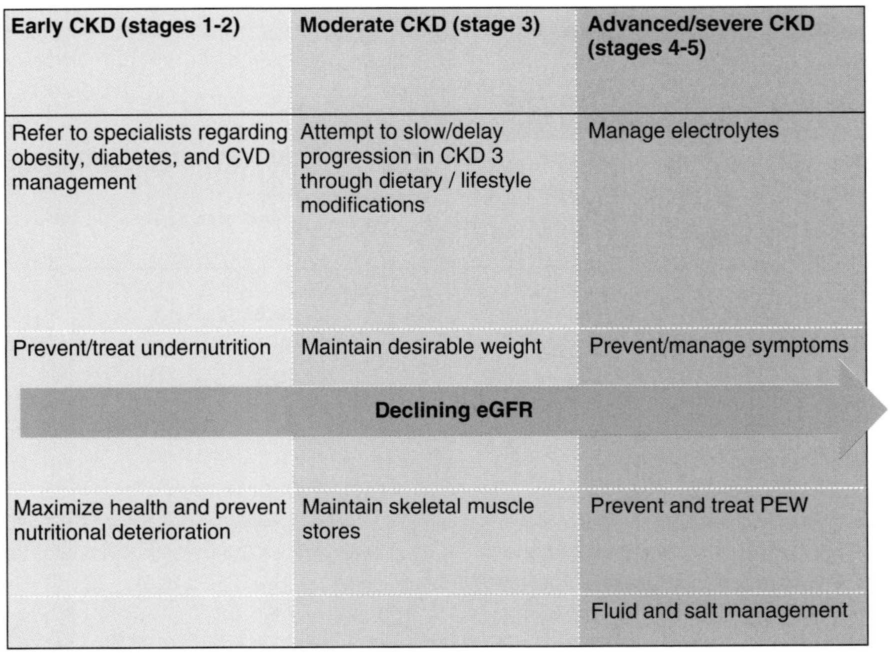

FIG. 13.1 Nutritional and lifestyle management goals and interventions for patients with declining kidney function. *CVD,* Cardiovascular disease; *eGFR,* estimated glomerular filtration rate; *PEW,* protein-energy wasting.

However, the optimal level and type of protein intake (animal vs. plant) remains unclear. Recent studies have suggested that plant proteins may be more protective than animal proteins in the primary prevention of CKD.[4] Nonetheless, confounding factors make drawing conclusions challenging given that plant protein is not consumed in isolation.[5] Fig. 13.2 illustrates the key differences in the nutritional profile of plant and animal proteins, highlighting that the benefits of consuming a plant-based diet probably go beyond the source of protein.

The efficacy and safety of a "low-protein diet" remain equivocal. The arguments for and against are illustrated in Table 13.2.

Use of a very-low-protein diet (0.3 g/kg IBW/day plus keto-analog of amino acid supplements) in patients with advanced CKD is regarded as an effective treatment to delay renal death by delaying commencement of dialysis for 1 to 2 years.[16] Switching to a very-low-protein diet should be carefully considered and managed to avoid nutritional inadequacies.[4]

Protein intake should be increased on starting dialysis, because those with higher protein intakes have had improved rates of survival.[17,18] Higher protein requirements are a result of dialysis-related protein loss,[13] greater energy expenditure,[19] and persistent inflammation.[20] PD protein loss can be considerable; however, variation among individuals in transporter status and energy and protein intake and choice of dialysate should also be considered.[13]

Nutritional recommendations tend to be made based on total nutrient intakes (i.e., total protein intake per day); however, the dietary pattern (timing and portion size) of protein intake may be an important consideration in the CKD population. In muscle metabolism research in healthy and older populations, there has been a shift away from total daily protein intake targets toward specific dose and timing recommendations. In healthy individuals, protein ingestion is a key stimulus for preserving skeletal muscle mass under rest and increasing skeletal muscle mass under exercise training conditions.[21] Although dependent on age and recent exercise stimuli, general recommendations suggest that each meal should contain approximately 0.25 g of high-quality protein per kilogram of body weight (or an absolute dose of 20 to 40 g) evenly distributed across three to four meals each day to

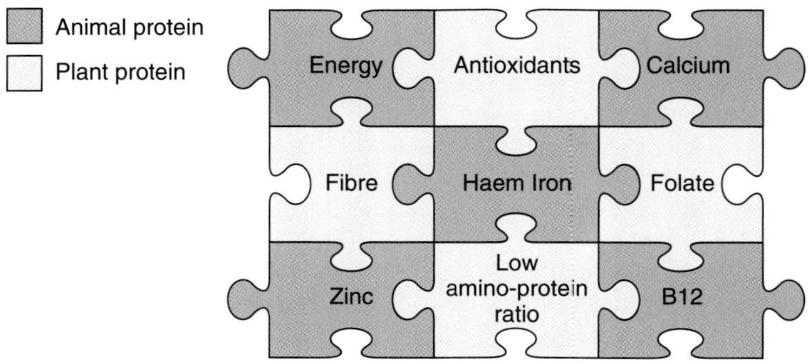

FIG. 13.2 Key differences in the nutritional profiles of plant and animal proteins. Nutrients are not consumed in isolation, but collectively in the foods. In light gray are shown nutrients frequently accompanying plant-based proteins and in dark gray nutrients frequently present with meat-based proteins. Accompanying nutrients can de facto impact on kidney function decline or preservation. (Adapted from Kelly JT, Carrero JJ. Dietary sources of protein and chronic kidney disease progression: the proof may be in the pattern. *J Ren Nutr.* 2017;27(4):221-224.)

TABLE 13.2 **Summary of Arguments For and Against the Implementation of a Low-Protein Diet in Patients With Non–Dialysis-Dependent Chronic Kidney Disease**

Rationale	For	Against
Efficacy of low-protein diet	Improves signs and symptoms of insulin resistance, osteodystrophy, and peripheral neuropathy.	Benefits reported in experimental models, but clinical evidence is lacking.
Slowing CKD progression rate	Findings are inconsistent findings because of variation in study design. Meta-analysis (Hahn et al., 2018, in press/under review, *Cochrane*) suggests very low protein diets (0.3–0.4 g/kg) may delay progression to end stage.	Benefits reported in experimental models, but publication bias favors positive results. Meta-analysis (Hahn et al., 2018 in press/under review, *Cochrane*) reported no difference in progression to end stage between low- (0.5–0.6 g/kg) and normal-protein (0.8–1.0 g/kg) diets.
Renoprotective effects	May help decrease albuminuria, proteinuria, and total sodium and phosphate intake.	No additional benefit beyond renin-angiotensin-aldosterone system blockade and blood pressure reduction.
Safety and lack of adverse effects	Supervised diet management preserves nutritional status, does not jeopardize survival, improves symptom score.	May induce or exacerbate malnutrition if unsupervised.
Adherence	Good adherence noted in a number of intervention studies.	Quality-of-life outcome measures have not been assessed.

Adapted from Chan M, Kelly J, Tapsell L. Dietary modeling of foods for advanced CKD based on general healthy eating guidelines: what should be on the plate? *Am J Kidney Dis.* 2017;69(3):436-450.

optimize muscle protein synthesis.[22] Furthermore, the amino acid content of dietary proteins should be considered, because leucine content appears to be a critical factor in postprandial muscle protein synthesis.[23] Studies are yet to be conducted in populations with CKD; however, it seems prudent to consider an even distribution of protein intake across each day when nutritional counseling or education is undertaken with patients.

Electrolytes

Sodium and Fluid Balance

Hypertension is a well-established cause and complication of CKD, and dietary interventions reducing salt intake have been found to be effective in reducing hypertension.[24] Sodium is thus an important nutritional consideration given its influence on blood pressure as well as fluid retention[8] and its role in exacerbating renal damage.[4] Dietary assessment should identify sources of packaged and preprepared foods (e.g., canned soups, processed meats, and ready-made meals) given that sodium is often added during manufacturing. In the early stages of CKD it is recommended to restrict salt intake to moderately low levels (<6 g/day of salt or <100 mmol of sodium). Furthermore, the restriction of salt may help manage thirst and thus aid compliance with fluid restrictions (Table 13.3).

Phosphorus

Those with renal impairment gradually lose the ability to excrete phosphorous, resulting in hyperphosphatemia, which has been found to be a strong predictor of mortality in patients with advanced stages of CKD.[25] The role of serum phosphate in the pathogenesis of vascular calcification and left ventricular hypertrophy might explain the link between elevated concentrations of serum phosphate and a higher mortality in dialysis patients.[26] Inorganic phosphorous found as an additive in processed foods is more biologically available compared with organic phosphorous found in plant and animal foods.[18] Excess consumption of phosphorus-rich food can be managed via dietary change targeting inorganic phosphorus and nutrient-poor foods first, then taking into account the phosphorous-to-protein ratio of animal and plant origin and the use of phosphorous binders and dialysis[4] (Table 13.4).

TABLE 13.3 Strategies to Aid Fluid Restriction Compliance

Strategies to Decrease Fluid Intake	Strategies to Decrease/ Manage Thirst
Spread out fluid allowance throughout day.	Avoid savory snacks.
Use smaller cups or tea cups.	Limit adding salt during cooking/at the table.
Use the jug method to aid awareness.	Hard-boiled sweets/mints/ chewing gum can stimulate saliva production.
Perform self-monitoring of intake and output.	Suck on frozen segments of lemon or lime.
	Administer artificial saliva spray.
	Sparingly use ice cubes.

Potassium

Individuals with CKD are at risk for hyperkalemia given the role of the kidneys in potassium homeostasis. Hyperkalemia has been associated with higher mortality in ESRD and dialysis patients because of its arrhythmogenic effects.[27] Recognizing nondietary causes, avoiding medications that might promote potassium retention (such as renin-angiotensin-aldosterone system inhibitors), and reducing intake of high-potassium foods with low nutritional value are recommended as initial steps to address and prevent hyperkalaemia[28] (see Table 13.4). Potassium is associated with healthy, desirable foods such as fruit and vegetables; hence, practitioners should prioritize the avoidance of foods with poor nutritional value first when considering food causes of hyperkalemia so as not to compromise the nutritional adequacy of the diet.

Dietary Quality

Traditionally, dietary management in CKD/ESRD has focused only on modifying single nutrients, such as protein, phosphorus, potassium, or sodium, that can accelerate kidney damage or result in adverse outcomes. It is possible that the overall dietary pattern may be more influential in the development and progression of CKD than an excess or deficiency of specific macro- or micronutrients. Recent observational studies have indicated that a diet rich in fruits, vegetables, fish, cereals, whole grains, dietary fiber, and polyunsaturated fatty acids (and low in saturated fatty acids), such as the Mediterranean and DASH (Dietary Approaches to Stop Hypertension) styles of eating, may be beneficial for patients with CKD.[4] Thus a shift away from interventions that focus on single nutrients toward the overall dietary picture may be advantageous given that healthy dietary patterns have been associated with lower mortality in observational studies.[29] In contrast, the "Western diet" is characterized by a high intake of red meat, animal fat, sweets, and desserts and a low intake of fruits, vegetables, and low-fat dairy products. Adherence to a Western diet has been associated with increased risk for albuminuria, more rapid kidney function decline, and increased inflammation.[30-32]

Several small studies using dietary pattern interventions, such as increasing fruit and vegetables and the Mediterranean diet pattern, have reported improvements in blood pressure and blood lipids; however, no dietary pattern intervention studies have yet examined mortality or CKD progression outcomes.[33]

PROTEIN-ENERGY WASTING IN CHRONIC KIDNEY DISEASE

Concept of Protein-Energy Wasting

PEW was proposed in 2007 by the International Society of Renal Nutrition and Metabolism[34] as a concept defining the multifactorial nature of metabolic processes and nutritional consequences of uremia in CKD. PEW involves a hypermetabolic state that promotes protein catabolism, attributed to

TABLE 13.4 **Possible Food and Nonfood Causes of Hyperkalemia and Hyperphosphatemia**

Electrolyte	Nonfood Causes	Food Causes
Potassium	Constipation	Salt substitutes
	Acidosis—bicarbonate	Chips, crisps, potato products
	Hyperparathyroidism	Nuts, chocolate
	Missed/inadequate dialysis	Fruit juice
	Insulin insufficiency	Not boiling vegetables
	Drugs	Excessive fruit consumption
	Potassium containing	
	Affecting potassium excretion (ACE inhibitors, ARBs, beta blockers, NSAIDs)	
	Potassium-sparing diuretics (spironolactone, amiloride)	
	Cellular trauma (hemolyzed blood samples, post–blood transfusion, infection, GI bleed, crush injury, gangrene)	
Phosphate	Binder compliance	Dark-colored carbonated drinks, chocolate drinks, condensed and evaporated milks, malted milk drinks, fudge
	Binder dose/regimen	Processed foods such as sausages, ham, corned beef, breaded chicken, cheese spread, processed cheese, and instant sauces (often contain phosphates or phosphoric acid)
	Parathyroid hormone/Ca^{2+} management	Organ meats (liver, kidney, heart, pate)
		Oily fish

ACE, Angiotensin-converting enzyme; *ARBs,* angiotensin II receptor blockers; *GI,* gastrointestinal; *NSAIDs,* nonsteroidal antiinflammatory drugs.

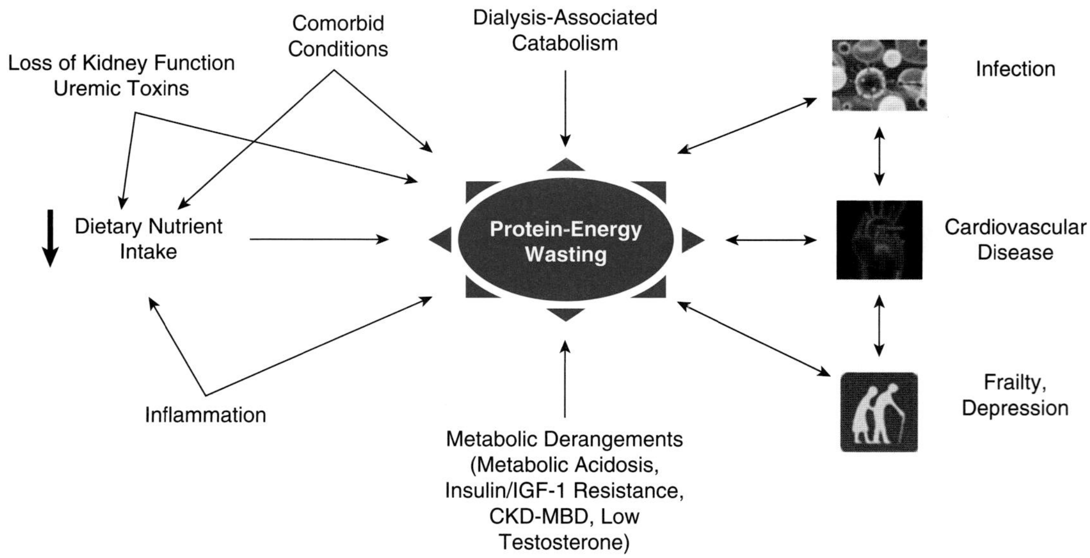

FIG. 13.3 The conceptual model for protein-energy wasting in chronic kidney disease. *CKD-MBD,* Chronic kidney disease–mineral bone disorder; *IGF-1,* insulin-like growth factor 1. (Adapted from Carrero JJ, Stenvinkel P, Cuppari L, et al. Etiology of the protein-energy wasting syndrome in chronic kidney disease: a consensus statement from the International Society of Renal Nutrition and Metabolism (ISRNM). *J Ren Nutr.* 2013;23(2):77-90.)

both metabolic consequences of CKD—including inflammation, oxidative stress, uremia, metabolic acidosis, diminished efficacy of anabolic hormones, and a multimorbid condition—and the catabolic nature of hemodialysis (HD), which can lead to protein losses and muscle and fat wasting (Fig. 13.3). Therefore the reduction in energy and protein intake associated with PEW is often secondary to other factors, rather than a primary consequence of inadequate access to adequate energy and protein to meet nutritional needs, as in primary malnutrition. In clinical practice the reduction in nutritional intake and causes may be difficult to separate because they are synergistic and may exacerbate each other.

BOX 13.1 Causes of Protein-Energy Wasting in Chronic Kidney Disease

1. Decreased protein and energy intake
   a. Anorexia, problems in organs involved in nutrient intake
   b. Dietary restrictions
   c. Depression, frailty, dependency
2. Hypermetabolism
   a. Increased energy expenditure
   b. Metabolic acidosis
   c. Inflammation
   d. Hormonal disorders
      i. Insulin resistance of CKD
      ii. Increased glucocorticoid activity
3. Decreased anabolism
   a. Resistance to GH/IGF-1
   b. Testosterone deficiency
   c. Low thyroid hormone levels
4. Comorbidities and lifestyle
   a. Comorbidities (DM, CHF, depression, CAD, PVD)
   b. Poor physical activity
   c. Unhealthy dietary pattern
5. Dialysis
   a. Nutrient losses into dialysate
   b. Dialysis-related inflammation and hypermetabolism

CAD, Coronary artery disease; *DM,* diabetes mellitus; *GH,* growth hormone; *IGF-1,* insulin-like growth hormone 1; *PVD,* peripheral vascular disease.
Carrero JJ, Stenvinkel P, Cuppari L, et al. Etiology of the protein-energy wasting syndrome in chronic kidney disease: a consensus statement from the International Society of Renal Nutrition and Metabolism (ISRNM). *J Ren Nutr.* 2013;23(2):77-90.

Causes of Protein-Energy Wasting in Chronic Kidney Disease

Understanding the features that contribute to the etiology of PEW is critical to inform appropriate assessment and treatment strategies. Box 13.1 lists the major contributing factors to PEW in CKD, and it is important to note that inadequate intake is just one of the five major causes of PEW. Furthermore, adequate nutritional intake will not alter some of the contributing factors, such as hypermetabolism secondary to inflammation, the reduction in anabolic response, the catabolic nature of HD, insulin resistance, or frailty associated with reduced physical activity. A multifaceted therapeutic approach for this complex syndrome is therefore necessary.

Decreased Protein and Energy Intake

Several observational studies have found that spontaneous protein intake decreases as CKD progresses.[36,37] In addition, the dietary modifications prescribed to reduce protein intake and to prevent hyperkalemia and hyperphosphatemia in CKD stages 4 and 5 may further contribute to poor nutrient intake if these modifications are presented as restrictions only and are not accompanied with counseling on alternative food choices and strategies to ensure adequate nutrient intake.[38] An important cause of undernutrition in CKD is reduced appetite, which decreases with declining estimated glomerular filtration rate and is reported by as many as 35% to 50% of dialysis patients.[36,39,40] Appetite is typically driven by the endocrine system; however, in HD patients, factors related to the dialysis and alterations in the gastrointestinal system, as well as hedonic and social implications, can reduce appetite, and meal times can be missed if eating is not permitted during dialysis.[41]

Hypermetabolism

Increased energy expenditure. REE is usually normal in stable maintenance dialysis or CKD patients. However, REE is increased during the HD procedure or in the presence of comorbidities such as cardiovascular disease, severe hyperparathyroidism, poorly controlled diabetes, inflammation, and PEW.[42,43] Higher energy intake may correct the energy deficit because of increased REE under these circumstances, although it will not reverse the cause of increased energy expenditure and higher intakes may need to be maintained over the long term to prevent unintentional weight loss.

Persistent inflammation. Increased concentration of inflammatory cytokines in CKD is the result of both reduced renal clearance and increased production, stimulated by comorbidities, dialysis, and genetic factors.[44,45] Inflammation induces appetite loss through central mechanisms blocking specific receptors in the melanocortin system, inhibiting feeding behavior and promoting energy expenditure and protein catabolism. Peripheral effects include mucosal inflammation in the mouth, periodontitis, gastritis, and bacterial infections,[46] which can also have a secondary effect via a reduction in nutritional intake as a result of pain or discomfort during or after eating.

Metabolic acidosis. Metabolic acidosis causes protein catabolism through a reduction in albumin synthesis contributing to hypoalbuminemia.[47] Correction of acidosis has been found to improve nutritional status,[48] likely through decreased protein turnover, improved appetite, and total protein intake. The mechanism of action through decreased protein degradation has been demonstrated in both HD[49] and PD.[50]

Decreased Anabolism

Resistance to insulin/insulin-like growth factor 1. Resistance to insulin, growth hormone (GH), and insulin-like growth factor 1 (IGF-1) are implicated in loss of muscle mass in adult patients with CKD. Insulin and IGF-1 normally bind distinct cell surface receptors to prevent loss of muscle protein.[51] Although current evidence suggests that myofiber shrinkage caused by accelerated protein degradation is the predominant mechanism for loss of muscle mass, both myofiber shrinkage and muscle cell fusion are regulated by insulin and IGFs. This has led to the hypothesis that the integrated outputs of these insulin/IGF–activated signaling pathways determines the balance between protein accretion and loss, determining overall changes in muscle mass.[35]

Testosterone deficiency and low thyroid hormone levels. Testosterone is an anabolic hormone that induces skeletal muscle hypertrophy by promoting nitrogen retention, stimulating fractional muscle protein synthesis, inducing myoblast

TABLE 13.5 Typical Comorbidities in Chronic Kidney Disease That Contribute to Protein-Energy Wasting

Comorbidity	Possible Effects Related to Cause of PEW
Diabetes	Gastroparesis, inflammation/oxidation, insulin deprivation (type I), insulin resistance
Cardiovascular disease/heart failure	Cachexia, inflammation, glucocorticoid release, sympathetic nerve overactivity, increased circulating angiotensin II, insulin resistance, decreased activity, pain
Peripheral vascular disease	Reduced activity, ulcers, inflammation, pain
Edema	Inflammatory cytokine release, gut edema, leg ulcers, decreased physical activity, pain
Hyperparathyroidism, CKD-MBD	Increased energy expenditure, glucose intolerance, hypovitaminosis D, muscle wasting, gastric ulcers, heart disease
Anemia	Frailty, decreased activity, iron deficiency, high-output heart failure
Infections	Inflammation, reduced appetite, increased REE, pain
Depression/dementia	Unwillingness to eat, anorexia, inability to obtain/prepare food, inflammation, decreased activity

CKD-MBD, Chronic kidney disease–mineral bone disorder; *PEW*, protein-energy wasting; *REE*, resting energy expenditure.
Adapted from Carrero JJ, Stenvinkel P, Cuppari L, et al. Etiology of the protein-energy wasting syndrome in chronic kidney disease: a consensus statement from the International Society of Renal Nutrition and Metabolism (ISRNM). *J Ren Nutr*. 2013;23(2):77-90.

differentiation, and augmenting the efficiency of amino acid reuse by the skeletal muscle. In CKD, more than 40% of dialysis patients are testosterone deficient. Testosterone deficiency in CKD patients has been associated with anemia and erythropoietin hyporesponsiveness, as well as with reduced muscle mass and strength.[52]

Available data cannot distinguish if low thyroid hormone levels in CKD patients with PEW are an adaptation that reduces energy expenditure and minimizes protein catabolism in PEW.[53] Low triiodothyronine (T3) levels in CKD correlate with systemic inflammatory markers, endothelial dysfunction, and both all-cause and cardiovascular mortality,[54] although the relationship with mortality is mediated through inflammation.[55] Correction of metabolic acidosis in dialysis patients improves these hormonal derangements.[56]

Comorbidities and Poor Physical Activity

Comorbidities. Common comorbidities that arise as a consequence of the failing kidney also contribute to catabolism, resulting in PEW. As Table 13.5 shows, these factors share common etiological mechanisms with PEW.

Poor physical activity. Reduced physical activity plays a major role in both the cause of PEW and the associated adverse outcomes. Individuals with poor physical activity are at higher risk for developing CKD as a result of associated obesity, diabetes, hypertension, and heart disease. Furthermore, complications of CKD, including anemia, edema, and muscle wasting, limit exercise capacity, which, at the extreme level, can affect the ability to perform usual activities of daily living.[57] In CKD stage 3 to 5, median peak oxygen consumption is decreased, which can limit exercise capacity, and muscle weakness is common, although exercise training can improve functional capacity and muscle strength.[57]

Dialysis

Hemodialysis. The HD procedure activates an inflammatory cascade,[58] and amino acid and protein losses occur during dialysis. This catabolic process together with low nutrient intake reduces nutrient availability for muscle synthesis and acute-phase reactant synthesis,[59] resulting in the breakdown of muscle protein.[60] Concurrent amino acid supplementation during the dialysis session can prevent or reverse these effects.[61] Further, optimizing dialysis provision or increasing the frequency of the dialysis procedure has been associated with improvements in nutritional markers because of a reduction in uremic factors.[62] Finally, HD results in a more rapid loss of residual renal function, which is also associated with poor nutritional status.[63]

Peritoneal dialysis. In PD, losses of amino acids into the dialysate of up to 60 g/week occur.[64] In addition, greater losses occur during an episode of peritonitis, as inflammation leads to muscle catabolism.[65] In both cases, these losses increase the protein requirement for dialysis patients. It has been found in PD patients that loss of residual kidney function contributes to PEW.[66]

Prevalence of Protein-Energy Wasting in Chronic Kidney Disease

The prevalence of undernutrition in CKD patients varies depending on the assessment methodology employed, geographical region, and criteria used to define nutritional status. There is no single measure of nutritional status in CKD, and a combination of biochemical anthropometric and nutritional intake assessment measures is recommended.

Few PEW prevalence studies have been done among nondialysis CKD patients. Those that used subjective global assessment (SGA) describe a prevalence of 12% to 18% in CKD stage 3 to 4 patients.[67,68] Those using serum albumin suggest that PEW is present in 20% to 40% of patients with CKD stage 3 to 5 who are not on dialysis,[7,69,70] although this suggests that inflammation is present, and may not be associated with a poorer nutritional status, which may account for the higher prevalence rates when albumin is used rather than a global measure of nutritional status.

PEW becomes much more common in the ESRD/dialysis patient.[71] Studies suggest prevalence rates of between 20% to 70% for PEW or undernutrition in patients undergoing either HD or PD, using malnutrition–inflammation score (MIS) or SGA methods to assess nutritional status and PEW.[72-82] Differences in nutritional status in dialysis patients across the world may be due to the adequacy of dialysis treatment in different countries, the usual diet, socioeconomic status, and the type of dialysis treatment used. Improvements in dialysis membranes and water purity over time are also likely to affect the inflammatory processes associated with dialysis and may have contributed to a reduction in the prevalence of undernutrition in more recent studies.

Consequences of Protein-Energy Wasting in Chronic Kidney Disease

Nutrients are the substrates for energy, tissue synthesis, and metabolism and are necessary for life. Undernutrition and hypermetabolism, the two features of PEW, lead to a number of metabolic abnormalities, such as inflammation,[83] oxidative stress,[84] and impaired immune function,[85] which per se or in addition to other factors increase the risk for poor quality of life, infection, hospitalizations, cardiovascular disease, and mortality.[72,73,86-88]

Mortality, Cardiovascular Events, Infections, and Hospitalizations

Most markers of PEW have been associated with adverse patient outcomes in HD patients,[72,86-88] including the incidence of hospitalizations,[89,90] increased healthcare costs,[89] and increased risk for infections, cardiovascular events, and death.[91-94]

An important aspect of epidemiological studies is their observational nature, which does not allow us to differentiate whether these associations with adverse outcomes are causal in nature. It is ethically difficult to design randomized controlled trials targeting treatment of PEW to assess the impact on mortality and quality of life. Several epidemiological studies have explored this issue based on the potential of providing oral nutritional support to hypoalbuminemic patients through quality improvement initiatives. In one study hypoalbuminemic individuals receiving nutritional support had a 34% reduction in 1-year mortality risk compared with those who did not receive it.[95] Nutritional support in persistently hypoalbuminemic HD patients reduced hospitalizations rates during the subsequent year by approximately 20%[96] versus those who did not receive it. Implementation of a protocol to provide nutritional support during HD on diagnosis of hypoalbuminemia and to maintain albumin within normal range was associated with a 30% reduction in mortality compared with similar patients not receiving nutritional support.[97]

Frailty and Poor Quality of Life

PEW plays an important role in the development and progression of frailty and poor quality of life in patients with CKD. Frailty and the individual components of frailty (unintentional weight loss, self-reported exhaustion, measured weakness, slow walking speed, low physical activity, and reduced muscle mass less than the 90th percentile for the age- and sex-matched general population) are common, closely related with PEW and muscle wasting, and associated with morbidities and mortality in patients with CKD, especially those requiring maintenance dialysis therapy.[98] The Chronic Renal Insufficiency Cohort study revealed that the prevalence of frailty in CKD stage 2 and stage 4 is 7% and 43%, respectively, indicating that muscle loss and frailty, as with PEW, may develop and progress during the course of CKD.[99] In a study of nondialysis CKD and incident HD patients, muscle mass, evaluated by multislice computed tomography, declined over time.[100] PEW also is strongly associated with a poor quality of life. In a cohort study of quality of life, as evaluated with the Short Form 36 questionnaire, and PEW, measured using the MIS, in 800 stable prevalent HD patients in the United States, PEW was associated with worse quality-of-life scores for general health and physical and mental health component scores.[73]

NUTRITION SCREENING AND ASSESSMENT

Systematic screening and assessment of nutritional status are essential in the management of patients with CKD. Nutrition screening aims to identify nutritional risk and initiates the systematic process of nutrition assessment. Nutrition assessment involves collecting and interpreting relevant information to identify nutrition-related problems, including PEW. This allows for the implementation and monitoring of an appropriate intervention.

There is no single measure that can provide a valid diagnosis of PEW in CKD given that its cause is multifactorial in nature. A range of measures should therefore be assessed, including anthropometric changes, biochemical parameters, and dietary intake. Data should, however, be interpreted with caution because nutritional markers such as albumin may be influenced by fluid status, inflammation, and renal replacement therapy. Furthermore, anthropometric measurements may be skewed by the presence of edema. Careful consideration of these confounding factors must be given before making a diagnosis.

Screening Tools

The goal of screening is to identify individuals who are at risk for undernutrition (and PEW) or who are malnourished and require nutrition intervention, including referral to a registered dietitian for nutrition assessment. Screening tools use measures that can be routinely collected in clinical practice, including body weight, other visual and palpable signs of muscle wasting,[101] and changes in food intake. Screening can virtually be performed by any healthcare professional. There is no consensus on the frequency of nutritional screening in chronic diseases such as CKD, although monthly to 3-month intervals have been proposed.[102] Table 13.6 describes several screening tools currently used in clinical practice. Is it important to screen patients for nutritional status, but the choice of screening tool is less important. These screening tools, however, are generic and may not be able to identify individuals with CKD who are at risk for malnutrition if changes in body weight are a key component of the tool, because often loss of body mass is masked by a concomitant increase in edema in advanced stages of CKD.

TABLE 13.6 Overview of Malnutrition Risk Screening Tools

Screening Tool	Description	Parameters Used
Malnutrition Screening Tool (MST)[103,104]	MST is a simple, quick-to-administer, two-question tool.	Unintentional weight loss Appetite
Malnutrition Universal Screening Tool (MUST)[105]	Developed for screening in the community, MUST is widely used in the United Kingdom and Europe.	Unintentional weight loss BMI Disease severity Food intake
Short Nutritional Assessment Questionnaire (SNAQ)[106]	SNAQ is a simple, easy-to-administer, three-question screening tool developed in the Netherlands for hospital screening.	Unintentional weight loss Appetite User of oral supplement or tube feeding
Nutritional Risk Screening 2002 (NRS-2002)[107]	Developed by ESPEN, this is a preferred tool to screen for malnutrition in European settings.	Unintentional weight loss BMI Disease severity Age Impaired general conditions
Mini-Nutritional Assessment (MNA-SF)[108]	MNA-SF was designed specifically for use with elderly patients (aged 65+).	Reduced food intake Weight loss Psychological stress Acute disease Neuropsychological problems BMI
Geriatric Nutritional Risk index (GNRI)[109]	GNRI is a dichotomous index designed for health-care assessment of elderly patients.	Serum albumin values Discrepancy between real and ideal weight

BMI, Body mass index; *ESPEN,* European Society for Clinical Nutrition and Metabolism.

Nutrition Assessment Tools

Anthropometry and Body Composition

Assessment of body weight and composition can be useful to assess the degree of fat and muscle change. Body weight measurements alone will not give any information about body composition[110] and may be influenced by alterations in fluid status. Caution is thus required when interpreting changes in body weight in patients with CKD. Surrogate measures of nutritional status may be applicable to help identify the nature of weight loss (i.e., subcutaneous fat loss versus muscle wasting) and can help monitor changes over time. For example, midarm circumference, calf circumference, and adductor pollicis muscle thickness may provide estimates of muscle mass and fat mass and have been found to predict prognosis in CKD.[101] Handheld dynamometers measure handgrip strength.[111,112]

Bioelectrical impedance analysis may be used to estimate body composition by measuring the resistance of body tissues to a small electrical current. Lean soft tissue (the sum of total body water, skeletal muscle mass, and fat-free parts of organs) is a good conductor, whereas fat, bone, and skin are poor conductors resulting in greater resistance to an electrical current. Because this technology is influenced by hydration status, repeated measures should be taken at a constant time after dialysis to obtain a more reliable assessment of body composition.[101] Dual-energy x-ray absorptiometry (DEXA) is another method used for assessment of body composition. DEXA is a reliable, noninvasive method to assess fat mass, fat-free mass, and bone mineral and density; however, it comes with a substantial cost and is thus not a practical tool for assessing body composition in daily clinical practice.[110,113]

Biochemistry

Laboratory biomarkers may be used to estimate nutritional status or nutrient intake and have the potential to be used in everyday clinical practice. However, laboratory biomarkers are influenced by factors such as uremic retention, fluid status, and inflammation. Therefore biochemical measurements should not be used in isolation but rather in the context of anthropometric, other biochemical, and dietary measures.[114]

Protein equivalent of nitrogen appearance. It is difficult to directly measure protein intake. Therefore an indirect marker used to estimate dietary protein intake is the protein catabolic rate or protein equivalent of nitrogen appearance (PNA). PNA is a valid and clinically useful measure and reflects the amount of protein that is catabolized beyond the amount synthesized per day. The total nitrogen appearance of the body should be equal to or slightly smaller than the nitrogen intake. An estimation of protein intake can be made on the fact that urea nitrogen appearance is highly correlated with total nitrogen appearance.[114] By use of regression equations, PNA can be assessed from the generation of urea nitrogen in blood or dialysate in HD and PD patients, respectively. PNA is usually normalized (nPNA), preferably to the urea distribution volume, which is highly correlated with fat-free or lean body mass. For a correct interpretation of nPNA, the clinician should be aware that nPNA may be affected by the use of corticosteroids and anabolic hormones. Furthermore, nPNA can only be used in a steady state with a relatively constant protein intake and a minimal influence of internal or external stressors.[113] Because of these limitations, PNA should not be used in isolation but together with other markers to evaluate patients' nutritional status[114] and is recommended to be assessed monthly in HD and every 3 to 4 months in PD.[113]

Albumin, prealbumin. Albumin is often considered a marker of nutritional status, albeit incorrectly, although it is highly correlated with mortality and morbidity.[113] Dietary protein intake directly affects serum albumin concentrations; however, its impact on albumin concentrations in the short term is minor because of a long half-life of 20 days.[115] Furthermore, inflammation results in reduced albumin synthesis and an increase in albumin breakdown, resulting in hypoalbuminemia.[113,116] Hypoalbuminemia is more likely to be reflective of an acute-phase response to inflammation or albumin dilution as a result of edema rather than nutritional status.[115]

Serum prealbumin, also known as *transthyretin*, has a shorter half-life (2 to 3 days) than albumin; therefore it can reflect subtle changes in protein status and may be a useful tool to monitor the efficacy of nutritional supplementation. However, prealbumin levels are also influenced by the presence of inflammation.[115]

Dietary Intake Assessment Methods

Patients with CKD may be required to modify their dietary intake. Registered dietitians are trained in assessing dietary intakes and may employ various methods to assess the adequacy of an individual patient's diet using recall methods and dietary records. Food frequency questionnaires (FFQs) are designed to collect information on nutritional intakes of populations and not for assessment of individual intakes.

Twenty-four-hour dietary recalls. The 24-hour diet recall method is a structural nutritional interview used to capture detailed information about the most recent food and drink intake. Patients are prompted to provide an accurate and chronological overview of the actual food and drinks they consumed over the previous 24 hours. Details including portion sizes and cooking methods (e.g., fried or boiled) are also obtained.[117] This is a quick method that results in minimal patient burden; however, it relies on patient recall, which may be subject to underreporting or limited memory, and a single interview may not be reflective of long-term dietary intakes and day-to-day variation.[117-119] In a research setting, multiple 24-hour recalls are used to assess dietary intake.

Food diaries and records. Food diaries or records provide self-reported information of all food and drinks consumed by an individual for several days (usually 3, 4, or 7 days).[120] Patients are provided with instructions and appropriate recording forms to assist in recording all relevant details of their food and drink consumption. Patients are usually instructed to record their intake in real time and may also be provided with scales for weighing food. The content of the diary may be reviewed by the patient together with a registered dietitian to improve its quality and gain greater detail through use of in-depth questioning.[117] This method can help obtain greater detail over extended periods; however, food diaries come with greater patient involvement and burden, which may result in inaccurate or missing recordings.[117]

Food frequency questionnaires. FFQs are used to quantify usual nutrient intakes.[120] The questionnaires consist of lists of foods with multiple choices of frequency and portion size. Some questionnaires add images to enhance reporting of portion size. The obtained data from an FFQ can be used to estimate usual total dietary intake or particular aspects of the diet in populations, such as in large epidemiological studies. FFQs tend to over- or underestimate nutrient intakes and are not suitable to estimate intake at the individual level.[117]

Nutritional Assessment Scores

Subjective global assessment. The SGA is a method using objective and subjective components to assess nutritional status. Trained assessors score four components of medical history (weight change, dietary intake, gastrointestinal symptoms, functional capacity, and three components of physical examination [signs of muscle wasting, signs of subcutaneous fat loss, and alterations in fluid balance]). Using an overall assessment, the patient is rated as A, well nourished; B, moderately undernourished; or C, severely undernourished; or rated similarly using a 7-point scale.[86] Presence of malnutrition as determined by SGA is associated with increased mortality. Over time, several versions of the original SGA have been made and validated to serve specific patient populations, and it is an appropriate method to assess nutritional status in both dialysis and nondialysis patients with CKD.[121-123]

Malnutrition-inflammation score. The MIS is a quantitative assessment tool designed specifically for the HD population[124] and has proven to be useful in the PD population as well.[125] It is based on seven original SGA components and three additional items (body mass index, serum concentrations of albumin, and total iron-binding capacity—an indirect measure of transferrin). Each individual component can be scored 0 (normal) to 3 (very severe), with a sum of all components between 0 and 30. Higher scores are associated with poorer nutritional status and greater hospitalization and mortality rates. These correlations were higher for MIS than for conventional SGA.[86,124]

TREATMENT OF PROTEIN-ENERGY WASTING IN CHRONIC KIDNEY DISEASE

Treatment of PEW in CKD should both aim to address the nutritional deficit and attempt to identify and reverse the cause (Table 13.7). Alterations in metabolic pathways caused by a reduction in kidney function and ultimately kidney failure can negatively affect nutritional status through changes to normal physiology and metabolism that can decrease spontaneous dietary intake. Chronic inflammation, gut flora dysbiosis, increased oxidative stress, acidosis, and changes in muscle metabolism that obstruct anabolic pathways can all contribute to PEW. Addressing the gap between nutritional requirements and actual intake requires physiological and

TABLE 13.7 Potential Causes of Protein-Energy Wasting in Chronic Kidney Disease and Strategies to Address Them

1. Reduced protein and energy intake	Relax potassium and phosphate and sodium restrictions to include a wider variety of foods Assess mood Assess dialysis adequacy and improve if required Assess ability to shop and prepare meals
2. Hypermetabolism	Increase energy and protein intake with energy-dense foods and/or supplemental nutrition Investigate and treat infection/inflammation
3. Metabolic acidosis	Treat with bicarbonate Consider increasing alkaline foods
4. Comorbidities	Optimize treatment of diabetes, heart disease, vascular disease; encourage physical activity as able
5. Dialysis	Optimize dialysis dose Optimize dialysis access
6. Uremic toxins	Consider taste changes, loss of appetite, early satiety, poor concentration, fatigue Increase dietary fiber

nutritional assessments and then implementation of a treatment plan with regular monitoring and reassessment.

In 2013 the International Society of Renal Nutrition and Metabolism published a consensus statement on the prevention and treatment of PEW in CKD[126] (Fig. 13.4).

Importantly, prevention of PEW is paramount, with ongoing nutritional counseling and regular assessment, together with optimal dialysis or management of CKD. Nutritional intervention should start early, when spontaneous energy intake is <30 kcal/kg/day and protein intake <1.2 g/kg/day in dialysis patients or <0.7 g/kg/day in those with CKD stage 3 to 4, or more simply, when signs and symptoms of PEW begin to be apparent. It is paramount to address PEW early, often before the full criteria of PEW are met, to prevent further nutritional decline. Evidence-based practice guidelines prescribing energy and protein intakes are important; however, they require expertise in dietary assessment to be useful and implemented successfully. Dietitians and those with skills in practical clinical nutrition have the expertise to assess nutritional intake for adequacy and implement these guidelines, yet dietitians may be a scarce resource in some countries. Hence more practical ways of assessing the adequacy of intake and providing additional nutrition may be required. Box 13.2 displays the early signs and symptoms of PEW, which can be assessed clinically and without a full assessment against energy and protein intake guidelines. It is important to note that body size is not always indicative of acute nutritional status. Acute undernutrition can occur in conjunction with excess fat stores—such as in obesity—when nutritional intake is reduced, and other early signs or symptoms of PEW are also present.

Dietary Counseling and Use of Oral Nutritional Supplements

Implementation of standardized guidelines for frequency of nutrition assessment, nutrition prescription, and dietary counseling is associated with an improvement in nutritional status in HD patients.[127] Dietary counseling is the cornerstone of nutritional interventions addressing energy and protein deficits and PEW. The Balance Wise study investigated problems related to poor nutritional intake in HD patients and found that having adequate time to prepare meals, changes in health, and feeling too tired to cook were associated with reduced energy intake.[128] The study also found that patients who had been having HD for longer had lower protein intake than those who had been on dialysis for fewer years. Therefore it is paramount to tailor the approach for individuals and their preferences, and strategies to address time management for meal planning and preparation, including easy cooking techniques and recipes, can be useful to improve nutritional intake. Table 13.8 outlines a range of dietary counseling strategies to improve nutritional intake from meals and snacks.

The use of oral nutritional supplements (ONS) in treating PEW in patients requiring dialysis has been studied in a series of small randomized controlled trials and also in several large cohort studies, which have been summarized in a review paper.91 Provision of ONS resulted in improved nutritional status, largely demonstrated as an increase in serum albumin and increased energy and or protein intake. Improvements in functional status,[129] nutritional status as measured by SGA, and quality of life have also been reported.[130] The limitations of the randomized controlled trials are the small sample sizes and short-term follow-up, with no studies to date reporting an impact on survival; however, the ethical limitations of this type of study are acknowledged, because it would be difficult to deny ONS to patients with evidence of PEW. With this limitation in mind, implementation of ONS during dialysis has been incorporated as standard care and the impact on mortality has been observed. Two large quasiexperimental cohort studies reported that a significant reduction in mortality was associated with ONS provided during dialysis,[96,131] suggesting that ONS has the potential to reduce PEW and may be able to decrease mortality associated with poor nutritional status in HD patients.

ONS can be used in conjunction with, or instead of, food-based strategies, depending on the individual situation and patient preferences. ONS comes in many formulations (Table 13.9) and can provide partial or total nutritional support, depending on the products and the amount able to be consumed by an individual.

There is very limited evidence for ONS in patients with CKD who are not on dialysis. In patients requiring dialysis, there are few well-conducted randomized controlled trials of nutritional supplementation, possibly because of the ethical implications of withholding available treatment to patients with identified malnutrition. In clinical trials and observational studies, ONS improves energy and protein intake by 20% to 50% and increases serum albumin, without evidence of increased potassium or phosphate. However, because studies

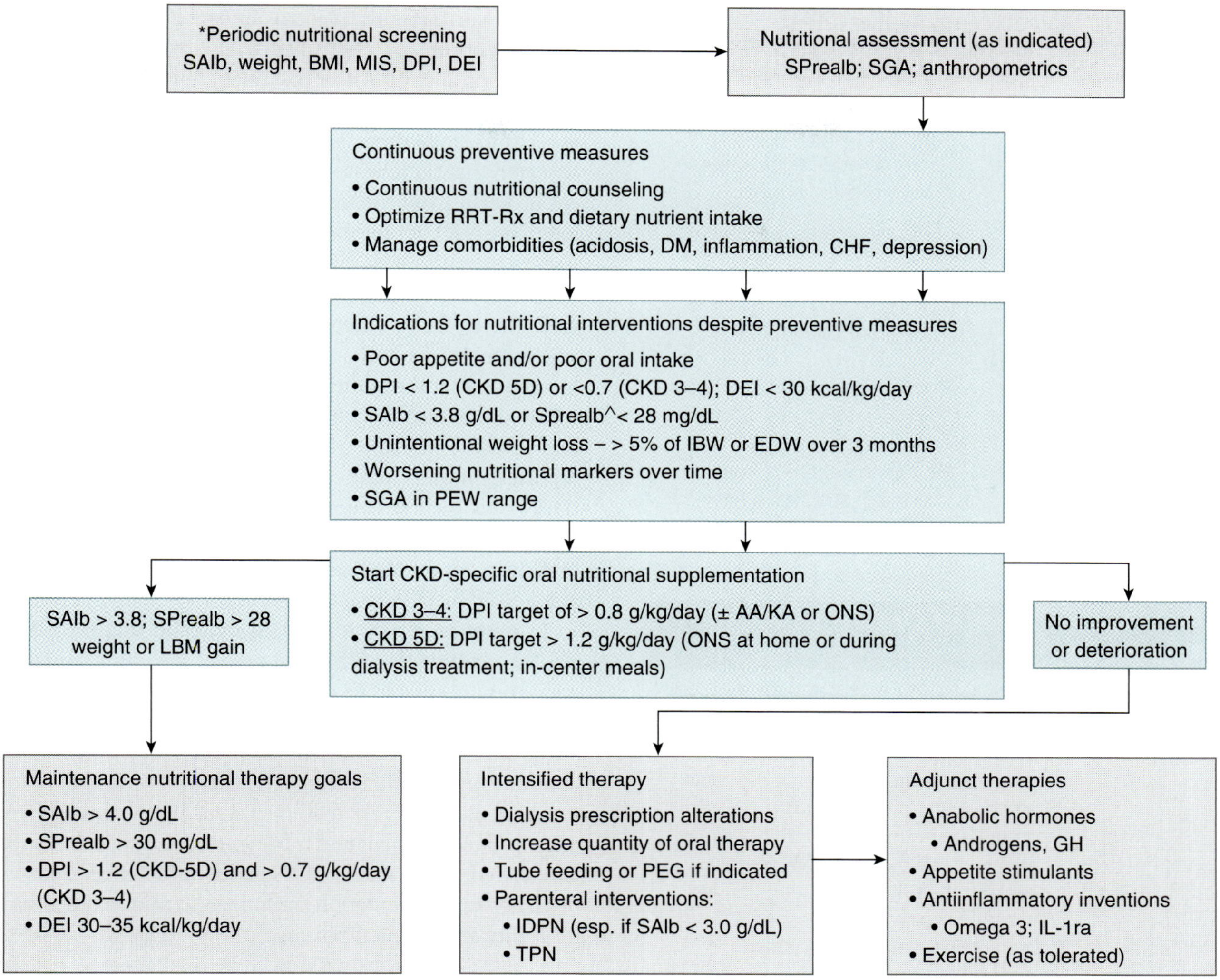

FIG. 13.4 An algorithm for detecting and treating PEW in CKD. *AA/KA,* aminoacids/ketoacids; *BMI,* body mass index; *CHF,* congestive heart failure; *DEI,* dietary energy intake; *DM,* diabetes mellitus; *DPI,* dietary protein intake; *EDW,* estimated dry weight; *GH,* growth hormone; *IL-1ra,* interleukin-1 receptor antagonist; *LBM,* lean body mass; *ONS,* oral nutritional supplements; *PEG,* percutaneous endoscopic gastrostomy; *RRT-Rx,* renal replacement therapy prescription; *SAlb,* serum albumin; *SPrealb,* serum prealbumin; *TPN,* total parenteral nutrition. (From Ikizler TA, Cano NJ, Franch H, et al. Prevention and treatment of protein energy wasting in chronic kidney disease patients: a consensus statement by the International Society of Renal Nutrition and Metabolism. *Kidney Int.* 2013;84(6):1096-1107.)

BOX 13.2 Early Signs and Symptoms of Protein-Energy Wasting

Poor appetite or loss of appetite, metallic/bitter taste
Eating less than ¾ of usual meals, or unable to finish usual meals
Weight loss, or a reduction in dry weight of 5% over 3–6 months, or stable weight with increasing edema
New fatigue or loss of strength/unable to perform usual tasks because of reduced food intake
Constipation, diarrhea, and/or nausea for >2 weeks
Reduced appetite for certain foods such as meat/eggs/dairy foods

were largely nonrandomized, had small sample sizes, and did not discriminate between different degrees of malnutrition, the effect on serum albumin could also be due to reduction in inflammation as a result of changing disease activity and hydration status. There is also insufficient evidence regarding the effect of ONS on clinical, economic, and metabolic outcomes in patients with CKD.[96,132-134]

Intradialytic Parental Nutrition

Intradialytic parental nutrition (IDPN) is a form of nutritional supplementation in which nutrients are administered through the extracorporeal circuit during HD. Because the provision of nutrition during HD is limited by the time of

TABLE 13.8 Dietary Counseling Strategies for Increasing Energy and Protein Intake

Consider individual preferences for energy-dense foods, such as puddings, sweets, cheese, meats, pastries, biscuits, cookies, crackers.	Fortify foods with added protein by adding skimmed milk powder, eggs, cheese, or vegetarian protein.
Recommend small meals and several snacks each day to provide frequent and regular protein intake.	Fortify foods with added fats by frying and adding oil, butter, or cream.
Cold foods may be better tolerated than hot foods.	Fortify foods with added sugars by adding jam, conserve, jelly, syrups, or sugar.
Offer recipes with few ingredients for simple meals.	Regular meal times help prompt food intake even when appetite is poor.

TABLE 13.9 Types of Oral Nutritional Supplements

Type of Product	Consideration in Patients With Chronic Kidney Disease
1 kcal/mL standard	May need high volume for adequate energy and protein; may be unsuitable for fluid restrictions; electrolytes usually appropriate
Low volume (2–2.4 kcal/mL)	Lower volumes may improve compliance; suitable when fluid restriction needed
Renal specific (lower electrolyte and energy dense)	Suitable if potassium or phosphate need modification despite poor intake
Powder style	May contain higher amounts of potassium or phosphate and usually high volume
High protein	May not be suitable if phosphate modification required
Amino acid supplement	Protein only

dialysis and its composition, it is considered a supplementary source of nutrition. At best, IDPN can provide around 25% of the energy and protein requirements of a 70-kg patient; therefore the effectiveness of IDPN to address PEW depends on difference between energy and protein deficits and amount of nutrition able to be provided being as small as possible.[135] European Society for Clinical Nutrition and Metabolism (ESPEN) guidelines suggest that IDPN should not be used as the first-line choice for nutritional therapy but rather when oral nutrition support and nutritional counseling do not result in an improvement in nutritional status or nutrient intake. Typically, studies investigating the provision of IDPN report an increase in serum albumin or prealbumin; however, clinical outcomes remain poorly studied. There are very few randomized controlled trials examining the effect of IDPN on nutritional status, and most are of a short duration and measure surrogate nutritional outcomes. A 2010 metaanalysis of randomized controlled trials investigated the effects of IDPN on nutritional status, quality of life, and survival.[136] Three studies were included in the systematic review, and few clinical outcomes were reported; therefore the authors reported that there was insufficient evidence to support benefit or harm from the use of IDPN in malnourished patients requiring HD.[136] In the largest and longest study in the review, patients on HD were given ONS with or without additional nutrition provided with IDPN for 12 months.[137] After 2 years there was no difference in survival between the groups, and both groups had an improvement in nutritional status, indicating that the addition of IDPN to ONS did not provide additional clinical benefit to ONS alone.[137] Since the publication of this systematic review, the German IDPN group has reported on their multicenter, randomized controlled trial of IDPN plus dietary counseling compared with dietary counseling only.[138] Provision of IDPN for 16 weeks resulted in an improvement in prealbumin but did not alter nutrition status as assessed by SGA and did not improve quality of life.[138]

In practice, IDPN is most likely to be useful in those at risk for malnutrition/PEW but not yet severely malnourished and who are unable to tolerate or access ONS. The optimal duration of treatment is not known; however, a trial of at least 3 to 6 months is recommended before a decision is made to continue or cease this therapy. It is also important to note that if a patient is severely malnourished, IDPN alone is not an appropriate treatment and more intensive nutritional support is required. More studies are needed to determine the effect of IDPN supplementation on longer-term outcomes such as mortality and hospitalizations.[135,136,139]

Nonnutritional Interventions

Interventions to Reduce Inflammation

Despite the many studies that associate systemic inflammation and the risk for mortality in CKD, there are few available strategies to reduce systemic inflammation. Probably the first step is to treat intercurrent illnesses that may induce inflammation, such as dental health, periodontitis, gastritis, and dyspepsia. There is also an antiinflammatory opportunity by improving aspects related to the dialysis technique, such as the use of central dialysis catheters, treating infectious complications of the HD access and thrombosed fistula or graft, use of biocompatible membranes, and so on.

The benefits of a healthy lifestyle and diet on systemic inflammation should not be underestimated. Supplementation with fish oil containing omega-3 polyunsaturated fatty acids significantly reduced C-reactive protein (CRP) level but not interleukin-6 or tumor necrosis factor α in patients requiring HD and PD.[140] Furthermore, supplementation with omega-3 fatty acids may also reduce the MIS in patients undergoing HD.[141] Systematic reviews of L-carnitine supplementation in HD patients report that treatment with L-carnitine reduces the inflammatory marker CRP, with studies of longer than 6 months more likely to report positive outcomes than studies of shorter duration.[142,143] A diet rich in fiber can also exert antiinflammatory effects directly or indirectly by improving dysbiosis in the intestinal flora.[144] There is some evidence regarding antiinflammatory effects of exercise in patients with CKD. Resistance and aerobic exercise performed during dialysis may induce a reduction in the levels of markers of inflammation.[145,146] In patients with stages 3 to 4 CKD, regular moderate-intensity aerobic exercise was found safe with regard to immune and inflammatory responses and has the potential to be an effective antiinflammatory therapy.[147] No adverse effect is to be anticipated from a healthier lifestyle, and it should always be encouraged in patients.

Finally, although some common pharmacological treatments in CKD have pleiotropic antiinflammatory effects, their use should be restricted to their main indication. For instance, statin therapy can decrease CRP in HD patients but does not affect serum albumin level.[148] Evidence on the safety and effectiveness of antiinflammatory drugs in CKD patients is currently small, hampered by short-term interventions in a limited number of patients.[149,150]

Megestrol Acetate

The use of megestrol acetate to reverse poor appetite and improve nutritional status and body weight and increase protein and energy intake has been studied in dialysis populations; however, most studies were of short duration and were limited by small sample sizes.[151] There are no studies in patients with nondialysis CKD. Studies have reported improvements in body mass, serum albumin, energy and protein intake, and appetite in patients with PEW undergoing dialysis treatment, with a high incidence of adverse events, including overhydration or excessive fluid gain, gastrointestinal disturbances, hyperglycemia, and death.[151,152] When studied, the use of megestrol did not improve quality of life.[153] The potential adverse effects of using megestrol in patients with CKD are significant and the long-term effects are unknown; therefore the use of megestrol should be considered only with extreme care and only when other treatments are not available.[151]

Exercise and Anabolic Agents

Resistance exercise training has been found to be safe, feasible, and well tolerated in outpatient settings,[154] home-based regimens,[155] and programs in connection with the dialysis session.[156] Although the acute muscle response to resistance exercise appears intact in ESRD,[157] long-term studies indicate a hampered effect of training compared with healthy older individuals.[158] This suggests that resistance exercise, despite being an effective acute anabolic stimulus in CKD patients, ought to be combined with other interventions aimed at normalizing protein homeostasis. Some studies suggest improved muscle strength after aerobic (or endurance) exercise training, most likely explained by the severely deconditioned state of the muscle in these patients. Such aerobic approaches may consider leg cycling during HD.[159] Combined approaches such as a 12-week/24-session aerobic and resistance exercise program in patients with CKD stages 3 to 4 improved physical capacity and quality of life.[160] Of note, these studies were done in well-nourished CKD patients. If exercise is to be recommended in patients with PEW, they will need to increase energy intake further when exercising.

Anabolic agents can also be effective in CKD patients with PEW. In a randomized controlled trial treatment in both male and female dialysis patients, supraphysiological dosages of nandrolone decanoate for 6 months resulted in a significant increase in muscle mass followed by functional improvement.[161] In HD patients, treatment with the androgenic steroid oxymetholone was associated with an increase in fat-free mass, handgrip strength, and muscle messenger RNA levels for several growth factors, together with a decrease in fat mass.[162] The combined approach of nandrolone decanoate and resistance exercise produced superior anabolic effects.[163] Other anabolic agents may involve recombinant human GH, which, administered at pharmacological doses, improved not only net muscle protein balance but also inflammation, cardiovascular status, lipid profile, and erythropoiesis.[164-166]

SUMMARY AND CONCLUSIONS

PEW is a relatively common metabolic complication inherent to CKD. A worsening of quality of life and an increase in the risk for comorbidities, hospitalizations, and death accompany the onset and progression of PEW. The cause of PEW is multifactorial, involving undernutrition (insufficient or inadequate nutrient intake) and excess protein catabolism that altogether favors the progressive and continuous loss of energy and fat fuels. This multifactorial nature makes diagnosis difficult; it must be based on the combined interpretation of complementary nutritional screening and assessment tools.

A full list of references is available at www.expertconsult.com.

14

Inflammation in Chronic Kidney Disease

Gabriela Cobo, MD, PhD, Magdalena Jankowska, MD, PhD, Peter Stenvinkel, MD, PhD, and Bengt Lindholm, MD, PhD

OUTLINE

Among the singular features exhibited by patients with chronic kidney disease (CKD), the high prevalence of persistent systemic inflammation and its association with poor outcomes stands out. It is now well established that systemic inflammation is a prominent, perhaps even inherent, feature of advanced CKD and a major culprit for the abysmal outcomes observed in this population as regards progression of cardiovascular disease (CVD), poor quality of life, and premature mortality. Although the pathophysiology associated with systemic inflammation in CKD is not fully understood, there is a broad understanding of many of the factors prompting it and also of the consequences associated with it. In this chapter, we review various aspects of this intriguing and challenging complication of CKD and its implications for the prognosis and management of patients with CKD.

CHRONIC INFLAMMATION: A MALADAPTIVE RESPONSE IN A PARTICULAR SETTING

Inflammation (Latin, *inflammatio,* to set on fire) is a complex process with a crucial role in mammalian physiology. The purpose of the inflammatory process is to provide host defence against infection, tissue-repair response, adaptation to stress and restoration of a homeostatic state.[1] A generic inflammatory pathway consists of inducers, sensors, mediators, and effectors, with each component determining the type of inflammatory response.[1] After the stimuli, the immune system prompts a complex orchestration of cells, cytokines, and other molecules that act in a paracrine, autocrine, or endocrine manner to protect the human organism; a successful acute inflammatory response should result in the elimination of the infectious agents (or other harmful factors) followed by a resolution and repair phase. Although the inflammatory process should be regarded as a protective mechanism, inflammation underlies a wide variety of not only physiological but also pathological processes.

It is generally understood that a controlled inflammatory response is favorable to remove injurious stimuli and to initiate the healing process for the tissue, but it can become detrimental if deregulated. Actually the pathological potential of inflammation is unprecedented for a physiological process, being associated with atherosclerosis, diabetes, and cancer, among others.[2]

Contrary to what happens with acute inflammation, the mechanisms leading to systemic chronic inflammatory states are in general poorly understood. It has been proposed that in certain conditions—other than infection and tissue damage—inflammation might presumably act as an adaptive response to tissue malfunction or homeostatic imbalance in order to restore homeostasis. In this sense, an adaptive change often provides short-term benefits; however, in a chronic phase, it can become maladaptive, as exemplified by a sustained decline in insulin sensitivity of the skeletal muscle or by squamous

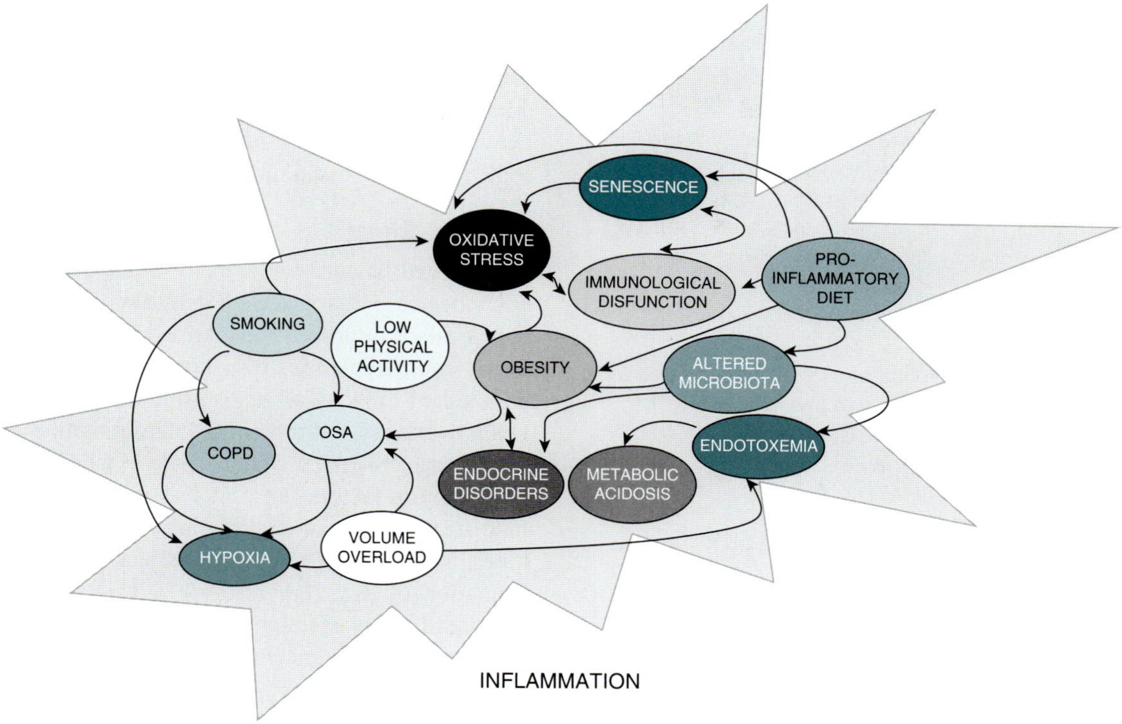

FIG. 14.1 Factors contributing to inflammation in CKD and their interrelationships. The effect of contributors to the inflammatory process in CKD is potentiated by their relationships. For example, immunological dysfunction, a feature of CKD, is further enhanced by premature senescence, another feature of CKD. On all of those contributors, complications of renal replacement therapy, genetic predisposition, and other comorbidities are frequently superimposed. *COPD*, Chronic obstructive pulmonary disease; OSA, obstructive sleep apnea.

metaplasia of the respiratory epithelium that may be consequences of sustained inflammation. Indeed, inducible adaptive changes generally occur at the expense of many other physiological processes and therefore cannot be sustained without adverse side effects caused by the decline in the affected functions.

CKD is a disease where a sustained chronic inflammatory state is often observed, and it has been associated with poor outcomes in this group of patients, being described as one of the most important causes of cardiovascular events, poor quality of life, and even all-cause mortality. Despite considerable progress in the understanding of the consequences of chronic inflammation in patients with CKD, more research is needed to fully recognise the cellular, molecular, and clinical events associated with this pathological process.

CHRONIC PERSISTENT INFLAMMATION IN CHRONIC KIDNEY DISEASE

Description of the Problem

Inflammation is a major feature in CKD patients, with increasing prevalence as renal function declines. In a report from the Chronic Renal Insufficiency Cohort (CRIC) including 3939 patients with different stages of CKD, all of the inflammatory biomarkers determined, such as C-reactive protein (CRP), interleukin (IL)-6, and tumor necrosis factor (TNF)-α, were inversely associated with measures of kidney function and positively associated with albuminuria.[3] Moreover, according to data from the National Health and Nutrition Examination Survey III (NHANES III; $n = 15{,}594$), approximately 54% of the patients with glomerular filtration rate (GFR) between 15 and 60 mL/min had some degree of inflammation (CRP > 2.1 mg/L). In addition, the age-adjusted probability of having elevated CRP (>2.1 mg/L) rose from 44% to 69% when estimated GFR (eGFR) was <60 and <30 mL/min, respectively.[4] Along the same lines, in a survey including 663 patients with CKD stage 5 (160 patients evaluated close to the start of dialysis and 503 patients on dialysis) from three different countries—Sweden, Germany, and Italy—approximately two-thirds of the patients showed CRP levels above 3.4 mg/L.[5]

The reasons behind the increased incidence of systemic inflammation in end-stage renal disease (ESRD) patients are complex and multifactorial and include a range of nondialysis and dialysis-related factors. The combination of an impaired immune response coupled with persistent immune stimulation may have a role in the low-grade chronic systemic inflammation and altered cytokine balance that characterize the uremic state and that may translate into increased morbidity and mortality. The close association between low-grade inflammation, comorbidities, and poor outcome highlights the importance of searching for strategies to ameliorate and avoid such conditions.

Etiology of Inflammation in Chronic Kidney Disease

The pathophysiology involved in the development of chronic inflammation in CKD has not yet been elucidated completely; however, it has been described as being the consequence of

TABLE 14.1 Immunocompetent Cell Alterations Associated With the Uremic State

Immunocompetent Cell	Alterations in Uremic State
Monocytes and macrophages	General expansion of circulating monocytes[248]
	Spontaneous activation and decreased phagocyte capacity[249]
	Overproduction of IL-1β, IL-6, IL-12, and TNF-α[250]
Polymorphonuclear leukocytes (PMNL)	Spontaneous activation[251]
	Decreased phagocytic capacity and reduced bactericidal capabilities[252]
	Altered apoptosis[253]
Lymphocytes B	B-cell lymphopenia[254]
	Impaired differentiation and maturation[254]
	Increased apoptosis[255]
Lymphocytes T	Decreased proliferation[256]
	Depletion of naive and central memory T cells[257]
	Increased apoptosis[258]
	Reduced ratio of CD4/CD8[257]
	Increased ratio of Th1/Th2[259]
Dendritic cells	Depletion of cells[260]
	Decreased antigen presentation capabilities[261]

a multifactorial etiology with interactions with a number of factors, some of which are shown in Fig. 14.1. The described factors include not only the decline of GFR and the noxious effect of uremic toxins but also several aspects usually present in this group of patients, such as comorbidities, superimposed illnesses, genetic predisposition, and therapeutic interventions, including the dialysis procedure itself. In this section we briefly describe the main etiological factors of inflammation in CKD.

Immune Dysfunction Proper of Chronic Kidney Disease

The uremic state in patients with kidney failure affects general immunity, with the two major branches—innate and acquired immunity—being altered in CKD patients. These alterations lead to a state of persistent systemic inflammation and acquired immunosuppression, circumstances that are manifested not only by increased risk for infections, which in turn associate with inflammation, but also by impaired response to vaccination and higher incidence of cancer.

In the uremic milieu, disturbances in the number and function of basically all immune cells have been described. Observed functional alterations include spontaneous activation, decreased phagocytic capacity, and increased apoptosis, altogether leading to increased generation and release of cytokines and reactive oxygen species (ROS), as well as diminished defensive capacity.[6] The main alterations of immunocompetent cells associated with the uremic state are listed in Table 14.1.

As a consequence of the altered function of the immune cells, a state of hypercytokinemia and elevated acute phase proteins are characteristic features of the uremic milieu, where the delicate equilibrium between proinflammatory cytokines and their inhibitors is clearly deregulated.[7,8] This topic will be discussed more in detail later.

Oxidative Stress

A disturbed balance between increased production of ROS and a decrease in antioxidant defenses is a hallmark of CKD. Specifically, a multifactorial increase in the production of ROS is not counterbalanced by a corresponding increase of the antioxidant capacity, which is profoundly disrupted in CKD. Oxidative stress and inflammation are manifested conjointly in uraemia, creating a vicious circle in which redox-sensitive transcription factors (e.g., nuclear factor kappa B [NF-κB]) mediate the activation of proinflammatory cytokines, chemokines, and adhesive molecules responsible for the excessive formation of ROS. For instance, NF-κB triggers a cascade of inflammatory reactions, activated directly but also indirectly as a consequence of enhanced formation of advanced glycation end products (AGEs).[9] The production of AGEs is increased in CKD, and AGEs are additionally retained due to the compromised kidney function. AGEs act via receptors for advanced glycation end products (RAGE), amplifying inflammation. This close relationship is reflected by the association between inflammation and oxidative stress markers in CKD.[10]

Increased markers of oxidative stress appear early in the course of CKD and remain uncorrected, or even deteriorate with dialysis initiation.[11] Moreover, inflammation and oxidative stress contribute to CKD progression.

The key role of NF-κB in the translation of the oxidative stress into inflammatory response explains the high potential of its antagonist, the nuclear factor erythroid 2-related factor (Nrf2), in enhancing the antioxidant barrier and protecting cells against inflammation.[12,13] Besides suppressing NF-κB, Nrf2 activates the transcription of several antioxidant enzymes such as superoxide dismutase, UDP-glucuronosyltransferase, NAD(P)H:quinoneoxidoreductase-1, heme oxygenase-1, glutathione S-transferase, and others. Accordingly, in experimental studies performed in Nrf2 knockout mice, the inflammatory response associated with NF-κB activation is much more pronounced compared with the wild-type mice.[14] Moreover, ablation of Nrf2 genes leads to the development of lupus-like nephritis and aggravates inflammation in diabetic kidney disease, highlighting the nephroprotective role of Nrf2.[15] Physiologically, Nrf2 expression is induced by oxidative stress and inflammation to counterbalance their potentially deleterious effects and to prevent cellular injury. However, in uremia this mechanism is altered, and, paradoxically, severe oxidative stress and enhanced inflammation are accompanied by reduced activity of Nrf2.[14] Consequently, downregulation of Nrf2 may play a role in the progression of CKD, and strategies to restore its activity seem to yield promising results in experimental models and may have an effect on retarding the progression of CKD in humans.[12] A phase

III clinical trial on bardoxolone methyl (an Nrf2-activating and nuclear factor-κn-inhibiting semisynthetic oleanane triterpenoid compound) in patients with type 2 diabetes mellitus and CKD stage 4 (BEACON) was terminated because of an increase in heart failure events in the bardoxolone methyl group.[16] However, the potential of gaining benefits from this treatment in patients with Alport syndrome is currently (2017) being investigated in a phase II/III trial (CARDINAL; https://clinicaltrials.gov/ct2/show/NCT03019185).

Fluid Overload and Sodium Expansion

Volume expansion is an important risk factor for increased mortality in CKD patients, especially in ESRD patients undergoing dialysis.[17] There is evidence linking volume expansion with the so-called malnutrition, inflammation, atherosclerosis (MIA) syndrome.[18,19] Interstitial accumulation of fluid in the lung, known as *pulmonary congestion*, is much more prevalent in patients with ESRD, than is generally presumed based solely on clinical observations.[20] Also, pulmonary congestion is associated with adverse outcomes and increased markers of systemic inflammation. The mechanisms underlying this association have yet to be elucidated; however, one of the apparent results of vascular congestion is increased permeability of membranes in the gastrointestinal tract and leakage of endotoxins into the vascular system, triggering systemic inflammation as described elsewhere in this chapter. Otherwise, the presence of the inflammatory status, resulting in increased vessel permeability and hypoalbuminemia, is sufficient to drive fluid shifts that result in volume derangements and congestion.

In addition, volume expansion could be a consequence of increased sodium loading. High sodium intake, sometimes enhanced by high dialysate sodium concentration in the dialysate targeted at reducing intradialytic complications, is commonly found in hemodialysis (HD) patients. The adverse effects of sodium are not limited to volume expansion; sodium excess is also responsible for oxidative stress and could be linked to systemic inflammation reflected by increased serum CRP in population-based studies.[21]

Metabolic Acidosis

Chronic positive acid balance contributes to numerous deleterious outcomes, including progression of CKD and increased mortality. There are several lines of evidence supporting a strong link between acidosis and inflammation, although the molecular mechanism underlying this relationship is not fully understood. The NF-κB transcription factor is likely to play a central role in this process because it regulates the transcription of genes encoding inflammatory cytokines, such as interferon (IFN)-β, TNF-α, and IL-1, IL-2, IL-6, and IL-8, and it could be influenced by low environmental pH. Accordingly, exposure of canine kidney cells to pH stress resulted in at least threefold upregulation of proinflammatory genes.[22] In another experimental study, environmental acidosis potentiated TNF-α synthesis and upregulated inducible nitric oxide (iNOS) activity in peritoneal macrophages.[23] In dialysis patients, correction of metabolic acidosis by the administration of sodium bicarbonate resulted in a decrease of TNF-α expression in peritoneal dialysis (PD) patients and changes in IL-10 secretion in patients treated with HD.[24,25] Moreover, correction of acidosis in patients treated with HD or PD resulted in a reduction of protein degradation because acidosis and inflammation are counterparts in the etiology of protein-energy wasting (PEW).[26]

Nevertheless some controversy exists around the real benefit of bicarbonate correction in these patients. Contrary to the results presented previously, in a cross-sectional study of HD patients, no significant difference in the inflammatory indices (CRP, IL-6) was observed among the different groups of serum bicarbonate concentrations.[27] In addition, results from the CRIC study showed that bicarbonate level was a better predictor of renal outcomes in participants with better preserved kidney function compared with those with more advanced CKD.[28] Moreover, the same study showed that increase in serum bicarbonate level above 24 mmol/L increased the risk of heart failure even in those without preexisting CVD.[28]

Thus although correction of metabolic acidosis in CKD patients may be an effective tool to slow the progression of kidney disease or reduce muscle wasting, there is not enough evidence supporting its general use in order to control inflammatory status, especially in view of possible adverse consequences of overcorrection of the serum bicarbonate level.

Comorbidities

Oral health and periodontal disease. Periodontitis is a dysbiotic inflammatory disease that is highly prevalent in patients with CKD. The risk of periodontitis was found to be several fold higher in the Renal Impairment In Secondary Care (RIISC) cohort study (odds ratio [OR], 3.8; 95% confidence interval [CI], 2.5 to 5.6) compared with a geographically matched control population.[29] In the mentioned study, the severe form of periodontitis—allegedly responsible for the systemic complications—affected about 50% of the RIISC cohort, whereas its prevalence in a general population reached only 1% to 1.5%. A plausible explanation for the high prevalence of periodontitis in this group of patients is the observed changes in the oral cavity accompanying CKD, usually described as xerostomia, and modifications in the microbial community.[30] These conditions, together with impaired immunity, poor oral hygiene, and malnutrition, enhance the manifestations of poor oral health in CKD patients.

In the course of periodontal disease, the presence of pathogens and bacterial lipopolysaccharides (LPS) activates the defenses of the oral mucosa, resulting in the release of proinflammatory cytokines and chemokines that attract inflammatory cells to the site of infection. Activated neutrophils are a source of ROS, contributing to local tissue destruction and allowing the translocation of proinflammatory factors, such as endotoxins (e.g., LPS) and ROS end products, to the blood circulation, resulting in systemic inflammation.[31,32] In fact, several studies have shown that patients with periodontitis have elevated levels of CRP and exert an adverse effect on general health.[33] Furthermore, an increasing body of evidence supports the hypothesis that poor oral health may constitute a risk factor for CKD progression through endothelial injury. It remains to be determined whether more successful management of poor oral health and periodontitis will reduce the risk of inflammation, infection, PEW, and atherosclerotic complications in CKD patients.

Bowel bacteria overgrowth and altered gut microbiota. The gut microbial community (microbiota) has an important role in the renal pathophysiology, with profound alterations of the gut microbial flora (called *dysbiosis*) typically found in CKD patients. The mutual interplay between microbiota and kidney has been acknowledged, and the term *gut-kidney axis* has been coined.[34] The high ammonia concentration responsible for lowering the pH in the gastrointestinal tract, the prolonged colonic transit, the dietary restrictions leading to decreased fiber intake, the fluid overload, and medication (phosphate binders, iron, antibiotics) are only a few of the numerous factors underlying the altered composition of the intestinal microbiota in uremic patients. There is a convincing body of findings in the literature demonstrating associations between systemic inflammation and gut dysbiosis in CKD. Dysbiosis disrupts the intestinal epithelial barrier structure and leads to increased gut permeability (leaky gut). This process allows the translocation of bacteria or bacterial LPS into the inner environment, as well as provokes the leak of gut-derived uremic toxins and their toxic derivatives into the systemic circulation. As a consequence, a cascade of proinflammatory response, targeted to eliminate the translocated pathogens, is activated with the enrollment of the innate immune system. Intestinal epithelial cells secrete IL-1, IL-6, and IL-18, and macrophages stimulate the development of effector $CD4^+$ T cells TH1 and TH17.[35] In addition, adaptive immunity might have a role in this process by changing the balance between Treg and T-effector cells.[36]

It is thought that gut-derived toxins might also play a role in the progression of kidney disease and in the pathogenesis of CKD-associated complications, including accelerated CVD. In past years, it has been described that toxins generated by colonic bacteria, including p-cresyl sulfate, trimethylamine-*N*-oxide, alfa-phenylacetyl-l-glutamine, and indoxyl sulfate, may accumulate in renal tubular cells, provoking their injury by production of inflammatory cytokines and profibrotic factors.

In this sense, the use of pre- and probiotics (living microorganisms that confer benefit to the host) to attenuate the imbalance in the microbiota has been proposed as a promising intervention to minimize inflammation that potentially could delay CKD progression in this group of patients.

Nutritional problems. Cachexia and obesity represent divergent manifestations of nutritional problems associated with CKD, and both may contribute to enhanced inflammatory activity. Obesity, a common finding in CKD patients—especially among those undergoing PD—is associated with a state of chronic, low-grade inflammation and insulin resistance (IR). Adipose tissue regulates food intake and energy expenditure and controls inflammation by secretion of adipokines and proinflammatory cytokines.[37] Considering the important effect that loss of renal function has on the clearance of these substances,[38] the systemic effects of adipokines in patients with CKD appear to be greater than in the general population. Also, it has been found that the production of proinflammatory molecules in the abdominal subcutaneous fat is increased in patients with CKD compared with patients who do not have the disease.[39] Moreover, the distribution of fat is important in the pathogenesis of inflammation; visceral fat appears to produce adipokines more actively than subcutaneous adipose tissue. Visceral abdominal fat is a main producer of IL-6. In a group of patients with CKD evaluated shortly before the start of renal replacement therapy (RRT), there was a significant association between serum IL-6 and truncal fat but not between IL-6 and nontruncal fat.[40] This association has also been seen in nondialyzed patients with CKD stage 3 to 5 and in PD patients where an increased amount of visceral fat correlated with higher levels of inflammatory parameters and increased coronary artery calcification.[41-44] Interestingly, an abnormal abdominal fat mass deposition in HD patients may associate not only with a higher prevalence of inflammation and increased mortality risk but also with PEW.[41] This circumstance may be mediated by the increased levels of TNF-α, one of the key mediators in a crosstalk between visceral fat and inflammatory response, which may originate in significant amounts from macrophages resident in the adipose tissue, having in fact an anorexic effect that is likely to induce cachexia.[45]

Sleep apnea and hypoxia. The lung-kidney link has received very limited attention to date, although the mutual interrelations between these two apparently distant organs are close and visible from the earliest stages of the human life. However, it is now accepted that CKD, hypertension, and obstructive sleep apnea (OSA) constitute a triad of mutually interrelated comorbidities with a deleterious effect on individuals' quality of life and mortality. Chronic obstructive pulmonary disease (COPD) and OSA are manifested frequently in patients with CKD.[46,47] COPD and OSA have a wide range of systemic effects, with inflammation, oxidative stress, and IR being some of their consequences. These findings support the role of hypoxia as a causative factor involved in the proinflammatory status of CKD individuals.[48]

It has been described that in hypoxic conditions an oxygen-dependent cell signaling reaction is activated, influencing the expression of adaptive, inflammatory, and apoptotic genes that lead to hypoxic inflammation.[49] The central role in this orchestration of transcription factors is played by the hypoxia-inducible factor (HIF). HIF, targeted to restore optimal cell oxygenation, manifests proinflammatory properties by promoting glycolysis in the inflammatory cells and affecting the expression of cytokines, adhesion molecules, and proinflammatory enzymes via NF-κB related pathways.[49] In parallel to its direct role in eliciting and maintaining inflammation, hypoxia influences the immune response by the activation of the sympathetic system, which promotes inflammation and oxidative stress and results in a vicious circle of mutually enhancing proinflammatory reactions. High sympathetic activity may also explain an association between hypoxia, proteinuria, and progression of CKD observed in some pulmonary diseases, but also in people who live at high altitudes.

Interestingly, in a recent study prolonged intradialytic hypoxemia was associated with high levels of laboratory indicators of inflammation and increased all-cause hospitalization and mortality.[48] Alarmingly, prolonged intradialytic hypoxemia was experienced by 10.2% of 983 individuals in a cohort of chronic HD patients,[48] and its prevalence may be even further enhanced in PD due to increase of intraabdominal pressure.[46]

Vitamin D deficiency. Intact kidney function plays a central role in vitamin D physiology, and low levels of 25-OHD and 1,25 dihydroxyvitamin D (1,25-OHD) accompany kidney disease from its earliest stages. Vitamin D acts as a key regulator of the immune system, and its deficiency has been proposed as a contributor to defective inflammatory response in CKD. There are several mechanisms by which vitamin D deficiency may promote inflammation, including NF-κB signaling, renal expression of the regulated on activation, normal T-cell expressed and secreted (RANTES) cytokine, activation of the renin-angiotensin-aldosterone system (RAAS), and activation of the TNF-α converting enzyme (TACE) with subsequent release of TNF-α, intercellular adhesion molecule (ICAM)-1, and vascular cell adhesion protein 1 (VCAM-1) into the circulation.[50]

Emerging evidence of the antiinflammatory effect of vitamin D suggest that vitamin D could be a promising tool for therapeutic purposes far beyond its established role in the treatment of secondary hyperparathyroidism.

Lifestyle Factors

Many lifestyle factors may potentiate the inflammatory status in CKD patients. Among them, diet may play a central role in the regulation of chronic inflammation because it is a source of both anti- and proinflammatory constituents.[51] In a recent study analyzing two community-based cohorts of elderly individuals, it was demonstrated that a proinflammatory diet is associated with systemic inflammation as well as reduced kidney function.[52] In this study, the proinflammatory effect of dietary constituents such as sugar and saturated fatty acids appeared to be mediated by CRP and linked to worsening kidney function.[52] In this regard, dietary habits and food patterns are probably targets of major relevance in modifying systemic inflammation.

On the other hand, physical inactivity, a common finding in CKD patients, has been found to be associated with higher values of inflammatory markers.[53,54] Moreover, physical exercise has been proposed as a valid antiinflammatory strategy. Among the several pathways and mechanisms by which physical activity may attenuate chronic inflammation, we can mention secretion of antiinflammatory cytokines, lowering of CD14 + CD16 + monocytes, reduction in the expression of TLR4, and reduction of oxidative stress.[55-57]

Likewise, cigarette smoking is regarded as one of most important modifiable lifestyle factors affecting general health. Cigarette smoke has been shown to alter both innate and immune systems, augmenting the production of numerous proinflammatory cytokines (such as TNF-α, IL-1, IL-6, IL-8, and granulocyte-macrophage colony-stimulating factor [GM-CSF]) and decreasing the levels of antiinflammatory cytokines (such as IL-10).[58,59] Moreover, cigarette smoking has been shown to enhance oxidative stress mediated by RAGE and its signaling pathways.[60] Among other known deleterious consequences to general health, tobacco consumption has been associated with increased incidence of kidney disease. The first report of a high risk for ESRD associated with smoking was reported in the Multiple Risk Factor Intervention Trial (MRFIT),[61] and consecutive studies supported this finding.[62,63] Interestingly, smoking cessation has not been proven to have an important effect on the risk of CKD; the risk of developing renal failure in smoking men remained significantly enhanced even after 9 years of cessation,[64] although the risk significantly decreased as the years elapsed.[65] Nevertheless, the effect of cigarette smoking on relevant clinical outcomes warrants focus on prevention of smoking initiation, as well as smoking cessation among current smokers in CKD individuals and in the general population.

Genetic Predisposition

Recent studies show that the inflamed uremic phenotype is also the result of genetic factors. The observation that Asian dialysis patients treated in the United States have a markedly lower adjusted relative risk of mortality than Caucasians[66] supports this statement. Indeed, a substantial heritability (35% to 40%) has been found for CRP and IL-10 production,[67,68] and many studies demonstrate a significant effect of genetic variations on the uremic inflammatory response.[69,70]

Our understanding of the genetic predisposition to inflammation in patients with CKD has increased enormously in the last couple of years, and undoubtedly variations in the genome play an important role for the development of specific phenotypes in CKD.[71-73] For instance, it is now known that the IL-6 gene has functional variants that affect inflammation and risk for CVD among dialysis patients, supporting a causal role for IL-6 in CVD.[74] Interestingly, the IL-6 gene variants, together with those from the lymphotoxin-α gene, independently predicted risk for CVD in a cohort of dialysis patients.[75] Moreover, genetic variations in the IL-6 gene seem to influence inflammatory and peritoneal transport parameters, thereby contributing to the interpatient variability in small solute transport rate at the start of PD.[76] Also, genetically determined interindividual differences in TNF-α,[77] IL-10,[78] myeloperoxidase,[79] and peroxisome proliferator-activated receptor (PPAR)-γ[80] release have been associated with the prevalence of inflammation, CVD, and survival in CKD

On the other hand, external and internal environmental stresses may affect the phenotype via changes in the epigenome. Aberrant DNA methylation—related to uremic dysmetabolism—may have complex interactions for the development of premature CVD. Shortening of telomeres (nucleoprotein complexes protecting the chromosome ends that are involved in chromosome stability and repair) has been associated with an inflammatory phenotype and increased mortality in dialysis patients.[81]

Dialysis Technique

In addition to the intrinsic inflammation accompanying CKD, patients undergoing dialysis are subjected to additional potential inflammation-activating factors. Indeed, there are several factors specific of the dialysis technique that are widely accepted as contributors to inflammation. Those factors include bioincompatible membranes, dialysate backflow, clotted access grafts, and catheter infections in HD, and peritonitis and bioincompatible glucose-based solutions in PD, as well as failed kidney transplant, and, in all types of techniques, endotoxemia and fluid overload.

Factors associated with hemodialysis technique. A number of factors related to the HD procedure promote inflammation. Although interestingly, dialysis-related inflammation seems to be associated with a specific genomic pattern,[82] several in vivo studies suggest that the membrane composition, the type and quality of dialysis, and the type of vascular access may contribute to inflammatory processes. It has been demonstrated in a randomized study that HD patients treated with polyamide membranes presented lower CRP levels compared with those exposed to cuprophane or polycarbonate membranes.[83] Accordingly, a significant relationship exists between membrane bioincompatibility and circulating levels of CRP, IL-6, and albumin.[84] Likewise, it has been proposed that the amount of convective transport and the frequency of dialysis might have an influence on inflammation.[85] The combination of better hemodynamic stability, high-flux synthetic and biocompatible membranes with ultrapure dialysis fluid that is offered by hemodiafiltration seems to reduce inflammatory activity and the production of proinflammatory cytokines compared with conventional HD.[86,87] Also, short daily HD (six sessions per week of 3 hours each) was associated with a reduction in left-ventricular hypertrophy and inflammatory mediators compared with conventional HD (three sessions per week of 4 hours each).[88]

It has been also postulated that exposure of blood to dialysate may contribute to chronic inflammation in addition to effects related to the immunogenic properties of the dialysis membrane. Cytokine production may be triggered by substances present in the dialysis fluid, which may penetrate intact dialyzer membranes.[89] Indeed, small bacterial DNA fragments in dialysis fluid can pass through dialyzer membranes and enter circulation.[90] In accordance, a switch from conventional to online-produced ultrapure dialysate resulted in lower bacterial contamination with a significant decrease in CRP and IL-6 blood levels in several studies. Apart from reducing levels of proinflammatory cytokines, changing from conventional to ultrapure dialysate improved nutritional status, decreased the need of erythropoiesis-stimulating agents (ESAs), and reduced the incidence of carpal tunnel syndrome.[91]

Furthermore, vascular access is a fundamental aspect in HD patients, and its dysfunction, and especially the use of central venous catheters, is among the most important sources of morbidity and mortality among HD patients. The type of vascular access has an important effect on inflammatory status and further outcomes.[92] In a study comparing arteriovenous fistulas with arteriovenous grafts versus central venous catheters, inflammatory mediators (IL-1, IL-1 β, and CRP, but not TNF-α) were significantly higher in the latter.[93] Clotted access grafts and access infections are both significant contributors to the inflammatory process in HD patients. It has also been speculated that biofilm formation is a cause of inflammation in this patient group.

Thus although adequate dialysis treatment to some extent can ameliorate some uremia-related proinflammatory factors, there are many dialysis-related factors that can contribute to the inflammatory state observed in CKD patients.

Factors associated with peritoneal dialysis technique. The PD procedure per se may exacerbate systemic inflammation, although to a lesser extent than the HD procedure. Moreover, inflammation promotes angiogenesis, an important constituent of morphological alterations in the peritoneal membrane that contribute to discontinuation of PD therapy. This relation is illustrated by the fact that alleviating inflammation reduces peritoneal angiogenesis.[94] Also, the most threatening complication of PD, encapsulating peritoneal sclerosis (EPS), is preceded by peritoneal inflammation, and patients who subsequently develop EPS have higher levels of inflammatory cytokines during PD.[95]

Conventional bioincompatible glucose-based PD solutions are important sources of inflammation, especially due to the content of glucose degradation products (GDPs) generated during heat sterilization. GPDs have shown to induce peritoneal inflammation and the formation of AGEs. In addition, glucose-based solutions lead to a substantial uptake of glucose, which may be associated with the induction of oxidative stress, dyslipidemia, and malnutrition, all of which are potent causes of inflammation.

Peritoneal transport status is another important fact to consider in PD patients. Patients presenting high peritoneal solute transport rates have worse clinical conditions, characterized by worse nutritional status and enhanced inflammation.[96] Although adverse clinical outcomes in the group of high transporters may be closely related to volume overload, analysis of the cytokine profile in effluent may predict altered transport characteristics.[97] Also, alterations of macrophage heterogeneity in peritoneal effluent were associated with different PD outcomes.[98] In addition, high incidence of overt peritonitis and exit-site and tunnel infections are important contributors to increased inflammatory response in patients undergoing PD. Moreover, an indwelling catheter potentiates inflammatory response through a foreign body reaction.[99]

CONSEQUENCES OF INFLAMMATION IN CHRONIC KIDNEY DISEASE

During the last few years and supported by a vast scientific basis, chronic inflammation has been acknowledged as a major culprit in a whole spectrum of pathological results associated with CKD. Poor outcomes, including CVD, diabetes, obesity, malnutrition, endocrine disruptions, and even premature aging, have been directly associated with a persistent inflammatory state. The specific pathways by which this association is mediated are still not fully understood; however, it is thought that inflammation, beside its own direct effect, potentiates other known risk factors, such as oxidative stress,[100] IR,[101] endothelial dysfunction,[102] vascular calcification,[103] bone mineral disorders,[104] and depression,[105] some of them previously described in this chapter. In this section we provide a brief review of some of the better-understood consequences of persistent inflammation in CKD patients.

Mortality

The association between inflammation and mortality in patients with CKD has been observed even in early stages of the disease. In patients with CKD stages 2 to 4, the multivariable-adjusted hazard ratio of death among those in the highest quartiles of IL-6 or CRP (and fibroblast growth factor-23 [FGF-23]) was several times higher than those in the lowest quartiles.[106] Both IL-6 and CRP, the most frequently used inflammatory biomarkers, have demonstrated high predictive value in the assessment of cardiovascular risk and all-cause mortality in this group of patients.[107,108] Moreover, other inflammatory markers, such as IL-1, IL-18, TNF-α, and P-selectin, have also shown mortality predictive value, although these markers have limited application in clinical practice.[109] However, it has been proposed that the use of combined inflammatory biomarkers (CRP, IL-1β, IL-6, IL-18, and TNF-α) could be a valid strategy to improve predictive accuracy.[110]

The link between inflammation and mortality is easily understood through the numerous complications associated with elevated inflammatory markers; nevertheless, it is interesting to highlight that the concurrent presence of inflammation with other pathologies such as PEW or CVD potentiates the mortality rates in ESRD patients. Namely, in a population of patients initiating dialysis (NECOSAD II study), the combination of inflammation, PEW, and CVD increased the mortality risk more than expected from the addition of their solo effects, implying additive interaction.[111]

Development and Progression of Chronic Kidney Disease

Multiple lines of evidence support the contribution of inflammation to the onset and progression of CKD. Epidemiological studies report association between the decline in eGFR and proinflammatory markers in both the general population and patients with CKD. Several mechanisms may interact in the development of renal injury in the inflammatory milieu, and CKD itself contributes to enhanced inflammation. Inflammation has been shown to aggravate glomerular injury; IL-6 regulates mesangial cell growth[112] and TNF-α contributes to endothelial damage[113] in various experimental models. Also, in transgenic mice, interstitial matrix synthesis was regulated by TNF-β,[114] and overexpression of IL-6 caused glomerulosclerosis and tubular damage.[115] Recently the associations between plasma levels of proinflammatory cytokines (IL-1, IL-1 receptor antagonist, IL-6, TNF-α, TGF-β, high-sensitivity CRP, fibrinogen) and the progression of CKD were investigated in 3430 participants of the CRIC study.[116] In this study, levels of fibrinogen, TNF-α, and albumin showed an association with rapid loss of kidney function,[116] reaffirming the previous findings from experimental models.

Protein-Energy Wasting

PEW, a state of nutritional and metabolic derangements characterized by loss of muscle mass and fuel reserves of the body,[117] is a common finding in patients with CKD.[118,119] Unequivocal evidence supports the causative relation between inflammation and PEW, with inflammation encompassed into the etiological model of PEW.[26]

Inflammation contributes to PEW by different mechanisms, among which anorexia is one of the better understood. Thus high serum concentrations of different inflammatory markers, including CRP and proinflammatory cytokines (IL-6 and TNF-α), have been associated with anorexia in HD patients.[120,121] Inflammatory cytokines have the capacity to regulate appetite through disturbing specific brain areas related to appetite regulation.[122] Specific cytokines access the brain and act directly on hypothalamic neurons and/or generate mediators, targeting both peripheral and/or brain target sites,[122,123] and, as a consequence, influence the size, duration, and frequency of meals.

On the other hand, inflammation in CKD patients paradoxically increases resting energy expenditure (REE), contributing to muscle loss. In an animal model, the infusion of inflammatory cytokines (TNF-α, IL-1, and IL-6) resulted in increase in the rate of muscle protein breakdown[124]; in humans, inflammatory markers are related to markers of muscle mass, indicating an important role of cytokines in the development of PEW and muscle catabolism.[125,126]

In addition, other features enhanced by inflammation, such as increased IR and activation of the adenosine triphosphate ubiquitin-proteolytic system, have proved to have a role in the pathogenesis of PEW.

Vascular Calcification

Large artery calcification (assessed by computer tomography or chest x-ray) is highly prevalent from the earliest stages of CKD, reaching a prevalence as high as 70% in individuals with ESRD[127,128] and even affecting as many as 15% of uremic pediatric patients.[129] Vascular calcification has catastrophic effects on the prognosis, raising cardiovascular mortality disproportionally and increasing the risk of sudden death.[130,131] Of note, elevated markers of inflammation (CRP and IL-6) in the presence of vascular calcification predict an even worse prognosis.[132]

In CKD, both intima and media arterial calcification are markedly increased.[133] Whereas intima and media calcification differ morphologically and their clinical consequences are also different,[131,134] both are associated with local and systemic inflammation.[135]

There is a substantial body of evidence supporting the involvement of the inflammatory response in the pathogenesis of vascular calcification. In a recent study in early CKD patients, biopsy-verified media calcification was associated with local upregulation of proinflammatory molecules but not with increased serum levels of phosphorous, calcium, or calcium x phosphorous index.[135] Also, in advanced CKD, only sclerostin—but not other circulating markers of bone metabolism—predicted biopsy-verified vascular calcification.[136]

Among the different inflammatory biomarkers in CKD patients, TNF-α and IL-1 promote the progression of vascular calcification,[137] whereas several other inflammatory markers, including IL-8 and IL-18, are associated with its occurrence.[138] In vitro studies have shown that TNF-α induces calcification of vascular smooth muscle cells (VSMCs),[139] and coculture of these cells with monocyte/macrophages can accelerate this process.[140] Moreover, two regulating molecules that belong to the TNF receptor superfamily, osteoprotegerin (OPG) and receptor activator of NF-κB ligand (RANKL), are probably key players mediating calcification of VSMCs. RANKL is one of the major osteoclast maturation factors, whereas OPG functions as a soluble decoy receptor for RANKL and inhibits its effects.[141] This finely regulated balance is profoundly disrupted in the presence of ESRD because OPG accumulates in such a setting, causing a decrease in circulating RANKL, which in turn constitutes a risk factor for unfavorable vascular outcomes.[141] This would explain the detrimental effects on survival of both increased inflammation and OPG levels observed in HD patients.[142]

Another important player involved in the process of extrabone calcification is fetuin-A. This inhibitor of ossification, which acts as a negative acute-phase reactant, has been shown to decrease with progression of CKD. Mice lacking the gene encoding for fetuin-A rapidly develop ectopic soft tissue ossification and die at an early age.[143] In CKD, low levels of circulating fetuin-A are associated with increased cardiovascular burden and mortality.[144-146]

Taken together, these data provide evidence for the existence of an active interplay between vascular calcification and inflammation and underscore its importance as a nonclassical cardiovascular risk factor in CKD.

Anemia and Erythropoiesis-Stimulating Agent Resistance

The pathogenesis of anemia in CKD is multifactorial, and resistance to ESA—a consequence of inflammation—is a key contributor. For instance, HD patients with increased CRP levels require as much as 80% higher doses of ESA compared with those with CRP below 20 ng/mL.[147]

Although the link between inflammation and ESA resistance and anemia is undoubted,[147-149] the exact pathophysiological mechanism underlying this phenomenon is not fully understood. Some possible mechanisms have been proposed, including reduced iron availability and deterioration in the red cell line.

Erythroid progenitors require coordination of iron acquisition and cell proliferation in the consecutive stages of maturation. In a pathway controlled by hepcidin, inflammation compromises the availability of iron for heme synthesis and, in consequence, impairs erythropoiesis.[150,151] Hepcidin is a peptide hormone that regulates iron absorption and its release from the macrophages. Due to increased hepcidin synthesis, iron is retained in enterocytes and macrophages, leading to functional iron deficiency. Hepcidin is known to increase in CKD, also independently of inflammation, and a decrease of hepcidin levels has been observed in response to administration of ESA.[152] There is also some evidence that ESA may decrease levels of inflammatory markers, especially IL-6, which in turn may explain its influence on hepcidin levels[152]

Recently a regulatory role of HIFs in hepcidin synthesis and iron metabolism has emerged.[153] This may constitute a new link in a relationship between inflammation and anemia, perhaps opening new perspectives for therapeutic use of HIF stabilizers in management of CKD.

On the other hand, inflammatory cytokines, TNF-α and IL-1, inhibit erythropoietin production, whereas TNF-α, INF-γ and IL-6 may directly suppress the erythroid progenitor cell proliferation.[154,155] Moreover, inflammatory cytokines (mostly TNF-α) are responsible for the shorter life span of mature erythrocytes because they provoke changes in erythrocyte membrane and enhance erythrophagocytosis.[156]

Depression and Cognitive Impairment

Depression is highly prevalent in CKD, with some reports describing the presence of depressive symptoms in up to 70% of HD patients. Depression is closely and directly associated with inflammation. Although this association may be a result of confounding, a causative relation is supported by the effect of antiinflammatory drugs on the course of depression and by a decrease of IL-6 levels in response to antidepressant treatment.[157] High serum levels of proinflammatory cytokines (IL-1, IL-6, TNF-α) and cell-mediated immune activation, typically found in CKD, led to increased activity of the hypothalamic–pituitary–adrenal (HPA) axis and decreased availability of tryptophan for serotonin and melatonin synthesis.[158,159] All of these immune-inflammatory crossed pathways contribute to depression and also to chronic fatigue, which may be a constituent of—or associated with—depressive disorders.[160] Not unexpectedly, poor health-related quality of life (HRQoL) associates with proinflammatory cytokines and their regulation in HD patients. Interestingly, despite the strong association between IL-6 and fatigue in HD patients, no such a relationship has been found in healthy individuals.[160]

On the other hand, in a cognitive study of the CRIC cohort, higher markers of inflammation (hs-CRP, fibrinogen, IL-1β) were associated with an increased risk of impairment in attention but not with other cognitive functions.[161] Depression, fatigue, and impaired cognition may undeniably contribute to a vicious circle of anorexia, physical inactivity, inflammation, and PEW.

Endocrine Disorders

The uremic state is associated with abnormalities of the endocrine system, affecting hormone production, metabolism, feedback regulation, and altered target tissue sensitivity. Evidence suggests that the observed hormonal dysmetabolism may be aggravated by persistent inflammation. Several hormonal axes are usually found to be altered in CKD patients, although the total implications of the disturbances in terms of outcomes are not completely clear.

Thyroid hormones. Inadequate kidney function, in addition to other factors accompanying CKD such as inflammation, exerts an influence on the thyroidal status of renal patients in whom alterations in thyroid hormones are observed in the absence of an underlying intrinsic thyroid disorder.[162,163] The most common observed thyroid disorder in this group of patients is the so-called low T_3 syndrome, characterized by a decrease in total (T_3) and free (fT_3) triiodothyronine plasma concentration, whereas thyroid-stimulating hormone (TSH) levels are usually normal. This condition, present in approximately one-fourth of patients with CKD,[164] is discussed in an ongoing debate regarding whether the observed thyroid alterations, like other hormonal alterations in CKD, represent a pathological condition or a physiological, adaptive, and protective mechanism against the disease. This question does not yet have a clear answer; however, some studies have reported worse outcomes associated to these hormonal derangements, suggesting that it is not a completely physiological process. In fact, previous studies have connected the state of subclinical hypothyroidism with low-grade persistent inflammation.[165] Indeed, IL-6 signaling has been reported to downregulate the peripheral conversion of total thyroxine (T_4) into T_3 in both experimental[166] and clinical[167] studies.

Sex hormones. Testosterone deficiency or hypogonadism is a common finding in men with CKD. Although the high prevalence of hypogonadism observed in this group of patients to a great extent might be a consequence of the failing kidney per se,[168] inflammation might have an important role in its physiopathology because it is known that inflammatory cytokines have a suppressive effect on the hypothalamic–pituitary–testicular axis.[169,170] In fact, several studies depict a strong inverse association between endogenous testosterone and surrogates of inflammation in various CKD populations.[171-174] Important to note is that testosterone also has immune-modulatory actions per se, as suggested by the suppression of cytokine production in hypogonadal men with diabetes, coronary heart disease, and metabolic syndrome after supplementation with testosterone.[175-177] The relationship between inflammatory markers and other sex hormones such as estrogen or prolactin in CKD patients has been less studied.

Hypothalamic–pituitary–adrenal. The HPA axis is a finely tuned neuroendocrine system that plays a main role in processes such as stress-response, energy balance, circadian rhythm, immunity, reproduction, emotions, and cognition. The HPA axis has been little studied in CKD. However, derangements in the functioning of HPA could be expected, as for other endocrine axes, and there is some evidence that deregulation of HPA function may be present in earlier stages of CKD (e.g., CKD stage 2).[178] The link between inflammation and alterations in the HPA axis is not well defined; however, it is known that increased levels of cortisol observed in CKD are related in part to decreased activity of the 11β-hydroxysteroid dehydrogenase type 2 (11b HSD2), which is responsible for the conversion of cortisol into cortisone, its inactive metabolite.[179] The activity of this hormone decreases in presence of inflammation.[180]

Other hormones. The inflammatory response inhibits the action of growth hormone (GH),[181] as supported by forearm perfusion studies demonstrating that resistance to pharmacological doses of GH is not related to uremia per se but rather to an increased inflammatory state.[182]

Insulin Resistance

IR, defined as a reduced sensitivity of the liver, skeletal muscles, and adipose tissue to insulin action, is a frequent finding in CKD from the earliest stages of the disease.[183,184] In ESRD, IR is believed to be present in virtually all patients,[185] although a direct correlation between insulin sensitivity and degree of decline of eGFR is weak or absent.[184] Inflammation, especially potentiated by oxidative stress, is one of the established causative factors predisposing CKD patients to IR. Proinflammatory cytokines may promote IR by inhibiting insulin-signaling pathways on the post receptor level in skeletal muscles (TNF-α) and liver (IL-6), whereas adiponectin mediates insulin-sensitizing effects.[186,187] Interestingly, immune cells do not develop IR. This protective mechanism, ensuring a sustained energy flow in acute inflammation, becomes debilitating in chronic and persistent conditions of immune stimulation. In cross-sectional studies, the homeostatic model assessment of insulin resistance (HOMA-IR) was positively associated with CRP, IL-6, fibrinogen, and TNF-α in different cohorts of dialysis patients.[188-190] Many factors typically coexisting with inflammation and CKD, such as physical inactivity, anemia, vitamin D deficiency, leaky gut, acidosis, and others, also contribute to IR and constitute a vicious circle of mutual interplay. IR profoundly influences outcomes because it is associated with cardiovascular events, mortality, and CKD progression. On the other hand, IR is a modifiable risk factor, and administration of angiotensin receptor blockade has shown promising results ameliorating IR and decreasing inflammatory markers in patients with CKD stages 2 to 4.[191]

Premature Senescence

Inflammation may determine the pace of aging; and their mutual relationship is reflected in the term *inflammaging*. The attrition of telomeres—the repetitive regions located at the end of chromosomes—is postulated to be a surrogate marker of cell senescence. There is considerable evidence linking the shortening of the length of telomeres to inflammatory response; it is observed in circulating macrophages exposed to enhanced expression of proinflammatory cytokines (IL-6, TNF-α, IFN-γ) and hyperactivity of NF-κB.[192]

CKD shares similarities with senescence and predisposes to premature aging via a variety of mechanisms.[193] Oxidative stress is likely to play a prominent role in this process. On the other hand, stress-induced premature senescence contributes reciprocally to the chronic inflammatory state of advanced CKD.[194] Senescence-associated secretory phenotype (SASP), understood as a proinflammatory drift resulting in release

TABLE 14.2 **Comparative Aspects of the Most-Used Inflammatory Biomarkers in Chronic Kidney Disease**

	CRP	IL-6	IL-10	TNF-α	ESR	PTX-3
Availability	High	Intermediate	Low	Low	High	Low
Cost	Low	Intermediate	High	High	Low	High
Interpretation	Easy	Easy	Difficult	Intermediate	Easy[b]	Difficult
Reliability in CKD	High	High	Unknown	Unknown	Low?[b]	High
Usefulness in clinical practice	High	High[a]	Low	Low	Low?[b]	Low

[a]Usefulness of IL-6 is potentially high, but IL-6 is still rarely used in clinical practice.
[b]Few studies have evaluated ESR in CKD.
CKD, Chronic kidney disease; *CRP*, C-reactive protein; *ESR*, erythrocyte sedimentation rate; *IL*, interleukin; *PTX-3*, pentraxin-3; *TNF*, tumor necrosis factor.

of a variety of proinflammatory cytokines, chemokines, and growth factors, may develop as a response to oxidative stress triggered by uremia.[195] The SASP contributes to reinforcement of senescence and can transmit the senescence to neighbor cells in a paracrine manner.[196]

Quality of Life

HRQoL is a subjective assessment of the effect of a disease on the physical, psychological, and social functioning dimensions of the patient's life. HRQoL is included in the World Health Organization's definition of health and is a strong, independent predictor of hospitalization and mortality in ESRD. In a study including patients with CKD stages 2 to 5 from the Stockholm region in Sweden, HRQoL scores deteriorated progressively with the loss of renal function and were the lowest in CKD stage 5.[197] However, CRP and not GFR had stronger predictive capacity of impaired HRQoL in this study. The results indicated that even a relatively moderate increase in CRP may affect HRQoL.[197] The relationship between proinflammatory cytokines and self-rated health and well-being was also reported in a cohort of women visiting a primary care unit in Sweden.[198] Poor self-rated health was associated mostly with higher levels of IL-6 and TNF-α, whereas impaired general well-being was related to increased TNF-α and IL-1β.[198] Further studies are needed to determine whether and to what extent treatments targeted toward decrease of inflammatory markers may affect HRQoL.

MEASURING INFLAMMATION IN CHRONIC KIDNEY DISEASE PATIENTS

With the diagnosis of inflammation, as with the diagnosis of other medical conditions, finding the right biomarker for this purpose is of utmost interest. The search for the perfect marker is complicated in patients with kidney disease, in whom some basic inflammatory markers (e.g., erythrocyte sedimentation rate, ESR) are affected by the decline of renal function.

In recent years, several novel inflammatory biomarkers have been described and tested; embracing a wide catalog of possibilities that go from plasma proteins, such as CRP; classical cytokines, such as IL-6, IL-10, and TNF; and cytokine receptors, such as TNF-receptors, to attractive new molecules such as pentraxin 3 (PTX3)[199] or soluble TNF-like weak inducer of apoptosis (sTWEAK).[200]

It has been advocated, often not based on conclusive evidence proving their superiority, that these more specific biomarkers are better determinants of inflammatory status and represent more independent indicators of disease severity. What is true is that despite many markers having been studied and suggested, only very few of them meet requirements that make them appropriate for use in clinical practice. In this section, we discuss some of the most studied inflammatory markers in CKD (Table 14.2).

C-Reactive Protein

CRP is an acute-phase protein first described in relation to its capacity to bind pneumococcal capsular polysaccharide. It is produced by the liver under the stimulus of inflammatory cytokines, in particular IL-6. CRP levels rise in about 2 to 8 hours after the injury, reaching their peak around 48 hours later, with a half-life of 18 to 19 hours. Apart from liver failure, there are few known conditions that interfere with CRP production, and kidney failure seems not to have an influence.

CRP has a suitable profile (i.e., stability over time, lack of circadian variation, and no effect of food intake) that makes it especially useful in renal care, and it is by far the most measured inflammatory marker in patients with CKD. Thus CRP remains the prototypic marker of inflammation.

Unlike what happens in the general population, in whom consensus has been made in terms of the established cut-off values for diagnosis of inflammation (i.e., undetectable or very low levels are considered normal, values between 1 and 10 mg/L are considered moderately elevated, and values over 10 mg/L are considered markedly elevated), little agreement exists regarding the optimal cut-off point to diagnose clinically significant inflammation in CKD patients, and usually arbitrary and nonconsensual cut-off values have been used. Some years ago, based on published data from pooled European cohorts, a cut-off point of 10 mg/L was proposed to define uremia-related inflammation,[5] and this value has become the most frequently used cut-off point in clinical research for the prediction of outcome. However, recent studies have shown a substantial increase in mortality risk associated with CRP concentrations >3 mg/L.[201]

Even though further research is needed to establish optimal the cut-off point for diagnosis and initiation of treatment in this group, the wide availability of CRP determination, its relatively inexpensive price, and the facility of interpretation make CRP a very favored inflammatory marker to be used in clinical practice.

Interleukins

Interleukins are a group of secreted proteins and signal molecules with fundamental regulatory roles in the immune system.

IL-6. IL-6 (MW 22 to 27 kD) is produced by numerous types of immune cells, including monocytes, mesothelial cells, fibroblasts, adipocytes, and lymphocytes, usually in response to physiological stimuli such as infection, trauma, or other tissue damage.

Among many other properties, IL-6 induces acute-phase reaction, being one of the starters of the inflammatory response. However, what is more interesting about IL-6 is that it acts as both a proinflammatory and an antiinflammatory cytokine. In addition, whereas most other cytokines function via paracrine/autocrine mechanisms, the major effects of IL-6 are a consequence of its presence in the circulation, and its effects can be exerted at sites distinct and distant from its origin.

IL-6 can be detected in the 1 pg/mL range in healthy individuals and is elevated in most, but not all, ESRD patients.[202] Although decreased elimination may be a major cause of elevated IL-6 levels in ESRD patients, increased cytokine generation also plays a role. For example, circulating concentrations of IL-6 increase after HD sessions, providing evidence of HD-induced delayed inflammatory response.[203]

Plasma IL-6 levels correlate with increased mortality and poor outcome in ESRD patients,[125,204] consistent with studies relating IL-6 to mortality in the elderly and in healthy men at risk for myocardial infarction.

IL-10. IL-10 (18 kD) is a product of immune-active cells, mainly monocytes and lymphocytes, and appears to have a critical role in suppressing the inflammatory response. Within the inflammatory response, the secretion of IL-10 is delayed and always follows that of proinflammatory factors with a latency of a few hours. IL-10 is mainly cleared through the kidneys, probably by glomerular filtration and tubular metabolism, so its plasma half-life is markedly increased in ESRD, leading to elevated plasma levels.[205]

Although some groups have speculated that subjects with the highest IL-10 levels have better immune balance, a recent study reported that patients with higher levels of IL-10 (above the median of the population) exhibited increased risk of CVD events and overall mortality,[206] probably as a reflection of an overall proinflammatory milieu. Although for the moment the lack of conclusive data about the role of IL-10 as a protective or risk marker does not make it a useful marker for the clinical practice, it is an interesting marker for research purposes.

TNF-. TNF, a proinflammatory cytokine (17 kD) originally associated with killing of tumoral cells, has a pivotal role in regulating both pro- and antiinflammatory mediators. It is produced mainly by activated macrophages, although many other cell types can produce it. TNF-α has been regarded as a key regulator of the cytokine cascade, providing a rapid form of host defence against infection; however, excessive TNF-α can be destructive. TNF influences lipid metabolism, coagulation, IR, and endothelial dysfunction. Interestingly, TNF-α levels have a rather weak correlation with CRP, suggesting that circulating levels of TNF may be influenced by a number of different factors,

Although a relationship between renal function and TNF-α and its soluble receptors has been demonstrated in patients with varying degrees of renal failure,[207] it is not clear to what extent reduction in renal function is directly responsible for increased levels of TNF-α. In CKD patients, higher levels of TNF have been related to poor outcomes, especially nutritional outcomes.

Other cytokines. Other cytokines have also been found to be increased in patients with CKD. IL-12 and IL-18 are elevated during the earlier stages of CKD but are not associated with arterial stiffness. IL-18 is associated with GFR, suggesting that its elevation in CKD is largely dependent on renal clearance.[208]

Other Biomarkers of Inflammation

A large number of other substances, including specific molecules involved in the inflammatory response, have been studied as potential inflammatory markers; however, due to less availability, difficulties in interpretation, and lack of additional predictive capacity over and above that of commonly used inflammatory markers, most of these are unsuitable at present to be used in clinical practice. Among commonly available biomarkers (which will not be further discussed here), white blood cell count and immunocompetent cells, including leukocytes, monocytes, and lymphocytes (see Table 14.1), ESR (see Table 14.2), and plasma albumin and fibrinogen levels are often used to assess presence and severity of inflammation.

Pentraxin 3. PTX3, a member of the pentraxin superfamily, is characterized by a cyclic multimeric structure with structural relation to other pentraxin molecules such as CRP. PTX3 is produced by a number of different cells, including endothelial cells, after primary inflammatory signals, activating the classic pathway of complement and having a dual role of protection against pathogens and control of autoimmunity.

However, it has been recognized that PTX3 has multifaceted properties extending beyond the fields of immunity and inflammation to CVD and other chronic conditions.

In normal conditions, pentraxin is detected in blood in very low levels, although it increases rapidly after noxious triggers.

In CKD patients, as in the general population, PTX3 represents a specific and sensitive marker connecting inflammation with CVD.[199] These data and epidemiological and clinical data support PTX3 as a valid biomarker for atherosclerosis and other poor outcomes.

Other, less commonly used inflammatory biomarkers in research protocols include, among others: high-mobility

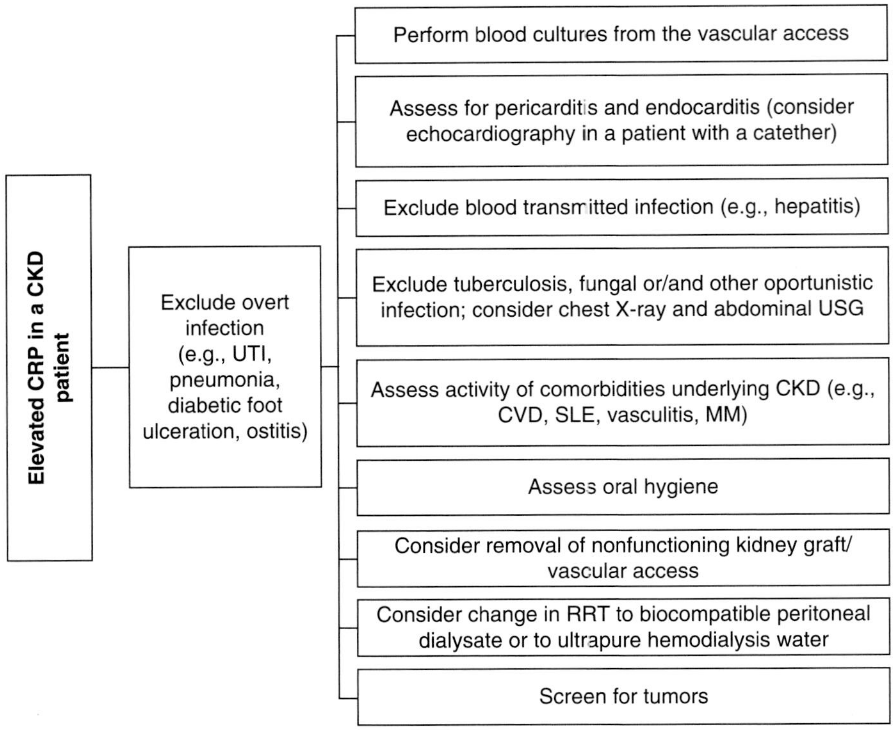

FIG. 14.2 Approaching a patient with inflammation. Consecutive steps in planning the diagnostic approach to ESRD patient with increased CRP. Routine examination allows confining the area of investigation to the most probable sites of infection, helping plan the next laboratory and imaging steps, and deciding about the urgency of an observed complication. *CKD*, Chronic kidney disease; *CRP*, C-reactive protein; *CVD*, cardiovascular disease; *MM*, multiple myeloma; *RRT*, renal replacement therapy; *SLE*, systemic lupus erythematous; *USG*, ultrasonography; *UTI*, urinary tract infection.

group box 1 protein (HMGB1), sTWEAK,[199] soluble TNF-related apoptosis-inducing ligand (sTRAIL), orosomucoid or α1-acid glycoprotein, soluble receptor for advanced glycation end-products (sRAGE), S100 calcium-binding protein A12 (S100A12; also called *calgranulin C*, or *EN-RAGE*). These—and many other biomarkers related to inflammation—reflect various specific aspects of inflammation that are relevant to its pathophysiology and downstream consequences.

MANAGING THE INFLAMED CHRONIC KIDNEY DISEASE PATIENT

Because persistent inflammation may be a silent reflection of various pathophysiologic alterations in CKD, and because its presence is associated with many deleterious outcomes in this population, it is essential that inflammatory markers are regularly monitored and therapeutic attempts are made to target inflammation. There is no consensus on how to manage inflamed CKD patients; however, based on the literature, measures have been proposed as possible valid therapeutic strategies in this group of patients. This section proposes some suggestions for the management of inflamed CKD patients.

Approaching a Patient With Inflammation

Regular assessment of inflammatory status is warranted in patients with advanced kidney failure. Data from the Dialysis Outcomes and Practice Patterns Study (DOPPS) registry shows that the monitoring of inflammation in dialysis units has increased considerably in the last decade in many parts of the world, and, in DOPPS III, CRP was examined in the majority of patients in nearly all countries except for the United States and Canada.[201] Centers where repeated CRP measurements are used routinely have reported better clinical outcomes. Thus DOPPS data showed that higher accessibility of CRP measurements in dialysis centers were associated with lower cardiovascular mortality.[201] Serial measurements of CRP in an individual patient should make it possible to detect and act on rapid or unexpected changes in the inflammatory response.

All unexpected changes in CRP should be meticulously investigated. The most important step in this investigation remains a detailed medical history and thorough physical examination. As depicted in Fig. 14.2, there are numerous contributors to increased CRP in CKD and especially in ESRD. The routine examination allows confining the area of investigation to the most probable sites of infection, helping plan the next laboratory and imaging steps, and deciding about the urgency of an observed complication. For instance, early diagnosis of ischemia of the intestinal wall, a complication quite frequently found in HD patients, might be critical for the patient's survival. Thus the first step in diagnostic procedure should be targeted at the exclusion of overt infection, which most frequently takes the form of pneumonia, urinary tract infections, infection of the dialysis access site, or osteitis in the course of diabetic foot pathology. More challenging remains investigating persistent inflammation of unknown origin. Attention should be directed to the vascular/peritoneal access in the first instance. In parallel, the volume status of the patient should be assessed and, especially, fluid overload excluded. Importantly, other laboratory indices should be analyzed, including persistent anemia, improper white blood cell and platelet counts, acid-base balance, parameters of dialysis adequacy, parameters of heart and muscle ischemia, coagulation, transaminases, and cultures. At this step, chest x-ray and abdominal ultrasound examination should be also performed if not attained earlier. Persistent anemia accompanying persistent inflammation in a patient with a vascular access should draw attention to suspicion of endocarditis, and performing echocardiography should be advocated.

As CKD entails profound changes in immunity, opportunistic infections are found relatively frequently in this population of patients, with a special prevalence of tuberculosis.

De novo hepatitis and activation of chronic infection are possible, although infrequent consequences of numerous medical procedures inscribed in the history of CKD, and these should be taken into account. At this stage of investigation, it is also important to exclude the exacerbation of concomitant comorbidities, especially of rheumatologic origin. Nonfunctioning kidney grafts and vascular accesses should be screened and removed if indicated. In the next step, screening for oncological processes should be implemented.

Poor oral hygiene is an important and frequent contributor to persistent inflammation and should be assessed during the initial physical examination. However, due to the high prevalence of poor oral health and the relatively prolonged time required for its treatment, relying on this finding as a main source of increased CRP may delay the diagnosis of more serious and perhaps life-threatening conditions, such as systemic lupus erythematosus flares, endocarditis, or lymphoma. This explains the low position of oral hygiene on the diagnostic ladder.

If the diagnostic process is unsuccessful, changes in the RRT procedure should be considered. Such changes could include attempts to inspect and, if necessary, change vascular access (especially avoiding HD catheters if possible), use ultrapure HD water, use more biocompatible HD dialyzers (including dialyzers with removal capacity of large uremic toxins including proinflammatory cytokines), or change the dialysis modality (e.g., from HD to PD), if possible, using biocompatible dialysis fluids.

Therapeutic Strategies in Inflamed Chronic Kidney Disease Patients

Treating the Basics

Documenting the presence of inflammation in a patient is crucial and should first of all lead to the diagnosis and appropriate treatment of comorbidities that may contribute to inflammation, such as heart failure, and especially local and systemic infectious processes. However, once the occurrence of an acute process has been treated or ruled out, other interventions are valuable in the clinical management of uremic inflammation (Table 14.3). These interventions include improvements in dialysis therapy and fluid status, as well as implementation of healthy lifestyle habits including diet modifications[209,210] and increased physical activity.[211]

Diet is an area involving a large number of potentially modifiable risk factors for CKD. Dietary supplementation or restriction of many different food compounds has shown beneficial effects on inflammation, although few studies so far have documented a positive effect on clinical outcomes. Among those with the strongest evidence we have:

a. *Salt restriction:* Dietary sodium restriction is associated with the attenuation of the inflammatory state depicted by a reduction in levels of CRP, IL-6, and TNF-α.[212]
b. *Omega-3 fatty acids*: Twelve-week fish oil supplementation decreased CRP in HD patients.[213]
c. *Gamma-tocopherol:* A small, randomized trial in HD patients showed an effect on IL-6.[214]
d. *Pomegranate juice*: One year of pomegranate juice intake yielded a significant time response reduction in the priming of polymorphonuclear leukocytes, protein oxidation, lipid oxidation, and levels of biomarkers of inflammation.[215]
e. *Probiotics:* In a randomized, double-blind, placebo-controlled trial including 39 PD patients, levels of serum TNF-α, IL-5, IL-6, and endotoxin significantly decreased after 6 months of treatment with probiotics, whereas levels of serum IL-10 significantly increased.[216] In addition, supplementation with prebiotics and probiotics, along with a low-protein diet over 12 months, resulted in delayed progression of CKD, in a small (n = 24) group of patients with CKD stages 3 to 5.[217]
f. *High fiber intake:* High dietary total fiber intake is associated with lower risk of inflammation and mortality.[218]
g. *Low-fructose diet:* Changing to a low-fructose diet decreased values of hs-CRP and soluble intercellular adhesion molecule 1 (sICAM), and hs-CRP values returned to baseline with resumption of the regular diet.[219]
h. *Green tea:* It reduces HD-induced production of hydrogen peroxide, hypochlorous acid, atherosclerotic disease risk factors, and proinflammatory cytokines.[220]
i. *Soy:* Lower prevalence of inflammation and better outcome in Asian HD patients have been suggested to reflect, in part, intake of products derived from soy beans; soy supplementation decreases CRP levels in HD patients.[221]
j. *Curcumin:* In an experimental model, curcumin exhibited salutary effects against adenine-induced CKD in rats by reducing inflammation and oxidative stress via upregulation of the transcription factor Nrf2.[222]

Concurrently, physical exercise has been shown to decrease hs-CRP and IL-6 levels[223] and improve cardiovascular outcomes[224] and dialysis efficacy[225] in patients undergoing HD. Although most of the best-quality evidence has been documented as regards HD individuals, the benefits of training have also been demonstrated in predialysis and transplant cohorts. The optimal form of physical training for CKD patients has not been determined; however, aerobic training is considered the most beneficial type of exercise for reducing hs-CRP levels.

TABLE 14.3 **Therapeutic Strategies in Inflamed Chronic Kidney Disease Patients**

Treating Underlying Causes of Inflammation	Pharmacological Treatment
Improving dialysis therapy	**Daily use drugs**
- Biocompatible membranes[83]	- Angiotensin-converting enzyme inhibitors, angiotensin receptor blockers, and renin inhibitors [276-278]
- Vitamin E–coated dialysis membranes[262]	- Statins[279]
- Ultrapure dialysate[89]	- Antidepressants[280]
- Haemodiafiltration[263]	- Allopurinol[281]
- Daily hemodialysis[88]	- Sevelamer[236,282]
- Avoid volume overload[264]	- Cholecalciferol[283]
- Avoid catheter usage[265]	- Paricalcitol[284]
	- Linagliptin[285]
Treating comorbidities	
- Periodontal disease[266]	**Potential antiinflammatory drugs**
- Bowel bacterial overgrowth[267]	- N-acetylcysteine[286]
- Relapsing vasculitis[268]	- Pentoxifylline[287]
- Hypogonadism[171]	- Bardoxolone[288]
- Silent cardiac ischemia[269]	- Anticytokine drugs (Tocilizumab,[289] Canakinumab,[247,290] Anakinra,[291] Etanercep[292])
- Calciphylaxis[270]	
- Failed kidney transplant271,272	
Improving diet and lifestyle	
- Diet modifications	
• Salt restriction[212]	
• Soy protein–containing isoflavones[221]	
• White wine and olive oil[273]	
• Omega-3[213]	
• Pomegranate juice[215]	
• Green tea[220]	
• Gamma-tocopherol[214]	
• Low-fructose diet[219]	
• Probiotics [216]	
• High fiber intake[218]	
- Promoting physical activity[211]	
- Cognitive-behavioral therapy for sleep disorders[274]	
- Smoking cessation[275]	

Pharmacological Interventions

Daily use drugs. Several drugs that are commonly used in the treatment of patients with CKD and other common pathologies have shown a potential favorable effect on inflammation. Some literature is available in this regard. For instance, statins use have been shown to have antiinflammatory actions[226,227] and antioxidative properties[228] in HD patients, besides their effect on cholesterol synthesis. However, no effect on survival was demonstrated in the Deutsche Diabetes-Dialyse (4D) randomized controlled trial.[229] In another study, aspirin consumption induced a reduction in IL-8, IL-6, and TNF-α levels in HD patients.[230] Angiotensin-converting enzyme (ACE) inhibitor treatment is associated with a reduction in IL-6 response to coronary artery graft surgery.[231] In accordance, we have found lower plasma levels of TNF-α, CRP,[232] and adhesion molecules[233] in patients with CKD treated using ACE inhibitors.

Other interesting approaches may include vitamin D, which effectively reduced the inflammatory milieu in a randomized, controlled trial performed in patients with chronic heart failure.[234] Sevelamer has also been suggested to exert favorable changes in lipids and inflammatory markers with potentially useful antiatherogenic effects in HD patients.[235] In addition, short-term sevelamer intake significantly increased fetuin-A levels and improved flow-mediated dilation in nondiabetic patients with CKD stage 4.[236] N-acetylcysteine could also be an interesting option to test, considering its effect on reducing atheroma progression (probably through a decrease in oxidative stress) in an animal model of uremia-enhanced atherosclerosis.[237] Finally, PPAR-γ activators such as rosiglitazone may be another interesting strategy to explore given their antiinflammatory effects in a group of PD patients.[238] However, because the myocardial ischemic risk associated with rosiglitazone treatment may be increased in patients with type 2 diabetes,[239] these drugs should be used with caution in dialysis patients.

Novel antiinflammatory drugs. Within the search of novel therapies for reducing inflammation, controlling or reducing the amount of cytokine production has been considered a major target. Although some studies in the general population are available, it remains unclear whether these results could be applied to the CKD population. Thalidomide, a drug with immunomodulatory, antiinflammatory, and antiangiogenic properties, exerts its therapeutic effects through the modulation of TNF-α. As thalidomide induces a Th2 response and has been associated with weight gain in other wasted patient groups, such as those with HIV or tuberculosis,[240] it would be of interest to test the effects of this drug in patients with ESRD. However, its teratogen effect is a major limitation. Pentoxifylline was recently shown to reduce TNF-α expression by more than 50% and to improve hemoglobin levels in a small group of HD patients with erythropoietin-resistant anemia.[241] Finally, treatment with IL-1-receptor antagonists has successfully reduced markers of systemic inflammation in patients with type 2 diabetes[242] and improved clinical arthritis in patients with acute gout.[243]

Specific antiinflammatory drugs (tocilizumab, canakinumab, pentoxifylline) have been used in other inflammatory diseases, such as giant cell arteritis,[244] familial mediterranean fever,[245] and Behcet's disease,[246] proving to be of value. A clinical trial of canakinumab, a therapeutic monoclonal antibody targeting IL-1β, involving 10,061 patients with previous myocardial infarction and high-sensitivity CRP >2 mg/L (at a dose of 150 mg every 3 months) led to a lower rate of recurrent cardiovascular events than placebo, independent of lipid-level lowering, whereas all-cause mortality was not affected.[247] However, there is still a lack of data regarding the safety and concrete benefits of this and other specific antiinflammatory drugs and other antiinflammatory medications in dialysis patients.

CONCLUSIONS

A persistent inflammatory state is a hallmark of CKD and especially ESRD, and is caused by a range of factors linked to loss of kidney function, such as immune dysfunction, oxidative stress, and retention of uremic toxins. It is worsened by genetic predisposition, inappropriate diets and lifestyles, common comorbidities such as CVD and infections, and iatrogenic factors: in particular, the dialysis procedure. It is essential that biomarkers of inflammation such as CRP are monitored in patients with inflammation and that potentially modifiable root causes of inflammation are identified and addressed in clinical practice by appropriate measures that today may be part of the available arsenal of tools. Further research is warranted to advance diagnostic procedures and specific antiinflammatory treatments, although risks of interfering with the inflammatory process must be carefully considered.

ACKNOWLEDGMENT

Baxter Novum is the result of a grant from Baxter Healthcare Corporation to Karolinska Institutet.

CONFLICT OF INTEREST

Bengt Lindholm is employed by Baxter Healthcare Corporation. The other authors do not declare any conflict of interest.

A full list of references is available at www.expertconsult.com.

15

Sleep Disorders in Chronic Kidney Disease

Maria-Eleni Roumelioti, MD, and Mark L. Unruh, MD, MS

OUTLINE

Sleep complaints are very common among patients with chronic kidney disease (CKD) with patients having end-stage kidney disease (ESRD) particularly at risk for sleep disorder-related symptoms. Drowsiness, fatigue, restless legs, and difficulty falling asleep are among the most common symptoms in ESRD.[1] Compared with the general population, CKD is characterized by a higher prevalence of sleep disorders that have a profound and well-documented impact on the overall health and quality of life (QOL) of these patients. The relationship between CKD and sleep disorders is complex and dynamic. Sleep disorders place an additional morbidity and mortality burden on patients suffering from CKD.[2] Sleep quality (SQ) is very important to patients with CKD as demonstrated by a survey reporting that fatigue and SQ were the most important justifications for more frequent dialysis.[3] The most commonly reported sleep disorders in this patient population are sleep apnea (SA), insomnia, restless legs syndrome (RLS), periodic limb movements in sleep (PLMS), and excessive daytime sleepiness.

Sleep is a key complex physiological and behavioral process playing a crucial role in wellness for the general population and patients with chronic health conditions. Sleep is crucial to avoid sleepiness and drowsiness. Adequate sleep is important for job performance[4] and avoiding catastrophic errors such as the Exon Valdez and Space Shuttle Challenger accidents. Sleep has important metabolic effects[5] and plays a role in energy conservation[6] as well as cardiovascular health.[7] Emerging research has linked poor sleep to obesity and increased risk of diabetes.[7] Sleep plays a role in immunological response with seminal work demonstrating a decreased immune response to vaccines among sleep deprived subjects.[8] For patients with complex care regimens such as CKD, sleep's role in memory and learning may be extremely important for long-term outcomes.

This chapter presents an overview of the studies investigating sleep disorders in CKD and will characterize the extent to which sleep disorders are found among adult and pediatric patients with CKD, ESRD on dialysis (hemodialysis [HD] or peritoneal dialysis [PD]), and kidney transplant recipients as well as their consequences on the patients' health, QOL, and kidney function. Finally, this chapter emphasizes the evidence-based interventional studies that attempted to alleviate the symptoms and health consequences of the various sleep disorders in patients with CKD.

SLEEP IN CHRONIC KIDNEY DISEASE

Assessment for sleep disorders should be considered when caring for CKD patients. This was shown in an ancillary sleep study conducted from 2003 to 2005 at the Chicago site of the Coronary Artery Risk Development in Young Adults (CARDIA) study with a 10-year follow-up. In this community-based cohort of young-to-middle aged black and white adults without a history of cardiovascular disease (CVD), CKD, proteinuria, or hypertension, parameters of poor objective and self-reported sleep may be novel and early indicators of adverse changes in kidney functioning.[9]

A retrospective cohort study examined the potential association between sleep duration and time to the development of proteinuria (defined as 1+ or higher by dipstick test). The study included 6834 employees of the Osaka University aged 20 to 65 years who visited the healthcare center for their mandatory annual health examinations between April 2006 and March 2010 and did not have estimated glomerular filtration rate (eGFR) <60 mL/min/1.73 m^2, proteinuria, or treatment for self-reported kidney disease. They found that short sleep duration, especially 5 hours or fewer, was a predictor of proteinuria, even after adjusting for clinically relevant factors.[10]

Information on melatonin rhythms and the relationships between melatonin, core body temperature, and cortisol in CKD is limited. The CREAM study aimed to characterize the rhythms of melatonin, cortisol, and temperature in relation to kidney function in 28 patients with various degrees of kidney dysfunction. The mean eGFR was 57 ± 30 mL/min. The subjects exhibited melatonin (n = 24) and cortisol (n = 22) rhythms. Estimated GFR was significantly correlated to melatonin amplitude ($r = 0.59$, $P = 0.003$) and total melatonin production ($r = 0.51$, $P = 0.01$), but not to core body temperature or cortisol rhythms. No association was found between the phases of the rhythms of melatonin, cortisol, and core body

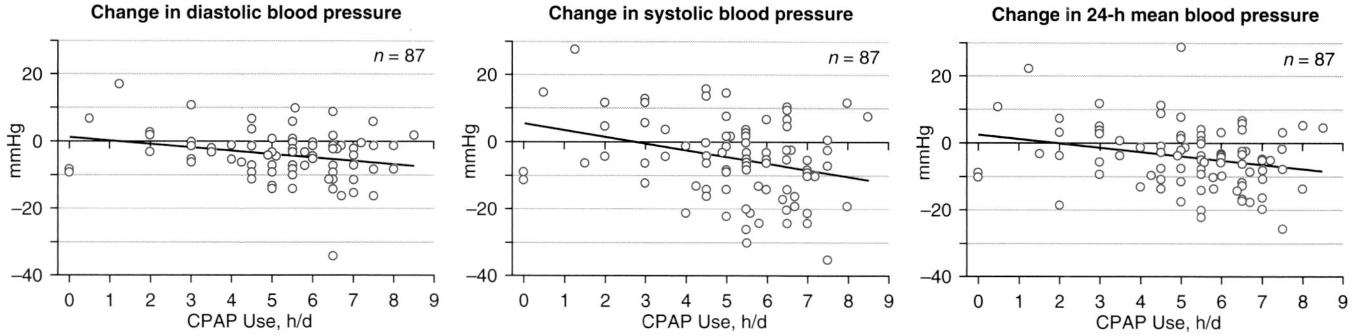

FIG. 15.1 Correlation between changes in 24-Hour mean, systolic, and diastolic blood pressure and number of hours of continuous positive airway pressure use. (From Martínez-García M, Capote F, Campos-Rodríguez F, et al., for the Spanish Sleep Network. Effect of CPAP on blood pressure in patients with obstructive sleep apnea and resistant hypertension. The HIPARCO randomized clinical trial. *JAMA*. 2013;310(22):2407-2415.)

temperature. As CKD progresses, follow-up research into circadian rhythms in these patients is warranted.[11]

Hypertension and obstructive sleep apnea (OSA) are highly prevalent among patients with CKD. SA is defined as repetitive prolonged cessation of airflow associated with sleep arousal and at times with oxygen desaturation. SA can be obstructive, in which respiratory effort persists during occlusion of the upper airway. SA may also be central, in which both respiratory effort and airflow cease, and mixed which combines a central and obstructive pattern.[12] The most common measure for SA severity is the apnea-hypopnea index (AHI), which is the number of apneas and hypopneas in 1 hour of sleep. These events lead to repetitive episodes of hypoxemia, hypercapnia, and sleep disruption as well as activation of the sympathetic nervous system. SA commonly produces daytime sleepiness[13] and decreased QOL[14] as well as impaired cognitive ability.[15] SA is an independent risk factor for hypertension[16] and is associated with CVD including stroke, myocardial infarction, and congestive heart failure after adjustment for obesity and other potential confounders.[17,18] In the general population, the treatment of SA with continuous positive airway pressure (CPAP) improves QOL,[19] vigilance, cognition, sexual performance, and restores nocturnal blood pressure (BP) dipping.[20]

This relationship between OSA and hypertension may be bidirectional, with high BP contributing to an increased risk and severity of OSA. The HIPARCO randomized controlled trial examined the effect of CPAP on BP in patients with OSA and resistant hypertension. This was an open-label, multicenter randomized controlled trial of parallel groups with blinded endpoint design conducted in 24 teaching hospitals in Spain involving 194 patients with resistant hypertension (an average of 3.8 antihypertensive drugs were taken per patient) and an AHI of 15 or higher between June 2009 and October 2011. The interventions were CPAP or no therapy while maintaining usual BP control medication. The primary endpoint was the change in 24-hour mean BP after 12 weeks. Secondary endpoints included changes in other BP values and in nocturnal BP patterns. Fig. 15.1 presents the correlation between changes in 24-hour mean, systolic, and diastolic BP and the number of hours on CPAP therapy in the patients of the CPAP group who finished the follow-up. At baseline, 25.8% of patients displayed a dipper pattern (a decrease of at least 10% in the average nighttime BP compared with the average daytime BP). When the changes in BP over the study period were compared between groups by intention-to-treat, the CPAP group achieved a greater decrease in 24-hour mean BP (3.1 mmHg [95% confidence interval (CI), 0.6 to 5.6]; $P=0.02$) and 24-hour diastolic BP (3.2 mmHg [95% CI, 1.0 to 5.4]; $P=0.005$), but not in 24-hour systolic BP (3.1 mmHg [95% CI, −0.6 to 6.7]; $P=0.10$) compared with the control group. Moreover, the percentage of patients displaying a nocturnal BP dipper pattern at the 12-week follow-up was greater in the CPAP group than in the control group (35.9% vs. 21.6%; adjusted odds ratio [OR], 2.4 [95% CI, 1.2 to 5.1]; $P=0.02$). There was a significant positive correlation between hours of CPAP use and the decrease in 24-hour mean BP ($r=0.29$, $P=0.006$), systolic BP ($r=0.25$; $P=0.02$), and diastolic BP ($r=0.30$, $P=0.005$).[21]

Another study explored the relationship between OSA and resistant hypertension in CKD and ESRD. Sleep parameters and BP were examined in 224 community-based, non-CKD participants from the Sleep-SCORE study, 88 nondialysis-dependent CKD and 95 ESRD participants. Unattended in-home polysomnography (PSG) with standardized scoring protocols and automated BP monitors were used. Resistant hypertension was defined as a BP ≥140/90 mmHg despite ≥3 antihypertensive agents. Mean systolic BP of the CKD and ESRD groups were significantly higher than that of the non-CKD group (148.2 [23.8], 144.5 [26.7] vs. 132.2 mmHg [26.7], respectively; $P < 0.0001$) despite the use of more antihypertensive medications. The CKD and ESRD groups had higher rates of resistant hypertension than the non-CKD group (41.4, 22.6 vs. 6.7%, respectively; $P < 0.0001$). The severity of SA was associated with a higher risk of resistant hypertension. Although resistant hypertension was associated with severe SA in participants with ESRD (OR 7.1; 95% CI, 2.2 to 23.2), there was no significant association in the non-CKD (OR 3.5; 95% CI, 0.8 to 15.4) or CKD groups (OR 1.2; 95% CI, 0.4 to 3.7) after accounting for case-mix.[22]

The treatment of hypertension to lower BP may improve SA by improving upper airway tone and by targeting hormone pathways (aldosterone, renin-aldosterone system) that may exacerbate OSA. The use of diuretics may also attenuate

SA by reducing the nocturnal rostral fluid shifts.[23] Therefore intensive BP and volume overload control may be a promising approach to treat OSA. A subsequent review and metaanalysis included 11 studies that reported changes in the severity of OSA objectively by using AHI or respiratory disturbance index. The pooled mean difference estimate (95% CI), based on a random-effects model, was −5.69 (95% CI , −10.74 to −0.65), consistent with an overall decrease in AHI or respiratory disturbance index attributable to antihypertensive medications. The effect size was even more pronounced, −14.52 (95% CI, −25.65 to −3.39), when only studies using diuretics were analyzed. There was no significant heterogeneity or publication bias among the studies. Metaregression indicated neither age, baseline AHI, nor change in systolic/diastolic BP influenced the results. They concluded that findings from these relatively small, short-term studies tended to support the contention that treatment with antihypertensive agents confers a statistically significant, albeit small, reduction in the severity of OSA, which may be more pronounced with the use of diuretics.[24]

In addition, CKD has been associated with increased fatigue and poor SQ. Fatigue with objective and subjective SQ was examined with a cross-sectional survey of 87 nondialysis-dependent CKD (eGFR ≤45 mL/min/1.73 m^2) and 86 ESRD patients using the Functional Assessment of Chronic Illness Therapy (FACIT-F) and the SF-36 vitality scale. Both advanced CKD and ESRD patients, experienced profound fatigue compared with the general population. Presence of CVD, low serum albumin, depressive symptoms, poor subjective SQ, excessive daytime sleepiness, and RLS were independently associated with greater fatigue in multivariable regression models.[25] Maintenance HD patients experience fatigue-sleepiness-exhaustion symptoms that demonstrate significant daily and diurnal variation. This was shown in a study by using of ecological momentary assessment.[26] This variability in symptoms may contribute to poor symptom awareness by providers and greater misclassification bias of fatigue related symptoms (e.g., exhaustion, feeling sleepy) in clinical studies.

SLEEP IN END-STAGE KIDNEY DISEASE

SQ is an important mediating factor in pain-related disabilities. Because pain is one of the most common symptoms experienced by HD patients, a study aimed to evaluate the experience of pain during dialysis, and at times when the patient was not receiving dialysis and to assess possible associations of perception of pain and sleep disturbance with survival in 128 HD patients. No association was found between survival and the presence of a sleep disorder or the duration of pain while off HD or any of the pain parameters while patients were on HD.[27]

Another study aimed to evaluate the prevalence and correlates of insomnia and OSA in 104 patients with stage 5 CKD or on chronic HD. Among these, 50% had chronic insomnia.[28]

RLS is a sensorimotor neurological disorder highly prevalent in ESRD patients. Uremic RLS is one of the most predominant types of secondary RLS and has been associated with further impairments in the already diminished QOL and health status of these patients. Both pharmacological and nonpharmacological treatment approaches have been used to improve uremic RLS symptoms (see Box 15.1). Currently, there are no specific published guidelines regarding the treatment of uremic RLS and the prescriptions given for uremic patients are based on the published instructions for the treatment of patients with idiopathic RLS.[29]

SA and PLMS often occur concurrently and may predict mortality in ESRD. A group of investigators examined

BOX 15.1 Therapeutic Interventions for Sleep Disorders in Chronic Kidney Disease and End-Stage Renal Disease

Sleep Apnea

Continuous positive airway pressure
Dental appliances
Oral surgery
Treating underlying medical conditions (such as obesity or hypothyroidism)
Lifestyle modifications (e.g., exercise, smoking cessation, no alcohol, loss of weight)
Optimal fluid volume control (low-sodium diet, diuretics, ultrafiltration)
Change of dialysis modality (e.g., switch from daily to nocturnal hemodialysis)

Insomnia/Mood

(a) Pharmacological
- Sedative antidepressants
- Anxiolytics
- Melatonin

(b) Nonpharmacological
- Cognitive-behavioral therapy
- Acupressure
- Relaxation therapy (yoga)
- Physical exercise (aerobic or resistance exercise programs)
- Change of dialysis modality
- Daily morning bright-light therapy (mood)

Restless Legs Syndrome

(a) Pharmacological
- Dopamine agonists (Das) (cabergoline, pergolide, ropinirole, pramipexole, rotigotine)
- Iron therapy
- Channel alpha-2-delta ligands (gabapentin, pregabalin)
- Opioids

(b) Nonpharmacological
- Aerobic exercise or resistance training
- Acupuncture
- Pneumatic compression devices
- Sleep hygiene improvement
- Pressure relieving mattress
- Near-infrared light
- Avoidance of alcohol, caffeine, and nicotine

Periodic Limb Movements

Pharmacological

Dopamine agonists

whether sleep fragmentation secondary to SA masks the underlying frequency or severity of PLMS in 16 patients with CKD, dialysis and not-on-dialysis, and if successful treatment of SA with CPAP results in the increased appearance of PLMS. All subjects had PSG-diagnosed SA. PLMS occur during uninterrupted nonrapid-eye-movement sleep. SA may mask the underlying incidence and severity of PLMS in CKD patients by disrupting nonrapid-eye-movement sleep. PLMS more than doubled during successful treatment of SA. The actual underlying prevalence and severity of CKD-associated PLMS are likely higher than appreciated and may often be masked by SA in the CKD population.[30]

Sleep in Hemodialysis

PLMS are a common disorder in HD patients and are described as repetitive, stereotypical, and unconscious leg movements that occur during sleep. PLMS are present in up to 80% of patients with RLS. PLMS cause significant sleep disturbance, result in nonrestorative sleep, and interfere with the expected sleep-associated dipping of BP. Therefore PLMS may constitute a risk factor for CVD and mortality. An interesting study investigated the association of PLMS with indices of heart structure and function in 19 HD patients with RLS. They found that severe PLMS seems to contribute further impairments in left ventricular mass and left ventricular internal diameter in diastole in HD patients with RLS. Therefore successful treatment of PLMS could result to reduced CVD risk and lower mortality rates in HD.[31,32]

In ESRD patients, the presence of OSA is associated with elevated BP, left ventricular hypertrophy, and increased mortality.[33-35] The high prevalence of OSA in ESRD has been attributed partly to instability of the respiratory control system due to uremia.[36] In patients with ESRD, fluid overload may contribute to their high prevalence of OSA by increasing the amount of fluid displaced from the legs into the neck overnight, and possibly compressing the upper airway. Indeed, in ESRD patients, the amount of overnight rostral fluid displaced from the legs is related to the frequency of apneas and hypopneas per hour of sleep (AHI).[37] Fluid overload via increased internal jugular vein volume, along with upper airway mucosal water content, contributes to the pathogenesis of OSA in ESRD patients.[38] This may explain the attenuation of OSA in association with nocturnal HD.[39] Fig. 15.2 depicts representative magnet resonance images of internal jugular veins from a subject with OSA (A) and another without OSA (B).

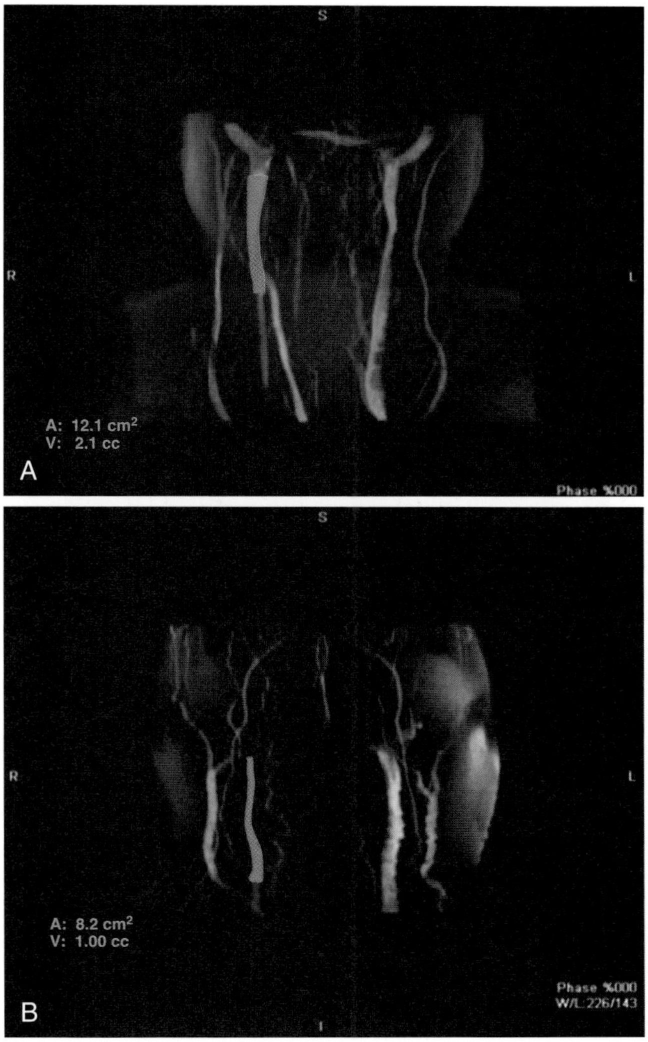

FIG. 15.2 Representative magnet resonance images of internal jugular veins from a subject with OSA (A) and another without OSA (B). The segment of the left internal jugular vein adjacent to the upper airway (UA) from the posterior aspect of the hard palate to the glottis is shown in green in both the subjects. Note that the internal jugular vein volume is greater in the subject with OSA (2.1 cm^3) than the subject without OSA (1.0 cm^3). (Reproduced with permission from Elias RM, Chan CT, Paul N, et al. Relationship of pharyngeal water content and jugular volume with severity of obstructive sleep apnea in kidney failure. *Nephrol Dial Transplant.* 2013;28(4):937-944.)

Poor SQ has been associated with both QOL and mortality risk among patients undergoing thrice-weekly HD. Data on SQ were collected from 11,351 patients in 308 dialysis units in seven countries in the Dialysis Outcomes and Practice Patterns Study (DOPPS) between 1996 and 2001 through a patient self-reported SQ scale, ranging from 0 (worst) to 10 (best). A score less than 6 reflected poor SQ. Nearly half (49%) of patients experienced poor SQ, which was independently associated with several QOL indices, medication use patterns, and mortality. Patients with poor SQ were more likely to be prescribed antihistamines, antidepressants, antiinflammatories, narcotics, gastrointestinal medications, antiasthmatics, or hypnotics. Physical exercise at least once a week (versus <1/week) was associated with 0.55 to 0.85 points lower odds of poor SQ ($P < .05$). Poorer SQ was associated with significantly lower mental and physical component summary scores (mental component summary scores 1.9 to 13.2 points lower and physical component summary scores 1.5 to 7.7 points lower when SQ scores were <10 vs. 10). The reduction ratio of mortality was 16% higher for HD patients with poor SQ.[40]

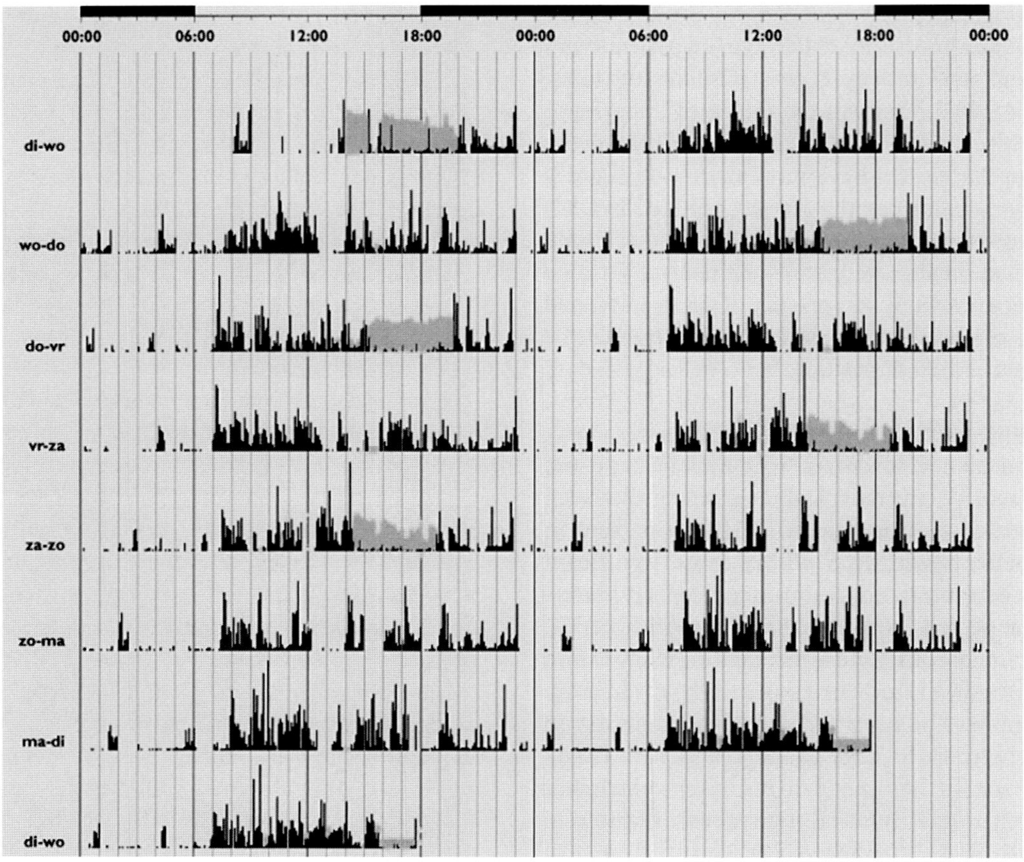

FIG. 15.3 Displays a week's actogram of a patient, at baseline. The graph shows the movements of the wrist during night and day. All days are double plotted, as on all lines two consequent 24-hour periods are shown. The black lines reflect the movement of the wrist. The lighter colored areas represent the light input on the Actiwatch of the patient. This patient dialyzed on Tuesday, Thursday, and Saturday afternoon. As can be seen, there are often low-light conditions during the day. Daytime napping does occur based on the absence of wrist movements, which can indicate sleep. (Reproduced with permission from Koch BC, Nagtegaal JE, Hagen EC, et al. The effects of melatonin on sleep-wake rhythm of daytime haemodialysis patients: a randomized, placebo-controlled, cross-over study (EMSCAP study). *Br J Clin Pharmacol.* 2009;67(1):68-75.)

The nocturnal endogenous melatonin rise is associated with the onset of sleep propensity and is largely absent in patients on thrice-weekly HD.[41] Exogenous melatonin administration can improve sleep in HD patients. One of the first studies examining the effects of exogenous melatonin on the sleep–wake rhythm of HD patients was the EMSCAP study.[42] This was a randomized, double-blind, placebo-controlled, crossover study of 3 × 6 weeks melatonin 3 mg at 22.00 hours every night. In the first 6 weeks melatonin 3-mg tablets or placebo tablets were taken. In the second period of 6 weeks, placebo and melatonin tablets were reversed. All patients received melatonin 3-mg tablets for the last 6 weeks. HD patients were asked to fill out a sleep questionnaire and wore a wrist actigraph to determine their sleep patterns. Melatonin concentrations in saliva were sampled the night after daytime HD and the consecutive night. On nights after daytime dialysis, objective sleep onset latency decreased significantly from a median of 44.5 (placebo) to a median of 15.5 min with melatonin ($P < 0.01$). Sleep efficiency increased from 67.3% to 73.1% with melatonin ($P < 0.05$). Actual sleep time increased from 376 min (placebo) to 388 min with melatonin ($P < 0.01$), and sleep fragmentation decreased from 4.5 to 3.1 ($P < 0.01$). Furthermore, subjective sleep parameters improved also. Patients reported less time needed to fall asleep ($P < 0.05$) and fewer wake periods ($P < 0.05$) on the nights with and without daytime dialysis and an increase in sleep time on the night of daytime dialysis ($P < 0.05$). Furthermore, the nocturnal melatonin rise was recovered. Fig. 15.3 displays a week's actogram of a patient from the EMSCAP study, at baseline.

Treatment with melatonin may improve objective sleep parameters, such as sleep fragmentation, sleep onset latency, and subjective SQ, and may recover the nocturnal melatonin rhythm. This finding was supported by a 6-week double-blind crossover randomized controlled trial, where 3 mg of melatonin or placebo were administered to 68 patients at bedtime. Lipid profile and the required dose of erythropoietin are also reported as secondary outcomes. Melatonin treatment significantly improved the global Pittsburgh Sleep Quality Index (PSQI) scores ($P < 0.001$), particularly subjective SQ ($P < 0.001$), sleep efficiency ($P = 0.005$), and sleep duration

($P < 0.001$). No differences in sleep latency and daytime sleepiness were observed. Melatonin also increased the high-density lipoprotein cholesterol ($P = 0.003$). The need for erythropoietin prescription decreased after melatonin treatment ($P < 0.001$).[43]

Many *nonpharmacological interventions* have been examined in HD patients to alleviate symptoms related to sleep disturbances. A randomized controlled trial evaluated the effects of a yoga-based exercise program (30 min session, twice per week for 3 months) on pain, fatigue, sleep disturbance, and biochemical markers in 37 stable HD patients. They found that a simplified yoga-based rehabilitation program is a complementary, safe, and effective clinical treatment modality in patients with ESRD and improved all those symptoms and parameters.[44] A noninvasive alternative therapy such as acupressure and its effects on SQ in 48 HD patients were investigated in another randomized controlled trial.[45] Patients who scored 5 points or higher on the PSQI were enrolled. The main outcome measures of this study were subjective SQ, latency and duration, habitual sleep efficiency, sleep disorders, daytime functional status, and use of sleeping medications. All outcome measures improved significantly in the acupressure group and the results supported the effectiveness of this therapy in improving SQ of HD patients.

Cognitive-behavioral therapy has also been shown to improve SQ and to reduce chronic inflammation.[46] Within this interventional randomized controlled trial, 37 sleep disturbed HD patients received tri-weekly cognitive-behavioral therapy lasting 6 weeks and the remaining 35 HD patients served as controls receiving sleep hygiene education. The adjusted posttrial primary outcome scores of the PSQI, the Fatigue Severity Scale, the Beck Depression Inventory, and the Beck Anxiety Inventory were all significantly improved from baseline by cognitive-behavioral therapy compared with the control group. High-sensitivity C-reactive protein, interleukin (IL)-18, and oxidized low-density lipoprotein levels also significantly declined with cognitive-behavioral therapy compared with the control group. Thus cognitive-behavioral therapy improved SQ, inflammation, and oxidative stress among HD patients with insomnia.

The beneficial effects of intradialytic aerobic exercise training were examined in a pilot study of 14 HD patients with RLS that aimed to evaluate the effect of 16-weeks supervised aerobic exercise training in the severity of RLS and QOL. Exercise training reduced the International RLS score by 42% and improved QOL and SQ. In this study, aerobic exercise training was safe and efficacious in reducing RLS symptoms and improving QOL and SQ in patients with RLS on HD.[47]

Five years later the same group of investigators conducted an exercise randomized controlled trial to investigate whether the reduction of RLS severity, often seen after training, is due to expected systemic exercise adaptations or it is mainly due to the relief that leg movements confer during exercise training on a cycle ergometer.[48] Twenty-four HD patients with RLS were randomly assigned to two groups: the progressive exercise training group ($n = 12$) and the control exercise with no resistance group ($n = 12$). The exercise session in both groups included intradialytic cycling for 45 min at 50 rpm. Only in the progressive exercise training group was resistance applied, at 60% to 65% of maximum exercise capacity, which was reassessed every 4 weeks to account for the patients' improvement. A 6-month intradialytic progressive exercise training program was found a safe and effective approach in reducing RLS symptom severity and improving SQ in HD patients. Because the exercise with no applied resistance protocol failed to improve the RLS severity status of the patients, it seems that resistance-applied exercise induced body adaptations that were largely responsible for the reduction in RLS severity score.

Another study evaluated the effects of aerobic training on SQ, inflammatory status, and serum leptin and C-reactive protein levels in 28 HD patients randomly assigned into control and training groups (14 patients per group). They found that aerobic exercise with moderate intensity during the first 2 hours of a dialysis session could improve SQ and inflammatory status of HD patients.[49]

One metaanalysis summarized and quantified the effects of three identified *nonpharmacological interventions* (cognitive-behavioral therapy, physical training, and acupressure) on SQ improvement in uremic patients on dialysis (HD, PD).[50] The primary outcome was the change of SQ before and after interventions (evaluated by PSG or subjective questionnaires such as the PSQI). They included 12 eligible randomized controlled trials and one prospective cohort study. All three interventions could result in a greater PSQI score reduction compared with controls: (1) cognitive-behavioral therapy versus sleep hygiene education (standardized mean difference 0.85; 95% CI, 0.37 to .34), (2) physical training versus no training (standardized mean difference 3.36; 95% CI, 2.16 to 4.57), and (3) acupressure (including other acupoints massages) versus control (standardized mean difference 1.77; 95% CI, 0.80 to 2.73). The finding of the cohort study suggested that intradialytic aerobic exercise training improved SQ in HD patients with RLS. This metaanalysis concluded that: (1) in dialysis-dependent patients, cognitive-behavioral therapy could shorten sleep latency, alleviate sleep disturbance, and reduce the use of sleep medications; and (2) acupressure and exercise training are promising interventions but the results in these subgroups should be interpreted cautiously due to the concern of methodological quality and potential confounding factors.

Sleep in Peritoneal Dialysis

Some sleep disorders may present differently depending on the dialysis modality used. Many important studies have attempted to evaluate sleep in PD patients (both in automated peritoneal dialysis [APD] and continuous ambulatory peritoneal dialysis [CAPD]) with objective and/or subjective measures and sometimes compared with HD patients as controls.

In a large cohort study,[51] data from the Comprehensive Dialysis Study (CDS) were used to examine the association of self-reported physical activity with self-reported symptoms of insomnia, RLS, and depression in 1678 patients new to dialysis (169 PD and 1509 HD patients). Sleep and mood disturbances were commonly reported (53% reported 1 of 3 insomnia symptoms, 29% symptoms of RLS and 28% symptoms of depression). Patients who reported lower levels of activity were more likely to report symptoms of insomnia, RLS, and depression.

In another interesting study, 166 clinically stable dialysis patients were randomly selected and divided into HD, CAPD, or APD. Self-administered questionnaires were collected for the investigation of insomnia, RLS, bruxism, rapid-eye-movement sleep behavior disorder, excessive daytime sleepiness, OSA syndrome, sleepwalking, sleep hygiene, depression, and anxiety. Insomnia was detected in more than 80% of patients in all three dialysis modalities. OSA syndrome was lower for patients on HD (36%) than on CAPD (65%) or APD (60%) and this was attributed most likely to their lower body mass indices. Patients on APD were more likely to have RLS compared with those on HD or CAPD (50% vs. 23% vs. 33%; $P < 0.04$) for unknown reasons. No differences among the modalities were found in bruxism, excessive daytime sleepiness, sleepwalking, sleep hygiene, depression, or anxiety.[52]

Another cross-sectional study aimed to investigate the association between SQ, health-related QOL, and depression, and to define independent predictors of SQ and depression in 64 PD and 90 HD patients receiving kidney replacement therapy for at least 3 months. This study showed that despite similar SQ scores between the two groups, HD patients had better health-related QOL and less depression than PD patients.[53] However, another study that assessed SQ in 90 HD and PD patients seemed to favor PD over HD. These investigators found that poor SQ was frequent in 86.6% of the cases in each group of HD and PD patients. Anxiety, depression, and being on HD were independent predictors of overall poor SQ.[54]

A cross-sectional study studied 42 CAPD patients and evaluated the relationship of SQ with RLS and depression and other potential risk factors. The prevalence of sleep disorders was 47.6% in the CAPD patients. RLS, depression, and low serum albumin were identified as risk factors for sleep disorders in this study.[55] A cross-sectional study explored the possible impact factors on excessive daytime sleepiness among 98 prevalent PD patients using both the PSQI and the Epworth Sleepiness Scale questionnaire. This study reported a high prevalence of poor SQ in PD patients and a correlation of excessive daytime sleepiness with low residual kidney function, poor nighttime SQ, and hypermagnesemia.[56] Another study attempted to assess the prevalence and relative risk factors of sleep disorders among 212 CAPD patients from a single center in southern China. PSQI was used to assess SQ. The average global PSQI score was 9.5 ± 5.2, with 171 (80.4%) poor sleepers (PSQI scores ≥5). This report demonstrated an important relationship of malnutrition and calcium to phosphate product with poor SQ in CAPD patients, which may partly explain the link between poor SQ and overall morbidity and mortality.[57] Finally, a descriptive study was performed to determine SQ, fatigue levels and related factors in 105 CAPD patients, as well as the effect of their SQ on fatigue. The investigators confirmed the high prevalence of poor SQ and increasing with age and fatigue in this patient population.[58]

A study from Sweden took a step further. These investigators aimed to describe the sleep–wake cycle, SQ, fatigue and health-related QOL measured with four questionnaires, actigraphy and a sleep diary during a 1-week period in 28 patients undergoing in-home PD. They also aimed to explore differences compared with 22 patients with coronary artery disease (CAD) and 18 individuals from the general population. Patients on PD had more fragmented sleep and worse sleep efficiency than patients with CAD or individuals from the general population. Pruritus (57%), RLS (46%), and fatigue (89%) were prevalent in PD patients. Pruritus correlated with fragmented sleep and sleep efficiency.[59]

SA has been evaluated in the past both by subjective (questionnaires) and objective (in-home PSG) measures in the PD population alone or in combination with HD patients. Sleep studies on CAPD and APD patients have also been performed. A cross-sectional study assessed the prevalence of SA and excessive daytime sleepiness in 227 ESRD patients (both PD and HD) using questionnaires. The overall prevalence of SA as defined by the Berlin Questionnaire was 37% in males and 34% in females, which was not a statistically significant difference ($P = 0.459$). SA was significantly associated with age, neck size, afternoon and evening HD shift, obesity, diabetes, and hypertension (P values: 0.001, 0.029, < 0.0001, < 0.0001, < 0.008, 0.002, and < 0.001, respectively). SA was also significantly associated with other sleep disorders such as RLS, insomnia, habitual snoring, and excessive daytime sleepiness (P values: < 0.001, < 0.001, < 0.001, and < 0.001, respectively). The prevalence of excessive daytime sleepiness was 44%, and excessive daytime sleepiness was significantly more prevalent in patients undergoing PD ($P < 0.001$); it was also associated with older age, diabetes mellitus, and other sleep disorders.[60]

An important study explored SA as a novel risk predictor of CVD events and death in patients receiving PD. This group of investigators prospectively followed the clinical outcome of 93 PD patients with baseline PSG. Of these, 51 were diagnosed with the syndrome defined by an AHI of at least 15 per hour. During a median follow-up of 41 months, there were 30 deaths, of which 17 were due to CVD causes. Patients with SA at baseline had significantly higher all-cause and CVD mortality during follow-up compared with those without SA. Minimal nocturnal saturation and desaturation indices were predictors of mortality and CVD events at univariate analysis. Multivariable Cox regression analysis identified significant SA syndrome at baseline as an independent predictor of increased all-cause mortality independent of age, male gender, and diabetes status. An absolute increase in the AHI was associated with an incremental risk of CVD events. Thus SA syndrome, detected at the start of PD, is a novel risk predictor for subsequent mortality and CVD events.[61]

It is well known that abnormal patterns of heart rate variability are associated with an increased risk of sudden cardiac death, stroke, and diabetes mellitus. In addition, dialysis patients and patients with CKD experience a substantial risk for abnormal autonomic function and abnormal heart rate variability. This was shown in a study where in-home PSG was performed in 95 patients with stages 4 to 5 CKD or ESRD on HD or PD. They found that patients with CKD and ESRD exhibited dysregulation of the autonomous nervous system tone manifesting as a failure to increase heart rate variability during wakefulness and sleep. Different patient characteristics were associated with changes in heart rate variability at different sleep stages. Patients with advanced CKD did not differ from dialysis patients in their inability to increase vagal tone during sleep.[62]

Another cross-sectional, descriptive study focused on estimating sleep disorders in APD patients by objective (PSG) and subjective (PSQI; Patient Health Questionnaire-9) measures. In this report, the investigators aimed to describe and compare the prevalence of sleep-disordered breathing (SDB), PLMS, poor SQ, and depression among 22 APD patients compared with 89 patients with CKD stages 3b to 5 and 75 patients treated by HD. In univariate analyses, APD patients had significantly lower AHI compared with HD patients (likelihood ratio test $P = 0.008$) and revealed the least proportion of total sleep time with nocturnal hypoxemia compared with CKD patients, respectively (likelihood ratio test $P = 0.01$). In multivariate analyses and after adjustment for age, gender, race, and body mass index, both APD and HD patients had higher average PSQI scores (worse SQ) than CKD patients, respectively (likelihood ratio test $P = 0.005$). They found that APD patients had similar sleep parameters and sleep architecture and as poor SQ and symptoms of depression as HD patients.[63]

Melatonin seems to play an important role in the sleep–wake rhythm of APD patients. It is well-known that this pineal hormone plays an important role in the synchronization of the circadian sleep–wake rhythm (defining periods of low and high sleep propensity), which may be negatively affected in dialysis patients, due to the pathology of ESRD and the dialysis process, causing daytime sleepiness and nocturnal insomnia.[64] An absence of the nocturnal rise in melatonin concentration in daytime HD patients has been described in the past.[65] Because little comparative data on sleep–wake rhythms in different dialysis groups existed, an innovative study aimed to investigate sleep–wake parameters measured with actigraphy and sleep questionnaires as well as melatonin rhythms in 6 APD, 20 conventional daytime HD, and 13 nocturnal HD patients. Melatonin in saliva was sampled at five time points (21:00, 23:00, 01:00, 07:00, and 09:00 hours). This study showed impaired sleep parameters in all dialysis patient groups. Conventional daytime HD patients had the worst sleep. In nocturnal HD patients, a normal nocturnal melatonin rise was found. In daytime HD and APD patients, this rise was absent.[64] As APD is also performed during night time, the same effect on normalized melatonin was anticipated as was found in nocturnal HD.

Are there any differences between APD and CAPD on sleep? A cross-sectional study aimed to determine any differences between these two PD modalities with respect to health-related QOL, depression, and SQ. Twenty APD and 48 CAPD patients were included. Moderate or severe sleep problems were found in 60% and 69% of the APD and CAPD patients, respectively. There were no significant differences between APD and CAPD in any of the studied parameters.[66] Similarly, a subsequent study compared 29 APD patients with 30 CAPD patients regarding their excessive daytime sleepiness and QOL. They found that the incidence of excessive daytime sleepiness was slightly higher in APD patients but not significantly different from the CAPD patients. Furthermore, the presence of excessive daytime sleepiness did not affect negatively daily activities or QOL.[67]

Both studies evaluated sleep by subjective means. However, our report regarding the contribution of uremia and volume overload to the pathogenesis of SA in ESRD has been supported by the improvement in SA with use of nocturnal APD. In a small study performed at two PD centers in Hong Kong, the investigators demonstrated a reduction in the severity of SA (AHI) with the use of nocturnal cycler-assisted PD in 23 patients that transitioned from APD to CAPD.[68] This hypothesis was further examined using MRI of the upper airway which demonstrated a reduction in cross-sectional space in the upper airway of 14 patients who transitioned from nocturnal PD to CAPD.[69]

Cognitive-behavioral therapy is effective for treating chronic insomnia in the general population and seems useful among the PD population as well. A pilot randomized controlled trial with parallel-group design investigated the effectiveness of cognitive-behavioral therapy in 24 PD patients with insomnia without active medical and psychiatric illness by assessing changes in SQ and inflammatory cytokines. The intervention group ($n = 13$) received cognitive-behavioral therapy from a psychiatrist for 4 weeks and sleep hygiene education, whereas the control group ($n = 11$) received only sleep hygiene education. Primary outcomes were changes in the PSQI and Fatigue Severity Scale scores, and secondary outcomes were changes in serum IL-6, IL-1β, and tumor necrosis factor-α levels during the 4-week trial. This study found that cognitive-behavioral therapy may be effective for improving SQ and decreasing fatigue and inflammatory cytokine levels in PD patients.[70]

Finally, a study evaluated the effects of nonpharmacological interventions; a pressure-relieving mattress and a 4-week individual sleep hygiene and sleep scheduling intervention on sleep, activity and fatigue in nine PD patients using both actigraphy and self-assessed questionnaires. Two women and seven men with sleep problems, 48 to 77 years old, treated with PD participated in a 17-week study. Physical activity advice was the element of the individual sleep hygiene and sleep scheduling intervention that yielded the most sleep improvements. This study demonstrated how a nonpharmacological treatment and self-management can be applied with kidney-supportive care to improve SQ in PD patients. This model can also reduce the pharmacological burden of these patients, because the current use of hypnotics can be replaced by sleep-hygiene self-care activities.[71]

SLEEP IN PEDIATRIC CHRONIC KIDNEY DISEASE

In the general pediatric population, nocturnal sleep disturbances have been associated with daytime behavioral problems, inattention, poor school performance, and reduced health-related QOL.[72,73] Sleep disturbances in children have also been linked to increased stress in parents, a negative effect on parental sleep, and even marital disruption.[74] In addition, a steady rise in the number of children and adolescents diagnosed with CKD has been observed with increasing CKD awareness. Despite these facts, only a small number of clinical studies have assessed the prevalence of sleep disturbances in pediatric CKD patients. In one of the first reports on the subject, an 85% prevalence rate of sleep disturbances among 21 children and adolescents on chronic dialysis (11 on PD and 10 on HD) was reported. Sleep disturbances in this report included the following: SDB (46%), excessive daytime sleepiness (60%), RLS (30%), and insufficient sleep time (25%).[75]

In 2009 the same group of investigators reported the results from a prospective, questionnaire-based, cross-sectional study that aimed to characterize the prevalence of sleep disorders among 49 children and adolescents (aged 6 to 18 years) with nondialysis-dependent CKD (including those with a kidney transplant for at least 3 months) using a validated pediatric sleep questionnaire. Four domains of sleep disturbance were assessed: SDB, RLS/PLMS, excessive daytime sleepiness, and insomnia. Positive responses to any of these signified the presence of a sleep disorder. Of the study participants, 37% were identified as having a sleep disorder (40% were in the nontransplant group and 32% in the transplant group). The most common type of sleep disorder was RLS/PLMS (27% in the nontransplant CKD group and 32% in the transplant CKD group). Other domains of sleep (e.g., SDB: 6%) did not seem to be a major problem and were only marginally higher than those in the general pediatric population. There was no correlation between stage of CKD and prevalence of sleep problems.[76]

In a subsequent report, the prevalence of sleep and fatigue issues was evaluated in 301 children with mild to moderate CKD from the Chronic Kidney Disease in Children cohort (CKiD). Symptoms of sleep problems (e.g., waking up early, falling asleep during the day, or decreased alertness) were reported from 12% of the study subjects. Those symptoms were associated with decreased overall health-related QOL.[77]

The prevalence of sleep disorder symptoms was described with a clinic-based survey in 159 school-aged patients with CKD. Three CKD patient groups were assessed: group 1, those not on dialysis and not transplanted; group 2, those on dialysis; and group 3, those with a functioning kidney allograft. Four symptom domains for sleep disorders were assessed: excessive daytime sleepiness, SDB, RLS symptoms, and insufficient sleep. Ninety-three patients (58.5%) had symptoms of a sleep disorder. The presence of a sleep disorder correlated with a decrease in health-related QOL scores that was independent of the CKD study group or eGFR.[78]

Although RLS is common among adults with CKD, RLS in children with CKD has not been extensively studied. The prevalence of RLS was evaluated in 26 children with CKD in different stages using a clinic-based or telephone survey. Definite or probable RLS was noted in 34.6% and, six of the nine patients with RLS had only mild CKD.[79] One publication tried to address conditions that might mimic RLS and can lead to overdiagnosis of this syndrome. In this prospective, cross-sectional study, RLS prevalence was compared between 124 pediatric CKD patients and 85 healthy children. RLS was assessed via a questionnaire that did not include mimics of the syndrome, such as nocturnal muscle cramps, arthritis, eczema, and positional discomfort, which may fulfill the diagnostic criteria for RLS and thus lead to overdiagnosis of the syndrome. Sleep characteristics and health-related QOL were also assessed. RLS was more prevalent in CKD patients than in normal children (15.3% vs. 5.9%; $P = 0.04$). Children with RLS were more likely to rate their SQ as "fairly" bad or "very" bad and to report the use of sleep medications. Finally, RLS was associated with lower health-related QOL by parent report.[80]

SDB in children may lead to serious and measurable end organ dysfunction. In the pediatric CKD population, the presence of SDB has been explored both using questionnaires as well as PSG findings, the gold standard for diagnosis of SDB. It remains unclear whether the prevalence of SDB in children correlates with the stage of CKD.[78,76] In the year 2013, a cross-sectional, control-matched group study assessed SQ in children on HD using a subjective sleep assessment and sleep questionnaire. Objective sleep evaluation was made using full night PSG. A total of 25 children with ESRD on HD were compared with 15 age-matched and sex-matched controls. Analysis of subjective data revealed markedly affected SQ in HD patients, as evidenced by excessive daytime sleepiness, night awakening, difficult morning arousal, and limb pains. Objective analysis showed less slow-wave sleep in HD children as well as increased SDB and PLMS.[81]

Another study aimed to ascertain the prevalence and type of SDB in 19 pediatric patients with severe CKD (stages 3 to 5 and seven were dialysis dependent, two on HD and five on PD) using overnight PSG. Study participants and/or their caregivers completed the pediatric modification of the Epworth Sleepiness Scale, the Patient Satisfaction Questionnaire, and the Pediatric Quality of Life Inventory at the time of the PSG. Based on the PSG results there was a 37% prevalence of SDB in this cohort. Central SA and OSA were found in three children each. The PSG and validated sleep questionnaires provided discordant results, highlighting the limitations of diagnosing SDB in pediatric CKD based solely on sleep questionnaires.[82]

In one short report, the authors reviewed two pediatric patients with CKD on PD and SDB in conjunction with their PSG results, and discussed the possible contributing factors. In PD patients such as these two children, the use of bicarbonate-containing solutions may predispose them to SDB as subsequent metabolic alkalosis can potentially lead to hypoventilation and hypercapnia. OSA, although commonly due to adenoidal/tonsillar enlargement, may be related to rostral fluid shifts and upper airway muscle weakness secondary to uremia.[83] More robust results about sleep disturbances in pediatric CKD patients on APD came from a group of investigators that conducted an observational and descriptive sleep study on eight children (up to 18 years of age) who had undergone APD for at least 3 months. PSG was performed while the children were on their usual cycler nocturnal dialysis regimen. A sleep questionnaire was completed on the same day as well. Sleep disruption was noted in five (62.5%) patients. The results of PSG showed decreased sleep efficiency and latency, increased awake time (23.08% of total sleep time), AHI (1.8 ± 1.9 per hour), and desaturation index (4.5 ± 3.7). Average periodic limb movement index was normal. Subjective data obtained by the sleep questionnaire underestimated the PSG findings.[84]

Finally, a review of publications on pediatric sleep in CKD (7 articles) identified indications of an increased prevalence of sleep disorders in children with CKD. The identification of sleep disorders should be based on PSG results or accomplished via structured interviews blinded to CKD state in studies with well-matched controls for age and gender. Pediatric CKD patients with sleep disorders are in need for longitudinal follow-up that would provide more insights on the underlying mechanisms and chronic health issues that arise. As sleep disorders may have serious consequences on a pediatric CKD patient's life, systematic sleep assessment should be considered an important part of the management and the therapeutic targets to achieve better clinical outcomes.[85]

SLEEP IN KIDNEY TRANSPLANTATION

Kidney transplant recipients are at increased risk for sleep disorders due to pharmacotherapy and multiple comorbidities. Numerous studies have evaluated sleep in kidney transplant recipients both by subjective and objective means. In most studies, sleep disorders improved after kidney transplantation. Langevin et al.[36] were among the first investigators reporting a significant improvement of both OSA and central SA in two HD patients after kidney transplantation. However, the prevalence of SDB remains high among kidney transplant recipients (27% vs. 33% of wait-listed patients) because it is dependent on risk factors of SDB (i.e., older age, male gender, obesity, lower educational status, use of hypnotic drugs, comorbidity) as well as on declining of kidney function.[86] The same group of investigators conducted a cross-sectional study of 100 kidney transplant and 50 wait-listed patients who underwent one-night PSG (SLEPT study).[87,88] In this study, the investigators assessed the prevalence of obstructive SA and its clinical correlates and compared the prevalence of this disorder between the two study groups. The prevalence of mild (AHI ≥5/h and <15/h), moderate (AHI ≥15/h and <30/h), and severe OSA (AHI ≥30/h) was 18%, 11%, and 14% in the kidney transplant group and 28%, 16%, and 10% in the wait-listed group, respectively. The AHI was significantly correlated with age (rho = 0.34), body mass index (rho = 0.45), neck circumference (rho = 0.4), abdominal circumference (rho = 0.51), and hemoglobin (rho = 0.24) in the kidney transplant group. The proportion of kidney transplant patients who were treated with three or more antihypertensive drugs was significantly higher in the OSA group (56 vs. 31%; $P = 0.022$). Despite taking significantly more antihypertensive drugs, the average systolic BP was still higher in patients with versus without OSA (147 ± 21 vs. 139 ± 18 mmHg; $P = 0.059$).[87]

Does kidney transplantation improve or even cure SA? Results from three different studies are inconclusive. The most optimistic study by Lee et al. examined 24 ESRD patients who were admitted for kidney transplantation and underwent a sleep study using a portable ventilation effort recorder on the night before transplantation. Of these patients, 20 could repeat the overnight monitoring 2 weeks after the transplantation. The median AHI of the 20 patients was 13.5 (range, 2 to 40), and significantly reduced to 4.5 (range, 0 to 20) after transplantation ($P = 0.003$). This reduction was most prominent in 12 patients with SA, for whom the median AHI fell from 22 (range, 10 to 40) to 6.5 (range, 1 to 20; $P = 0.010$). SA improvement, defined as an AHI ≥50% and/or reduced to <10/h, was observed in 8 of the 12 apneic patients. However, two other studies supported a different takeout message. In the first study by Beecroft et al., 18 dialysis-dependent patients awaiting kidney transplantation and predialysis patients with an identified living donor kidney had overnight PSG, which was repeated several months after successful kidney transplantation. Patients were divided into apneic and nonapneic groups based on an AHI >10/h during pretransplant PSG and, after transplantation, apneic patients were further divided into responders and nonresponders based on >50% reduction in AHI and/or AHI <10/h. Pretransplant SA was present in 11 of 18 (61%) patients. Although transplantation was associated with a significant reduction in blood urea nitrogen and serum creatinine, there were no significant changes in AHI (pre vs. post: 20.2 ± 15.1 vs. 23.5 ± 21.3). Among the 11 patients with SA, only 3 met the criteria for a significant improvement ("responder"). There were no patient characteristics, SA indices, or renal function changes that distinguished responders from nonresponders. Therefore the investigators concluded that SA improves in a minority of patients with ESRD after successful kidney transplantation, but specific determinants of improvement were not identified. Finally, Rodrigues et al. studied 34 nondiabetic patients with ESRD. Clinical, laboratory test, and PSG features were determined and compared before and after transplantation, and between groups with or without SDB, defined as having an AHI ≥5. An AHI ≥5 was present in nine patients (26.5%) before and seven (21%) after transplantation, and no significant reduction of mean AHI was found between study phases (5.3 ±7.3 vs. 3.1 ± 4.5; $P > 0.05$). This study concluded that kidney transplantation is associated with an improvement in sleep architecture, but does not cure SDB in all patients.[89-91]

Persistent SDB may contribute to the risk of CVD and death-censored graft loss in these patients. Transplanted patients with OSA had higher BP despite taking more antihypertensive medications compared with wait-listed patients.[87] However, the same investigators did not find an association between inflammatory markers (C-reactive protein, serum albumin, white blood cell count, IL-6, tumor necrosis factor-α) and objectively assessed sleep disorders (OSA, PLMS) in a large sample ($n = 100$) of kidney transplant recipients.[92]

In addition, high risk of OSA is a risk factor of death censored graft loss in these patients. This was shown in an observational cohort study that investigated the association of "high-risk OSA" with death-censored graft loss and mortality in 1067 prevalent kidney transplant recipients by using a questionnaire.[93] However, the same group of investigators developed subsequently a prospective cohort study of 100 prevalent kidney transplant recipients who underwent one-night PSG at baseline and were followed for a median 75 months. No association was found between the presence of OSA and the rate of progression of CKD or all-cause mortality.[94]

SQ in kidney transplant patients has been reported as poor. Poor sleep is observed not only in dialysis but may be secondary to different factors, like comorbidities linked to kidney diseases or psychological problems.[95] The fact that poor sleep in kidney transplant recipients is related to anxiety, some dimensions of health-related QOL, medical comorbidity, and sexual relationships was also shown in a subsequent study.[96] The etiology of ESRD seems to affect SQ in these patients. A study investigated the correlation between ESRD secondary to hypertension and SQ among 201 kidney transplant recipients. They found that SQ and sleep duration scores were poorer among transplanted patients with ESRD secondary to hypertension (group 1) compared with transplanted patients with ESRD secondary to other causes (group 2).[97] ESRD duration before transplant is also significantly associated with SQ in this patient population.[98] Another cross-sectional study aimed to characterize fatigue and sleep disturbances in 100 wait-listed and 100 transplanted patients and examined their association with psychological functioning and QOL. Wait-listed patients had more difficulty with SQ, latency, duration, efficiency, and disturbance and were more likely to have "poor" SQ compared with posttransplant patients. Poor SQ was predicted by high body mass index and mood disturbance.[99]

Furthermore, another study investigated the prevalence of changes in SQ and their outcomes in kidney transplant recipients and analyzed the variables affecting SQ in the first years after transplantation. Kidney transplant recipients were evaluated at two time points after successful transplantation: between 3 and 6 months (Phase 1) and between 12 and 15 months (Phase 2). The prevalence of poor sleep was 36.7% in Phase 1 and 38.3% in Phase 2 of the study. There were no significant differences between patients with and without changes in SQ between the two phases. No changes in sleep patterns were found throughout the study.[100]

Kidney transplantation significantly improves kidney function and alleviates many uremic symptoms and complications. RLS is one of the most troublesome sleep disorders that has been thought to improve substantially after a successful kidney transplantation. One of the initial reports on this subject was a single case report that showed an improvement in RLS symptoms after restoration of kidney function by a successful transplantation.[101] A case series described the clinical course of RLS symptoms and the frequency of remission in 11 HD patients with RLS who received a kidney transplant. In all patients, RLS symptoms disappeared within 1 to 21 days posttransplant. At follow-up visits, four patients with well-functioning grafts were still free of RLS symptoms up to the longest follow-up period of 9 years. In three other patients, RLS symptoms gradually reappeared. In three patients, the transplant failed and RLS symptoms reoccurred within 10 days to 2 months.[102]

The effects of kidney transplantation on RLS in dialysis patients was evaluated in a subsequent study as well. The clinical course of RLS was investigated in 30 HD patients who underwent kidney transplantation. Patients were given a standardized questionnaire evaluating details of RLS at baseline and twice after kidney transplantation. Biochemical and hematological indices were measured at each time. In this study, kidney transplantation was associated with reduced RLS symptoms.[103]

Another study aimed to evaluate the prevalence of OSA and RLS in 200 kidney transplant recipients. Kidney transplant recipients had a higher prevalence of RLS (51.5%) and OSA (26%) compared with the general population. Mostly interesting there was a significant association between OSA and RLS in these patients. OSA was observed in almost 42% of patients with positive RLS, compared with 9% of patients with negative RLS.[104]

Another cross-sectional study analyzed the complex relationship between RLS, insomnia, and health-related QOL in kidney transplant recipients by using questionnaires. At a single transplant center, 1067 patients were invited to participate and 785 had complete datasets. Patients with RLS were three times more likely to have insomnia than patients without RLS (29% vs. 9%), and the presence of RLS was a significant and independent predictor of insomnia in multivariate analysis. RLS was also associated with impaired QOL in kidney-transplanted patients, due to both sleep-related and sleep-independent factors.[88]

Furthermore, a study tested the hypothesis that kidney transplantation improves PLMS in patients with ESRD. Attended overnight PSG was performed before and after kidney transplantation on 18 patients. Study participants were divided based on a periodic limb movement index >15 events per hour during sleep. Kidney transplantation was associated with a significant reduction in periodic limb movement index in all patients and this reduction was greatest in the seven patients with a periodic limb movement index >15 events per hour. Therefore successful kidney transplantation has been associated with decreased PLMS.[105]

There are several biological, psychological, and social factors that may predispose this patient group to develop insomnia. The prevalence and correlates of insomnia in the kidney transplant population was explored in the following two cross-sectional studies. In the first study, the Athens Insomnia Scale was used to assess the prevalence of insomnia in a large sample of kidney transplant recipients compared with wait-listed dialysis patients and a matched group obtained from a nationally representative sample of the Hungarian population. The prevalence of insomnia was 15% in wait-listed patients, whereas it was only 8% in transplant recipients ($P <$ 0.001), which, in turn, was not different from the prevalence of insomnia in the general population study sample (8%). Insomnia was significantly and independently associated with treatment modality (transplantation vs. wait-listing), as well as the presence of depression, RLS, and high risk for OSA syndrome, and with self-reported comorbidity.[106] The second study describes the prevalence and frequency of self-reported sleep disorders in 249 kidney transplant patients using questionnaires. Their findings show high prevalence and incidence of insomnia, with negative effects on daytime functionality.[107]

Even though the prevalence of depression is lower in kidney transplant recipients (22%) than in wait-listed patients (33%),[108] 20% of transplant patients are still at high risk of clinically significant depression. Many psychological and behavioral factors, including negative mood, QOL, napping, and caffeine consumption, are related to sleep disturbance among pre- and postkidney transplant patients. Many of these factors have different relationships with sleep disturbance when comparing these two groups. Such factors may be worthwhile areas for intervention in treating insomnia symptoms among pretransplant patients and posttransplant recipients.[109]

Undoubtedly, kidney transplantation provides the best outcome for patients with ESRD in terms of health-related QOL, which has been recognized as an important outcome measure in patients with many different chronic medical conditions. Sleep disorders are one of the many factors impacting negatively QOL in kidney transplant patients.[110] This was shown in a cross-sectional study that examined by subjective means (questionnaires) the SQ and health-related QOL in patients after kidney transplantation and explored the relationship between SQ and health-related QOL. They found that SQ and health-related QOL were lower than the norm in these patients and that poor sleep was associated with lower health-related QOL.[111]

In multivariate regression models adjusting for clinical and sociodemographic characteristics, sleep disorders, and depressive symptoms, the modality of kidney-replacement therapy (wait-listed vs. transplantation) remained independently associated with three (general health perceptions, effect, and burden of kidney disease) of the eight health-related QOL dimensions analyzed. Poor sleep seems to be a part of depressive symptomatology that negatively affects health-related QOL in these patients.[112]

A multicenter wait-list randomized controlled trial evaluated the effect and feasibility of implementing a daily morning bright light therapy intervention on sleep, circadian rhythms, subjective feelings, depressive symptomatology, and cognition of 30 kidney transplant recipients with diagnosed sleep–wake disturbances. Study participants were randomly assigned one-to-one to either 3 weeks of bright light therapy or a wait-list control group. Morning bright light therapy (10,000 lux) was individually scheduled for 30 minutes daily for 3 weeks. Wrist actimetry for sleep and circadian rhythms, validated instruments for subjective feelings and cognition, and melatonin levels for circadian timing were assessed. Among the 26 kidney transplant recipients that completed the study, the intervention group showed a significant get-up time phase advance and a small but significant bedtime phase advance from intervention to follow-up. Overall, bright light therapy shows preliminary evidence of benefit on sleep–wake disturbances in these patients.[113]

In a subsequent report on the same study group, the investigators assessed salivary melatonin levels and found that a large proportion of study participants had low melatonin levels, which precluded calculation of the dim-light melatonin onset as a circadian marker. In this study, 29 kidney transplant recipients were retrospectively grouped into two groups: those with measurable dim-light melatonin onset ($n = 11$) and those with not-measurable dim-light melatonin onset ($n = 18$). Those with measurable dim-light melatonin onset differed from those without dim-light melatonin onset in that they were younger and had higher hemoglobin levels, less anxiety, and a better overall sense of coherence. In conclusion, those with measurable dim-light melatonin onset had fewer health impairments, underlying the relevance of a stable circadian rhythm.[114]

An inadequate fall in nocturnal BP ("nondipping" profile) persists after kidney transplantation[115,116] and is associated with impaired nocturnal endogenous melatonin secretion in hypertensive patients.[117] The effects of kidney transplantation on sleep, melatonin levels, circadian rhythm, and QOL in recipients and living donors was examined by assessment of saliva melatonin concentrations, SQ and daytime sleepiness before and at 2 weeks and 3 months after transplantation in 23 kidney transplant recipients. In 23 living donors, they assessed the same parameters before and at 3 months after donation. In addition, they assessed 24-hour core body temperature, 24-hour BP profile, and QOL. Regarding sleep, the amount of nighttime awake minutes tended to be reduced in recipients after kidney transplantation. Nocturnal melatonin concentrations did not change with transplantation or donation. The BP dipping profile and two circadian markers (dim-light melatonin onset and time of core body temperature minimum) also did not change. Nevertheless, kidney transplant recipients reported that daytime sleepiness and QOL had improved. Objectively, nocturnal SQ marginally improved after transplantation. Subjectively, patients reported improved QOL and daytime sleepiness scores. Changes in kidney function were not associated with modified melatonin secretion or circadian rhythmicity.[118]

Another study evaluated a different intervention: the effect of a period of exercise training, as a nontherapeutic interventional method, on quality and quantity of sleep and lipid profile in kidney transplant patients. Forty-four kidney transplant recipients were selected to participate in the study and were randomized into exercise ($n = 29$) and control ($n = 15$) groups. The exercise group participated in a cumulative exercise program (3 days per week for 10 weeks in 60 to 90 min exercise sessions). In the exercise training group, SQ of the subjects was improved by 27% and the sleep quantity was increased by 30 minutes. In this study, exercise activity improved SQ and sleep quantity, as well as several sleep-related physiological parameters, in kidney transplant recipients and could be an effective approach to sleep-related disorders in these patients.[119]

Subsequently the Exercise in Kidney Transplant Trial (ExeRT Trial) was a 12-week pilot randomized controlled trial that examined the potential effect of aerobic training or resistance training on vascular health and indexes of CVD risk in kidney transplant patients. Sixty participants were randomly assigned to aerobic training (n = 20), resistance training (n = 20), or usual care (n = 20) and 46 completed the study (aerobic training, n = 13; resistance training, n = 13; and usual care, n = 20), resulting in a 23% attrition rate. Participants were included if they had a kidney transplant within 12 months before baseline assessment. Patients were excluded if they had unstable medical conditions or had recently started regular exercise. Aerobic training and resistance training were delivered 3 days per week for a 12-week period. Pulse wave velocity, peak oxygen uptake, sit-to-stand time, metric quadriceps force, and inflammatory biomarkers were assessed at baseline and after 12 weeks. Analyses of covariance, adjusted for baseline values, age, and dialysis vintage pretransplantation, revealed significant mean differences between aerobic training and usual care in pulse wave velocity of −2.2 ± 0.4 (95% CI, −3.1 to −1.3) m/s (P < 0.001) and between resistance training and usual care of −2.6 ± 0.4 (95% CI, −3.4 to −1.7) m/s (P < 0.001) at 12 weeks. Secondary analyses indicated significant improvements in peak oxygen uptake in the aerobic training group and in peak oxygen uptake, sit-to-stand 60, and isometric muscle force in the resistance training group compared with usual care at 12 weeks. There were no reported adverse events, cardiovascular events, or hospitalizations as a result of the intervention. Kidney transplant recipients have an increased risk of CVD and could benefit from such posttransplant exercise-based interventions.[120]

CONCLUSIONS

CKD usually coexists with other common comorbid conditions. Therefore the identification, diagnosis, and treatment of various sleep disorders is complex and complicated. The practicing physician must be aware of multiple concurrent and interactive processes, such as: (a) psychological disorders, (b) lifestyle factors, (c) treatment-related factors, and (d) ESRD-specific symptoms and complications. Inevitably, the therapeutic approach calls for a multilayered and comprehensive treatment of sleep disorders in these patients. Because sleep disorders may be treated by pharmacological and nonpharmacological approaches, the diagnosis and management of sleep disorders in CKD provides an opportunity to improve both the QOL and long-term outcomes.

A full list of references is available at www.expertconsult.com.

16

Depression and Neurocognitive Function in Chronic Kidney Disease

Daniel Cukor, PhD, Deborah S. Rosenthal Asher, PhD, and Paul L. Kimmel, MD, MACP

OUTLINE

A biopsychosocial perspective on patients with renal disease compels the clinician to consider the context and take the patient's reactions into account. Although the psychological landscape of renal disease is, in some ways, similar to other chronic health conditions, it also represents a novel combination of physical, emotional, and social changes. The high treatment burden, chronicity, and course are all unique, and patients respond to these demands in a variety of ways based on personality, psychological functioning, social context, resources, and personal experience. Stress and the response to stress may be key in determining the ability of the patient to cope with and adapt to the challenges of illness and its treatment. The scientific literature, heretofore, has focused on the two most common psychiatric challenges to the patient with renal disease: depression and neurocognitive impairment.

PART I. DEPRESSION IN CHRONIC KIDNEY DISEASE

ETIOLOGY OF DEPRESSION

Depression has long been identified as the primary mental health issue for patients with chronic kidney disease (CKD) and specifically end-stage renal disease (ESRD).[1-6] It is unclear what etiological factors contribute to the increased vulnerability to depression, but understanding the biological, psychological, and social context in which the depression develops is essential. The biopsychosocial model[7] proposes that various etiological factors play roles in establishing vulnerability to depression. The diathesis-stress model[8] posits that depression results when preexisting vulnerability is activated by stressful life events. This predisposition can be either genetic,[9] implying an interaction of nature and nurture, or cognitive,[10] involving a lasting influence of attitudes and beliefs formed in childhood, or perhaps both.

Several biological theories for vulnerability to depression have been proposed, including a monoamine hypothesis,[11-13] abnormalities in neurogenesis,[14-18] known side effects of commonly prescribed medications for ESRD or common comorbid illnesses,[19] an overactive hypothalamic-pituitary-adrenal (HPA) axis,[20] hormonal dysregulation,[21] as well as certain vitamin deficiencies.[22] Although all these theories have a substantial basis, none have emerged as a singular explanation for the increased biological vulnerability. At core of these theories is the concept of stress[23] and the ability to achieve stability through change, or "allostasis."[24,25] McEwen and Stellar[26] developed the construct of allostatic load to express the vulnerability to disease that continuous physiological and psychological demand creates. The stress response of the CKD or ESRD patient may be impaired or overwhelmed due to the biochemical milieu created by renal disease or by the broad range of psychosocial threats the ESRD patient encounters.[27] The expressed psychological reaction can be viewed as the combination of the biological and psychosocial threats in the context of the patient's resources to cope with these increased demands.[27]

Another way to conceptualize the psychological vulnerability to depression may be through noxious learning experiences. Beck and colleagues developed the cognitive model of depression in which he proposed three concepts as the hallmarks of depression: a triad of negative thoughts that comprise a negative bias about oneself, one's world, and one's future; distorted information processing and recurrent patterns of depressive thinking; and distorted cognitive schema.[28] These patterns of maladaptive thinking often begin in childhood or adolescence and serve as a risk factor for the future development of the full depressive syndrome.[29]

What these theories share in common is predicated on the acknowledgment that life on dialysis for patients with ESRD is demanding. Although kidney disease shares similarities with other chronic disorders, there may be other substantial losses associated with ESRD, beyond the loss of kidney function. Patients can undergo profound changes in role functioning, work status, autonomy, intimate relationships, and body image.[1] The treatment burden of hemodialysis (HD) is also demanding. The weekly time demand is substantial and lifelong, without successful transplantation. Patients with ESRD report fatigue, pain, sexual dysfunction, gastrointestinal symptoms (nausea, vomiting, and anorexia), dermatological changes, and appetite changes.[30,31] These ongoing challenges of living with ESRD can serve as the trigger that interacts with the person's previous vulnerabilities and induce depression. There are a variety of psychological pathways in which the challenges of ESRD can affect a person. It is possible that patients with ESRD are put into a state of "learned helplessness" because treatment options are limited, and they are forced indefinitely to remain in their difficult situations with little hope for improvement or control over their outcomes.[32] Threats to the patient's autonomy and control[27] as a result of the demanding course of treatment can serve as the precipitating stressor for a depressive episode.

The onset of depressive symptoms and depression can also be associated with changes in interpersonal factors, including strained or critical personal relationships. Patients with ESRD may experience changes in social role functioning, relationships with a spouse or adult children as a result of the transition to a caregiving or care-needing role, the death of a significant other, or the availability or quality of social relationships with friends because of their own health-related life events.[33] These types of change have been associated with late-life depression.[34]

One new integrative theory of depression, the social signal transduction theory of depression,[35] posits that life stressors, particularly ones that involve interpersonal threat initiate a cascade of neural, physiological, molecular, and genomic processes that lead to the development and maintenance of depression.[36-39] The stress response is not specific but initiates survival mechanisms in which proinflammatory cytokines upregulate components of the immune system, which then can lead to profound changes in behavior, which can be essential in the face of immediate physical threat, but maladaptive in the chronic state or in the context of prolonged social stress.

EPIDEMIOLOGY OF DEPRESSION

The precise definition of *depression* as a construct, mood state, or a clinical syndrome is difficult because the feelings of sadness and hopelessness are ubiquitous and are not unique to depression or even any specific mental health problem.[40] *The Diagnostic and Statistical Manual of Mental Disorders* (*DSM*)[41] defines depression by the presence of specific symptoms in the absence of a range of other symptoms presenting for a specified duration. The hallmark symptoms of depression are low mood and loss of interest or pleasure in formerly enjoyable activities. In the fifth edition of the *DSM* (*DSM-V*), mood disorders with depression are divided into unipolar and bipolar depression. The latter includes a manic component. The most common form of depression is major depressive disorder, characterized by the presence of a major depressive episode in the absence of mania. The hallmark features of a depressive episode must occur during the same 2-week period but are often difficult to distinguish from the common symptoms of uremia (Table 16.1).[42]

To diagnose a major depressive episode, the clinician must determine whether the depressed mood has been of a significant intensity for a 2-week duration. The clinician should explicitly inquire about each of the symptoms in Table 16.1 and then must use his or her *clinical judgment* to determine whether the symptoms meet the criteria. A major depressive episode represents a significant change in the patient's functioning. Other diagnoses, such as chronic depression or an adjustment disorder, may be more appropriate for more-chronic or less-severe presentations.[41]

TABLE 16.1 Symptom Overlap Between Criteria for a Major Depressive Episode and Uremia

***DSM-V* Major Depressive Episode**	**Uremia**
Depressed mood	Irritability, cognitive changes, encephalopathy, drug effects
Decreased interest in activities	Decreased libido, cognitive dysfunction
Weight change	Anorexia, edema, cachexia, volume overload
Sleep changes	Insomnia, sleep apnea
Psychomotor agitation	Encephalopathy
Fatigue	Fatigue, anemia
Diminished ability to concentrate	Cognitive dysfunction, malaise
Feelings of worthlessness	—
Thoughts of death/suicide	—

DSM, Diagnostic and Statistical Manual of Mental Disorders.

DIFFERENTIATING DEPRESSION FROM MEDICAL ILLNESS

The task of distinguishing depression from subclinical mood dysregulation is made more complex by the overlap of the symptoms of depression and advanced CKD.[42-44] The clinician must pay careful attention to the etiology, nature, and timing of the presentation, because there is considerable overlap between the somatic symptoms of depression and those of uremia. The depressive symptoms of psychomotor agitation or retardation, decreased appetite or weight change, sleep disturbance, and aches and pains are often difficult to distinguish from the uremic symptoms of encephalopathy, anorexia, day/night reversal, and neuropathy, respectively, adding to the difficulty of making an accurate diagnosis (see Tables 16.1 and 16.2).[1,42,43]

PREVALENCE

The difficulty in defining and identifying depression has led to challenges in its standard measurement. There is still no universal standard for the most appropriate screening technique. Different studies in patients with CKD use the Beck Depression Inventory (BDI), the Hamilton Depression Rating Scale (HAM-D), The Patient Health Questionnaire (PHQ), the Zung Self-Rating Depression Scale, subscales from the SF-36, and questions from the Kidney Disease Quality of Life (KDQOL) Instrument.[1] To provide a validating clinical diagnosis, researchers have used the Structured Clinical Interview for the *DSM-IV* (SCID), the Diagnostic Interview Schedule (DIS), or the Primary Care Evaluation of Mental Disorders (PRIME-MD). The field still needs to achieve consensus regarding the appropriate screening and diagnostic tools for the broad population of patients with ESRD. Furthermore, there is an urgent need to precisely identify appropriate screening measures' cutoff scores that have meaningful prognostic value in varying ESRD samples.

A few studies have begun this task by validating the BDI against structured psychiatric interviews to determine meaningful cutoff scores for ESRD populations. In a sample of 99 white HD patients, Craven and colleagues[45] found a 45.4% prevalence of depression using the BDI cutoff score of 10, but found a BDI score of 15 or greater had better sensitivity and specificity for the diagnosis of depressive disorders in dialysis patients when the DIS was used as the criterion. Watnick and colleagues[46] validated the BDI and the PHQ-9 against the SCID as depression assessment tools in an ethnically diverse dialysis population in several dialysis centers. Twenty-six percent of the sample were diagnosed with a depressive disorder. The optimal BDI cutoff value that maximized sensitivity and specificity was 16, whereas the optimal cutoff for the PHQ was 10. Hedayati and colleagues[47] compared the BDI and the Center for Epidemiological Studies Depression Scale (CES-D) to the SCID.[48] The prevalence of depression was 27% in their sample of 98 ethnically diverse patients. About one-quarter of the subjects were veterans. A BDI cutoff score of 14 and a CES-D score of 18 had the most predictive value. These studies indicate there is agreement between the BDI and clinician administered diagnostic tools, and a BDI score of 14 to 16 suggests the presence of a depressive disorder.

Other studies report varying rates of depression, depending on the sample population and the measurement tool. A study of mostly white patients starting home dialysis in the Midwest United States found the prevalence of depression to be 18% using diagnostic criteria.[49] Kimmel and colleagues studied primarily African American patients with ESRD in HD centers in Washington, D.C. About one-half of the patients scored greater than 10 on the BDI.[50-53] When the more conservative cutoff of 15 was used, about 25% of the patients screened positive.[54] In their sample of primarily African Americans in Brooklyn, New York, Cukor and colleagues[54] found that more than 70% of HD patients had a psychiatric diagnosis by the SCID, and 29% of the sample had a current depressive disorder.

To develop an accurate picture of depression in patients with chronic medical illnesses, such as CKD, it is possible that longitudinal assessments provide valuable information. As a follow-up study, Cukor and colleagues reassessed subjects 16 months later, and three different clinical pathways emerged.[55] About one-half of the patients did not have a psychiatric diagnosis at either baseline or follow-up, 21% had a variable or intermittent course, and 11% had a persistent course, with depression diagnoses at both evaluations. The persistent course of depression was associated with significantly lower quality of life and more reported health problems. Kimmel and colleagues[51] and Boulware and colleagues[56] demonstrated that associations with outcomes existed with multiple measurements of depression that did not exist with baseline data. These data suggest a single measure of depression at a specific time might not be as meaningful as measuring depression over the course of a time span.

Beyond the timing of the assessment, the demographics of the patient need to be taken into account. Specifically, the patient's gender and race need to be evaluated. In community samples, women have higher rates of depression and present for treatment more frequently.[57,58] It is unknown whether this pattern holds true in the US ESRD population. Race and age have been identified as factors in the likelihood of depression developing in patients with diabetes,[59] a primary cause of ESRD. Ethnicity has been associated with a variety of barriers to care,

TABLE 16.2 Beck Depression Inventory-II Items With Somatic Items *Italicized*

1. Sadness	12. Loss of interest
2. Pessimism	13. Indecisiveness
3. Past failure	14. Worthlessness
4. Loss of pleasure	15. *Loss of energy*
5. Guilty feelings	16. *Changes in sleep*
6. Punishment feelings	17. *Irritability*
7. Self-dislike	18. *Changes in appetite*
8. Self-criticalness	19. *Concentration difficulty*
9. Suicidal thoughts or wishes	20. *Tiredness or fatigue*
10. Crying	21. *Loss of interest in sex*
11. Agitation	

leading to mental health disparities.[60,61] There is some evidence in the ESRD literature that quality of life,[62-64] perceptions of religious support,[65,66] and quality of social support vary according to race and might contribute to depression. One study[67] compared 78 black and 82 white HD patients, and found no differences in their levels of depressive affect. They did, however, find a stronger emphasis on religion/spirituality as a coping tool within a group of black patients. As the new Medicare QIP requirement to screen for depression goes into effect, the provider community will need to decide the appropriate measures, frequency, and follow-up for depression evaluation.

SEQUELAE OF DEPRESSION

Patients with ESRD who are also depressed are at risk for consequences that extend beyond disordered mood. Depression can affect the course of disease progression through direct and indirect pathways.

Suicide

The most acute danger that depression presents is the increased risk of suicide. Patients with ESRD may be particularly at risk because they can commit suicide through passive means, by no longer receiving dialysis or by manipulating a functional vascular access site. This makes suicide in this population readily available and complicates assessment and intervention strategies. Increased levels of depression have been associated with higher levels of suicidality.[68] Patients with ESRD had an 84% increased rate of suicide compared with the general US population.[69] Important risk factors for suicide in the ESRD population include a previous history of mental illness, recent hospitalization, age greater than 75 years, male gender, white or Asian race, and alcohol or drug dependence. Because of the increased prevalence and the relative ease with which patients with ESRD can commit suicide, screening for depression and suicidal ideation should be an essential part of the treatment plan in depressed patients with ESRD.[70]

Malnutrition

A possible route through which depression could influence the course of ESRD is malnutrition. Some exploratory studies have found negative correlations between BDI scores and serum albumin levels, protein catabolic rate, and nutritional status scores in small samples,[71-73] whereas others have not.[74,75] The reasons for these disparate findings remain unclear, but may be related to differences in composition of the study samples, cultural and socioeconomic factors, or treatment conditions.[75] The causal pathways between increased depressive affect and decreased appetite or nutrition have not yet been determined but may be bidirectional. Careful longitudinal or interventional studies will be needed to establish causal relationships.

Treatment Compliance

Another route through which depression can exert an influence on ESRD outcomes is through impairing treatment compliance. Better adherence to the HD prescription has been associated with improved survival.[52,76,77] Studies[78-80] have indicated a relationship between depressive affect and laboratory and behavioral markers of poor compliance in dialysis patients. Decreased behavioral compliance with the dialysis prescription correlated with increased depressive affect is prevalent HD patients.[78,80] Initial findings suggest that successful treatment of depression may, at least temporarily, be associated with improved fluid compliance.[79]

Social Support

Patients with depression may be more likely to feel less connected to their existing relationships and isolated from social connections. In chronic illness, this can lead to deleterious consequences. Several studies have shown an association between survival and perception of social support in patients with ESRD of different ethnic backgrounds.[52,76,81-85] McClellan and colleagues used a prospective design and demonstrated that social support predicted survival of HD patients.[85] Christensen and colleagues showed that a social support indicator, measured by family cohesion, predicted survival in HD patients.[83] The result of these studies remain tentative, because the effects of medical and treatment parameters were not controlled. Kimmel and colleagues showed increased perception of social support, measured by the Multidimensional Scale of Perceived Social Support, predicted survival even when variation in age, severity of comorbid illness, serum albumin concentration, dialysis membrane type, and study site were controlled.[52] In an analysis of the Dialysis Outcomes and Practice Patterns Study (DOPPS) on over 30,000 patients from a multinational sample,[86] higher mortality rates were found among patients reporting less social support. Lower levels of perceived family support were also associated with decreased adherence to fluid and weight gain recommendations. It is unclear to what extent the quality of one's social support is mutable and whether interventions designed to promote social support will have an effect on other outcomes such as mood, adherence, and survival.

Immunological Response

Depression may affect the course of ESRD through its impact on immunological factors and inflammation. Stress has long been linked to the dysregulation of the HPA axis,[1,25] and depression has long been associated with abnormal glucocorticoid metabolism in healthy people.[87] The precise mechanisms through which depression may modulate the immune system are still unclear, but one proposed theory is that depression increases cytokine activity, which may disrupt the HPA axis by impairing negative feedback of circulating corticosteroids.[20,88]

There is also some evidence that inflammatory biomarkers, such as proinflammatory cytokines and C-reactive protein, are dysregulated and predict outcome in patients with ESRD.[89,90] In one small study,[91] there was an association between genetic predisposition to produce low levels of interleukin (IL)-10 (A/A genotype for the IL-10—1082 polymorphism) and increased chance of depression. The reasons for the increased risk of chronic inflammation in ESRD are complex; however, it has been suggested that a proinflammatory state is intrinsic to ESRD and is related to the higher-than-expected rates of cardiovascular disease and other causes of increased mortality in this population.[92] Antiinflammatory agents may be a new frontier in treating depression in comorbid medical illnesses.[93]

Mortality

There has been a great deal of scientific discussion regarding the association between depression and mortality in patients with ESRD. Some initial studies in ESRD patients[94-97] found associations between depressive affect and mortality. However, these studies were preliminary and used comparisons of means between groups of deceased and surviving patients, without accounting for confounding medical and demographic factors. Other studies have been unable to detect simple associations between depression or depressive affect and survival in patients with ESRD.[52,75,82,98,99] The Dialysis Outcomes and Practice Patterns Study,[100] an observational study on a large multinational sample, has provided information regarding screening questions related to depressive affect and survival in patients with ESRD treated with HD. They used statements from the KDQOL regarding depressive affect and found that those who answered affirmatively to having more frequently experienced depressive affect had a higher risk of mortality, withdrawal from dialysis therapy, and hospitalization. Despite the nature of their nonstandard assessment, the study findings seem to indicate a robust relationship between depressive affect and medical sequelae. One prospective longitudinal study[101] found that when subjects were divided by affect severity based on a single depression score, those with severe depressive affect had significantly shorter time to death. Kimmel and colleagues were initially unable to demonstrate a relationship between increased level of baseline depressive affect and mortality in a sample of almost 300 HD patients. They did report associations between the perception of increased burden of illness and mortality and between the perception of a high level of social support and improved survival.[52] The group subsequently performed longitudinal assessments of the study population, evaluating BDI scores up to six times over a period of 20 months to 5 years (mean 38.6 months). The data were analyzed using Cox regression models to predict the length of survival. They found that an increased level of depressive affect over time was associated with an increased risk of mortality, even when the analysis was controlled for medical parameters.[51] Boulware and colleagues generated similar results when they evaluated baseline and longitudinal data from the Choices for Healthy Outcomes in Caring for End-Stage Renal Disease (CHOICE) study, a large cohort of incident patients starting dialysis.[56] They determined that levels of depressive affect, measured by nonvalidated mood questions from the SF-36, at the beginning of the study were not associated with increased overall mortality. However, similar to Kimmel's findings, using several different time-dependent analyses, the investigators demonstrated that persistently higher levels of depressive affect over time were associated with increased risk of death and cardiovascular events in both adjusted and unadjusted analyses.

There is also evidence that the repeated measurement of a depression diagnosis is more informative than cross-sectional assessments. Patients with ESRD who were depressed at two diagnostic interviews, spaced 16 months apart, exhibited correlations with lower quality of life and more reported health problems.[52] Although the limited study duration prevented these results from being extended directly to mortality, it appears that a persistent course of depression represents an increased risk of morbidity and mortality for patients with ESRD treated with HD.

Hedayati and colleagues[102] reported on time to death or hospitalization in an ESRD sample. They found a hazard ratio of about 2 for patients with ESRD with depression, compared with patients with ESRD without depression. A metaanalysis concluded that the conflicting research reports are likely due to the use of different depression scales and the ability of the studies to meaningfully correct for illness variables, but that there appears to be need to elucidate the mechanisms underscoring such relationships.[103]

Marital Issues

Depressed ESRD patients may be at particular risk for marital difficulty.[104] In addition to the typical strain that the development of a chronic illness places on a couple,[105] the depressed patient could feel more easily overwhelmed and can be perceived as not being invested in the relationship. Role changes can be profound[33,106] because spouses can now become caregivers or wage earners, which may promote further depression or resentment. There have been only a few studies that assess marital relationships in patients with ESRD, with one study reporting that greater than 50% of couples that included a patient with ESRD experienced marital discord.[106] In a study of Indian HD patients and their spouses, marital discord was reported in about one-third of the sample, which had a strong relationship to either individual's depression.[107] Marital support and conflict may also be associated with the degree to which a patient adheres to the dialysis prescription.[83,99]

COMORBIDITIES OF DEPRESSION

Depression often presents with other common coexistent psychiatric conditions. It is important to carefully evaluate each presenting patient for the co-occurrence of these other conditions.

Substance Use

All ESRD patients should be carefully screened for substance abuse because of the potentially nephrotoxic effects of some illicit drugs.[108] Patients with depression are often unsure regarding how to effectively cope with their mood and may turn to drugs or alcohol to "self-medicate". One study found that in a sample of 145 HD patients, 28% were judged to have a problem with chronic alcohol abuse.[109] The study further found that the alcoholic group had poorer nutritional markers than the nonalcoholics.

Little is known about the effect of intravenous drug use on dialysis or vascular access; however, active substance abuse should be considered an acute situation, and coordination of care with addiction specialists should be undertaken. In a systematic review of opioid and benzodiazepine use, the authors found wide variability between centers, due to varying assessment techniques. They concluded that more precision in substance research and overall, more attention is required to further elucidate rates of substance use, the reasons for use and the consequences of use/over use.[110] Recent findings suggest prescription of opioid medication in ESRD dialysis patients is common and associated with increased morbidity and mortality.[111]

Anxiety Disorders

Anxiety is a complicating comorbid diagnosis for many patients with medical illness.[112,113] Anxiety often occurs with depression in ESRD populations.[54,55,114] Anxiety is consistently ranked as a major cause of years lost to disability in the United States.[115] There is relatively little anxiety research specific to ESRD patients, but it appears that an anxiety diagnosis exerts a powerful negative effect on quality of life.[116-118] Compound depression and anxiety might represent a clinical entity that has a synergistic, negative effect on patients' perception of quality of life.[118] One must consider that anxious patients can have characteristics on a spectrum from the more classic worried and withdrawn to agitated or angry.[114]

When disruptive behavior presents in ESRD patients, it is important to try to understand the cause of the patient's distress and to explore whether stress and anxiety may lead to undesirable outcomes. Similarly, excessive anxiety might lead to somatic vigilance, a discomfort with changes in bodily sensations. This may be particularly important to evaluate in patients who often prematurely end dialysis sessions because pain or discomfort might be a concomitant of anxiety.

Dementia/Delirium

Neurocognitive disorders are common in patients with ESRD.[119] Depression can be a precipitant for neurocognitive decline, and the evaluation of any patient who reports a change in his or her mental acuity should include screening for depression. Withdrawal from dialysis is relatively common, especially in elderly patients or patients who fail to thrive,[120,121] and the physician should try to determine the patient's wishes before the patient's mood and mental status may compromise his or her ability to provide a meaningful directive.[122] A full discussion of neurocognitive changes in ESRD is in the following section.

TREATMENT OF DEPRESSION

The difficulties in identifying and assessing depression should not serve as barriers to the successful treatment of depression. Although there has been relatively little clinical research on the treatment of depression in ESRD patients, the literature that does exist has been encouraging. The main treatment options for depression include psychotherapy and pharmacotherapy.

Psychotherapeutic Options

There are several forms of psychotherapies (cognitive-behavioral, interpersonal, supportive, group therapy) that have demonstrated consistent and substantial efficacy in the treatment of depression in general populations, which may well be effective tools for patients with ESRD as well.[123] In comparison to pharmacological interventions, psychotherapy has the advantage of few deleterious side effects, frequently introducing benefits such as improved sleep, improved interpersonal relationships, and improved regimen compliance. However, a significant disadvantage is that therapy typically requires the patient to be motivated to change. The first step in wanting to change is acknowledging the presence of a problem. Denial, an unconscious mental operation that allows the person to avoid facing harsh realities, is a considerable obstacle. Incorporating a mental health evaluation as a standard of care is one strategy to reduce barriers to psychological care and to minimize patients' resistance to psychotherapeutic interventions. In addition, referring clinicians should explain their biopsychosocial[7] conceptualization of disease and how treating psychological components is essential for good medical care.

There is an insufficient amount of literature on psychotherapeutic intervention in HD populations,[70,124] but there is increasing interest in psychotherapeutic interventions for ESRD patients treated with HD.[125,126] There is increasing literature indicating that psychosocial interventions, such as cognitive behavioral therapy, are effective for treating depression. In two small randomized controlled trials (RCTs) cognitive-behavioral therapy was shown to be effective in reducing depression when administered in both individual[79] and group formats.[127] Although this initial evidence is encouraging, larger scale trials are needed, and some are underway.[128]

Pharmacotherapy

In today's healthcare environment, nephrologists have, in many ways, become primary care providers for ESRD patients and often find themselves prescribing medications usually prescribed in primary care or other settings. When considering a psychotropic medication for patients with ESRD, it is important for nephrologists to balance their familiarity with the pharmacokinetics of psychotropic agents against the probability of the patient accepting a psychiatric referral, attending the appointment, and following through on the recommendations. Nephrologists must be aware of whether a drug is cleared through renal or hepatic metabolism and whether the drug clearance is affected by HD or peritoneal dialysis (PD). Most psychotropic medications are protein-bound, lipid soluble, penetrate the blood–brain barrier, and are cleared by the liver, with the notable exception of lithium. Protein binding may be impaired in ESRD, which can affect drug metabolism.[129] Therefore, to reduce the potential for overdosing, consideration should be given to the reduction of the initial dose of psychotropic medications in this patient population. Clinical responses should be carefully monitored as doses are increased, and drug levels should be obtained if available.

Antidepressants have a potentially essential role in treating unipolar depression in patients with ESRD, with selective serotonin reuptake inhibitors (SSRIs) being the first line of pharmacological treatment.[129] Tricyclic antidepressants (TCAs) and SSRIs are typically cleared by the liver, and therefore require only a minimal dose adjustment in patients without liver disease. For patients with ESRD, the initial dose of an SSRI is often one-half to two-thirds the usual dose. Typically, treatment with SSRIs should be continued for at least 4 to 6 weeks before deciding whether there has been a therapeutic benefit. If improvement is not achieved after 3 to 4 months, then consideration should be given to switching to another antidepressant. Establishing an appropriate antidepressant regimen may involve trial and error. The nephrologist and patient should expect that adjustments will need to be made to identify the optimal medication and dosing.[129]

There is some evidence that SSRIs are effective in the treatment of depression in patients with ESRD. An early study found a treatment advantage in 12 depressed patients with ESRD treated with the SSRI fluoxetine over those given a placebo.[130,131] Wuerth and colleagues found that depressive symptoms were markedly ameliorated in PD patients who completed a 12-week course of treatment with sertraline, bupropion, or nefazodone, despite low rates of compliance overall.[132,133] Researchers in Korea found that fluoxetine significantly reduced HAM-D scores in patients with ESRD.[72]

For a variety of reasons, SSRIs are the preferred medication for the treatment of ESRD patients with depression. SSRIs typically cause fewer anticholinergic symptoms than TCAs, are not associated with cardiac conduction abnormalities, and are less lethal in large doses compared with TCAs, which are lethal in large doses and can be used in suicide attempts. An additional benefit of SSRIs in this patient population is that they may reduce postural hypotension, presumably through effects on vascular tone.[129] Fluoxetine, the first available SSRI, is the best-studied drug in this family.[130,131] Other medications in this family include paroxetine, sertraline, and citalopram.

Venlafaxine and bupropion hydrochloride are examples of a different class of antidepressants called *selective norepinephrine reuptake inhibitors* (SNRIs). The SNRIs should be used with caution in ESRD patients because these drugs are primarily cleared by the kidneys.[131] Bupropion has active metabolites that are almost completely excreted through the kidney. These may accumulate in dialysis patients, predisposing them to developing seizures.

Monoamine oxidase inhibitors (MAOs) have numerous side effects and should be avoided if possible in ESRD patients because of their potential to cause hypotension. All medications carry the risk of adverse effects, and patients' regimens need to be carefully selected and then closely monitored. If the nephrologist does not believe that the regimen is sufficiently improving the depression, or he or she is not comfortable with the multiple iterations that are often required in gaining efficacy from antidepressants, a psychiatric consultation is warranted.

The literature has highlighted the challenges in having patients effectively accept an SSRI prescription at the dialysis center. Wuerth and colleagues[132,133] documented some of the barriers to patient acceptance, but data from two studies emphasize the significant role of the patient's willingness to take the medication.[134,135] Successfully prescribing a medication for depression includes appropriate diagnosis, appropriate selection of an agent and dose, as well as patient education regarding the need for and potential benefits and harms of the intervention choice.

CASE PRESENTATION

A 63-year-old African American man with diabetes recently transferred into an HD center. He was employed as a bus driver and approaching retirement, and, after 6 months on dialysis, he had to stop working because of a disability. The patient was married to his second wife, who was many years younger. The majority of his friends and social interactions were centered at his job with the Transit Authority.

The nutritionist was concerned over the change in the patient's dietary compliance and excessive interdialytic weight gain. The patient dismissed the dietician's attempts at intervention, and a psychological consult was obtained. The psychologist found that the patient had been functioning quite well before stopping work, and then a chain of events transpired that developed into a vicious circle, promoting greater depression and poorer health (Fig. 16.1). The patient confided that, since he began dialysis, he had been experiencing erectile difficulty. This, coupled with his discontinuation of work, had him feeling like he was "less of a man." He began avoiding conversations with his wife during the day and ceased sleeping alongside her at night. He also was less social with his friends at work.

The psychologist proposed an intervention that included family sessions to promote open communication, a referral to discuss the use of sildenafil, and "behavioral activation," a series of exercises designed to enable the patient to reengage in pleasurable activities despite his lack of desire. Simultaneously, the patient's beliefs about what it means to "be a man" were challenged. After some time, he was able to redefine his role from being a "provider" to that of a "partner." After 6 months of treatment, the patient was enjoying a modified lifestyle with his wife and friends that provided them with satisfaction and fulfillment. The patient's medication and diet compliance improved.

SUMMARY OF DEPRESSION IN CHRONIC KIDNEY DISEASE

Depression has a multifaceted etiology that can interact with the substantial burden of ESRD. The true prevalence rates for depression are difficult to establish because of the overlap of depressive and uremic symptoms. The rate of depression in pre-ESRD CKD patients is not well known, and whether depression rates increase with the progression through CKD stages is also unclear. Using a clinician-administered, semistructured interview, the rates for a diagnosis of depression in ESRD patients treated with HD appear

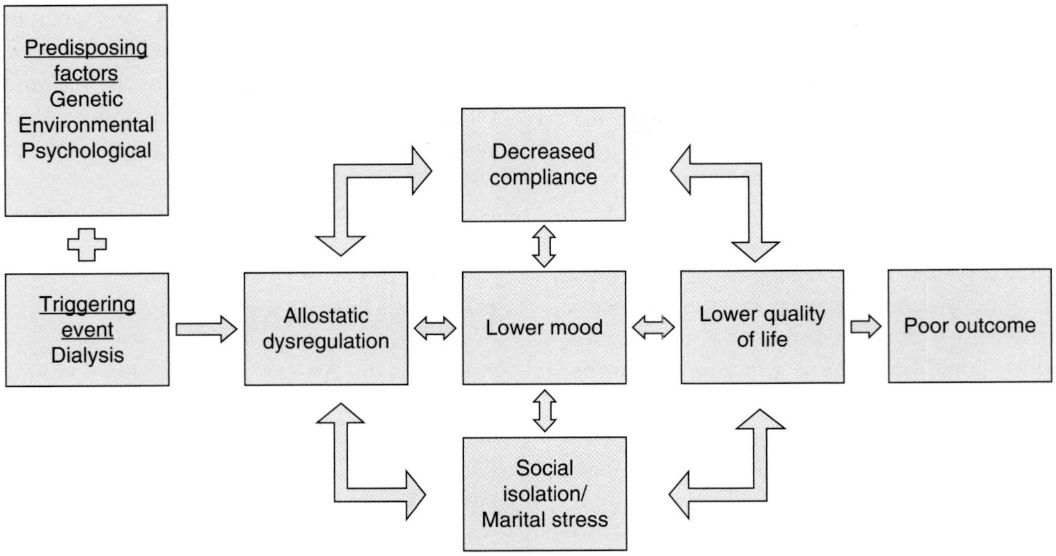

FIG. 16.1 Proposed map of interaction between depression and ESRD.

to be 20% to 30%. ESRD patients report elevated levels of depressive affect at a rate approaching 40%. Longitudinal assessment of depression has revealed stronger associations with outcomes. Depression's deleterious effects may extend to higher rates of poorer nutrition, poorer treatment compliance, decreased social support, and mortality. It is also possible that depression is associated with changes in immunological or inflammatory responses. Depression may be comorbid with substance abuse, anxiety disorders, or dementia, which complicates treatment. The literature on treatment of depression in the setting of ESRD is still developing, but both psychotherapy and psychopharmacological strategies appear to be efficacious. The initial dose of an SSRI in patients on HD is typically one-half to two-thirds the usual dose for patients with ESRD. Great care should be extended in engaging the patient as partner in depression care; otherwise, the likelihood that he or she will take medications as directed is greatly reduced. Cognitive-behavioral therapy shows promise as a possible first-line treatment for depression at the dialysis center, but larger clinical trials are needed.

PART II. NEUROCOGNITIVE FUNCTION IN CHRONIC KIDNEY DISEASE

ETIOLOGY OF NEUROCOGNITIVE IMPAIRMENT

Cognitive impairment poses many challenges to the CKD or ESRD patient, their caregivers, and their families. Depending on the severity of impairment, activities of daily living, such as ability to manage medications or even driving to medical appointments may become unsafe. Remembering to take one's medication or even attend dialysis sessions may become problematic. The burden of impairment often falls on those who take on caregiving responsibilities, and the stress of witnessing a loved one undergo cognitive decline can be devastating.

The assessment of neurocognitive functioning is a vital part of the comprehensive care of the CKD patient.[136] Aside from the impact on activities of daily life, cognitive dysfunction can be associated with disease progression[137] and affect the likelihood of adherence to the medical regimen,[138,139] or it can serve as a gross measure of adjustment.[140] Tables 16.3 and 16.4 provide, respectively, lists of cognitive domains and tests that can be used in the evaluation of cognition. Cognitive impairment can range from subtle, with only minor impairment in a circumscribed domain, to gross diffuse dysfunction. Major neurocognitive disorder, or "dementia," is used when there is a decline in cognitive functioning in one or more areas of cognition that affects independence in daily activities, such as remembering to pay bills and managing medication.[141] If the cognitive decline is transient and abrupt, and there is a change in attention or awareness, the impairment is referred to as *delirium*. Delirium may occur with a concurrent neurocognitive disorder.[141] The most common type of dementia is Alzheimer disease.[142] Alzheimer disease can be progressive and, in advanced stages, result in profound impairment in memory and language and visuoperceptual ability.[141,143] Another common cause of dementia is vascular neurocognitive disorder, which is often characterized by significant impairment in executive functioning.[144]

Manifestations of cognitive dysfunction may include difficulties within the domains of behavior, cognition, and affect.[141,144] Dysfunction in these areas may result from difficulty with memory, receptive and expressive language, communicating information, planning and organizing information, motivational and attention difficulties, personality changes, mood disturbances, paranoia, agitation, or a decrease in goal-directed behavior.[141] Cognitive dysfunction may be a result of various factors. Certain levels of cognitive dysfunction are associated with normal aging. Traumatic brain injury and stroke are two common causes of dysfunction. Viral and bacterial infections can also cause impairment. Cognitive dysfunction has been associated

TABLE 16.3 Cognitive Domains Evaluated by Neurocognitive Testing

Intelligence	
• Full scale IQ (FSIQ)	Overall intellectual functioning
• Verbal scale IQ (VIQ)	Verbal comprehension and working memory
• Performance scale IQ (PIQ)	Perceptual reasoning and processing speed
Attention	
• Sustained attention	Attention for an extended duration of time
• Divided attention	Attention to multiple tasks or multiple task components
• Alternating attention	Ability to shift attention on tasks
Memory	
• Short-term (working memory)	Retaining information for a relatively short duration of time
• Sustained attention	Attention for an extended duration of time
• Divided attention	Attention to multiple tasks or multiple task components
• Alternating attention	Ability to shift attention on tasks
• Long-term	Retaining information for a longer duration of time
• Episodic	Recall of past personal events, autobiographical memory
• Semantic	Recall of information regarding factual world events, learned information
Executive functioning	Cognitive functions involving goal-directed behavior, organization, planning
Processing speed	A measure of speed in which a person performs intake and output of information

with various medical illnesses, including acquired immunodeficiency syndrome (AIDS),[145] multiple sclerosis,[146] lupus,[147] and Lyme disease.[148] Toxic exposure to alcohol or environmental fuels has also been associated with cognitive dysfunction.[141] Malnutrition, such as folic acid or vitamin B_{12} deficiency, may also alter neurocognitive functioning.[141] In addition, hypothyroidism has been associated with cognitive impairment.[149,150]

Uremia, as well as age, can contribute to impairment in cognitive functioning. HD patients are often elderly and are therefore at greater risk for cognitive difficulties.[121] Uremia has a significant impact on cognitive ability, with symptoms such as fatigue, nausea, drowsiness, irritability, decreased libido, and sleep disturbances[151-154] associated with reduced concentration, memory impairment, and decrease in intellectual functioning.[155-158] Anemia may also result in cognitive impairment,[159] particularly in those with neurological or cerebrovascular diseases.[137,160] One study, however, did not find an association between anemia and cognitive functioning in an adult CKD population aged 55 years and older.[161]

TABLE 16.4 Frequently Used Neurocognitive Tests to Assess Cognitive Functioning

Neuropsychological Test	Cognitive Abilities Measured
Wechsler Adult Intelligence Scale (WAIS-IV)	Intellectual functioning comprising verbal and performance domains
Wechsler Intelligence Scale for Children (WISC-V)	Intellectual functioning comprising verbal, performance, memory, and processing speed domains
Wechsler Memory Scale (WMS-IV)	Verbal memory, visual memory, attention
California Verbal Learning Test (CVLT)	Verbal memory, immediate and delayed recall
Trail Making Test, Forms A and B	Psychomotor speed, attention, visual scanning, and planning skills
Mini-Mental State Examination (MMSE)	Overall cognitive function, including attention, orientation, attention, language, and memory
The Modified Mini-Mental State (3MS)	Overall cognitive function, including attention, orientation, language, and memory
The Symbol Digit Modalities Test (SDMT)	Immediate visual memory, learning, hand-eye coordination, and reading-writing ability
The Controlled Oral Word Association Test (COWAT)	Verbal fluency, planning and organization, and semantic memory
Rey Auditory Verbal Learning Test (RAVLT)	Verbal learning, immediate memory, and retrieval from long-term storage
Conners' Continuous Performance Test (CPT)	Attention, processing speed, and psychomotor ability
Wisconsin Card Sorting Task	Attention and executive functioning (mental flexibility)
Cognitive Abilities Test (CAT)	Processing speed, memory, and stimulus discrimination
Paced Auditory Serial Addition Test (PASAT)	Attention, processing speed, and working memory
Stroop Color-Word Test	Selective and focused attention
Rey-Osterrieth Complex Figure	Memory, attention, and visuospatial ability
Montreal Cognitive Assessment (MoCA)	Attention, executive functioning, memory, language, visuoconstructional skills, orientation

Treatment of anemia with recombinant human erythropoietin (rHuEPO) for 3 months improved cognitive functioning in patients with renal failure.[162] Cognitive assessments were administered at three intervals: before erythropoietin treatment and after 3 and 12 months of treatment. Subjects completed each assessment approximately 24 hours after dialysis. After 3 months of treatment, patients showed improvement on the Symbol Digit Modalities Test (SDMT). This test requires learning, memory, psychomotor speed, and scanning efficiency skills. After 12 months of treatment, patients evidenced significant improvement on the Trail Making Test Part

B. Temple and colleagues[163] assessed cognitive changes in 18 HD patients: 9 treated with rHuEPO and 9 controls. There was a significant 8.7-point, increase in IQ scores in the group that received rHuEPO treatment, compared with a nonsignificant change of 2.5 IQ points in the group that did not receive rHuEPO treatment. Singh and colleagues evaluated the impact of rHuEPO treatment on cognitive status using P300 event related potentials (ERPs) as a marker of cognitive dysfunction.[164] Thirty anemic patients with CKD, 15 of whom were on HD and 15 patients with less-severe renal failure, were examined. All 30 patients received rHuEPO treatment and were compared with a control group of 30 healthy individuals who did not receive rHuEPO treatment. The authors found a reduction in P300 latency in both groups that underwent rHuEPO treatment and a significant increase in the P300 amplitude in the HD group, both markers of improved cognitive function. The control group did not demonstrate any significant change in ERPs.[164]

Psychological factors, such as depression, have also been found to affect cognitive functioning.[165] Depression affects memory in the general population.[165,166] Depression is highly prevalent among patients with CKD and therefore may contribute to neurocognitive impairment.

Tyrell and colleagues[167] assessed cognitive functioning and depression in a sample of older dialysis patients. Depression was assessed using the Montgomery-Asberg Depression Rating Scale (MADRS). Forty-five percent of patients were both depressed and cognitively impaired, as measured by the Mini-Mental State Examination (MMSE).[167] Pliskin and colleagues[156] tested whether cognitive functioning was associated with depression, as measured by the BDI. Results indicated significant differences in cognitive functioning when comparing a depressed group (mean BDI = 18.4) to a nondepressed group (mean BDI = 6.1). Those who were less depressed had higher full scale and verbal IQ scores.[156] Agganis et al. used the CES-D and a neuropsychological battery to assess cognitive functioning and depression in 241 HD patients. Those with increased depressive symptoms demonstrated greater impairment in processing speed, attention, and executive functioning.[168] In a study of 458 PD patients, Dong et al. found that those who evidenced mild to moderate or severe depressive symptoms had increased risk of cognitive impairment, and performed more poorly on tasks of executive function, immediate memory, and delayed memory compared with individuals who were not depressed, even after controlling for demographic, clinical, and biomarker data.[169]

Other common comorbid disorders associated with kidney disease may also contribute to the development of cognitive impairment. Hypertension and diabetes have been associated with compromised cognitive ability. Hypertension is a risk factor for developing vascular dementia and Alzheimer disease,[141] hypothesized to be the result of the effect of elevated blood pressure on the vasculature of cerebral white matter and promotion of atherosclerosis.[141] Obisesan and colleagues[170] reported hypertension to be negatively associated with cognitive functioning in the general population, as measured by the MMSE. Hanon and colleagues[171] studied the impact of the antihypertensive medication, Eprosartan, on cognitive functioning in hypertensive patients across 28 countries. Antihypertensive treatment was associated with significant improvement in cognitive functioning, as measured by MMSE, after 6 months of drug treatment. Interestingly, the largest effect was found among the elderly.[171] A later meta-analysis demonstrated that in a hypertensive population without a history of neurological or cerebrovascular disease, antihypertensive treatment across drug classes benefitted cognitive functioning.[172] Use of antihypertensive medication was also associated with a reduction in risk for the development of dementia, although this finding did not remain significant when only including RCTs in the analysis.[172] The extent to which different antihypertensive medications are effective is an important area for further study.

Diabetes has also been associated with impairment in cognitive functioning. Almost one-half of ESRD cases in the United States are associated with diabetes.[173] Individuals with diabetes are at increased risk for cardiovascular and cerebrovascular disease.[174] Saczynski and colleagues reported that processing speed was reduced among individuals with diabetes compared with normoglycemic subjects. In addition, patients with at least 15 years since diabetes diagnosis were found to be significantly more cognitively impaired than subjects more recently diagnosed with diabetes.[174] Arvanitakis and colleagues reported that diabetes mellitus was associated with decreased semantic memory and perceptual speed.[175] Furthermore, Sinclair and colleagues found that those with lower MMSE scores, and thus lower cognitive functioning, were less involved with self-management of their diabetes than individuals who scored higher on the MMSE.[176] These findings highlight the possible impact that cognitive functioning may have on the adherence to medical regimens.

The relationship between cognitive decline and stage of CKD is not well understood. Assessing cognitive impairment in a sample of 80 patients with CKD not receiving dialysis treatment and 80 patients with ESRD receiving HD, Kurella and colleagues[177] found an association between stage of CKD and degree of cognitive impairment. Seliger and colleagues reported that participants with moderate CKD were 37% more likely to develop dementia over a median of 6 years.[178] Yaffe et al. found in 825 individuals with CKD over the age of 55, those with worse kidney functioning (estimated glomerular filtration rate [eGFR] <30 mL/min/1.73 m^2) demonstrated greater cognitive impairment compared with individuals with mild or moderate CKD (eGFR 45 to 59 mL/min/1.73 m^2).[179] In a later study, Weiner et al. assessed whether urine albumin-to-creatinine ratio (ACR) and eGFR were associated with cognitive impairment in a sample of individuals with cardiovascular disease, elevated cardiovascular disease risk, or CKD. Increased ACR and reduced eGFR were associated with worse cognitive functioning.[180]

It is unclear whether the HD procedure modifies cognitive functioning in patients with ESRD. Hemodynamic shifts resulting from dialysis treatment may cause short-term cognitive fluctuations[155] because changes in blood volume may cause cerebral edema or reduce intracerebral blood pressure and blood flow.[137] It is also possible that as dialysis treats uremia, there is a commensurate improvement in cognitive processing. One study identified such improvement in cognitive functioning 24 hours after HD.[181] Lewis and colleagues reported an increase in reaction time and visual-motor speed and accuracy 24 hours after receiving dialysis treatment.[182] Najafi and colleagues assessed attention and reaction time and did not find any changes in these variables before and after HD treatment in 45 HD patients.[183] Williams and colleagues measured cognitive functioning, specifically attention and memory, 1 hour, 24 hours, and then 67 hours after HD, and found subjects performed significantly more poorly 67 hours after dialysis compared with the earlier measurements.[155] Cukor et al. used a computer-based neuropsychological assessment battery to measure cognitive functioning before and after HD treatment in 25 HD patients and 6 PD patients used as controls. Cognitive functioning improved after a single session in the HD group compared with the control group.[184] Kurella Tamura et al. assessed the impact of initiating dialysis on cognitive functioning in 212 advanced CKD patients.[185] Cognitive functioning was assessed via a telephone battery over a 2-year period. Results revealed an association between initiation of dialysis treatment and poorer performance on executive functioning tasks. The study did not find any significant changes in global cognitive functioning.[185] These studies suggest that HD can have varying effects on cognitive performance, and neurocognitive performance may differ depending on the timing of the assessment.

Studies that examined differences in cognitive functioning between HD and PD patients have demonstrated inconsistent results.[177] Yount and colleagues reported that those receiving PD had a greater attention ability than those receiving HD.[186] Wolcott and colleagues also reported better cognitive functioning among PD patients compared with those receiving HD.[187] In contrast, Rozeman and colleagues[188] did not find significant differences in cognitive functioning comparing patients treated with the two modalities. Williams et al. found that patients receiving PD exhibited stable cognitive performance over 67 hours after dialysis, compared with HD patients, who demonstrated decline in cognitive functioning.[155] One metaanalysis[189] found that those receiving HD performed more poorly on tasks assessing executive functioning compared with PD, although this finding was based on only two studies. The authors concluded there was insufficient information to show that cognitive functioning differed between HD and PD patients.[189] Differing neurocognitive performance between HD and PD groups may, in part, be the result of patient selection or intrinsic differences in the treatment modalities.[159] HD is typically performed three times per week and can create abrupt hemodynamic shifts. In contrast, PD provides more stable control of uremia and electrolytes because of its continuous nature.[190] There also may be some inherent differences in baseline cognitive functioning in patients who choose one treatment method over the other, or other unmeasured differences in patient characteristics.

The long-term impact of nocturnal daily hemodialysis (NHD) on cognitive functioning has been investigated. Jassal and colleagues[191] examined cognitive functioning in patients treated with NHD at a baseline assessment and after an average of 8.3 months. Patients showed significant improvement in processing speed and attention at the second evaluation.[191] Vos et al. compared cognitive functioning of individuals who received conventional HD to those who received HD for 2 hours, 6 times per week. The investigators did not find improvement in cognitive functioning.[192] Similarly, a later study did not find improvement in executive functioning or overall cognitive functioning with more frequent HD treatment and more frequent home nocturnal HD treatment of 6 days per week versus 3 days per week.[193]

Cognitive functioning has also been studied in children with CKD. Bawden and colleagues[194] assessed cognitive functioning in 22 children with ESRD and 22 sibling controls. All participants with ESRD were either currently receiving dialysis treatment or waiting to begin dialysis. Children with ESRD scored significantly lower on domains of intellectual functioning compared with their siblings.[194] The study did not find significant differences on memory tasks between children with ESRD and their matched controls. Duquette and colleagues[195] examined intellectual functioning in 30 children with CKD. Fifteen participants were dialysis patients, and 15 participants received conservative forms of treatment. The CKD group was matched with 41 control participants. The two groups differed significantly on intelligence, with the control group performing better than the CKD group. In addition, the CKD group had a significantly higher percentage of individuals with Full Scale IQ scores lower than the 25th percentile.[195] In addition, Mendley et al. found that in a sample of 340 children and adolescents with mild to moderate CKD, increased duration of CKD was associated with a greater likelihood of poorer performance on tasks that measure attention regulation and inhibitory control.[196]

The findings have generally been mixed when cognitive functioning is measured in patients with CKD.[197] Earlier studies are hard to evaluate because the amount and frequency of dialysis provided were often not reported. Dialysis administration may significantly affect cognitive results.[156] Furthermore, many studies did not consider cognitive assessments relative to the time of dialysis.[198] Another study questioned whether cognitive testing results may be generally biased in a CKD population, given the many limitations patients frequently endure.[199] Visual or physical impairments, as well as depression, all common in ESRD patients, may negatively affect testing ability and therefore results. Impairments may also result in exclusion from studies, thereby limiting the generalizability of findings.[199]

PREVALENCE OF NEUROCOGNITIVE IMPAIRMENT

Although the number of incident cases of ESRD is leveling off in the United States, the ongoing need to decrease incidence and prevalence rates of the disease is paramount.[200] It has been estimated that the prevalence of cognitive impairment in patients with stage 5 CKD is 30% to 60%.[121] Seghal and colleagues concluded that 22% of HD patients evidenced mild cognitive impairment (MMSE 18 to 23), and 8% had more severe impairment (MMSE 0 to 17).[201] Fazekas and colleagues examined cognitive functioning in 30 HD patients and 30 matched controls. Sixty percent of the HD patients evidenced cognitive impairment as measured by *DSM-III* criteria for the diagnosis of dementia or deficits, according to neuropsychological testing.[202] In addition, MMSE scores were significantly different between the two groups, with HD patients demonstrating cognitive impairment. Another study[177] compared the prevalence of cognitive impairment in 80 patients with CKD and 80 patients with ESRD. In the combined sample, 17% evidenced global cognitive impairment. Twenty-seven percent of patients with ESRD demonstrated global cognitive impairment, whereas 15% of CKD patients evidenced impairment. Interestingly, only patients with advanced stage CKD demonstrated impairment.[177] Murray and colleagues assessed cognitive functioning in 338 HD patients. Based on their cognitive test battery results, patients were divided into mild, moderate, or severe impairment groups, with 14% categorized as having mild impairment, 36% moderate dysfunction, and 37.3% with severe impairment.[121] Overall, there is evidence that cognitive dysfunction is common in ESRD patients. There is less evidence that the stage of CKD may be an important determinant of degree of impairment. However, the specific cognitive domains that are affected by CKD are less clear. In general, small sample sizes limit the ability to generalize findings.

NEUROCOGNITIVE FUNCTIONING AFTER TRANSPLANTATION

Cognitive changes after kidney transplantation have also been the subject of scientific inquiry. Kramer and colleagues[203] assessed neurocognitive functioning in HD patients before and after kidney transplantation. These patients were compared with healthy control subjects. Cognitive functioning was measured using evoked potentials, the MMSE, and the Trailmaking Test. Before transplantation, evoked potentials of the dialysis patients were significantly delayed and smaller in amplitude compared with healthy subjects. In addition, before transplantation, dialysis patients performed significantly more poorly on the two neuropsychological tests compared with healthy subjects. After transplantation, dialysis patients did not differ on the MMSE or Trailmaking Test compared with healthy subjects. However, latency between evoked potentials decreased and amplitude of evoked potentials increased, suggesting an improvement in cognitive functioning.[203]

Mendley and Zelko[204] assessed neuropsychological functioning in children with ESRD before and after kidney transplantation. There were significant improvements after transplantation in processing speed, discriminatory ability, and working memory. Other cognitive functions assessed did not differ before and after transplantation.[204]

A study in which participants were assessed on cognitive domains before transplantation and 6 months after transplant also demonstrated an increase in memory performance.[205] Psychomotor performance and attention, however, did not significantly improve after transplantation.[205] Mendley and Zelko[204] also found improvement in memory functioning after kidney transplantation.

The affect of immunosuppressive medications on cognitive functioning after kidney transplantation is also of interest. Long-term glucocorticoid use has been associated with atrophy of the hippocampus, an area of the brain associated with memory.[206] One study demonstrated impairment in long-term memory, more specifically delayed memory recall, in 50 kidney transplant patients taking immunosuppressive medication compared with normative scores.[206] Immunosuppressive medications have also been associated with various side effects, including tremors, weakness, seizures, and difficulty with sleep.[158] Contemporary kidney transplant recipients, however, often do not experience these symptoms, possibly as a result of efforts to minimize immunosuppressive therapy.[198] Cognitive impairment related to glucocorticoid treatment may improve by reducing dosages or with steroid-free immunosuppressive regimens.[198,206]

SEQUELAE OF NEUROCOGNITIVE IMPAIRMENT

Impairment in cognitive functioning in those with kidney disease may affect levels of compliance with dialysis treatment, medication adherence, and fluid and dietary restrictions.[78,138] Rates for nonadherence to the dialysis prescription range from 30% to 60%.[78,207] Nonadherence to the medical regimen has been associated with increased mortality.[77,78] In addition, nonadherence to immunosuppressive medication in kidney transplantation is a primary cause of rejection.[208] One metaanalysis found that nonadherent transplant patients were seven times more likely to have graft failure than those who were adherent.[209]

One study sought to examine the association between cognitive impairment and levels of adherence in 63 older adults receiving HD treatment.[138] Cognitive impairment was assessed using the 3MS, with a score lower than 80 marking impairment. Approximately 39% of the sample was found to have cognitive impairment. Of those with cognitive impairment, 58% were found to be nonadherent, measured by serum phosphate levels.[138] A limitation of this study was that it focused on adherence in those who were cognitively impaired and did not measure adherence in those who were cognitively intact. Griva et al.[210] found an increased risk for mortality in dialysis patients who had cognitive impairment compared with those who were not cognitively impaired. The authors excluded individuals with severe cognitive impairment from the study. The 7-year survival rate for individuals who met criteria for impairment was 49%, compared with 83.2% for those who were not impaired.[210] Cognitive deficits involving attention, memory, processing speed, and other functions may compromise the understanding of medical procedures and treatment regimens.[78,144]

Expectations that patients with CKD are able to manage the complex demands of medical management may not be realistic, especially given the common occurrence of cognitive impairment in this population. Addressing cognitive impairment is critically important for overall adjustment to chronic illness and prognosis in CKD. Quality of life and well-being may be favorably influenced if cognitive ability can be maintained.

TREATMENT OF NEUROCOGNITIVE IMPAIRMENT

Despite the high prevalence of cognitive impairment in CKD, studies that describe intervention methods for this population are not available. Medications such as cholinesterase inhibitors are available for treatment of neurocognitive disorders, although the safety of these medications in ESRD is not well established.[211] There are several strategies that have been used in other populations with chronic illness, which may be applicable to CKD patients. For example, computer-based strategies have been used to improve attention, memory, and executive functioning.[212] One group used computer retraining to increase attention in a group of patients with multiple sclerosis.[213] Other cognitive rehabilitation strategies are compensatory in nature, such as using calendars and logs for recording activities such as taking medications or dietary regimens. These techniques are often useful for individuals with memory impairment. Breaking tasks into smaller parts may help decrease inattention and reduce overwhelmed feelings. Involving the patient's supportive network in managing activities of daily living is another helpful strategy. Neurological rehabilitation is a field still in its infancy, but it holds much promise, especially for those with less severe impairment. Compromised cognitive functioning in patients with CKD often goes undetected.[138] Routine screening of cognitive function should be a component of regular care for the ESRD patient. An efficient way to monitor cognitive function is to regularly test gross neurocognitive performance using a simple tool, such as the MMSE. Patients can be referred for further assessment if a substantial change in function occurs.

CASE PRESENTATION

A 60-year-old HD patient was diagnosed with ESRD 5 years ago. She had a long-standing history of hypertension and was compliant with dietary, medication, and clinic attendance goals. Recently, however, there was an increase in the variability of the patient's blood pressure. She admitted to having difficulty remembering to take her medications. Her nephrologist requested neuropsychological testing, which included the MMSE, memory tasks, and the Trail Making Test. She obtained a score of 22 on the MMSE, indicating obvious cognitive impairment. Specifically, the patient had difficulty recalling new information (verbal and nonverbal) and with control of attention. She performed considerably worse on working memory and immediate memory scales and demonstrated compromised processing speed and attention relative to her overall neurocognitive performance. Neurological examination, imaging of the brain, and biochemical assessments revealed no apparent reason for her impairments other than ESRD. Urea clearance (Kt/V) was adequate, and the vascular access functioned efficiently.

Compensatory strategies were identified to help her better manage her medical regimen. She was advised to use external cues, such as an alarm watch, to alert her when to take her medications. Her family was encouraged to assist the patient by placing her medications into a week-long pill case. A food diary log was also suggested to help her record her food intake more specifically and monitor her diet. It was also recommended to the patient's healthcare team that they relay information to her in a simple and slow-paced manner to accommodate her impaired information processing ability. Verbal information should also be supplemented by simple, legible written instructions. Within a few weeks, the patient was taking her medication more regularly, and her diet improved. She appreciated the extra help and felt less overwhelmed by her medical problems. The patient's neurocognitive deficits may have been related to aging, vascular complications, or uremia. Regardless of the etiology, her neurocognitive deficits were addressed by basic behavioral strategies that allowed her to regain some of the lost functions.

SUMMARY OF NEUROCOGNITIVE FUNCTION IN CHRONIC KIDNEY DISEASE

Possible etiologies of impaired neurocognitive functioning in CKD patients include aging, vascular disease, diabetes, uremia, anemia, depression, toxin exposure, and malnutrition. The impact of hemodynamic changes on acute neurocognitive processing is still unclear. The prevalence of impairment in dialysis patients ranges from 30% to 60%, depending on assessment methodology and population factors. Deficits appear in global intellectual functioning, memory, attention, executive functioning, and processing speed. It appears that neurocognitive function improves mildly after transplantation. Cognitive impairment may negatively affect treatment compliance. There are only limited data on treatment strategies for cognitive impairment in CKD or ESRD patients.

A full list of references is available at www.expertconsult.com.

17

Improving Drug Use and Dosing in Chronic Kidney Disease

Wendy L. St. Peter, PharmD, Lori Wazny, BSc, PharmD, and Joanna Q. Hudson, PharmD

OUTLINE

Assuring safe, effective, and convenient drug therapy for patients with chronic kidney disease (CKD) is challenging from multiple perspectives. Many drugs are partially or wholly excreted by the kidneys; these drugs are typically dose-reduced to produce similar blood or plasma concentrations as in patients with normal kidney function. Often, compendia such as Micromedex, AHFS, and Lexicomp recommend dosing based on categories of creatinine clearance (CrCL) or glomerular filtration rate (GFR). In the United States, most creatinine assays used by US clinics or hospitals have been calibrated to an isotope dilution mass spectrometry (IDMS) reference (creatinine standardization) so results are consistent across laboratories. However, this creates a dilemma for dosing adjustment. The pharmacokinetics of most marketed US drugs that require dosage adjustment in CKD patients have been evaluated using the Cockcroft–Gault (CG) estimated CrCL (eCrCL) formula (including patient weight), which was developed before creatinine standardization. However, most clinics and hospitals automatically report estimated GFR (eGFR) normalized to body surface area (BSA) with each serum creatinine level, that clinicians use to determine drug dosage adjustments. We discuss the implications of creatinine standardization and use of eCrCL or eGFR in drug dosing assessment in CKD patients and in special CKD populations (obese and elderly).

Kidney dysfunction decreases elimination of drugs that are mainly cleared by the kidney, but kidney dysfunction can also affect drug absorption, distribution, and metabolism, as well as drug targets or effector proteins. Thus kidney dysfunction can greatly alter drug pharmacokinetics and pharmacodynamics, causing variable drug efficacy and toxicity in CKD patients compared with patients with normal kidney function. We discuss key principles that all clinicians should be aware of when prescribing medications for patients with CKD and present pharmacokinetic and dosing information on selected newer drugs (direct oral anticoagulants, newer diabetes agents).

Clinicians seeing maintenance dialysis patients face added complexities related to the effects of dialysis therapy when determining drug dosage adjustments. We discuss drug- and dialysis-related characteristics that predict dialyzability and where to find updated information on drug dialyzability, and we provide an example of how to assess a new drug for dialyzability and initial dosing in a patient receiving renal replacement therapy (RRT).

Patients with CKD are very complex with regard to disease, comorbidity, number of medications, and dosage regimens. Consequently, hospitalizations are frequent and healthcare costs are high. We review the evidence to suggest best practices for team care, transitions of care, and informatics approaches or tools that may improve health outcomes and reduce costs.

ASSESSMENT OF KIDNEY FUNCTION FOR DRUG DOSING, INCLUDING SPECIAL POPULATIONS

Assessment of kidney function is important for drug regimen design with drugs that depend on renal clearance. Although direct measurement of GFR using a marker such as iothalamate is most accurate, it is not practical in the clinical setting. Estimating equations include the CG,[1] Modification of Diet in Renal Disease (MDRD), and Chronic Kidney Disease-Epidemiologic Prognosis Initiative (CKD-EPI) equations (with and without cystatin C).[2-5] (See Chapter 2 for detailed information on measurement and estimation of kidney function.) The CG equation estimates CrCL, a surrogate marker of GFR. The MDRD and CKD-EPI equations were developed using measured iothalamate clearance, and they estimate GFR. The eGFR has become a standard laboratory result reported by most clinical laboratories when serum creatinine level is available; eGFR has been recommended for determining and classifying CKD and for drug dosing.[6] The most recent Kidney Disease: Improving Global Outcomes (KDIGO) CKD guideline recommends the CKD-EPI equation as the eGFR method for routine clinical practice.[7] As it replaces the MDRD equation, clinicians should consider its specific performance for drug dosing.

Regardless of the method used, the limitations of these estimates for drug dosing must be considered. Creatinine standardization began in 2005 and was fully implemented by most US laboratories by 2010. Before assay standardization, serum creatinine values were overestimated by approximately 10% to 20%.[6] Standardization led to less variability in creatinine results; however, only newer equations such as the reexpressed MDRD equation, CKD-EPI equations, and Schwartz equation for children, use standardized creatinine.[3-5,8] For many drugs, manufacturer dosing recommendations are based on eCrCL using the CG equation, as this was the method used to assess kidney function in the pharmacokinetic studies. As many of these studies were performed before creatinine standardization, measured serum creatinine values were, on average, higher (leading to lower eCrCL values). Although adjustment methods have been suggested, valid reexpression of the CG equation is not possible, as plasma creatinine samples used to develop it are no longer available to be assayed by a standardized method. Controversially, the National Kidney Foundation recently recommended the CG equation only for research purposes, given that it cannot be reexpressed using standardized creatinine values and the potential for inaccurate results.[9] At present, however, not enough data support replacing the CG equation exclusively with eGFR methods, and the CG equation remains widely used in clinical practice for drug dosing.[10] The eGFR has been recommended for use in pharmacokinetic studies for new drugs being developed.[11] The US Food and Drug Administration (FDA) 2010 draft of the Guidance for Industry related to pharmacokinetic studies in patients with impaired renal function recommended that pharmacokinetic studies be conducted using both eGFR and eCrCL.[12] If such studies become standard and new evidence regarding drug dosing with eGFR becomes available, support may increase for use of eGFR for drug dosing in clinical practice.

A key study that led to the recommendation to use eGFR for drug dosing compared differences in dosing recommendations based on FDA-approved dosing for 15 drugs eliminated by the kidney.[13] Discrepancies in recommended doses using measured GFR were compared with recommendations using MDRD eGFR and CG eCrCL using total and ideal body weight (TBW, IBW) for 5504 individuals. Agreement was highest for the MDRD eGFR (88%), followed by the CG eCrCL TBW (85%) and the CG eCrCL IBW (82%). Of note, one controversy about this study relates to dosing recommendations for the drugs evaluated being based on measured GFR, not measured or estimated CrCL, which was the method used by the manufacturers in the initial pharmacokinetic studies. Several other studies have compared dosing recommendations based on estimates using eGFR and CG eCrCL; however, they vary with regard to the equations used and the reference method for dosing comparison. Most discrepancies occur in patients at extremes of body weight and the elderly.[14-18] For most of these studies, the clinical significance has not been determined, but discrepancies clearly exist. Findings such as these have led practitioners to question whether these estimates can be used interchangeably for drug dosing.

Discrepancies in dosing recommendations for obese patients using eGFR versus eCrCL highlight body size as an important factor to consider with current assessment equations for drug dosing. The MDRD and CKD-EPI equations, when developed, were normalized to a BSA of 1.73 m^2, and their values are reported in mL/min/1.73 m^2.[2,4] This differs from the CG eCrCL, which is reported in mL/min. In general, when using the MDRD or CKD-EPI equation for drug dosing, the result should be multiplied by the patient's BSA divided by 1.73 m^2 to convert the values to mL/min. This is particularly important for underweight or overweight individuals whose BSA differs substantially from 1.73 m^2. With regard to body size, the weight to use in the CG equation is somewhat controversial. Creatinine is a metabolic by-product of muscle metabolism derived from creatine, and its production and release are affected by muscle mass, not fat, which makes use of TBW in overweight/obese individuals a less-reliable body size descriptor in the CG equation. Other body size descriptors that have been used include IBW, lean body weight (LBW),[19,20] or an adjusted body weight (ABW).[21] Using LBW in the CG equation provided the most unbiased, precise, and accurate estimate of measured CrCL in 54 morbidly obese individuals.[20] However, based on the performance of ABW in the CG equation compared with measured CrCL in over 2800 individuals with body mass index (BMI) ≥25 kg/m^2, use of the "TIA" method was recommended: use TBW in the CG equation when BMI is <18.5 kg/m^2 (underweight), IBW when BMI is 18.6 to 24.9 kg/m^2, and ABW when BMI is ≥25 kg/m^2 (Table 17.1).[21] Of note, adjustment of eGFR for BSA has been shown to overestimate kidney function in morbidly

TABLE 17.1 "TIA" Method to Calculate CrCL Using the Cockcroft–Gault Equation[21]

Weight Descriptor	Calculation
ABW (kg)	IBW + 0.4 (TBW − IBW)
BMI (kg/m²)	Weight/height²
IBW for males (kg)	50 + 2.3 kg (for every inch over 5 feet)
IBW for females (kg)	45.5 + 2.3 kg (for every inch over 5 feet)
TBW (kg)	Actual weight in kg

TIA method = use TBW when BMI <18.5 (underweight), IBW when BMI is between 18.6 and 24.9, and ABW when BMI is ≥25.
ABW, Adjusted body weight in kg; *BMI,* body mass index; *IBW,* ideal body weight; *TBW,* total body weight.

obese (BMI >40 kg/m²) patients[22]; the CG equation with the TIA method may provide a more reasonable estimate for drug dosing for such patients.

Variations in drug dosing recommendations are also notable in elderly patients, emphasizing the importance of considering age. Unfortunately, when available estimating equations were developed, relatively few elderly individuals were included. The CG equation was developed using data from 249 predominantly male veterans with 45% aged 60 years or older (oldest, 92 years).[1] The MDRD equation was developed using data from 1070 individuals with a mean age of 51 ± 13 years and 22% aged older than 65 years.[2,23] The CKD-EPI population included 5504 individuals of whom 15% were aged older than 65 years, and the CKD-EPI creatinine-cystatin C 2012 population included 5352 individuals of whom 13% were older than 65 years.[4,5] More variation among subgroups based on age occurred in the MDRD study in individuals with eGFR ≥60 mL/min/1.73 m². At these higher eGFR levels, eGFR overestimated measured GFR in individuals aged older than 65 years.[23] In subsequent analysis of the MDRD and CKD-EPI equations, the CKD-EPI equation performed similarly to the MDRD equation in individuals aged older than 65 years.[24] The challenges with using estimating equations for drug dosing in elderly patients relate to whether differences in the eGFR and CG with increasing age are recognized. In the mathematical simulation study described by Delanaye et al.,[25] CG eCrCl results were progressively lower than CKD-EPI eGFR results with increasing age. After age 60 years, CKD-EPI results began to exceed CG results, and by age 95 years, the CKD-EPI result was 40% higher than the CG result. The Berlin Initiative Study equation has been proposed as a better estimate of kidney function in the elderly[26]; however, this equation showed no significant advantage over the CKD-EPI creatinine-cystatin C equation for estimating gentamicin clearance in 99 individuals older than 70 years.[27] The European Renal Best Practice Group noted the limitations of using the available estimating equations in elderly patients with eGFR <45 mL/min/1.73 m² and risk for kidney function misclassification and recommends measuring GFR or using the CKD-EPI equation with both creatinine and cystatin C when more precise estimation is needed.[28] Because serum creatinine becomes less reliable as a marker of kidney function as muscle mass declines (as in the elderly), some practitioners suggest that serum creatinine be rounded up to 1.0 in elderly individuals with a measured creatinine <1 to avoid overestimating kidney function. However, this practice has not been shown to improve the performance of the estimate and is not recommended.[17,29]

Clearly, choice of body size descriptor (i.e., TBW, IBW, ABW) in the CG equation and individualizing the eGFR estimate for BSA (i.e., multiplying by BSA/1.73 m²) has a substantial effect on estimates of kidney function. Table 17.2 shows an example of the differences in estimates based on the method used. In scenario 1, the individual is close to IBW; therefore the weight used in the CG equation has little effect on the results and his eCrCL is approximately 40 mL/min. The CKD-EPI eGFR without adjustment for BSA is 27 mL/min/1.73 m², but 35 mL/min when adjusted for BSA. Although the difference in adjusted and unadjusted CKD-EPI results is relatively minor, these estimates straddle a typical dosing threshold of 30 mL/min. The dosing decision for a drug requiring adjustment or discontinuation with a GFR or CrCL <30 (e.g., enoxaparin, metformin, dabigatran) would become more challenging. In this case, the adjusted value of 35 mL/min is more appropriate. This example highlights the similarity of the CKD-EPI estimate in mL/min and the CG eCrCL estimate, and drug dosing recommendations would not differ based on method because the estimates are 30 to 40 mL/min. In scenario 2, the individual is obese. Now the eCrCL ranges from 41 mL/min with IBW to almost 60 mL/min with TBW. ABW would give a result close to 40 mL/min. The CKD-EPI unadjusted eGFR remains 27 mL/min/1.73 m² as in the first scenario, but adjusting for BSA yields a value of 40 mL/min. If the CKD-EPI equation is not adjusted for BSA, a drug with a dosing threshold at 30 mL/min could be underdosed. It could be overdosed by using the eCrCL with TBW, as results of 59 mL/min may be above another common dosing threshold of 50 mL/min.

As an example of age-related differences, scenario 3 in Table 17.2 shows CG eCrCL and CKD-EPI eGFR for a 90-year-old white woman with serum creatinine 1.4 mg/dL who is below her IBW. The CKD-EPI adjusted eGFR is 30 mL/min; however, the eCrCL based on TBW is 22 mL/min. Scenario 4 is this same individual with serum creatinine 0.7 mg/dL. The difference in eCrCL and the adjusted CKD-EPI result is 25 mL/min, which has substantial implications with a dosing threshold at 50 to 60 mL/min. Whether the serum creatinine is a reliable marker in this 90-year-old individual with reduced muscle mass would have to be determined. In this case, a measured CrCL or GFR may be reasonable if the drug has a narrow therapeutic index. The general implications of scenarios 3 and 4 are that older individuals would be prescribed higher doses of a given drug using the eGFR result as opposed to the CG result. This has been shown in several studies evaluating hypothetical dosing differences for drugs eliminated by the kidney when the CG results (using varying body weights) were compared to eGFR.[16-18,30]

Clinicians should be well aware of the potential difference in estimates of kidney function in populations that include

TABLE 17.2 **Estimates of Kidney Function Using the Cockcroft Gault Equation With Differing Weight Adjustments and CKD-EPI Equation With and Without Adjustment for Body Surface Area (in mL/min/1.73 m² and mL/min) in Four Scenarios**

Scenario	CG-TBW (mL/min)	CG-IBW (mL/min)	CG-ABW (mL/min)	CKD-EPI (mL/min/1.73 m²)	CKD-EPI Adjusted (mL/min)
58-year-old white male; SCr 2.5 mg/dL; Ht 76 in; Wt 90 kg; IBW = 87 kg; BSA 2.21 m²	41	40	40	27	35
Scenario 1 with wt = 130 kg BSA = 2.58	59	41	47	27	41
90-year-old white female; SCr 1.4 mg/dL; Ht 65 in; Wt 52 kg; IBW = 57 kg; BSA 1.56 m²	22	*	*	33	30
90-year-old black female; SCr 0.7 mg/dL; Ht 65 in; Wt 52 kg; IBW = 57 kg; BSA 1.56 m²	44	*	*	76	69

*Not appropriate to use because the patient's weight is below her IBW.
ABW, Adjusted body weight; *BSA,* body surface area; *CG,* Cockcroft–Gault; *CKD-EPI,* Chronic Kidney Disease-Epidemiologic Prognosis Initiative; *IBW,* ideal body weight; *TBW,* total body weight.

overweight and underweight individuals and the elderly and should take into account the effect on drug dosing decisions. Careful consideration of the method used to estimate kidney function, the method used to develop dosing recommendations for the drug, and the risk–benefit profile is warranted when designing a drug regimen in patients with reduced kidney function. The limitations of applying estimating equations for the purpose of drug dosing in obese individuals or in elderly individuals with reduced muscle mass are acknowledged by KDIGO and the National Kidney Disease Education Program (NKDEP). NKDEP states that "neither eGFR nor creatinine clearance will be accurate in individuals with extremes of body size or muscle mass . . . the limitations in creatinine-based estimating equations are particularly relevant for populations with reduced muscle mass, including the frail and elderly."[6]

Fortunately, more objective data are becoming available that support eGFR-based equations. Examples include vancomycin and gentamicin. Some studies have shown that CKD-EPI equations incorporating both creatinine and cystatin C (e.g., the CKD-EPI cr-cys C equation) are better predictors of drug clearance than other estimates.[27,31,32] As additional evidence to support eGFR equation results for drug dosing becomes available and manufacturers incorporate eGFR into pharmacokinetic studies, practitioners may feel more comfortable with eGFR over eCrCL for assessing drug dosing. Until then, clinical judgment is important, considering the implications of overdosing or underdosing the specific drug in question. For example, if a drug eliminated by the kidney with a narrow therapeutic index or potential for serious toxicity (e.g., enoxaparin) is prescribed to an elderly individual, a measured CrCL or GFR may be warranted if therapeutic drug monitoring with plasma levels is not available. The method used when dosing recommendations were developed should also be considered. The package labeling for the recently approved direct oral anticoagulant (DOAC) betrixaban includes dosing adjustments for individuals with reduced kidney function, but specifically states that the method used to derive dosing recommendations was the CG equation with TBW. Since this drug was approved by the FDA in 2017, standardized creatinine was likely used to derive CG results. In this case, the CG equation with TBW should be used to estimate kidney function until newer evidence suggests otherwise. Clinical monitoring for desired effects and avoidance of adverse effects for any drug, particularly those with narrow therapeutic indices such as DOACs (e.g., apixaban, rivaroxaban), is essential to prevent medication-related problems in patients with CKD.

GENERAL PHARMACOKINETIC AND PHARMACODYNAMIC PRINCIPLES

Pharmacokinetics describes the disposition of a drug in the body and is affected by a drug's absorption, distribution, metabolism, and elimination (often referred to as *ADME*), whereas pharmacodynamics describes the physiological effect of a drug. The effect of a drug is typically related to its concentration at the site of action. Although ideally the concentration would be measured at the receptor site, this is not practical. Therefore, the blood or plasma concentration of a drug is used as a surrogate to predict activity at the site of action for drugs with good correlation between the pharmacological response and the plasma concentration. In clinical practice, plasma concentration is generally measured for drugs with a narrow therapeutic index, meaning there is a narrow margin between a therapeutic and a toxic concentration, and for drugs for which the desired effect cannot be measured by any other practical method (e.g., hemoglobin response with epoetin alfa). For example, the concentration of phenytoin at its site of action in the central nervous system cannot be measured to make clinical decisions. Instead, plasma concentrations are measured with the goal of sustaining a concentration within the therapeutic range that correlates with the desired tissue concentration (e.g., free [unbound] phenytoin concentration 1 to 2 mg/L). Achievement of these concentrations at steady state (when the rate of drug input equals the rate of drug metabolism and/or elimination) depends on the pharmacokinetic characteristics or the ADME. In individuals with kidney disease, pharmacokinetic parameters are most often altered, as opposed to the pharmacodynamic effects. These parameters and the potential changes with CKD are reviewed here.

Absorption

Absorption is a process of drug movement from its site of delivery into the bloodstream. The bioavailability of a drug is the fraction of an administered dose that reaches the systemic circulation. The bioavailability for a drug administered intravenously is 100%, but is often less with oral administration. This is because oral drug absorption is affected by gastrointestinal (GI) transit time, edema of the GI tract, gastric pH, GI metabolism, and liver metabolism as the drug makes its first pass through the liver from the GI tract to reach systemic circulation. Metabolism occurs due to the activity of the cytochrome P450 enzymes in the GI tract and liver, which may be altered in individuals with kidney disease. Reduced activity of these enzymes can result in greater bioavailability of the parent drug or active metabolites, which may be clinically significant for drugs with a narrow therapeutic index that are extensively metabolized by these enzymes (e.g., cyclosporine). The activity of uptake and efflux transporters present in the GI tract, including P-glycoprotein (Pgp) and organic anion transporters (OATs), also affects bioavailability. Pgp on intestinal epithelial cells is responsible for efflux of certain drugs (e.g., apixaban, digoxin) and limits cellular uptake and absorption into enterocytes. These transporters are not necessarily changed in patients with CKD, but the patients may be taking drugs or other substances that are inhibitors (e.g., amiodarone, omeprazole, grapefruit juice), resulting in increased bioavailability, or inducers (e.g., St. John's wort, phenytoin), resulting in decreased bioavailability. In addition, gastric pH may be altered by other drugs (e.g., proton pump inhibitors, H2-receptor antagonists) and high salivary urea concentrations (urea is converted to ammonia). Delayed gastric emptying due to gastroparesis in patients with diabetes and CKD may also delay the time to reach a maximum plasma concentration after orally ingesting a drug.

Distribution

The extent to which a drug distributes to body fluids and tissue is indicated by the volume of distribution (Vd), often expressed in L or L/kg. This is a theoretical volume necessary to account for the total amount of drug if it were present throughout the body at the same concentration as in the plasma. The Vd depends on the drug characteristics, including plasma protein binding (only unbound drugs may distribute extravascularly), total body water, and tissue binding. The plasma compartment is the smallest volume in which a drug may distribute, and drugs with a very small Vd (e.g., <10 L; warfarin) are mainly confined to this intravascular space. Drugs with low lipid solubility may distribute throughout total body water in the extracellular compartment and have a relatively small Vd (12 to 20 L; gentamicin), whereas more lipophilic drugs can distribute into other body fluids and tissue and have a large Vd (>50 L; duloxetine). In individuals with kidney disease, protein-binding changes may occur, specifically with acidic drugs that bind to albumin. Decreases in serum albumin concentrations (due to malnutrition or nephrotic syndrome) and changes in plasma protein binding due to conformational changes or displacement of acidic drugs from protein binding sites with the accumulation of acidic "uremic toxins" lead to an increase in unbound drug.[33,34] Phenytoin is an example of a drug with altered protein binding in advanced kidney disease.[35] Unbound free fraction ratio (unbound concentration/total concentration) increases from approximately 10% to 20%[35]; however, unbound (active) phenytoin plasma concentrations remain similar to concentrations in patients with normal kidney function and normal albumin levels, as unbound phenytoin clearance by the liver increases and unbound phenytoin distributes outside the vascular system. Total phenytoin concentrations are often decreased, but this does not warrant an increased phenytoin dose because the unbound concentration that determines drug exposure and response does not appreciably change. Dosing changes should be based on unbound phenytoin concentrations (unbound or free phenytoin therapeutic range, 1.0 to 2.0 mg/L) and clinical response. Available estimating equations based on total phenytoin concentration (e.g., Winter–Tozer equation) that attempt to account for decreased serum albumin level and presence of uremia have not been shown to accurately predict free phenytoin concentrations in patient settings such as critical care, inpatient medicine or neurology services, or hemodialysis.[36,37] Thus, estimating equations based on total phenytoin concentration should not be used if unbound phenytoin assays are available. The acidic protein that binds basic drugs, α1-acid glycoprotein, may be increased in patients with advanced CKD, resulting in increased binding of basic drugs and a decrease in the unbound fraction. Examples of alkaline drugs that may be affected include clonidine and propranolol.[34]

Metabolism

Nonrenal drug metabolism occurs primarily in the liver but also in the intestine and lungs. Phase I drug metabolism involves oxidation, reduction, and hydrolysis to convert drugs to metabolites that are eliminated by the kidney or excreted by the biliary system. Phase II metabolism involves conjugation reactions of the parent drug or phase I metabolite (e.g., by glucuronidation or *N*-acetylation). The cytochrome P450 isoenzymes (e.g., CYPs 1A2, 2C9, 2C19, 2D6, 3A4), conjugative enzymes (e.g., uridine diphosphate-glucuronosyltrans-ferase [UGT] and *N*-acetyltrans-ferase [NAT]), and intestinal and hepatic transporters are responsible for the metabolic biotransformations that occur. Influx and efflux transporters, including Pgp, OATs, and multidrug resistance–associated proteins also play a key role.

Decreased clearance of CYP3A substrates observed in CKD animal models may not be due to reduced CYP3A4 activity, but to changes in transporter activity, as demonstrated in clinical studies including patients with end-stage renal disease (ESRD).[38] Reduced non-renal clearance and/or increased oral bioavailability of over 70 drugs has been reported in patients with CKD (Table 17.3).[39] Whether the changes in metabolism or transporter activity are specifically due to CKD or to other factors has not been determined in many cases; Fig. 17.1 summarizes what is currently known about the effects of uremia on drug metabolism and transport. The potential for accumulation of active or toxic metabolites cleared by the kidney is important to consider in patients with advanced kidney disease. Examples of drugs metabolized to active and/or toxic metabolites by the liver that accumulate in patients with kidney disease include allopurinol (to oxypurinol), meperidine (to normeperidine), and morphine (to morphine-6-glucuronide and morphine-3-glucuronide).

TABLE 17.3 Currently Used Drugs Reported to Exhibit Reduced Non-Renal Clearance and/or Increased Oral Bioavailability in Chronic Kidney Disease Patients[a]

Acyclovir	Dihydrocodeine[b,c]	Nortriptyline
Aliskiren	Desmethyldiazepam	Oxprenolol[b,c]
Alfuzosin	Duloxetine	Procainamide[d]
Aprepitant	Encainide	Propoxyphene[b]
Aztreonam	Eprosartan	Propranolol[b]
Bupropion	Erythromycin[b]	Quinapril
Captopril	Felbamate	Raloxifene
Caspofungin	5-Fluorouracil	Ranolazine
Carvedilol	Guanadrel	Reboxetine
Cefepime	Imipenem	Repaglinide
Cefmenoxime	Isoniazid[d]	Rosuvastatin
Cefmetazole	Ketoprofen	Roxithromycin
Cefonicid	Ketorolac	Simvastatin
Cefotaxime	Lanthanum	Solifenacin
Ceftibuten	Lidocaine	Sparfloxacin
Ceftizoxime	Lomefloxacin	Tacrolimus
Cefsulodin	Losartan	Tadalafil
Ceftriaxone	Lovastatin	Telithromycin
Cibenzolin	Metoclopramide	Valsartan
Cilastatin	Minoxidil	Vancomycin
Cimetidine	Morphine[c]	Vardenafil
Ciprofloxacin	Moxalactam	Verapamil[b]
Cyclophosphamide	Nefopam	Warfarin
Darifenacin	Nicardipine[b]	Zidovudine[c]
Diacerein[c]	Nimodipine	
Didanosine	Nitrendipine	

[a]Except where noted, nearly all the listed drugs undergo oxidative metabolism mediated by CYPs.
[b]Drugs known to exhibit an increase in oral bioavailability as well as reduced nonrenal clearance.
[c]Drugs that mainly undergo *O*-glucuronidation.
[d]Drugs that mainly undergo *N*-acetylation.
(Printed with permission from Yeung CK, Shen DD, Thummel KE, et al.: *Kidney Int* 2014;85(3): 522–528.)

Elimination

Overall clearance or elimination of a drug is the sum of kidney and non-renal (e.g., hepatic) clearance. Kidney clearance is the net result of glomerular filtration plus active tubular secretion minus reabsorption. Insulin is a drug that undergoes metabolism in the kidney. Determinants of kidney clearance include GFR and the contribution of tubular transporters: organic cationic transporters, OATs, and Pgp. Drug transporters are significant contributors, and the FDA has proposed that important drug transporters be identified in vitro for new drugs that undergo substantial elimination by the kidney.[40] Drugs not bound to protein may be freely filtered at the glomerulus unless restricted by molecular weight. Secretion is the primary elimination process for high-molecular-weight drugs or those that are highly protein bound. The relative contribution of filtration, secretion, and reabsorption may be estimated by calculating the Eratio for a drug [Eratio = Renal clearance/(unbound fraction × 125 mL/min)]. An Eratio <1 indicates the drug is filtered and undergoes net reabsorption; >1 indicates the drug is filtered and undergoes net secretion; 1 indicates the drug is filtered and reabsorption is equal to secretion or the drug is exclusively filtered. These primary processes may be altered in individuals with kidney disease; the alterations are more important for drugs that depend primarily on kidney versus non-renal clearance. The relative contribution of kidney clearance to overall clearance is important in determining whether dosing adjustments are warranted.

Pharmacokinetic parameters that characterize drug disposition and are helpful for drug regimen design in patients with kidney dysfunction include the half-life, or the time required for the drug's plasma concentration to decrease by one-half, and the fraction of the drug that is eliminated by the kidney, or fe. Gabapentin is an example of a drug that is exclusively dependent on kidney function for elimination (fe = 1). If prescribing gabapentin to a patient with advanced CKD, a prolonged half-life is predictable; therefore a dose reduction or extended dosing interval would be warranted to prevent drug accumulation and adverse drug effects (e.g., dizziness, ataxia).

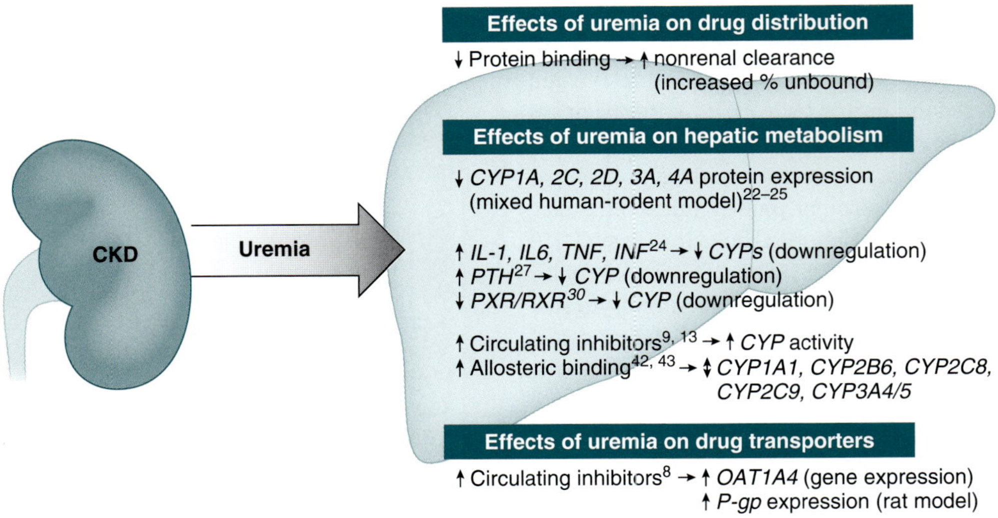

FIG. 17.1 Summary of the recognized effects of uremia on drug metabolism and transport. (Reprinted with permission from Yeung CK, Shen DD, Thummel KE, et al.: *Kidney Int.* 2014;85(3):13.)

GENERAL APPROACH FOR DRUG REGIMEN DESIGN IN CHRONIC KIDNEY DISEASE

Some general steps may help guide clinicians in determining a dosing regimen for patients with CKD. Once a drug is selected based on the indication, available resources should be used to determine if dose adjustments are warranted. This question may be answered by evaluating the drug's pharmacokinetic parameters. This information may be included in the approved package labeling and/or in other drug references such as Lexicomp[41] or Micromedex. Parameters of interest include the fe, half-life, and Vd. An fe >30% generally indicates that a dosing adjustment is likely warranted for a patient with advanced kidney disease, depending on the drug. More caution is warranted if the drug has a narrow therapeutic index (e.g., enoxaparin) rather than a wider index (e.g., cephalosporins). The patient's kidney function should be assessed using available estimating equations and considering the caveats for special populations (e.g., elderly, obese). Based on the assessment of kidney function, the dose for reduced kidney function provided by the manufacturer or other available resources may be used as a reasonable starting dose. Unfortunately, dosage adjustment recommendations from various resources often conflict, which is a source of frustration for clinicians. *Renal Pharmacotherapy* is a textbook[42] of compiled drug dosage adjustment information from multiple sources, including FDA-approved product labeling and alternative dosage adjustments from primary literature and compendia such as "Drug Prescribing in Renal Failure: Dosing Guidelines for Adults and Children."[43] Renal Pharmacotherapy provides comments when dosing information is contradictory or not supported by evidence. References are provided for the various recommendations. Micromedex and Lexicomp also provide references for many drug dosage recommendations.

For any agent prescribed, its adverse effects should also be considered. The effect of RRT (e.g., intermittent hemodialysis, peritoneal dialysis) on drug disposition must also be assessed (see the section Considerations for Drug Removal by Renal Replacement Therapies).

A dosing regimen typically includes a loading dose (LD) and a maintenance dose (MD) to "maintain" drug concentrations within a therapeutic range at steady state. An LD is administered when the goal is to achieve a target concentration sooner than four to five half-lives, which is the time required to reach steady-state conditions. This is an important consideration for patients with CKD, as the half-lives of many drugs (and thus time to steady-state) are prolonged. The LD can be calculated as LD = desired concentration (mg/L) × Vd (L/kg) × patient weight (kg) × bioavailability. The bioavailability may range from 0 to 1; it is 1 for drugs administered intravenously. Typically, the LD for a patient with kidney disease does not differ from that for a patient with normal kidney function (some exceptions are aminoglycosides, vancomycin, digoxin). The MD is the dose needed to maintain the concentration within the therapeutic window when the drug reaches steady-state conditions and is taken consistently at constant intervals. Options for dosage regimen changes for drugs eliminated by the kidney in patients with CKD include lowering the dose, prolonging the dosing interval, or both, depending on the drug. For example, for drugs dependent on concentration for therapeutic effect (e.g., aminoglycosides, quinolones), the better option is to use the same dose as for a patient with normal kidney function, but prolong the dosing interval. For drugs dependent on time above a certain concentration (e.g., cephalosporin antibiotics depend on time above the minimum inhibitory concentration for therapeutic efficacy), maintaining the same dosing frequency but lowering the dose is more appropriate.

For many drugs, information on drug disposition (the ADME) is limited for patients with advanced CKD (eGFR/CrCL <30 mL/min), and manufacturers often recommend to "avoid use" in such patients. Duloxetine is one example.

It is a serotonin/norepinephrine reuptake inhibitor used for depression, anxiety, and select chronic pain disorders, and is metabolized by the liver with <1% of unchanged drug found in the urine and most eliminated as metabolites. Although elimination by the kidney is not a clinically significant elimination pathway for the active drug, there was a twofold higher maximum concentration and area under the plasma concentration versus time curve (AUC) after oral administration of this drug to 12 individuals with ESRD.[44] This is an example of a drug predominantly cleared by non-renal mechanisms that exhibits reduced metabolism in CKD. This increase in overall drug exposure warrants cautious use in individuals with eGFR/CrCL <30 mL/min as described in the labeling. When deciding whether or how to use such agents in individuals with kidney disease, the approved prescribing information in the drug labeling must be evaluated, along with any subsequently published pharmacokinetic studies and reports regarding use and outcomes (desired and undesired). Clinical judgment should be employed when prescribing agents with limited information for patients with advanced kidney disease, particularly those who, based on assessment of kidney function, are on the borders of dosing thresholds (e.g., eGFR/CrCL 30 mL/min or 50 to 60 mL/min).

DOSING OF SELECT NEWER AGENTS IN CHRONIC KIDNEY DISEASE

Direct Oral Anticoagulants

DOACs make up a class of drugs that deserves special attention due to the risk/benefit profile in individuals with low kidney function. Drugs in this class include apixaban, betrixaban, dabigatran, edoxaban, and rivaroxaban. These agents inhibit factor Xa (apixaban, betrixaban, edoxaban, rivaroxaban) or thrombin (dabigatran) and are approved for prevention and treatment of venous thromboembolism (VTE) and atrial fibrillation (Table 17.4).[45] Betrixaban is the agent most recently approved for VTE prophylaxis.[45] Some data support the efficacy and safety of DOACs in CKD patients not treated by dialysis, although primarily from subanalysis of larger studies and metaanalyses.[46-50] With regard to safety, use of DOACs resulted in a 19% decrease in risk for major bleeding compared with warfarin in individuals with atrial fibrillation and non–dialysis-dependent CKD (eGFR/CrCL 25 to 80 mL/min) based on a metaanalysis of three randomized controlled studies.[47] This was supported by another metaanalysis of eight studies including over 10,000 individuals with CrCL 30 to 50 mL/min receiving a DOAC for atrial fibrillation or VTE compared with warfarin.[46] Similar efficacy outcomes (stroke, systemic thromboembolism, recurrent thromboembolism, thromboembolism-related death) and safety outcomes (major bleeding, clinically relevant nonmajor bleeding) were reported. Furthermore, significantly reduced stroke and systemic embolism and reduced major bleeding compared with warfarin were reported in a metaanalysis of 13,878 individuals with CKD (CrCL <50 mL/min, CG equation) and atrial fibrillation treated with a DOAC.[48] Although these studies are encouraging, data regarding efficacy, safety, and pharmacokinetics are lacking overall for individuals with stage 4 to 5 CKD or ESRD. Patients with CrCL <30 mL/min were excluded from clinical trials for dabigatran, rivaroxaban, and edoxaban, and those with <5 mL/min for betrixaban. Apixaban studies excluded individuals with CrCL <25 mL/min or serum creatinine above 2.5 mg/dL.

Pharmacokinetics and Pharmacodynamics in Chronic Kidney Disease

The fe for approved DOACs ranges from ≈6% for betrixaban to 80% for dabigatran (see Table 17.4); therefore there is concern for accumulation in patients with advanced CKD or ESRD, most notably with dabigatran.[51] Dosing recommendations depend on the drug, indication, kidney function, and use of concomitant Pgp inhibitors (due to the potential for drug interactions). Dosing criteria for all DOACS are based on eCrCL, a possible cause for concern if eGFR is used for dosing in individuals with kidney disease.[52] Apixaban, betrixaban, edoxaban, and rivaroxaban specifically state that the CG equation was used to calculate CrCL; clinical trials with betrixaban and rivaroxaban used actual body weight in the equation. These agents are not recommended below some eGFR thresholds due to a paucity of evidence (see Table 17.4). The exception is apixaban, which is approved at a dose of 5 mg twice daily (the dose for an individual with normal kidney function) across the eGFR spectrum unless weight is ≤60 kg or age is ≥80 years.[45] But this dosing recommendation is based on a single-dose pharmacokinetic and pharmacodynamic study of eight patients with ESRD on hemodialysis.[53] In this study, a 36% increase in the AUC occurred for hemodialysis patients compared with individuals with normal kidney function. Due to concern about accumulation, a subsequent study evaluated the pharmacokinetics of apixaban at steady-state in patients with ESRD with a 2.5-mg, twice-daily dose followed by the 5-mg, twice-daily dose (each administered for 8 consecutive days) in seven and five patients, respectively.[54] The 5-mg, twice-daily dose resulted in an AUC above the 90th percentile for individuals without kidney dysfunction—which is concerning, given that this dose is recommended in the drug labeling. However, the AUC for the 2.5-mg dose was similar to the AUC for non-ESRD patients in the initial apixaban studies requiring reduced dose based on weight and/or age. Canadian labeling does not recommend use in dialysis patients. The pharmacokinetics of rivaroxaban have also been studied in patients with ESRD.[55] A 15-mg dose administered 3 hours postdialysis resulted in a 56% increase in AUC, and decrease in drug clearance was estimated at 35% compared with individuals with normal kidney function. The authors concluded that these changes are consistent with those observed in individuals with moderate to severe kidney dysfunction and recommended a 15-mg dose for ESRD patients. The FDA label for rivaroxaban does not recommend a specific dose adjustment, but does reference this pharmacokinetic study. Unfortunately, there are no safety or efficacy data in a large ESRD population to support any specific dose in ESRD patients.

The overall lack of evidence with DOACS in patients with CKD stage 4 to 5 or ESRD warrants caution when considering their use. The risk versus benefit compared with warfarin must be considered. These agents should be discontinued and other anticoagulants used (e.g., heparin) in patients who develop acute kidney injury (AKI). Except for dabigatran, DOACs are not removed by hemodialysis and thus are not a viable reversal method for patients with bleeding complications associated with DOACS other than dabigatran. Dabigatran has a reversal agent, idarucizumab, a monoclonal antibody fragment that binds to dabigatran and its metabolites to neutralize the anticoagulant effect; however, a reversal agent's availability does not warrant dabigatran use in patients with a CrCL <15 mL/min (for nonvalvular atrial fibrillation) or <30 mL/min (for VTE) (see Table 17.4).[45] Dabigatran is contraindicated for any use in individuals with CrCL <30 mL/min based on Canadian labeling. Antidotes for DOACs other than dabigatran are currently being developed.

TABLE 17.4 FDA-Approved Dosing of Direct Oral Anticoagulants (DOACS) for Nonvalvular Atrial Fibrillation and Venous Thromboembolism Treatment

Drug	fe	Indication	CrCL (mL/min) or sCr (mg/dL)	Dose
Apixaban[a] (reduce dose by 50% if patient receiving dual strong CYP 3A4 and Pgp inhibitors and apixaban dose is ≥2.5 mg twice daily)	0.27	Nonvalvular AF	sCr <1.5	5 mg twice daily
			(if weight ≤60 kg AND age ≥80 y)	(2.5 mg twice daily)
			sCr ≥1.5 and either weight ≤60 kg or age ≥80 y	2.5 mg twice daily
			Hemodialysis[b]	5 mg twice daily
			(if weight ≤60 kg OR age ≥80 y)	(2.5 mg twice daily)
		VTE treatment	All patients	10 mg twice daily × 7 d, then 5 mg twice daily
		VTE prevention	All patients	2.5 mg twice daily after 6 mo of treatment
Betrixaban	0.05–0.07	VTE prevention	>30	160 mg followed by 80 mg once daily for 35–42 d
			≥15–≤30	80 mg followed by 40 mg once daily for 35–42 d
Dabigatran	0.80	Nonvalvular AF	>30[c]	150 mg twice daily
			15–30[d]	75 mg twice daily
			<15	No recommendations provided
		VTE treatment and prevention	>30[e]	150 mg twice daily after 5–10 d of parenteral anticoagulation
			≤30 or on dialysis	No recommendations provided
Edoxaban[a]	0.50	Nonvalvular AF	>95	Not recommended
			>50–95	60 mg daily
			15–50	30 mg daily
			<15	Not recommended
		VTE treatment	>50	60 mg daily after 5–10 d of parenteral anticoagulation
			(if weight ≤60 kg or on concomitant Pgp inhibitors)	(30 mg once daily)
			15–50	30 mg daily
			<15	Not recommended
Rivaroxaban	0.36	Nonvalvular AF	>50	20 mg once daily
			15–50	15 mg once daily
			<15	No recommendations provided
		VTE treatment	≥30	15 mg twice daily × 21 d, then 20 mg once daily
			<30	Avoid use

[a]Patients with a CrCL <25 mL/min (for apixaban) and <30 mL/min (for edoxaban) were excluded from clinical trials.
[b]Based on single-dose pharmacokinetic and pharmacodynamic study performed in eight patients with end-stage renal disease.[53]
[c]Reduce dose by 50% if CrCL 30 to 50 mL/min and patient is on concomitant Pgp inhibitors.
[d]Do not give if CrCL less than 30 mL/min and patient is on concomitant Pgp inhibitors.
[e]Do not give if CrCL less than 50 mL/min and patient is on concomitant Pgp inhibitors.
Postoperative VTE prophylaxis dosing not included in table.
AF, Atrial fibrillation; *CrCL,* creatinine clearance; *DOAC,* direct oral anticoagulant; *ESRD,* end-stage renal disease; *Pgp,* P-glycoprotein; *sCr,* serum creatinine; *VTE,* venous thromboembolism.

Agents for Type 2 Diabetes Mellitus—Sodium–Glucose Cotransporter 2 Inhibitors

Sodium–glucose cotransporter 2 (SGLT-2) inhibitors block the SGLT-2 protein involved in 90% of glucose reabsorption in the proximal renal tubule, resulting in increased renal glucose excretion and lower blood glucose levels; they also likely increase insulin sensitivity, decrease gluconeogenesis, and improve insulin release from pancreatic beta cells.[56] By reducing glucose and sodium reabsorption in the proximal tubule, these agents decrease glomerular hyperfiltration and reduce glomerular hypertension by reducing tubuloglomerular feedback.[57] They also lead to modest decreases in blood pressure and weight gain through these natriuretic effects and have a negligible risk for hypoglycemia when used as a monotherapy.

Pharmacokinetics and Pharmacodynamics in Chronic Kidney Disease

As a class, SGLT-2 inhibitors share similar pharmacokinetic characteristics with excellent oral bioavailability, long elimination half-life allowing once-daily administration, metabolism mainly via glucuronidation to inactive metabolites, and low renal elimination of the parent drug.[58] Plasma AUC for the active parent drug has been shown to increase at lower levels of kidney function (Table 17.5). In vitro studies with dapagliflozin have demonstrated that the kidney, in addition to the liver, is involved in the glucuronidation to inactive metabolites.[59] The increased AUC with empagliflozin is attributed to decreased clearance by the kidney.[60] Although increases in plasma exposure less than twofold are commonly used criteria, suggesting that no dose adjustment is required in

TABLE 17.5 Pharmacokinetics of Newer Diabetes Medications

Drug	Bioavailability (%)	Volume of Distribution (L)	*Plasma Protein Binding (%)	Metabolism	Renal Excretion	Comments
SGLT-2 Inhibitors						
Canagliflozin	65	84	99	Hepatic and renal: extensive via O-glucuronidation to two inactive metabolites	33% (<1% as parent drug)	Single dose canagliflozin 200 mg increased parent drug AUC 15% (eGFR 60–<90); 29% (eGFR 30–<60); 53% (eGFR 15–<30) but no AUC increase in HD vs. normal kidney function.
Dapagliflozin	78	118	91	Hepatic and renal: extensive via O-glucuronidation to 1 inactive metabolite. In vitro data show that dapagliflozin 3-O-glucuronide is formed in both the kidney and liver.	75% (<2% as parent drug)	Dapagliflozin 20 mg for 7 d increased parent drug AUC 32% (CrCl 51–80); 60% (CrCl 30–50); 87% (CrCl <30) vs. normal kidney function.[59] Not studied in dialysis.
Empagliflozin	78	74	85% normal kidney function, 81% CKD	Limited via hepatic glucuronidation to three minor metabolites with unknown activity (<10% each metabolite); 41% eliminated as parent drug in feces	54% (11%–19% as parent drug[58]	Single dose empagliflozin 50 mg increased parent drug AUC 18% (eGFR 60–<90), 20% (eGFR 30–<60), 66% (eGFR <30), 48% (dialysis).[60]
DPP-4 Inhibitors						
Alogliptin	≈100	417	20	Hepatic: limited metabolism, via CYP2D6 and CYP3A4 to active metabolite (<1%)	76%, (60%–71% parent drug)	

Continued

TABLE 17.5 **Pharmacokinetics of Newer Diabetes Medications—cont'd**

Drug	Bioavailability (%)	Volume of Distribution (L)	*Plasma Protein Binding (%)	Metabolism	Renal Excretion	Comments
Linagliptin	30	1110	70–99	Hepatobiliary: limited to an inactive metabolite	<7% parent drug	Linagliptin is the only DPP-4 inhibitor not primarily excreted by the kidneys but via hepatobiliary excretion. A PK study of linagliptin and post hoc analyses of trough plasma levels with linagliptin 5 mg daily for 24–52 wk showed that decreased GFR has negligible effects on total drug exposure.[148,149]
Saxagliptin	75	198	Negligible	Hepatic: primarily via CYP450 3A4/5 enzyme subsystems to an active metabolite.	60%, 24% parent drug; 36% as active metabolite	Saxagliptin is also metabolized to an active metabolite, 5-hydroxy-saxagliptin, which exerts significant DPP-4 inhibition (half as potent as the parent compound), and both are excreted primarily by the kidneys.[74]
Sitagliptin	87	198	38	Hepatic: minimal, primarily CYP3A4 with contribution from CYP2C8.	87%, 79% parent drug	
GLP-1 Receptor Agonists						
Albiglutide	ND	11	ND	Protein catabolism degradation to amino acids.	ND	Once-weekly albiglutide assessed in a pooled analysis of four phase III, randomized, active, or placebo-controlled, multiple-dose studies of patients with CKD[150] (eGFR ≥15–<90) showed modest increases in albiglutide plasma concentrations and a trend for a more potent glucose-lowering effect as eGFR decreased.
Dulaglutide	47 (1.5-mg dose)–65 (0.75-mg dose)	17.4–19.2	ND	Protein catabolism degradation to amino acids.	ND	

TABLE 17.5 Pharmacokinetics of Newer Diabetes Medications—cont'd

Drug	Bioavailability (%)	Volume of Distribution (L)	*Plasma Protein Binding (%)	Metabolism	Renal Excretion	Comments
Exenatide	ND in humans 65–76 (animal data)	28.3	ND	Protein catabolism degradation to amino acids.	Predominantly renal: glomerular filtration with subsequent proteolytic degradation	Baseline CrCL was determined to be the most significant predictor of steady-state concentration of exenatide once-weekly formulation.[74]
Liraglutide	55	13	>98	Protein catabolism degradation to amino acids.	6%, 0% parent, 6% degraded	Liraglutide half-life was not increased and clearance was not decreased in 30 subjects with varying stages of CKD administered a single dose of 0.75 mcg SQ supporting observation that the kidneys are not a major site for elimination or degradation.[151]
Lixisenatide	ND in humans	100		Protein catabolism degradation to amino acids.	Predominantly renal: glomerular filtration with subsequent proteolytic degradation	Limited PK data in patients with CKD are available.

AUC, Area under the curve; *CKD,* chronic kidney disease; *CrCL,* creatinine clearance; *DPP-4,* dipeptidyl peptidase 4; *eGFR,* estimated glomerular filtration rate; *GFR,* glomerular filtration rate; *ND,* no data; *PK,* pharmacokinetic; *SQ,* subcutaneously.

patients with kidney disease,[61] the higher AUC might explain the increase in adverse effects when these drugs are given to patients with eGFRs 30 to 60 mL/min/1.73 m^2 (Table 17.6). Also of note, patients receiving dialysis either do not have an increase in plasma AUC versus individuals with normal kidney function (canagliflozin), or the increase is less than for those with very low eGFRs (empagliflozin) (see Table 17.5). Dialysis may remove uremic substances that inhibit metabolic enzymes and transporters.[62,63] Despite the increase in parent drug AUC, the pharmacodynamic response to SGLT-2 inhibitors as assessed by urinary glucose excretion declines with increasing severity of kidney impairment, as the kidneys can no longer promote glucose excretion into the urine.[58] After 7 days of treatment with 20 mg dapagliflozin, steady-state renal glucose clearance was reduced by 42%, 83%, and 84% in type 2 diabetes (T2DM) patients with CG eCrCl 51 to 80 mL/min, 30 to 50 mL/min, and <30 mL/min not receiving dialysis, respectively, leading to progressive attenuation of the glucose-lowering effect.[64] In Japanese patients with T2DM, 24-hour urine glucose excretion increased after administration of 100-mg and 200-mg canagliflozin doses, but in patients with eGFR 31 to 49 mL/min/1.73 m^2, the increase was only about 70% of that in patients with normal kidney function or with mildly decreased eGFR (≥ 80 mL/min/1.73m^2).[65]

The expected HbA1C decrease with these agents in patients without CKD is 0.5% to 0.7%, but effects were attenuated to about 0.4% with canagliflozin and empagliflozin in stage 3 CKD.[57] Canagliflozin also lowered body weight and blood pressure versus placebo in stage 3 CKD over 52 weeks in a phase III trial.[66]

In 252 T2DM patients with stage 3 CKD, dapagliflozin did not improve glycemic control but reduced body weight and blood pressure compared with placebo when used as add-on therapy.[67] Dapagliflozin is not recommended for patients with eGFR <60 mL/min/1.73 m^2 (see Table 17.6). Empagliflozin efficacy has been evaluated in stage 2 to 4 CKD

TABLE 17.6 **Recommended Dosing of Diabetes Medications in Chronic Kidney Disease**[57]

Drug	Usual Dose	Renal Dose	Dialysis Dose	Removal by Dialysis	Comments
SGLT-2 Inhibitors					
Canagliflozin (Invokana) 100, 300 mg tabs	• 100 mg once daily before first meal • May ↑ to max dose of 300 mg once daily	• eGFR ≥60: no dose adjustment • eGFR <60: *do not initiate* therapy • if eGFR persistently falls to 45–59 during therapy, do not exceed 100 mg once daily • eGFR <45: *use contraindicated but CANVAS trial allowed participants with eGFR >30*	Contraindicated	Negligible (hemodialysis)	Patients with eGFR 30–<50 had higher occurrence of kidney adverse events (↓eGFR, ↓ intravascular volume) and less glycemic efficacy. Not studied at eGFR <30 mL/min/1.73 m^2, including dialysis.
Dapagliflozin (Forxiga) 5, 10 mg tabs	• 5 mg once daily may ↑ to max dose of 10 mg once daily	• eGFR ≥60: no dose adjustment • eGFR 30–59: not recommended for initiation or ongoing use when eGFR is persistently between 30 and <60 • eGFR <30: contraindicated	Contraindicated	ND	Patients with eGFR 30–<60 had more renal adverse events, more bone fractures, and no improvement in glycemic control.
Empagliflozin (Jardiance) 10, 25 mg tabs	• 10 mg once daily may ↑ to max dose of 25 mg once daily	• eGFR ≥45: no dosage adjustment • eGFR <45: not recommended but EMPA-REG; allowed participants with eGFR ≥30.[71] • eGFR<30: contraindicated	Contraindicated	ND	Patients with eGFR 30–60 had higher risk for kidney impairment, volume depletion, and urinary tract infection related adverse reactions and reduced glucose lowering.
DPP-4 Inhibitors					
Alogliptin (Nesina) 6.25, 12.5, 25 mg tabs	• 25 mg once daily • Max 25 mg once daily	• CrCl ≥30–<60: 12.5 mg once daily • CrCl <30: 6.25 mg once daily	-CrCl <15 or requiring HD: 6.25 mg once daily without regard to timing of HD - Drug not studied in PD	Negligible <7% removed over 3 h (HD)	In CKD caused by immunological conditions and treated with steroids, alogliptin improved steroid-induced hyperglycemia by decreasing glucagon levels via increasing plasma GLP-1 levels.[152]
Linagliptin (Tradjenta) 5 mg tab	• 5 mg once daily • Max 5 mg once daily	No dosage adjustment necessary	No dosage adjustment necessary	No (HD) No (PD)	MARLINA – T2D and RENALIS trials are assessing whether linagliptin attenuates progression of diabetic CKD.[86]
Saxagliptin (Onglyza) 2.5, 5 mg tabs	• 2.5–5 mg once daily • Max 5 mg once daily	• CrCl >50: no dosage adjustment • CrCl ≤50: 2.5 mg once daily	Suggested dose 2.5 mg once daily after dialysis (US prescribing information)	Yes (HD), 23% removed over 4 h	Saxagliptin 2.5 mg versus placebo in HD patients showed no significant reduction in HbA1C and is not recommended for use in HD population in some countries.[153]
Sitagliptin (Januvia) 25, 50, 100 mg tabs	• 100 mg once daily • Max 100 mg once daily	• CrCl ≥50: no dosage adjustment • CrCl ≥30–<50: 50 mg once daily • CrCl <30: 25 mg once daily	Recommended dose in HD or PD patients is 25 mg once daily without regard to timing of dialysis	Yes (HD), 13.5% removed over 3–4 h	Studies of sitagliptin have shown that it is frequently administered at inappropriate doses in patients with CKD.[154,155]

GLP-1 Agonists					
Albiglutide (Tanzeum) 30 mg and 50 mg prefilled pens	• 30 mg SQ once weekly; may ↑ to 50 mg once weekly	No dosage adjustment necessary; use caution when initiating/escalating	No recommendations	ND	Patients with eGFR ≥15–<30 had higher frequency of gastrointestinal events (e.g., diarrhea, constipation, nausea and vomiting) and hypoglycemic events compared with patients with eGFR ≥30–<90.[150]
Dulaglutide (Trulicity) 0.75 mg/0.5 mL and 1.5 mg/0.5 mL prefilled pens	• 0.75 mg SQ once weekly, may ↑ to max 1.5 mg SQ once weekly	No dosage adjustment necessary; use caution when initiating/escalating	No recommendations	Unlikely	AWARD-7 trial in Stage 3-4 CKD.[150a]
Exenatide (Byetta) 250 mcg/mL (1.2 and 2.4 mL prefilled pens) Exenatide extended-release dose form (2 mg/dose) (Bydureon)	• 5 mcg SQ bid within 60 min before meal; after 1 mo can ↑ to max 10 mcg bid • Extended-release 2 mg SQ once weekly	• CrCl ≥50: no dosage adjustment • CrCl 30–50: no adjustments provided but use with caution. Clinical experience with exenatide twice-daily formulation[156] or exenatide once-weekly formulation[157] in CKD is very limited. • *CrCl <30: use is not recommended*	Not recommended	ND	In ESRD, exenatide clearance was reduced by about 70% and a single 5-mcg dose of exenatide was not well tolerated.[158] Based on these PK studies, currently available exenatide dosages may not be suitable for use in patients with CrCl <30 mL/min or receiving dialysis.
Liraglutide (Victoza) 6 mg/mL (3 mL prefilled pens)	• 0.6 mg SQ once daily × 1 wk, then 1.2 mg SQ once daily (smaller initial dose intended to ↓GI symptoms, does not provide effective BG control) • Max 1.8 mg SQ once daily	• CrCl ≥30: no dosage adjustment • CrCl <30: *use is not recommended (limited experience, 115 subjects with eGFR <30 received liraglutide in the LEADER trial*[91]	Not recommended	No (HD)	A metaanalysis of six LEAD clinical trials showed a trend toward increased nausea in patients with CrCl <60 mL/min receiving liraglutide compared with other CrCl groups.[159]
Lixisenatide (Lyxumia) 50 or 100 mcg/mL (3 mL prefilled pen)	• 10 mcg once daily × 14 d then increase to 20 mcg once daily	No dose adjustment required for eGFR 60–89 No dose adjustment required for eGFR 30–59, but patients should be monitored for adverse effects and changes in kidney function. Lixisenatide may elicit a significant reversible decline in GFR.[160] Exposure is increased and clinical experience is limited with eGFR 15–29; patients should be monitored for adverse effects and changes in kidney function. Avoid if eGFR <15 (has not been studied).	Not recommended	ND	Incidence of gastrointestinal adverse events (diarrhea, nausea and vomiting) 14% higher in CKD (CrCl <30–89 mL/min) vs. normal kidney function group.[161] ELIXIRS trial for treatment of diabetic kidney disease in progress.[94]

AWARD-7, Study Comparing Dulaglutide With Insulin Glargine on Glycemic Control in Participants With Type 2 Diabetes and Moderate or Severe Chronic Kidney Disease trial; *BG,* blood glucose; *CANVAS,* Canagliflozin Cardiovascular Assessment Study; *CKD,* chronic kidney disease; *CrCl,* creatinine clearance; *eGFR,* estimated glomerular filtration rate; *ELIXIRS,* Effect of Lixisenatide on the Renal System trial; *EMPA-REG OUTCOME,* Empagliflozin, Cardiovascular Outcomes and Mortality in Type 2 Diabetes trial; *max,* maximum; *ND,* no data; *HD,* hemodialysis; *LEAD,* Liraglutide Effect and Action in Diabetes; *LEADER,* the Liraglutide Effect and Action in Diabetes: Evaluation of Cardiovascular Outcome Results; *MARLINA – T2D,* Evaluation of Linagliptin in Patients With Type 2 Diabetes and Albuminuria trial; *PD,* peritoneal dialysis; *RENALIS,* Renal Effects of Linagliptin in Type 2 Diabetes trial; *SQ,* subcutaneously.

patients. Mean placebo-subtracted change from baseline in HgbA1C at week 24 with 25 mg was −0.68%, −0.42%, and no significant reduction in stage 2, 3, and 4 CKD, respectively.[58]

Kidney-Related Outcomes and Drug Safety

In addition to a reduction in death and cardiovascular outcomes with empagliflozin[68] and cardiovascular outcomes with canagliflozin[69] (cardiovascular outcome data for dapagliflozin are pending[70]), clinical trial data are available for each currently available SGLT-2 inhibitor showing reduced albuminuria with treatment.[57] Post hoc analyses of the empagliflozin (EMPA-REG) trial showed beneficial kidney effects, including reduced albuminuria, slowed eGFR decline, and a 50% reduced risk for progressing to ESRD; benefits were consistent in patients with eGFR <60 and ≥60 mL/min/1.73 m^2.[71] The CREDENCE trial (NCT02065791) is assessing whether canagliflozin treatment reduces diabetic kidney disease progression, with expected completion in 2019.[72] The Dapa-CKD trial will assess the effects of dapagliflozin on renal outcomes and cardiovascular mortality in patients with eGFR ≥ 25 to ≤ 75 ml/min/1.73 m^2, with expected completion in 2020 (NCT03036150).

In subjects with T2DM and stage 3 CKD, slightly higher rates of urinary tract infections and AKI related to osmotic diuresis and reduced intravascular volume occurred with canagliflozin 300 mg compared with canagliflozin 100 mg and placebo.[73] Canagliflozin is associated with a dose-dependent increase in serum potassium that is more pronounced in patients with kidney impairment. In a pooled population of patients with eGFR 45 to <60 mL/min/1.73 m^2, increases in serum potassium to >5.4 mEq/L and 15% above baseline occurred in 5.3%, 5.0%, and 8.8% of patients treated with placebo, canagliflozin 100 mg, and canagliflozin 300 mg, respectively. Hyperkalemia ≥6.5 mEq/L occurred in 0.4% of patients treated with placebo, no patients treated with canagliflozin 100 mg, and 1.3% of patients treated with canagliflozin 300 mg. However, 84% of these patients were taking medications that interfere with potassium excretion, such as potassium-sparing diuretics, angiotensin-converting enzyme inhibitors and angiotensin receptor blockers.[45]

Agents for Type 2 Diabetes Mellitus—Dipeptidyl Peptidase-4 Inhibitors

Dipeptidyl peptidase-4 (DPP-4) inhibitors inhibit inactivation of both endogenous glucagon-like peptide-1 (GLP-1) and glucose-dependent insulinotropic polypeptide, resulting in higher GLP levels with stimulation of insulin secretion and reduction of glucagon secretion in a glucose-dependent manner. These drugs produce clinically relevant improvement in overall and postprandial glucose control without inducing hypoglycemia or weight gain.[74]

Pharmacokinetics and Pharmacodynamics in Chronic Kidney Disease

Pharmacokinetics of DPP-4 inhibitors are summarized in Table 17.5. All DPP-4 inhibitors, except linagliptin, undergo extensive metabolism by the kidney and require dose adjustments. Recommended dose adjustments based on GFR are in Table 17.6.

The DPP-4 inhibitors are expected to decrease HbA1C by about 0.7% in the general T2DM population; however, clinical efficacy is attenuated to about 0.6% in stage 3 to 5 non–dialysis-dependent CKD patients.[75] In patients with T2DM and eGFR ≥30 to 49 or <30 mL/min/1.73 m^2 CKD, sitagliptin and glipizide provided similar reductions in HbA1C. Sitagliptin was generally well tolerated, with a lower risk for hypoglycemia (6.2% vs. 17.0%) and weight loss (−0.6 kg) versus weight gain (+1.2 kg), relative to glipizide.[76] In patients with T2DM receiving hemodialysis or peritoneal dialysis, sitagliptin 25 mg daily was almost as effective in reducing HbA1C as glipizide, with lower incidence of symptomatic hypoglycemia (6.3% vs. 10.8%) and severe hypoglycemia (0% vs. 7.7%).[77] However, this study suffered from underenrollment, high drop out (40%), and significant differences in baseline characteristics between the sitagliptin and glipizide groups, calling into question comparative efficacy results.[78] Alogliptin 6.25 mg/day as monotherapy or in combination with other oral antidiabetic agents improved glycemic control and was generally well tolerated in hemodialysis patients over a 48-week period.[79] These results were confirmed in a longer 2-year study with alogliptin monotherapy, suggesting its efficacy as a new treatment strategy in diabetic patients with ESRD treated with hemodialysis.[80]

New-onset diabetes after kidney transplant is a serious complication. In these patients, sitagliptin increased insulin secretion and reduced fasting and postprandial plasma glucose and was well tolerated.[81,82]

Cardiovascular Outcomes

DPP-4 inhibitors have demonstrated neutral effects versus placebo in cardiovascular outcome trials conducted to date.[57] However, the SAVOR-TIMI 53 trial reported an increase in hospitalization for heart failure with saxagliptin compared with placebo,[83] which could be problematic in a CKD population. A metaanalysis of randomized clinical trials of DPP-4 inhibitors could not confirm whether this increased risk for hospitalization was a class effect or a specific effect of saxagliptin.[84] However, an observational study of congestive heart failure admissions from Canada, the United Kingdom, and the United States did not demonstrate increased hospitalizations with either DPP-4 inhibitors or GLP-1 receptor agonists.[85]

Kidney-Related Outcomes

All currently available DPP-4 inhibitors appear to reduce the onset of albuminuria. Whether this effect is independent of blood pressure or glycemic changes is unknown.[57] Two ongoing trials are investigating the kidney-protective effects of linagliptin.[86,87]

Agents for Type 2 Diabetes Mellitus—Glucagon-Like Peptide-1 Receptor Agonists

GLP-1 receptor agonists mimic the action of endogenous GLP-1 to enhance insulin secretion and inhibit glucagon secretion from pancreatic islet cells.[57] As a monotherapy, these agents reduce HbA1C by about 1.0% in individuals with normal kidney function, with negligible risk for hypoglycemia. They improve postprandial blood glucose control and are associated with significant weight loss resulting from increased satiety due to delayed gastric emptying and central anorectic activity by GLP-1.[74] The experience with GLP-1 agonists in patients with CKD is more limited than the experience with DPP-4 inhibitors. AWARD-7, a clinical trial comparing once-weekly dulaglutide to basal insulin glargine in study participants with CKD stages 3 to 4, found similar efficacy in terms of change in HbA1C over 52 weeks. However, dulaglutide treatment was associated with 50% lower rates of hypoglycemia and weight loss of 2-3 kg versus weight gain with insulin glargine.[95]

Pharmacokinetics and Pharmacodynamics in Chronic Kidney Disease

GLP-1 receptor agonists are catabolized to amino acids. Exenatide and lixisenatide (parent drugs) are primarily eliminated by the kidney, but only a minimal amount of liraglutide is eliminated through the kidney route. There are no renal elimination data for albiglutide or dulaglutide (see Table 17.5). The pharmacokinetics of GLP-1 receptor agonists are summarized in Table 17.5. Current dose recommendations based on kidney function for all currently marketed GLP-1 agonist are provided in Table 17.6.

Kidney-Related Outcomes and Safety

In a large retrospective observational study, changes in GFR or albuminuria at 1 year did not differ significantly in patients treated with exenatide twice daily or insulin glargine as administered in routine practice.[88] Studies of patients with diabetic kidney disease have shown that liraglutide reduces albuminuria, and improved glycemic control with liraglutide does not adversely affect eGFR in patients with stage 3 CKD.[89,90] Data from the liraglutide (LEADER) study and clinical trials of semaglutide and dulaglutide show reduced risk for macroalbuminuria onset and progression.[91-93] The mechanisms of action are believed to be multifactorial, including better glycemic control, reduced body weight, and/or direct kidney effects.[57] The dulaglutide (AWARD-7) trial noted a significantly smaller decline in eGFR versus insulin glargine over 52 weeks. This was most evident in patients with macroalbuminuria. Dulaglutide also led to a significantly greater decrease in the albumin to creatine ratio in participants with baseline macroalbuminuria. This effect was dose-related. These benefits were observed despite background treatment with angiotensin-converting enzyme inhibitors or angiotensis receptor blockers in >90% of participants.[95]

Postmarketing reports of AKI have been described with GLP-1 receptor agonists, likely triggered by dehydration due to GI adverse events. However, AKI has not been consistently observed in clinical or observational studies.[88,91,96,97] Most case reports of altered kidney function with exenatide have also reported at least one contributory factor, such as chronic heart failure, pancreatitis, infection, volume depletion, and/or use of concomitant medications, such as diuretics, renin-angiotensin-aldosterone system inhibitors, or nonsteroidal antiinflammatory drugs.[57]

Metformin

Metformin is one of the oldest and most frequently prescribed antidiabetic medications, and is the preferred pharmacological agent to treat T2DM.[98] Reevaluation of safety data has led to its more liberal use. Metformin is excreted unchanged in the urine (fe of 0.9 to 1), primarily by active tubular secretion by organic cationic transporters, with a half-life of approximately 5 to 6 hours.[45,99] Metformin-associated lactic acidosis, a rare yet potentially fatal adverse reaction, is more likely in individuals with reduced kidney function. A recent review by researchers conducting pharmacokinetic and safety studies of metformin at various CKD stages reported that metformin can cause lactic acidosis (alone or with other factors), but frequently it may not play a causal role.[100] These researchers suggest more specific terminology to categorize lactic acidosis accompanied by metformin therapy to improve diagnosis, prognosis, and quality of reporting. Until recently, package labeling for metformin suggested that it should be contraindicated based on serum creatinine cutoff levels: >1.5 mg/dL for men, >1.4 mg/dL for women. Thus, a likely beneficial drug was not given to many patients with T2DM. Based on a review of available safety information for metformin in patients with kidney impairment, the FDA recommended expanding its use.[101] For example, based on prior metformin dosing recommendations, it would not be prescribed for a 55-year-old black man with serum creatinine 1.6 mg/dL; height 5 feet, 10 inches; weight 90 kg; CKD-EPI eGFR 55 mL/min/1.73 m^2, and CKD-EPI BSA-adjusted eGFR 66 mL/min. With recent dosing recommendations using eGFR, not serum creatinine, to guide dosing, metformin would be indicated in this patient. In current FDA recommendations, the risk versus benefit of continuing metformin should be considered for patients whose eGFR falls below 45 mL/min/1.73 m^2. Initiation of metformin is not recommended for individuals with eGFR 30 to 45 mL/min/1.73 m^2, and is contraindicated for patients with eGFR <30 mL/min/1.73 m^2. These guidelines are consistent with KDIGO recommendations.[8] Of note, other countries, including Australia, Canada, and some in Europe, have also adopted more liberal use of metformin in individuals with reduced kidney function.

DRUG DOSING IN DIALYSIS PATIENTS

For the purpose of drug dosing, estimation of kidney function using available estimating equations is not necessary for individuals with ESRD on dialysis. Dialysis removes serum creatinine, and thus eGFR will overestimate residual native kidney function. These patients are assumed to have an eGFR/CrCL <15 mL/min and, in general, drug dosing recommendations for patients with this degree of kidney dysfunction may be followed. However, residual kidney function in hemodialysis patients has been shown to materially affect cefepime levels.[102] Researchers showed that a recommended dose of 1 or 1.5 g after high-flux dialysis before a 48- or 72-hour interval, respectively, maintained adequate levels in anuric hemodialysis patients, but not in those with significant residual kidney function. Thus they advised that 1.5 or 2.0 g be administered before the 48- or 72-hour interval, respectively, in hemodialysis patients with significant residual kidney function and less susceptible pathogens. Other cephalosporin or penicillin antibiotics typically dosed after each dialysis session should be similarly investigated.

The main factor to consider is the effect of dialysis on drug removal. Adjustments in the drug regimen should be made for drugs with characteristics conducive to transport across the dialyzer (for hemodialysis patients) or the peritoneal membrane (for peritoneal dialysis patients).

Most patients with ESRD who require hemodialysis receive conventional hemodialysis, usually administered 3 days per week for 3 to 5 hours. More frequent hemodialysis regimens of varying duration are also offered by many dialysis centers. Variations include short daily hemodialysis (less than 3 hours per session, six times per week), standard daily hemodialysis (3 to 5 hours per session, six times per week), and long daily hemodialysis (more than 5 hours per session, six times per week). Sessions may occur during the day or at night, in-center (i.e., in a dialysis facility) or at home. Other variations in frequency include every other day and four or five times per week. For drugs removed by hemodialysis, most dosing recommendations apply to thrice-weekly sessions; therefore a regimen that includes higher or more frequent doses (i.e., reduced intervals between doses) may be warranted. Importantly, dialysis dosing recommendations are not available for many drugs, and dosing regimens are often based on theoretical considerations if a drug has characteristics that make it likely to be removed. For drugs removed by hemodialysis (e.g., levetiracetam, metoprolol), a general recommendation is to administer the prescribed dose after the session. An alternative is to give a supplemental dose after the session, but this may present adherence challenges. Many antibiotics are removed by dialysis, and this should be considered when developing dosing regimens, particularly for dialysis facilities that administer antibiotics during the last 30 minutes to 1 hour of the session to avoid keeping patients at the facility solely for antibiotic administration.

Automated peritoneal dialysis (APD) is becoming more common and more widely used than continuous ambulatory peritoneal dialysis (CAPD). Continuous cycling peritoneal dialysis (CCPD) is the most common form of APD; it requires frequent exchanges of 1 to 3 liters of dialysate over an extended period (usually overnight). Most dosing recommendations for drugs removed by dialysis apply to CAPD. Dose regimen modifications are warranted to account for differences in the dialysis regimen. The most common agents requiring specific dosing considerations for peritoneal dialysis patients are antibiotics used to treat peritonitis. Antibiotics administered systemically reach the peritoneal cavity and may diffuse across the peritoneal membrane into the dialysate and be removed. Similarly, antibiotics administered interperitoneally (i.e., in the peritoneal dialysate fluid) may diffuse from the dialysate to blood during the dwell time, and blood concentrations of a given antibiotic increase over the dwell time and may be therapeutic for peritonitis over an extended period. Also, with peritonitis, solute transport may increase when the peritoneal cavity is inflamed. This is the reason vancomycin may be administered every 3 to 5 days through the intraperitoneal route to treat peritonitis.

CONSIDERATIONS FOR DRUG REMOVAL BY RENAL REPLACEMENT THERAPIES

Determining safe and effective drug dosage regimens in patients with CKD can be challenging. Add the effect on drug clearance of maintenance dialysis or continuous RRT (CRRT) in a patient with AKI, and the exercise can become very complex. Often, little information on drug dialyzability can be found. Relatively few drugs have undergone formal pharmacokinetic assessment in patients receiving various RRT modalities. One reliable information source on drug dialyzability is "Dialysis of Drugs."[103] This reference, updated annually, evaluates dialyzability of medications with hemodialysis using conventional or high-permeability membranes and peritoneal dialysis, and an app is available for iPhone and iPad. Its limitation is that it does not include information on the extent of removal with other dialysis modalities, so it is less useful for determining dose adjustments. When no clinical studies have assessed drug elimination during dialysis, the authors use drug characteristics to determine whether a drug is likely to be significantly dialyzable.

Clinicians can use the same strategy to determine the likelihood of significant dialysis clearance with drugs that have not had formal pharmacokinetic studies conducted during RRT by simply assessing key drug-related factors (Box 17.1) that affect dialyzability. Information on molecular weight, Vd, water or lipid solubility, and protein binding can be found in product information or in compendia such as Micromedex or Lexicomp. Drugs with molecular weights >20,000 daltons are unlikely to be significantly cleared by conventional or

BOX 17.1 Key Factors for Clinicians to Consider When Making Drug Dose Adjustment Decisions With Kidney Replacement Therapy

- Patient residual kidney function
- Drug-related factors
    - Molecular weight
    - Volume of distribution (in CKD, if known)
    - Water or lipid solubility
    - Plasma protein binding (in CKD, if known)
- Kidney replacement therapy factors
    - Modality
        - Hemodialysis (conventional intermittent in-center hemodialysis, short daily hemodialysis, standard daily hemodialysis, long daily hemodialysis)
        - Peritoneal dialysis (continuous ambulatory peritoneal dialysis, automated peritoneal dialysis, including continuous cycling peritoneal dialysis)
        - Continuous renal replacement therapy (CVVH, CVVHD, CVVHDF)
        - Other
    - Membrane (high permeability or high flux versus conventional or low flux), if applicable

CKD, Chronic kidney disease; *CVVH,* continuous venovenous hemofiltration; *CVVHD,* continuous venovenous hemodialysis; *CVVHDF,* continuous venovenous hemodiafiltration.

high-permeability dialysis membranes, but may be cleared by peritoneal dialysis. Drugs that are not soluble in water (are lipid-soluble) are less likely to be removed by diffusive clearance because they will not readily diffuse from plasma water into dialysate, which is mainly water. However, as noted later, some lipid-soluble drugs can be substantially removed over time with CRRT using high-flux filters and high-convective-clearance dialysis prescriptions.

As drugs must reside in plasma to be cleared by any form of dialysis, drugs with high Vd (>1 L/kg) are less likely to be significantly cleared by RRT[104]; however, the absolute amount removed may be greater with dialysis techniques involving longer sessions (e.g., nocturnal hemodialysis, CRRT, peritoneal dialysis), as drugs continuously redistribute from tissue sites into plasma. Albumin and other large plasma proteins are not removed by currently available RRT membranes. Highly plasma protein bound (PPB) drugs, >80%, are typically not significantly dialyzable by RRT membranes, as only free (unbound) drug can be removed.[104] However, in CKD, the bound fraction of acidic drugs decreases as albumin levels decline, and the affinity to albumin is reduced due to accumulating organic acids that may displace drugs from albumin binding sites or induce conformational changes in albumin that reduce the affinity of drug to albumin. Phenytoin is the classic example of a drug that is highly (90%) bound to albumin in patients with normal kidney function, but the percentage bound can be as low as 75% in CKD patients and even lower with concurrent use of displacer drugs such as valproic acid. In this case, more unbound (free) drug is presented to the dialyzer membrane, increasing the likelihood that a significant amount may be removed. Phenytoin is also highly lipid soluble, reducing its potential to be cleared by diffusion into water-based dialysate. However, in the right circumstances (decreased PPB in CKD, high-flux filter, and CRRT methodology using high-convective clearance), even a drug like phenytoin can be significantly cleared; two case reports demonstrate that up to 30% of a daily phenytoin dose can be removed each day with modern continuous venovenous hemofiltration.[105] Clinicians should closely monitor unbound phenytoin concentrations in patients receiving CRRT therapies with high convective clearance to ensure therapeutic levels. Highly PPB drugs, like phenytoin, may be cleared through peritoneal dialysis techniques, because albumin and other plasma proteins can pass through the peritoneal membrane into dialysate.[106]

These general rules can guide decisions about whether dosage regimen changes are needed with dialysis. However, knowing whether a drug is likely dialyzable is not sufficient to determine a reasonable dosage regimen around dialysis sessions. A helpful resource is the textbook *Renal Pharmacotherapy*,[42] which focuses on dosage adjustment of medications eliminated by the kidneys. When information is available, it includes dosing suggestions for hemodialysis, CAPD, and CRRT. The main strength of this reference is that it includes information from multiple sources, including FDA-approved product labeling–suggested dosage adjustments and alternative dosage adjustments from other sources, including primary literature and compendia such as "Drug Prescribing in Renal Failure: Dosing Guidelines for Adults and Children."[43] One limitation is that much of the pharmacokinetic information on removal during intermittent hemodialysis was gathered from studies conducted before high-permeability (high-flux) hemodialysis membranes were widely used. Because dose recommendations are not connected directly to a specific reference, it is not clear what hemodialysis conditions (membrane type, length of dialysis, blood flow rate, dialysate flow rate) were used to establish the dosing recommendations. Similar issues arise with CRRT recommendations from this source. CRRT studies have been performed in <20% of currently marketed drugs.[107] CRRT methodologies vary much more by clinical site than do intermittent hemodialysis methods, and most existing data on CRRT drug removal are from small, single-center, investigator-initiated studies that are inconsistently executed.[107] Effluent flow rate (QE) is the most important parameter in determining drug removal during CRRT. QE varies markedly by CRRT modality and by site, even with the same modality. Golightly's CRRT dosing recommendations do not include CRRT modality or information on CRRT prescription (QE, dialysate, blood flow rate).

Use of CRRT prescription with high convective clearance (effluent flow rate) increases the likelihood of inadequate dosing, and this undoubtedly contributes to sepsis/infection as the primary cause of death in AKI patients.[108] The Kidney Health Initiative recognized the problems with current CRRT dosing guidelines and assembled a working group of stakeholders, including the FDA, to review the evidence. They recommended a standardized assessment of pharmacokinetics of drugs in CRRT, which clinician-investigators and the pharmaceutical industry can use to study drug pharmacokinetics in patients with AKI receiving CRRT.[107]

Several groups have compiled dosing recommendations for antibiotics commonly used in AKI patients on CRRT.[108-110] Scoville and Mueller compared their dosing recommendations for five antibiotics to those of Heintz and Aronoff,[108] based on a standard effluent rate of 25 mL/kg/h, which is consistent with KDIGO clinical practice guidelines.[111] In general, Scoville and Mueller's dosing recommendations are higher than those of Aronoff and Heintz,[109,110] who compiled their data 8 to 10 years ago and certainly included studies using old CRRT methods (arteriovenous access and smaller, low-permeability hemodiafilters). Because CRRT prescriptions are highly variable, a one-size-fits-all approach to drug dosing is not useful. A case example of determining an initial starting dose of a new drug, brivaracetam, in hemodialysis or CRRT is given next.

Case Example: Dosing Brivaracetam in Hemodialysis and Continuous Kidney Replacement Therapy

A 40-year-old male black patient with a history of partial-onset seizures and ESRD receiving intermittent hemodialysis Monday, Wednesday, and Friday for 4 hours with a polysulfone high-flux dialyzer, BSA 2.0 m^2, blood flow rate 350 mL/min, dialysis flow rate 500 mL/min. His neurologist decides to add brivaracetam 50 mg twice daily to a phenytoin regimen of 200 mg phenytoin sodium (Dilantin) every 12 hours to better control partial-onset seizures. Patient is 5 feet 11 inches tall and weighs 80 kg. Steady-state trough phenytoin concentrations are free (unbound) 1.7 mg/L, total 7.5 mg/L. Serum albumin level is 3.5 g/dL. Brivaracetam was recently approved by the FDA for use as adjunct therapy to control partial-onset seizures

Q1: Should Brivaracetam Dosing be Altered in This End-Stage Kidney Disease Patient?

Package labeling information for FDA-approved medications are online at DailyMed.[45] The package labeling for brivaracetam (as for other drugs) includes a required section on pharmacokinetics. Brivaracetam is primarily metabolized to three inactive metabolites. Metabolism (hydroxylation) is primarily mediated by the CYP2C19 pathway. One study of individuals with CrCL <30 mL/min (not on dialysis) showed that the plasma AUC of the active drug (brivaracetam) was moderately increased (21%), whereas AUCs of the three inactive metabolites were increased 3-fold to 21-fold. Based on this information, the package labeling suggests no need for dose alterations in severe CKD. In this patient, the starting dose was 50 mg twice daily, the usual initial dose in patients with normal kidney function.

However, importantly, the information cited in the package label comes from a single pharmacokinetic study of 18 subjects: 9 healthy controls, 6 subjects with CrCL 15 to 29 mL/min, and 3 subjects with CrCL <15 mL/min.[112] There are two important considerations. First, this patient is receiving hemodialysis, so his CrCl/GFR is likely <15 mL/min. The single pharmacokinetic study in CKD patients (CrCl <30 mL/min, not on dialysis) showed that both non-renal and kidney clearance of brivaracetam were reduced; although the AUC of brivaracetam increased by only 21%, on average; importantly 6/9 participants with CKD had CrCL >15 mL/min. Average drug clearance would be expected to be reduced further in patients on dialysis. Second, the patient is also on phenytoin, which according to the package label, has an interaction with brivaracetam. Phenytoin decreases brivaracetam AUC by 21%, but concomitant brivarecetam can also increase phenytoin plasma concentrations up to 20%. Thus taking into consideration that reduced CrCL leads to increased brivaracetam AUC but concomitant phenytoin decreases brivaracetam AUC, starting this patient on the usual dose of 50 mg twice daily would be reasonable. Starting at a lower dose of 25 mg twice daily would also be reasonable. Brivaracetam has a relatively short half-life of about 8 hours, so steady-state levels will be achieved in about 2 days. At that point, the patient can be evaluated for efficacy and safety endpoints, and the dose can be titrated upward as needed to maximum dose. Phenytoin-free (unbound) concentrations should be monitored to assure levels stay within the free phenytoin therapeutic range of 1 to 2 mg/L, as phenytoin levels are likely to increase with concomitant brivaracetam.

Q2: Is Brivaracetam Dialyzable?

There is no information on pharmacokinetics of brivaracetam in patients receiving dialysis or in patients with AKI on CRRT. Thus clinicians can evaluate the physical and relevant pharmacokinetic characteristics of brivaracetam (see Box 17.1) to determine if it is likely to be dialyzable. The package labeling gives the following information:

- Molecular weight is 212.29 daltons
- Vd is 0.5 L/kg (close to total body water)
- Rapidly and evenly distributed in most tissues
- Weakly bound to plasma proteins (≤20%)
- Very soluble in water

As the molecular weight of brivaracetam is small (<500 daltons), it is potentially dialyzable by conventional (low-flux) or high-permeability (high-flux) membranes. The Vd is <1 L/kg (relatively small), and the drug rapidly distributes in tissues, which means that it will be present in plasma, available to be cleared by any dialysis or CRRT modality, and will redistribute back to plasma as it is cleared by dialysis. In addition, brivaracetam is not highly PPB, so the free drug is available to be cleared. It is very soluble in water, so it would be expected to be removed by either diffusion or convective clearance. Based on its physical characteristics, brivaracetam is likely to be highly dialyzable by dialysis or CRRT modalities.

Q3: How Should Brivaracetam Dose be Altered in This Patient With Intermittent Hemodialysis?

Although we predict that brivaracetam would be significantly dialyzable by any dialysis or CRRT modality based on physical and pharmacokinetic characteristics, the extent of removal should be evaluated by well-designed pharmacokinetic studies using current high-permeability membranes and standard prescriptions for intermittent hemodialysis. Given our prediction of significant dialyzability, it would be prudent to administer the first dose (or second, depending on the time of day of the hemodialysis session) after dialysis on Monday, Wednesday, and Friday. Drug doses can be titrated up or down based on efficacy endpoints (reduction in partial-onset seizures) and safety endpoints (somnolence, sedation, dizziness, fatigue).

Q4: What If This Patient had Acute Kidney Injury and was Receiving Continuous Venovenous Hemofiltration With the Following Continuous Kidney Replacement Therapy Prescription: Postfilter Replacement Fluid, 1500 mL/h; Ultrafiltrate, 250 mL/h; Blood Flow Rate, 180 mL/min.

This CRRT prescription would result in a QE of 1750 mL/h (or approximately 29 mL/min of clearance). This is within the range of CrCL that was evaluated in the single pharmacokinetic trial of brivaracetam in CKD patients. Although we predict that brivaracetam would be significantly dialyzable by any CRRT modality based on physical and pharmacokinetic characteristics, the extent of removal should be evaluated by well-designed pharmacokinetic studies using current high-permeability membranes and standard effluent rate (QE) targets of 25 or 35 mL/kg/h.[107] Even without standard pharmacokinetic studies, initiating a usual dose of 50 mg twice daily with titration upward based on seizure frequency and adverse effects is reasonable.

DRUG INTERACTIONS IN CHRONIC KIDNEY DISEASE

The risk for drug interactions is considerable in the CKD population, since these patients are prescribed an average of 11 to 12 medications and take 17 to 25 medication doses daily.[113] There is the potential for interactions with other drugs (drug–drug interaction), diseases (drug–disease interaction), or foods (drug–food interaction). Online databases and smart phone apps with information on these interactions include Micromedex, Lexicomp, and ePocrates, among others.[41,114,115]

There is also a potential decrease in cytochrome P450 drug metabolism in patients with ESRD.[39] This is believed to be due to the effect of uremia milieu on specific cytochrome P450 enzymes, as the decrease in drug metabolism noted after oral administration of propranolol and telithromycin in patients was normalized after a regular dialysis session. The Flockhart Table of Clinically Relevant P450 Interactions provides useful information for practicing clinicians on P450 drug interactions and may be accessed free online.[116]

Limited publications have addressed specific drug–drug interactions comprehensively in patients with CKD. A recent study conducted in a nephrology inpatient unit reported that drugs most frequently implicated in drug–drug interactions were cardiovascular (beta blockers, calcium-channel blockers), antidiabetic (insulin), antimicrobial (fluoroquinolones), and vitamin/mineral classes.[117] The reported interactions led to clinically inappropriate increases or decreases in blood pressure or blood glucose and/or reduced drug efficacy. Authors noted that interactions generally exhibited a delayed onset, which could lead to their underidentification. A recent study evaluated drug–disease interactions in older patients, including patients with CKD.[118] Medications identified in drug–disease interactions in CKD patients were nonsteroidal antiinflammatory drugs and triamterene. These limited studies suggest the need to more fully evaluate potential drug–drug and drug–disease interactions in patients with CKD.[119] Fortunately, the FDA appears to have taken note of older drugs lacking extensive drug–drug interaction information. The FDA recently required the manufacturer of sodium polystyrene sulfonate (Kayexalate) to conduct drug interaction studies after their review of patiromer (Veltassa), another cation exchange polymer, for treatment of hyperkalemia.[120] In vitro binding studies showed that sodium polystyrene sulfonate bound significantly to the following tested drugs: warfarin, metoprolol, phenytoin, furosemide, amlodipine, and amoxicillin.[45] It is now recommended that patients take orally administered prescriptions and over-the-counter medicines at least 3 hours before or 3 hours after sodium polystyrene sulfonate. The time should be increased to 6 hours for patients with gastroparesis or other conditions resulting in delayed emptying of food from the stomach into the small intestine.[120] The recommended spacing interval is based on the expected amount of time it would take for either sodium polystyrene sulfonate or the other drugs to pass through the stomach.[120] Further in vivo studies were not required by the FDA. Patiromer was tested for interactions with 28 drugs and was shown to decrease systemic exposure in vivo to ciprofloxacin, metformin, and levothyroxine, likely due to drug binding to patiromer in the GI tract, resulting in decreased absorption. No drug interactions were observed when these medications were taken 3 hours apart from patiromer. The current labeling of patiromer states that all oral medications should be administered 3 hours before or 3 hours after patiromer.[45] Similar binding interactions have been found for phosphate binders (calcium acetate, sevelamer hydrochloride and carbonate, lanthanum carbonate, ferric citrate, sucroferric oxyhydroxide) and a number of drugs. Clinicians should consult package labeling for each drug for specific interactions.[45] This is especially important for antibiotics, such as ciprofloxacin, where reduced absorption may lead to uncontrolled infection and severe sequelae.

IMPORTANCE OF INTERDISCIPLINARY TEAMS IN IMPROVING CHRONIC KIDNEY DISEASE CARE

A metaanalysis of interdisciplinary team care (ITC) in adult patients with stage 3 to 5 CKD found that it was associated with significantly lower risks of all-cause mortality, dialysis initiation, and catheterization for hemodialysis. In this analysis, ITC was not associated with a higher chance of choosing peritoneal dialysis or a lower chance of hospitalization for dialysis.[121] However, a randomized trial (not included in the metaanalysis), found that ITC over 2 years was associated with significantly fewer hospitalizations and a lower overall cost of care versus primary care with nephrologist consultation.[122] Pediatric CKD studies have also demonstrated significantly slower declines in GFR and shorter hospital stays with ITC versus usual care.[123,124] To become the standard of care, ITC must be cost-effective.[125] Estimates indicate that the additional salary costs of an interdisciplinary team consisting of a pharmacist, nurse, social worker, dietitian, and data manager could be recovered in 1 year if dialysis were delayed by 1 year for only 2% of pediatric CKD patients.[126] It has been suggested that administrative data be used to determine a minimum standard for healthcare funding needed to provide a reasonable ratio of allied healthcare professionals to CKD patients that is associated with acceptable outcomes.[126] Where interdisciplinary CKD teams are readily available, such as in Canada, 91% of nephrologists report using them for patient care.[127] A unique way to obtain a no-cost or low-cost pharmacist, and potentially other allied health support, in outpatient clinics is to partner with local universities and request an allied health professor who will precept students within the clinics. This approach has been employed successfully in rheumatology and endocrinology outpatient settings.[128]

Future research in ITC should focus on the optimal composition of the interdisciplinary team. Nephrologists, dietitians, and nurses have been included in most studies, and pharmacists, diabetes educators, or social workers in many others.[121] More research is also needed to identify which subset of patients is most likely to benefit from ITC. Future studies should include patients with glomerulonephritis receiving complex immunosuppressive regimens.[125]

IMPROVING CHRONIC KIDNEY DISEASE CARE DURING TRANSITIONS

Transitions of care from hospital to home or other setting (nursing home, rehabilitation center) are notoriously vulnerable to medication errors and development of medication-related problems. Under The Joint Commission standards, US hospitals are responsible for conveying specific information about the care, treatment, and services provided during hospitalizations to service providers who will provide care after discharge. Information should include the reason for discharge and a summary of care, treatment and services provided, and progress toward goals at the time of discharge.[129] Although hospital discharge planning teams in the United States do a reasonable job of conveying discharge-related information to primary care clinics, they do not always convey information to dialysis centers or specialists (e.g., nephrologists or nephrology clinics). It is incumbent on dialysis centers to establish teams to communicate with area hospital discharge planners. Wingard and colleagues implemented a novel patient information exchange between hospitals and several dialysis clinics in West Virginia, Ohio, and Kentucky.[130] Admission and postadmission checklists were provided to nurses in phase I to remind them to transmit or obtain key pieces of information. A Care Transitions Report (including a home medication list) was sent to the hospital on patient admission using information obtained from the dialysis center electronic medical record. After discharge, the posthospitalization checklist included items that nurses needed to address or facilitate, including medication review. Telephonic case managers (registered nurses) were added in phase II; they contacted patients within 72 hours of discharge and then every week, reviewing medication changes. In phase III, call center support was added for centralized information exchange and prompt notification of hospital admission and discharge. The Care Transitions Report was sent to the inpatient dialysis program and others on request. On discharge, the call center obtained hospital discharge records and securely transmitted them to providers involved in posthospital care. Dialysis clinics with these resources (Right TraC clinics) were matched to control clinics without Right TraC resources. Thirty-day all-cause readmissions significantly declined for Right TraC clinics, but not for controls.[130] Investigators did not evaluate which interventions (e.g., medication review, target weight adjustment) in the care bundle had the largest effect.

A hospital National Patient Safety Goal focuses on the process of medication reconciliation.[131] In medication reconciliation, an appropriately trained clinician compares the medications a patient is supposed to be taking (and is actually using) with new medications ordered on discharge and resolves any discrepancies. The reconciled list must be documented in patient medical records and dialysis records. Medication reconciliation is not performed routinely in most dialysis clinics due to limited data sharing between care facilities (dialysis centers, hospitals, skilled nursing facilities, rehabilitation centers) and lack of trained staff or pharmacists to in the dialysis unit.[113] A small randomized controlled trial demonstrated that dialysis patients assigned to receive medication reconciliation and management of medication-related problems by a clinical pharmacist used fewer medications and were hospitalized less than to a usual care group after 2 years.[132] Recognizing the safety issues related to medication errors and medication-related problems, the Kidney Care Quality Alliance advanced a measure on Medication Reconciliation for Patients Receiving Care at Dialysis Facilities to the National Quality Forum, which endorsed it. A Centers for Medicare & Medicaid Services (CMS) technical expert panel is reviewing evidence to support the proposed measure and recommend draft final measure specifications.

INFORMATICS APPROACHES TO IMPROVE CHRONIC KIDNEY DISEASE CARE

Given the complexity of medication use and care in patients with CKD, well-designed electronic health records (EHRs) that allow for efficient and secure exchange of health data among practitioners, patients, administrators, and researchers, and that incorporate screening and decision support for healthcare teams, could potentially reduce medication-related problems in patients with CKD. Development of informatic tools that can assist healthcare professionals to safely use medications in patients with CKD is critical. Essential to safe and effective drug use is current and past information on kidney function in the perspective of current drug use. Most hospitals and clinics increasingly use EHR and informational technology to integrate data to aid clinical decision making. The data necessary to define and stage CKD and AKI are readily available. The NKDEP Health Technology Working Group reviewed several organizations that had implemented various CKD-related tools to aid in CKD identification, staging, or management through EHR.[133] The Working Group noted that all were implemented at single institutions, at significant cost, and had not been replicated elsewhere. Challenges to implementing these systems more widely include legacy coding systems and EHRs customized for each organization. Thus laboratory data needed to diagnose CKD (serum creatinine with eGFR and method of estimation, urine albumin excretion), data related to CKD risk factors (e.g., diagnoses, medications, laboratory measurements, nephrology referral), patient education and preferences regarding dialysis modality, and patient-reported outcomes (e.g., quality of life) should be structured using standard code systems and units. CMS created incentives for eligible professionals or hospitals who see Medicare or Medicaid patients to demonstrate meaningful use of certified EHR technology.[134] This incentive program increased use of structured data fields within EHR for diagnoses, laboratory data, medications, and other clinical data, making development of CKD-specific flow sheets easier.

Once a flow sheet is developed, decision support tools, clinical reminders, and links to references or clinical guidelines can be embedded to improve CKD medication and clinical management. These CKD-related data can be aggregated to develop a CKD registry, which could facilitate reporting on quality measures such as the percentage of diabetic patients with CKD and hypertension who are being treated with angiotensin-converting enzyme inhibitors or angiotensin receptor blockers.

Several studies have evaluated physician computer order entry (CPOE) and implementation of clinical decision support systems (CDSS) regarding outcomes in patients with CKD. Leung and colleagues evaluated the effect of various CPOE systems with or without clinical decision support tools on kidney-related adverse drug events (ADEs). This study is particularly relevant because it showed a decrease in the rate of preventable ADEs in all sites after CPOE and/or CDSS implementation, but the magnitude of effect was related to the level of decision support. Four hospitals that had basic CPOE only with no CDSS (two sites) or had basic CPOE with display of serum creatinine when kidney-related drugs (cleared by the kidney or potentially nephrotoxic) were used had nonsignificant reductions in preventable ADEs. However, at the single site with basic CPOE, laboratory checks and physicians were provided with suggested doses for drugs cleared by the kidney or nephrotoxic medications and appropriate monitoring for narrow therapeutic index medications (e.g., suggested vancomycin doses and automated laboratory monitoring), and rates of preventable ADEs were reduced from 12.4 to 0 per 100 admissions.[135] Level of decision support mattered, as borne out in another study evaluating the effectiveness of an alert that was triggered if patients with kidney impairment were prescribed 1 of 24 targeted drugs that required adjustment as GFR declined. The alert included a table with drug dosage adjustments for all drugs. There was no significance difference in this study between control and intervention periods.[136] This is in contrast to a study by Chertow et al., in which the CDSS interfaced with laboratory data to estimate kidney function or changes in kidney function in real time and presented the prescriber with default adjusted medication doses and dosing frequency, together with an alert that suggested that changes were necessary in patients with CKD or AKI.[137] Appropriate doses and dosing frequency were prescribed in 54% and 35% of cases in the control period versus 67% and 59% in the intervention period, respectively ($P < 0.001$ for both measures). Few studies have evaluated the effect of CPOE or CDSS on hard patient outcomes in CKD. A small nonrandomized study evaluated the effect of CPOE and CDSS on frequency of antithrombotic medication errors in 80 patients with CKD admitted for acute coronary syndrome.[138] Physicians could choose to use standard paper-based orders following American Heart Association/American College of Cardiology guideline recommendations for antithrombotic therapy selection and dosing or CPOE with CDSS (standard orders), with patient thrombotic and bleeding risk profiles calculated and specific drug recommendations and dosing based on clinical risk, weight, and calculated CrCL. Contraindicated antithrombotics were given to zero patients in the CPOE group and to eight (17%) in the standard orders group. In-hospital bleeding occurred in 5 of 8 patients (63%) receiving contraindicated antithrombotics versus 8 of 72 (11%) receiving appropriate medications. Hospital stays were 4.3 days longer in the standard order group compared with the CPOE group. A better-designed study should be done to validate these findings, but positive patient and cost effects are expected if these results stand up.

The Acute Dialysis Quality Initiative recently conducted an evidence review to assess best practices and characteristics of optimal electronic (e)-alert systems to identify AKI. Hoste et al. found 14 studies that used e-alerts for AKI detection and also measured outcomes. Eleven of these showed positive changes in process of care (eight studies) or reduced risk for AKI, AKI progression, or mortality from AKI (six studies). Process of care improvements included earlier medication adjustment, more adequate antibiotic or medication prescription, more adequate medication dosing, and higher use of prophylaxis for contrast.[139] The authors also outlined the technological and human factors and delivery methods that should be considered before initiating an alert system. Overall, they showed that e-alerts for AKI can improve outcomes, but type of alert matters. Goldstein et al. implemented an EHR screening and decision support trigger in a hospital for noncritically ill pediatric patients receiving an intravenous aminoglycoside for more than 3 days or concurrent use of more than three nephrotoxic medications.[140] Before implementing the automated EHR-generated screening report, pharmacists manually screened patient lists and EHR records daily to detect patients with high-risk nephrotoxic medication regimens.[141] Once patients meeting criteria were identified, daily serum creatinine monitoring was recommended by the pharmacist and substitution of less nephrotoxic medications and/or pharmacokinetic monitoring was implemented. After the automated EHR screening reports were implemented, Goldstein et al. observed a 42% decrease in AKI intensity (using four measures), due to more rapid recognition of AKI and reduced nephrotoxic medications. A follow-up study showed that results were sustained over 3 years; nephrotoxic medication exposure rates decreased by 38% and AKI rates by 64%.[140] Thus medication-related AKI is avoidable when healthcare personnel are apprised in near-real time regarding high-risk patients.

Despite mounting evidence suggesting that CPOE and CDSS can improve patient care and safety, implementation of these systems has been slow and organization specific. The most widely cited barriers are financial and cultural.[142] Field et al. found that it cost $48,688 and 925 man-hours to develop a CDSS for CKD medication dosing (94 alerts for 62 drugs),[143] daunting amounts for smaller health systems or physician offices. A return on investment analysis by Brigham and Women's hospital revealed net savings for CPOE of $16.7 million over 10 years.[144] One of four CPOE system elements that resulted in the greatest savings was kidney-related dosing guidance. Although this information is compelling, individual health system administrators may require estimated cost savings based on their patient population. The NKDEP Health Technology Working Group has taken on this issue.

The goal of the NKDEP Health Technology Working Group is to "enable and support the widespread interoperability of data related to kidney health among healthcare software applications to optimize CKD detection and management." To that end, one of its subgroups developed a draft set of CKD care plan data elements with currently available standardized codes.[145] Although there are no standardized codes for some key CKD healthcare goals, including managing risks and key laboratory values, this is a start to helping healthcare organizations create a CKD-specific flow sheet. Another NKDEP subgroup developed a draft financial model to help decision makers realize the positive financial effect that CKD population health programs can have. This model is available in an Excel format and can be downloaded for testing.[145] It may be helpful in the future to make a case for health organizations or systems to invest money in developing tools to support the electronic infrastructure necessary to reliably detect CKD and provide optimal medication therapy management to patients with this condition.

Informational technology strategies have shown positive benefits for other chronic conditions. The TRANSLATE (set your Target, use Registry and Reminder Systems, get Administrative buy-in, Network information systems, Site coordination, Local physician champion, Audit and feedback, Team approach, and Education) model has been shown to be effective in diabetes.[146] Investigators are comparing the effects of adding this 9-point action plan to CDSS tools with CDSS tools alone in a large cluster-randomized trial of CKD stage 3 and 4 patients within primary care practices. Investigators are testing if the TRANSLATE model encourages more evidence-based care for CKD than CDSS only, if use of the model reduces mortality compared with CDSS alone, and whether intervention is cost-effective. This study is in the data analysis phase.[147]

A full list of references is available at www.expertconsult.com.

18

The Pathophysiology of Uremia

Tariq Shafi, MBBS, MHS, and Eugene P. Rhee, MD

OUTLINE

In a monograph on the history of uremia research, Richet wrote, "one hundred and fifty years after its birth, 'uremia' remains a clinico-chemical enigma."[1] This description remains apt to this day and summarizes some of the key features of the topic that will be discussed in more detail in this chapter. First, uremia is a clinical syndrome, with a wide range of signs and symptoms, rather than a well circumscribed disease. Second, because uremia arises with advanced kidney failure, it is characterized by the accumulation of numerous organic chemicals that would normally be cleared by healthy kidneys. Indeed, the etymology of uremia derives from the Greek *ouron* (urine) and *haima* (blood), or urine in the blood. And third, despite an ever expanding catalog of retained chemicals, or uremic solutes, a fundamental understanding of the specific cause(s) of uremia remains elusive.

Although the essence of Richet's comment endures, two notes on evolving terminology warrant mention. First, uremia was historically understood to subsume all of the signs and symptoms that arise with kidney failure. Over time, its meaning has shifted such that the term is now often used to signify only the adverse effects of renal failure that cannot be explained by derangements in volume, inorganic ions, or known renal endocrine functions (i.e., calcitriol and erythropoietin synthesis).[2] For the purpose of this chapter, we will largely adhere to this narrower conception of uremia, recognizing that signs and symptoms in patients can be multifactorial and difficult to parse. For more comprehensive discussions of these topics, the reader should refer to Chapter 9 and Chapter 10. The second note on terminology relates to the impact the advent of widespread renal replacement therapy has had on the uremic syndrome. Dialysis prevents immediate death and attenuates some of the acute symptoms of uremia. However, despite achieving adequate dialysis as defined by current standards of care, many patients continue to manifest some signs and symptoms of uremia, a phenomenon Depner described as the "Residual Syndrome."[3] This chapter will address both variants of uremia, before and after dialysis initiation, highlighting commonalities and differences when appropriate.

We will begin with a consideration of uremia as a clinical syndrome, highlighting the burden of symptoms and reduced health-related quality of life (HRQoL) experienced by patients with end-stage renal disease (ESRD) on dialysis. Next, we will examine the widely held hypothesis that retained uremic solutes are the fundamental cause of uremia. For consistency we will favor the term *uremic solute* throughout; this term is sometimes used interchangeably with *uremic toxin* in the literature, although the latter term is more properly reserved for solutes that are known to exert adverse biological effects. Because the list is always expanding, we do not provide an exhaustive survey of all or even most published uremic solutes. Rather, our goal is to provide a conceptual framework for categorizing different solute types, appreciating why they accumulate with kidney disease, and understanding the limitations of current extracorporeal approaches to their removal. In addition, we discuss factors beyond retention, including diet, the gut microbiome, and oxidative stress, that contribute to increased solute levels in ESRD. Throughout, we review how impactful clinical trials and emerging technologies have modified our understanding of uremia and identified new areas for future inquiry.

TABLE 18.1 Common Manifestations of Uremia

Anorexia	Uremic component includes reduced appetite and altered taste and smell; compounded by dietary and fluid restrictions, medications, and comorbidities (e.g., diabetic gastroparesis).
Nausea and vomiting	In conjunction with anorexia, a very common trigger for dialysis initiation; uremia can affect both central (CNS chemoreceptor) and gastrointestinal (delayed emptying) mechanisms.
Fatigue	Often with significant contributions from comorbid illness such as anemia and cardiovascular disease as well as deconditioning; reduced muscle mass and resultant frailty are common.
Neuropathy	Distal polyneuropathy characterized by sensory symptoms, initially paresthesias, but also pain with progression; more advanced neuropathy can also cause motor symptoms.[130]
Altered mental status	Can range from subtle cognitive deficits to coma; often accompanied by fine action tremor, asterixis, or hyperreflexia.[131] Most common EEG finding is prominence of slow waves.
Insomnia	Includes difficulty initiating sleep, maintaining sleep, and waking too early; ESRD disturbs circadian sleep–wake rhythm; exacerbated by sleep-disordered breathing, restless legs syndrome, and pruritus, all of which are common with uremia.[132]
Pruritus	Large variation in presentation; can be generalized or localized to the back, face, arms, etc.; often worse at night, but in some patients most severe during dialysis.[133]
Bleeding	Primarily due to platelet dysfunction, typically with normal platelet count and normal prothrombin and partial thromboplastin times.[134]
Pericarditis	Sometimes subdivided into "uremic" (develops before or shortly after dialysis initiation) or "dialysis-associated"; can be serous or hemorrhagic; classic ECG manifestations of diffuse ST elevations uncommon.[135]
Amenorrhea and sexual dysfunction	Includes disturbances in menstruation and fertility in women, erectile dysfunction in men, and loss of libido in both; associated with disruption in hypothalamic–pituitary–gonadal axis.[136]

CNS, Central nervous system; *ECG*, electrocardiogram; *EEG*, electroencephalogram; *ESRD*, end-stage renal disease.

UREMIA: THE CLINICAL SYNDROME

Classic Signs and Symptoms

Uremia affects nearly every organ system (Table 18.1). The term often connotes prolonged illness, but uremia can arise with either acute or chronic renal failure. Common manifestations include loss of appetite, altered smell and taste, nausea, vomiting, progressive weakness and fatigue, neuropathy, impaired sleep, altered mentation, pruritus, and reduced platelet function. Uremic frost, which reflects the excretion of urea through the skin, and uremic fetor, which reflects the breakdown of urea to ammonia in saliva, are now rare as dialysis is usually initiated before these signs develop. Similarly, uremic stupor, coma, and death are uncommon in modern healthcare settings, except when dialysis is deferred in the context of palliation.

Clinical context matters a great deal when evaluating uremia's contribution to a patient's presentation. For example, uremia is sometimes invoked as the cause of coma in the intensive care unit, when in fact hypoxic or ischemic brain injury, infection, hypercarbia, liver disease, and sedating medications may play a more significant role. The confounding effects of medications always require careful consideration. For example, the accumulation of renally cleared medications, such as morphine, oxycodone, gabapentin, and pregabalin, can cause nausea, sedation, or abnormal neurological findings that may be mistaken for uremia.[4,5] Patient-specific factors such as age, frailty, cognitive and cardiopulmonary reserve, and other comorbidities affect how uremia manifests. In addition, although we outline a conceptual distinction between uremia and derangements in fluid, electrolytes, and renal endocrine functions, this compartmentalization is often not feasible in clinical practice. For example, fatigue in uremic patients is often compounded by congestive heart failure and anemia. There is no gold standard for isolating the effects from uremia or grading its severity. Thus the recognition and assessment of this protean syndrome can only be performed at the bedside, on an individualized basis.

Variability with the timing of uremia onset adds to this complexity. Uremia exists along a continuum of kidney failure, with subtle deficits detectable at relatively modest levels of kidney dysfunction. In clinical practice, however, the term is generally reserved for the appearance of signs and symptoms severe enough to trigger consideration of dialysis initiation. This generally does not occur until the estimated glomerular filtration rate (eGFR) is less than 15 mL/min/1.73 m^2. The results of an important clinical trial provide valuable perspective on this transition period. The IDEAL Study randomized 828 adults with eGFR 10 to 15 mL/min/1.73 m^2 to early (eGFR 10 to 14 mL/min/1.73 m^2) or late (eGFR 5 to 7 mL/min/1.73 m^2) dialysis initiation.[6] For the early-start group, the median time to dialysis initiation was 1.8 months compared with 7.4 months for the late-start group. Notably, 322 (75.9%) of the late-start group initiated dialysis before their eGFR had reached the target range, such that the mean eGFR at dialysis initiation was 9.8 mL/min/1.73 m^2. The reasons for starting dialysis at an eGFR >7 mL/min/1.73 m^2 in the late-start group are informative: 234 for uremia, 28 for fluid overload, 25 for physician discretion, and 4 for hyperkalemia. Thus among individuals randomized to late-start, uremia was the major indication for dialysis initiation and was evident in the majority of patients by the time eGFR had fallen to ~7 mL/min/1.73 m^2. During a median follow-up of 3.6 years, there was no difference in mortality between the early- and late-start groups, supporting the use of uremic symptom onset as a major criterion for dialysis initiation.

TABLE 18.2 **Residual Uremic Symptoms**

Symptoms	Prevalence
Anorexia	49%
Nausea	33%
Pruritus	55%
Excessive daytime sleepiness	44%
Difficulty concentrating	54%
Fatigue	71%
Pain	47%

(From Murtagh FE, Addington-Hall J, Higginson IJ. The prevalence of symptoms in end-stage renal disease: a systematic review. *Adv Chronic Kidney Dis.* 2007;14:82-99; Novak MJ, Sheth H, Bender FH, et al. Improvement in Pittsburgh Symptom Score index after initiation of peritoneal dialysis. *Adv Perit Dial.* 2008;24:46-50.)

Uremia After Dialysis Initiation

Dialysis attenuates, but does not eradicate uremic symptoms in most patients. This "residual syndrome" is characterized by high symptom prevalence among patients on dialysis, with rates for individual symptoms ranging from 30% to 70% (Table 18.2).[7,8] This burden of *persistent uremic symptoms* contributes significantly to poor HRQoL, with additional contributions from the physiological and psychological burden of dialysis therapy as well as other comorbid illnesses. Individual self-reported symptoms, including anorexia,[9] sleep quality,[10] and pruritus,[11] as well as reduced HRQoL have all been associated with increased mortality in ESRD. Independent of these associations, symptoms and HRQoL are clearly important outcomes in and of themselves.[12] Indeed, HRQoL is often a greater concern than survival for patients; in one study, when asked about the possibility of improvement in HRQoL or survival by switching to intensive HD, 94% would consider it for improving energy, 57% for improving sleep, but only 19% would consider it for improving survival by 3 years.[13]

In addition to a syndrome of attenuated yet persistent symptoms, uremia after dialysis initiation is characterized by *chronic end-organ toxicity.* Two examples that have received significant attention, both independent predictors of mortality in ESRD, are uremic cardiovascular disease (CVD) and uremic alterations in energy metabolism.[14] For both topics, the reader is also referred to more comprehensive discussions in Chapter 12 and Chapter 13.

Uremic Cardiovascular Toxicity

CVD is highly prevalent in patients with ESRD, with a risk for CVD mortality 10- to 100-fold higher than in the general population.[15] In part, this reflects shared risk factors for CVD and chronic kidney disease (CKD), particularly diabetes and hypertension. However, traditional risk factors do not fully account for this excess mortality, and clinical trials have shown no benefit to standard CVD treatments such as angiotensin-converting enzyme inhibitors or statins in dialysis patients.[16,17] Derangements in erythropoiesis and mineral metabolism that arise with progressive kidney failure likely play a role in the pathogenesis of CVD in ESRD, but raising hemoglobin or lowering parathyroid hormone levels have also shown no benefit.[18,19] Thus there is significant interest in understanding how the uremic milieu contributes to accelerated CVD pathogenesis. From a clinical perspective, uremic CVD is characterized by left ventricular hypertrophy, myocardial fibrosis, medial vascular calcification, endothelial dysfunction, and sympathetic nervous system derangements.[20,21] Left ventricular hypertrophy is particularly common, present in up to 80% of individuals at dialysis initiation.[22] Approximately 50% of CVD mortality in dialysis patients is due to sudden death, although the relative contribution of malignant ventricular arrhythmias, bradyarrhythmias, asystolic arrests, or other events is unknown.[23]

Uremic Metabolic Toxicity

Protein-energy wasting (PEW) is the term endorsed by the International Society of Renal Nutrition and Metabolism to describe the syndrome of reduced protein and energy reserves in ESRD.[24] It has consequences throughout the body, but can be conceptualized at least in part as chronic toxicity to skeletal muscle and adipose deposits. Common features of PEW include hypoalbuminemia, low body mass index, and low serum cholesterol levels. PEW is often also characterized by insulin resistance, increased resting energy expenditure, and inflammation, all of which are believed to contribute to its pathogenesis. Anorexia, acidosis, and decreased physical activity are additional etiological factors. Despite amino acid losses of 4 to 8 g/day with peritoneal and hemodialysis,[25,26] the initiation of maintenance dialysis can improve nutritional status in uremic patients.[27] However, increasing the intensity or frequency of treatment above standard adequacy goals does not further improve nutritional indices.[28,29]

In summary, uremia is a clinical syndrome that arises with severe acute or chronic kidney failure. It can affect nearly every organ system, but there is no objective indicator of its onset or severity. How and when uremia manifests depends on patient-specific factors, and significant uremic symptoms are a major impetus for dialysis initiation. Although dialysis improves some features of uremia, many patients continue to experience both persistent uremic symptoms and chronic end-organ toxicity.

UREMIA AND SOLUTE RETENTION

Several observations suggest that retained solutes are the primary cause of uremia. First, uremia occurs with severe renal failure regardless of the etiology of kidney disease. Thus it is an *acquired* syndrome attributable to the loss of kidney function itself, rather than a specific manifestation of long-standing diabetes mellitus, systemic lupus erythematosus, autosomal dominant polycystic kidney disease, and so on. Second, severe renal failure leads to the accumulation of numerous solutes that are usually cleared by healthy kidneys, sometimes many-fold above normal levels. Third, solute clearance with dialysis improves, but does not fully ameliorate the uremic syndrome. Fourth, unlike dialysis, kidney transplantation results in dramatic improvement, even normalization, of both uremic solute levels and uremic symptoms.

Normal Kidney Function

Understanding solute retention requires an understanding of normal kidney function. The kidneys generate ~140 L/day of glomerular filtrate, and then subsequently reabsorb the vast majority of filtered sodium and water, glucose, amino acids, and other urinary constituents required to maintain volume and nutritional homeostasis. Second only to the heart in mitochondrial abundance, the kidney consumes an enormous amount of energy for this reclamation across electrochemical gradients. Although this cycle of filtration and reabsorption seems energetically wasteful, it permits very high rates of clearance of freely soluble waste products such as creatinine (~120 mL/min/1.73 m^2). In addition to glomerular filtration, normal renal excretory function includes tubular secretion, a critical mechanism for the excretion of protein-bound waste products that do not readily cross the glomerular filtration barrier. As with tubular reabsorption, tubular secretion is energy-intensive and is mediated by specific apical and basal membrane spanning transporters. Studies in knock-out mice have begun to map the secretion of specific uremic solutes to specific organic anion transporters (OATs) expressed in the renal tubular epithelium.[30] Finally, the kidneys also take up and catabolize some circulating small molecules, such as asymmetrical dimethylarginine (ADMA) and S-adenosylhomocysteine, as well as numerous peptides.[31-33] Thus, through a combination of *filtration*, *reabsorption*, *secretion*, and *metabolism*, the kidneys have a broad and heterogeneous impact on circulating solute levels, minimizing the loss of desired nutrients while facilitating the clearance of waste products.

Renal Failure and Solute Retention

Solutes normally cleared by the kidneys accumulate as kidney function declines. Indeed, kidney dysfunction is most often detected and monitored on the basis of serum creatinine levels, a marker of glomerular filtration. However, the relative rise in creatinine does not necessarily predict the relative rise in other uremic solute levels.[34] This discrepancy is magnified among patients with ESRD on dialysis. Both hemodialysis and peritoneal dialysis, which are discussed in detail in Section III, differ fundamentally from endogenous kidney function. For both, the rate of clearance of *freely-soluble solutes*, such as creatinine, is substantially less than normal, with standard thrice-weekly hemodialysis and continuous ambulatory peritoneal dialysis achieving creatinine clearances of <10 to 15 mL/min/1.73 m^2 per day. The rate of clearance of *protein-bound solutes* is even worse because it is free rather than total solute levels that drive the diffusion gradient across the hemodialysis or peritoneal membrane. For example, one study showed predialysis elevations of phenylacetylglutamine (122-fold), hippurate (108-fold), indoxyl sulfate (116-fold), and p-cresol sulfate (41-fold), four solutes normally cleared by tubular secretion, significantly greater than for urea (5-fold) and creatinine (13-fold).[35] Dialysis is also less effective for the clearance of relatively *large molecules* (often referred to as *middle molecules*), generally composed of peptides or small proteins. Some of these molecules, such as β_2-microglobulin (11.8 kDa), cystatin C (13.3 kDa), leptin (16 kDa), and select advanced glycation end-products (AGEs) undergo glomerular filtration followed by uptake and catabolism within tubular epithelial cells, and thus can accumulate substantially with renal failure.[36,37] Finally, a limitation specific to hemodialysis is the intermittency of treatment, which stands in contrast to the continuous clearance provided by endogenous kidney function. Whereas hemodialysis removes waste products from circulating blood, its access to the intracellular space or different tissue beds is contingent on rapid equilibration of levels across these different compartments.[38] Thus for *sequestered solutes*, or solutes that do not rapidly equilibrate across compartments, hemodialysis may transiently lower plasma concentrations without making a large impact on total body solute excess.

Residual Clearance

Due to the relative inefficiency of dialysis in replicating the excretory function of the kidney, residual kidney function (RKF) in dialysis patients can make an important contribution to solute clearance. For example, among individuals on hemodialysis with a mean residual urea clearance of 2.5 mL/min, RKF provided 20% of total urea removal, 34% of the total p-cresol sulfate removal, and 66% of the total hippurate removal.[39] In addition, nonrenal clearance may also be an important route for the excretion of some uremic solutes in patients with renal failure. Creatinine excretion through the gastrointestinal tract is known to increase with advancing renal failure, attributable to increased degradation by gut microbes.[40,41] To what extent similar mechanisms augment the nonrenal clearance of other uremic solutes is poorly characterized. Conversely, uremia may reduce the nonrenal clearance of some solutes by impairing the expression or function of hepatic and intestinal solute transporters.[42]

In summary, "normal" kidney function includes glomerular filtration, tubular absorption and secretion, and metabolism. Acting continuously and cooperatively, these functions both retain valuable circulating nutrients as well as excrete waste products with a range of physiochemical properties, including protein binding, size, and sequestration. With kidney failure, loss of these functions results in solute retention, with relative levels of accumulation that may not correlate with the levels of filtration markers such as creatinine and urea. Because renal replacement modalities are best suited for small, soluble solutes, the accumulation of large and/or protein-bound solutes can be very high, for example, >100-fold above normal. Even a low level of RKF can have a large impact on uremic solute burden.

SOLUTE PRODUCTION

Solute Production From Food

Carbohydrates, lipids, and protein are largely composed of glucose, fatty acids, and amino acids, respectively. The catabolism of these molecules converge on the citric acid cycle (Fig. 18.1), also known as the *tricarboxylic acid cycle* or *Krebs cycle*. This series of chemical reactions receives carbon

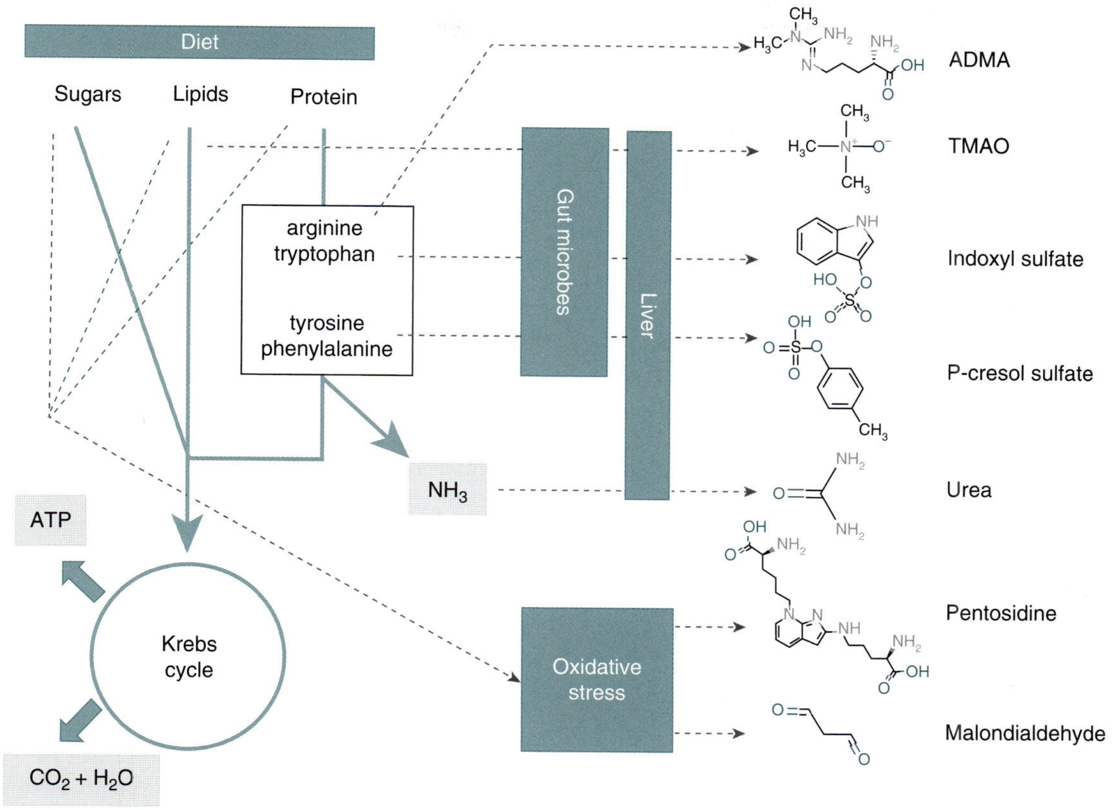

FIG. 18.1 Uremic solute production. Diet is a major source of uremic solutes, with ingested compounds often modified by enzymatic actions of the gut microbiome and/or liver. Protein-derived solutes are particularly notable because of the kidney's fundamental role in the excretion of nitrogenous waste products. Oxidation of macromolecules, with subsequent macromolecule degradation, is a mechanism for endogenous solute production. *ADMA*, Asymmetrical dimethylarginine; *TMAO*, trimethylamine-*N*-oxide.

end-products from glycolysis, the β-oxidation of fatty acids, and various amino-acid catabolic pathways, ultimately yielding CO_2, H_2O, and reducing equivalents that drive adenosine triphosphate (ATP) production via oxidative phosphorylation. Despite this convergence of biochemical pathways, amino acid metabolism differs in two important ways. First, unlike glucose and fatty acids, which are composed entirely of carbon, oxygen, and hydrogen, every amino acid has a nitrogen-containing amino group. Second, unlike glucose and fatty acids, which can be stored as glycogen or triglyceride when ingested in excess of energetic needs, amino acids cannot be stored (muscle is a reservoir of amino acids that can be catabolized under starvation conditions, but muscle mass does not increase simply as a function of protein intake). Thus the daily ingestion and break down of amino acids necessitates ongoing nitrogen excretion to maintain net balance. Most aquatic species simply release ammonia into their surroundings. Because free ammonia is toxic, humans and other mammals shuttle tissue derived amino groups as glutamine or alanine to the liver where the amino groups are converted to urea, which is then excreted by the kidneys.

Given the kidneys' fundamental role in maintaining whole-body nitrogen balance, nitrogenous waste products represent a large fraction of the uremic solutes identified to date. This includes urea as well as numerous amino acid derivatives. Because the underlying ring structure of tryptophan, phenylalanine, and tyrosine make these amino acids hydrophobic, many of their derivatives are protein-bound. As will be discussed in more detail, gut microbes perform key enzymatic steps in the production of some of these compounds. In addition to protein, other dietary sources contribute to the pool of nitrogen that must be excreted to maintain whole-body balance. For example, uric acid, an end-product of purine nucleotide breakdown, and creatinine, a break-down product of muscle-derived creatine phosphate are abundant nitrogenous waste products in urine.[43] Trimethylamine is synthesized from dietary nutrients such as choline and carnitine.

Finally, nonnitrogen-containing dietary constituents also produce uremic solutes. Because of odd carbon number, side chains, or other structural features, some organic acids cannot be fully metabolized to CO_2 and H_2O and thus require renal excretion. Acidosis in the context of methanol or ethylene glycol poisonings illustrate this possibility, with dangerous accumulation of metabolites, such as formic acid and oxalic acid, even in individuals with normal kidney function. More commonly, oxalate is derived from plants or from the catabolism of ascorbic acid (vitamin C) and can reach very high levels in ESRD. Sugar alcohols such as sorbitol, mannitol, and myoinositol can also reach high levels in ESRD; myoinositol in particular can accumulate significantly, as it is normally degraded by the kidney.

Solute Production and the Gut Microbiome

Modern sequencing methodologies have enabled a more comprehensive assessment of the gut microbial community, circumventing the bias imposed by traditional culture-based methods.[44] One approach has been targeted sequencing of 16S ribosomal DNA in stool or other gut-derived samples. This gene is present in all living organisms, but slight differences in sequence provide information about microbial diversity at the family, genus, and sometimes even species level. Complementary with 16S ribosomal DNA-based taxonomic profiling, another approach has been to sequence as many fragments of DNA as possible in a given biological sample in a nontargeted fashion. This latter, "metagenomic" approach is more computationally challenging, but provides information about the full breadth of genes, and thus the range of enzymatic capabilities in a given microbial community. Studies using these tools have affected many areas of biomedicine, with several common themes: the gut microbial community is abundant and diverse, it harbors metabolic capacities that are distinct from the host, it varies across individuals and disease states, it has diverse impacts on host metabolism, and it represents a potential target for therapeutic intervention.[45,46]

The gut microbiome plays a large role in shaping the biochemicals absorbed from diet.[41,47] Indeed, a major evolutionary driving force for harboring large microbial communities is that they can degrade dietary substances that are otherwise nondigestible, maximizing host nutrition. Perhaps quantitatively most important is the gut microbial digestion of polysaccharides, such as cellulose and starch, yielding short-chain fatty acids, which can then be absorbed and utilized by the host. The gut microbiome also affects amino acid and lipid metabolism. The effect on amino acids is at least twofold. First, amino acids synthesized de novo by bacteria are absorbed and contribute to the host amino acid pool. This effect can be enormous in ruminant animals, which can survive with ammonia and urea as their only sources of dietary nitrogen.[48] In humans, the quantitative importance of microbial amino acid synthesis is much less, ranging from 1% to 20% for select amino acids.[49] Second, bacterial metabolism of luminal protein yields amino acid derivatives that are then absorbed into the host circulation. Bacterial metabolism of tryptophan and phenylalanine/tyrosine, followed by additional conjugation steps in the liver, yield uremic solutes such as indoxyl sulfate and p-cresol sulfate, respectively. One study elegantly underscored the requirement of gut microbes for this process, demonstrating normal levels of indoxyl sulfate and p-cresol sulfate among ESRD patients who had undergone a colectomy.[50] Using mass spectrometry (MS), this study showed that many other compounds, most of which remain unidentified, were elevated only among ESRD patients with intact colons, implicating colonic microbes in their production. Similar results have been demonstrated in mice with renal failure in germ-free (no gut microbes) versus control conditions.[51] Gut microbes have also recently been identified as a potential mediator of the proatherosclerotic effects of dietary lipids. More specifically, they convert dietary choline into trimethylamine, which is then oxidized in the liver to yield trimethylamine *N*-oxide (TMAO), a potential cardiovascular toxin.

Thus the gut microbiome participates in the production of some, and perhaps many, uremic solutes (see Fig. 18.1). In turn, the uremic milieu appears to modify the gut microbiome, with small studies suggesting bacterial overgrowth in the small intestine.[52] One study utilizing 16S rRNA gene analysis showed marked differences in the taxonomy of stool microbes in individuals with ESRD compared with healthy controls.[53] ESRD could modify the gut flora via several mechanisms, including alterations in diet, increased delivery of nitrogenous compounds into the gut lumen, increased frequency of antibiotic use, other medications such as iron, and reduced integrity of the gut epithelial barrier.[54] Given the gut microbiome's impact on host metabolism, as well as its contribution to uremic solute production, understanding how the microbiome and its functional capacity changes as kidney function declines warrants further investigation.

UREMIC INFLAMMATION AND OXIDATIVE STRESS

Progressive loss of kidney function results in increased systemic inflammation and oxidative stress, which in turn may contribute to various features of the uremic illness, particularly chronic toxicities such as CVD and PEW. Thus uremia is both a cause and consequence of inflammation and oxidative stress. Here, we discuss how this interrelationship overlaps with the solute-centric approach outlined in this chapter while also providing an alternative perspective on uremia.

The etiology of increased inflammation and oxidative stress in ESRD is likely multifactorial, and remains incompletely understood (see Chapter 14, Inflammation in Chronic Kidney Disease, for a more comprehensive discussion). Ikizler and Himmelfarb have shown that biomarkers of inflammation and oxidative stress increase in patients with CKD stage 3 to 5, remain persistently elevated despite initiation of hemodialysis, and fall substantially after renal transplantation, supporting a causal role for the loss of kidney function in triggering these alterations.[55-57] These observations align with the rise, persistent elevation, and fall of poorly dialyzed uremic solutes across these clinical scenarios, raising the possibility that *solute retention* may contribute to the genesis of inflammation and oxidant stress in patients with CKD. Indeed, middle molecules normally cleared by the kidney include cytokines, for example, interleukin-6 (IL-6), as well as complement peptides and AGEs; loss of renal clearance can result in the retention and subsequent accumulation of these proinflammatory molecules. In addition, and as discussed in more detail later, other uremic solutes such as p-cresol sulfate and indoxyl sulfate may induce aberrant inflammation and oxidative stress, either through tissue injury or by stimulating immune cells.

In turn, this milieu can itself drive *solute production*, creating a deleterious cycle. This process of self-amplification is exemplified by AGEs, a heterogeneous group of compounds derived from the nonenzymatic ligation of proteins and other macromolecules with carbonyl compounds.[58] These carbonyl compounds include sugars (hence the term *glycation*) as well as small carbonyl precursors produced from the oxidation of sugars and lipids.[59] AGEs can come from diet or be produced endogenously. The increase in oxidative stress in ESRD can significantly increase endogenous AGE production, even in the absence of hyperglycemia or diabetes mellitus, compounding the loss of renal AGE clearance.[60,61] AGEs can accumulate in cells and tissue, where they cross-link with proteins and interfere with macromolecule function. In addition, AGEs can signal through the receptor for advanced glycation end-products (RAGE), activating proinflammatory and proo-xidant signaling pathways. In addition to AGE formation, oxidative stress produces other macromolecule modifications as well, including lipid peroxidation, protein thiol oxidation, protein tyrosine nitration, and DNA strand breaks.[62] Although most glycated or oxidized macromolecules are not cleared by the kidney, their breakdown products, such as pentosidine and *N*-carboxymethyllysine (AGEs), 4-hydroxynonaneal and malondialdehyde (lipid peroxidation), and 3-nitrotyrosine (tyrosine nitration), are solutes that can accumulate in ESRD (see Fig. 18.1).

Although the burden of inflammation and oxidation in ESRD can be considered through the framework of solute retention and production, it also provides a different perspective on the uremic illness.[63] The toxicity of these processes is likely mediated primarily through their effects on macromolecule structure and function, in circulation and within tissue, rather than the inherent toxicity of the smaller solutes derived from macromolecule degradation. For example, oxidation of lipoproteins has been hypothesized to enhance the atherogenicity of low-density lipoprotein (LDL) cholesterol and impair high-density lipoprotein (HDL)-mediated reverse cholesterol transport, accelerating the development of CVD.[64] Further, mechanisms beyond solute retention and production contribute to inflammation and oxidative stress in ESRD. Increased exposure to infectious agents, either from overt infection or with subclinical pathogen exposure due to periodontal disease, biofilms on hemodialysis or peritoneal dialysis catheters, or impaired gut epithelial-barrier integrity are all potential culprits, as are exposure to bioincompatible hemodialysis membranes or impure dialysate.[65] Whatever the etiology, the cumulative burden of inflammation and oxidative stress correlates strongly with adverse outcomes in ESRD.[66]

CURRENT CATALOG OF UREMIC SOLUTES

Hemodialysis was initially performed using membranes that provided limited clearance of solutes with molecular weights (MWs) >1 kDa. Because these treatments could improve some symptoms of uremia, for example waking comatose patients or relieving vomiting, there is wide acceptance that some important uremic toxins are small. However, the incomplete resolution of uremia with dialysis raised the question of whether increased clearance of small molecules like urea or increased clearance of relatively larger "middle molecules" would be beneficial.[67] The Hemodialysis (HEMO) study was a landmark randomized clinical trial of 1846 prevalent hemodialysis patients that used a two-by-two factorial design to examine the effects of standard or high-dose dialysis (as defined by urea clearance, Kt/V) and low-flux or high-flux dialyzers (with the latter providing enhanced clearance of some middle molecules).[68] Unfortunately, neither higher dose (spKt/V_{urea} of 1.71 ± 0.11 vs. 1.32 ± 0.09) nor use of a high-flux membrane (β_2-microglobulin clearance of 34 ± 11 mL/min vs. 3 ± 7 mL/min) improved the primary outcome of all-cause mortality over a mean follow-up of 2.84 years, reinforcing the need to identify and target the actual uremic solutes that cause uremia.

Because a detailed mechanistic understanding of uremia is lacking, a common approach is to classify solutes according to the physical characteristics that affect solute retention and dialytic clearance, such as solubility, protein binding, and size. For example, in a 2003 report of the European Uremic Toxin Work Group, Vanholder and colleagues summarized the existing literature at that time on 90 uremic compounds, dividing them into water-soluble low molecular weight solutes (MW <500 Da), protein-bound solutes, and middle molecules (MW ≥500 Da).[69] This compendium has been updated over time and is available online (http://www.uremic-toxins.org/); of the ~130 compounds currently listed, approximately half are categorized as water-soluble, one-quarter are categorized as protein-bound, and one-quarter are categorized as middle molecules.[70] Table 18.3 highlights select solutes representative of each class of molecules. As already discussed in the overview of solute production, many of these solutes are nitrogenous waste products. Among water-soluble solutes, these include arginine derivatives (guanidines), nucleotide breakdown products, and TMAO, whereas protein-bound solutes include tryptophan (indoles) and phenylalanine/tyrosine derivatives (phenols). By contrast, middle molecules are composed almost entirely of peptides or small proteins. Markers of inflammation and oxidative stress are represented in all three categories.

The advent of high-throughput analytical approaches has expanded the list of known uremic solutes. Nevertheless, the fundamental question of proving which solutes are toxic remains, and significantly less progress has been made in this regard. In this section, we provide an overview of emerging approaches to solute discovery, the challenge of proving causality in uremia, and strategies to prioritize among a multiplicity of solutes. Finally, we provide a focused discussion of potential mechanisms of solute toxicity.

Metabolomics Studies

Metabolomics refers to the systematic analysis of small molecules, typically <1500 Da, in a biological specimen.[71] Nuclear magnetic resonance (NMR) spectroscopy and MS have served as the two main workhorses in metabolomics. NMR uses the magnetic properties of select atomic nuclei (^1H, ^{13}C, or ^{31}P) to determine the structure and abundance of metabolites in a biological specimen. MS methods resolve compounds on the basis of their mass, or more precisely their mass-to-charge ratio after ionization, and are typically coupled to up-front separation techniques including gas

TABLE 18.3 Representative Uremic Solutes

Class	Name	Comment
Water-soluble	Urea	Used to measure dialysis adequacy
	ADMA	Guanidine; inhibits NO synthase
	TMAO	Produced by gut bacteria
	Pseudouridine	Nucleoside
	Oxalate	Organic acid
	Myoinositol	Sugar a cohol
	Malondialdehyde	From degradation of oxidized lipids
Protein-bound	P-cresol sulfate	Phenol; produced by gut bacteria
	Indoxyl sulfate	Indole; produced by gut bacteria
	Pentosidine, *N*-carboxymethyllysine	Advanced glycation end-products
Middle molecules	β_2-microglobulin	Causes dialysis-related amyloidosis
	Parathyroid hormone, fibroblast growth factor-23	Hormones that regulates bone and mineral metabolism
	Leptin, ghrelin	Hormones that regulates appetite and energy homeostasis
	Interleukin-6, tumor necrosis factor alpha	Cytokines

ADMA, Asymmetrical dimethylarginine; *TMAO*, trimethylamine-*N*-oxide.

and liquid chromatography. Although all of these analytical tools have been in use for decades in uremia research,[72] recent advances have increased their speed, sensitivity, and specificity, enabling the simultaneous measurement of hundreds to thousands of analytes in a given blood sample. Metabolomics studies of ESRD, spearheaded by Niwa and others, have identified dozens of novel uremic solutes, rapidly expanding the total list to >270 molecules.[73-76] Although offering clear advantages for solute discovery, metabolomic approaches also have notable limitations. Current platforms do not provide comprehensive coverage of the metabolome, and for any given method there is heterogeneity in how well individual analytes are measured. Further, metabolomics usually provides semiquantitative results, such that follow-up studies are required to determine the absolute concentrations of newly identified uremic solutes. Proteomics, the comprehensive study of proteins in a biological specimen, has also been utilized in uremia research.[77] Given some technical restraints, however, these studies have been limited to relatively smaller numbers of patient samples, although this is likely to change with emerging, higher-throughput proteomic approaches.[78]

Proving Causality in Uremia

In analogy with Koch's postulates for identifying infectious pathogens, Bergstrom suggested that proof of a solute's toxicity requires a demonstration that reducing its concentration improves uremia (or some specific feature of uremia), and that raising its concentration in normal people recapitulates the illness. No purported uremic toxin has met this standard. In a classic study, investigators added urea to the dialysate of three patients to maintain blood concentrations between 181 and 600 mg/dL, for periods of 7 to 90 days.[79] Serial electromyography and electroencephalography did not show evidence of progressive neuropathy or encephalopathy during urea loading. A blood urea nitrogen concentration of less than 300 mg/dL was generally well tolerated, and symptoms such as malaise, vomiting, headache, and bleeding only emerged with urea levels exceeding this threshold, providing compelling evidence that urea alone is not responsible for the uremic illness.

Although Bergstrom's framework is intellectually appealing, it is unclear whether the approach it embodies is either realistic or appropriate for the investigation of causality in uremia. First, the uremic illness is multifaceted, and it is likely that different solutes are responsible for different symptoms. Second, uremic symptoms are difficult to quantify, and symptoms such as fatigue are multifactorial with contributions from comorbid illness. Third, uremia subsumes both acute and chronic complications. Long-term studies of chronic end-organ toxicities rather than acute symptoms would be difficult to conduct, and in some cases would be unethical. Fourth, some uremic solutes may need to act in combination, or in the setting of advanced kidney failure, to exert toxicity. For example, solutes might coactivate common pathways or displace each other from protein binding, yielding higher free concentrations. Finally, ideal animal models for the study of uremia are lacking. In vivo assessment of uremic symptoms such as fatigue, nausea, change in taste, or pruritus is difficult. Arguably, model systems are more helpful for the study of end-organ toxicities, such as left ventricular hypertrophy, vascular calcification, or alterations in energy metabolism. Even these studies, however, are limited by an inability to faithfully recapitulate the uremic milieu in small animals. For all of these reasons, the goal of mapping uremic symptoms and end-organ toxicities to individual solutes or groups of solutes in humans is a formidable challenge.

Uremic Solutes Associated With Adverse Clinical Outcomes

One approach to prioritizing among numerous uremic solutes is to identify which solutes predict adverse clinical outcomes. In general, these epidemiological studies comprise of dialysis cohorts with stored specimens at baseline and longitudinal follow-up on clinical outcomes. Some issues unique to dialysis patients include timing of sampling in relation to dialysis (day of the week; pre- or posthemodialysis session),

TABLE 18.4 **Epidemiological Studies of Selected Uremic Toxins and Cardiovascular Outcomes in Dialysis Patients**

Solute	Year	N	Plasma Concentration Mean ± SD or Median [IQR]	Outcome Adjudication	Association With CVD Outcomes	Ref
P-cresol sulfate	2012	112	Total: 2.8 [0.1, 9.9] mg/dL Free: 0.22 [0.001, 2.56] mg/dL	Not described	Total: No Free: Yes	137
	2013	521	Total: 3.2 ± 1.8 mg/dL	Yes	No	138
	2015	394	Free: 0.20 ± 0.13 mg/dL	Yes	Yes	139
	2017	1273	Total: 3.3 ± 1.7 mg/dL	Yes	No	In press*
Indoxyl sulfate	2013	521	Total: 1.8 ± 1.1 mg/dL	Yes	No	138
	2015	394	Free: 0.13 ± 0.10 mg/dL	Yes	No	139
	2015	258	Total: 3.5 ± 1.8 mg/dL	Yes	Yes	140
	2017	1273	Total: 2.5 ± 1.2 mg/dL	Yes	No	In press*
ADMA	2001	225	2.5 [1.6, 3.9] μmol/L	Yes	Yes	141
	2014	259	0.8 ± 0.2 μmol/L		Associated with all-cause mortality (NO CVD events)	142
	2017	1276	0.9 ± 0.2 μmol/L	Yes	Yes	143
TMAO	2015	235	50 ± 32 μmol/L	No	No	144
	2017	1232	102 ± 64 μmol/L	Yes	Yes	145

*Shafi T, Sirich TL, Meyer TW, et al. Results of the HEMO study suggest that p-cresol sulfate and indoxyl sulfate are not associated with cardiovascular outcomes. *Kidney Int.* 2017;92(6):1484–1492.
ADMA, Asymmetrical dimethylarginine; *CVD*, cardiovascular disease; *IQR*, interquartile range; *SD*, standard deviation; *TMAO*, trimethylamine-*N*-oxide.

frequent administration of heparin (which activates lipoprotein lipase, releasing free fatty acids that can displace bound uremic solutes and increase their free concentrations), and dialysis facility level factors that can introduce confounding (facilities with poor sample handling techniques may have deficiencies in other process measures that cause poor outcomes).[80] In addition, CVD is common in dialysis patients but may be undiagnosed or not captured at baseline, such that new CVD "events" may simply represent preexisting disease. In longitudinal follow-up, cause-specific event rates may be inaccurate, particularly among the substantial fraction of individuals who succumb to sudden death.

Notwithstanding these challenges, several studies have sought to identify solutes associated with CVD outcomes or mortality in ESRD (Table 18.4). Elevated levels of p-cresol sulfate, indoxyl sulfate, ADMA, and TMAO have been associated with these outcomes in some, but not all studies performed to date. Typically, only one or a handful of molecules were examined in any given study, making it difficult to compare the relative strength of associations. Metabolomic approaches enable simultaneous measurement of many solutes. One study examined the association of 165 metabolites and 1-year cardiovascular mortality among 500 incident dialysis patients.[81] Long-chain acylcarnitines were significantly associated with death, but there was no association for the 24 uremic solutes measured, including p-cresol sulfate, indoxyl sulfate, ADMA, and TMAO. The different results across these studies may relate to whether free or total solute levels were measured, how outcomes were defined, differences between incident and prevalent dialysis patients, and differences in duration of follow-up.

Importantly, examining the association between uremic solutes and hard clinical endpoints overlooks symptoms as a fundamental feature of uremia that require elucidation. As already noted, improving HRQoL is a major priority for patients with ESRD, and it is possible (or even likely) that the solutes responsible for chronic end-organ toxicities are different from the solutes that cause uremic symptoms. To date, the study of individual solutes (or the metabolome) in relation to uremic symptoms has received far less attention than studies of mortality, in part because of the challenge of quantifying symptom burden. One study used scores on validated tests of executive function to identify several metabolites associated with impaired cognitive function in ESRD.[82] Leveraging similar test or survey-derived measures may provide an opportunity to more systematically study the association between solutes and symptoms in uremia.

Although linking solutes with clinical outcomes is of interest, it is insufficient to prove causality. Confounding variables may underlie the association between select solutes and outcomes, and there are no studies demonstrating a benefit to reducing the solutes highlighted in Table 18.4. Mendelian randomization leverages human genetics to test the causality of associations between biomarkers and clinical outcomes.[83] The logic of this approach is illustrated by the two following examples. Plasma levels of C-reactive protein (CRP) have consistently been associated with CVD. If circulating CRP is deleterious, genetic variants that increase CRP levels would be expected to be enriched among individuals with CVD compared with individuals without CVD. In fact, genetic variants that modulate CRP levels have no association with CVD, arguing that CRP is only a marker of underlying atherosclerosis.[84] By contrast, genetic variants that increase LDL cholesterol levels are more common among individuals with CVD than individuals without CVD, consistent with LDL cholesterol's established causal role in atherogenesis.[85] Important preconditions for mendelian randomization analyses are that the genetic determinants of the biomarker of interest have been identified, that the genetic determinants have a clinically meaningful impact on biomarker levels, and that the genetic determinants only affect disease status via their effect on the biomarker. Because many uremic solutes are commonly measured in metabolomics studies of large, extensively genotyped cohorts, this approach may be used to test whether they are causally implicated in adverse outcomes. However, it is also possible that causal gene–biomarker–disease relationships established among individuals with normal kidney function will not be generalizable to ESRD. After all, despite incontrovertible evidence that LDL cholesterol causes CVD among individuals with normal kidney function, randomized clinical trials of statins among individuals with ESRD have shown no benefit despite substantial LDL lowering.[86,87] Similarly, negative (noncausal) gene–biomarker–disease results among individuals with normal kidney function may not rule out causality in ESRD. Uremic solute levels can be markedly elevated relative to normal, that is, orders of magnitude above the range of variation attributable to genotype; further, some uremic solutes may need to act in combination to exert toxicity. Thus, as a quintessential *acquired* disease state, uremia may be relatively sidelined from the causal inferences enabled by human genetics.

Potential Mechanisms of Solute Toxicity

In lieu of summarizing the extensive literature on uremic solutes that spans innumerable clinical, animal, and in vitro studies, we provide a general overview of different potential mechanisms of solute action in uremia. In some cases, the mechanisms outlined here may be overlapping or even redundant, but nevertheless are delineated to provide the reader with a nuanced perspective of uremic toxicity.

Direct Cellular Toxicity

As circulating molecules, uremic solutes have wide access to different tissues, with the potential to exert direct cellular injury. A common approach has been to test the effect of exogenous solute administration on cells or animals. P-cresol sulfate and indoxyl sulfate have been studied extensively, with studies demonstrating their ability to cause adverse effects on endothelial cells, smooth muscle cells, leukocytes, cardiomyocytes, renal tubular cells, and adipocytes, as well as in vivo in animal studies.[88] Readouts of interest have varied widely, including cell proliferation, cell senescence, fibrosis, and inflammation/oxidative stress (see later). Many of these experiments have been performed using free solute concentrations consistent with levels observed in ESRD, supporting their potential relevance to human uremia. The precise molecular mechanisms triggered by these solutes, however, is unclear.

Inflammation and Oxidative Stress

As noted, retention of select molecules, such as cytokines and AGEs, promote inflammation and oxidative stress in ESRD. Uremic solutes such a p-cresol sulfate and indoxyl sulfate may also contribute, with studies demonstrating their ability to increase leukocyte activation and adhesion, increase leukocyte free-radical production, enhance renal cell cytokine expression, and reduce endothelial cell glutathione levels.[88] To what extent the increase in inflammation and oxidative stress observed in ESRD is ultimately attributable to retained solutes, and hence might improve after reduction of their circulating levels is not known.

Hormonal Functions

Some retained middle molecules are hormones. Parathyroid hormone provides an example of both the magnitude and complexity of effects that elevated hormone activity can have in ESRD. Elevations in other hormones have drawn considerable interest in the pathogenesis of PEW. For example, leptin is frequently elevated in ESRD, in part because the kidneys play a significant role in its clearance.[36] Leptin is an adipocyte-derived peptide with broad effects, including in the hypothalamus where it acts to suppress appetite and increase energy expenditure.[89] Elevations in leptin, as well as cholecystokinin, des-acyl ghrelin, and visfatin, have all been correlated with anorexia in dialysis patients.[90-92] In mice, neutrophil gelatinase-associated lipocalin (NGAL) has also been shown to act in the hypothalamus to suppress appetite,[93] but elevations in serum NGAL appear to be inversely correlated with malnutrition in ESRD patients.[94]

Enzyme Inhibition

As substrates and products of defined biochemical reactions, some uremic solutes may exert toxicity by modulating specific enzyme actions. For example, ADMA is an endogenous inhibitor of nitric oxide synthase, preventing the synthesis of NO from arginine. Consistent with this, increasing or decreasing ADMA levels results in increased and decreased blood pressure in mice, respectively. Thus elevated ADMA is a potential mediator of the widespread endothelial dysfunction observed in ESRD.[95]

GPCR (G-Protein Coupled Receptor) Signaling

Traditionally, metabolites have been defined in terms of their intracellular bioenergetic functions. More recently, however, several metabolites have emerged as extracellular signaling molecules that can act as ligands at specific GPCRs, similar to many hormones.[96] For example, the citric acid cycle intermediate succinate binds GPR91 to modulate various physiological processes, including blood pressure, lipolysis, and cardiac hypertrophy in mice.[97] Similarly, gut microbe-derived short-chain fatty acids bind to Olfr78, a receptor expressed in the renal juxtaglomerular apparatus, to mediate renin secretion.[98] Kynurenic acid, an established uremic solute generated from tryptophan degradation, signals through GPR35 to modulate monocyte function.[99] Historically, research on uremic toxicity has focused on the most significantly elevated solutes; that some circulating metabolites have cognate cell-surface receptors raises the possibility that even relatively modest alterations in their levels may be biologically meaningful.

Central Nervous System Activity

The presence of organic ion transporters at the blood–brain barrier, in some cases the same as expressed in renal tubules,[100, 101] suggests that the two sites may act in concert to maintain very low levels of uremic solutes in the central nervous system.

In turn, accumulation of these compounds, in blood and cerebrospinal fluid, are hypothesized to alter mental status; although the identity of these neurotoxic compounds is unknown, solutes that undergo significant tubular secretion are attractive candidates.[102] Whether these compounds exert toxicity through direct tissue injury, by interfering with the transit of other compounds across the blood–brain barrier, by disrupting osmolarity, or by acting as false neurotransmitters (even if a given solute is not the natural ligand for a given neuroreceptor, it may have a biological effect at very high concentrations) is unknown.

Protein Modification

As already discussed, alterations of protein structure, such as glycation and oxidation, increase in uremia and may cause toxicity by altering protein structure and function, both in circulation and within tissues. Carbamylation is another covalent protein modification that has gained interest as a potential cause of uremic toxicity. Carbamylation results from the nonenzymatic reaction between free amino groups in proteins with cyanate, a dissociation product of urea. Thus it may provide a time-averaged indicator of urea concentration. Increased carbamylated serum albumin levels have been associated with an increased risk for death among both incident and prevalent hemodialysis patients.[103-105] Whether this represents chronic toxicity due to elevated urea levels or is a marker for some other process, such as inflammation, is unknown.

Tissue Deposition

Retention of β_2-microglobulin can result in its deposition as amyloid fibrils, particularly in bone and connective tissue, resulting in spondyloarthropathy, bone cysts, and carpal tunnel syndrome. Although the comparison of low-flux and high-flux dialyzers in the HEMO study did not demonstrate an overall difference in mortality, the widespread adoption of high-flux dialyzers in clinical practice has coincided with a reduction in the incidence of clinically overt dialysis-related amyloidosis. Calcium oxalate deposition in skin, heart, and other tissues has also been reported in ESRD (among individuals who do not have primary hyperoxaluria).[106]

Solute Depletion

Uremia is primarily a condition of small molecule excess, but reduced dietary intake, increased dialytic clearance, or loss of renal biosynthesis can result in the depletion of some solutes relative to healthy controls. Because carnitine is required for fatty-acid oxidation, its depletion has been hypothesized to contribute to skeletal and cardiac muscle dysfunction in ESRD. Carnitine supplementation, however, does not improve outcomes. Metabolomics studies expanding the list of metabolites depleted in ESRD may identify additional opportunities for therapeutic repletion.[74]

Although we highlight several mechanisms by which solutes may exert toxicity, decisive proof of causation for any given solute is lacking in humans. In some cases, uremic solutes associated with adverse outcomes in ESRD are unlikely to be directly toxic, but rather serve as markers of an underlying deleterious process. For example, an association between long-chain acylcarnitine levels and uremic cardiovascular risk may reflect the significance of underlying mitochondrial dysfunction, as these molecules deliver fatty acids across the mitochondrial membrane and are known to increase in blood secondary to inborn errors of mitochondrial β-oxidation.[81]

In summary, despite an expanding catalog of uremic solutes, the specific molecules responsible for the uremic illness are unknown. Proving causality in uremia is challenging for several reasons, including the multiplicity of solutes and symptoms and the lack of ideal model systems. Studies that seek to link uremic solutes with hard endpoints, such as CVD outcomes, may help prioritize among candidate toxins, but no unequivocal signal has emerged from these efforts to date. Further, these studies do not address the pathogenesis of uremic symptoms. Uremic solutes have the potential to exert toxicity through a wide range of mechanisms. Improved understanding of which solutes are toxic and why they are toxic is required to improve therapeutic options for uremia.

TREATMENT OF UREMIA

The treatment of ESRD encompasses a number of strategies to compensate for loss of kidney function. This includes control of extracellular fluid volume and inorganic ions, replacement of renal calcitriol and erythropoietin synthesis, and reduction of uremic solute levels. In this section, we will focus on the management of uremic solutes, considering both extracorporeal and nonextracorporeal approaches.

Extracorporeal Methods

Hemodialysis and peritoneal dialysis are the most widely used extracorporeal methods for the treatment of uremia. Both hemodialysis and peritoneal dialysis are prescribed to achieve a target urea clearance, recognizing that urea itself is not the cause of uremia and that its clearance on dialysis may not reflect that of other solutes. In general, large, protein-bound, and sequestered solutes are poorly removed by conventional dialysis. Approaches to increase clearance of large solutes such as β_2-microglobulin include the use of more permeable (high-flux) hemodialysis membranes and convection strategies such as hemofiltration and hemodiafiltration. Approaches to enhancing the clearance of protein-bound solutes, such as p-cresol sulfate and indoxyl sulfate, include increasing dialysate flow rate, dialyzer membrane surface area, and treatment duration. Removal of highly sequestered solutes requires increasing the frequency and duration of dialysis treatments.[107] Although each has theoretic merit, clinical trials to date have failed to demonstrate a conclusive benefit to these strategies.[29,68,108]

The failure of more intensive dialysis to improve outcomes does not necessarily argue against the toxicity of retained solutes, as increased clearance of uremic solutes has not consistently translated into large reductions in blood levels. For example, a 10-fold increase in β_2-microglobulin clearance using high-flux membranes only reduced plasma β_2-microglobulin levels by ~20% in the HEMO study.[109] Hemodiafiltration also reduced plasma β_2-microglobulin by 25% compared with low-flux hemodialysis but had minimal benefit in reducing β_2-microglobulin compared with high-flux hemodialysis.[110] A separate post hoc analysis of the HEMO study examined the effect of dialysis dose, as measured by urea clearance, on several small uremic solutes.[111] Compared with individuals achieving an spKt/V_{urea} of ~1.3, individuals who achieved a 30% higher spKt/V_{urea} of ~1.7 had only an ~11% reduction in indoxyl sulfate, ~9% reduction in TMAO, and no change in ADMA (+ 0.5%) or p-cresol sulfate (+ 2.2%), such that all remained significantly elevated compared with normal. Similarly, a post hoc metabolomics analysis of the Frequent Hemodialysis Network Daily (FHN) trial comparing 53 individuals who received standard thrice-weekly dialysis and 30 individuals who received six-times-per-week dialysis found that increased treatment frequency resulted in a mean 15% reduction in uremic solute levels, with no changes in p-cresol sulfate and indoxyl sulfate.[112] Smaller studies focused on p-cresol sulfate have shown that the removal of this protein-bound solute can be increased by 66% to 100% by increasing dialysate flow rate and dialyzer membrane surface area, but with no significant reduction in predialysis plasma levels.[113-115] This discrepancy between dialytic clearance and predialysis solute levels is incompletely understood. Reduced nonrenal solute clearance and increased solute production are possible mechanisms that could counteract the effects of dialysis intensification. Similar explanations have been invoked to explain why indoxyl sulfate and p-cresol sulfate levels are similar in hemodialysis and peritoneal dialysis patients, even though hemodialysis provides higher clearance of these solutes.[116] Other extracorporeal techniques for further enhancing solute removal (Table 18.5), such as newer membranes with greater permeability or adsorptive properties, remain experimental at this time and await confirmation that they can substantially reduce uremic solute burden.

Nonextracorporeal Methods

Given the challenge of recapitulating the efficiency of endogenous renal clearance via extracorporeal methods, nonextracorporeal therapies may be required to successfully treat uremic toxicity. For example, preclinical studies have targeted solute transporters in the kidney and heart to enhance renal excretion and reduce cardiac toxicity, respectively, but await demonstration of efficacy in human studies.[117,118] To date, most human studies have been devoted to reducing solute production, either by modifying diet or the gut microbiome. Increased dietary fiber, prebiotics, and an alpha-glucosidase inhibitor have all been shown to reduce microbiome-derived solutes such as p-cresol sulfate and indoxyl sulfate.[119-121]

TABLE 18.5 Conventional and Novel Therapeutic Options for Uremia

Extracorporeal Therapies	Nonextracorporeal Therapies
Conventional (increase time or frequency)	Colonic microbiome (probiotics, inulin, acarbose, fiber, ketoacids)[119-121,146-155]
Hemofiltration and hemodiafiltration[156-160]	Organic anion transporters (cardiac, renal)[117,118]
New membranes (permeability, surface area, biocompatibility)[161-167]	Oral adsorbents (AST-120)[125]
Adsorption (beads, microparticles)[167-184]	Antioxidants Antiinflammatory agents Specific uremic toxin antagonists

AST-120, an oral adsorbent, also lowers blood levels of these solutes, with smaller studies suggesting that it can slow the rate of CKD progression or improve malaise in CKD.[122,123] However, a large randomized control trial of 2035 CKD patients did not demonstrate a benefit in slowing progression to ESRD.[124] Among patients already on hemodialysis, AST-120 administration lowers uremic solute levels and is associated with lower inflammatory and oxidative stress markers, but its effect on hard clinical endpoints in ESRD have not been examined.[125,126]

Finally, some studies have directly targeted inflammation and oxidative stress in uremia. One trial randomized maintenance hemodialysis patients to oral antioxidant therapy, composed of a combination of tocopherols plus α-lipoic acid, or placebo. After 6 months, there was no difference in mortality or hospitalization, as well as no difference in biomarkers of inflammation or oxidative stress, contrary to an earlier positive study of vitamin E in dialysis patients.[127,128] In a smaller study not powered for clinical events, 4 months of coenzyme Q10 reduced plasma concentrations of F2-isoprostanes, a marker of oxidative stress.[129] To target inflammation, a pilot study randomized dialysis patients to subcutaneous injections of a recombinant IL-1 receptor antagonist or placebo. After 4 weeks, active treatment significantly reduced high-sensitivity CRP and IL-6 levels. These changes were accompanied by a significant increase in adiponectin levels, suggestive of a salutary effect on metabolism. Whether treatments directed toward inflammation and oxidative stress can improve survival requires additional long-term studies.

CONCLUSIONS

In the conclusion of their classic review on uremia, Meyer and Hostetter note that "Maintenance of life in patients without kidney function is a remarkable achievement of modern medicine. But current treatment with dialysis carries a high price and leaves a persistent burden of disability."[185] The pairing of these sentiments is exactly right. Despite real limitations, current approaches to extracorporeal solute removal help sick patients feel better and live longer, and it is important not to overlook these substantial gains while also acknowledging that there is more to be learned. Retained solutes remain the primary etiological suspect; although large trials of dialysis intensification have been negative, post hoc analyses demonstrate minimal impact of these interventions on uremic solute levels, leaving this fundamental hypothesis only partially tested. Emerging insights about the gut microbiome, previously unanticipated signaling roles for circulating metabolites, and the functional consequences of solute-induced protein modification have expanded the scope of uremia research and have outlined new therapeutic targets. As knowledge continues to expand on new solutes, their origins, and their potential mechanisms of toxicity, the development of effective treatments informed by this knowledge remains the defining challenge in the field.

A full list of references is available at www.expertconsult.com.

19

Timing, Initiation, and Modality Options for Renal Replacement Therapy

Matthew B. Rivara, MD, and Rajnish Mehrotra, MD, MS

OUTLINE

Chronic kidney disease (CKD), defined as a reduction in the level of estimated glomerular filtration rate (eGFR) to <60 mL/min/1.73 m^2 of body surface area, or by the presence of markers of structural or functional abnormalities of the kidney, affects a significant proportion of the population in the United States and across the globe.[1] Globally it is estimated that the prevalence of CKD of all stages is approximately 13%, with the majority of this burden comprising individuals with CKD stages 3 through 5 (i.e., eGFR <60 mL/min/1.73 m^2).[2] In the United States, the overall prevalence of CKD among the adult population is approximately 30 million individuals, and continues to grow annually.[3,4] Among this group are >670,000 US individuals with kidney failure requiring treatment with renal replacement therapy (RRT), defined as either dialysis or kidney transplantation.[5] Although from 2006 to 2012 the incidence rate for new cases of kidney failure requiring RRT, or end-stage renal disease (ESRD), leveled off for the first time in nearly two decades, the period from 2012 to 2014 again saw a rise in new ESRD cases. In 2014, the number of incident newly reported ESRD cases exceeded 120,000 for the first time. This included 106,097 individuals who initiated dialysis (either hemodialysis or peritoneal dialysis [PD]), and 3102 patients who received a preemptive kidney transplant.[5] This growth in new ESRD cases has translated into a doubling of the prevalent dialysis population in the United States over the past 20 years. A recent report from the Global Burden of Disease project indicates that the growth in the provision of maintenance dialysis seen in the United States has been mirrored by similar growth in many other parts of the world, in particular in Australasia, Asia, and western Europe.[6]

For patients with newly diagnosed kidney failure, the transition to RRT is a time characterized by exceptionally high risk for adverse outcomes. The mortality rate for patients with stage 5 CKD and ESRD approaches 20 per 100 patient-years, and the first 120 days after dialysis initiation represents the period of greatest risk, with an annualized mortality rate approaching 50%.[5,7] In addition, the ESRD transition period is characterized by increased risks for other adverse patient-important outcomes, including high rates of hospitalization, heart failure exacerbations, and new strokes.[8-10] Furthermore, ESRD care is extraordinarily costly to the US healthcare system.[11] In 2012 spending for ESRD patients in the United States exceeded $28 billion, representing 5.6% of total Medicare costs, although the ESRD population represents <1% of the total Medicare population.[12] For this plurality of reasons, optimizing the transition to ESRD care represents a critical challenge to the nephrology community, and one that encompasses timely and adequate preparation for RRT, as well as determining the appropriate timing for initiation of dialysis or kidney transplantation. In addition, optimizing the transition to ESRD also includes patient-centered modality selection and consideration of nondialytic conservative management of kidney failure. This chapter will review these important aspects of timing of RRT, selection of dialysis modalities, and transplantation for ESRD.

INDICATIONS FOR INITIATION OF DIALYSIS IN CHRONIC KIDNEY DISEASE

Nephrologists have long agreed on a number of "absolute" indications for initiation of maintenance dialysis in patients with advanced CKD.[13] These strong indications represent emergent life-threatening complications of kidney failure, and include electrolyte disturbances such as hyperkalemia refractory to medical management accompanied by electrocardiogram changes, severe metabolic acidosis, volume overload refractory to diuretic therapy and leading to respiratory compromise, and certain manifestations of the uremic syndrome including uremic pericarditis, uremic encephalopathy, or severe uremic nausea and vomiting.[14,15] The vast majority of patients with incident end-stage kidney failure, however, do not initiate RRT due to one of these classic and life-threatending complications.[16] Instead, the decision on the part of the nephrologist to recommend initiation of dialysis to a patient with advanced CKD is usually determined by a complex integration of clinical and laboratory data elements reflecting the fluid, electrolyte, hormonal, and metabolic abnormalities that develop as kidney function deteriorates. These elements include biochemical markers of filtration function such as serum creatinine and blood urea nitrogen concentrations, blood concentrations of other markers of uremia such as low blood hemoglobin, high serum phosphorus and parathyroid hormone concentrations, complications of fluid retention including hypertension and volume overload, and also includes assessment of physical examination signs and symptoms consistent with the uremic syndrome. In addition to the clinical manifestations of uremic stated previously, other frequent manifestations include fatigue, lethargy, anorexia, pruritis, sleep disturbances, bleeding diathesis associated with platelet dysfunction, memory impairment and other neurocognitive dysfunction, headaches, musculoskeletal pain, melanosis, muscle wasting, weight loss and protein-energy wasting (PEW), and sexual dysfunction.[17-21]

Adding to the complexity regarding optimal timing of initiation of dialysis based on assessment of uremic complications is uncertainty about which signs and symptoms of advanced kidney disease consistently improve with the start of dialysis, and whether such improvement may vary based on patient demographic or clinical characteristics.[22,23] A number of studies published over the past decade have indicated that patients undergoing maintenance dialysis suffer from a high prevalence and severity of residual physical, psychological, and emotional symptoms, and in many cases the symptom complex shares a high degree of similarity with the classic constituent components of the uremic syndrome.[24-26] In addition, although it was previously thought the uremic symptom complex did not consistently manifest until late stage 4 or stage 5 CKD, more recent data have suggested that uremic symptoms may present at earlier stages of CKD.[27,28] The central task of the nephrologist in assessing the optimal timing of initiation of dialysis for a patient with advanced CKD is to balance the risk for exposing the patient to complications of untreated kidney failure against the potential for harm from the dialysis procedure itself, along with the burden of dialysis therapy. Delaying the start of dialysis to too great a degree may lead to frequent hospital admissions or emergency department visits for uncontrolled hypertension, pulmonary edema, or hyperkalemia, or may lead to PEW, weight loss, and malnutrition.[29] Conversely, initiation of dialysis at too early a stage may expose the patient unnecessarily to complications of dialysis therapy. Potential mechanisms of harm from dialysis include hemodynamic fluctuations leading to regional cardiac wall motion abnormalities, potentially arrhythmogenic electrolyte flux, oxidative stress, or risk for infection related to dialysis access.[30-33] Finally, the significant and potentially adverse effect of daily or thrice-weekly dialysis treatments on patients' ability to work, travel, socialize, and accomplish other activities of daily living cannot be overstated.[34,35]

EVOLUTION OF CLINICAL PRACTICE GUIDELINES FOR INITIATION OF DIALYSIS

Given the inherent limitations of the subjective assessment on the part of clinicians of the presence of components of the uremic syndrome in patients with advanced kidney disease, there has long been an interest on the part of the nephrology community in identifying less subjective and more standardized guidelines for the timing of initiation of maintenance dialysis.[14,36,37] This interest and an underlying understanding of the importance of optimizing the transition to ESRD has led to the publication of numerous clinical practice guidelines for the timing of initiation of dialysis in patients with advanced CKD.

Past Kidney Disease Outcomes Quality Initiative Recommendations for Timing of Initiation of Dialysis

In the 1990s, in efforts to identify less subjective markers of uremia, a number of studies were carried out that highlighted the strong correlation between various markers of PEW and progression and outcomes of advanced CKD. These studies showed that not only did dietary protein intake decrease linearly with a decrease in native kidney creatinine clearance, but also that markers of PEW, such as serum albumin, at the time of dialysis initiation strongly predicted subsequent mortality risk.[36,38] Furthermore, it was demonstrated that dietary protein intake increased significantly over the first 3 to 6 months after initiation of dialysis, presumed secondary to at least partial correction of uremic toxicity.[39] These observations and others led to an early strong interest in objective measures of PEW as a complement to clinical assessment of uremia in timing initiation of maintenance dialysis in advanced CKD. In 1997 the Dialysis Outcomes Quality Initiative (DOQI, now Kidney Disease Outcomes Quality Initiative [KDOQI]), working group on dialysis adequacy released its first set of recommendations synthesizing many such observations about the association of advanced CKD with uremic PEW. In this early clinical practice guideline, the group recommended that patients with advanced CKD be advised to initiate some form of dialysis when the weekly renal Kt/V_{urea} falls <2, unless either edema free body weight is stable or increased, the normalized protein catabolic ratio is ≥0.8 g/kg of body weight per day, or there is an absence of clinical signs or symptoms attributable to remia.[40] This recommendation to assess patients' native kidney weekly renal urea clearance as the primary criterion used to determine when to initiate dialysis was based on expert opinion, and corresponded to a threshold of eGFR of approximately 10.5 mL/min/1.73 m^2. Nearly a decade later, in 2006, the KDOQI clinical practice guidelines for hemodialysis adequacy were updated to reflect a growing emphasis and understanding of the importance of focusing on patients' symptoms and functional status in determination of the optimal timing for dialysis initiation among patients with advanced CKD. The 2006 KDOQI guideline update omitted discussion of calculation of the weekly renal Kt/V_{urea}, reflecting contemporary changes in clinical nephrology that included widespread adoption of serum creatinine–based equations for estimation of glomerular filtration. Instead, the guideline stated that nephrologists should evaluate the benefits, risks, and disadvantages of initiation of RRT when patients reach stage 5 CKD, corresponding to an eGFR threshold of 15 mL/min/1.73 m^2.[41] Furthermore, the guideline recommended that certain clinical considerations or complications may prompt initiation of therapy *before* stage 5, including decline in functioning or patient well-being, gastrointestinal dysfunction, or weight loss/malnutrition.

Initiation Dialysis Early and Late (IDEAL) Trial

Although early clinical practice guidelines such as those written and published by KDOQI working group members provided recommendations to practicing nephrologists regarding thresholds of glomerular filtration at which to consider initiation of RRT, such recommendations were based on accumulated clinical experience and expert opinion of the members of the guideline committees rather than on the results of observational or interventional studies. During the first decade of the 21st century, numerous observational studies were conducted to investigate the association between eGFR at dialysis initiation with subsequent risk for adverse outcomes.[42-47] The results of these studies consistently demonstrated that initiation of RRT at higher levels of GFR calculated using serum creatinine-based estimating equations were associated with higher mortality risk. In contrast, studies employing timed urea or creatinine clearances rather than serum creatinine–based estimating equations to calculate GFR demonstrated little to no association with mortality risk.[48,49]

Given persistent uncertainty regarding the optimal timing for initiation of RRT in patients with advanced CKD, the results of the Initiation Dialysis Early and Late (IDEAL) trial, published in 2010, were welcomed by the nephrology community.[50] The IDEAL study was the first (and to date only) large randomized trial to study the effect of estimated glomerular filtration function at the time of dialysis initiation with subsequent patient-centered outcomes such as mortality, hospitalization, and health-related quality of life (HRQoL). The IDEAL study was conducted between July 2000 and November 2008, and ultimately enrolled 828 adults with advanced CKD, defined as an eGFR (calculated by the Cockcroft-Gault method) of <15 mL/min/1.73 m^2 body surface area. Patients were recruited from 32 centers in Australia and New Zealand and were randomized to initiation of dialysis at eGFR of 10 to 15 mL/min/1.73 m^2 ("early start") or eGFR of 5 to 7 mL/min/1.73 m^2 ("late start"). The median follow-up period was 3.6 years. Results of the primary analyses, published in a landmark paper in 2010, showed that there was no significant difference between the randomized groups in any clinically important outcome, including mortality, hospitalization risk, or cardiovascular events.[50] A follow-up economic analysis of the IDEAL study demonstrated no significant difference in overall healthcare costs or HRQoL between the treatment groups.[51]

The IDEAL trial, although groundbreaking and successful at bringing high-quality clinical trial data to bear on the question of the optimal time for initiation of maintenance dialysis in patients with advanced CKD, was not without a number of important limitations. Among patients randomized to the early-start group, approximately 20% initiated dialysis with eGFR <10 mL/min/1.73 m^2. Conversely, among individuals assigned to the late-start group, 76% started dialysis with eGFR >7 mL/min/1.73 m^2. The effect of these protocol deviations was that the difference in eGFR at the time of dialysis initiation between the two treatment groups was only 2.2 mL/min/1.73 m^2, which some commentators have identified as a major contributor to the trial's null results.[52-54] In addition, participants in IDEAL were predominantly white and with lower burden of coexisting medical illnesses compared with the typical patient with ESRD in the United States, raising a concern about generalizability of the IDEAL trial findings. Finally, the majority of patients in early-start treatment group in IDEAL initiated dialysis with PD, making comparisons difficult with ESRD patients in the United States, where >90% of patients are treated with conventional in-center hemodialysis, and >80% initiate dialysis with a central venous catheter (CVC). Notwithstanding these limitations, in the few short years since its publication, the legacy of the IDEAL trial has profoundly influenced clinical nephrology practice and clinical practice guidelines regarding the timing and initiation of maintenance dialysis in patients with advanced CKD.

Current Kidney Disease Outcomes Quality Initiative Recommendations for Timing of Initiation of Dialysis

As previously stated, the influence of the results of the IDEAL trial was profound. The interpretation of the IDEAL results by many nephrologists and commentators was that among asymptomatic patients with advanced CKD without clinical appearance of uremia or its various complications, initiation of dialysis may be safely postponed until signs, symptoms, or complications of uremia are evident. What follows from this interpretation, but what is less commonly discussed, is that dialysis should not be delayed in patients in whom adverse effects from chronic kidney failure have appeared simply

TABLE 19.1 Current Clinical Practice Guidelines (CPGs) on the Timing of Initiation of Maintenance Dialysis for Patients With End-Stage Renal Disease

Guideline	Statement
NKF-KDOQI (2015)[58]	The decision to initiate maintenance dialysis in patients who choose to do so should be based primarily upon an assessment of signs and/or symptoms associated with uremia, evidence of protein-energy wasting, and the ability to safely manage metabolic abnormalities and/or volume overload with medical therapy rather than on a specific level of kidney function in the absence of such signs and symptoms.
Canadian Society of Nephrology (2014)[60]	For adults (aged > 18 yr) with an eGFR of less than 15 mL/min/1.73 m^2, we recommend an "intent-to-defer" over an "intent-to-start-early" approach for the initiation of chronic dialysis. With the intent-to-defer strategy, patients with an eGFR of less than 15 mL/min/1.73 m^2 are monitored closely by a nephrologist, and dialysis is initiated with the first onset of a clinical indication or a decline in the eGFR to 6 mL/min/1.73 m^2 or less, whichever of these should occur first. Clinical indications for the initiation of dialysis include the following: symptoms of uremia, fluid overload, refractory hyperkalemia or acidemia, or other conditions or symptoms that are likely to be ameliorated by dialysis. In the absence of these factors, the eGFR should not serve as a sole criterion for the initiation of dialysis unless it is 6 mL/min/1.73 m^2 or less.
ERA-EDTA/ERBP Advisory Board (2011)[59]	In patients with a GFR <15 mL/min/1.73 m^2, dialysis should be considered when there is one or more of the following: symptoms or signs of uremia, inability to control hydration status or blood pressure, or a progressive deterioration in nutritional status. It should be taken into account that the majority of patients will be symptomatic and need to start dialysis with GFR in the range 9–6 mL/min/1.73 m^2. High-risk patients (e.g., diabetics and those whose renal function is deteriorating more rapidly than eGFR 4 mL/min/year) require particularly close supervision. Where close supervision is not feasible and in patients whose uremic symptoms may be difficult to detect, a planned start to dialysis while still asymptomatic may be preferred. Asymptomatic patients presenting with advanced CKD may benefit from a delay in starting dialysis in order to allow preparation, planning and permanent access creation rather than using temporary access.
KDIGO (2012)[1]	We suggest that dialysis be initiated when one or more of the following are present: symptoms or signs attributable to kidney failure (serositis, acid-base or electrolyte abnormalities, pruritus), inability to control volume status or blood pressure, a progressive deterioration in nutritional status refractory to dietary intervention, or cognitive impairment. This often but not invariably occurs in the GFR range between 5 and 10 mL/min/1.73 m^2.

CKD, Chronic kidney disease; *eGFR*, estimated glomerular filtration rate.
(Reprinted from Rivara MB, Mehrotra R. Timing of dialysis initiation – what has changed since IDEAL. *Semin Nephrol.* 2017;37(2):181-193. Copyright 2017, with permission from Elsevier.)

because the level of eGFR has not declined below a preconceived threshold.[15] Further observational studies published since IDEAL using advanced statistical methods such as casual inference modeling with inverse probability weights and marginal structural models have confirmed the results of IDEAL through examination of existing clinical cohorts and demonstration that there is no significant survival impact of initiation of dialysis at higher versus lower eGFR.[55-57]

The most recent iteration of the KDQOI guidelines for hemodialysis adequacy were published in 2015 and contain guidance for practicing nephrologists regarding the timing of dialysis initiation that reflect the message and lessons learned from IDEAL, as well as continued clinical experience and observational data from the past decade. These latest KDOQI guidelines recommend that rather than focusing on a specific level of kidney function, the decision to initiate maintenance dialysis should be based primarily on an assessment of attributable complications of kidney failure, including signs and symptoms of uremia, PEW, and development of metabolic or volume disturbances refractory to medical therapy (Table 19.1). Although straightforward at first glance, the authors of this guidance statement acknowledge that the subjective assessment of signs and symptoms attributable to kidney disease can be quite challenging in patients with multiple coexisting illnesses, many of which may cause systemic symptoms that may mimic the quality and severity of those caused by kidney failure.[58]

Other Clinical Practice Guidelines for Timing of Initiation of Dialysis

In addition to clinical practice guidelines published by the National Kidney Foundation (NKF) KDOQI working group on hemodialysis adequacy, numerous other guidelines have been published in recent years providing different perspectives and recommendations for clinicians facing the decision of when to recommend initiation of dialysis for their patients. The Kidney Disease Improving Global Outcomes (KDIGO) initiative released its own guideline in 2012 that, similar to the KDOQI guidance document, also endorses an approach to the timing of dialysis initiation that focuses on assessment of signs and symptoms attributable to kidney failure (see Table 19.1). Unlike KDOQI, the KDIGO guidance does identify a range of eGFR at which signs and symptoms of kidney failure are likely to appear (i.e., between 5 and 10 mL/min/1.73 m^2), but does not specifically recommend using this eGFR threshold as the basis for dialysis initiation.[1] Similarly, the European Dialysis

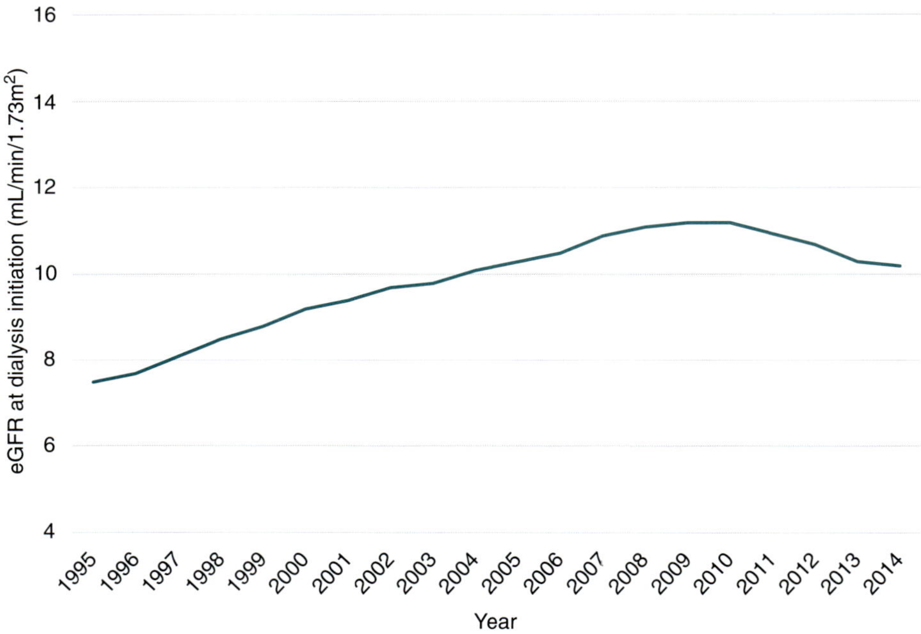

FIG. 19.1 Trends in mean estimated glomerular filtration rate at initiation of dialysis in the United States, 1995 to 2014. (Adapted from United States Renal Data System Annual Data Reports from 2007, 2010, 2013, 2015, and 2016.)

and Transplant Association updated its position statement in 2011 regarding timing of dialysis initiation, and although it provides a range of eGFR at which uremic symptoms are likely to appear, the guidance document specifically cautions against the use of eGFR as the primary guide to dialysis decision making (see Table 19.1).[59] In contrast, the Canadian Association of Nephrology's updated 2013 clinical practice guideline for timing the initiation of chronic dialysis identifies a threshold of 6 mL/min/1.73 m^2 as the absolute threshold below which dialysis should be initiated (see Table 19.1).[60] This threshold was determined through consideration of the median eGFR targeted in the "late-start" arm of the IDEAL trial.

TRENDS IN TIMING OF INITIATION OF DIALYSIS

From the mid-1990s through the end of the first decade of the 21st century, the mean eGFR at dialysis initiation for patients with incident ESRD in the United States rose steadily from 7.7 mL/min/1.73 m^2 to a peak of 11.2 mL/min/1.73 m^2 in 2009 (Fig. 19.1).[5] Evidence from population-based cohort studies in Canada and Europe has revealed a similar trend of increasing eGFR at dialysis initiation over that period outside of the United States as well.[11,61,62] Although definitive evidence regarding the cause of these secular trends is lacking, there are multiple potential contributing factors. First, before the clinical trial results from IDEAL, conventional wisdom was that earlier use of dialytic clearance to complement native kidney clearance would provide enhanced clearance of uremic toxins that were associated with adverse cardiovascular outcomes, improved control of metabolic complications of advanced kidney disease, and further prevent hospitalizations related to volume overload as extracellular volume accumulated.[63] The assumption was that such enhanced clearance and volume control would undoubtedly translate into improved patient-centered outcomes, such that earlier dialysis was indicated for most patients. Further potential contributing factors may have included changes in the demographic makeup of the ESRD population areound the world, implementation of automated reported of eGFR by laboratory facilities around the world, and changes in the predialysis practice characteristics such as duration of predialysis nephrology care and presence of a permanent dialysis access.[64-67]

The year 2010 represented an inflection point in the secular trend of eGFR at dialysis initiation for patients with incident ESRD in the United States. From 2010 through 2014, the mean eGFR at dialysis initiation has decreased from 11.2 mL/min/1.73 m^2 to 10.2 mL/min/1.73 m^2, its lowest point since 2004.[5] Although representing a small absolute change in mean GFR, this fall marks a shift from the inexorable upward trend seen over the preceding two decades. Although data are limited, evidence from international data sources suggests that such recent shifts in practice have occurred outside the United States as well.[68] The basis for these changing trends are uncertain and likely numerous, but have mirrored the publication and widespread dissemination of the results from the IDEAL trial as well as the revisions to clinical practice guidelines for timing of dialysis initiation that were discussed earlier in this chapter.

We recommend a patient-centered approach to dialysis initiation decision making that incorporates broad assessment of a patient's clinical status including markers of metabolic and volume complications of advanced kidney disease, the presence of uremic signs and symptoms, as well as incorporation of patients' values and preferences regarding RRT (Fig. 19.2). Our recommendation is in line with the most recently revised KDOQI

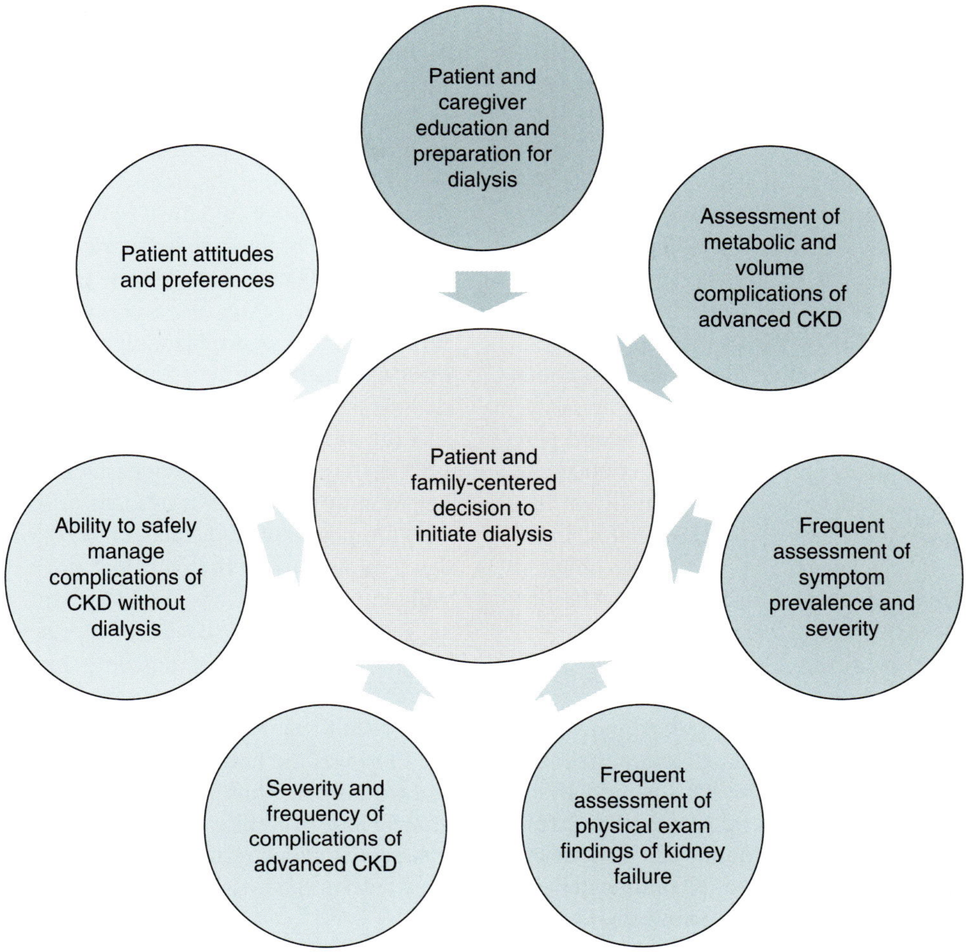

FIG. 19.2 An example of a comprehensive patient-centered approach to decision making regarding timing of dialysis initiation.

guidelines. Furthermore, we agree with the KDOQI guidelines that clinicians should avoid using a specific level of eGFR as a threshold for recommending that patients initiate dialysis. A reasonable approach is to defer initiation of dialysis until the development of signs and symptoms that could reasonably by attributed to kidney failure, and which would be likely to improve with the initiation of dialysis. It is important to recognize that such symptoms may not be overt, and patients may adapt to a lower level of functioning without conscious recognition of this adaptation. Similarly, patients may experience the effects of PEW leading to weight loss and malnutrition without recognition, and thus clinicians should be vigilant in frequent assessment of weight and functional capacity. To adopt this approach, patients must be seen and assessed by the clinician on a frequent and ongoing basis, and the principles of shared decision making should be employed to ensure that the decision of whether and when to start dialysis is patient- and family-centered.

PREPARATION FOR RENAL REPLACEMENT THERAPY

Timeliness of Nephrology Referral

A critical component of optimizing the transition from medical management of advanced kidney disease to the initiation of RRT is timely referral to a kidney specialist. Unfortunately, in the United States, available data show that only 30% of incident ESRD cases received care from a nephrologist before the onset of ESRD of >12 months.[5] Nearly 25% of all patients with incident ESRD never saw a nephrologist before the initiation of RRT. Racial and ethnic disparities in late referral also are evident, with blacks and Hispanics less likely to have had pre-ESRD care than whites and non-Hispanic individuals.[12] Late referral to a nephrologist has been found to be an independent risk factor for early death on dialysis, even after adjusting for demographic and healthcare utilization factors.[69] Conversely, earlier nephrology referral has been associated with lower mortality and hospitalization, greater uptake of home dialysis modalities, lower utilization of CVCs at dialysis start, and better HRQoL.[70,71] The KDIGO recommendations for referral of patients to specialist kidney care services for individuals with CKD include referral for an abrupt or sustained fall in GFR, eGFR <30 mL/min/1.73 m^2, persistent albuminuria, or in whom the risk for kidney failure within 1 year is >10%.[1] We recommend that early predialysis nephrology care be the goal for most individuals with stage 3 or greater CKD, in particular for individuals with evidence of progressive loss of kidney function,to allow adequate medical and psychosocial preparation for the initiation of RRT.

Predialysis Chronic Kidney Disease Education

Current KDOQI and KDIGO guidelines suggest that dialysis-related education should begin at stage 4 CKD, allowing adequate preparation for consideration of initiation of RRT once patients develop signs or symptoms consistent with kidney failure, generally when patients reach stage 5 CKD. Dialysis-related education should include dietary counseling, education regarding different RRT options including preemptive kidney transplantation, vascular or PD access options, and consideration of the psychosocial and medical effects on the patient of the transition to ESRD. We also recommend consideration of maximum conservative management without provision of dialysis. CKD patient education programs have been shown to be associated with greater objective and perceived kidney disease knowledge by patients, higher uptake of home dialysis modalities, better self-reported quality of life, and survival after dialysis initiation.[72-77] CKD education initiatives empower patients, facilitate patient- and family-centered shared decision making, and embrace current national health-care priorities for care to be patient-centered.

Timing of Dialysis Access Placement

The most recent NKF KDOQI clinical practice guidelines suggest that all patients should have a functional permanent access at the initiation of dialysis therapy.[41] For hemodialysis, this means timely placement of an arteriovenous (AV) fistula or AV graft. For patients planning to initiate PD, this means timely placement of a PD catheter. Current recommendations are for an AV fistula to be placed at least 6 months before the anticipated start of hemodialysis, with the goal to allow adequate time for fistula maturation and the potential for access intervention and revision of necessary. An AV graft should be placed at least 6 weeks before the anticipated start of hemodialysis, although in many cases grafts can be used sooner than this conservative estimate. A PD catheter should ideally be placed at least 2 to 4 weeks before the anticipated need for initiation of dialysis to allow for adequate time for healing and to avoid the risk for pericatheter leaks. An alternative strategy for PD access is to implant a PD catheter far in advance of the anticipated need for dialysis, but instead of leaving a portion of catheter externalized, this portion is embedded under the skin in the subcutaneous space. When kidney function declines and the patient is felt to have a clinical need to initiate dialysis, this portion of the catheter is exeernalized through a small skin incision allowing immediate use of the catheter for full-volume PD exchanges. Studies have demonstrated that PD catheters can be embedded for prolonged periods and still result in functional dialysis access at the time the patient requires initiation of RRT.[78,79]

Unfortunately, notwithstanding current clinical practice guideline recommendations, >80% of patients initiating hemodialysis in the United States were using a CVC rather than a permanent AV access, a figure that has remained steady for more than a decade. A large body of literature has demonstrated that the use of CVCs for dialysis access is associated with greater risk for adverse clinical outcomes, including higher risk for hospitalization, infection-related morbidity, cardiovascular events, and mortality.[80-84] The United States and Canada have higher rates of catheter use at dialysis initiation than other industrialized countries, despite multiple vascular access initiatives implemented over the past two decades aimed at increasing the use of permanent AV access and decreasing the use of CVCs for dialysis access.[81,85,86] Most notably, the Fistula First Breakthrough Initiative (FFBI) was jointly developed and implemented by the Centers for Medicare & Medicaid Services and the ESRD networks with the goal to encourage AV fistulas as the primary vascular access for ≥50% of all new patients initiating maintenance hemodialysis, and to reduce the prevalence of catheter use for >90 days to <10% of prevalent hemodialysis patients.[85] However, recognition over the past 5 years that the proportion of incident ESRD patients using catheters for dialysis access remains persistently and unacceptably high has recently led to a shift in focus of the FFBI to include not only promotion of AV fistulas, but a coprimary aim of discouraging catheter use in both incident and prevalent hemodialysis patients.[87] This shift has coincided with a growing literature suggesting that for particular subgroups of patients (in particular the elderly), AV graft outcomes may equal those achieved by patients using AV fistulas, in part due to the high rate of primary fistula maturation failure in these groups.[88-91] Recently, the FFBI was the Fistula First Catheter Last (FFCL) Coalition as a symbol of its shifting focus. In contrast to the 2006 KDOQI guidelines for vascular access, the FFCL Coalition has recommended fistula placement ≤12 months before the anticipated need for hemodialysis initiation.

Timing of Referral for Kidney Transplant Evaluation

Preemptive kidney transplantation is considered the preferred method of RRT for the majority of patients, given the well-demonstrated improved morbidity, mortality, and patient-reported outcomes in transplant recipients compared with those undergoing dialysis.[92,93] Wait times from listing to transplantation vary considerably in the United States based on patient characteristics and geography, and in some areas can approach 10 years. The median wait time nationally is approximately 4.5 years.[94] Thus we believe that all patients with advanced kidney disease should be considered by their providers for early kidney transplant evaluation. Although there are a few agreed-upon absolute contraindications to kidney transplantation, such as active malignancy and severe active cardiovascular disease, inclusion and exclusion criteria for patients vary widely between transplant programs. Thus we believe that referral for transplant should be the default plan for most patients with advanced CKD. In general, all patients with stages 4 and 5 CKD (i.e., with eGFR <30 mL/min/1.73 m^2) are appropriate for referral. In some select cases of patients with rapidly progressive CKD, referral at even higher levels of eGFR may be appropriate.

DIALYSIS MODALITY SELECTION

The choice of dialysis modality should be based on the principle of patient-centeredness, and should be made via shared decision making among the patient, family members and other caregivers, and the provider. Such decision making should incorporate patient values and preferences, clinical appropriateness, and local and regional availability of dialysis modality options. As previously reviewed, early predialysis CKD education should incorporate review of different dialysis modalities so that patients can make informed decision regarding dialysis modality, if preemptive kidney transplantation is not an option. Options for RRT modalities, including in-center dialysis, home dialysis modalities, and kidney transplantation, are reviewed next.

IN-CENTER DIALYSIS MODALITIES

Conventional In-Center Hemodialysis

In 2014 approximately 88% of all patients with incident ESRD in the United States began RRT with conventional in-center hemodialysis.[5] This figure has decreased somewhat since 2010, largely due to the increase in the proportional use of home dialysis modalities. The vast majority of patients treated with conventional center-based hemodialysis are treated three times weekly for between 3 and 4.5 hours per session.[95] Recent data suggests that patients in facilities routinely initiating hemodialysis with session durations of ≥4 hours may have substantially lower mortality relative to patients dialyzing in facilities where initial treatment times are 3 hours.[96] A typical conventional hemodialysis prescription uses a high-flux dialyzer, standard blood flows of between 300 and 450 mL/min, and standard dialysate flows of between 500 and 800 mL/min. Patients initiating in-center hemodialysis may start with one or more shorter runs with lower blood and dialysate flows to prevent complications associated with rapid changes is blood solute concentrations, including development of the dialysis disequilibrium syndrome. With adequate preparation, patients initiating RRT with conventional in-center hemodialysis can safely start dialysis at an outpatient dialysis facility rather than in the inpatient setting.[16,97]

Extended-Hours Dialysis

Recently, an increasing number of patients with ESRD in the United States have been able to gain access to in-center extended-hours hemodialysis, a modality consisting of substantially longer treatment times than conventional thrice-weekly in-center hemodialysis. Extended-hours dialysis has been used for decades by groups in Canada and Europe, with observational studies from these centers reporting higher than expected survival and, in particular, excellent control of blood pressure with low rates of use of antihypertensive medications.[98,99] Although there is no established definition of extended-hours hemodialysis, patients are typically treated three times per week for between 6 and 10 hours per session. In most cases, patients are treated overnight while they sleep at the dialysis facility. Thus many investigators and clinicians have termed this *nocturnal in-center hemodialysis*. Recent observational data suggests that extended-hours hemodialysis is associated with a 25% to 45% lower risk for mortality than conventional in-center hemodialysis, and is further associated with a lower risk for hospitalization.[100-102] In addition, patients undergoing extended-hours hemodialysis have lower serum phosphorus and lower blood pressures than in-center hemodialysis patients.[100,102] However, extended-hours hemodialysis does increase the burden of dialysis treatment for patients, and it is currently uncertain as to what degree this is outweighed by improved clinical outcomes.

FREQUENT IN-CENTER HEMODIALYSIS

Frequent in-center hemodialysis consisting of conventional dialysis session durations delivered typically five to six times weekly is used for some patients with ESRD. Similar to extended-hours hemodialysis, frequent in-center hemodialysis consists of substantially longer total weekly dialysis treatment times than conventional thrice-weekly in-center hemodialysis. Interest in frequent in-center hemodialysis originally stemmed from observational studies in the first decade of the 21st century showing an association with better laboratory and patient-reported outcomes.[103] In addition, the results from the landmark National Institutes of Health-funded Frequent Hemodialysis Network (FHN) Daily Trial showed that in-center hemodialysis six versus three times a week was associated with an improved composite outcome of death and change in left ventricular mass or death and change in a physical-health composite score.[104] Interest in frequent in-center hemodialysis has been tempered somewhat by the recognition that frequent treatment is also associated with an increase in vascular access complications requiring intervention, as well as an increase in the burden of treatment on the lives of patients living with ESRD. In addition, the recently published ACTIVE trial, which randomized patients with ESRD to extended-hours (≥24 h/wk) or standard hemodialysis (12–15 h/wk) for 12 months, found no effects of extending weekly hemodialysis hours through increasing session duration and/or frequency on overall HRQoL scores.[105]

HOME DIALYSIS MODALITIES

Peritoneal Dialysis

PD has been available as a therapy for chronic kidney failure since the refinement of the PD catheter for permanent peritoneal access by Tenchkoff in the 1960s.[106] PD involves infusion of dialysate into the peritoneal space such that salt, water, toxins, and other solutes can be dialyzed out of the body using the peritoneum as the dialysis membrane. There are a variety of forms of PD, the most common of which are continuous ambulatory PD (CAPD) and automated PD (APD). In CAPD, patients or their caregivers perform manual fills and drains of the abdomen generally three to five times daily, with 2 to 2.5 L of dialysate. In APD, which includes continuous cycling PD, patients use an automated cycler machine overnight to perform exchanges often while sleeping, with no to two daytime manual exchanges for additional solute and water clearance. In contrast to ultrafiltration accomplished via mechanical means as in hemodialysis, ultrafiltration in PD is accomplished using an osmotically active substance in

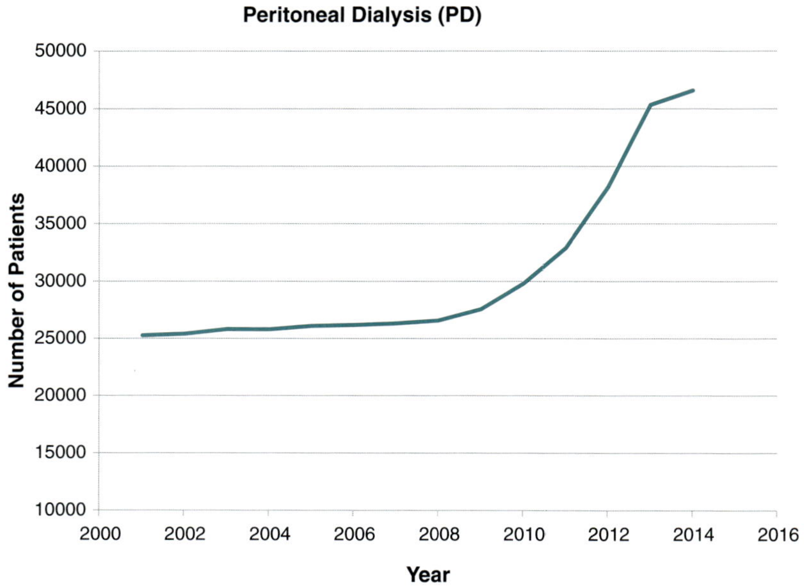

FIG. 19.3 Prevalence of use of peritoneal dialysis in the United States, 2001 to 2014. (Adapted from United States Renal Data System Annual Data Reports from 2007, 2010, 2013, 2015, and 2016.)

the dialysate, which acts to pull water and solute across the peritoneal membrane into the peritoneal space. In the United States, this osmotically active substance is either dextrose in varying concentrations (generally 1.5%, 2.5%, or 4.25%), or icodextrin, a starch-derived glucose polymer that is much more slowly absorbed relative to dextrose. Addiitonally, in areas outside of the United States, PD solutions using amino acids to compensate for protein losses are available for use in clinical practice.[107]

The past decade has seen a remarkable resurgence in interest in and adoption of PD by both incident and prevalent dialysis patients in the United States (Fig. 19.3). In 2008, <7% of the total prevalent dialysis population were treated with PD. By 2014, this number had risen to nearly 10%, representing >46,000 patients across the United States.[5] The majority of studies conducted over the past 15 years that have sought to compare clinical outcomes among patients treated with PD and those treated with conventional in-center hemodialysis have either demonstrated no difference in overall survival, or in some cases a lower risk for death in patients treated with PD.[108-111] Treatment with PD also is associated with higher satisfaction with care and higher HRQoL than conventional in-center hemodialysis.[112,113] However, studies show that only between one- and two-thirds of incident ESRD patients are presented with PD as a modality option.[114,115] We recommend that all medically eligible patients with advanced CKD be educated about home dialysis modality options, including PD. For many patients, PD has the potential to enhance patient-centeredness of care by encouraging self-management and allowing flexibility in travel and work, and furthermore can potentially reduce overall healthcare costs.

Home Hemodialysis

Like PD, home hemodialysis has seen a remarkable resurgence in growth over the past decade in the United States. In 2006 there were <1700 patients undergoing home hemodialysis in the United States, representing only 0.7% of the total US dialysis population. In 2014 the last year for which there are data available through the USRDS, >8500 patients were treated with home hemodialysis, making up nearly 2% of the US dialysis population (Fig. 19.4). Although the absolute number of patients treated with home hemodialysis remains substantially less than the number of individuals treated with either conventional hemodialysis or PD, the proportional growth of home hemodialysis over the past decade is the greatest of any dialysis modality. Multiple factors have contributed to the recent growth in adoption of home hemodialysis in the United States, including the advent of simple-to-operate home systems such as the NxStage System One machine and a growing body of literature suggesting that patients undergoing home hemodialysis have similar or better outcomes than patients treated with conventional in-center hemodialysis.[116-120]

Home hemodialysis can be performed using conventional dialysis equipment, typically with the aid of a trained dialysis helper. Modifications to patients' home plumbing and electrical system typically need to be made to ensure that traditional reverse osmosis water systems can be installed and work properly. Dialysis schedules with conventional home hemodialysis typically mimic those for in-center patients. Alternatively, patients dialyzing at home using conventional equipment may choose to perform nocturnal home hemodialysis three or more times per week for 6 to 8 hours nightly using low dialysate and blood flows. Frequent nocturnal home hemodialysis has been shown to result in improved phosphate, reduced left ventricular mass, better blood pressure control, and higher HRQoL than thrice-weekly hemodialysis, at least over the short term.[121,122] Since the advent of the NxStage System One machine, which employs a low dialysate flow and volume approach using a patient-friendly interface, an increasing number of patients are being treated with short

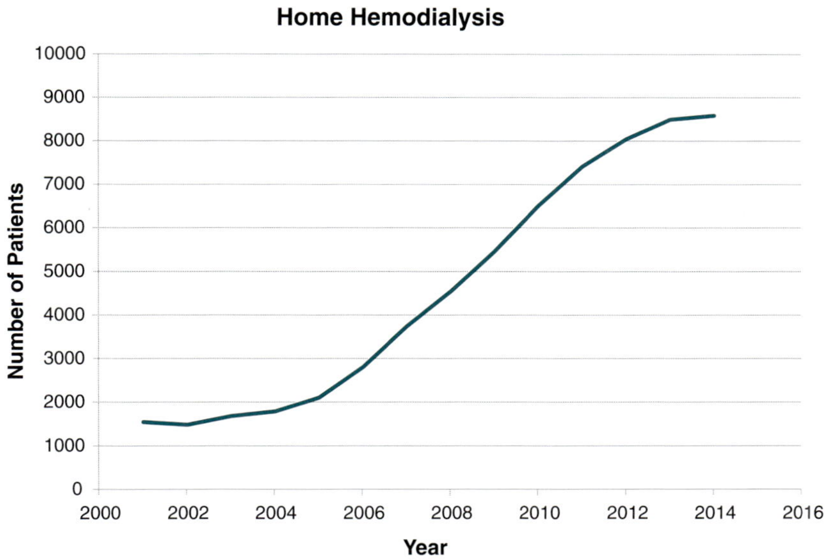

FIG. 19.4 Prevalence of use of home hemodialysis in the United States, 2001 to 2014. (Adapted from United States Renal Data System Annual Data Reports from 2007, 2010, 2013, 2015, and 2016.)

daily home hemodialysis, in which they undergo dialysis for ≥2 hours 5 to 6 days per week. The shorter sessions associated with short daily home hemodialysis can allow patients to fit their dialysis treatments to their daily schedules, even varying on and off times from day to day to maximize flexibility and autonomy.

TRANSPLANTATION

Kidney transplantation remains the preferred method of RRT for patients approaching the need for dialysis, as well as those currently undergoing dialysis, whether in-center or at home. Relative to dialysis, kidney transplantation is associated with better survival for all patients, regardless of race or underlying comorbid conditions.[123] As of 2014, >200,000 individuals in the United States were living with a functioning kidney transplant, an increase in 2.9% from the prior year.[5] The overall probability of 1-year survival for deceased-donor kidney transplant recipients exceeds 95%, and for living-donor recipients approaches 99%.[5] However, access to kidney transplantation continues to be limited by the number of deceased-donor kidneys available (12,328 in the United States in 2014) as well as by the lack of availability of living donors.[5] Fewer than 6000 kidney transplants using living-donor kidneys were performed in the United States in 2015. Given these factors, the number of patients on the waitlist in 2017 for kidney transplantation (>96,000) far exceeds the supply of donor organs.[94] Living-donor transplantation affords the best long-term patient and graft survival, and the transplant community continues to promote the importance of kidney donation. Donors may be related, unrelated, or altruistic. Increasingly, transplant centers are employing methods such as paired kidney exchange or even longer kidney transplant chains to increase the availability of live-donor organs for transplantation for patients living with advanced CKD or ESRD.[124]

In 2014 the kidney allocation system in the United States underwent a major change with the stated purpose to decrease racial/ethnic disparities in kidney transplantation and to promote longevity matching between kidney transplant donors and recipients. As part of this overhaul, the Kidney Donor Profile Index (KDPI) was introduced, replacing the previous system of categorization of donors as standard criteria or extended-criteria donors (ECDs). Similarly, the KDPI implemented a score for potential kidney recipients called the Expected Post-Transplant Survival (EPTS) score, with the goal of matching patients with the best EPTS scores to donor organs with the best KDPI scores, thus promoting longevity matching. The new kidney allocation system also gives increased priority for "sensitized" patients with a high burden of panel-reactive antibodies, who may have experienced extremely long wait times under the older system. Although early reports suggest that the new allocation system has resulted in higher rates of transplantation to blacks, younger, and sensitized patients, with similar overall graft and patient survival, the full effect of the new system is not yet evident.[125]

CONCLUSIONS

The population of individuals with kidney failure requiring the initiation of RRT in the United States and around the world continues to grow. The optimal timing for the initiation of maintenance dialysis in patients with incident ESRD is currently unknown. Data from the IDEAL study have challenged the established paradigm of using eGFR as the primary guide for initiation of dialysis, and recently published clinical practice guidelines now emphasize the importance of a patient-centered approach to dialysis decision making based primarily on the assessment of signs and symptoms attributable to kidney failure and the ability to medically manage metabolic and volume complications of advanced kidney disease. Options for RRT for patients with established ESRD include in-center hemodialysis, home hemodialysis, PD, and kidney transplantation. Preemptive kidney transplantation remains the preferred method of treatment for ESRD, but a large and growing imbalance exists between the supply of donor kidneys and the number of patients approaching and living with ESRD. Finally, home dialysis modalities, including both PD and home hemodialysis, have seen resurgent growth in the United States over the past decade, but remain underused. Home dialysis modalities are associated with equivalent or better patient-centered clinical outcomes compared with conventional in-center hemodialysis, and may enhance patient-centeredness of ESRD care through promoting patient self-management, autonomy, and independence.

ACKNOWLEDGMENTS

Some data reported in this chapter have been supplied by the United States Renal Data System (USRDS). The interpretation and reporting of these data are the responsibility of the authors and in no way should be seen as an official policy or interpretation of the US government. Dr. Rivara is supported in part by funding from the Extramural Grant Program (EGP) by Satellite Healthcare, a not-for-profit renal care provider.

A full list of references is available at www.expertconsult.com.

20

Ethical Challenges and the Role of Palliative Care in Kidney Disease

Michael J. Germain, MD, and Lewis M. Cohen, MD

OUTLINE

"The moral unity to be expected in different ages is not a unity of standard, or of acts, but a unity of tendency. ... At one time the benevolent affections embrace merely the family, soon the circle expanding includes first a class, then a nation, then a coalition of nations, then all humanity, and finally, its influence is felt in the dealings of man with the animal world."

Weh Lecky 1869.[1]

ETHICAL PRINCIPLES

Medical ethics derive from the basic concept of human ethics. The word *ethics* is derived from the Greek word *ethos*, meaning "custom." Accordingly, medical ethics are a set of changeable principles for what is considered "good, right or wrong behavior".[1a]

Ethics addresses the fundamental question, "How should I live my life?"

Ethics are based on accepted standards of behavior. For example, in virtually all societies and cultures, it is wrong to kill or steal property from someone. These standards have developed over time and have been memorialized in religious, philosophical, and legal thought.

Moral standards are based on emotions and reason and lead to altruism. Altruism is likely a genetically based drive developed through evolution. For example, when a hunter/gatherer kills or gathers a large amount of food, that person will share it with the group rather than waste the food. Over time there was an evolutionary advantage to this behavior. [2]

Bioethics speak to how we, as medical personnel, treat our patients. In Western (and increasingly global) society, the accepted principles are autonomy, justice, beneficence, and nonmaleficence (Boxes 20.1 and 20.2).

Autonomy, especially in the United States, is a core value. But even this principle is strained when the question of euthanasia or physician-assisted suicide/dying is discussed. Interestingly, preservation of life at all costs is not a principle of medical ethics, so there are no medical ethical issues raised by these death-hastening practices. Withholding or withdrawing dialysis can similarly be viewed in this context.

MEDICAL ETHICS IN NEPHROLOGY

The renal replacement therapy of dialysis is one of the first life-sustaining treatments and since its inception, nephrology has had to consider the ethics of withdrawing or withholding life support. The dilemmas that early nephrologists had to deal with are discussed in depth by Blagg in his 1999 article about the Seattle "selection committee."[3]

After dialysis became more universally available in the United States, ethical dilemmas shifted from justice (who will get a scarce resource?) to nonmaleficence (who will be more likely to be harmed than to benefit?). The Clinical Practice Guideline "Shared Decision-Making in the Appropriate Initiation of and Withdrawal from Dialysis"[4] (The Guidelines) were the first comprehensive attempt to provide an ethics-based guideline for nephrology's difficult decisions. We will refer to the guidelines where we mention "Recommendations."

In the second edition of the Guidelines (2010), the authors state: "Ethical decisions should be analyzed by means of four topics: medical indications, patient preferences, quality of life (QoL), and contextual features (i.e., the social, economic, legal, and administrative context in which the decision occurs). Every case can be viewed in terms of these four topics; no case can be adequately discussed without reference to them" (see Box 20.2).

BOX 20.1 Six Medical Ethics Principles

1. Respect for autonomy: The patient has the right to refuse or choose their treatment (voluntas aegroti suprema lex).
2. Beneficence: A practitioner should act in the best interest of the patient (salus aegroti suprema lex).
3. Nonmaleficence: "First, do no harm" (primum non nocere).
4. Justice: Concerns the distribution of scarce health resources and the decision of who gets what treatment (fairness and equality).
5. Respect for persons: The patient (and the person treating the patient) has the right to be treated with dignity.
6. Truthfulness and honesty: The concept of informed consent.

From http://en.wikipedia. org/wiki/Medical_ethics#Values_in_medical_ethics.

BOX 20.2 The 7-Step Process of Ethical Decision-Making in Patient Care

1. **What are the ethical questions?**
2. **What are the clinically relevant facts?**
3. **What are the values at stake?**
4. **List options.** What could you do?
5. **What should you do?** Choose the best option from the ethical point of view.
6. **Justify your choice.** Refer back to the values and give reasons why some values are more important in this case than others.
7. **How could this ethical issue have been prevented?** Would any policies/guidelines/practices be useful in changing any problems with the system?

A recent Kidney Disease: Improving Global Outcomes (KDIGO) Controversies Conference, Supportive Care in Chronic Kidney Disease: Developing a Roadmap to Improving Quality Care,[5] endorsed the Guidelines and expanded them globally.

ESTIMATING PROGNOSIS

Although all patients with a potentially life-threatening disease should engage in advance care planning (ACP), it is helpful for programs to prioritize these discussions for patients with a poor prognosis. Estimating prognosis for a 6- to 12-month time frame has been studied as a way to facilitate ACP.[6-8] We systematically discuss goals of care and completing advanced directives such as Physician Orders for Life-Sustaining Treatment (POLST) with the top quintile 6-month mortality risk of our population. We use a clinically useful tool to identify high-risk hemodialysis patients with limited prognoses. The tool was validated in the dialysis population,[9] and a mobile app is available (https://qxmd.com/calculate/calculator_135/6-month-mortality-on-hd).

Estimating prognosis is not meant to predict the future for any given patient. Instead, it is used to identify patients who are at high risk for early death, and more importantly for frequent and extended hospitalization with often-unnecessary invasive procedures. Although a patient may not want to know a "number" in terms of risk for early death, studies have shown that they do want to be told their "prognosis."[10] Often, that means an honest explanation by the doctor of what the patient is likely to experience in the near future in terms of medical complications (Box 20.3).

BOX 20.3 Suggested Steps for Implementing Recommendation 3

- For ESRD patients, estimate prognosis based on patient's age, functional status, medical condition, including comorbidity and recent sentinel events, and the "surprise" question. The website http://touchcalc.com/calculators/sq provides a calculator for use of the surprise question response and other variables to estimate prognosis in dialysis patients. The same degree of precision does not exist for tools that estimate prognosis for patients with AKI.
- Present the prognosis in a manner that is considerate of the patient's emotional condition. Balance the patient's desire for QoL and length of life and provide reassurance that the physician has kept the patient's best interest in mind. With the patient's permission, strongly encourage the patient's legal agent/family to participate in the discussion of prognosis and treatment options. See Recommendation 10 for suggested approaches to discussing prognosis, treatment options, and goals of care with AKI, CKD, and ESRD patients.
- Identify the patient's wishes and goals for treatment at the onset of dialysis and again after any irreversible change in medical condition.
- For ESRD patients, reassess and communicate prognosis on at least an annual basis, and more often as indicated by any major change in status.
- For CKD and ESRD patients, during each annual Comprehensive Assessment and Plan of Care discussion, communicate appropriate options based on the patient's condition, prognosis, and goals for care. Regardless of choice, palliative care should be offered for pain and symptom management and advance care planning. Hospice referral is appropriate for ESRD patients stopping dialysis.
- Provide recommendation to withhold/stop dialysis in patients who are not likely to benefit.
- If conflicts arise in shared decision making, consider palliative care or ethics consultation (see Recommendation 8).

ADVANCE CARE PLANNING

ACP has progressed since the days when dialysis and do not resuscitate (DNR) orders were felt to be incompatible and withdrawal from dialysis was considered suicide. ACP is now a condition of coverage in dialysis facilities. POLST, also known as Medical Orders for Life-Sustaining Therapy (MOLST), or its equivalent form, is legal in all but one state (polst.org/programs-in-your-state/).

Normalizing and starting these discussions early in the disease process is considered a key part of the comprehensive clinical management of patients with CKD.[11-13] Staff

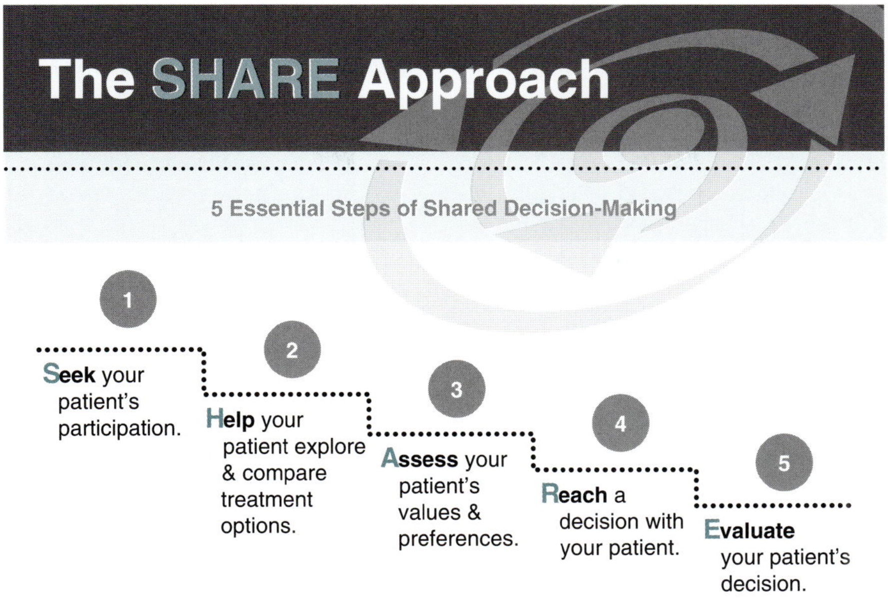

FIG. 20.1 The steps for shared decision-making.

members in dialysis facilities experience time restrictions, and the most pragmatic approach to initiating such conversations entails taking advantage of the team approach.[14-16] For example, the Patient-Centered Outcomes Research Institute (PCORI) sponsored a study at Baystate Medical Center and the University of New Mexico Medical Center to assess how dialysis social workers and nephrologists can be trained to collaboratively deliver ACP.

SHARED DECISION-MAKING

Shared decision-making is recognized as the preferred approach to medical management. It involves the patient and their family/loved ones/legal healthcare proxy. The patient (or their proxy if they lack decision-making capacity) first must be engaged to share their values, goals, and the things that are important to them (Fig. 20.1). They also need to determine who they want involved in their care and in decision-making. In some cultures, the patient will defer the decisions and discussion to a family member (Boxes 20.4 and 20.5).

In the field of nephrology, shared decision-making is especially complex because of the option for life-sustaining therapy with dialysis in ESRD and acute kidney injury (AKI). The Guidelines make clear that not all patients should receive dialysis when they reach ESRD or when they have AKI: **Recommendation 5.**

If Appropriate, Forgo (Withhold Initiation or Withdraw Ongoing) Dialysis for Patients with AKI, CKD, or ESRD in Certain, Well-Defined Situations.

These situations include:

- Patients with decision-making capacity who, after being fully informed and making voluntary choices, still refuse dialysis or request that dialysis be discontinued.
- Patients who no longer possess decision-making capacity but who previously indicated refusal of dialysis in an oral or written advance directive.
- Patients who no longer possess decision-making capacity and whose properly appointed legal agents/surrogates refuse dialysis or request that it be discontinued.
- Patients with irreversible, profound neurological impairment such that they lack signs of thought, sensation, purposeful behavior, and awareness of self and environment.

Recommendation 6

Consider Forgoing Dialysis for AKI, CKD, or ESRD Patients Who Have a Very Poor Prognosis or for Whom Dialysis Cannot be Provided Safely

Included in these categories of patients are:

- Those whose medical condition precludes the technical process of dialysis because the patient is unable to cooperate (e.g., advanced dementia patient who pulls out dialysis needles) or because the patient's condition is too unstable (e.g., profound hypotension).
- Those who have a terminal illness from nonrenal causes (acknowledging that some in this condition may perceive benefit from and choose to undergo dialysis).
- Those with stage 5 CKD older than 75 years of age who meet two or more of the following statistically significant very poor prognosis criteria (see **Recommendations 2 and 3**): (1) clinicians' response of "No, I would not be surprised" to the surprise question; (2) high comorbidity score; (3) significantly impaired functional status (e.g., Karnofsky Performance Status score less than 40); and (4) severe chronic malnutrition (i.e., serum albumin less than 2.5 g/dL using the bromocresol green method).

CONFLICT RESOLUTION

Often there can be disagreement among the stakeholder as to what the care plan should be. The nephrologist might recommend against dialysis treatment believing that dialysis would

BOX 20.4 Suggested Steps for Implementing Recommendations 1 and 2

- Identify provider(s) who will coordinate communication with the patient or legal agent and family (e.g., nephrologist in conjunction with the primary care provider for ESRD patients or intensivists for AKI).
- Assess patient decision-making capacity and whether it is diminished by major depression, encephalopathy, or other disorder (see Tool 4 in Section 9: Tool Kit for helpful instruments). Obtain psychiatric and/or neurological consultation as appropriate, and institute treatment for conditions impairing decision-making capacity.
- Communicate diagnosis to patient (or legal agent) and family (if the patient agrees).
- Discuss prognosis based on patient's medical condition, comorbidities, functional status, and age (see Tools 6-1–6-3 in Section 9: Tool Kit for tools for assessing functional status and quality of life, and estimating prognosis).
- Identify the patient's wishes.
- Communicate options, taking advantage of educational resources such as other patients or videotapes and brochures.
- If the patient wants to forgo dialysis, determine why.
  - Are the patient's perceptions about dialysis accurate? Does the patient know what to expect if dialysis is not started or is discontinued?
  - Does the patient really mean what he or she says or is the decision to refuse or stop dialysis made to get attention, help, or control?
  - Are there changes that might improve quality of life and would the patient be willing to start or continue dialysis while the factors responsible for the patient's request are addressed?
  - Are there persons (e.g., social worker, chaplain) with whom the patient would be willing to discuss the decision?

(Also, see Tool 8-2 in Section 9: Tool Kit for NKF checklist on withdrawing dialysis.)

- Reach decision based on medical indications and patient's preferences.
- Encourage patient to discuss end-of-life issues with others such as family, friends, or spiritual advisors (see Tool 5-1 in Section 9: Tool Kit for helpful questions to use).
- Refer for palliative care and hospice as appropriate.

BOX 20.5 Developing Goals of Care and Advanced Care Planning (ACP)

- Assess decision-making capacity (see Tool 4-1 in Section 9: Tool Kit).
- Include ACP in the Comprehensive Assessment and Plan of Care for each individual patient.
- Inform dialysis patient of his or her right to complete an advance directive and of the dialysis facility's policy with regard to advance directives as required by the 2008 Conditions for Coverage.
- Encourage patient-centered ACP among patients and families; raise the issue of ACP with each patient at the initiation of dialysis (earlier is preferred) and on at least a yearly basis. Hospitalizations and/or significant changes in medical, physical, or functional status should prompt reconsideration of ACP.
- Discuss ACP by asking:
  - If you become unable to make decisions for yourself, whom do you want to make decisions for you?
  - If you had to choose between being kept alive as long as possible regardless of personal suffering or living a shorter time to avoid suffering, which would you choose?
  - Under what circumstances, if any, would you want to stop dialysis?
  - If your heart stops beating or you stop breathing, would you want to allow a natural death?
  - Under what circumstances, if any, would you not want to be kept alive with medical means such as cardiopulmonary resuscitation, a feeding tube, or mechanical ventilation?
  - Where do you prefer to die and who do you wish to be with you when you die?
- Determine whether the patient has an appointed legal agent through a written advance directive.
- If the patient lacks decision-making capacity and has not completed an advance directive, arrange for or initiate the process for appointing a surrogate according to state law.
- Encourage patients to be specific about their preferences with legal agent, family, friends, and providers.
- Document provider's discussion and understanding of patient's preferences, show the patient the documentation, and offer to assist the patient in documenting the patient's agreement or modification of the documentation. Where available, complete a Physician Orders for Life-Sustaining Treatment (POLST) or similar form to translate patients' wishes into medical orders (see www.polst.org).
- Place a copy of advance directives, DNR order card, and/or POLST form in multiple medical records as appropriate, including dialysis facility, commonly attended clinics, hospital, nursing home, and home.
- Encourage the patient, family, and/or legal agent to carry a current copy of the patient's advance directive, DNR order card, and/or POLST form whenever traveling or being admitted for overnight medical care.

result in more harm than benefit to the patient. An example is a patient with advanced dementia who would be emotionally and physically distressed by dialysis treatment without any appreciation of the benefits. The family may understandably want dialysis because they do not want the patient to die, but staff may justifiably object to administering treatment that causes suffering. The Guidelines have excellent recommendations for conflict resolution **(Recommendation 8)** (Box 20.6; Fig. 20.2) in such complex cases.

In some instances, the Guidelines call for initiation of a time-limited trial **(Recommendation 7)**. It is recommended that the duration of the trial be understood by all parties and

BOX 20.6 Suggested Steps for Implementing Recommendation 8

Engage in extended conversation for either request for dialysis when not recommended or refusal of dialysis when recommended:

- Why does the patient or legal agent desire dialysis when it is not recommended by the renal care team?
- Does the nephrologist misunderstand the patient's or legal agent's reasons for requesting dialysis?
- Does the patient or legal agent misunderstand the diagnosis, prognosis, and treatment alternatives and why dialysis is not recommended?
- Why does the patient or legal agent refuse dialysis when it is recommended by the renal care team?
- Is the patient's refusal of recommended dialysis based on an accurate understanding of the likely benefits of dialysis?
- Is the patient's refusal of recommended dialysis consistent with the patient's values and goals?
- Does the nephrologist understand the psychosocial, cultural, or spiritual concerns and values the patient or legal agent has?
- Has the nephrologist consulted a psychologist, social worker, or chaplain for assistance in fully understanding the concerns of the patient or legal agent/family? Have strategies in the Decreasing Provider Patient Conflict project been used as appropriate? (http://esrdnetworks.org/resources/special-projects/copy_of_DPPCProviderManual.pdf)

For circumstances in which the patient/legal agent requests dialysis when it is not recommended, the following process may be helpful to resolve the conflict:

- Consult with other physicians.
  - Do other physicians agree or disagree with the attending physician's recommendation to withhold or withdraw dialysis?
  - Is the request for dialysis by the patient or legal agent medically appropriate?
- Consult with an ethics committee or ethics consultants.
  - Has the patient or legal agent been informed that the purpose of the ethics consult is to clarify issues of disagreement, and ideally, to enable resolution?
  - Has the patient or legal agent met with the ethics committee or ethics consultants to explain their perspective and reasoning behind their request for dialysis?
  - Can the ethics committee identify the reasons why the patient or legal agent is resistant to the physician's recommendation to forgo dialysis?
  - Can the ethics committee identify the reasons why the healthcare provider is resistant to the patient's or legal agent's desire to begin or continue dialysis?
  - Has the ethics committee explained in understandable terms to the patient or legal agent its conclusions and the reasoning behind them?
  - Can the impasse be resolved with accommodation, negotiation, mediation, or a time-limited trial of dialysis?
- Document.
  - The physician must document the medical facts and his or her reasons for the recommendation to forgo dialysis and the decision not to agree to the request by the patient or legal agent.
  - The consultants also should document their assessment of the patient's diagnosis, prognosis, and their recommendations in the chart.
- Attempt to transfer the patient's care.
  - If reconciliation is not achieved through the above procedure and the physician in good conscience cannot agree to the patient or legal agent's request, the physician may ethically and legally attempt to transfer the care of the patient to another physician.
  - Another physician and/or institution may not be found who is willing to accept the patient under the terms of the family's request. Physicians and institutions that refuse to accept the patient in transfer and their reasons should also be documented in the medical record.
- Consider consultation with a mediator, extramural ethics committee, or the ESRD network in the region.
- Request regional ESRD network to assist with arranging dialysis.
- Notify the patient, legal agent, and/or family.
  - If no other physician or institution can be found in the community or region by the treating nephrologist to provide dialysis as requested, the physician may inform the patient or legal agent that the nephrologist will cancel the patient's dialysis orders and the dialysis center will no longer provide dialysis to the patient. The nephrologist is obligated to give the patient sufficient advance notice and the names and addresses of other nephrologists and other dialysis facilities in the area.
- Communicate options.
  - The options of filing a grievance with the ESRD network (chronic patients only) or seeking legal or regulatory recourse by the patient or legal agent should be communicated.

that milestones be agreed upon in advance. If the milestones are not met by the end of the trial, dialysis is discontinued. Ideally a written "contract" is signed by the parties.

If the clinician feels that dialysis will result in more harm than good or that the situation meets the criteria for withholding dialysis outlined in the Guidelines, the clinician should not feel obligated to order dialysis even if requested by the family (Guideline Recommendations 5–8).

Providing Supportive (Palliative) Care

A generally accepted definition of supportive care is "Care given to improve the quality of life of patients who have a serious or life-threatening disease. The goal of supportive care is to prevent or treat as early as possible the symptoms of a disease, side effects caused by treatment of a disease, and psychological, social, and spiritual problems related to a disease or its treatment. [It is] also called comfort care, palliative care, and symptom management."[17]

Supportive care is not focused on extending or shortening the length of time until death occurs. It is informed by the concept of death as a natural and inevitable process. The goal is to allow death to happen on the patient's and family's terms and to provide symptom relief and maintenance of the best QoL possible. The concept of supportive care grew

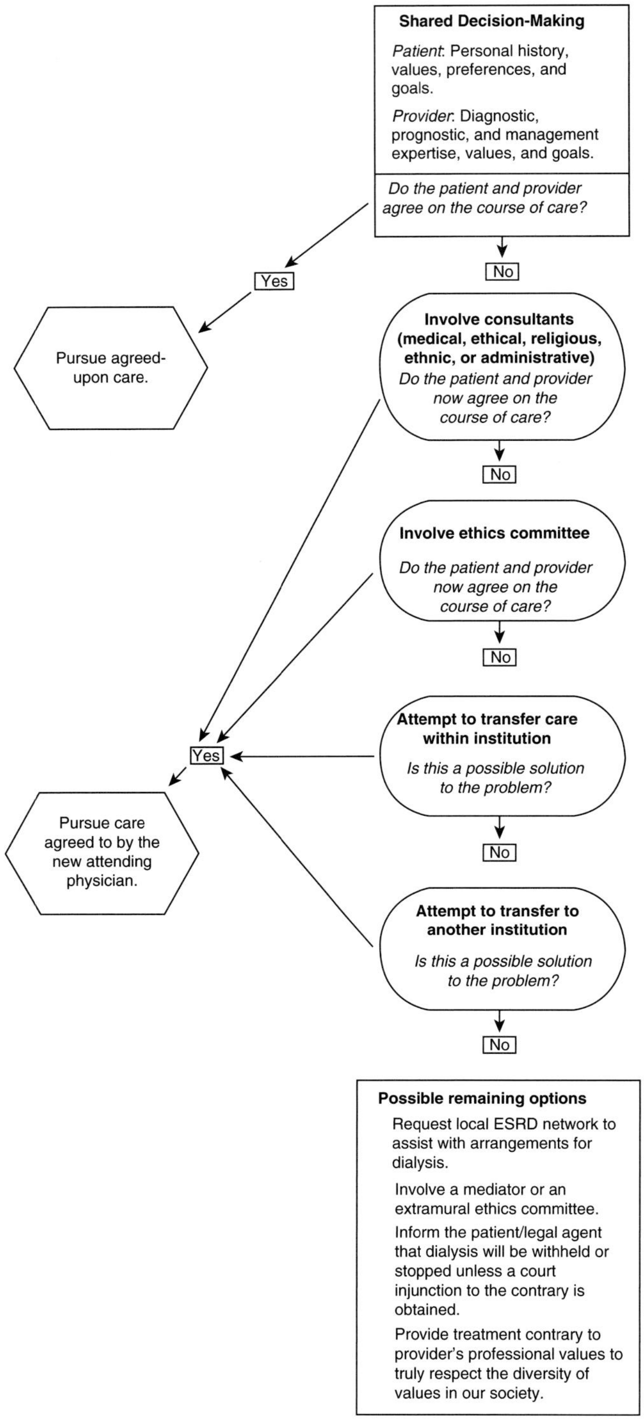

FIG. 20.2 Suggested steps for conflict resolution.

out of the realization that traditional palliative care services could be provided throughout the patient's disease and could be used alongside restorative/curative treatments (Fig. 20.3; Box 20.7). An example is the use of supportive care in conjunction with dialysis. The renal replacement therapy of dialysis can sometimes be viewed as a "palliative" treatment. Some studies have shown that supportive care can result in longer survival.[18]

Renal supportive care has been based on the work of the Robert Wood Johnson Foundation's (RWJF) Promoting Excellence in End of Life Care Program.[19] RWJF supported the nephrology community in developing key work products and sustained these programs in the community. RWJF funding to Baystate Medical Center facilitated the formation of a model program.

The following principles are outlined:

1. Symptom assessment and treatment algorithms
2. Estimating prognosis, ACP, shared decision-making, communication skills, cultural sensitivity
3. Transition to end-of-life (EOL) care including withdrawal from dialysis, conservative management, and hospice
4. Imminent EOL symptom management
5. Spiritual/existential support
6. Memorial–bereavement programs

(Boxes 20.8 and 20.9)

The work products for these initiatives and other resources are found at the Coalition for Kidney Supportive Care (http://www.kidneysupportivecare.org/Home.aspx). Many excellent programs have been developed around the world, in particular in the United Kingdom, Australia, and western Canada. Educating providers in communication skills to facilitate ACP and EOL care also have been championed through the NephroTalk project. The Guidelines have likewise been incorporated into an iPad app that allows providers to work through the steps for conservative management, withdrawal from dialysis, and EOL care (http://www.kidneysupportivecare.org/Files/Press-Release-for-SDM-App-2014-final.aspx).

Chapter 5 has a detailed discussion of many of these topics.

End-of-Life Care

Conservative care is common in the United Kingdom and Australia, and is becoming more available in the United States and Canada. Research suggests that conservative management in elderly patients with comorbidities does not result in any significant decrease in survival and can result in better QoL and dialysis.[20-22]

An early investigator of dialysis withdrawal received death threats because some felt this was the equivalent of physician-assisted suicide or murder (personal communication, Carl Kjellstrand, MD). Withdrawal from dialysis has been well studied,[23-26] and recent US Renal Data System data show an increasing incidence of withdrawal over the past 16 years. Patients older than 85 years of age have close to a 40% withdrawal rate from dialysis, which raises the question of whether dialysis may not have been the appropriate choice for many of these patients.[25] Withdrawal has been shown to be compatible with a good death[26] (see Box 20.9), especially when hospice care is provided.[27-31] The flow chart in Fig. 20.4 is a guide, and more resources are available at the Coalition for Supportive Care for Kidney Patients website.[31]

Use of time-limited trials of dialysis have not been well studied but are recommended by the Guidelines.[32,33] Time-limited trials are performed when there is equipoise between the clinician, patient, and family as to whether dialysis will do more harm than good. If a time-limited trial is contemplated, agreement should be documented as a written contract with milestones and a firm timeline that is agreed upon by all parties (Box 20.10).

"Palliative dialysis,"[34,35] although controversial, is an option when dialysis withdrawal or not starting dialysis are not the best choices. Palliative dialysis is prescribed for the patient with

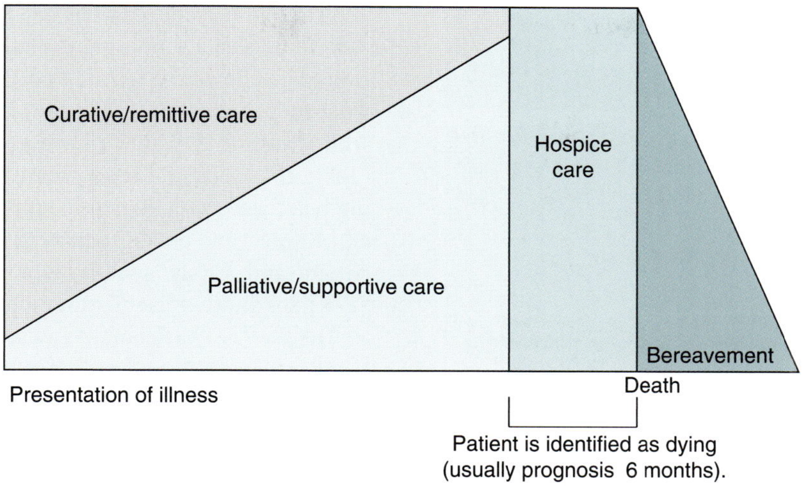

Conceptual framework for supportive care in chronic kidney disease (CKD).

FIG. 20.3 A model for supportive care.

BOX 20.7 Principles of a Renal Palliative Care Program

1. Identify patients who would benefit from palliative care interventions.
   a. Those who are being managed medically, i.e., a glomerular filtration rate ≤15 mL/min/1.73 m^2 with no dialysis.
   b. High risk for death within the next year. Consider using an integrated prognostic model (see Tool 6-1 in Section 9: Tool Kit) and/or the "surprise" question, "Would I be surprised if this patient died in the next year?"
2. Screen for and manage pain and other physical symptoms routinely.
   a. A simple tool such as the Edmonton Symptom Assessment Scale (ESAS) is appropriate and has been validated in CKD. See also Tools 9-1 and 9-2 in Section 9: Tool Kit.
3. Screen for and manage emotional, psychosocial, and spiritual distress; refer to allied health professionals as appropriate.
   a. The ESAS is also appropriate for screening for anxiety and depression.
   b. A simple question such as "Do you have any spiritual needs or concerns that your healthcare providers may help address?" may be appropriate for screening for spiritual distress.
4. Assess patients' desire for prognostic information.
5. Enhance predialysis education.
   a. Educate regarding active medical management without dialysis option as appropriate.
   b. Describe available palliative care and hospice services.
6. Provide routine advance care planning as described in Recommendation 5.
   a. Ensure patients and families are aware of the relevance of these discussions (i.e., have an understanding of their overall health state and prognosis).
   b. Consider initiating advance care planning at the time that patients are being educated with respect to renal replacement options.
   c. Include discussions of patients' goals of care, health states for which the patients would no longer want dialysis, and preferred location of death.
   d. Establish a surrogate decision maker.
   e. Ensure that family and other important people (as identified by the patient) are present for these discussions, especially the surrogate decision-maker.
7. Increase access to specialist palliative care, including hospice.
8. Develop relationships with hospice providers that focus on transition of care from dialysis to hospice, bridging patients into hospice by decreasing frequency of dialysis treatments, and having the patient be in control of when they are ready to stop palliative dialysis.
9. Provide bereavement support to patients' families where necessary.
10. Incorporate palliative care training for all nephrology fellows with an emphasis on symptom management, advance care planning, and communication about prognosis and treatment options.

a limited prognosis where the benefits of dialysis (living longer) outweigh the risks and harms. Instead of aiming for a KT/V of 1.2 to 1.4 as is the standard of care, the dialysis time and frequency are prescribed according to the patient's choice and comfort. It may be twice-weekly or less, or treatment time may be shortened. An example of palliative dialysis would be the patient with cancer who wants to remain alive as long as possible and is balancing a poor prognosis with the benefits and hardships of dialysis.

Hospice care is underused in dialysis patients but for the past 10 years has been used more frequently.[29,31,36,37] The hospice Medicare benefit can be provided concurrently with the ESRD Medicare benefit only if there is a separate hospice diagnosis such as cancer or terminal heart disease. In practice, there are considerable barriers to receiving a hospice benefit when patients wish to continue their maintenance dialysis. Although the Medicare hospice benefit can be paid concurrently with the Medicare ESRD benefit, this is not always easy to arrange because of the requirement for a terminal illness diagnosis distinct from that of ESRD.[37] "Medicare patients can receive care under both the ESRD benefit and the hospice benefit. The key is

BOX 20.8 A Systems Approach in Developing a Renal Supportive Care Program

1. Normalize ACP and EOL discussion in the dialysis unit and office. All members of the team should feel comfortable discussing these issues with patients and family. Teach simple communications skills.
2. Start discussion early in the disease process.
3. Have a champion.
4. Integrate into the workflow.
5. Carry out continuous quality improvement on the process.
6. Learn best practices from other programs and adapt to your site.

BOX 20.9 Expected Outcomes of Good Supportive Care

- Enhance patient and family understanding about their illness and end-of-life issues, including prognosis and likely outcomes of alternative plans of care.
- Define the particular patient's key priorities in end-of-life care and develop a care plan that addresses these issues and identifies the patient's overall goals of care.
- Enhance patient autonomy by shaping future clinical care to fit the patient's preferences and values.
- Improve the process of healthcare decision-making generally, including (1) patient and family satisfaction with the advance care planning process; (2) healthcare provider understanding of advance care planning and advance directives; and (3) provider comfort in participating in advance care planning.
- Help patients find hope and meaning in life and achieve a sense of spiritual peace.
- Explore ways to ease the emotional and financial burdens borne by patients and families.
- Strengthen relationships with loved ones.
- Complete written advance directives, particularly those identifying a legal agent, do not resuscitate documents, and POLST documents where available.
- Honor advance directives, do not resuscitate orders, and POLST orders at the end of life.

whether or not the services are related to ESRD. If the patient's terminal condition is not related to ESRD, the patient may receive covered services under both the ESRD benefit and the hospice benefit. Hospice agencies can provide hospice services to patients who wish to continue dialysis treatment. However, remember that when services are being provided to the beneficiary, that in the physician's opinion would extend the prognosis past 6 months, the beneficiary would not be considered eligible to receive services under the Medicare hospice benefit."[37]

Doctor–Patient/Family Communication

Patient–clinician communication is at the core of providing shared decision-making and palliative care to patients. It is part of an expert skill set needed for the nephrologist to develop and maintain. Several methods have been developed and studied.[38] NephroTalk is a nephrology-specific program. Ask-Tell-Ask is a simple guide that emphasizes that the patient should be allowed to talk first and tell the healthcare provider what they understand, what they want to know, and how and with whom they want to have a shared decision discussion (Table 20.1). NURSE is another valuable mnemonic reminding healthcare providers to Name the emotions, Understand and Respect the patient perspective, Provide Support for the patient and family, and Explore the emotions (Table 20.2). SPIKES is another useful mnemonic (Boxes 20.11 and 20.12).

The Renal Physicians Association, American Society of Nephrology (https://www.asn-online.org/education/distancelearning/curricula/), National Kidney Foundation, and KDIGO have encouraged the employment of supportive care in the comprehensive management of patients with CKD, and many resources are currently available to help clinicians obtain necessary skills and knowledge (http://www.kidney-supportivecare.org/Home.aspx). Guidelines also are available that detail processes to develop a sustainable program.[39,40] There also are robust, ongoing research programs throughout the world. In the United States, the PCORI currently is sponsoring a number of research projects.[41]

Symptom Assessment and Treatment

Key to supportive/palliative care is symptom assessment and treatment. Patients with advanced CKD, especially ESRD, are highly symptomatic both in terms of the number of distressing symptoms and their severity. Dialysis, and particularly kidney transplant, ameliorates symptoms, but many remain burdensome. In hemodialysis patients, the symptoms that are most prevalent and interfere with QoL are fatigue (71%); pruritus (55%); and anorexia, pain, anxiety, sleep disturbances (all 50%). Pain, when present, is moderate to severe in 82% of these patients.[16] Depression is very common (27%) and has significant overlap with the prevalent symptoms.[42] These symptoms correlate with mortality and poor QoL.[43] The Edmonton Symptom Assessment System a simple, short tool that is well validated in ESRD patients.[44] Once the problematic symptoms are identified, there are excellent evidence-based algorithms for treatment (Box 20.13). Advances in management of pruritus, a very prevalent and distressing symptom,[45] are actively being tested and likely soon to be available for use.[46]

Pain management needs to be adapted for the impaired clearance of many pain medications in CKD.[47] The World Health Organization's pain ladder has been modified for CKD[48-50] (Fig. 20.5; Table 20.3). Cannabinoids are poorly studied but may be safe and effective for chronic pain and do not have adverse effects in CKD patients. Finally, at the end of life, patients with CKD have special palliative care needs related to volume overload and uremic symptoms[51,52] (see Box 20.13).

Summary

Since its inception, the specialty of nephrology has compelled ethicists to grapple with the complex issue of artificially prolonging life after organ failure. In turn, bioethics has had a profound effect on the field and nephrologists have needed to be flexible as dialysis went from being rationed to being legislated

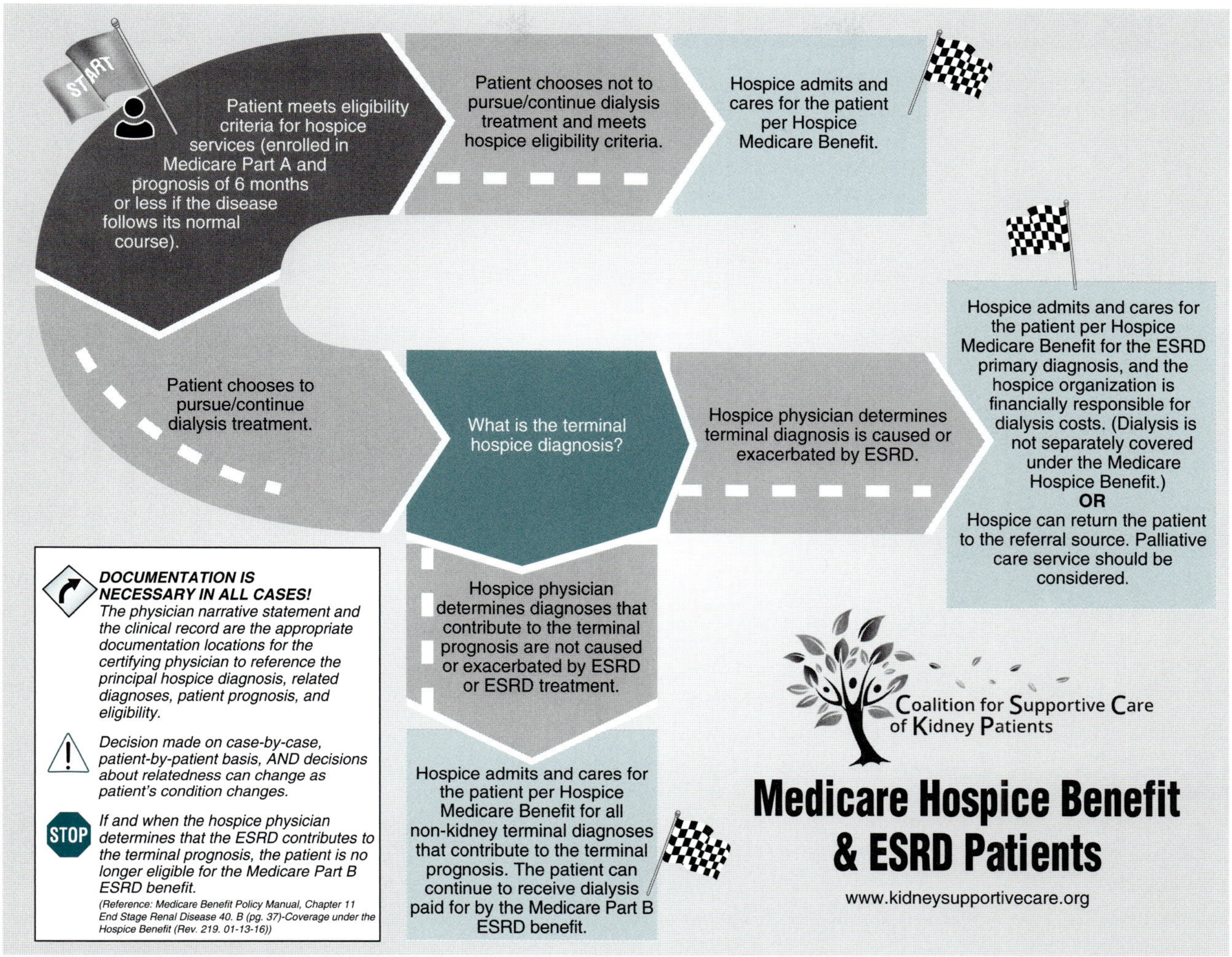

FIG. 20.4 Steps to facilitate hospice coverage in dialysis patients. Redrawn from www.kidney-supportivecare.org.

BOX 20.10 Key Elements of Time-Limited Trials

Elements

- Define clinical problems and prognosis
- Achieve consensus among all involved physicians
- Set limits on invasive treatments if unlikely to be beneficial

Identify the patient's goals and life values

- Review previous advance care planning decisions
- Assess the patient's competency and identify surrogate decision maker if necessary

Clarify clinical measures of improvement or treatment failure

- Obtain physician consensus for these measures
- Link markers to signs readily apparent to patients and families
- Provide regular family updates
- Make a time frame
- Consider patient's condition, proposed interventions, and patient/family needs; reassess time frame as patient's clinical condition changes
- Identify possible consequences at the conclusion of the time-limited trial
- Consider a written contract signed by all parties and list symptoms, functional status, nutritional parameters, and comorbid conditions at initiation

as a Medicare entitlement. As a result, a treatment that was originally available to only a few young patients is now offered to a sizeable, predominantly elderly population. Nephrology professionals have needed to shift from carefully selecting candidates for dialysis and transplantation to focusing on a host of geriatric and EOL issues. Accordingly, much of this chapter focused on what is now called renal palliative care or renal supportive care. The past decade has seen initiatives to improve communication and advance directives, research investigations, model programs, and the development of sensitive guidelines. All of these efforts are being informed by bioethics, and they will continue to greatly affect the practice of nephrology.

Funding acknowledgment: This work was supported through a Patient-Centered Outcomes Research Institute Program Award (CD-1304-7360).

Disclaimer: All statements in this report, including its findings and conclusions, are solely those of the authors and do not necessarily represent the views of the Patient-Centered Outcomes Research Institute, its Board of Governors or Methodology Committee.

A full list of references is available at www.expertconsult.com.

TABLE 20.1 **Ask-Tell-Ask Model**

Step	What to Do
1. Getting the setting right	Choosing a setting with privacy and without interruptions. • Find out if the patient wants other(s) present. • Confirm medical facts. • Plan what you will say. • Think about your own emotional reaction to giving the news.
2. Patient perception, ASK (#1)	What does the patient know? • Sometimes patients give or already know the bad news. Consider open-ended questions.
3. Invitation	Find out what the patient wants to know. Find out what the patient already knows. Explore how much detail the patient would like. Consider cultural variation. Allow the patient to decline voluntarily to receive information. Allow the patient to designate someone to communicate on his or her behalf. Give the patient control over hearing the news.
4. Giving knowledge, TELL	Foreshadow. Prepare for bad news. Say it – then stop. Provide clear, patient-specific information. Avoid jargon. Provide small bits of information. Pause frequently. Check for understanding. Use silence and receptive body language.
5. Addressing emotions, ASK (#2)	Anticipate emotional reactions. Resist the temptation to try to make the bad news better than it is. Employ techniques to respond to patient emotions. Use NURSE statements (Back et al., 2009) • Name an emotion. • Understand fears, concerns, and other emotions. • Respect the patient's experiences, emotions. • Support; continue to help the patient, identify resources • Explore; clarify.
6. Summary and strategy	Ask about the patient's concerns and fears: • What are your concerns? Do you want to talk about them? Plan for next steps (e.g., tests, treatment).

Based on information from Back AL, Arnold RM, Baile WF, et al. Efficacy of communication skills training for giving bad news and discussing transitions to palliative care. *Arch Intern Med.* 2007;167:453-460.

TABLE 20.2 **NURSE Model**

Name	• Identify the underlying emotion in a suggestive manner, e.g., "I wonder if you are feeling angry," "Sounds like you were really frightened when you got that news…" [2,6]
Understand	• Confirm that you understand what the person is feeling by discussing their experience, listening actively (do not be planning what you next want to say), and allowing silence. • Do not provide simple reassurance, disagreement, advice, clinical information, or justification without definitely understanding what the patient's true concern is. • Do not try to convey that you understand what someone is feeling by saying, "I know how you are feeling" because their reaction is often negative, with the person thinking, "How can you possibly know how I'm feeling?" Rather, consider using phrases like, "People going through your situation often report experiencing … Is this how you feel?"
Respect	• Give verbal and nonverbal evidence that their reaction is important.[2] • Match the level of your response to their level of emotion, i.e, a strong emotion needs to receive strong acknowledgment and respect.[2] • Accept their perspective without judgment and validate their input. Acceptance of their view is not the same as agreement with it.[2]
Support	• Give a variety of help sources, provide opportunities to participate in decision-making, and validate their efforts to cope. • State your availability for them, preferably in a way that demonstrates a partnership.[2,12]
Explore	• Target questions to the specifics of what the person has said and show explicit interest in their emotions.

BOX 20.11 SPIKES Model

Setup
- Prepare yourself with the medical facts.
- Determine who will participate in the conversation.
- Determine the location of the discussion, preferably a quiet location.
- Obtain a translator if needed.
- Let other staff know what you are going to be doing to avoid interruptions.

Perception
- Determine the participant's current perception about the situation.

Invitation
- Determine how much information the participants want to find out.

Knowledge
- Give a warning shot; for example, "I have some serious news to tell you."
- Deliver information in small parts.
- Avoid medical jargon.
- Allow time for comprehension.

Empathize
- Address participants' emotions and allow time for participants to understand their emotions (NURSE mnemonic; see Table 20.2).
- Resist the temptation to make things better.

Summary
- Summarize everything discussed and allow time for questions.

(From Back AL, Arnold RM, Baile WF, et al. Approaching difficult communication tasks in oncology. *CA Cancer J Clin.* 2005;55(3):164-177; Rodrigueq V. Communication: the most valuable palliative care tool. 2015. Available at https://www.quantiamd.com/player/yemeuzwgd?cid = 1818.)

BOX 20.12 Principles of a "Good Death"

A Good Death
- Anticipate death and know what to expect.
- Retain control of choices and have those wishes respected (advance care planning).
- Maintain dignity.
- Control of pain and other troublesome symptoms.
- Choose where death occurs.
- Easy access to needed care and expertise (palliative care).
- Spiritual and emotional support as needed.
- Access to hospice at all locations (home, hospital, nursing home).
- To have those present at death that one chooses.
- To have time to say goodbye and choose the time of death (withdrawal from dialysis if appropriate).
- Bereavement services for those left behind.

BOX 20.13 Treatment of Common Symptoms in Chronic Kidney Disease

Symptom Treatment

Cramps

Quinine 260–325 mg PO prn; give before symptoms; limit to 3 doses/d
Carnitine 1000-2000 mg IV during dialysis
Also used for myopathy, cardiomyopathy, refractory anemia

Restless Legs Syndrome

Clonazepam 0.5–2.0 mg hs prn
Carbidopa-levodopa 25/100 mg hs prn
Pergolide 0.05–0.2 mg qd
Pramipexole 0.3 mg qd

Pruritus

Skin moisturizer; limited effectiveness
Hydrourea cream

continued

BOX 20.13 Treatment of Common Symptoms in Chronic Kidney Disease—cont'd

Gabepentin start low and slow; 100 mg bid up to 800 mg qid (pregabalin also effective)
Capsaicin 0.025% cream qid; burning sensation may be problematic; expensive. therefore, not practical for generalized pruritus
Antihistamines
Clemastine
Ketotifen
1–3 mg bid prn
2 mg bid prn
Trial any H1 antagonist; inexpensive, safe, but often poor clinical response
Ultraviolet B light 2–3 times/wk
Effective but potentially noxious in the long term, impractical, and often not available
Ondansetron 2–4 mg bid
High cost, constipating
IV lidocaine 100 mg IV during dialysis
Potential seizures
Activated charcoal 6 g qd for 8 wk
Impractical, poorly tolerated
Plasmapheresis 3–4 exchanges
Impractical

Dialysis Symptoms

Hypotension, intradialytic or persistent
Alterations to the dialysis bath, temperature, sodium, ultrafiltration
Midodrine 1–10 mg tid prn or predialysis
Oral α-adrenergic agonist
Sertraline 25–50 mg predialysis
Anorexia Megestrol 40–400 mg
Has been used in ESRD
Dronabinol 2.5–5.0 mg bid/tid
Cannabinoid
Lethargy, fatigue
Methylphenidate 5–10 mg AM and noon
Psychostimulant, limited use and effectiveness in ESRD

Symptoms at the End of Life

Symptom Treatment

Retained secretions
Scopolamine
Shortness of breath
Fan, oxygen, patient position (upright), opioids
Agitation (includes involuntary twitching)
Ensure that pain and psychosocial issues addressed, haloperidol, methotrimeprazine (effective for anxiety, restlessness, nausea, and pain), and benzodiazepines
Nausea and vomiting
Metaclopramide, prochlorproperazine, ondansetron
Hiccups
Chlorpromazine, haloperidol, metoclopramide
Pruritus, cramps, neuropathic pain
Gabepentin

Addiction Facts

1. The incidence of addiction in patients receiving opioid therapy for acute pain relief is <1%. The incidence of addiction in patients receiving opioid therapy for chronic pain is less clear but is felt to be <5%.
2. Patients will become physically dependent when treated with opioids for a time and therefore will have effects of withdrawal if the opioid is stopped suddenly.
3. Physical dependency is easily managed by a slow taper of the opioid when pain has resolved.
4. Physical dependency is not synonymous with addiction.
5. Addiction is a psychological problem rather than a physical one and is characterized by patients engaging in manipulative behaviors to secure the drug.
6. Individuals who are addicted use opioids for reasons other than pain. Taking drugs for pain management is different from taking them for pleasure.

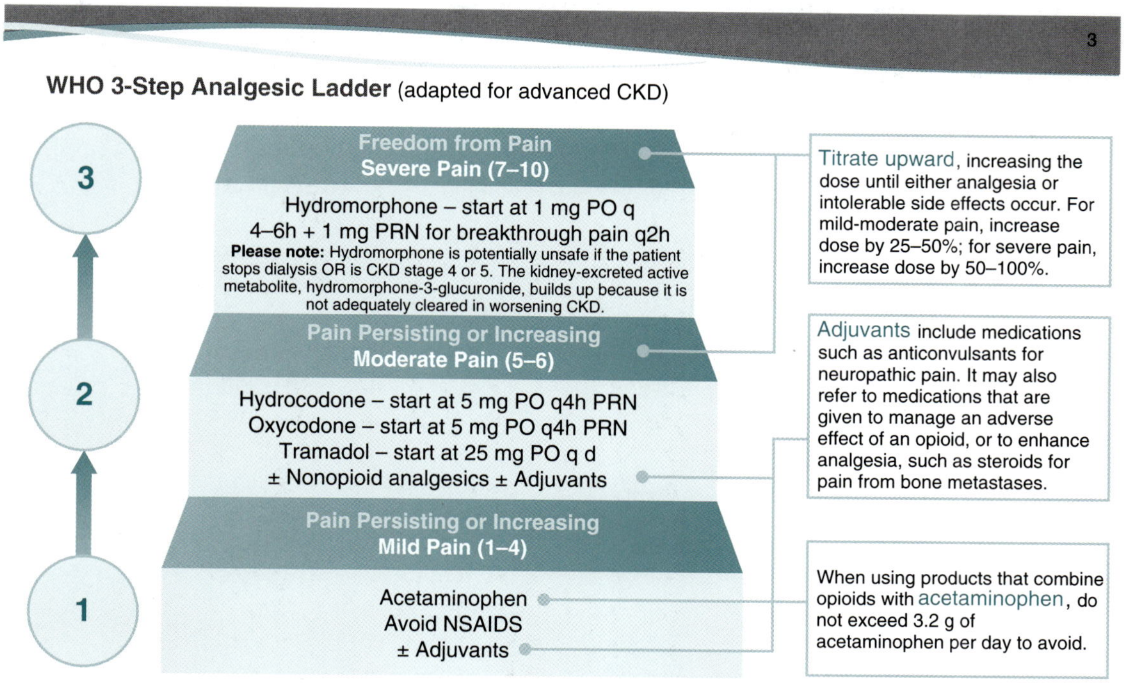

FIG. 20.5 Modified World Health Organization 3-step analgesic ladder for patients with chronic kidney disease. *NSAID*, Nonsteroidal antiiflammatory drug. (From Barakzoy AS, Moss AH. Efficacy of the World Health Organization analgesic ladder to treat pain in end-stage renal disease. *J Am Soc Nephrol.* 2006;17:3198-3203.)

TABLE 20.3 Pain Medications in Chronic Kidney Disease

Recommended	Use With Caution	Do Not Use
Acetaminophen	**Tramadol** Limit dose to 50 mg bid. Higher doses have been used but caution needs to be taken as pharmacokinetics are not well established.	**Morphine**
Hydromorphone Hydromorphone is potentially unsafe if the patient stops dialysis OR is CKD stage 4 or 5. The kidney-excreted active metabolite, hydromorphone-3-glucuronide, builds up because it is not adequately cleared in worsening CKD.	**Hydrocodone/Ocycodone** Insufficient pharmacokinetic evidence to establish safety in CKD, but literature reports use without major adverse effects.	**Codeine**
Fentanyl	**Desipramine/Nortriptyline.** Alternative to treat neuropathic pain, but more adverse effects than gabapentin and pregabalin.	**Meperidine**
Methadone		**Propoxyphene**
Gabapentin Doses in ESRD up to 300 mg/d are generally considered safe, but higher disease should be used with caution; note that gabapentin use for neuropathic pain is off-label but effectiveness has been documented.		Renally excreted metabolites accumulate in CKD, causing neurotoxicity.
Pregabalin Doses up to 100 mg/d are generally considered safe in ESRD.		

CKD, Chronic kidney disease; *ESRD*, end-stage renal disease.

SECTION III

Dialysis

21

Dialysis and End-Stage Kidney Disease: Epidemiology, Costs, and Outcomes

James B. Wetmore, MD, MS, and Allan J. Collins, MD

OUTLINE

End-stage renal disease (ESRD), defined as loss of kidney function such that life is unsustainable in the absence of renal replacement therapy (RRT), is an enormous public health challenge. RRT, provided in the form of a transplanted kidney (renal allograft) or, much more commonly, long-term ("maintenance") dialysis, exacts an immense toll on the affected individual, the healthcare system, and society in general. Dialysis, as an "organ replacement therapy," has been rightly hailed as one of the greatest advancements in the history of medicine[1]; however, it is expensive, burdensome, and far from an ideal solution to kidney failure. Since ESRD is no longer limited to industrialized countries, nations at all levels of economic development will struggle to meet the growing worldwide need for RRT.[2] One positive development is that ESRD, which has long been recognized within the nephrology community as a problem of immense proportions, has gradually come into greater focus in the broader public health community. The US Healthy People (HP) 2020 initiative,[3,4] for example, outlines specific public health targets for both chronic kidney disease (CKD) and ESRD. In this chapter, we discuss the epidemiology, outcomes, and costs of ESRD, particularly as they pertain to maintenance dialysis.

DEVELOPMENT OF END-STAGE RENAL DISEASE: CONCEPTUAL CONSIDERATIONS

Ongoing loss of functioning renal parenchyma has been termed the *sine qua non* of progressive kidney disease leading from CKD to ESRD.[5] CKD does not inevitably lead to ESRD, and ESRD is not invariably a consequence of CKD. For example, for some patients, CKD is only slowly, if at all, progressive, as can occur due to a transient renal insult earlier in life. In contrast, some patients can develop ESRD after acute kidney injury (AKI) resulting from a serious illness or trauma, perhaps via a hastening of progressive CKD.[6-12] Although CKD progression and advancement to ESRD are by no means inevitable, especially in people with less-advanced CKD, ESRD is generally the result of chronic processes that characterize CKD and that lead to progressive nephron loss.[13-15] Nephron loss results in compensatory hyperfiltration in the remaining nephrons, an injurious process that itself contributes to CKD advancement.[5] Depending on the underlying cause of CKD, proteinuria often is manifest, which itself is injurious to the kidney through a variety of biological mechanisms.[16]

The risk that CKD will advance to ESRD can be underappreciated because mild to moderate CKD generally produces no signs or symptoms, and compensatory nephron hyperfiltration makes estimated glomerular filtration rate (eGFR) a "lagging indicator" of disease. Once serum creatinine levels have overtly increased (i.e., once eGFR has manifestly decreased), more than half of nephron mass may have been lost. The unfortunate reality is that the symptoms associated with kidney failure often occur only when ESRD is impending. An additional difficulty is that CKD progression is variable and often unpredictable for individual patients,[17] so the urgency to act and the calculation of risks and benefits for particular therapies may be uncertain for patients and their healthcare providers.

EPIDEMIOLOGY OF END-STAGE RENAL DISEASE

Causes of End-Stage Renal Disease and Indications for Maintenance Dialysis

The cardinal causes of CKD are diabetes, hypertension, glomerulonephritis, and polycystic kidney disease. As would be expected, the major causes of CKD are also the major causes of ESRD. Large ESRD registries, such as the United States Renal Data System (USRDS), provide information about causes of ESRD. As noted in the USRDS Annual Data Report, attempting to determine the cause of ESRD at the level of the individual patient or at the population level presents considerable difficulties.[18] First, attribution of the cause of ESRD, which must be reported to the USRDS, relies on the physician's best judgment, and it can be difficult to determine with confidence that hypertension, for example, is the specific cause. This issue is particularly acute when a patient's condition (such as hypertension or diabetes) rarely results in a renal biopsy, or when a patient has received little pre-ESRD care. Second, presence of a comorbid condition, such as diabetes, does not mean that it is the sole or even major cause of ESRD. Finally, many patients have more than one medical condition that can contribute to ESRD, so choosing a single condition as the primary cause is a somewhat artificial exercise.

With these important caveats, the USRDS Annual Data Report provides information on temporal trends in the major causes of ESRD. As shown in Fig. 21.1, the adjusted rate of diabetes as a cause of ESRD declined between 2001 and 2014, from 175.2 to 156 per million per year (PMPY), whereas the rate of hypertension was relatively stable (102.3 PMPY, 2001; 100.9 PMPY, 2014). The rate declined substantially for glomerulonephritis (from 38 to 27.2 PMPY), and only slightly for cystic disease. As the overall adjusted rate of ESRD in 2014 was approximately 354 PMPY, diabetes is attributed to 44% of individuals who develop ESRD and hypertension to 29%; the two leading causes therefore contribute to nearly three-quarters of the total.

Although much is known about the causes of ESRD, at least in the United States and other developed countries where standardized forms are completed for new dialysis initiates, information about the indications for dialysis initiation is surprisingly sparse.[19] Data from large registries or other administrative data sets are unlikely to provide granular detail about bedside indications for dialysis, making the generation of broad-based epidemiological conclusions problematic. However, a recent systematically conducted chart review of >450 dialysis initiates from a single center between 2004 and 2012 rendered important insights.[20] Development of uremic symptoms was the largest primary indication for dialysis initiation, at 47%, followed by volume overload/hypertension (21%) and laboratory evidence of abnormalities (18%); the indication was uncertain for 14%. Initiation for volume overload/hypertension was associated with the highest unadjusted risk for subsequent (postinitiation) mortality (hazard ratio [HR], 2.2 compared with the referent group of laboratory abnormalities); HRs were 1.2 for both uremic symptoms and unknown indications. After full adjustment, the magnitude of the HRs was much attenuated and significant differences ablated between the groups, yet the adjusted point for volume overload/hypertension remained notably higher than for the other etiologies. Although 69% of all initiations were judged as being urgent, this was the case for 88% of the patients initiating for volume overload but only 55% of the patients initiating for laboratory abnormalities. With the caveat that the study was a relatively modestly sized sample of US patients, this report appears to be the first to rigorously quantify the percentage distribution of indications for dialysis initiation and their associations with outcomes.

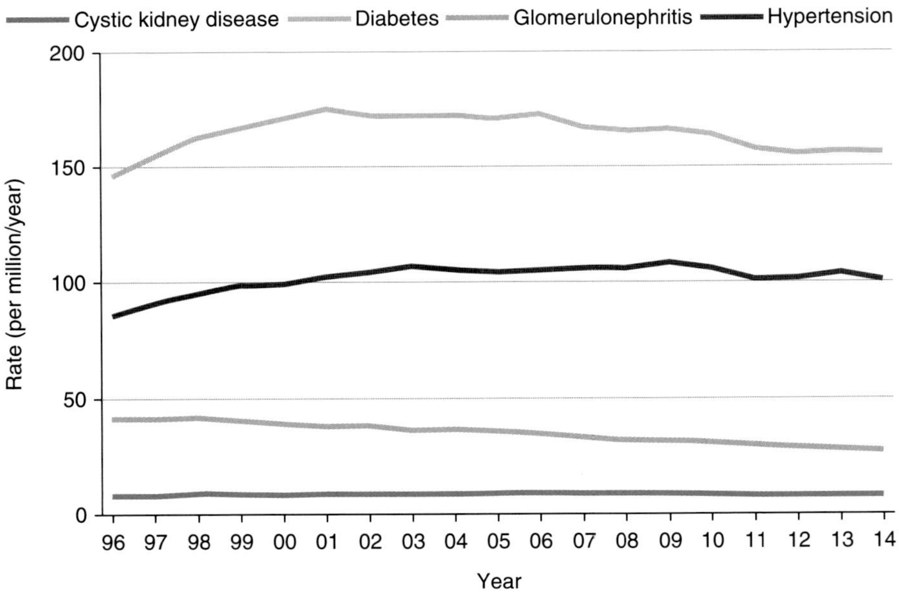

FIG. 21.1 Trends in adjusted ESRD incidence rate (per million/year), by primary cause of ESRD, in the US population, 1996 to 2014. Adjusted for age, sex, and race. (From United States Renal Data System. *2016 USRDS Annual Data Report: Epidemiology of Kidney Disease in the United States*. Bethesda, MD: National Institutes of Health, National Institute of Diabetes and Digestive and Kidney Diseases; 2016.)

Incidence and Prevalence of End-Stage Renal Disease

The epidemiology of disease is best considered using the familiar concepts of incidence and prevalence. Incidence is classically defined as the new diagnosis or other manifestation of disease in individuals previously without evidence of disease, and prevalence as the number of individuals who have the disease in the general population at any one time. Incidence is typically expressed as the number of new cases divided by person-time at risk, and prevalence as the number of individuals with a disease divided by the number alive at any given point in time (point prevalence) or the number diagnosed within a certain period of time (period prevalence). Prevalence often is expressed as a percentage, and therefore can be considered a cross-sectional perspective of how common a disease is. Prevalence is the product of disease incidence multiplied by disease duration. Disease duration reflects the natural history of the disease, the effectiveness of treatment for it (both the "inherent" effectiveness of treatment and how effectively it is rendered, in real-world settings, to individuals with the disease), and other diseases and factors that contribute to death.

Consideration of ESRD incidence differs from that of many other diseases. As with many medical conditions, ESRD incidence depends in part on the presence and severity of ESRD risk factors (hypertension, diabetes, vascular disease, etc.). However, ESRD is an unusual disorder in that the treatments—dialysis or kidney transplant—often are electively withheld. Information on ESRD incidence therefore reflects not true incidence, but rather treated incidence. In countries where maintenance dialysis therapy is universally available, decisions to forgo dialysis initiation are likely driven primarily by personal choice, comorbidity burden, and a conversation between patient and physician about the utility of dialysis compared with the burden it imposes on the patient. As detailed more fully later, however, in countries where dialysis is a limited healthcare resource, ESRD is infrequently treated.[21,22] Thus registries that track patients initiating maintenance dialysis or undergoing kidney transplant identify only patients for whom ESRD treatment is offered, not those for whom a decision is made not to offer RRT. Even in developed countries, the number of individuals who develop ESRD and are not offered RRT is uncertain, meaning the true ESRD incidence is unknown.

Incidence of Treated End-Stage Renal Disease

Establishing the incidence and prevalence of treated ESRD is not especially difficult in industrialized countries due to comprehensive registries, typically funded by governments, such as the USRDS,[18] the United Kingdom Renal Registry,[23] the Canadian Organ Replacement Register,[24] the Japanese Society for Dialysis Therapy Renal Data Registry,[25] the Australia and New Zealand Dialysis and Transplant Registry,[26] and others.[27] As the definition of ESRD includes not only patients receiving maintenance dialysis (in-center hemodialysis, home hemodialysis, or peritoneal dialysis [PD]), but also those who have undergone kidney transplant (preemptively or after initiating dialysis), estimates of ESRD are incomplete in the absence of data on transplant recipients.

The USRDS, which contains near-universal identification of patients receiving dialysis or undergoing kidney transplant, provides important information. Even this registry is imperfect, however,[28] as approximately 2% of patients are thought to be missing from it. In particular, early death (i.e., death soon after initiating maintenance dialysis before registration can occur) appears to be missed.[29] An additional source of difficulty for any such registry is ambiguity concerning recovery of renal function (i.e., misclassification of AKI that subsequently recovers as ESRD); however, these challenges likely do not seriously undermine the broad conclusions drawn from research endeavors or, ultimately, the formation of public policy.

Data from the most recent USRDS registry demonstrate that, in the United States, approximately 121,000 patients developed ESRD in 2014, representing an unadjusted rate of 370 persons PMPY and a demographically adjusted rate of 354 PMPY.[18] Of these, slightly >106,000 initiated hemodialysis, >11,000 initiated PD, and slightly >3000 underwent preemptive kidney transplant. Since 2006, when adjusted incidence rates peaked at 387 PMPY, adjusted rates declined to about 354 PMPY over 2012 to 2014 (Fig. 21.2).

Incidence of ESRD varies by demography.[18] Rates are higher for older than for younger individuals: 1556 PMPY, aged ≥75 years; 1265, ages 65 to 74; 573, ages 45 to 64; and 129, ages 22 to 44 years. Rates are much higher for blacks/African Americans (877 PMPY) than for whites (286 PMPY); values are intermediate for Asians (357 PMPY) and Native Americans (333 PMPY). Adjusted incidence rates are substantially higher for individuals of Hispanic ethnicity (466 PMPY) than for non-Hispanics (346 PMPY). Rates are substantially higher for men than for women.

Comprehensive examination of the demography of ESRD incidence is incomplete, however, without an examination of temporal trends. Incidence rates have been declining more for older than for younger individuals (Fig. 21.3); more for members of racial minorities, with little change for whites (Fig. 21.4); and more for Hispanic than for non-Hispanic individuals.

Incidence rates vary substantially by geography, from a low of 250 PMPY in New England (Connecticut, Rhode Island, Massachusetts, New Hampshire, Vermont, and Maine) to 432 PMPY in Texas, a nearly 1.4-fold difference.[18] As these rates are adjusted, demographic case mix alone, at least as determined by traditional variables, cannot account for the difference. Gross geographical location, such as a crude division into north versus south, also cannot fully account for the difference; rates in Pennsylvania and Delaware are 352 PMPY, for example, but 325 PMPY in North Carolina, South Carolina, and Georgia. The reasons for this are not fully understood, but likely relate to socioeconomic, historical, cultural, and perhaps even geographical differences, and to systems of care delivery.

One notable trend in ESRD incidence is the eGFR at which patients initiate dialysis. Since the late 1990s, the mean eGFR at maintenance dialysis initiation has increased. In 2001 for example, approximately 22% of patients initiated dialysis with

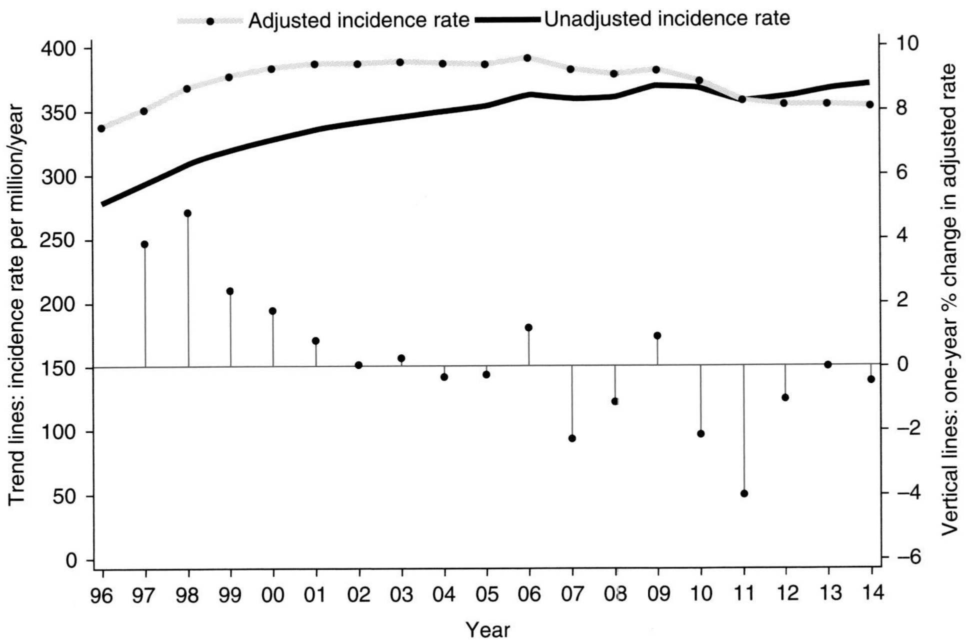

FIG. 21.2 Trends in the unadjusted and adjusted incidence rates (per million/year) of ESRD (trend lines; scale on left), and annual percent (%) change in the adjusted incidence rate of ESRD (vertical lines; scale on right) in the US population, 1996 to 2014. Adjusted for age, sex, race, and ethnicity. (From United States Renal Data System. *2016 USRDS Annual Data Report: Epidemiology of Kidney Disease in the United States.* Bethesda, MD: National Institutes of Health, National Institute of Diabetes and Digestive and Kidney Diseases; 2016.)

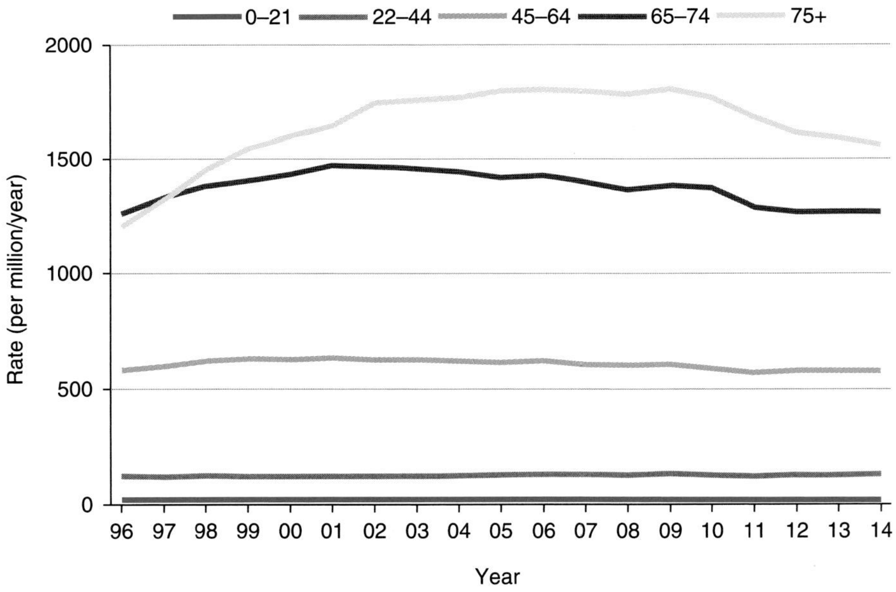

FIG. 21.3 Trends in adjusted ESRD incidence rate (per million/year), by age group, in the US population, 1996 to 2014. Adjusted for sex and race. (From United States Renal Data System. *2016 USRDS Annual Data Report: Epidemiology of Kidney Disease in the United States.* Bethesda, MD: National Institutes of Health, National Institute of Diabetes and Digestive and Kidney Diseases; 2016.)

eGFR <5 mL/min/1.73 m^2; this decreased to 14% in 2014. The percentage of patients initiating with eGFR 10 to <15 mL/min/1.73 m^2 increased from 18% to 27%, whereas the percentage initiating with eGFR ≥15 mL/min/1.73 m^2 increased from 8% to 12%. This trend appeared to peak in 2010, and has moderately reversed in the years since (Fig. 21.5), possibly influenced in part by clinical trials and observational studies, as discussed later in this chapter.

Prevalence of ESRD

In contrast to incidence, prevalence counts and rates continue to increase substantially, due primarily to increasing longevity

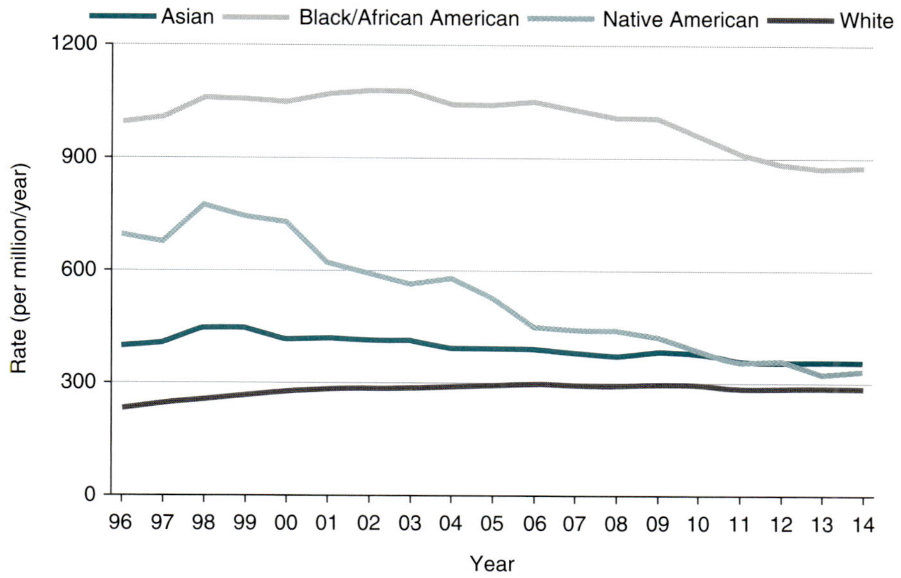

FIG. 21.4 Trends in adjusted ESRD incidence rate (per million/year), by race, in the US population, 1996 to 2014. Adjusted for age and sex. (From United States Renal Data System. *2016 USRDS Annual Data Report: Epidemiology of Kidney Disease in the United States.* Bethesda, MD: National Institutes of Health, National Institute of Diabetes and Digestive and Kidney Diseases; 2016.)

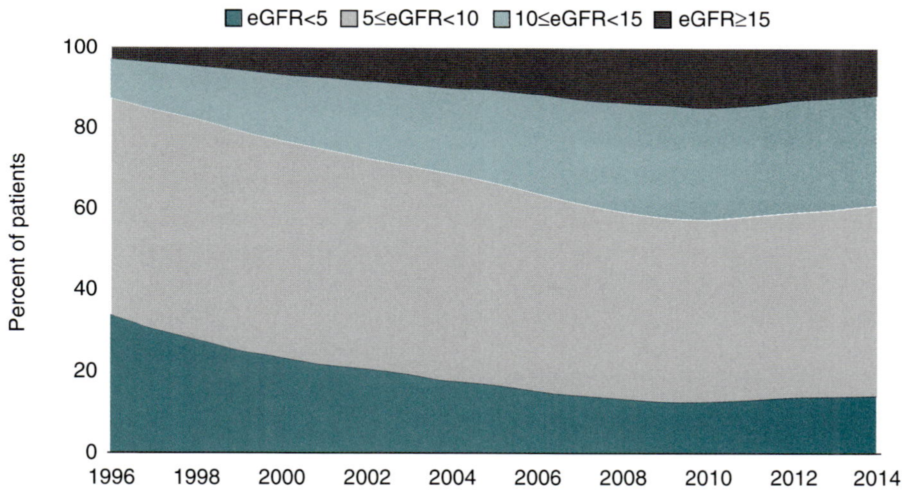

FIG. 21.5 Trends in the distribution (%) of eGFR (mL/min/1.73 m^2) among incident ESRD patients, 1996 to 2014. (From United States Renal Data System. *2016 USRDS Annual Data Report: Epidemiology of Kidney Disease in the United States.* Bethesda, MD: National Institutes of Health, National Institute of Diabetes and Digestive and Kidney Diseases; 2016.)

for ESRD patients, especially those receiving maintenance dialysis.[18] Prevalence counts increased from approximately 570,000 in 2009 to 678,000 a mere 5 years later. Adjusted prevalence rates increased from 1598 PMPY in 2001 to 1977 in 2014 (Fig. 21.6), a 19% increase over that period, with year-on-year increases averaging 1% to 2%.

Of prevalent ESRD patients in 2014, approximately 429,000 were receiving maintenance hemodialysis, 47,000 were receiving PD, and 201,000 had undergone kidney transplantation (Fig. 21.7). Prevalence is higher for blacks/African Americans than for whites, for older than for younger individuals, for Hispanics than for non-Hispanics, and for men than for women. As would be expected, prevalence rates vary by geography: Adjusted rates are lowest in the Pacific Northwest (Alaska, Washington, Oregon, Montana, and Wyoming), at 1419 PMPY, and highest in the South Central region (Tennessee, Alabama, and Mississippi), at 2339 PMPY, a roughly 1.5-fold difference.

Temporal trends demonstrate important findings. Between 2001 and 2014, adjusted prevalence rates increased more for older than for younger individuals (from 4284 PMPY to 6243, or about 46%, aged ≥75 years; 2973 PMPY to 3658, or about 23%, ages 45 to 64 years) and for whites than for blacks/African Americans (from 1108 to 1507 PMPY, or 36%, whites; 4839 to 5605 PMPY, or 16%, blacks/African Americans).[18]

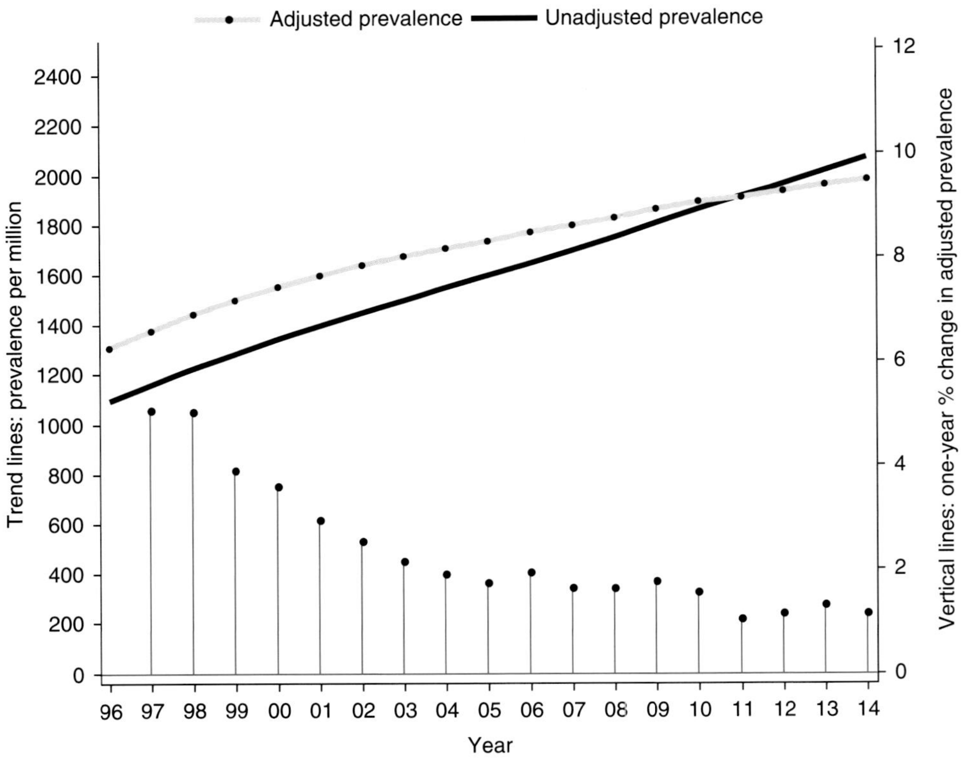

FIG. 21.6 Trends in the unadjusted and adjusted ESRD prevalence (per million) (trend lines; scale on left), and annual percent change in adjusted prevalence of ESRD (vertical lines; scale on right), in the US population, 1996 to 2014. Adjusted for age, sex, race, and ethnicity. (From United States Renal Data System. *2016 USRDS Annual Data Report: Epidemiology of Kidney Disease in the United States.* Bethesda, MD: National Institutes of Health, National Institute of Diabetes and Digestive and Kidney Diseases; 2016.)

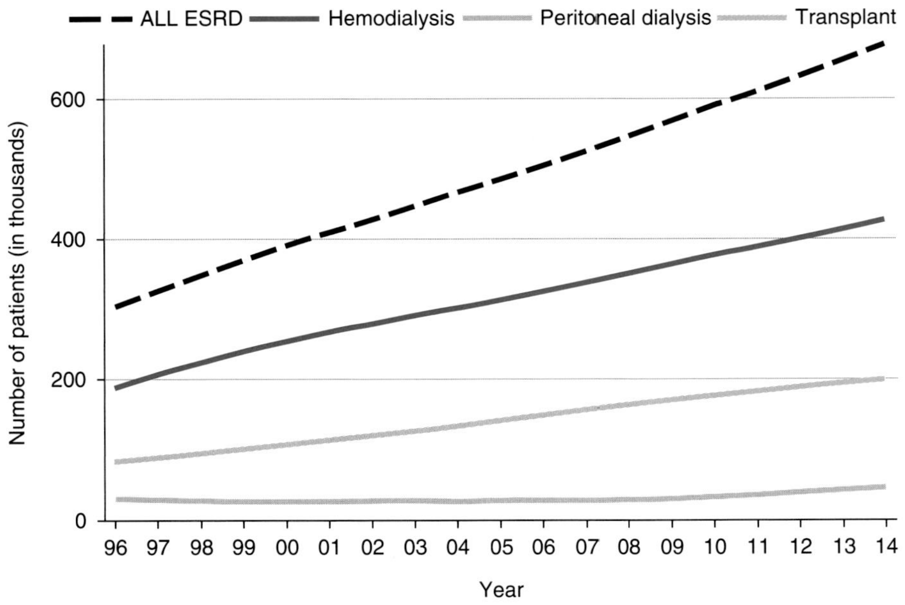

FIG. 21.7 Trends in the number of ESRD prevalent cases (in thousands) by modality, in the US population, 1996 to 2014. (From United States Renal Data System. *2016 USRDS Annual Data Report: Epidemiology of Kidney Disease in the United States.* Bethesda, MD: National Institutes of Health, National Institute of Diabetes and Digestive and Kicney Diseases; 2016.)

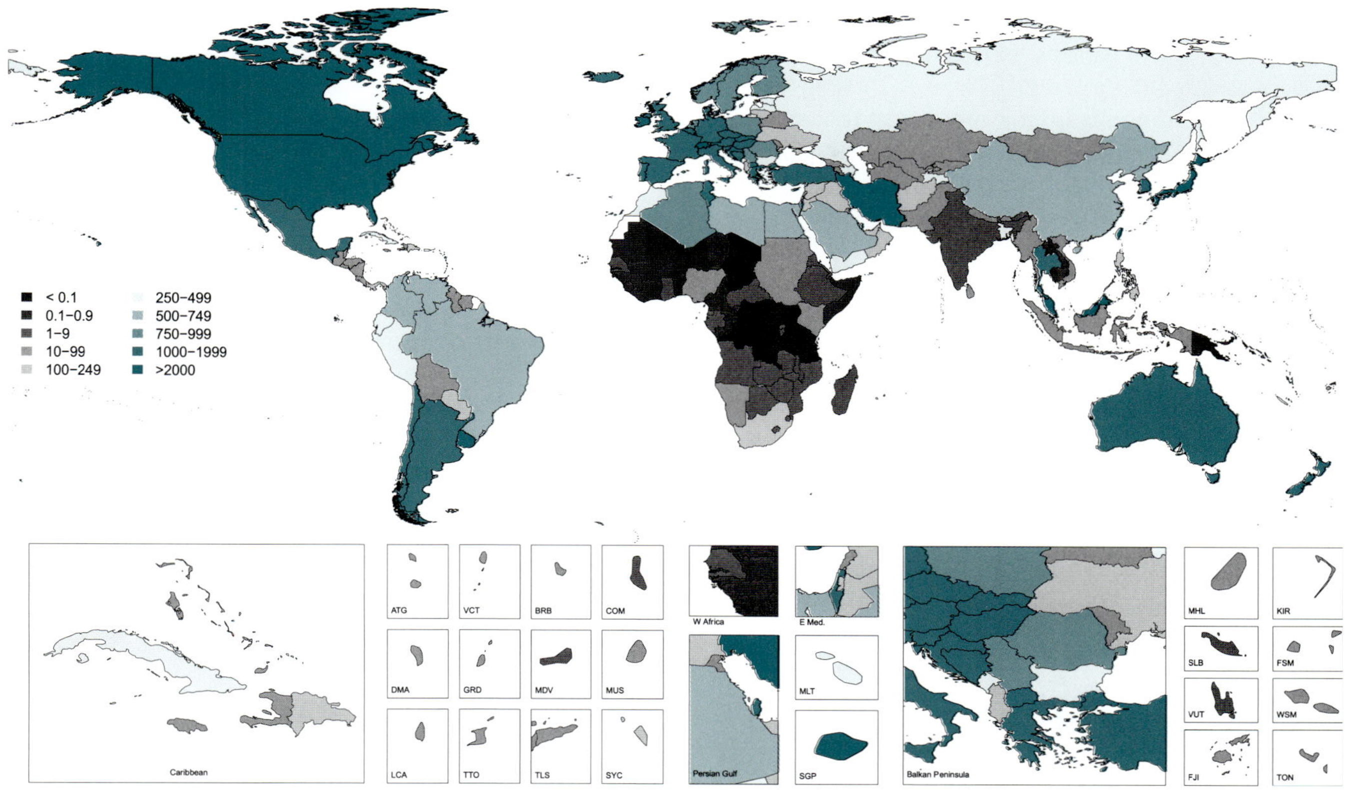

FIG. 21.8 Worldwide prevalence of ESRD. (From Thomas B, Wulf S, Bikbov B, et al. Maintenance dialysis throughout the world in years 1990 and 2010. *J Am Soc Nephrol.* 2015;26:2621-2633.)

Several recent studies have investigated the prevalence of maintenance dialysis worldwide[21,22] (Fig. 21.8). Because only a small minority of patients with ESRD undergo kidney transplant, especially in developing countries, receipt of maintenance dialysis is generally a good proxy for ESRD, or what might be more precisely termed the need for RRT. One study reported a 70% increase in prevalent dialysis patients between 1990 and 2010 alone.[21] The authors estimated that 284 persons per million population received dialysis as of 2010, or roughly 2 million people worldwide. This estimate was comparable to that of another recent study.[22] Global incidence of ESRD more than doubled during this period, from 44 to 93 per million population, corresponding to roughly 700,000 new cases per year. Interestingly, this increase appears not to be fueled so much by population growth and structure (mainly aging), estimated to have been responsible for about one-third of the increase, or by increases in diabetes or hypertension (two main drivers of ESRD), as by increases in the availability of maintenance dialysis. This would suggest a substantial increase in governmental support of maintenance dialysis programs around the world, including in developing countries, constituting a major welcome development. However, this also indicates a likely huge unmet need for RRT, and as governmental programs expand, many more patients will be recognized as requiring RRT. These authors projected the need for RRT out to 2013, by region (Fig. 21.9). This likelihood is highlighted by estimates of the number of people who die prematurely because they cannot access RRT; using conservative and liberal approaches, between 2.3 and 7.1 premature deaths have likely occurred because patients need maintenance dialysis that has not been provided. In Asia alone, at least 1.9 million people have likely died due to lack of access to RRT. The RRT gap could grow dramatically as China, India, and other nations develop.

Timing of Dialysis Initiation

Timing of dialysis initiation has long been a matter of great uncertainty in nephrology, but work published since 2010 has greatly improved understanding and, it seems, palpable trends recently observable in the epidemiological data. The timing of dialysis initiation typically involves consideration of the symptom burden associated with uremia, fluid status (volume overload) and its consequent hypertension, and laboratory-based values (eGFR usually derived from creatinine, blood urea nitrogen [BUN], potassium, and, perhaps to a lesser degree, other analytes such as albumin and bicarbonate). From 1996 to 2007, the mean eGFR at which patients initiated maintenance dialysis increased from approximately 7.7 to 11.2 mL/min/1.73 m^2,[18] a trend that does not seem to be accounted for by changes in case-mix,[30] even when markers of frailty[31] or detailed assessments of symptomology[32] are explicitly considered. The potential reasons for this increase are unknown. The widespread introduction of automated eGFR laboratory reporting, an obvious potential explanation, does not appear to be responsible,[33] nor do reimbursement incentives, regional variation in the nephrology workforce, or regional differences in dialysis facility practice patterns.[34-36]

However, this trend appears to be reversing; as of 2013, the mean eGFR at which patients initiated maintenance dialysis had decreased to 10.3 mL/min/1.73 m^2.[18] This may be due to a confluence of results from a key clinical trial and multiple observational studies. In 2010 the Initiating Dialysis Early and Late (IDEAL) trial was published.[37] This trial randomized patients to initiate dialysis at 10 to 15 mL/min/1.73 m^2 or much later, at 5 to 7 mL/min/1.73 m^2. Although the control arm did initiate within the range intended (12 mL/min/1.73 m^2), the late-start group initiated at a mean eGFR of 9.8 mL/min/1.73 m^2; a major reason appeared to be the perceived threat of hyperkalemia in the patients randomized to start at lower eGFRs. Nevertheless, this seemingly small difference of slightly over 2 mL/min/1.73 m^2 represented a nontrivial difference in start times of fully 6 months between the two groups. The main finding was no difference in all-cause mortality a mean of 3.6 years later, providing strong support for the benefits of initiating dialysis later rather than earlier.[38] The study found no major differences in secondary endpoints such as cardiovascular events or hospitalizations,[37] markers of cardiac structure or function,[39] or overall costs.[40] Gratifyingly, these results are largely concordant with multiple large observational studies,[41-46] many of which used advanced design and analytical techniques such as stratification, propensity-score matching, inverse probability of treatment weighting, and marginal structural models.[47]

As a result of this evidence, clinical practice guidelines from the United States, Canada, and Europe have become

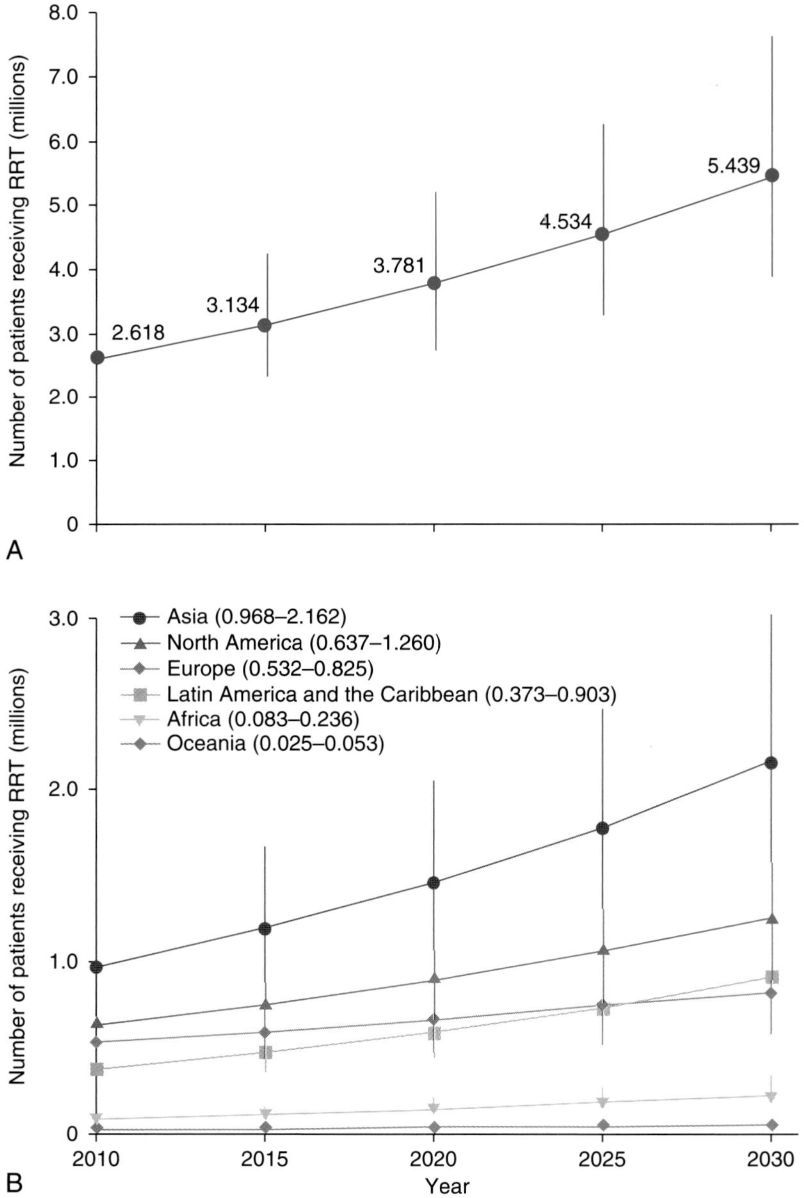

FIG. 21.9 Projections in the growth in need for renal replacement therapy from 2010 to 2013, overall and by world region. (From Liyanage T, Ninomiya T, Jha V, et al. Worldwide access to treatment for end-stage kidney disease: a systematic review. *Lancet.* 2015;385:1975-1982)

much more favorable toward initiating maintenance dialysis on the basis of signs, symptoms, and laboratory values other than creatinine, BUN, and eGFR, and generally appear to condone later dialysis initiation.[48-51] Only in the Canadian guidelines is an eGFR threshold for initiation (specifically, 6 mL/min/1.73 m^2) explicitly recommended.[50]

OUTCOMES IN END-STAGE RENAL DISEASE

Mortality Trends in Patients Receiving Maintenance Dialysis

Since the late 1990s, mortality rates have declined substantially for maintenance dialysis patients and kidney transplant recipients, easily exceeding the HP 2020 goal.[4] Adjusted mortality rates in 2014 for these populations were 166 and 30 per 1000 patient-years, respectively, representing decreases of 32% and 44%, relative to 1996[18] (Fig. 21.10). Changes in mortality by dialysis modality over several eras are shown in Fig. 21.11. In all four cohorts, death rates for hemodialysis patients are high immediately after initiation and decline precipitously thereafter, reflecting the fact that the sickest, and likely frailest, patients die soon after initiation. This can be conceptualized as the first stage of a "survivor cohort effect." Death rates then increase progressively until about 8 years after dialysis initiation, as shown by the oldest two cohorts (1996 and 2001); this will likely be the case for younger cohorts, such as the 2008 cohort, which is likely close to a leveling off in mortality rates. After approximately 8 years, death rates decline and perhaps even show a small annualized decline, likely representing continued survival of only the healthiest or most resilient patients. However, the number of survivors 8 years after dialysis initiation is, unfortunately, only a small fraction of the initiating cohort.

Changes in the unadjusted (crude) death rates are somewhat smaller, primarily because the mean ages of dialysis patients and transplant recipients have increased. The rate of decrease in adjusted mortality has not been monotonic; for hemodialysis patients, for example, adjusted mortality rates declined by 4% from 1996 to 2003, but by fully 24% from 2004 to 2014. Overall, during this period, adjusted mortality rates decreased by 29% in hemodialysis patients and by 44% in PD patients.[18]

Mortality in the first year after maintenance dialysis initiation deserves special scrutiny. As noted, death rates among hemodialysis patients are highest soon after initiation. Because of a marked interaction of mortality with age, it is most useful to consider patients aged ≥65 years separately from those aged <65 years. For example, for patients aged ≥65 years incident to hemodialysis in 2013, the mortality rate was highest in the second month after initiation, at 620 deaths per 1000 patient-years, decreasing to 297 by month 12; corresponding values for patients aged <65 years were 214 and 117.[18] However, the death rate in the first month of dialysis is almost certainly a substantial undercount, as deaths in the first month are likely not fully identified if they occur before patients are registered with the Centers for Medicare & Medicaid Services (CMS) as having ESRD.[29]

The pattern of deaths for PD patients is quite different, as rates increase throughout the first year, from 32 to 54 per 1000 patient-years among patients aged <65 years, and from 115 to 214 for patients aged ≥65 years. These differential patterns of first-year deaths may be attributable to the fact that patients initiating PD are generally healthier than those initiating hemodialysis, and are likely to have greater social support.

Mortality rates also differ by race, with an interaction with age. Death rates are similar between younger whites and blacks/African Americans (aged ≤22 years) but are substantially lower for blacks/African Americans than for whites in older age groups. Regarding age and sex, death rates are lower

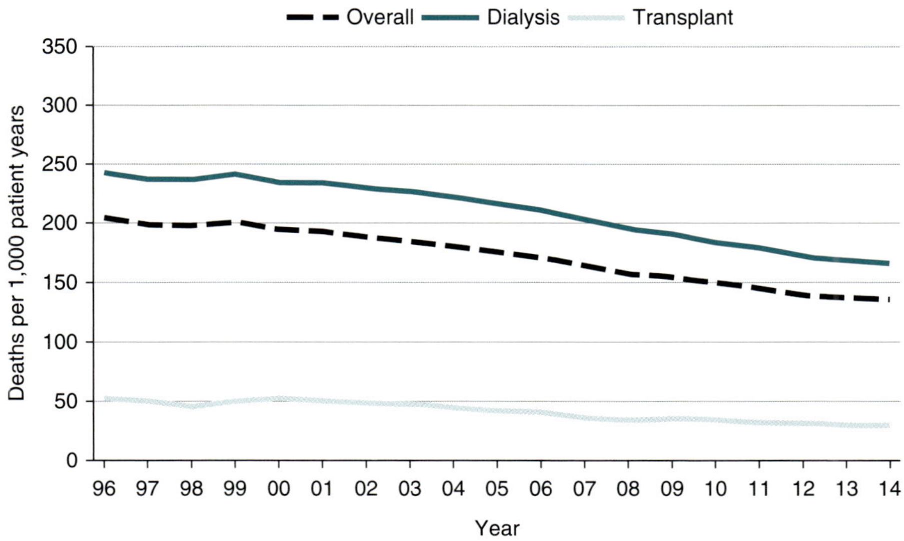

FIG. 21.10 Adjusted all-cause mortality (deaths per 1000 patient-years) by treatment modality: overall, dialysis, and transplant, period-prevalent patients, 1996 to 2014. (From United States Renal Data System. *2016 USRDS Annual Data Report: Epidemiology of Kidney Disease in the United States*. Bethesda, MD: National Institutes of Health, National Institute of Diabetes and Digestive and Kidney Diseases; 2016.)

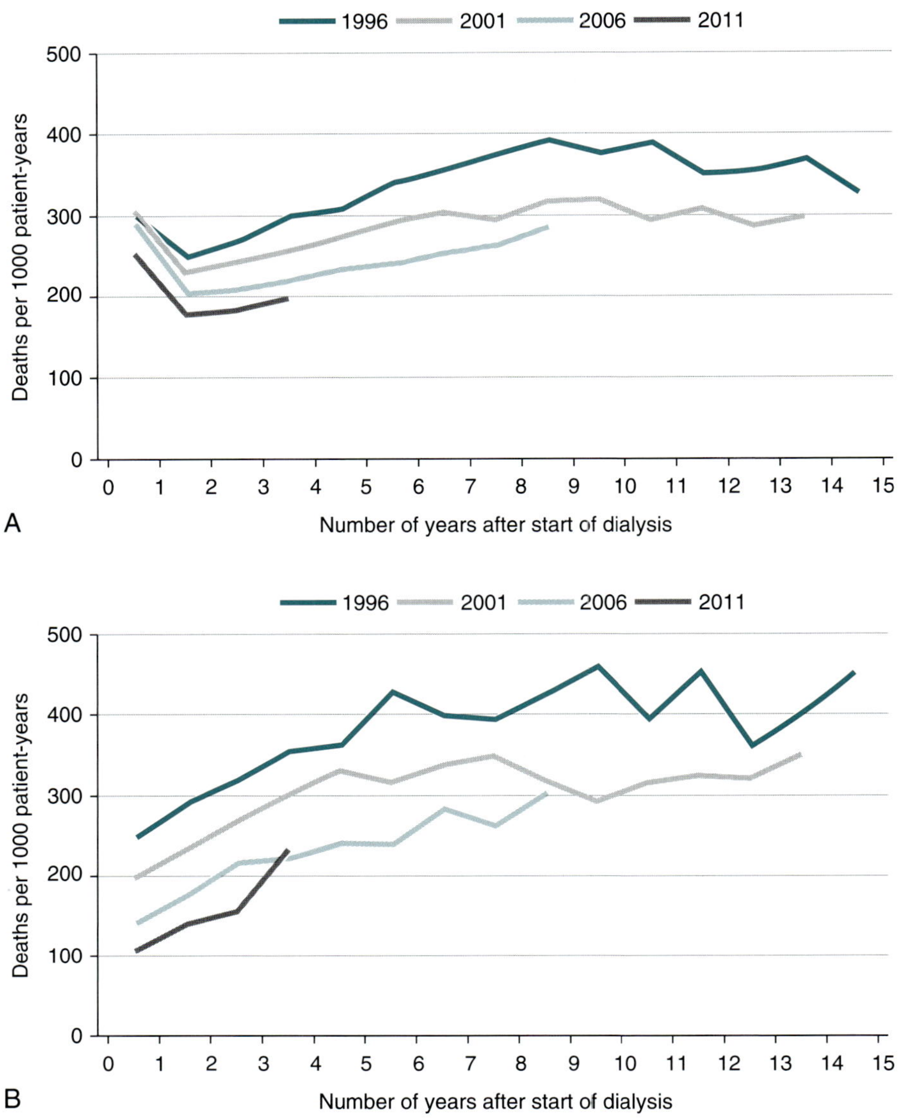

FIG. 21.11 Adjusted all-cause mortality (deaths per 1000 patient-years) by treatment modality, cohort (year of ESRD onset), and number of years after start of dialysis among incident (A) hemodialysis patients and (B) peritoneal dialysis patients, 1996, 2001, 2006, and 2011. Adjusted for age, sex, race, and primary diagnosis. (From United States Renal Data System. *2016 USRDS Annual Data Report: Epidemiology of Kidney Disease in the United States*. Bethesda, MD: National Institutes of Health, National Institute of Diabetes and Digestive and Kidney Diseases; 2016.)

for men than for women aged ≤44 years, comparable for ages 45 to 64 years, and higher for men than for women aged ≥65 years.[18] These rates are shown in Table 21.1, which demonstrates the age-×-race and age-×-sex interactions in death rates among prevalent dialysis patients in 2014.

Two related quantities, survival probabilities and expected remaining years of life, may constitute intuitive ways of conceptualizing dialysis survival, at least compared with annualized mortality rates. The associated unadjusted increase in life span can be graphically illustrated, as in Fig. 21.12, which represents unadjusted increases in life span for prevalent dialysis patients between 2004 and 2010. Life spans increased for all age groups. On a relative scale, 5-year survival probabilities increased by approximately 17% for hemodialysis patients and 31% for PD patients between 2001 and 2009. However, in absolute terms, 5-year survival probabilities remain low, increasing from 36% to only 42% for hemodialysis patients and from 39% to 51% for PD patients over this period. Younger individuals experienced both higher absolute mean increases and higher proportional increases, but this would be expected since they have more potential remaining years of life than older individuals do. However, in absolute terms, the increases have been modest; this is especially concerning regarding younger individuals, who, were it not for ESRD, could expect many decades of remaining life.

Expected remaining years of life for patients receiving maintenance dialysis can be compared with the general population or with relevant disease-specific populations. The former comparison strikingly demonstrates the reality of lower survival among dialysis patients relative to the general

TABLE 21.1 Adjusted All-Cause Mortality (Deaths Per 1000 Patient-Years) by Age and Race, and by Age and Sex, Among End-Stage Renal Disease Patients in the United States, 2014

Age (y) and Race	ESRD	Dialysis	Transplant
0–21			
White	10	33	4
Black/African American	18	35	6
Other	8	26	4
22–44			
White	33	64	9
Black/African American	43	54	11
Other	20	37	4
45–64			
White	108	155	35
Black/African American	98	112	34
Other	77	102	20
65–74			
White	209	249	80
Black/African American	171	185	79
Other	139	161	59
≥75			
White	357	377	136
Black/African American	270	276	143
Other	233	240	111
Age (y) and Sex			
0–21			
Male	9	31	3
Female	12	36	4
22–44			
Male	34	56	9
Female	39	66	10
45–64			
Male	105	141	36
Female	107	144	31
65–74			
Male	205	245	83
Female	196	224	74
≥75			
Male	357	379	140
Female	330	342	129

ESRD, End-stage renal disease.
(From United States Renal Data System. *2016 USRDS Annual Data Report: Epidemiology of Kidney Disease in the United States.* Bethesda, MD: National Institutes of Health, National Institute of Diabetes and Digestive and Kidney Diseases; 2016.)

population. As expected, survival probabilities are far worse than for age- and sex-matched individuals in the general population; overall 3-year survival is 56% and 67% for hemodialysis and PD patients, respectively, but 92% to 94% for the general population. The difference in expected remaining years of life is >43 years for women aged 20 to 24 years (16.4 vs. 59.5 years), and >6.5 years for men aged 75 to 79 years (3.2 vs. 9.8), to illustrate two possible examples from among all age groups (Table 21.2).

However, the differences reflect more than the effects of kidney failure, as patients receiving maintenance dialysis have a much higher nonrenal comorbidity burden than individuals in the general population. As such, a more appropriate comparison might be with other populations with major medical conditions such as diabetes, heart failure, coronary artery disease status-post acute myocardial infarction, cerebrovascular disease status-post stroke or transient ischemic attack, cancer, and others. Although modest improvements in survival have occurred for most such conditions since 1996 (Fig. 21.13), the improvements in survival for dialysis patients have been substantially greater, at least since about 2004.

Cause-Specific Mortality

The major causes of death for prevalent dialysis patients are shown in Fig. 21.14. Sudden cardiac death (SCD) is responsible for approximately 30% of deaths and other cardiovascular disease (CVD) for 11%, meaning that CVD is the cause of death for more than two in five prevalent dialysis patients. The findings are similar for incident patients throughout the first years of dialysis. However, because the cause of death is unknown for roughly 25% of patients, and because many such deaths are likely cardiovascular in nature, the overall proportion of deaths attributable to CVD may well be more than half. In comparison, infection is responsible for approximately 8% of deaths. Withdrawal from dialysis is technically the cause of death for roughly 14% of patients, but some misclassification in this attribution is possible since any elective cessation of dialysis before death, even if it occurs before imminent death from other causes, can often be classified as withdrawal. Approximately one in eight deaths are attributable to other causes.

In the first year of dialysis, death rates decline steeply immediately following initiation, as noted. However, rates of certain causes of death decline more steeply than others. Fig. 21.15 depicts trends in cause-specific mortality by month in the first year after dialysis initiation. SCD rates are strikingly high immediately after initiation, but decline dramatically in the ensuing 3 months. The pattern of deaths from unknown cause is similar to the pattern for SCD, providing circumstantial evidence that many unknown deaths are likely due to SCD. Infectious causes of death also decline over the first year, but the decrease is not as large in either absolute or relative terms as the decrease in SCD. Withdrawal is a relatively common cause of death throughout the first year. The rate of deaths due to withdrawal may well be underestimated within the first month after dialysis initiation, as many patients afforded a "trial" of dialysis may elect not to pursue it, especially patients who are very old, very frail, were initiated in the hospital (particularly in critical care units), or have other life-limiting medical conditions.

Morbidity and Hospitalizations

Overall Trends

Hospitalizations are common in patients receiving maintenance dialysis, as might be expected. In 2014 the adjusted

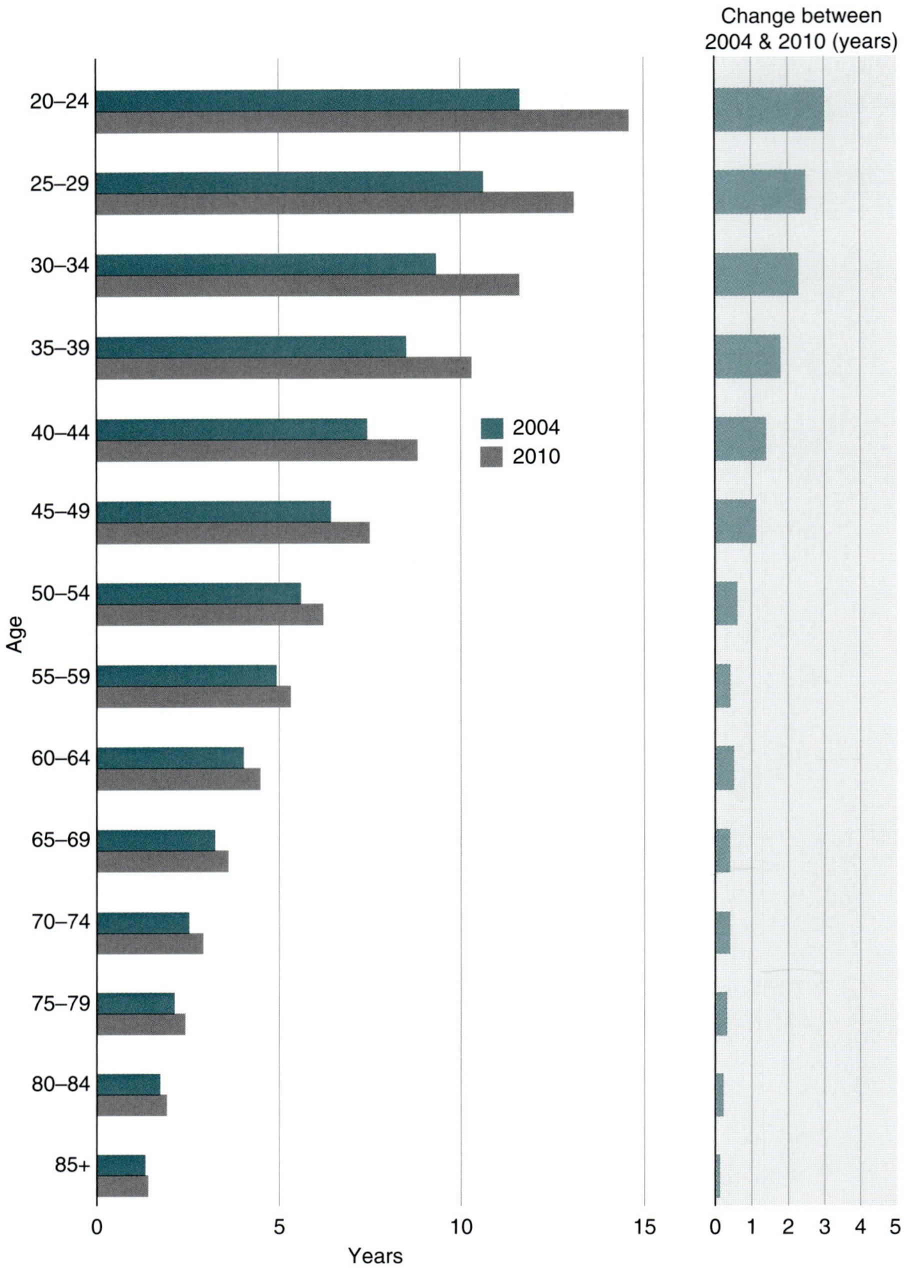

FIG. 21.12 Increase in expected remaining lifetimes in incident dialysis patients, by age group, between 2004 and 2010. (From Peer Kidney Care Initiative, Peer Report: Dialysis Care and Outcomes in the United States, 2014. Available at http://www.peerkidney.org/wp-content/uploads/2016/10/peer-kidney-full-report.pdf. Chapter 3, Mortality, page 104.)

all-cause hospitalization rate was approximately 1.8 per year among hemodialysis and among PD patients. Most admissions, comprising a combined total of about 45%, are for cardiovascular- and infection-related causes among hemodialysis and PD patients. Hospitalization rates have declined steadily over the past decade (Fig. 21.16), from more than two per person per year in 2005; most of the decrease appears to have occurred in 2010 and thereafter. Roughly 50% of this decline likely represents a broad shift in site of care from inpatient to outpatient settings (e.g., observation stays) that is occurring throughout the US healthcare system, but approximately 50% of the decline likely represents a true improvement in the rate of healthcare encounters.[52] Time spent in the hospital decreased from about 15 to 11 days for hemodialysis patients and from about 16 to 11 days for PD patients from 2005 to 2014; however, the total does not include increasingly used observation stays and so is likely an underestimation. While reductions in hospitalization days are undoubtedly real, approximately half of the decrease in days during which a patient is formally admitted to the hospital is offset by an increase in days spent under observation status. In addition, hospitalization rates demonstrate substantial geographical variation (Fig. 21.17), even after adjustment for basic demographic characteristics.

TABLE 21.2 Expected Remaining Lifetime (y) by Age, Sex, and Treatment Modality of Prevalent Dialysis Patients and Transplant Patients in the United States, and the General US Population, 2013

	AGE (Y)															
	0–14	15–19	20–24	25–29	30–34	35–39	40–44	45–49	50–54	55–59	60–64	65–69	70–74	75–79	80–84	≥85
ESRD patients, 2013																
Dialysis																
Male	22.6	21.6	18.5	16.2	14.3	12.6	11.0	9.2	7.9	6.6	5.5	4.5	3.8	3.2	2.6	2.2
Female	23.3	19.0	16.4	14.3	13.0	11.6	10.4	8.9	7.8	6.6	5.7	4.8	4.0	3.5	2.9	2.4
Transplant																
Male	60.1	47.9	43.4	39.2	35.1	31	27.2	23.4	19.9	16.7	13.8	11.4	9.5	7.7*		
Female	59.8	48.5	44.2	40.2	36.4	32.8	28.9	25.2	21.7	18.3	15.3	12.6	10.4	8.7*		
General US population, 2013																
Male	70.7	59.7	55.0	50.3	45.7	41.0	36.4	31.9	27.7	23.7	19.8	16.2	12.8	9.8	7.1	3.7
Female	75.4	64.4	59.5	54.6	49.7	45.0	40.3	35.6	31.1	26.8	22.6	18.5	14.7	11.3	8.4	4.4

*Cell values combine ages ≥75 years.
ESRD, End-stage renal disease.
(From United States Renal Data System. *2016 USRDS Annual Data Report: Epidemiology of Kidney Disease in the United States.* Bethesda, MD: National Institutes of Health, National Institute of Diabetes and Digestive and Kidney Diseases; 2016.)

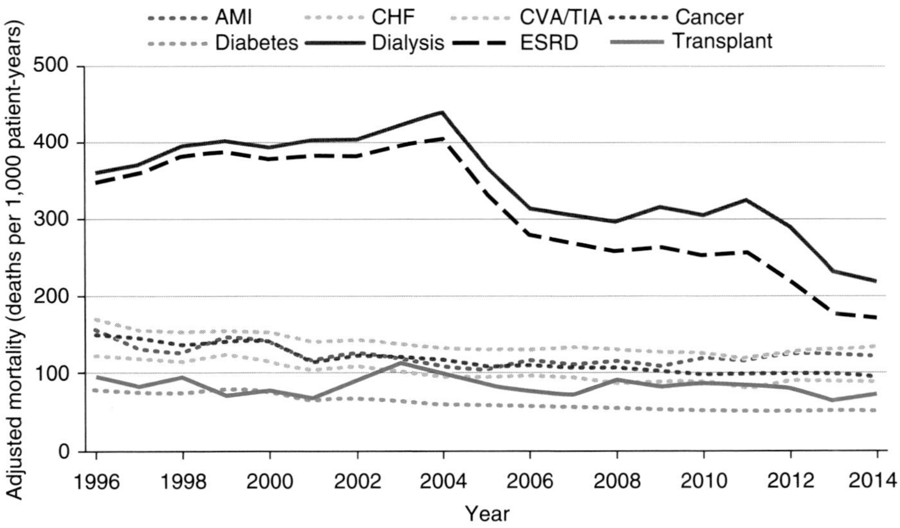

FIG. 21.13 Adjusted mortality (deaths per 1000 patient-years) by calendar year, treatment modality, and comorbidity among ESRD patients and comorbidity-specific Medicare populations ≥65 years of age, 1996 to 2014. Adjusted for sex and race. (From United States Renal Data System. *2016 USRDS Annual Data Report: Epidemiology of Kidney Disease in the United States.* Bethesda, MD: National Institutes of Health, National Institute of Diabetes and Digestive and Kidney Diseases; 2016.)

Readmissions, typically defined as an admission within 30 days of a hospital discharge, remain a vexing problem for dialysis patients. Readmission data at the patient level are shown in Fig. 21.18, which contrasts rehospitalization patterns in ESRD and CKD patients and the general population. Several studies from the United States and Canada[53,54] recently examined all-cause, infection-related, and cardiovascular-related readmissions among dialysis patients. Although study designs differ, the findings have been consistent. Roughly one in three hospitalizations is followed by a readmission within 30 days, regardless of the indication (cardiovascular, infection, or all-cause); this is more than half again as much as in the general population, where approximately 22% of patients are readmitted within 30 days.[55] Table 21.3 depicts unpublished data on readmissions in the United States after an index cardiovascular admission. Remarkably, half of readmissions (representing about one-sixth of all index admissions) result in hospital readmission within a mere 10 days. These figures actually underestimate healthcare encounters after an index admission, since nearly 25% of admissions result in an observation stay or emergency department encounter (i.e., an encounter not resulting in a readmission) within 30 days. Notably, roughly 50% of readmissions involve a disease category nonconcordant with the initial reason for admission; that

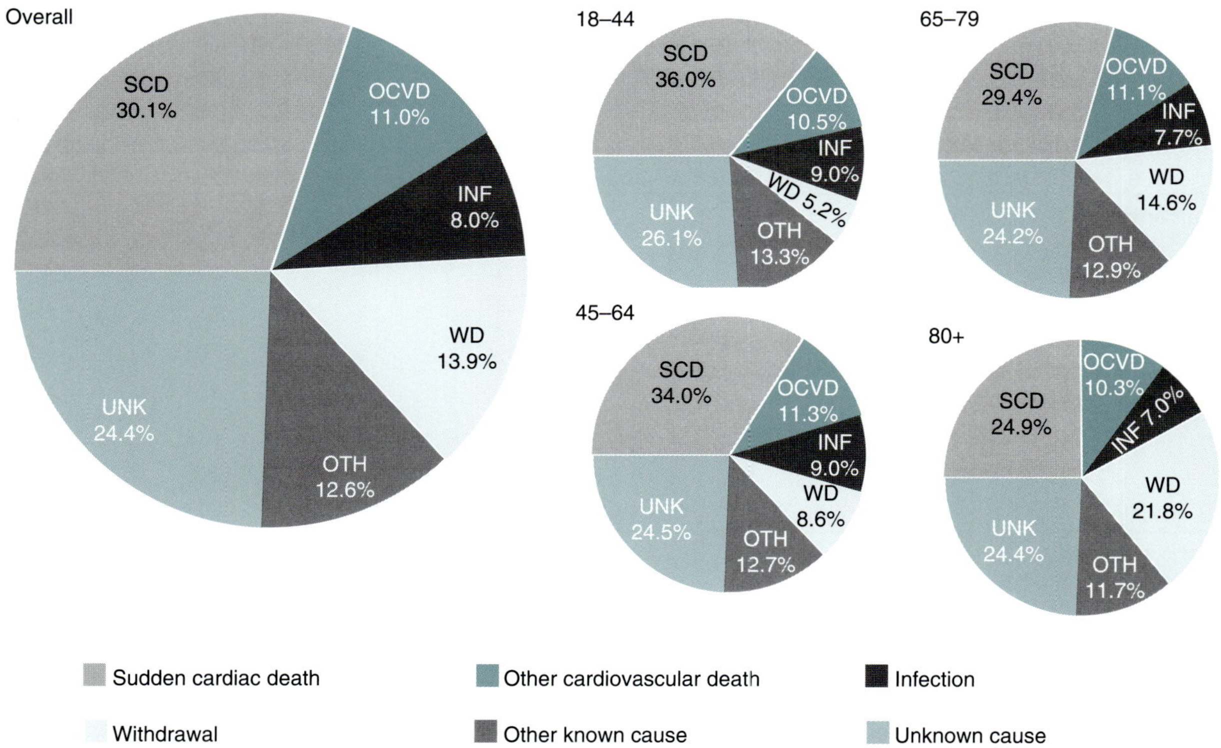

FIG. 21.14 Distribution of causes of death in prevalent dialysis patients, according to the Death Notification form; patients prevalent on January 1, 2013, ≥18 years of age. (From Peer Kidney Care Initiative. Peer Report: Dialysis Care and Outcomes in the US, 2016. Available at http://www.peerkidney.org/. Fig. 3.8.)

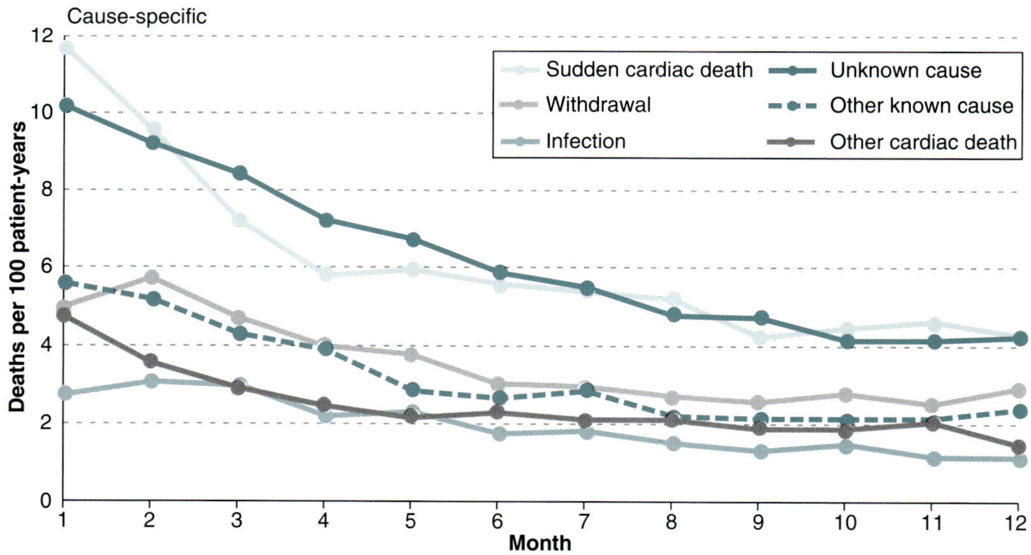

FIG. 21.15 Cause-specific, first-year mortality rates in incident dialysis patients, according to the Death Notification form; incident patients in 2012 ≥18 years of age. (From Peer Kidney Care Initiative. Peer Report: Dialysis Care and Outcomes in the US, 2016. Available at http://www.peerkidney.org/. Fig. 3.11.)

is, following an index admission for a cardiovascular or infectious indication, half of readmissions within 30 days are for a noncardiovascular or noninfectious indication, highlighting the overall medical instability that characterizes many dialysis patients. A cardiovascular indication for an admission is particularly ominous, since nearly 1 in 20 admissions (4.5%) will result in death within 30 days, regardless of whether a readmission occurs. Age tends to be inversely associated with risk for readmission after a cardiovascular event, an apparent paradox that has nevertheless been observed in the nondialysis population. Although readmission rates do not vary substantially between whites and blacks/African Americans,

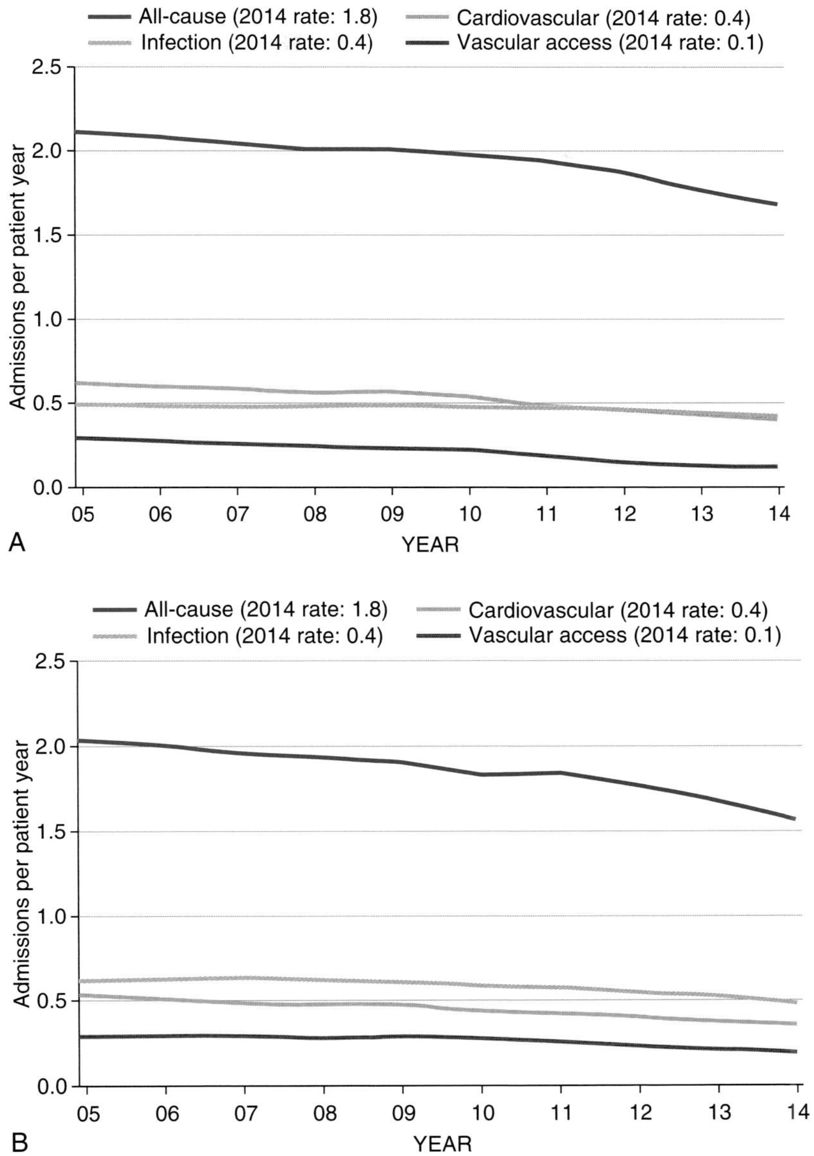

FIG. 21.16 Adjusted all-cause and cause-specific hospitalization rates for ESRD patients, by treatment modality, 2005 to 2014. (A) hemodialysis; (B) peritoneal dialysis. Adjusted for age, sex, race, primary cause of kidney failure, and their two-way interactions. (From United States Renal Data System. *2016 USRDS Annual Data Report: Epidemiology of Kidney Disease in the United States.* Bethesda, MD: National Institutes of Health, National Institute of Diabetes and Digestive and Kidney Diseases; 2016.)

the latter are roughly half as likely to die within 30 days of a cardiovascular readmission as are whites, a finding that should be further studied. As in the general population, there is evidence of geographical variation in readmission rates, likely reflecting differences in access to and delivery of care.

CVD and infectious disease, therefore, remain the two largest sources of morbidity and mortality in dialysis patients, and so are deserving of special scrutiny.

Cardiovascular Disease: Implications for Morbidity and Mortality

The importance of CVD in kidney disease patients has long been appreciated.[56] The relationship between these entities is complex: The processes that cause CVD can contribute to kidney disease, but CVD also can exist contemporaneously with kidney disease (regardless of the underlying cause of the latter) and, as such, contribute to cardiovascular morbidity and mortality. In addition, uremia itself contributes to processes intrinsic to CVD development.

CVD manifestation is shown by ESRD category (hemodialysis, PD, transplant) in Fig. 21.19. For all categories of CVD except venous thromboembolic disease (including pulmonary embolism), rates of CVD are higher for hemodialysis than for PD patients, whose rates are generally higher than for transplant patients. When any manifestation of CVD is considered, >70% of hemodialysis patients, 60% of PD patients,

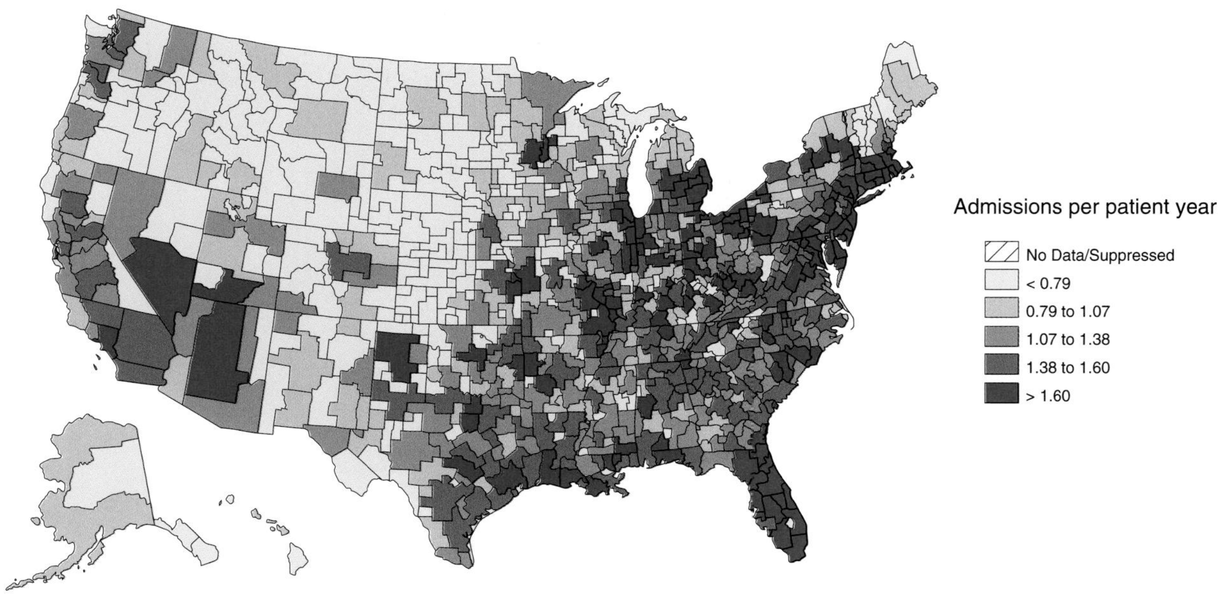

FIG. 21.17 Map of the hospitalization rates of ESRD, by Health Service Area, in the US population, 2014, adjusted. (From United States Renal Data System. *2016 USRDS Annual Data Report: Epidemiology of Kidney Disease in the United States*. Bethesda, MD: National Institutes of Health, National Institute of Diabetes and Digestive and Kidney Diseases; 2016.)

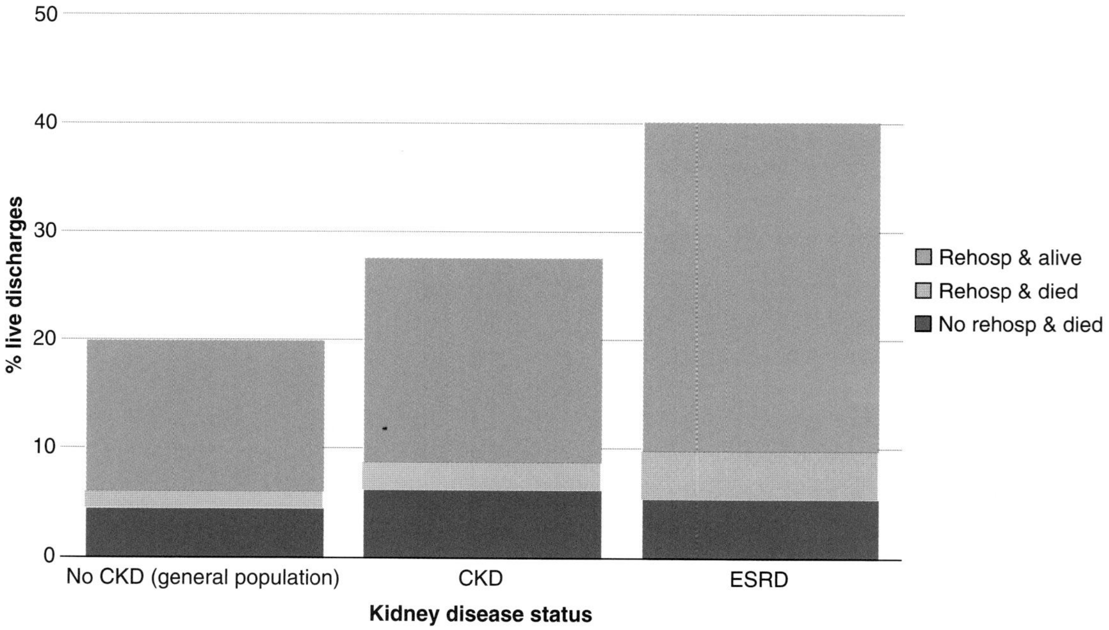

FIG. 21.18 Proportion of patients at ≥66 years of age discharged alive from the hospital who were either rehospitalized or died within 30 days of discharge, by kidney disease status, 2014. (From United States Renal Data System. *2016 USRDS Annual Data Report: Epidemiology of Kidney Disease in the United States*. Bethesda, MD: National Institutes of Health, National Institute of Diabetes and Digestive and Kidney Diseases; 2016.)

and 55% of transplant patients carry at least one diagnosis. Importantly, the effect of these modalities on CVD cannot be informed by these data; patients receiving hemodialysis often are sicker than those offered, or capable of undertaking, PD, whereas patients capable of undergoing kidney transplant are the healthiest.

Presence of congestive heart failure (CHF) can immensely complicate dialysis patient treatment. Volume removal is a key overarching goal for dialysis patients with CHF, yet this can be challenging in patients with little or no residual renal function. Recently, interest in diastolic heart failure has been growing. Its prevalence has likely been historically underestimated in the general[57] and in the dialysis population, and it has few, if any, evidence-based therapies. Determining the relative contributions of diastolic and systolic heart failure in dialysis patients is difficult. Although systolic heart

TABLE 21.3 Outcome Events After Discharge From Index Hospitalization, by Type of Index Cardiovascular Admission, Within 10 or 30 Days in the United States

	EVENTS					
Hospitalizations, N = 142,210	**All-Cause Readmission**	**Cardiovascular Readmission**	**Death, No Readmission**	**Death and Readmission**	**Death***	**ED visit/Obs. Stay**
30-d outcomes, %						
All cardiovascular hospitalizations	34.2	14.7	1.8	2.6	4.5	24.6
Acute coronary syndrome	37.0	16.8	2.6	3.8	6.4	24.4
Arrhythmia	31.2	13.3	1.9	2.9	4.8	22.9
CHF†	34.6	16.1	1.8	2.8	4.6	23.7
Stroke	29.1	9.8	3.0	3.3	6.3	23.0
Other cardiovascular disease	34.5	14.0	1.5	2.1	3.6	26.1
10-d outcomes, %						
All cardiovascular hospitalizations	15.6	6.6	0.9	0.6	1.5	11.6
Acute coronary syndrome	19.0	8.7	1.3	1.0	2.3	12.0
Arrhythmia	15.1	6.6	0.9	0.6	1.5	10.8
CHF†	15.1	6.9	0.9	0.6	1.5	10.6
Stroke	14.5	4.8	1.8	0.7	2.4	11.4
Other cardiovascular disease	15.5	6.2	0.8	0.5	1.2	12.5

*Regardless of readmission.
†Comprising heart failure, fluid overload, and cardiomyopathy.
CHF, Congestive heart failure; *ED*, emergency department; *Obs.*, observation.

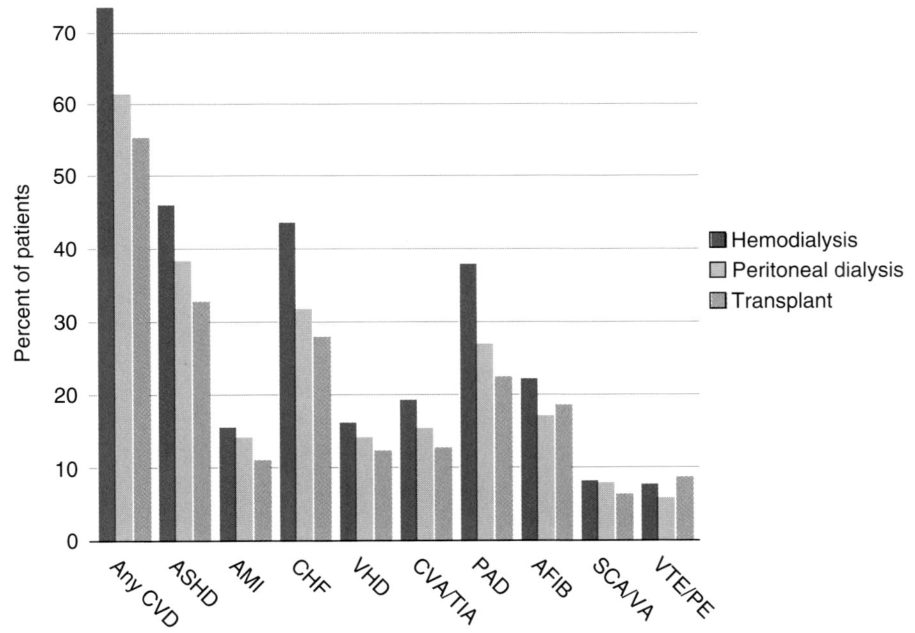

FIG. 21.19 Prevalence of cardiovascular disease in adult ESRD patients by treatment modality, 2014. (From United States Renal Data System. *2016 USRDS Annual Data Report: Epidemiology of Kidney Disease in the United States.* Bethesda, MD: National Institutes of Health, National Institute of Diabetes and Digestive and Kidney Diseases; 2016.)

failure appears to be relatively more common in hemodialysis and, especially, PD patients, diastolic heart failure may be a more-common cause of CHF than appreciated (Fig. 21.20). In the analysis presented, patients were designated as having systolic heart failure whether or not diastolic heart failure was present, an approach that would tend to inflate rates of systolic, compared with diastolic, heart failure. In addition, the largest single contributor is unspecified heart failure, severely limiting any conclusions about the relative importance of these two entities and demonstrating the importance of specificity when recording clinical data to inform epidemiological conclusions.

From an epidemiological perspective, the past decade has witnessed both the advent of welcome developments and the

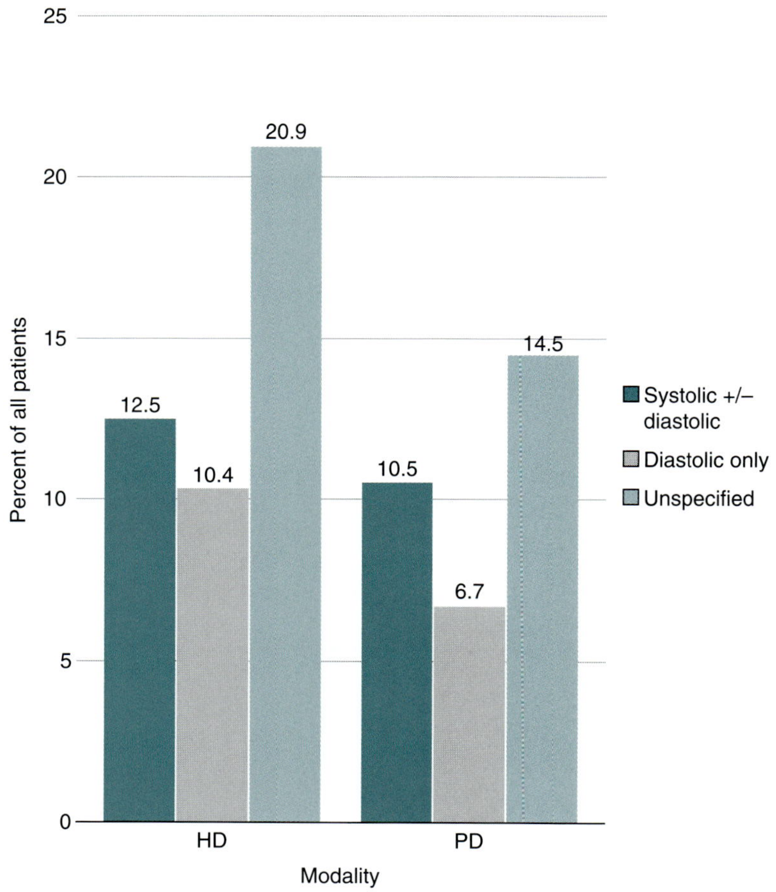

FIG. 21.20 Heart failure in adult ESRD patients by modality, 2014. (From United States Renal Data System. *2016 USRDS Annual Data Report: Epidemiology of Kidney Disease in the United States*. Bethesda, MD: National Institutes of Health, National Institute of Diabetes and Digestive and Kidney Diseases; 2016.)

persistence of vexing challenges. Overall, cardiovascular-related mortality rates have declined substantially. Trends in rates of death due to the various manifestations of CVD are shown in Fig. 21.21. The HP 2020 project set a goal of 10% improvement in cardiovascular mortality in prevalent patients,[3] corresponding to an annual improvement of about 0.8% per year. However, between 2001 and 2013, realized annual cardiovascular mortality improvement was more than 4%, far exceeding the annual goal.

However, progress also lags in key areas of CVD, namely arrhythmias, SCD, and heart failure/fluid overload. SCD and its antecedents (atrial and ventricular arrhythmias and asystolic events) remain major problems. Hospitalization rates for arrhythmias have remained virtually unchanged over the past decade, at about five events per 100 patient-years, with a slightly higher overall first-year rate for incident patients (5.7 per 100 patient-years, on average) compared with the overall annual rate for prevalent patients (4.6 per 100 patient-years, on average).[52] Lack of improvement in hospitalization rates for arrhythmias may be due to the prevalence of atrial fibrillation, which has been increasing in both the general[58] and dialysis[59] populations. As the dialysis population ages, this problem is likely to become more acute, since atrial fibrillation in dialysis patients,[60] as in the general population,[58,61] is strongly related to age. Notably, for hyperkalemia (a disorder related to arrhythmias), hospitalization rates have also failed to improve, at about 3.8 per 100 patient-years for prevalent patients and 2.4 for incident patients.[52]

Perhaps as a result, SCD as a proportion of total cardiac-related deaths has increased. SCD was responsible for approximately 53% of cardiac-related deaths in 1996, but this increased to 73% in 2013 (Fig. 21.22). The aforementioned lack of decrease in hospitalization rates for arrhythmias is likely related to this. To decrease arrhythmia-related morbidity and mortality, several issues merit further exploration, including the timing of these events across days of the dialysis week, the risk for hyperkalemia over the long dialytic interval, and the risk for postdialysis hypokalemia or other electrolyte changes induced by dialysis. Avoidance of low-potassium baths and optimal use of drugs such as β-adrenergic blockers, guided by improved understanding of the dialyzability of these medications,[62] could be studied in future clinical trials.

Hospitalizations for CHF and volume overload also require specific attention. Hospitalizations for CHF among prevalent dialysis patients declined nearly 40% over a decade, from roughly 15.6 per 100 patient-years in 2004 to 9.5 in 2013.[63] At the same time, however, hospitalizations for

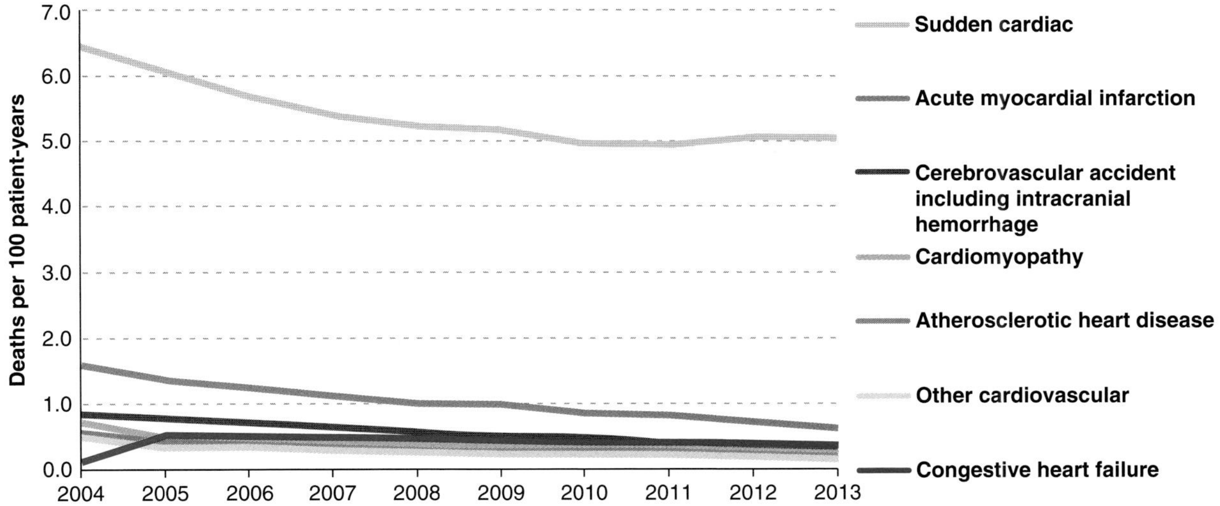

FIG. 21.21 One-year cardiovascular mortality rates, by primary cause of death, according to the Death Notification form, patients aged 18 years or older. (From Peer Kidney Care Initiative. Peer Report: Dialysis Care and Outcomes in the US, 2016. Available at http://www.peerkidney.org/. Fig. 4.5.)

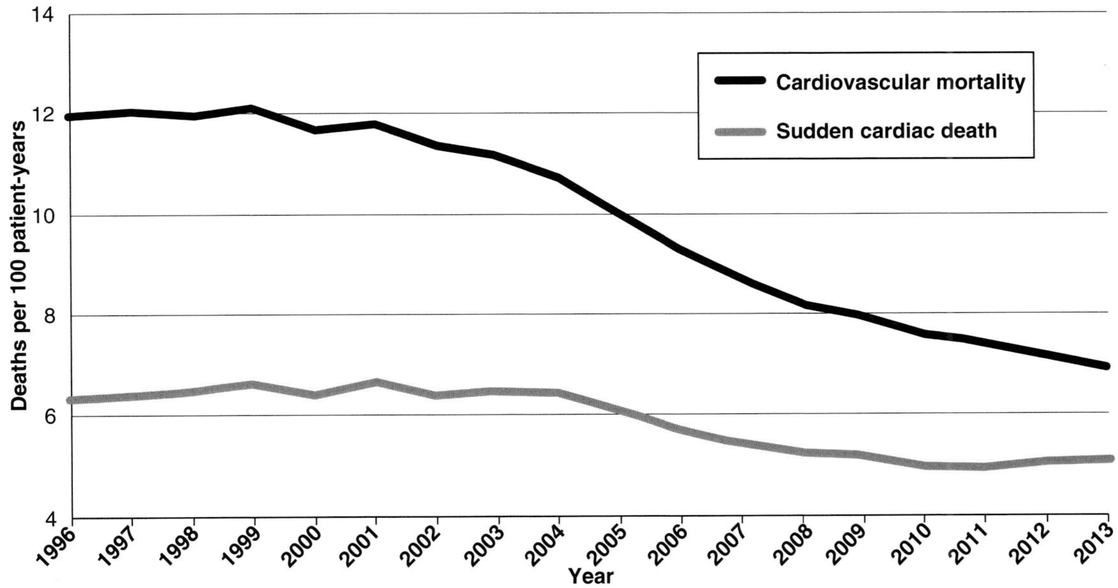

FIG. 21.22 Annual rates of all-cause cardiovascular mortality and sudden cardiac death in maintenance dialysis patients. (From Wetmore JB, Li S, Molony JT, et al. Insights from the 2016 Peer Kidney Care Initiative Report: still a ways to go to improve care for dialysis patients. *Am J Kidney Dis.* 2018;71:123-132.)

volume overload (fluid overload, pleural effusions, and pulmonary edema) doubled among prevalent patients, from 3 to 6.1 per 100 patient-years from 2004 through 2013, attenuating the apparent decline attributable to CHF from billing codes by roughly half. Given the intense scrutiny Medicare affords hospital readmission rates for CHF,[55] observed trends may be due to regulatory changes, whereby hospitalizations previously labeled as CHF may be increasingly labeled as "volume overload" by hospital coders, a phenomenon known as *coding drift*. Unfortunately, little improvement in volume management has occurred since the turn of the millennium; data from Dialysis Outcomes and Practice Patterns Study (DOPPS) suggest that only small decreases in interdialytic weight gains (amounting to only about 0.4% of postdialysis dry weight) occurred worldwide between 2002 and 2014.[64] For continued improvement in admission rates for CHF and volume overload, nontraditional methods of dialysis delivery, such as long-duration, nocturnal, home-based, and/or more-frequent hemodialysis (e.g., true every-other-day hemodialysis, eliminating 72-hour interdialytic intervals), should be explored, especially if undertaken with the aim of persistently reducing volume overload.

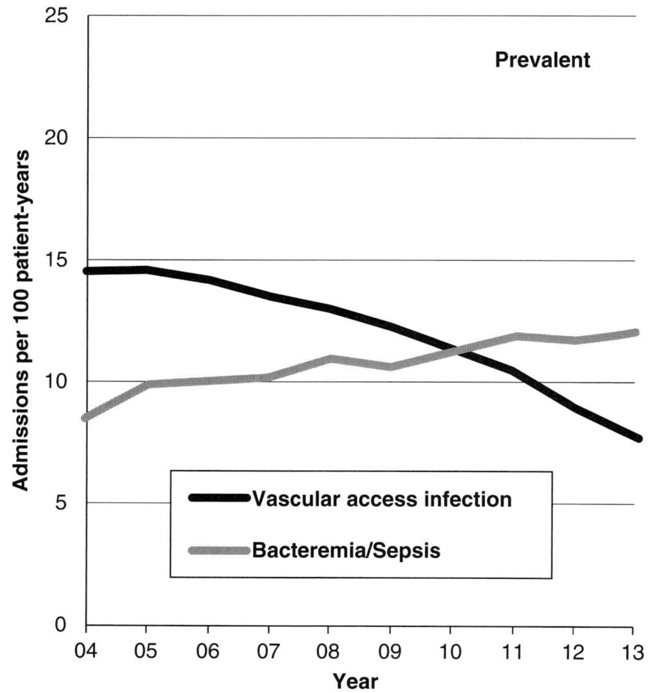

FIG. 21.23 Annual rates of hospitalizations with primary discharge diagnosis of vascular access infection or bacteremia/sepsis for prevalent maintenance dialysis patients. (From Wetmore JB, Li S, Molony JT, et al. Insights from the 2016 Peer Kidney Care Initiative Report: still a ways to go to improve care for dialysis patients. *Am J Kidney Dis.* 2018;71:123-132.)

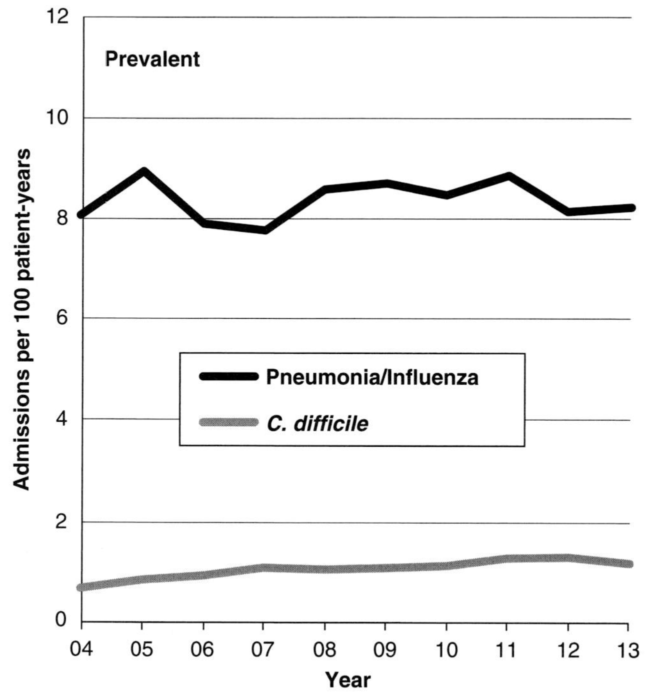

FIG. 21.24 Annual rates of hospitalizations with primary discharge diagnosis of pneumonia/influenza or *Clostridium difficile* for prevalent maintenance dialysis patients. (From Wetmore JB, Li, S, Molony JT, et al. Insights from the 2016 Peer Kidney Care Initiative Report: still a ways to go to improve care for dialysis patients. *Am J Kidney Dis.* 2018;71:123-132.)

Infectious Diseases: Implications for Morbidity and Mortality

The dramatic overall decrease in cardiovascular-related hospitalizations in prevalent patients means that they now approach rates of infection-related hospitalizations, each at about 40 per 100 patient-years as of 2013. A similar phenomenon is occurring for incident patients. Thus infection-related hospitalizations remain a persistent problem for patients receiving maintenance dialysis.

One major source of infection-related morbidity in hemodialysis patients is infection of vascular accesses. Rates of vascular access infection hospitalizations have decreased in incident and in prevalent patients, from approximately 22.3 to 15.6 per 100 patient-years in the former and 14.5 to 7.8 in the latter, decreases of 30% and 46%, respectively.[63] Rates of bacteremia/sepsis, however, have shown an opposite trend, increasing by 38% (from 12.9 to 17.8 per 100 patient-years) in incident patients and by 40% (from 8.6 to 12 per 100 patient-years) in prevalent patients (Fig. 21.23). Vascular access infections often result in bacteremia and systemic inflammatory response syndrome, colloquially termed *sepsis*. The rise in hospitalizations for bacteremia/sepsis along with decreasing rates of vascular access infections suggests that hospitalizations previously coded for access-related infections are likely now being coded as bacteremia, and that assessing true progress in vascular access infections is difficult.

Rates of hospitalization for pneumonia and influenza, another common source of infection-related morbidity, have remained relatively unchanged over the past decade, at approximately eight hospitalizations per 100 patient-years (Fig. 21.24). Regarding prevention of these disorders, the role of vaccines will need further examination before hospitalization rates are likely to decrease. The optimal way to vaccinate dialysis patients for influenza, for example, is unknown.[65] Although the US Centers for Disease Control and Prevention (CDC) recommended influenza vaccinations for high-risk populations such as patients with kidney disease,[66] and although providers have responded by increasing vaccination rates, little is known about the antibody responsiveness to single-dose vaccines. Because response to the influenza vaccine may wane before the end of an influenza season, it has been suggested that patients on dialysis should receive high-dose or adjuvanted influenza vaccines.[67,68] The answers to these and other questions will come only from completion of clinical trials.

One potentially underappreciated contributor to infection-related modbidity, and likely even to mortality, is *Clostridium difficile* infections. *C. difficile* infections among incident and prevalent patients have increased over the past decade; rates increased by 61%, from approximately 1.4 to 2.2 per 100 patient-years, for incident patients, and by 68%, from 0.7 to 1.2 per 100 patient-years, for prevalent patients.[63] *C. difficile* infections are a substantial source of morbidity in dialysis patients, and treatment can be challenging because patients often experience recurrence,[69] sometimes related to treatment with antibiotics for other indications. One key question is whether these rates may be driven, in part, by growing awareness of the importance of this disorder, or represent a true increase. *C. difficile* rates may be increasing due to administration of antibiotics in dialysis units or as a result of suspected sepsis syndrome and administration of "preemptive" antibiotics, raising issues of antibiotic stewardship for the nephrology community.

In appreciation of the importance of infections in dialysis patients, the CDC has joined with the American Society of Nephrology to create a new initiative, the Nephrologists Transforming Dialysis Safety program.[70] This public health agenda is designed to decrease the burden of infection-related morbidity and mortality in dialysis patients. Such efforts are likely to be critical in continuing the downward trend in infection rates, as infection likely constitutes the largest potentially preventable source of morbidity and mortality in dialysis patients.

Dialysis Modality

Selection of the optimal dialysis modality for a given patient is a long-standing issue in nephrology. The single most compelling question facing the practitioner is whether a given patient would derive greater benefit from hemodialysis or PD. This question can be further extended: Within the realm of hemodialysis, for example, choices include in-center versus home hemodialysis, "intensive" in-center versus traditional thrice-weekly hemodialysis, and longer-duration therapies (e.g., nocturnal hemodialysis) versus traditional hemodialysis. Somewhat analogous questions arise in the realm of PD, such as the relative benefits of traditional continuous ambulatory PD versus regimens using the nocturnal cycle (augmented by manual daily exchanges where needed). This question is critically important because, with the growth of treated (and, presumably, untreated) ESRD worldwide, virtually all nations face a major challenge in delivering RRT to their citizens. The model pursued for a half-century by the United States, namely relying on a widely dispersed network of expensive "bricks-and-mortar" dialysis units delivering traditional thrice-weekly hemodialysis to >90% of patients, may not be sustainable, especially in developing countries, countries with large rural populations, and countries with poor infrastructure.[2]

In principle, this question could be answered with a randomized clinical trial comparing, for example, incident patients randomized to hemodialysis versus PD. If sufficiently powered and adequately conducted, such a trial could examine the relative effects of the therapies in subgroups such as older patients, those with diabetes, and those with heart failure. However, randomization would require selection of patients who are equally suitable medical candidates for either therapy, and who have no social barriers to either therapy. In addition, strong patient preferences would make recruitment a major challenge. Thus, no satisfactory trial has yet been conducted. The Netherlands Cooperative Study on the Adequacy of Dialysis (NECOSAD), designed and originally powered as a survival trial, was terminated when only 38 patients were randomized after 3 years.[71] A randomized clinical trial in China, the China Q study, was undertaken several years ago, but low initial event rates reportedly threatened its ability to yield conclusions on mortality.[72] Although it is thought that this trial is completed, no results are available.

A number of well-performed observational studies have been conducted to examine mortality and hospitalization differences between hemodialysis and PD and between in-center and home hemodialysis. A complete examination of the findings is beyond the scope of this chapter, but they have been well-reviewed.[72] Although this issue has been studied since at least mid-1990s,[73-79] interest has continued from 2010 onward, with later studies using more advanced design and analytical approaches than earlier ones. Because hemodialysis is effectively the "default" treatment modality in the United States, patients who select (or who are selected for) PD may differ fundamentally in ways that cannot be accounted for in large observational studies. Advanced design and analytical techniques have been increasingly employed to attempt to account for nonrandom treatment allocation. Weinhandl et al.,[80] employing propensity-score matching in an analysis of patients from the USRDS, reported that PD was associated with a very modest survival advantage from day 1 of initiation (HR 0.92; 95% confidence interval, 0.86 to 1.00), but, when survival was counted from day 90, there was no such difference. This finding may be accounted for by the reality that a substantial number of patients initiate maintenance hemodialysis in an urgent or emergent setting, and these patients are at increased risk for early death. Other studies that have attempted to account for the "orderliness" of the transition to maintenance dialysis also have suggested that survival implications are similar for hemodialysis and PD. For example, Quinn et al.,[81] using comprehensive provincial data from Canada, found, after analyzing only patients who initiated dialysis electively as outpatients and accounting for duration of predialysis care (a putative marker of the orderliness of the transition), no differences in survival between modalities. A study using the Canadian Organ Replacement Registry[82] provided compelling evidence that use of hemodialysis catheters may, in large measure, be responsible for the inferior outcomes for hemodialysis compared with PD patients; comparison of PD patients only with catheter-free hemodialysis initiates demonstrated no survival difference between modalities. A particularly novel analytical approach was used by Mehrotra et al.,[83] who employed marginal structural modeling to mitigate confounding, and found no differences in survival among patients initiating in the recent eras they studied.

However, some investigators have more recently suggested that PD may be associated with a lower risk for death in the longer term that cannot be accounted for by differential events in the initiation period, such as frequency of urgent starts and percentages using suboptimal dialysis access.

Lukowsky et al.,[84] using data from a large national dialysis provider in the United States, employed marginal structural modeling to examine survival over 2 years. They also accounted for time-dependent variables, including laboratory values, and for censoring due to modality switches and transplant. They found a lower death risk ostensibly attributed to PD far larger than in other studies, with a HR of 0.52. A large (more than twofold) effect size for PD also was found for ≤2 years after initiation in a study using data from a large, closed health maintenance organization,[85] that does not seem to be accounted for by access to care or hemodialysis access (i.e., catheter vs. graft or fistula). Furthermore, a study of 20 years' worth of dialysis initiates in Denmark[86] found that, although survival for hemodialysis and PD patients improved over time (concordant with other data), the improvement was relatively larger for PD than for hemodialysis patients. A novel survival pattern was noted, such that PD was superior to hemodialysis for a full 4 years after initiation, but hemodialysis trended toward better survival thereafter.

When considering the relative potential benefit of one therapy over another, one important consideration is that modality use varies by race. Members of racial minorities are substantially less likely than whites to use home-based therapies such as PD and home hemodialysis (Fig. 21.25).[87] Notably, adjustment for potential (known) confounders does little to change the odds of being prescribed home-based therapies, and in some instances, even noticeably accentuates them. This suggests that patient, provider, or healthcare system effects may "channel" racial and ethnic minorities into traditional in-center hemodialysis. This affect appears to be independent of insurance status (appropriately adjusted for by the authors, as one might hypothesize that lower rates of private health insurance among nonwhites might contribute to such a proposed channeling effect). Whether this is

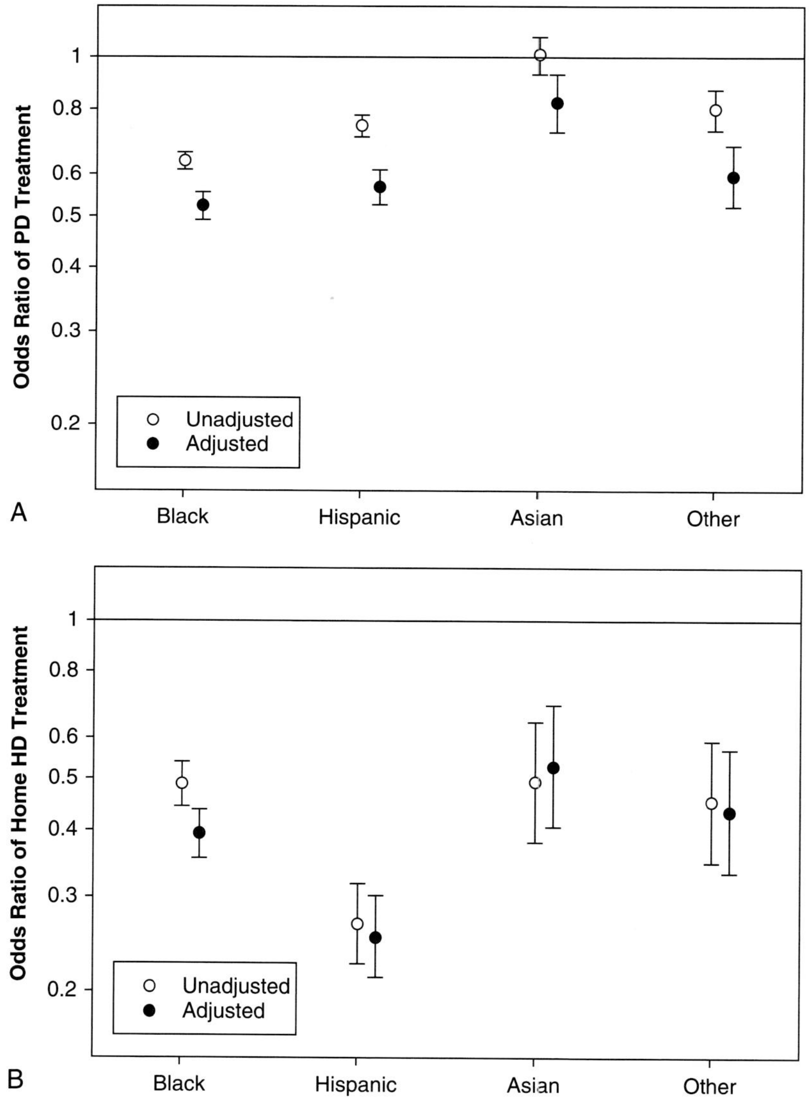

FIG. 21.25 Association of race/ethnicity with treatment with peritoneal dialysis or home hemodialysis. (From Mehrotra R, Soohoo M, Rivara MB, et al. Racial and ethnic disparities in use of and outcomes with home dialysis in the United States. *J Am Soc Nephrol.* 2016;27:2123-2134.)

justifiable on clinical grounds alone is uncertain; patient preference, systems of social support, socioeconomic factors, or other bedside-level factors known only to patients and their providers may well be responsible, as acknowledged by the authors. One potential explanation for a putative channeling effect is that historically, black patients have tended to dialyze in units where PD was relatively less available.[88] However, this finding is paradoxical on several fronts. First, nonwhite patients had significantly fewer comorbid conditions than whites, a characteristic that would typically increase the likelihood of receiving PD. In a further paradox, survival was better for black patients receiving both PD and home hemodialysis than for whites (Fig. 21.26). The survival advantage was greater than for blacks receiving in-center hemodialysis, but the course on PD was also more "adverse" for black patients with regard to (greater) likelihood of transition to hemodialysis and (lesser) likelihood of undergoing kidney transplant. Clearly, more study of how race and, more broadly, socioeconomic and geographical factors, influence selection of dialysis modality is needed.

The evidence for an overall modality-wide advantage is therefore conflicting, at present, on several fronts. PD may be associated with lower early (<1 year) death risk compared with hemodialysis, but studies disagree regarding whether preinitiation factors such as duration of predialysis nephrology care, urgency and location (inpatient vs. outpatient) of initiation, and hemodialysis access type can account for these differences. Whether the lower death risk persists beyond

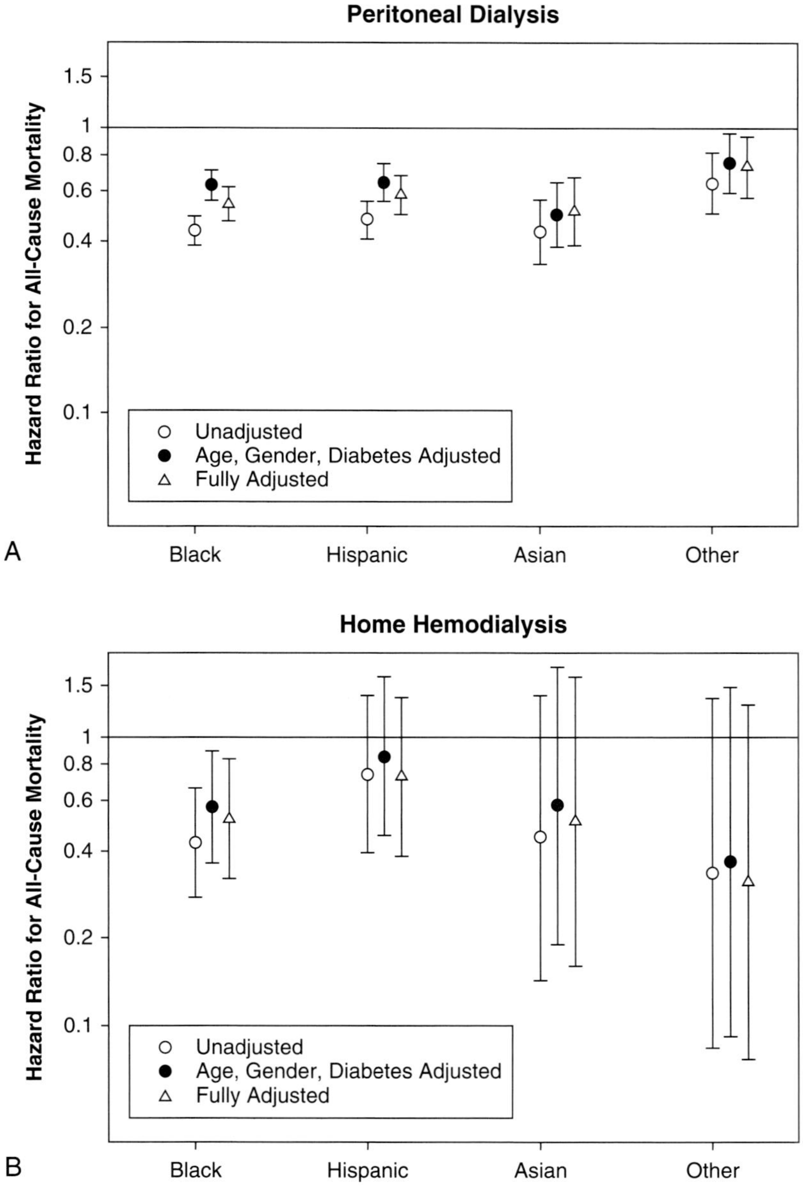

FIG. 21.26 Association of race/ethnicity with mortality among patients undergoing peritoneal dialysis or home hemodialysis. (From Mehrotra R, Soohoo M, Rivara MB, et al. Racial and ethnic disparities in use of and outcomes with home dialysis in the United States. *J Am Soc Nephrol.* 2016;27:2123-2134.)

6 months (e.g., to 2–4 years) also is uncertain. Whether hemodialysis might be associated with a lower death risk at many (e.g., >4) years out is unknown, but PD may become more challenging over time due to changes in the peritoneal membrane. Even whether hemodialysis is associated with a lower death risk in patients with diabetes is uncertain. Although several studies have suggested this,[83,86,89] a recent review concluded that the balance of evidence does not support it.[90] Thus, available evidence suggests that presence of diabetes should not be considered an absolute contraindication to PD for motivated patients who are otherwise good candidates.

Different forms of hemodialysis have been compared in clinical trials and observational studies. Traditional thrice-weekly in-center hemodialysis, serving as the "reference" modality, has been compared with home hemodialysis (which often duplicates the in-center hemodialysis prescription) and with intensive hemodialysis; that is, hemodialysis involving greater frequency of treatment sessions, more contact time with the dialysis membrane, or both. Intensive hemodialysis encompasses more frequent in-center hemodialysis (e.g., treatments four or more times per week), home hemodialysis with more than three treatments prescribed (often five or six per week), and nocturnal dialysis (in which treatment sessions typically exceed 6 hours, and are usually performed in-center). Thus, comparisons of in-center hemodialysis with "nontraditional" hemodialysis regimens encompass three cardinal issues: treatment frequency, treatment duration, treatment location. A relatively early trial of increased dialysis clearance, the Hemodialysis Study (HEMO), found no difference in mortality for patients treated to higher versus lower Kt/V targets.[91] This study cast considerable doubt as to whether increasing dialysis dose could improve mortality, but did not explicitly test issues of dialysis treatment length and frequency.

The Frequent Hemodialysis Network (FHN) group tested these very issues. The parent FHN trial, which tested six versus three times per week in-center hemodialysis for a composite outcome of mortality and reduction in left ventricular hypertrophy, found that frequent hemodialysis was associated with a HR of 0.61 for the coprimary endpoints.[92] Risk for mortality tended to favor frequent in-center hemodialysis, although absolute numbers of deaths were small. Over a median 3.6-year long-term follow-up period, in which deaths were frequent enough to examine as an individual endpoint, risk for mortality favored frequent in-center hemodialysis patients, with a HR of 0.54. However, the Nocturnal Trial component of FHN found no initial benefit of six-times-weekly nocturnal hemodialysis (vs. conventional hemodialysis) using the same combined primary endpoint.[93] In a long-term (median 3.7 years) follow-up study, risk for death increased in the nocturnal group in both intention-to-treat and as-treated analyses (HR, 3.99 and 3.06, respectively).[94] Although the authors appropriately urged caution in interpretation due to an unexpectedly low death rate in the traditional hemodialysis arm, modest statistical power, and substantial modality switching, the results nevertheless stand in striking contrast to the Daily trial. Observational studies provide some evidence for benefits of home hemodialysis. For example, in a large study comparing patients undergoing traditional in-center hemodialysis versus six-times-per-week home hemodialysis, Weinhandl et al.[95] used a conscientious matching strategy to attempt to reduce confounding; they found a 13% lower mortality in patients receiving home hemodialysis, an effect that appeared to be homogenous by subgroup. Their follow-up work suggested that overall hospitalization rates did not differ by modality, but that home hemodialysis patients had lower rates of cardiovascular-related, but higher rates of infection-related, hospitalizations.[96]

Insights into comparative effectiveness between the major PD modalities have come almost exclusively from observational studies. Traditional continuous ambulatory PD (CAPD), in which a patient performs manual exchanges throughout the day typically consisting of perhaps four dwells of 4 hours each, has been increasingly displaced by automated PD (APD, sometimes referred to as *continuous cycling PD*), in which a nocturnal cycler is used to deliver shorter-duration automated dwells over 8 to 10 hours. Although APD was historically considered suitable only for rapid or high transporters, patients of all transport characteristics can, in most cases, be successfully treated with it, especially when it is augmented with a daily exchange performed manually.[97] The great benefit of APD is that it confers much greater liberty for patients during waking hours. This, rather than a medical or scientific reason, appears to have been the main driving force in a shift from CAPD to APD in developed countries[98]; more than 70% of US and 60% of Canadian PD patients are now treated with APD.[18,99] A recent comprehensive narrative review concluded that there is no convincing evidence that either modality confers a benefit in preservation of residual renal function, volume management, or risks for peritonitis, technique failure, or mortality.[97]

In the United States, attempts recently have been undertaken to encourage greater use of home-based therapies, driven, in large measure, by efforts at cost containment, as home-based therapies are generally less expensive than in-center hemodialysis. These incentives, contained in what is known as the revised Prospective Payment System (PPS),[100] include bundling payments for previously separately billable injectable medications (expenses that are generally higher for in-center hemodialysis patients than for patients on home-based therapies), earlier initiation of reimbursement for patients who select home dialysis (at day 1 of dialysis, rather than day 91 as for in-center hemodialysis), and, more recently, a 50% increase in reimbursement for home dialysis training.[101] Collectively, these measures are expected to substantially increase the incentives for healthcare providers to encourage home-based therapies in the United States.[102,103] However, use of PD is variable around the world; for example, in Japan and much of Europe, usage has actually decreased.[104] Financial incentives, although important, are not the only factor that could influence use of PD; training nephrologists in prescribing PD, full embrace by the dialysis community, and, crucially, the ability to generate and deliver supplies locally, chiefly peritoneal dialysate and the sterilized components required to conduct the therapy, are all critical.

Vascular Access

Considerable attention has been devoted to vascular access in hemodialysis patients. The National Kidney Foundation Kidney Disease Outcomes Quality Initiative (NKF KDOQI) guidelines recommend initiating a permanent vascular access when dialysis is anticipated to commence in the next 6 months.[105] Despite concerted effort in nephrology to adequately prepare hemodialysis initiates with permanent vascular accesses, particularly arteriovenous (AV) fistulas, roughly four in five hemodialysis patients initiate with a catheter, either a catheter only (in roughly three of five patients) or a catheter with a developing fistula or graft (roughly one in five).[18] This represents a major failing, as CKD is almost always a long-term, slowly progressive disease that presents adequate opportunity for access placement. The true percentage of patients initiating with a catheter is likely higher because catheter use is associated with mortality and, as noted, early mortality among dialysis patients appears to be underreported. Exclusive catheter use upon initiation is highest for patients aged ≤21 years, at 81%, but is comparable across the older age groups, ranging from 60% for ages 65 to 74 years to 66% for ages 22 to 44 years. Women have only slightly higher catheter-only use than men, at 63% versus 60%, and differences by race are also modest (e.g., ranging from a low of 59% in Asians to a high of 62% in whites). Regarding cause of ESRD, only in cystic kidney disease, the archetypal slowly progressive kidney disease often involving consistent long-term follow-up, is catheter initiation much less common (at 37%, compared with 58% for diabetes and 62% for hypertension). Failure of access placement is therefore broad-based. A recent study suggested that roughly two-thirds of the risk of initiation with a catheter can be traced to patient-related factors, with only one-third likely due to system-related factors.[106]

Unfortunately, fistula use is not equivalent to fistula placement, since fully one-third of fistulas appear never to be used, presumably due to lack of maturation.[18] As creation of an AV fistula is not a trivial surgical procedure, this raises the possibility that fistulas may not be the best option for all patients, and that tailored strategies designed to match the access most appropriately to the patient profile might prove valuable. Another difficulty is that fistulas require a long maturation time, at least in the United States: Mean time to maturation averages nearly 4 months (mean, 114 days).[18] Although use of a catheter in prevalent patients falls to roughly one in five at 1-year postinitiation,[18] this number is less optimistic than it first appears, as patients with catheters are more likely to die in the first year, leaving a "survivor cohort" enriched in use of permanent accesses.

COSTS OF END-STAGE RENAL DISEASE

Costs associated with ESRD in the United States are immense, constituting $33 billion in 2014. These include costs of dialysis (in-center hemodialysis, home hemodialysis, PD) and of all associated hospitalizations, creation and maintenance of dialysis accesses, medications to manage anemia (principally erythropoiesis-stimulating agents and iron) and secondary hyperparathyroidism, and all renal transplant-related costs (including immunosuppressive medications). This accounts for 7.2% of the overall Medicare budget for a population comprising approximately 0.9% of Medicare beneficiaries. Thus, patients with ESRD are eight times more costly to care for than the average beneficiary. Costs associated with ESRD as a proportion of all Medicare costs have remained relatively stable since the turn of the millennium. Broadly speaking, inpatient costs are responsible for slightly less than one-third of the total costs, and outpatient costs for about one-third; of the remaining one-third, physician/supplier and Medicare Part D medication costs are the largest contributors. Regarding hospitalizations for dialysis patients, infection-related events were responsible for approximately 27% of spending and cardiovascular events for 25%.[18]

Hemodialysis costs in the United States were responsible for approximately $26 billion of the ESRD total in 2014, representing per patient per year (PPPY) spending of approximately $88,000. PPPY costs for kidney transplant recipients are far less, approximately $33,000. Although total ESRD costs increased 3.3% between 2011 and 2013, the PPPY increase was only 0.3%, meaning that the growth in total costs was due primarily to the increase in lives covered. The small PPPY cost increase is likely due, in large measure, to implementation of the ESRD PPS in 2011.

Medications also represent substantial costs for dialysis patients. Part D prescription drug plans covered 77% of ESRD patients in 2014, compared with 69% of the general Medicare population; 80% of hemodialysis patients are covered. The largest contributors to these costs were oral phosphate binding agents ($841 million, 37% of total Part D costs), cinacalcet ($480 million, 21%), and insulins ($161 million, 7%).

The US experience is in many ways exceptional. Healthcare delivery systems differ vastly by country, making cost comparisons with the United States difficult, but per-person costs appear to be less, and in many cases far less, in other countries compared with the United States. Nevertheless, care of patients with kidney disease, especially those receiving maintenance dialysis, is inevitably expensive. In Sweden, annual per-person cost was estimated as €87,000 (US $107,273) for hemodialysis and €59,000 (US $72,748) for PD[107]; these costs included provision of RRT and medications, hospitalizations, and outpatient care. In the United Kingdom, hemodialysis provision alone was estimated to cost £33,000 to 35,000 (US $46,064 to $48,848; depending on whether care was rendered at a hospital-based unit or a less expensive satellite unit) and £16,000 (US $22,331) for CAPD on a per-person basis.[108] In Spain, direct per annum costs were estimated as €38,000 (US $46,856) for hemodialysis and €26,000 (US $32,060) for PD.[109] In Australia, annual costs were estimated as $AUS 49,000 (US $38,443) for hemodialysis and $AUS 57,000 (US $44,719) for PD.[110] Notably, there appears to be little relationship between countrywide annual healthcare expenditure per capita and annual expenditure per ESRD patient once the United States is removed from consideration (Fig. 21.27).

Comparatively little work has been undertaken on this issue in middle- and low-income countries. A recent

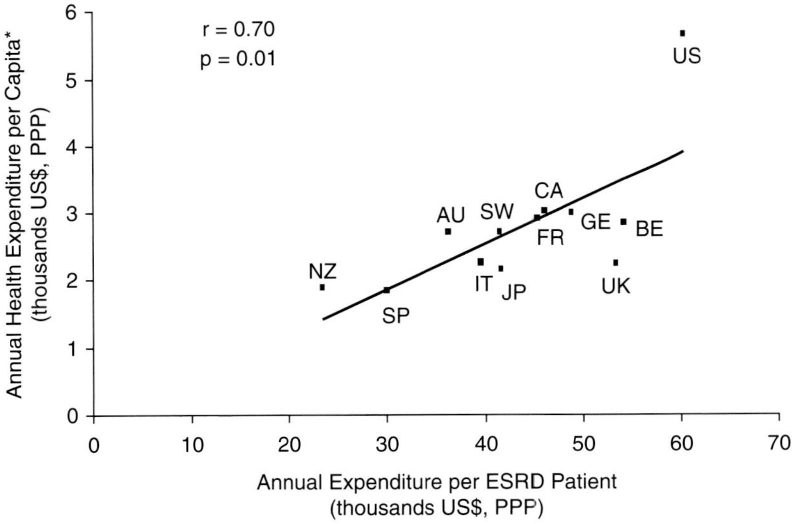

FIG. 21.27 Annual expenditure per ESRD patient relative to annual per-capita health expenditure, by country. (From Dor A, Pauly MV, Eichleay MA, et al. End-stage renal disease and economic incentives: The International Study of Health Care Organization and Financing (ISHCOF). *Int J Health Care Finance Econ.* 2007;7:73-111.)

meta-analysis[111] yielded only 18 published reports suitable for analysis. This review converted costs into international dollars ($Int), according to World Bank convention, to encompass the concept of purchasing power parity (thereby making comparisons between vastly different countries more meaningful). Study methodology to estimate assessed costs differed substantially. For high–middle-income countries such as Turkey, Iran, Chile, and Brazil, where dialysis is relatively widely available, annual costs ranged from about $Int13,000 to $Int30,000 (Turkey, $Int28,000 for hemodialysis and PD[112]; Iran, $Int13,000 for hemodialysis[113]; Chile, $Int24,000 for hemodialysis and PD[114]; Brazil, $Int30,000 for hemodialysis, $Int29,000 for PD).[115] In lower–middle-income countries, where dialysis is far less widely available, costs for hemodialysis were generally $Int4000 to $Int9000: Sri Lanka, $Int9000[116]; Indonesia, $Int 7000[117]; Egypt, $Int8000.[118] Finally, in low-income countries, where access to dialysis is poor, dialysis remained expensive, especially relative to the per-capita gross domestic product (GDP): Sudan, $11,000 for hemodialysis, $12,000 for PD[119]; Bangladesh, $5000 for hemodialysis.[120] Notably, the association between annual per-person hemodialysis cost and per capita GDP appears weak. Perhaps more paradoxically, increased GDP per capita and a higher percentage of GDP spent on health care were inversely associated with survival on dialysis; posited explanations include the strong possibility that greater healthcare expenditure is a sign that sicker patients, who are more likely to die, are treated more intensively. The implication is that countries that spend a great deal on health care are more likely to support dialysis initiation in very sick patients whose life expectancy is poor.[121] The Global Burden of Disease research group recently attempted to estimate costs associated with prevalent maintenance dialysis as a percentage of total healthcare costs, relative to the United States[21] (Fig. 21.28).

Costs associated with the transition to dialysis are also substantial. As the USRDS reports,[122] costs rise gradually from about 6 months before dialysis initiation until about 2 months before, increase more steeply in the next month, and grow prodigiously in the final month before initiation, peaking in the period immediately surrounding initiation. Costs then begin to drop, but never to predialysis levels (Fig. 21.29).

Several studies have found that predialysis care may decrease initial dialysis-related costs and mortality in incident patients. In a study examining US Department of Veterans Affairs patients, increasing intensity of predialysis care was associated with a substantial decrease in savings. Care was expensive; costs associated with the first year of dialysis in individuals who received no predialysis care (37% of the cohort) averaged $104,000, compared with $90,000 for individuals who received the most-intense care (23% of the cohort); although these savings were likely lost once the intensity of predialysis care was considered, a mortality benefit was demonstrated, since 43% of the patients who received little or no predialysis care died in the first year, compared with only 25% of those who received the most intense care.[123] A small study from Taiwan, where CKD-related costs appear to be more contained than in the United States, suggested that intensive predialysis care management, although more expensive than traditional care, resulted in lower costs after dialysis initiation and in lower combined (i.e., pre- and postinitiation) costs.[124] A Canadian study demonstrated even more substantial savings between "optimally" initiated patients, whose costs averaged approximately $CAD 39,000 (US $30,712), and "suboptimally" initiated patients, whose costs averaged more than $CAD 63,000 (US $49,611).[125] However, savings appear to attenuate over time. A retrospective study from Korea demonstrated that patients referred early for nephrology care accrued fewer costs before initiation and in the month after, but costs reached parity, on a per-month

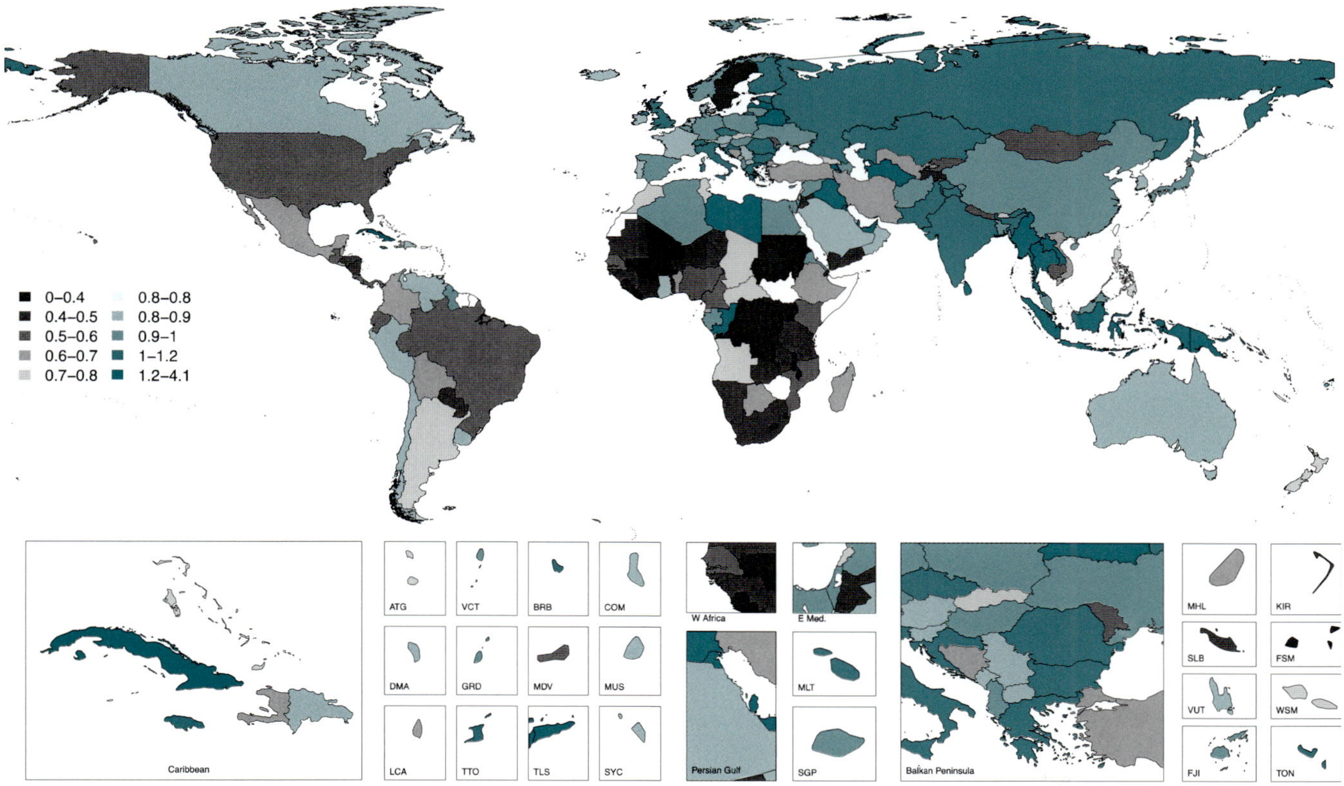

FIG. 21.28 Estimated percentage of country-specific total health expenditure allocated to prevalent maintenance dialysis using the US reimbursement model. (From Thomas B, Wulf S, Bikbov B, et al. Maintenance dialysis throughout the world in years 1990 and 2010. *J Am Soc Nephrol.* 2015;26:2621-2633.)

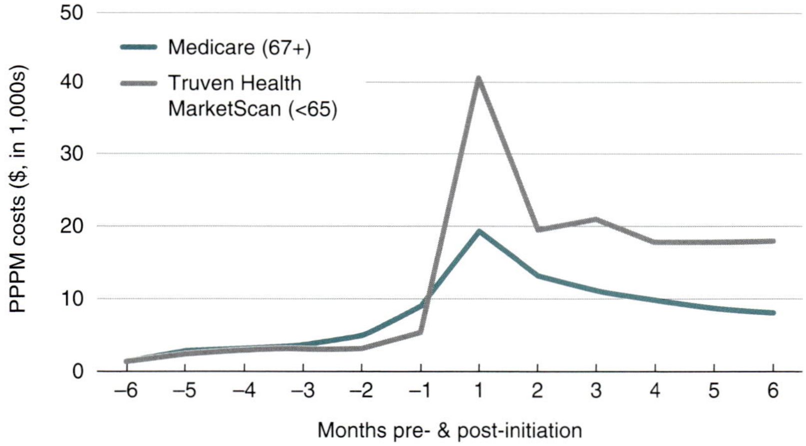

FIG. 21.29 Per-person per-month expenditures during the transition to ESRD, in Medicare and Truven Health MarketScan employer group health plan, 2011. (From US Renal Data System. *2016 USRDS Annual Data Report: Epidemiology of Kidney Disease in the United States.* Bethesda, MD: National Institutes of Health, National Institute of Diabetes and Digestive and Kidney Diseases; 2016.)

basis, by only the second month of dialysis.[126] One potentially important determinant of cost savings in the peri-initiation period may be prompt placement of AV fistulas,[127] although fistula placement rates may reflect, in large measure, patient characteristics that may be only weakly modifiable.[106]

Slowing the rate of progression of CKD to ESRD may produce substantial savings. Slowing the rate of GFR decline in stage 3 CKD patients by 10% was projected to save the US healthcare system $19 billion[128]; although dated, this study provided a conceptual model by which such savings could be estimated. Early dialysis initiation, a trend present in the United States[18] despite studies suggesting lack of association with improved clinical outcomes, does not appear to save money.[40]

Conclusions

Annual rates of dialysis initiation appear to have stabilized in recent years in the United States. Over this period, prevalent patients have experienced survival gains, meaning that they are living longer on dialysis than ever before. Thus, the growth in the ESRD population in the United States has mainly been among prevalent patients. A vast and growing unmet need for RRT remains, most of which will undoubtedly be in the form of maintenance dialysis, in developing countries. In many developed countries, large networks of centers delivering in-center hemodialysis may not be feasible or even appropriate. Cardiovascular mortality rates have declined substantially over the past decade, in keeping with trends in the general population, but SCD remains a major problem, especially early after initiation. Infections remain a persistently important source of morbidity and mortality, requiring concerted effort by the nephrology community.

Evidence is generally lacking to support one maintenance dialysis modality over another, with the possible exception that hemodialysis may be associated with a lower risk for death compared with PD in diabetic patients. Nevertheless, patient ability and commitment to perform PD appears to be the dominant factor in modality selection. Despite increasing incentives for therapies other than traditional thrice-weekly in-center hemodialysis, it will likely be the most widely used modality for the foreseeable future in the United States and in most developed countries. For patients choosing hemodialysis, placing an access before initiation is important, as use of central venous catheters is associated with mortality. New avenues to secure care for patients with advanced CKD are critical, since timely placement of a permanent access, which is associated with lower mortality after initiation, is a major challenge. Dialysis is extremely costly in the United States especially, prompting governments to attempt to contain costs without sacrificing care. Developing countries will have to confront how to render care for a growing population with recognized ESRD, and will likely have to explore models that are more cost-effective than those in the United States.

A full list of references is available at www.expertconsult.com.

22

Principles of Hemodialysis

Jane Y. Yeun, MD, Thomas A. Depner, MD, and Shubha Ananthakrishnan, MD

OUTLINE

More than 2 million people require life-sustaining renal replacement therapy worldwide, including dialysis and transplantation.[1] This dependence on an extracorporeal blood device is both the fulfillment of hopes by some and the dashing of dreams by others and highlights the need for an in-depth understanding of all aspects of hemodialysis, including the human reactions to it. Before one can configure hemodialysis optimally, one must understand its target, the uremic syndrome. In this chapter we review the physical, chemical, and clinical principles of hemodialysis as they relate to the treatment of uremia, starting with historical milestones and ending with projections for the future. The discussions include brief notes of comparison with other modalities, such as peritoneal dialysis and hemofiltration, that are reviewed more extensively in other chapters.

FUNDAMENTAL CONCEPTS

Historical Development

Hemodialysis was originally termed *extracorporeal dialysis* because it was performed outside the body.[2] Several early pioneers laid the foundation for therapeutic dialysis. Graham (1805–1869), a professor of chemistry in Scotland, invented the fundamental process of separating solutes using semipermeable membranes in vitro and coined the word *dialysis*.[3] In 1916 Abel dialyzed rabbits and dogs in the United States with a "vividiffusion" device using celloidin membranes and a leech extract called *hirudin* as an anticoagulant.[4] Abel was the first to apply dialysis to a living organism and to use the term *artificial kidney*. In Germany, Haas first used the artificial kidney to dialyze a human in 1924.[5] His attempts were only marginally successful because toxicity from his crude anticoagulant limited his ability to prolong flow in the extracorporeal circuit.

In view of these previous failures, it was not at all certain in 1944 that Kolff's use of extracorporeal dialysis as a human lifesaving treatment for patients with kidney failure would be successful. Three major advances aided his efforts in the nearly 20 years since Hass's work: the invention of cellophane, the discovery of antibiotics, and the availability of heparin as an anticoagulant. Through his keen interest in kidney failure and his aptitude for mechanics, Kolff and his patients ultimately met with success.[2] Kolff is often called the "father of hemodialysis" because his method became accepted as the standard for temporary replacement of kidney function in patients with short-duration acute kidney failure.[6,7]

Attempts to apply hemodialysis to patients who had more prolonged or permanent loss of kidney function were limited because the artery and vein used for blood access had to be tied off after each treatment. In 1960 Scribner, working with Quinton and Dillard at the University of Washington in Seattle, developed a blood access device for repeated dialysis using plastic tubes inserted into the artery and vein.[8] This device, known as the *Scribner shunt*, and the more permanent arteriovenous (AV) fistulas later introduced by Brescia and Cimino allowed hemodialysis to be repeated for many years as a life-sustaining treatment.[9] For their pioneering work in the field of artificial organs, Kolff and Scribner were granted the prestigious Lasker Clinical Medical Research Award in 2002.[10]

Kidney Replacement Therapy

The goals of extracorporeal kidney replacement therapy include clearance of solutes and to maintain normal volume status. Several methods to achieve this exist, including hemodialysis, hemofiltration, and hemodiafiltration. The most successful intracorporeal modality has been peritoneal dialysis. The most promising replacement therapy is kidney transplantation because it can restore normal or near-normal kidney function, including potential functions not yet discovered, with the least inconvenience to the patient. The kidney is also an endocrine organ involved in the metabolism of hormones such as erythropoietin, calcitriol, prostaglandins, and renin. Overall care of the patient requiring renal replacement therapy also requires anticipation and management of problems; current approaches include attempts to reverse the psychological effects of kidney loss, preventing anemia and bone disease, monitoring the patient for signs of protein-energy wasting, monitoring the function of peripheral AV access devices, expecting hypotension during dialysis in patients with concentric ventricular hypertrophy, adjusting medication doses appropriately, and monitoring the quality of dialysate water (detailed in various chapters). Clinical practice guidelines and practical recommendations have been published and are now available in several countries, each with the ultimate goal of improving quality of life.[11-13]

Definitions

Dialysis is the passage of molecules in solution by *diffusion* across a *semipermeable membrane*. Essential elements of this process are the *solvent*, which contains dissolved *solutes*, and the membrane that contains *pores* through which some or all of the solutes move by diffusion (Fig. 22.1A). The molecular kinetics of diffusion are both solute and membrane specific. Solute characteristics that affect movement across a particular membrane include its concentration, molecular weight, shape, charge, and lipid solubility. Membrane characteristics that determine permeability to a particular solute include the average effective pore size; the number, geometry, and distribution of pores within the membrane; membrane surface area and thickness; and surface characteristics, such as charge and hydrophilicity. The solvent itself may also move by diffusion if its chemical activity is not balanced across the membrane. Although solutes may move in both directions across the membrane, it is customary to refer to the compartment containing more vital substances that one wishes to preserve as the *dialyzed compartment* and to the solution in the other, usually larger, compartment as the *dialysate*.

The concept of molecular diffusion is critically important to the definition of dialysis. Solutes pass through the membrane down an *electrochemical gradient* caused primarily by a difference in concentration across the membrane (see Fig. 22.1A). This concentration gradient, which is the driving force for diffusion, may also be dissipated by the dialysis (i.e., the molecular concentration gradient tends to fall with dialysis).

In the absence of an electrochemical gradient, solutes may also pass through pores in the membrane by filtration, a process of convection. The driving force for filtration is pressure, either hydraulic or osmotic, that is unbalanced across the membrane (Fig. 22.1B) and independent of dialysis. During filtration, solute passively accompanies the solvent from one compartment to the other, causing no change in solute concentration. Convective movement may occur in the opposite direction to diffusive movement, and even in the same direction, convective movement may interfere with dialysis (i.e., the two fluxes may not be additive when they occur simultaneously).

Hemodialysis means literally "dialysis of the blood." This form of dialysis is distinguished by its location outside the body and by the continuous flow of blood across the dialyzer membrane. Therapeutic hemodialysis is most often used to treat kidney failure by equilibrating the blood against an isoosmotic dialysate. Vital solutes are added to the dialysate at concentrations designed to mimic those normally maintained in the blood by the native kidney (Table 22.1; see Fig. 22.1A). The resulting dialysate is essentially a physiological salt solution that, in addition to creating a gradient for removal of unwanted solutes, reproduces another vital function of normal kidneys, that of maintaining a constant physiological concentration of extracellular electrolytes.

UREMIA: THE TARGET OF HEMODIALYSIS

Uremia is the clinical state or syndrome that is reversed by dialysis therapy, and it literally means "urine in the blood." Whether or not urine output falls, all patients with uremia accumulate solutes, collectively known as *uremic toxins*. It is this accumulation of solute, the most abundant of which is urea, that prompted the application of dialysis as a treatment for uremia.[5] From another perspective, the concept of uremia as a state of intoxication by substances normally eliminated by the kidney is supported by the success of therapeutic dialysis. The kidney separates large from small solutes by filtration, powered by the heart and accomplishing much the same function as the dialyzer, which also depends on cardiac output to deliver solute for elimination but is not powered by the heart. Some have likened dialysis to the original elimination mechanism of organisms that evolved in the infinite "dialysate" of the primordial sea. Conserved adaptation to diffusive removal of solute might explain the marked success of therapeutic dialysis compared with other artificial organ replacements.[14]

Clinical Syndrome

Although not all patients exhibit all the symptoms and signs of uremia, the monotony of the clinical syndrome

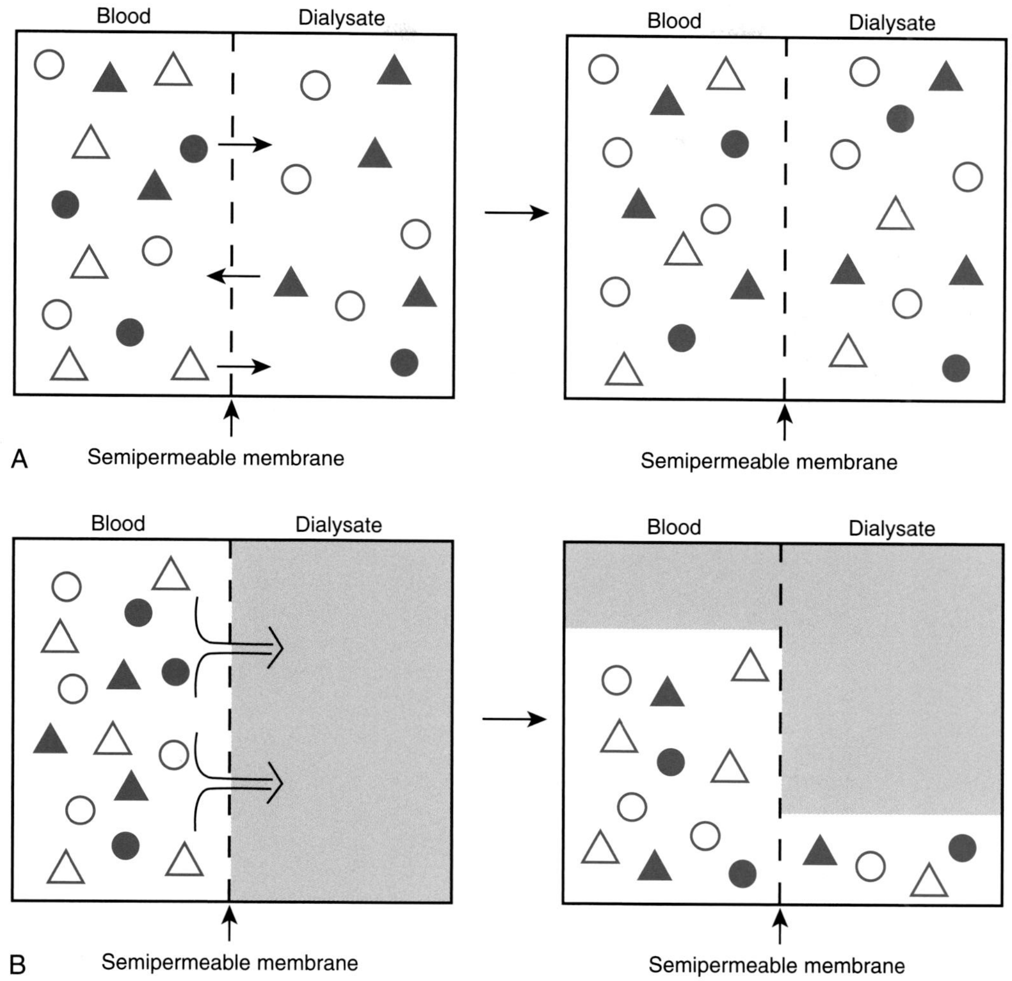

FIG. 22.1 (A) Diffusion across a semipermeable membrane. Solutes with higher concentrations in the blood compartment, such as potassium *(solid circles)* and uremic toxins *(open triangles)*, diffuse through the membrane into the dialysate compartment. Conversely, solutes with higher concentration in the dialysate, such as bicarbonate *(closed triangles)*, diffuse into the blood compartment. Solutes such as sodium and chloride *(open circles)*, with concentrations nearly equivalent in the two compartments, move little across the membrane. (B) Convection across a semipermeable membrane. Hydrostatic pressure applied to the blood compartment causes the solvent to flow across the membrane into the dialysate compartment, bringing along solutes. As a result, for solutes with a sieving coefficient close to 1, there is no change in concentrations in the blood compartment with time.

TABLE 22.1 Solutes Present in Dialysate

Component	Concentration (mEq/L)
Sodium	135–145
Potassium	0–4.0
Chloride	102–106
Bicarbonate	30–39
Acetate	2–4
Calcium	0–3.5
Magnesium	0.5–1.0
Dextrose	11
pH	7.1–7.3

in patients with widely divergent causes of kidney failure indicates that the syndrome is the consequence of the kidney failure per se, not the underlying disease. Nearly every organ system is involved, but the most highly targeted are the gastrointestinal tract and the central nervous system. Early symptoms include dysgeusia, loss of appetite, nausea, weight loss, inability to concentrate on a mental task, lethargy, daytime sleepiness, pruritus, and menstrual irregularity in women. Unfortunately, these symptoms are not specific and are sometimes mistaken for an unrelated infection or can be confounded by coexisting anemia. They appear in most patients only at an advanced stage of kidney damage (80% to 90% loss of nephrons). Far advanced symptoms and signs include uremic serositis with pericarditis, once the harbinger of death as a result of uremia; central nervous system suppression leading to uremic coma; overt peripheral neuropathy; and uremic fetor caused by volatile amines emitted in the breath. Fluid accumulation, which is subtle in most patients, contributes to hypertension that eventually leads to cardiac hypertrophy and diastolic dysfunction.

TABLE 22.2 Solutes That Accumulate in Uremia and Their Proposed Toxicity (If Known)

Solute	Proposed Toxicity
Free Water Soluble, Low Molecular Weight	
Sodium	Volume overload
Potassium	Arrhythmia, muscle weakness
Hydrogen ion (metabolic acidosis)[226]	Degrades protein (activates ubiquitin proteasome); alters vitamin D and parathyroid hormone levels
Urea	None
Creatinine	None
Guanidines[33]	Immune dysfunction; neurotoxicity
Oxalate[227]	Tissue deposits; inhibits endothelial cell replication and migration
Asymmetrical dimethylarginine[228-230]	Cardiovascular disease; inhibits inducible nitric oxide synthase
3-carboxyl-4-methyl-5-propyl-2-furanproprionic acid[227]	Displaces drugs bound to albumin; inhibits erythropoiesis; inhibits mitochondrial oxidation
4-hydroxybenzoic acid (phenolic acid)[227]	Platelet dysfunction; shortened red cell survival; neurological symptoms
Trimethylamine-N-oxide (TMAO)[231]	Cardiovascular disease
Protein Bound	
Hippuric acid[227]	Muscle weakness; neurological symptoms; decreases drug binding to albumin
Indoxyl sulfate[33,227,232]	Displaces drugs bound to albumin; oxidative stress; cardiovascular disease
p-Cresol[33,232-234]	Immune dysfunction; cardiovascular disease; oxidative stress
Quinolinic acid[227]	Inhibits erythropoiesis; seizures in mice
Homocysteine[24]	Cardiovascular disease
Pentosidine[235]	Cardiovascular disease
Leptin[33,236]	Cardiovascular disease
Sequestered	
Phosphate	Osteodystrophy; cardiovascular disease
Magnesium	Muscle weakness
Middle (500–5000 Da) and High (5000–50,000 Da) Molecular Weight	
Parathyroid hormone[237,238]	Inhibits mitochondrial oxidation; hypertrophic cardiomyopathy; cardiac fibrosis; immune dysfunction
β_2-Microglobulin[239,240]	Dialysis amyloidosis
Carbamylated proteins[241]	Possible cardiovascular disease
Advanced glycation end products[239,242]	Dialysis amyloidosis; cardiovascular disease; oxidative stress

Uremic Toxins

The most life-threatening solutes known to accumulate in uremia (Table 22.2) are low in molecular weight and consequently are dialyzable. A host of other substances have been found to accumulate in renal failure, and data on their potential toxicity are emerging. As the list of uremic retention solutes grows steadily, approaches to analyze these solutes more systematically are underway and realization that a significant number of uremic retention solutes may not be amenable to removal with conventional dialysis is dawning (Fig. 22.2).

Despite its importance as a measure of dialysis adequacy, urea itself has been found to have little toxicity, as reported in experiments where toxicity was alleviated despite addition of urea to the dialysate to prevent its removal.[15,16] Similarly, although all other solutes mentioned accumulate in patients with kidney failure, their levels are well less than that necessary to evoke toxic responses in animals and in humans, even when measured in patients with end-stage renal disease (ESRD).[17,18] Even after decades of research, investigators are unable to identify a single toxin or a group of toxins responsible for the immediate life-threatening uremic syndrome that is quickly reversed by dialysis.[19,20] Because dialysis does little more than remove fluid and dialyzable solutes, the uremic syndrome must result from accumulation of known and unknown toxins in aggregate, perhaps each at subtoxic levels.

Residual Syndrome

It is now clear that the amount of dialysis necessary to sustain life is not enough to maintain a high quality of life. A challenge to investigators is the development of techniques for analyzing and treating this “residual syndrome,” which affects some patients more than others but reduces the quality of life despite apparently adequate dialysis.[20] Several components of the syndrome can be identified, such as anemia, osteodystrophy, dialysis amyloidosis, accelerated atherosclerosis, anorexia, disordered sleep, and fatigue, some of which are treatable (see relevant chapters). The proposed uremic toxins discussed previously may account, in part, for the residual syndrome, but almost certainly other components remain to be defined. These components include (1) the causes of inflammation and malnutrition and the interactions among malnutrition, inflammation, and atherosclerosis in dialysis

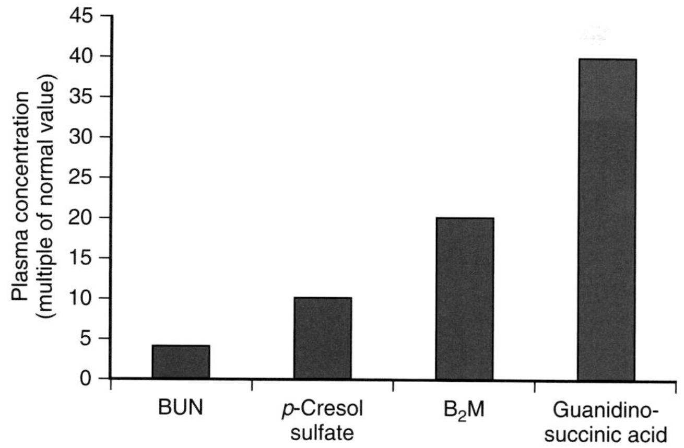

FIG. 22.2 Effect of protein binding, molecular weight, and sequestration on solute concentrations in hemodialysis patients. Conventional thrice weekly dialysis removes blood urea nitrogen (BUN) effectively, rendering the average urea level in a hemodialysis patient about 4 times the normal value. Binding of *p*-cresol to albumin and the large molecular size of β_2-microglobulin limit the ability of conventional dialysis to remove them. Thus their levels are about 10 to 20 times that of normal, respectively. Plasma guanidinosuccinic acid levels are even higher at 40 times that of normal because of increased production in kidney failure and sequestration within cells, thereby limiting its removal during dialysis. Although plasma levels of solutes other than urea are several orders of magnitude higher than normal, their absolute levels are much lower than that of urea. In addition, it is unclear if they exert any toxicity or are simply retained because of kidney failure. (Modified from Meyer TW, Hostetter TH. Uremia. *N Engl J Med.* 2007;357(13):1316-1325.)

patients[21,22]; (2) the cause of accelerated atherosclerosis[21-23]; (3) the role of hyperhomocysteinemia in accelerated atherosclerosis[24,25] and graft thrombosis[26]; (4) the role of hyperphosphatemia in cardiovascular disease[27,28]; and (5) the role of endothelial dysfunction as a mediator of cardiovascular disease.[29-32] Other proposed underlying causes of the residual syndrome include accumulation of toxins that are poorly dialyzable because of their larger molecular size,[33] protein binding in the blood or tissues,[17,18,34] and sequestration with slow release from compartments other than the blood.[35,36] A complete understanding of the basis for the residual syndrome remains elusive, but several concepts are emerging, based on evidence from clinical studies. The Hemodialysis (HEMO) Study[37] (see Goals of Hemodialysis) found that increasing the clearance of middle molecules (MMs) such as β_2-microglobulin using high-flux dialyzers did not alter survival in hemodialysis patients. Subsequent studies reported that the clearance of some protein-bound solutes can be increased by increasing both dialyzer surface area and dialysate flow,[34] postdilution online hemodiafiltration,[38] addition of sorbent to dialysate,[39] and fractionated plasma separation and adsorption.[40] Increasing the frequency of dialysis to 6 days per week may also improve weekly removal of larger or sequestered molecules.[41-43] An interesting study[44] also found that increased dietary fiber reduces levels of some colon-derived protein-bound solutes in hemodialysis patients. Despite many such developments in our understanding of the contributors to the residual syndrome, clinical outcome studies on the impact of reducing these various uremic toxins are either limited or nonexistent.

Goals of Hemodialysis

The primary goal of hemodialysis is the replacement of kidney excretory function. There is no doubt that hemodialysis can sustain life in patients who have no kidney function. Survival for as long as 30 years has been documented for hemodialysis alone, a treatment that does nothing more for the patient than remove solute.[45] Earlier experience indicates that the most life-threatening toxins are easily dialyzable. Precise goals and standards of dialysis adequacy have been defined, based on outcome studies in large populations, in terms of the clearance of small-molecular-weight, easily dialyzed solutes, the marker for which is urea.

A prospective interventional study of dialysis adequacy in the late 1970s, the US National Cooperative Dialysis Study (NCDS), provided clear-cut evidence for a level of urea clearance that was inadequate.[46] Later uncontrolled experience suggested that more dialysis might be better for the patient.[47-50] Analysis of solute kinetics, however, indicated that the benefit of dialysis is logarithmically related to the dose and that, depending on the frequency of treatments, a point is reached beyond which more dialysis does nothing more than inconvenience the patient, potentially worsening the quality of life. This theoretical construct was confirmed by the National Institutes of Health (NIH)–sponsored HEMO Study, a multicenter prospective clinical trial that randomly assigned 1846 patients to receive thrice weekly hemodialysis with a target equilibrated Kt/V (where K is dialyzer clearance of urea, t is dialysis time, and V is volume of distribution of urea) of 1.05 (equivalent to single-pool Kt/V of 1.25, the generally accepted minimal standard at the time of the study) versus 1.45 (equivalent to single-pool 1.65).[37] After the publication of uncontrolled studies indicating possible beneficial effects of more frequent dialysis on several outcomes, such as blood pressure, patient-reported outcomes, and laboratory parameters,[51,52] a randomized trial was needed to definitively determine the optimal dose of hemodialysis. This led to the Frequent Hemodialysis Network (FHN) trial, sponsored mainly by the National Institute of Diabetes and Digestive and Kidney Diseases and the Centers for Medicare and Medicaid Services (CMS).[53] The trial compared standard three-times-a-week hemodialysis to six-times-a-week hemodialysis. The frequent hemodialysis group (which had a standard Kt/V [see later] of 3.54 compared with the standard group Kt/V of 2.49) had beneficial effects on the composite endpoint of death or change in left ventricular mass. The FHN trial also included a nocturnal hemodialysis arm, which achieved a standard Kt/V of 4.5. Patients in the nocturnal group had better control of hyperphosphatemia and blood pressure, but the trial failed to find a beneficial effect on either of the two coprimary endpoints of death or left ventricular mass.[54] One should also bear in mind that more frequent hemodialysis has potential adverse effects as well, such as more frequent vascular access procedures,[55] more rapid loss of residual kidney function,[56] and both patient and caregiver burnout.[57] Long-term post-trial follow-up of the two FHN trials were published in 2015 and 2016, reporting a significant reduction in mortality in patients randomly assigned to frequent in-center hemodialysis[58] but a surprisingly *increased* mortality risk in the patients randomly assigned to the home nocturnal arm in the FHN Nocturnal study.[59] For now, the dose of dialysis as measured by single-pool Kt/V (sp Kt/V [see later]) of at least 1.2 per dialysis is recommended for three treatments per week,[60] and this is also a CMS clinical performance measure of dialysis facilities. However, the ultimate goal of dialysis should not rely solely on achievement of a "universal target" of Kt/V[61] but also take into account adequate control of uremic symptoms, achievement control of fluid balance and blood pressure, resolution of the "residual syndrome," and prolonging survival while achieving quality of life for the patient.[62]

DIALYSIS

As defined previously, dialysis is a process of diffusion of molecules in solution across a semipermeable membrane. Forces that govern the pattern and rate of diffusion have been defined in precise mathematical terms that include properties of the molecule, the solvent, and the membrane. The salient points of the physics applicable to dialysis are discussed here because a detailed analysis is beyond the scope of this chapter. For detailed analysis of the physical laws that govern dialysis, the reader is referred to formal texts on kinetic modeling.[63-65]

Laws of Diffusion

Diffusion is a consequence of random molecular movements *(molecular kinetics)* that follow the laws of probability and are driven by temperature, pressure, and concentration. Because temperature and pressure are relatively constant during therapeutic dialysis and among dialysis centers (see later), the major clinical variable that affects diffusion is the solute concentration. Fick's law of diffusion, derived from mathematical laws of statistical probability, indicates that the rate of diffusion is linearly dependent on the *concentration gradient* (i.e., the driving force for diffusion):

$$-j = (DA/X)\,\Delta C \tag{1}$$

J is solute flux (mg/min), which, when applied to a membrane, can be viewed as the unidirectional rate of movement of a solute across the membrane (see Fig. 22.1). ΔC is the concentration gradient across the membrane (mg/mL), A is the membrane area (cm^2), X is the membrane thickness (cm), and D is a constant, called the *coefficient of diffusion* or diffusivity (cm^2/min). The last mentioned item is a measure of the permeability of the membrane material to the measured solute, independent of solute concentration, area, and thickness. Conventionally, a minus sign is placed on the left side of Eq. 1 to indicate that solute moves away from the dialyzed compartment (opposite to the direction of the gradient). Eq. 1 reflects the intuitive concept that diffusion across a membrane varies directly with the membrane area and solute concentration gradient and inversely with the membrane thickness.

Dividing both sides of Eq. 1 by ΔC results in an expression for *solute dialysance*:

$$-J/\Delta C = \text{dialysance} = DA/X \tag{2}$$

Eq. 2 indicates that dialysance is always independent of concentration and is constant throughout a static dialysis despite changes in concentration on both sides of the membrane. Clinicians rarely use the concept of dialysance, opting instead to describe dialysis in terms of *clearance.* This is reasonable because clearance is derived from measurements only on the blood side of the membrane, where solute concentrations are easily measured. The only difference between dialysance and clearance is the substitution of blood side C for ΔC in Eq. 2:

$$-J/C = \text{clearance} = K \tag{3}$$

When the concentration of solute on the dialysate side is zero, ΔC = C and clearance is equal to dialysance. This condition exists at the start of a dialysis procedure and during all therapeutic single-pass dialyses (see Hemodialysis). For all other conditions, ΔC < C, so clearance is lower than dialysance.

If the volume of the dialyzed compartment (V) is constant, dividing both sides of Eq. 3 by V shows that the fractional rate of change in concentration is constant:

$$-(J/V)\,C = K/V = K \tag{4}$$

The symbol k is called the *rate constant.* The constantly changing term *J/V,* when expressed at any given instant, is dC/dt and therefore (J/V)/C is (dC/C)/dt. The latter can be viewed as the fractional change in concentration over an initial short period (dt):

$$-(dC/C)/dt = K/V = K \tag{5}$$

Eq. 5 indicates that concentration-dependent diffusion is a first-order process; that is, despite the minute-to-minute changes in concentration within the dialyzed compartment, the fractional rate of change is constant when the dialysate concentration remains zero. Flux of solute across the membrane, which is the goal of dialysis, is both driven by the concentration and expressed as a change in concentration. When the rate of change is factored by the driving force ([dC/dt]/C), the resulting fractional rate of change is constant.

The rate constant (k) in Eq. 5 has units of time^{-1} or a fraction per unit of time and is a function of both the molecular properties of size, shape, charge, and interaction with the membrane and of the membrane itself, including its surface area, porosity, and thickness. Large molecules, those with complex shapes, and those with an electrical charge diffuse less readily across the membrane. Membranes that are more porous, have a larger surface, and are thinner favor passage of solutes by diffusion. Although the rate constant is useful to demonstrate the first-order concept, it has less practical value than the expression for clearance depicted in Eq. 3.

The difference between the rate constant (k) in Eq. 4 and the clearance (K) shown in Eq. 3 is V, the volume of solute distribution. Eq. 3 has the advantage of expressing the dialysis effect as a volume equivalent of solute diffusing across the membrane per unit of time. The volume transferred per unit of time is constant; that is, a milliliter equivalent of solute is transferred per unit of time regardless of how much solute is contained in that milliliter. The rate of diffusion is directly proportional to the membrane surface area, which is constant for any given model of dialyzer.

Effects of Temperature, Pressure, and Molecular Weight

Diffusion is a consequence of molecular motion, which is affected by pressure and heat energy and by molecular mass. The rate of diffusion is proportional to the absolute temperature, which is approximately 273°K at room temperature. Within the range of temperatures experienced in the dialysis center, the proportionate change in absolute temperature (260°K to 280°K) is so small that its influence on diffusion across the dialysis membrane is negligible. More important are the physiological effects of temperature on blood flow and body water compartmentalization, which have significant effects on solute kinetics within the patient (see Quantifying Hemodialysis). Similarly, pressure effects have little influence on diffusion within the range of pressures recorded in modern dialyzers.

Molecular mass plays a more significant role in determining the rate of diffusion because at a given temperature and pressure, the heavier molecules move more slowly and collide with the semipermeable membrane less frequently. Small-molecular-weight substances, such as urea and creatinine, diffuse readily across a semipermeable membrane, whereas larger substances, such as β_2-microglobulin or albumin, diffuse slowly or not at all. The larger size of the heavier molecules further impedes diffusion through small pores.

Dialysate

Preparation of the dialysate and the resulting composition are critical to the success of dialysis. For hemodialysis the solution must be prepared from properly treated water and contain the solutes listed in Table 22.1 in concentrations comparable to those of plasma. Dialysate must have a low concentration of endotoxin to prevent pyrogen reactions in the patient, but, in contrast to peritoneal dialysate, sterility is not a requirement because the semipermeable membrane excludes large particles, such as bacteria and viruses. Vital electrolytes and glucose are added to the dialysate to reduce or abolish their concentration gradients, whereas bicarbonate or a bicarbonate precursor is added in higher concentrations to promote accumulation in the patient. Dialysate glucose concentrations are near those of plasma; thus in contrast to peritoneal dialysis, osmotic forces do not play an important role in removing fluid.

In practice, solute concentrations in the dialysate are fairly standard. The most common concentrations that may be individualized are those for potassium, calcium, and bicarbonate (see Table 22.1). In many dialysis centers, the bicarbonate concentration is fixed at 35 or 39 mEq/L, although many centers may err on the side of a lower dialysate bicarbonate concentration, after the observation of higher all-cause mortality with higher dialysate bicarbonate concentrations.[66] One should also take into account the contribution of the acid concentrate (acetate) to the total alkali exposure to the patient during a dialysis session, given the conversion of the acetate to bicarbonate.[67] Potassium ranges from 0 to 4 mEq/L, depending on the patient's serum concentration before dialysis. A compelling reason must exist, however, to use dialysate potassium concentrations of 0 or 1 mEq/L because of the dangers associated with a precipitous drop in the serum concentration. In particular, patients on digoxin must be dialyzed against at least 2 mEq/L of potassium. Calcium concentrations vary from 1 to 3.5 mEq/L. At the lower concentration, calcium is removed from the patient, whereas at the higher concentration, calcium diffuses into the patient during dialysis. (A calcium concentration of 2.5 mEq/L is equal to 5 mg/dL, which is roughly the amount of ionized calcium in plasma—equaling about 10 mg/dL of total calcium.) The concentration of sodium had until recently been fixed at 140 mEq/L, which is the middle of the normal range in whole plasma. More recently, with evidence suggesting that lowering the dialysate sodium level to the range of 134 to 138 mEq/L may be beneficial and avoid intradialysis sodium loading, an increasing number of dialysis facilities are using 135 to 137 mEq/L as the standard dialysate.[68] Results of ongoing clinical trials will hopefully clarify the optimum dialysate sodium levels.

HEMODIALYZERS

A *hemodialyzer,* synonymous with *dialyzer,* is often called an "artificial kidney." It is configured to allow blood and dialysate to flow, preferably in opposite directions, through individual compartments, separated by a semipermeable membrane. By convention, blood entering the hemodialyzer is designated *arterial,* whereas blood leaving the hemodialyzer is *venous.* The principal differences among the many available hemodialyzers are the membrane composition, membrane configuration, and membrane surface area. Hemodialyzers affect the efficiency and the quality of dialysis by virtue of their membranes, which determine their K_OA value, and by the rates of blood and dialysate flow, which determine their clearance values (see later discussion of K_OA) (Box 22.1).

Membrane Composition, Configuration, and Surface Area

Composition of the Membrane

Two major classes of membrane material are available commercially: (1) cotton fiber, or *cellulose-based membranes,* and (2) *synthetic membranes.* Cellulose-based membranes range from unmodified cellulose to substituted cellulose membranes. Unmodified cellulose membranes have many free hydroxyl groups, which are thought to be responsible for their bioincompatibility and propensity to activate white blood cells, platelets, and serum complement. In an effort

BOX 22.1 Key Factors That Affect the Solute Clearance of a Hemodialyzer

Properties of the membrane
- ↑ Membrane porosity
- ↓ Membrane thickness
- ↑ Membrane surface area

Properties of the solute
- ↓ Molecular weight and size
- ↓ Shape
- ↓ Charge

Blood side
- ↓ Unstirred blood layer
- ↑ Blood flow

Dialysate side
- ↓ Dialysate channeling and unstirred layer
- ↑ Dialysate flow
- ↑ Countercurrent direction of flow

↑, Increases clearance; *↓*, decreases clearance.

to improve membrane biocompatibility while keeping costs down, the cellulose polymer is treated with acetate and tertiary amino compounds to form a covalent bond with the hydroxyl groups (e.g., cellulose acetate and animated cellulose [Cellosyn or Hemophan]).

The major polymers in commercial synthetic membranes are polyacrylonitrile, polysulfone, polycarbonate, polyamide, and polymethylmethacrylate. Despite their increased thickness, these membranes can be rendered more permeable than the cellulose membranes, allowing for greater fluid and solute removal. They are also more biocompatible. Because the pore sizes in the synthetic membranes can be made wider, larger-molecular-weight substances, such as β_2-microglobulin, can be removed more efficiently.[69] High-flux synthetic membranes also clear phosphate more efficiently, although the effect on serum phosphate levels is minimal. Despite their higher cost, synthetic hemodialyzers are increasingly preferred.

Hollow-Fiber Dialyzers

Current hemodialyzers are constructed with a plastic casing, usually polycarbonate that encloses several thousand hollow-fiber semipermeable membranes stretched from one end to the other, embedded at each end into a plastic *potting compound*, usually polyurethane, that serves as the headers.

The blood compartment fiber bundle volume of the hollow-fiber dialyzer is 60 to 120 mL, which, in contrast to older dialyzer designs, does not expand during dialysis. Each fiber has an inside diameter of approximately 200 μm. The potting material separates the blood compartment from the dialysate compartment where dialysate flows between and around each fiber in the direction usually opposite to blood flow. Blood flows to or from the open end of each fiber through a removable header attached to the blood tubing. In addition to a lower blood-priming volume, the hollow-fiber design increases the area of contact between blood and dialysate, allowing for the most efficient exchange of solutes. Recent efforts to prevent loss of surface area by fiber-to-fiber contact include insertion of spacer yarns between fibers and a wavy moiré configuration of the fibers. Major disadvantages of the hollow-fiber design are thrombosis and the potting compound, which can absorb chemicals used to disinfect newly manufactured dialyzers (e.g., ethylene oxide) or reused dialyzers (e.g., formaldehyde, peracetic acid, or glutaraldehyde). These chemicals can leach slowly from the material and potentially enter the patient's blood during dialysis.

Surface Area Considerations

Most hemodialyzers have a membrane surface area of 0.8 to 2.1 m^2. As the area increases, solute transport, often called *efficiency of the dialyzer*, increases. To maximize membrane surface area, one can increase the length of the hollow fiber, increase the number of hollow fibers, or decrease the diameter of the hollow fiber while holding other parameters constant.[70] Each of these maneuvers, however, has undesirable effects when carried too far. Increasing the fiber length increases shear rate and magnifies the pressure drop between blood entering and exiting the dialyzer. Increased shear rate increases ultrafiltration, whereas the pressure drop decreases ultrafiltration because the transmembrane pressure (TMP) gradient dissipates at the venous end of the dialyzer. Any decrease in ultrafiltration decreases its contribution to solute clearance and offsets the potential advantage of the increased surface area. Increasing the number of hollow fibers increases the volume of extracorporeal blood and may eventually compromise hemodynamic stability. Finally, as the diameter of the hollow fiber decreases, the increase in resistance to blood flow enhances filtration and backfiltration, but clotting is also enhanced. As fibers thrombose, effective surface area for diffusion decreases and solute clearances fall. Because of these adverse consequences, the minimal acceptable internal fiber diameter is 180 μm.[71] The design and geometry of the hollow-fiber dialyzer represent a delicate balance among these factors.

The composition and the thickness of the membrane varies considerably and is often more important than the surface area in determining dialyzer efficiency. In general the thinner the membrane, the more efficient the transport of solutes and fluid across the membrane.

Effects of Flow on Clearance

Blood Flow

Dialyzer blood flow (Q_b) is driven by a roller pump and generally ranges from 200 to 500 mL/min, depending on the type of vascular access. Blood flow influences the efficiency of solute removal (see Box 22.1).

As Q_b increases, more solute is presented per unit of time to the membrane, and solute removal increases. Urea removal rises steeply as Q_b increases to 300 mL/min, and although urea removal continues to rise as Q_b approaches 400 to 500 mL/min, the slope is less steep. For larger-molecular-weight substances, removal is slower and more time dependent rather than flow dependent because diffusion across the membrane is limited, as discussed previously.

Dialysate Flow

Most dialysis equipment generates a single pass of dialysate; that is, the dialysate is discarded after one passage through the dialyzer. For sorbent dialysis, however, only about 5 L of water are used and dialysate is constantly regenerated by cycling through a cartridge system to remove the undesirable solutes (e.g., urea, creatinine, and potassium).

Countercurrent flow maximizes the concentration gradient between blood and dialysate throughout the length of the dialyzer (see Box 22.1). When blood flow and dialysate flow are in the same direction *(cocurrent),* small solute clearance decreases by about 10%. In addition to decreasing boundary layers and streaming effects (see later discussion), increasing Q_d minimizes the accumulation of waste products in the dialysate, providing a higher solute gradient between blood and dialysate for optimal diffusion. However, even for highly diffusible solutes, the benefits progressively diminish as the dialysate flow rate is increased higher than the blood flow rate. In fact, increasing dialysate flow rate beyond 600 mL/min offers no additional benefit to delivered Kt/V_{urea}.[72]

K_0A, the Mass Transfer Area Coefficient

K_OA is the product of the *mass transfer coefficient,* K_O, which has units of centimeters per minute, and the membrane area, A. K_O is specific for a particular molecule and membrane type, including the membrane's pore size and thickness, but is independent of solute concentration and membrane surface area. It can be considered the solute flux per unit of area per unit of concentration gradient and is equivalent to D/X in Eq. 2. Because solute flux per unit of concentration gradient is defined as dialysance, K_O may also be expressed as the dialysance per unit of membrane area. K_OA, which is the mass transfer area coefficient, therefore has units of milliliters per minute and is equivalent to the dialysance of a membrane with a fixed area during static dialysis (no flow). In addition to being independent of solute concentration, K_OA is also independent of blood and dialysate flow within certain limits (see later text). Therefore K_OA is the most specific constant that describes the efficiency of a dialyzer for removal of a particular solute and is the best parameter for comparing dialyzers. Higher values indicate more efficient solute removal.

K_OA has the same units of measurement as clearance and, in practical terms, can be considered the maximum clearance achievable for a particular dialyzer and solute. Maximum clearance is achieved at the beginning of dialysis when blood solute concentrations along the length of the dialyzer are equal (no flow) and dialysate concentration is 0 or, at the opposite extreme, when blood and dialysate flow rates are infinite. Under these two conditions, the only factor governing a solute's clearance is the dialysis membrane.

Conversely, when Q_b and Q_d are finite, the clearance is lower than K_OA because both flow rates govern diffusion, as discussed previously and because of the way clearance is expressed, as the solute removal rate divided by the inflow concentration. The net driving force for removal is the mean concentration gradient across the membrane, which is a complex function of Q_b and Q_d (see next section). The increase in clearance caused by an increase in Q_b is the result of a flow-dependent increase in the mean concentration gradient across the membrane, driving more solute into the dialysate. Because the inflow concentration does not change with increased Q_b, the conventional measure of clearance as defined previously increases with increasing Q_b.

Boundary Layers and Streaming Effects

Despite a rapid flow along the membrane, the solvent tends to adhere to the membrane, creating a boundary layer, or unstirred layer, that adds to the diffusive pathway on both sides of the membrane.[64] This layer of solvent adjacent to the membrane tends to thin out as flow is increased or as turbulence is produced at the membrane surface. In addition to forming boundary layers, dialysate tends to move along the path of least resistance or channel, leading to nonuniform flow and bypassing some of the membrane area. This streaming effect is more pronounced at lower dialysate flow rates, especially in large dialyzers.[73] Both boundary layer and streaming effects cause K_OA (the resistance to solute diffusion across the membrane) to increase as dialysate flow increases,[71] although the effect is less in vivo than in vitro.[74,75] Recent changes in the shape of hollow fibers and the insertion of inert spacer yarns have improved dialyzer performance further through reducing the effects of channeling and unstirred layers.[76,77] Both effects are less prominent on the blood side of hollow fibers because of the geometrical advantages of flow within hollow fibers, the scrubbing effects of red blood cells, and less variance in Q_b.

High-Efficiency and High-Flux Dialyzers

Initial hemodialyses were limited by low dialyzer membrane permeability, requiring more than 6 hours for each treatment. Although treatment times were shortened to 4 hours or less three times a week as dialyzer design improved, the time spent attached to the dialysis machine was still unacceptable to many patients. The next major advancement came in the late 1980s, when the technical problems with bacteriological contamination of bicarbonate dialysate, inadequate blood flow, imprecise ultrafiltration control, and continued low dialyzer solute clearance were solved.

The distinction between *high-efficiency* and *high-flux* dialyzers is not always made clear, and sometimes these terms are used interchangeably. In essence, both terms address improved solute and fluid clearance compared with standard hemodialyzers, taking advantage of higher blood and dialysate flow rates to decrease dialysis time while maintaining an adequate dose. The two dialyzer designs are not mutually exclusive and in fact often overlap (Table 22.3). The high-efficiency dialyzer contains either a synthetic or a modified cellulose membrane and has a higher clearance of small molecules, such as urea, compared with a standard dialyzer. The high-flux dialyzer always has a highly permeable synthetic or modified cellulose membrane that removes larger molecules. By their nature, high-flux dialyzers have a higher ultrafiltration coefficient (K_{Uf}) compared with high-efficiency dialyzers but not necessarily high urea clearances. Conversely, high urea clearance defines high-efficiency dialysis, but the clearance of larger molecules is variable (see Table 22.3).

TABLE 22.3 Characteristic Values for Standard, High-Efficiency, and High-Flux Dialyzers[a]

	Standard	High Efficiency	High Flux
Blood flow rate (mL/min)	250	≥350	≥350
Dialysate flow rate (mL/min)	500	≥700	≥700
K_oA urea	300–500	600–1000	Variable
Urea clearance (mL/min)	<200	250–400	Variable
Urea clearance/body weight (mL/min/kg)	<3	>3	Variable
Vitamin B_{12} clearance (mL/min)	30–60	Variable	>100
Ultrafiltration coefficient (mL/h/mmHg)	3.5–5.0	<15	>15
Membrane	Cellulose	Variable	Variable

[a]See section High-Efficiency and High-Flux Dialyzers.

The advent of substituted cellulose and synthetic membranes improved dialyzer permeability because substituted cellulose membranes can be made thinner to increase porosity and surface area, whereas synthetic membranes can be manufactured with more and larger pores. Both high-efficiency and high-flux dialysis require the use of bicarbonate dialysate and volume-controlled filtration. Because the high-efficiency and high-flux dialyzers have a higher K_{Uf}, precise control of ultrafiltration is also mandatory to prevent massive volume depletion (see Mechanics of Hemodialysis).

Because of their greater porosity, high-flux dialyzers can remove larger molecules.[69,78] Use of these membranes to improve β_2-microglobulin removal has been associated with a reduction in the risk for carpal tunnel syndrome in long-term patients treated with high-flux dialysis.[79,80] Other benefits that derive possibly from removal of large molecules are an improved lipid profile,[81] a greater response to erythropoietin,[82] and perhaps lower mortality and hospitalization rates.[79,80,83] Potential adverse consequences from increased removal of larger molecules, however, include greater removal of drugs such as vancomycin,[84] amino acids,[85] and albumin,[86] although the last mentioned is disputed.[69] The presence of backfiltration during high-flux dialysis has been postulated to increase the risk for exposing patients to endotoxin from the dialysate, although this potential problem has not been clearly identified in clinical studies.[87,88] One other potential issue with high-efficiency dialyzers is that even at low blood flows, urea clearances are substantial compared with clearances achieved with low-efficiency membranes, which might pose a risk to critically ill acute-dialysis patients because of rapid removal of urea.[89]

Only a few studies have evaluated the comparative efficacy of standard dialysis versus high efficiency and high flux. Nearly all high-flux dialyzers also have high efficiency, so most studies focus on high-flux versus standard hemodialysis. Randomized controlled or crossover trials using bicarbonate dialysate found no difference in the incidence of hypotension and intradialysis symptoms[69,90] or in the control of blood pressure[91] among the three modalities. In a small number of patients treated with high-flux dialysis versus standard dialysis, neuropsychological function[92] was comparable. The best data available come from the HEMO Study, which detected no significant difference in mortality or morbidity between patients treated with standard versus high-flux dialysis and only a slight difference in subgroup analyses.[37] A smaller study in Europe (the Membrane Permeability Outcome Study) found a small but significant improvement in mortality but only in the subgroup with low serum albumin levels (<4.0 g/dL).[93] A Cochrane review of high-flux versus low-flux membranes concluded that high-flux membranes had no effect on all-cause mortality but may reduce cardiovascular mortality.[94]

HEMODIALYSIS

Using dialysis as a form of therapy for the patient vastly complicates this otherwise simple procedure. Factors that complicate the delivery of dialysis include the access device, the patient's adherence with the dialysis prescription and diet, and solute disequilibrium. Developing standards of adequacy requires detailed studies of large populations, with careful attention to the multiple variables that, in addition to the dialysis itself, influence outcome. Achieving target solute concentrations in the patient during and between treatments requires complex mathematical models with multiple variables to account for differences among patients, including differences in size and solute generation rate. These factors add considerable complexity to the relatively simple laws of diffusion and flow discussed earlier, so that the solutions to patient problems are often approximations at best.

Types of Clearance

As noted in the discussion of dialysis and depicted in Eq. 2, dialyzer clearance is the solute removal rate (flux) factored by the blood inflow concentration. During single-pass dialysis, the flux of urea is directly proportional to the inflow concentration, so that urea clearance tends to be constant despite the fall in blood concentration with time. The simplest type of clearance is the *instantaneous dialyzer clearance*, which can be measured by sampling blood on both sides of the dialyzer while recording Q_b at any instant in time. Although the dialyzer urea clearance tends to remain constant, it may fall during treatment because of loss of surface area from clotting or because of changes in Q_b or Q_d. The *effective clearance*, or *integrated dialyzer clearance*, accounts for these changes by linking the measurement of clearance to the predialysis and postdialysis blood urea nitrogen (BUN). This clearance is essentially the answer to this question: What average urea clearance would be required to drive the BUN down to the measured postdialysis value from the measured predialysis value?

The mathematical solution requires a process known as *urea modeling* (see Quantifying Dialysis). It can be calculated

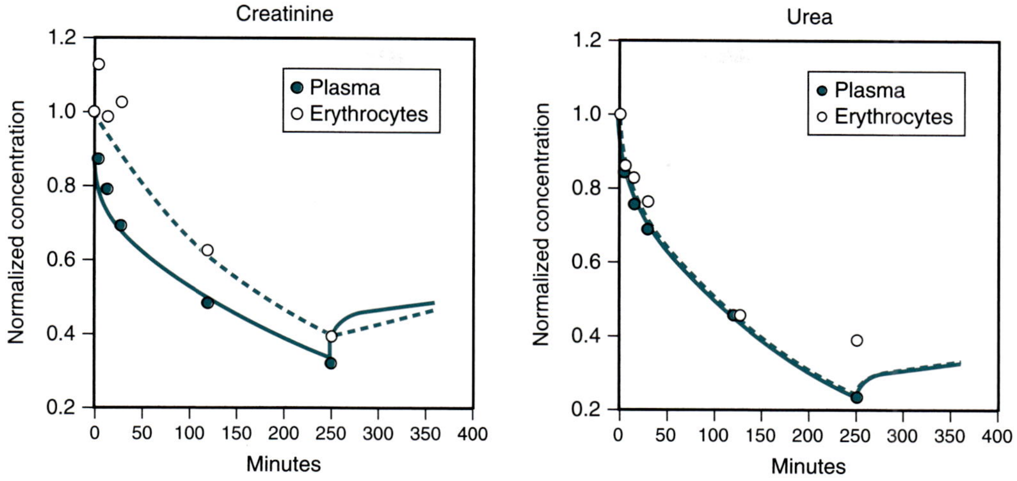

FIG. 22.3 Disequilibrium within the dialyzer itself. Normalized concentrations predicted by a complex mathematical model are shown as *solid lines* (plasma) and *dotted lines* (erythrocyte); measured values are shown as *solid circles* (plasma) and *open circles* (erythrocyte). Urea is efficiently removed from erythrocytes within the dialyzer, but creatinine is not. (Modified from Schneditz D, Platzer D, Daugirdas JT. A diffusion-adjusted regional blood flow model to predict solute kinetics during haemodialysis. *Nephrol Dial Transplant.* 2009;24(7):2218-2224.)

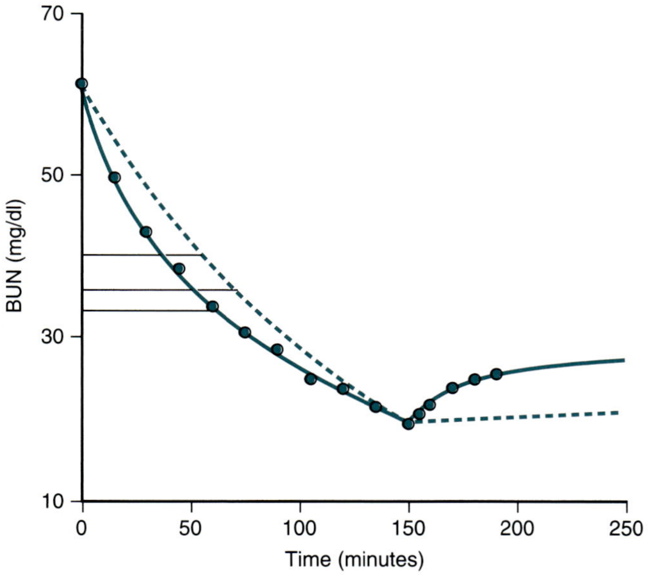

FIG. 22.4 Changes in BUN concentrations during and after dialysis. Measured BUN levels during and immediately after dialysis fit best into a two-compartment variable-volume mathematical model *(solid line)*. The single-compartment variable-volume model *(dashed line)* overestimates BUN levels during the dialysis and fails to predict the rebound. The *upper dotted horizontal line* at 40 mg/dL is the simple arithmetic mean of the predialysis and the postdialysis BUN. The *middle dotted horizontal line* at 36 mg/dL represents the log mean BUN during the treatment, as predicted by the single-compartment model. The *lower dotted horizontal line* at 34 mg/dL is the true mean BUN, obtained from actual measurements throughout dialysis.

using either a single-compartment or a two-compartment urea kinetic model, entering a predialysis and immediate postdialysis BUN in the former case and multiple intra dialysis and postdialysis BUN in the latter case. In either case, the result is a dialyzer urea clearance that is not affected by urea disequilibrium. The integrated dialyzer clearance is often called the *delivered clearance* to distinguish it from the prescribed clearance.

During dialysis, solutes must diffuse from body tissues into the blood to reach the dialyzer. Even within the dialyzer as blood passes through it, solutes must diffuse from within red cells to the plasma before diffusion can take place across the dialyzer membrane into the dialysate. The striking difference between the ability of urea and creatinine to traverse red cell membranes shown in Fig. 22.3 explains in part why urea is preferred to creatinine as a marker for small-solute clearance.[95] Such compartmentalization of body fluids adds complexity to the concept of clearance because different values may be chosen for the denominator of Eq. 3. Even for urea, which diffuses easily across cell membranes from tissue to blood, some disequilibrium still develops among the various body compartments during dialysis, as reflected in the postdialysis urea rebound shown in Fig. 22.4. As a result, the patient's clearance, or *whole body clearance,* defined as the urea removal rate divided by the average urea concentration in total body water, is always less than the dialyzer clearance. Whole body clearance is a virtual clearance (not instantaneously measurable) that can be derived from single-compartment modeling (see Mathematical Models of Urea Kinetics) of the predialysis and *equilibrated* postdialysis BUN. Like dialyzer clearance, it is also a mean clearance integrated over time on dialysis, but it accounts for the presence of solute disequilibrium.

Adding further complexity to the concept of clearance are the frequency and duration of dialysis. Because residual native kidney clearance (K_r) exerts most of its effect between dialyses when dialyzer clearance is zero, it cannot be directly added to dialyzer clearance (see Quantifying Hemodialysis). Intermittent clearance, as obtained with

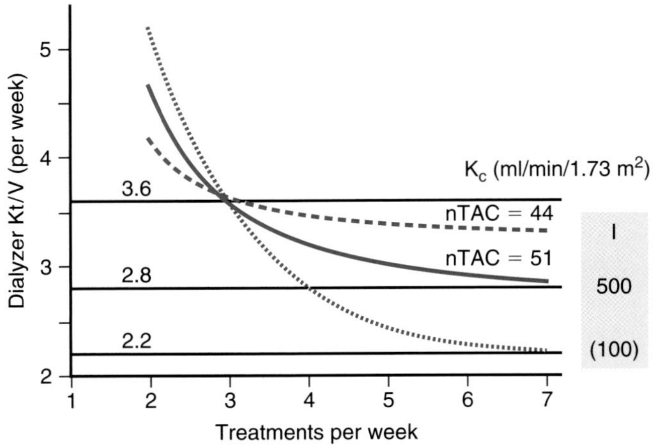

FIG. 22.5 Urea kinetics value (Kt/V) required to maintain the same timed average urea concentration (TAC) of urea. To achieve the same mean blood urea nitrogen concentration, the dose of dialysis provided per week may be reduced as the frequency of dialysis increases. The *upper solid line* shows the required weekly Kt/V for urea based on an intercompartment mass transfer coefficient (K_C) of 500 mL/min. Even a simple single-compartment model with no resistance to diffusion in the patient (*dashed line* = infinite K_C) shows a dependence of weekly Kt/V on dialysis frequency. The discrepancy in weekly Kt/V between intermittent and continuous dialysis is even greater for a theoretical substance that dialyzes as well as urea but exhibits greater disequilibrium within the patient (*dotted line* = K_C of 100 mL/min). (Modified from Depner TA. Quantifying hemodialysis and peritoneal dialysis: examination of the peak concentration hypothesis. *Semin Dial.* 1994;7:315-317.)

hemodialysis, is inherently less efficient than the continuous clearance of native kidneys or continuous peritoneal dialysis. There are two explanations for this reduced dialysis efficiency.

First, although dialyzer clearance is not compromised by an intermittent schedule, total solute removal is reduced because blood solute concentrations decline logarithmically and not linearly during dialysis (see Fig. 22.4).[63,96] Because solute levels do not change during continuous dialysis, this effect is absent and solute removal is maximal at all times. Therefore to reduce solute levels to a similar value, intermittent dialysis must be more intense when averaged over a week of treatment, as shown by the uppermost line in Fig. 22.5. This explanation applies even in the absence of solute disequilibrium.

The second explanation applies to the more realistic situation in which solute concentration in the blood compartment is less than that in other compartments as solute disequilibrium develops during dialysis. Here again, dialyzer clearance is unaffected but solute access to the dialyzer is limited (see later further discussion in Solute Disequilibrium). For continuous replacement modalities and native kidney function, the blood solute concentration is stable and the effect of solute disequilibrium is minimal, so clearances are easy to calculate:

$$\text{Native kidney urea clearance} = K_r = (U_{urea} \times V)/(P_{urea} \times t) \quad (6)$$

$$\text{Peritoneal urea clearance} = (D_{urea} \times V)/(P_{urea} \times t) \quad (7)$$

where U_{urea} is urinary urea concentration, P_{urea} is blood urea concentration, D_{urea} is peritoneal dialysate urea concentration, t is time, and V is 24-hour urinary volume for Eq. 6 and 24-hour dialysate volume for Eq. 7. Continuous clearances are easier to calculate but more difficult to measure than intermittent clearances. For hemodialysis, the clinician can take advantage of the dialysis-induced perturbations in urea concentrations to measure clearance and other patient variables that are not readily measurable by other means.

It is apparent from the previous discussion that the clearances measured during intermittent forms of dialysis are not directly comparable to native kidney clearance or clearances measured in patients undergoing continuous dialysis. The previous observations also help to explain the significant difference between the minimum recommended weekly dose of dialysis (Kt/V) for hemodialysis (1.2 per dialysis × 3 dialyses per week = 3.6/week) and for peritoneal dialysis (1.7/week). To allow a direct comparison, the following formulas adjust for intermittence by calculating the continuous equivalent of intermittent clearance (*equivalent* Kt/V or EKR). For intermittent therapy during a steady state of urea nitrogen balance,[97]

$$EKR_{mean} = \frac{\text{removal rate}}{\text{mean concentration}} = \frac{\text{generation rate}}{\text{mean concentration}} = \frac{G}{TAC} \quad (8)$$

$$EKR_{mean} = \frac{\text{generation rate}}{\text{peak concentration}} = \frac{G}{\text{Av Peak BUN}} \quad (9)$$

G and TAC (time-averaged concentration) are derived from formal urea modeling. Using Eq. 8 and adjusting for time and patient volume, the quantity of hemodialysis necessary to keep a patient's time-averaged BUN constant falls from a weekly Kt/V of 3.6 for thrice-weekly treatments to an EKR of 2.8 for continuous treatment.[98] If mean peak urea is substituted for TAC in Eq. 9, the EKR falls to approximately 2.0, consistent with the previously clinically accepted minimum adequacy for peritoneal dialysis.[99] Although the EKR_{peak} values defined by Gotch as "standard clearance" better match clinical experience, the argument that peak urea levels mediate uremic toxicity does not naturally follow because urea is relatively nontoxic. Instead the relationship likely reflects a fortuitous difference between the diffusibility of urea and the true uremic toxins.[35]

Quantifying Hemodialysis

Dialysis is a treatment born out of empiricism. Solute mass transport during dialysis has been described in precise mathematical terms but only after dialysis was established as a life-sustaining treatment for patients with advanced kidney failure. Much of the effort to describe the kinetics of solute transport has been devoted to determining how to best quantify the amount of dialysis prescribed and delivered. Because it is easy to measure and because the exact uremic toxins are not known, mathematical models of urea kinetics have been used to quantify dialysis.

Mathematical Models of Urea Kinetics

Because urea is a highly water-soluble molecule with little binding to proteins, it distributes only in aqueous environments. Its small size and lack of an electric charge in concert with specific pathways for membrane transport allow it to diffuse rapidly among the various body water compartments. The rate of diffusion is so rapid that a single space of distribution (total body water) can be assumed for most approximations. Between dialyses, when urea accumulates at a slow, constant rate and there is ample time for distribution among the compartments, this assumption is reasonable and the single-pool or *single-compartment kinetic model* is appropriate. During dialysis, however, when blood concentrations change rapidly, urea gradients appear. Serum concentrations fall lower than predicted by the single-compartment model and rebound after dialysis, as shown in Fig. 22.4. Because of this disequilibrium, more complicated mathematical models were developed to explain better the behavior of urea during dialysis.

The *two-compartment model* (Fig. 22.6) assumes that the body is divided into two pools of water, with a finite resistance to diffusion between them. The resistance is expressed inversely as the intercompartment mass transfer coefficient (K_C), which is a measure of the average solute conductivity among compartments for the particular solute. K_C is analogous to K_OA, is solute specific, and has units of measurement that are similar to K_OA (mL/min). The mathematical solution in most cases suggests that the two compartments are the intracellular and extracellular pools separated by cell membranes, but the model does not require this assumption.

For solutes of larger molecular weight, varying charge, and bulkier configuration than urea, disequilibrium among the various compartments is even more pronounced, K_C is lower, and the solute gradients are even larger. Urea is unique in its ability to diffuse across cell membranes, especially the red cell membrane, where urea transporters have been found.[100,101] Most other solutes, even in the same range of molecular weight as urea, probably require a more complex kinetic model.

Kt/V_{urea}

The greatest lesson learned from the NCDS was that patient outcome correlates best with dialyzer urea clearance (K_d). When the level of any known solute is compared with urea clearance, the latter is better able to predict morbidity and mortality in dialysis populations.[102] To allow comparisons among patients and patient populations, a standard expression of clearance must be used, normalizing variables such as the frequency and duration of dialysis and patient size. Adjustment for size is most conveniently done using the patient's volume of urea distribution (V) as

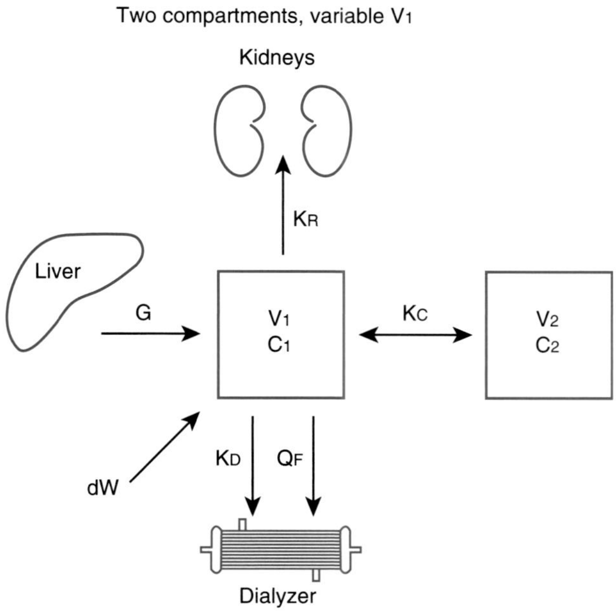

FIG. 22.6 Two-compartment, variable-volume urea kinetic model. This model assumes that urea is distributed in two compartments *(subscripts 1 and 2). V* and *C* are the volume and concentration of urea in each of the two compartments. *G*, Urea generation rate; K_C, intercompartment mass transfer coefficient; K_R, residual native kidney clearance; K_D, dialyzer clearance; Q_F, rate of fluid removal during dialysis. (From Depner TA. *Prescribing Hemodialysis: A Guide to Urea Modeling.* Boston, MA: Kluwer Academic Publishers; 1991.)

the denominator instead of the patient's surface area, commonly used for native kidney clearance. Standards for adequacy are available for hemodialysis delivered three times weekly. If K_d/V is multiplied by the duration of each dialysis (t), the result ($K_d \times t/V$) is a normalized or fractional clearance expressed per dialysis instead of per unit of time. During dialysis, total clearance is the sum of native kidney clearance and dialyzer clearance ($K_r + K_d = K$), so the fractional clearance per dialysis is more often expressed as Kt/V.

Eq. 5 shows that simple first-order diffusion across a dialyzer membrane can be expressed as a constant fractional removal rate if the dialysate concentration remains zero. For hemodialysis with a constant blood flow and a constant single-pass flow of dialysate, fractional solute removal (dC/C) is also constant. Integration and log transformation of Eq. 22.5 gives a powerful expression for the normalized clearance:

$$Kt/V = \ln (C_0/C) \qquad \textbf{(10)}$$

Eq. 10 shows that the normalized clearance (Kt/V) can be determined simply by measuring a predialysis BUN (C_0) and a postdialysis BUN (C). This eliminates the need to measure or estimate the dialyzer clearance, the native kidney clearance, the patient's urea volume, or even the duration of each dialysis to obtain this most powerful correlate to patient survival.

Residual Clearance

Because native kidney function is continuous and occurs between as well as during dialysis treatments, K_r cannot be simply added to K_d. To do so would grossly underestimate the contribution of K_r to overall excretory function. Methods have been proposed to combine the two clearances to represent overall excretory function as a single clearance.[65] Several observational studies have suggested that residual kidney clearance should be included in an expression of total clearance.[103,104] In a 15-year outcomes study of 650 incident patients in a renal unit in the United Kingdom, patients treated with incremental dialysis (accounting for residual kidney urea clearance) had better survival than patients with insignificant residual kidney function.[105] The 2015 update of the Kidney Disease Outcomes Quality Initiative (KDOQI) provided a recommendation to target a standard weekly Kt/V of 2.3 (with a minimum *delivered* weekly Kt/V of 2.1) for hemodialysis schedules other than three times weekly, using calculations that incorporates residual kidney function.[60]

Dialysate Methods

The single-pool kinetic model discussed earlier estimates mass balance of urea across the dialyzer from changes in blood concentration. It makes several incorrect assumptions that cause the errors shown in Fig. 22.4, but the two largest errors are in opposite directions and tend to offset each other.[63] This fortuitous balancing of errors has justified continued use of the single-compartment model to monitor dialysis adequacy. The indirect measurement of urea removal on the blood side, however, has been criticized by some who favor more direct measurements on the dialysate side to avoid these errors. However, use of instruments that measure dialysate urea concentrations either continuously (e.g., by urea electrode) or at multiple times intermittently[106,107] is important to ensure the accuracy of the dialysate method.[108] With these instruments, the dialysate curve-fitting method can be used, which is more accurate than the dialysate/volume method.[108] Dialysate monitoring offers additional advantages, including elimination of blood removal from the patient and avoidance of exposure to the patient's blood, eliminating this potential risk to the patients and staff.

Volume of Urea Distribution

The total body water volume is equal to the volume of urea distribution (V) and can be calculated using various methods, including indicator dilution,[63] bioimpedance,[109] or urea kinetic modeling.[63] V is most easily estimated from anthropometric formulas that are based on the patient's height (centimeters), weight (kilograms), sex, and age (years).[110-112] The most commonly used is the Watson formula[110]:

$$\text{Males}: V\,(\text{liters}) = 2.447 - 0.09516 \times \text{age} + 0.1074 \times \text{height} + 0.3362 \times \text{weight} \quad (11)$$

$$\text{Females}: V\,(\text{liters}) = -2.097 + 0.1069 \times \text{height} + 0.2466 \times \text{weight} \quad (12)$$

Eqs. 11 and 12 were designed to apply to all people and thus to people with widely differing anatomy, but because V can vary independently of height and weight,[112] the anthropometric estimates of V have a large coefficient of variation.[110] V can be measured more precisely in individual patients by modeling urea kinetics because the model makes none of the assumptions found in the anthropometric formulas and because repeated modeling further reduces the variance. The resulting modeled V is analogous to V measured by indicator dilution methods, using urea as the indicator. The HEMO Study Group found that kinetically modeled V was consistently 13% to 19% lower than that derived from the Watson equation.[113] It is unclear whether this difference indicates a reduction in total body water or a difference in the volume of water compared with the volume of urea distribution in patients with ESRD.

Urea Generation and Protein Catabolism

In anuric patients, serum urea concentrations reflect urea generation from net protein catabolism and removal of urea by dialysis. Virtually all urea derives from breakdown of amino acids, and conversely protein nitrogen is catabolized mostly to urea. Under steady-state conditions, only 10% of amino acid nitrogen is converted to nonurea nitrogenous wastes.[114,115] Furthermore, the net protein catabolic rate (PCR) approximates protein intake during a steady state of nitrogen balance. Therefore the measurement of the urea generation rate (G), provided by formal urea modeling, allows an easy estimate of PCR and protein intake. In practice, PCR is usually normalized (divided) by V (PCRn) to allow comparison among patients of different size.

Based on independent detailed studies of two separate groups of patients, one group receiving dialysis[114] and the other with chronic kidney disease but not receiving dialysis,[115] the relationship between PCR (g/day) and G (mg/min) can be described with the following equation:

$$PCR = 9.35 \times G + 11 \quad (13)$$

Eq. 13 shows that the majority of nitrogen released from excess catabolism of dietary and endogenous protein is converted to urea; only 11 g of protein per day are converted to nonurea nitrogenous compounds, such as creatinine, uric acid, hippurate, and amino acids. The generation of nonurea nitrogenous compounds varies with patient size but not with daily protein intake, whereas the generation of urea depends on protein intake. Adjusting the production of nonurea nitrogenous compounds for the average body size in these studies, using urea volume, and normalizing the entire expression to V,

$$PCRn = 5420\,(G/V) + 0.17 \quad (14)$$

where PCRn is normalized PCR in g/kg/day and V is the patient's urea volume (total body water) in liters.

The importance of PCR, PCRn, and G cannot be overemphasized. The NCDS found that a consistently high BUN resulted in a poor outcome, but low BUN levels resulting from low urea generation rates (low PCRn) were associated with even higher morbidity and mortality.[116] A subsequent large population study,[117] as well as the Modification of Diet in Renal Disease study (MDRD), confirmed that patients with low protein intake and PCRn, and therefore low G, had high morbidity and mortality rates, possibly as a result of severe protein-energy wasting, although other disease states may have suppressed the patients' appetites. These studies illustrate that it is not enough to know the BUN level; one must know how it got there. A low BUN from protein-energy wasting is bad, but a low BUN from vigorous dialysis is good. Urea kinetic modeling allows the clinician to separate nutritional influences from the dialysis effect by examining both the absolute urea concentrations and the urea clearance derived from the fall in urea concentrations sampled immediately before and after dialysis.

The causes of low PCRn are myriad, including inflammation, cardiovascular disease, and malignancy, often unrelated to kidney failure or dialysis and in most cases not responsive to increasing the dose of dialysis (Kt/V). In this regard, it is important to be aware of the spurious association in population studies between modeled Kt/V and PCRn because of mathematical coupling. Because both measurements are derived from the same predialysis and postdialysis BUN, a spurious positive correlation occurs as a result of mathematical coupling of BUN measurement errors.[118,119]

Solute Disequilibrium

Solute disequilibrium is defined as a concentration difference or gradient for dissolved solutes among body compartments. This problem develops during dialysis and slowly dissipates over several minutes to hours after the end of dialysis (see Fig. 22.4). Solute disequilibrium caused by resistance to diffusion across cell membranes is called *diffusion-dependent disequilibrium* (see Fig. 22.6). When disequilibrium is caused by differences in blood flow among various vascular beds, it is termed *flow-dependent disequilibrium* (Fig. 22.7).

Solute disequilibrium among body compartments is at least partially caused by variances in tissue perfusion.[120,121] In fact, mathematical models have been developed that fully describe urea disequilibrium using purely flow-dependent disequilibrium.[122] These models assume that solutes diffuse instantly between compartments, so the observed gradients are attributed to differences in relative blood flow/volume served by the vascular bed. In reality, both mechanisms likely contribute, but their relative importance remains to be determined.

Vascular access recirculation may cause a decrease in effective solute clearance[123,124] and is a special case of flow-dependent disequilibrium. Access recirculation occurs in about 5% of patients when blood that has just been dialyzed returns immediately to the dialyzer in the reverse direction through the access device. Multiple causes have been identified, including venous outflow stenosis, central venous stenosis, close proximity of the dialysis needles, and accidental reversal of the arterial and venous needles. Although dialyzer clearance is preserved, total solute removal decreases because the recirculated venous blood dilutes the solute concentration of the incoming arterial blood, thus lowering the solute concentration gradient across the dialyzer membrane. When 100% recirculation exists, all the dialyzed blood returns to the dialyzer and the patient derives no benefit from dialysis.

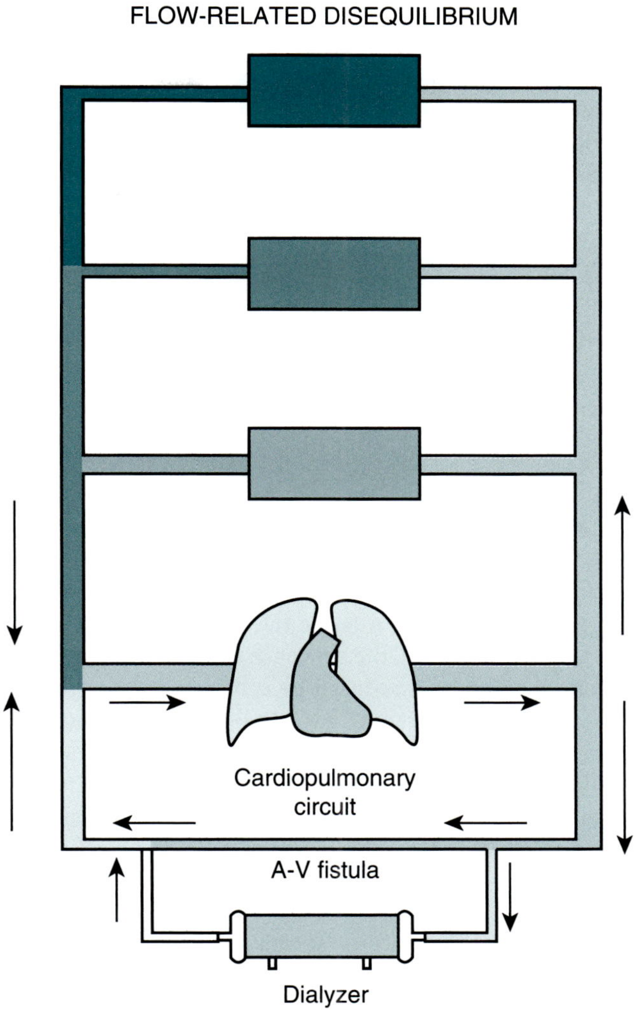

FIG. 22.7 Urea disequilibrium as a consequence of differences in regional blood perfusion. Differing simultaneous concentrations of urea throughout the body can develop solely as a consequence of differences in regional blood perfusion, shown here as a parallel arrangement of tissue compartments. Although the consequences are similar to urea disequilibrium resulting from membrane-limited diffusion, the mechanism is entirely different because this model assumes an absence of diffusion barriers. Instead the rapid changes in blood urea levels at the beginning and end of treatment are caused by the differing blood perfusion rates. Blood in the more rapidly flowing circuits comes into contact with the dialyzer more frequently, so it has a lower urea and solute concentration and essentially dilutes the solute concentration from slower-flowing blood pools. The proximal and most rapidly flowing blood pathway is the cardiopulmonary circuit through the peripheral AV access device. (From Depner TA. Approach to hemodialysis kinetic modeling. In: Henrich WL, ed. *Principles and Practice of Dialysis*. 4th ed. Baltimore, MD: Williams & Wilkins; 1999.)

With a model of multiple parallel circuits,[125] differences in blood flowing to various parts of the body have been invoked to explain the differences in solute concentration among these vascular beds during dialysis (see Fig. 22.7). Blood from the rapidly flowing circuits is exposed to the dialyzer more frequently and dilutes the solute concentration of blood flowing to the dialyzer. This essentially limits the access to the dialyzer of slower-flowing circuits that have higher solute concentrations. Thus differences in blood flow within the blood pool reduce the solute concentration entering the dialyzer and the average concentration in the patient. This reduces the efficiency of dialysis, decreases solute removal, and invalidates the use of solute concentration in peripheral venous blood for calculating vascular access recirculation.[125-127]

Cardiopulmonary recirculation, present in dialysis patients with AV shunts[128] (see Fig. 22.7), is a specific example of one of these multiple parallel circuits. Because the vascular shunt has low resistance and routes blood directly from the arterial to the venous circulation, blood flowing through this circuit returns to the heart at a faster rate. Although the dialyzer clearance is unaffected, the concentration gradient across the dialyzer membrane is reduced by cardiopulmonary recirculation so that solute removal is impaired. Cardiopulmonary recirculation contributes to the rebound in blood solute (urea) concentration after dialysis is completed, since the various blood compartments equilibrate. Cardiopulmonary recirculation is not present in patients with central venous catheters for vascular access because blood drawn from the central vein is returned to the same vein and the shunt circuit is absent. However, it is important to note that significant recirculation can exist in central venous catheters because of shorter lengths, especially in the femoral location.[129,130]

Body Size and Dialysis Adequacy

Current standards factor the dose of hemodialysis according the patient's urea volume (V), which is equated to total body water volume. This is a departure from the usual body surface area (BSA) denominator but has the tremendous advantage of convenience, as outlined earlier. Use of V is also logical if the goal is to maintain concentrations equal among different-sized patients. This logic, however, depends not on V but on toxin generation rates that are proportional to V. Although we have little understanding of toxins, as discussed earlier, it is likely that generation rates, much like other physiological functions, correlate more closely to BSA than V. Variability in the slope of outcomes related to dose also suggest that another denominator would be more appropriate, especially in population studies.[131] Clinical concerns include the potential for underdosing small patients and women.[132,133] This issue has been subject to scrutiny, and methods for converting the denominator have been proposed but are not yet a standard of care.

Adequacy of Hemodialysis: Current Recommendations

Before the NCDS, absolute blood urea concentrations were used to monitor the efficacy of dialysis and to determine the frequency of dialysis. Kinetic modeling gained popularity and increasing acceptance after the NCDS reported that both high and low blood urea concentrations were associated with increased mortality,[102,116] highlighting the fact that the absolute blood urea concentration is a poor marker of uremia and dialysis dose. Using absolute blood urea levels risks setting in motion the vicious cycle of providing less dialysis to patients who have protein-energy wasting, causing a further reduction in BUN. Assessing dialysis adequacy with kinetic modeling avoids this vicious cycle because kinetic modeling determines the clearance of urea based on the change in urea concentration.

The NCDS data indicated that maximal benefit from dialysis was obtained with a Kt/V_{urea} greater than 1 per dialysis administered three times a week.[116] Subsequent data from uncontrolled studies suggested that further benefit may be derived from increasing Kt/V_{urea} to 1.2 or greater.[47-50] Based on the available data, the NIH, the Renal Physicians Association, and the National Kidney Foundation established the minimum Kt/V_{urea} at 1.2 per dialysis administered three times a week in their respective consensus conferences. The HEMO Study results support this minimum Kt/V_{urea} because increasing single-pool Kt/V_{urea} from an average of 1.32 to 1.71 did not further reduce mortality or morbidity.[37] The 2015 update to the KDOQI clinical practice guidelines for hemodialysis adequacy recommended a *target* Kt/V of 1.4 and a *delivered* Kt/V of 1.2 for patients on thrice weekly hemodialysis and also makes recommendations (as noted in the preceding sections) regarding reducing dose of dialysis for patients with residual kidney function. For patients on more frequent dialysis regimens, a standard Kt/V of 2.3 is targeted for a minimum delivered dose of 2.1.[60]

Filtration and Dialysis

Because fluid nearly always accumulates in patients between therapeutic hemodialyses, net ultrafiltration must be a part of each treatment to maintain fluid balance. In a sense, water is also a toxin that accumulates and must be removed on a regular basis. The mechanism of water removal during hemodialysis is not diffusion but pressure filtration of the blood as it passes through the dialyzer. Although filtration also removes solute, and solute removal by filtration is also a first-order process, the additional clearance from filtration is often less than expected. Conversely, one can remove solute with filtration alone (see Hemofiltration and Hemodiafiltration Therapy). If no dialysis takes place and the sieving coefficient is close to 1, the clearance is simply the filtration rate (see Quantitative Contribution of Filtration to Solute Removal). The sieving coefficient is the fractional concentration of the solute in dialysate compared with blood water.

Dialyzer Ultrafiltration Coefficient

The same membrane properties (i.e., thinner, more porous membranes with a large surface area) that improve solute clearance also improve hydraulic fluid removal. In addition, membrane tensile strength plays a role in determining the maximum pressure that can be applied. Dialyzers are rated by their ultrafiltration coefficient (K_{Uf}), with units of mL/h/mmHg. Typical K_{Uf} values for standard and high-flux dialyzers are listed in Table 22.3.

Quantitative Contribution of Filtration to Solute Removal

As plasma water moves from the blood compartment to the dialysate, solutes dissolved in plasma follow passively. Convective clearance thus augments diffusive transport, and the contribution can be quantified mathematically. When ultrafiltration is present during dialysis, blood flow into the dialyzer (Q_{bi}) can be expressed as the sum of blood flow out of the dialyzer (Q_{bo}) and the ultrafiltration rate (Q_f):

$$Q_{bi} = Q_{bo} = Q_f \quad (15)$$

From the previously described definition of dialyzer clearance and considering mass balance, dialyzer clearance (K_d) can be expressed as a function of solute concentrations and blood flow rates through the dialyzer:

$$K_d = J/C_{in} = [(C_{in} \times Q_{bi}) - (C_o \times Q_{bo})]/C_{in} \quad (16)$$

where J is the solute flux, C_{in} the inlet (arterial) solute concentration, and C_o the outlet (venous) solute concentration. Combining and rearranging Eqs. 15 and 16 yields the following:

$$K_d = Q_{bi}(C_{in} - C_o)/C_{in} + Q_f(C_o/C_{in}) \quad (17)$$

Eq. 17 shows that dialyzer clearance of a particular solute is the sum of solute clearance in the absence of ultrafiltration ($Q_{bi} = Q_{bo}$) and a fraction of the ultrafiltration rate. At one extreme, when all the solute is removed by diffusion (C_o = 0), there is no contribution from ultrafiltration. At the other extreme, when no diffusion is present ($C_{in} = C_o$), the dialyzer clearance is the ultrafiltration rate. This latter case occurs in the setting of hemofiltration (to be discussed further), where all solute clearance results from filtration. During the usual hemodialysis treatment, the contribution of convective clearance to the total dialyzer clearance is small. Even at high rates of ultrafiltration (2 L/h or 33 mL/min), the relative contribution of ultrafiltration to total urea clearance is only about 10 mL/min or 5%, assuming C_o/C_{in} for urea of 0.3 to 0.4 and dialyzer urea clearance of 200 mL/min.

In clinical practice, outlet solute concentration is rarely measured, limiting the usefulness of Eq. 17. With further mathematical manipulation,[63] C_o can be eliminated, yielding

$$K_d = K_{d0} + Q_f(1 - K_{d0}/Q_{bi}) \quad (18)$$

where K_{d0} is the dialyzer clearance without ultrafiltration and can be calculated from Q_{bi} and the dialyzer K_OA. Q_f is readily calculated from the weight loss during dialysis divided by the duration of dialysis or directly measured by volume-controlled dialysis machines.

Hemofiltration and Hemodiafiltration Therapy

Up to now, we have discussed the principles of filtration in the context of hemodialysis, using filtration mainly for removing excess fluid, while relying on diffusion for solute removal. Hemofiltration alone can also be used to remove both solute and solvent. As discussed earlier and as evident from Eq. 18, in the absence of diffusion (K_{d0} = 0), dialyzer clearance is the ultrafiltration rate. Therefore to achieve solute clearance comparable to that of hemodialysis, large amounts of fluid must be removed, on the order of 30 to 80 L during each treatment, with simultaneous replenishment using a pyrogen-free physiological salt solution.[134,135]

Larger-molecular substances are removed more effectively by hemofiltration because convection has a greater effect of enhancing the relatively slow diffusive movement of larger molecules compared with small molecules (see earlier discussion of convection and diffusion). Hemofiltration requires a highly permeable (high flux) membrane to achieve the high filtration rates (30 to 80 L per dialysis). During filtration, peripheral vascular resistance has been reported to increase in part because of a cooling effect,[136] which helps support blood pressure. The primary disadvantage of hemofiltration is the large amount of sterile replacement fluid required, but equipment designed to simplify hemofiltration and produce sterile replacement fluid online is available in some countries.[137]

Hemodiafiltration is the combination of hemodialysis and hemofiltration (i.e., addition of dialysate flow to the hemofiltration circuit). Solute removal is accomplished by both diffusion and filtration, but, in contrast to traditional hemodialysis, the filtration component contributes much more because of its higher magnitude relative to dialysis. Although intermittent hemofiltration and hemodiafiltration are not widely used in the United States for treating ESRD, these two modalities have been adapted for wide use in intensive care units to treat patients with acute kidney injury.[138,139] Outcome benefits of hemofiltration and hemodiafiltration compared with hemodialysis have been conflicting. Some small studies have suggested a comparative benefit,[140] but larger studies have not found a clear mortality benefit of hemodiafiltration compared with hemodialysis.[141,142] In aggregate, current data do not seem to justify one modality over the other.[143]

Filtration Effects on Blood Pressure, Regional Blood Flow, and Solute Removal

Blood pressure falls as fluid is removed in part because the normal response of vasoconstriction to fluid removal is impaired in dialysis patients. Use of bioincompatible membranes and acetate as sources of bicarbonate during hemodialysis can cause vasodilation and further predispose the patient to hypotension. To aggravate the situation further, solute removal decreases blood osmolarity, causing slight fluid shifts from the intravascular compartment into the intracellular compartment. In patients at high risk for hypotension during dialysis, separating filtration (isolated ultrafiltration) from dialysis may improve their hemodynamic stability.

Although theoretically filtration may account for a significant fraction of solute removal during hemodialysis, in practice it can also interfere with solute removal by diffusion. In addition, the development of intravascular volume depletion during dialysis causes vasoconstriction in the skin and skeletal muscle and shunts blood through more central vascular circuits (such as the AV shunt), enhancing flow-related solute disequilibrium.

Middle and Large Molecule Removal

MMs were originally defined by Scribner and his associates[144] as poorly dialyzable solutes that might account for the

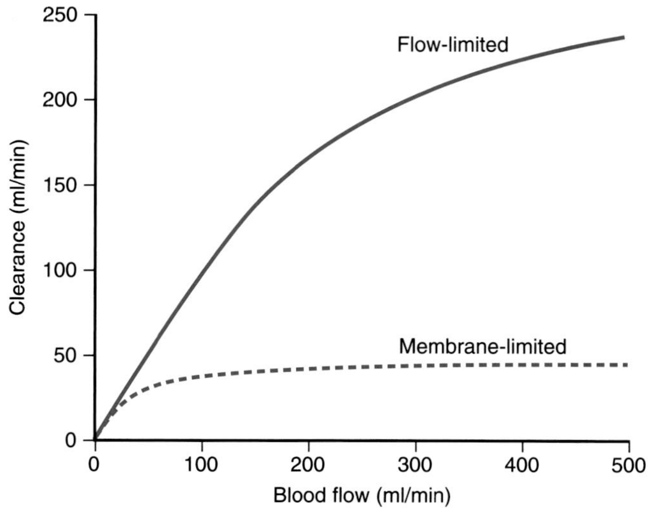

FIG. 22.8 Clearance of larger solutes tends to be membrane limited, as depicted in the *lower curve,* unaffected by changes in blood or dialysate flow within the usual therapeutic range. For the smaller, more diffusible solutes like urea, an increase in blood flow causes a near-proportionate increase in clearance within the therapeutic range of blood flow.

failure of more intense dialysis to restore health. They imagined that these solutes were "membrane restricted," meaning that their clearances were limited by membrane porosity and surface area independent of blood and dialysate flow rates (Fig. 22.8). An increase in MM clearance requires larger and more porous membranes or an increase in treatment time. These theoretical solutes were considered to be dialyzable by the membranes available at the time, but clearances were low. Because the available cellulosic membranes had an effective size cutoff of 10 kDa, the molecular weights of MMs were postulated to range from 500 to 3000 Da. More recent investigators have attempted to redefine the upper MM size limit to the 20 to 30,000 Da range to accommodate the greater porosity of modern high-flux dialyzers.[33] However, it is important to recall that anuric patients treated with these older cellulosic dialyzers survived, sometimes for more than a decade. This observation diminishes but does not eliminate the potential impact of MMs on survival or quality of life.

The middle molecule theory was popular in the 1960s and 1970s, spurred by the failure of biochemists to identify specific uremic toxins in the low-molecular-weight range. Many thought that small polypeptides accounted for the uremic syndrome, and they encouraged membrane manufacturers to improve MM removal by developing high-flux dialyzers. Biochemists were similarly encouraged to look for toxic polypeptides that depended on renal elimination and that were retained in ESRD.[145,146] Polypeptides in the 500 to 3000 Da range are not abundant in the urine but are nonetheless dependent on kidney function for elimination by filtration and reabsorption. The popularity of the MM theory at the time of the design phase of the NCDS likely had an influence on the decision to include dialysis treatment time as one of the two interventions, because high-flux membranes were not yet available. The hypothesis tested by the NCDS was that retention of low-molecular-weight solutes, reflected in urea TAC, was more important than retention of MMs, the surrogate for which was treatment time. Because the results overwhelmingly favored TAC as the primary determinant of outcome, the popularity of the MM hypothesis diminished and more emphasis was subsequently placed on improving small-molecule clearances in the form of Kt/V_{urea}.[102] The quest for middle- and larger-molecular-weight toxins is still ongoing, but the rationale has shifted to their potential contribution to the residual syndrome.

Importance of Treatment Time

In the early 1990s emphasis was placed on shortening the treatment time while maintaining an "adequate" Kt/V. It soon became apparent, however, that the effective clearance was treatment time dependent (see previous discussion of eKt/V)[99,147] and that outcomes were adversely affected by shortening dialysis time.[148-150] Shortening the treatment time will predictably decrease efficiency because it accentuates the effects of intermittence and exacerbates solute disequilibrium (see Solute Disequilibrium and Fig. 22.4). In addition, as discussed earlier, the shorter duration of high-efficiency hemodialysis may not allow sufficient time to remove larger molecules, such as β_2-microglobulin, for which removal is more time dependent.[151] Advocates of longer treatment times pointed to the more prolonged treatments in Europe and Japan, where outcomes are better than in the United States,[148] and to the borderline significant effect of treatment time in the NCDS.[152] Results of the Time to Reduce Mortality in End-Stage Renal Disease (TiME) Trial, a pragmatic trial of hemodialysis session duration, are awaited.[153] Another potential problem with shortening time is the required increase in the filtration rate.[90,154] Most patients can tolerate up to 0.35 mL/min/kg of filtration (1.5 L/h in a 70-kg person) without developing nausea, cramping, or hypotension.[154] Therefore an average-sized patient whose weight gain exceeds 4 to 5 kg is a poor candidate for short-duration dialysis and will experience a progressive rise in end-dialysis weight, eventually leading to pulmonary edema. Finally, once patients are accustomed to the shorter time, it might be challenging to accept prolonging dialysis time when conditions such as large fluid gains, inadequate clearance of larger molecules, poorly functioning access, or loss of residual kidney function occur.

MECHANICS OF HEMODIALYSIS

Twenty to thirty years ago, hemodialysis equipment for a single patient occupied the greater part of an entire room. Now hemodialysis machines are about the size of a 3- to 4-drawer filing cabinet and can be transported easily by one person. In addition to the reduction in size, advances have included more reliable dialysate delivery systems, monitoring devices, and automated safety mechanisms. Several online devices allow dynamic monitoring of the vascular access, the hematocrit, and the adequacy of the treatment.

Dialysate Delivery Systems

The most commonly used system discards the dialysate after a single passage through the dialyzer (*single-pass* delivery). Most dialysis clinics also use *single-patient* delivery systems in which a machine at each patient station continuously prepares dialysate by mixing a liquid concentrate with a proportionate volume of purified water. To dilute the concentrates safely, the dialysis machine has many built-in safety monitors. Some clinics use a central multipatient delivery system in which either the concentrated dialysate is mixed in an area away from patient care and then piped to each dialysis station or the concentrate is piped to each station before mixing. The advantages of these centralized systems are lower patient care costs and fewer staff back injuries from carrying the individual concentrate jugs, but a major disadvantage is inflexibility in modifying the dialysate concentration of electrolytes, such as calcium and potassium, to suit individual patient needs.

Mechanical and Safety Monitors

The dialysis machine draws up and warms purified water to physiological temperatures. The heated water then undergoes deaeration under vacuum to prevent dissolved air from coming out of solution as negative pressure is applied during dialysis. Air bubbles in the dialysate cause the blood leak detector and the conductivity detector to malfunction. They also "lock" part of the dialysate pathway, increasing channeling and masking parts of the membrane surface area.

The heated and deaerated product water is then mixed with the concentrate to produce dialysate. To ensure proper proportioning, the *conductivity monitor* downstream from the proportioning pump continuously measures the electrical conductivity of the product solution. Because malproportioned dialysate may cause severe electrolyte disturbances in the patient, leading to death, the conductivity monitor has a narrow range of tolerance and is usually redundant. Dialysate conductivity may be altered by temperature, the presence of air bubbles, or malfunction of the sensor, usually an electrode. Periodically, the conductivity monitor must be calibrated using standardized solutions or by laboratory measurements of electrolytes in the dialysate.

Because the patient is exposed to 100 to 200 L of dialysate during each treatment, the dialysate must be heated to near body temperature to avoid hypothermia. If the dialysate is too hot, however, protein denaturation (>42°C) and hemolysis (>45°C) occur. In practice the dialysate temperature is maintained at 36ºC to 37ºC and falls slightly in transit from the proportioning device to the patient. The *temperature monitor* within the dialysate circuit sets off an alarm if the dialysate temperature is outside the limits of 36ºC to 42°C, and dialysate is pumped directly to the drain, automatically bypassing the dialyzer.

Located downstream from the dialyzer, the dialysate pump controls dialysate flow and generates negative dialysate pressure. The dialysate circuit must be able to generate both negative and positive dialysate pressures within the dialyzer because, although many dialyzers require a negative dialysate pressure for filtration, dialyzers with high K_{Uf} or conditions that increase pressure in the blood compartment require a positive dialysate pressure to limit filtration. The dialysate circuitry controls the pressure by variably constricting the dialysate outflow tubing while maintaining a constant flow rate. The dialysate delivery system also monitors the filtration rate, either indirectly by controlling the TMP (*pressure-controlled* ultrafiltration) or directly by controlling the actual filtration (*volume-controlled* ultrafiltration). Earlier dialysate delivery systems used pressure-controlled filtration, requiring dialysis personnel to calculate the TMP, enter the TMP into the machine, closely monitor the filtration rate, and recalculate and adjust the TMP as needed. To prevent excessive fluid removal when using dialyzers with K_{Uf} greater than 6 mL/h/mmHg, dialysate delivery systems capable of performing volume-controlled filtration are mandatory. Such systems have built-in balance chambers and servomechanisms that accurately control the volume of fluid removed during dialysis once the desired goal is set.[155]

The blood leak monitor is situated in the dialysate outflow tubing and is designed to alarm and shut off the blood pump when blood is detected. The presence of blood in the dialysate usually indicates membrane rupture and may be caused by a TMP exceeding 500 mmHg. Although a rare complication, membrane rupture can be potentially life threatening because it allows nonsterile dialysate to come into contact with blood. In this era of dialyzer reuse, the potential for membrane rupture is increased because both bleach and heat disinfection can damage the dialyzer membrane. Intravascular hemolysis with hemoglobin in the dialysate as well as hydroxocobalamin used in cyanide poisoning, [156] may also trigger the blood leak alarm.

Bicarbonate Delivery

Dialysate previously contained acetate as a source of bicarbonate. Advantages of acetate included the low incidence of bacterial contamination, no precipitation with calcium, and ease of storage. However, acetate is a hemodynamic stressor especially during high-efficiency and high-flux dialysis,[157-159] when the rate of acetate diffusion into blood can exceed the metabolic capacity of the liver and skeletal muscle. Acetate accumulation leads to acidosis, vasodilation, and hypotension. All clinics using high-flux dialysis and the majority using standard-flux dialysis now use bicarbonate-based dialysate to prevent these complications.

The major complications of bicarbonate dialysate are bacterial contamination and precipitation of calcium and magnesium salts. Gram-negative halophilic rods require sodium chloride or sodium bicarbonate to grow and thus thrive in bicarbonate dialysate.[160,161] When bicarbonate containers are disinfected, these bacteria have a latency period of 3 to 5 days, have an exponential growth phase at 5 to 8 days, and achieve maximum growth at 10 days,[160] compared with a latency of 1 day, exponential growth phase at 2 to 3 days, and maximum growth by 4 days in a contaminated container. Mixing bicarbonate and disinfecting the containers daily help prevent bacterial contamination. Alternatively, commercially available dry powder cartridges can circumvent this problem.

Recognition of the risks from microbiological contamination and the subsequent steps taken to prevent contamination have greatly reduced the incidence of pyrogen reactions reported during the early application of high-flux dialysis. Although the risk is theoretically increased by back filtration during high-flux dialysis, few reports of this complication have appeared.[87,162]

To prevent formation of insoluble calcium and magnesium salts with bicarbonate, the final dialysate is mixed from two separate components: the bicarbonate concentrate and the acid concentrate. The acid concentrate contains all solutes other than bicarbonate and derives its name from the inclusion of a small amount of acetic acid (4 mEq/L in the final dilution). The dialysate delivery system draws up the two components separately and mixes them proportionately with purified water to form the final dialysate. This process minimizes but does not eliminate the precipitation of calcium and magnesium salts, so the dialysate delivery system must be rinsed periodically with an acid solution to eliminate any buildup.

Water Quality

Treatment of the water used to generate dialysate is essential to avoid exposure during dialysis to harmful substances, such as aluminum, chloramine-T, endotoxin, and bacteria. Accumulation of aluminum in the body may cause dialysis dementia, microcytic anemia, and osteomalacia. Chloramine-T, a product of chlorine and organic material, causes acute hemolysis during dialysis. Endotoxin and bacteria cause febrile reactions and hypotension. Good water quality is even more imperative when dialyzers are reused because the blood compartment is exposed to unsterile water and any accompanying bacteria or endotoxin. To avoid these complications, tap water is first softened, then exposed to charcoal to remove contaminants such as chloramine, then filtered to remove particulate matter, and then filtered under high pressure (reverse osmosis) to remove other dissolved contaminants.

Blood Circuit Components

The steady flow of blood required for dialysis may be drawn from a central vein, from the ports along the sides of a double-lumen catheter (arterial lumen), and returned through the port at the distal tip (venous lumen). Alternatively, the blood may be drawn from an AV fistula or graft through an "arterial" needle and returned through a second "venous" needle. The blood pump is usually a peristaltic roller pump, which sequentially compresses the pump segment of the blood tubing against a curved rigid track, forcing blood from the tubing. After the roller has passed, the elastic tubing recoils and refills with blood, ready for the next roller. As a result, blood flow through the dialyzer is pulsatile. Most pumps have two or three rollers. The greater the number of rollers, the less pulsatile the flow but the higher the risk of hemolysis and damage to the pump segment.

Alternatively the dialysate delivery system can be configured with one blood pump and two pressure-controlled blood-line clamps or two pressure-controlled blood pumps that will allow the delivery of dialysis through a single needle in the vascular access or a single-lumen catheter.[163,164] This configuration offers less trauma to the vascular access but suffers from an increase in recirculation and hemolysis[164] and potentially a decline in adequacy, although this is debated.[163-165]

When the upper or lower limits are exceeded, pressure monitors sound an alarm and turn off the blood pump. An arterial pressure monitor should be located proximal to the blood pump and a venous monitor located distal to the dialyzer. Accepted ranges for arterial inflow pressures are −20 to −80 mmHg but may be as low as −200 mmHg when Q_b is high. Accepted ranges for venous pressures are +50 to +200 mmHg. Kinks in the tubing, improper arterial needle position, hypotension, or arterial inflow stenosis can cause excessively low arterial pressures. High venous pressures should prompt an investigation for blood clotting in the dialyzer, kinking or clotting in the venous blood lines, improperly positioned venous needles, infiltration of a venous needle, or venous outflow stenosis. Accurate measurements of both the arterial and venous pressures are essential to determining the TMP. Excessive positive pressures anywhere in the blood compartment may rupture the dialyzer membrane or cause the blood circuit to disconnect. An abrupt fall in pressure anywhere in the blood circuit may signal an accidental disconnection of the blood circuit, which can result in exsanguination if not corrected promptly.

Two other important safety devices, located in the blood line distal to the dialyzer, are (1) the *venous air trap* and (2) the *air detector.* The venous air trap prevents any air that may have entered the blood circuit through loose connections, improper arterial needle position, or the saline infusion line from returning to the patient. If air is still detected in the venous line after the venous air trap, the machine alarms and turns off the blood pump. Excessive foaming of blood will also trigger the air detector. These safety features prevent air embolism, which carries a high mortality rate, especially when the problem is not immediately recognized.[166]

Computer Controls

As discussed earlier, solute removal during hemodialysis decreases plasma osmolarity, favors fluid shift into the cells, and makes fluid removal more difficult. Increasing the dialysate sodium concentration helps to preserve plasma osmolarity and allows continued fluid removal[167,168] but may lead to increased thirst, excessive weight gain, and hypertension.[167,169] Computer-controlled sodium modeling allows the dialysate sodium concentration to change automatically during dialysis according to a preselected profile, usually 150 to 160 mEq/L at the beginning of dialysis to 135 to 140 mEq/L near or at the end of dialysis. Theoretically this sodium modeling offers the benefit of greater hemodynamic stability while minimizing thirst and interdialysis hypertension. To date, a few small studies support this theory,[169-173] but the results are not conclusive.[174,175] Most authorities advise against sodium modeling.[176]

Ultrafiltration modeling, like sodium modeling, provides a variable rate of fluid removal during dialysis, according to a preprogrammed profile (linear decline, stepwise changes, or exponential decline of filtration rate with time). Altering the filtration rate during dialysis theoretically allows time for the blood compartment to refill from the interstitial compartment, leading to improved hemodynamic stability and less cramping. As with sodium modeling, ultrafiltration modeling must be individualized. In fact, the effects of the two are difficult to distinguish because they are often used together.[170,173,174,177]

Technological advances include the development of dialysis machines with feedback control systems that allows for computer-controlled adjustments of the ultrafiltration rate and dialysate conductivity to prevent the blood volume from dropping to less than a preset value throughout the dialysis session.[178,179] Studies in small groups of hemodialysis patients have reported that this device reduces symptoms in both hypotension- and non–hypotension-prone patients.[178,180,181] The ability to monitor plasma conductivity throughout dialysis also ensures sodium balance during treatment despite constant modifications to the dialysate conductivity and may reduce the problem of thirst and interdialytic hypertension reported with sodium modeling.[178] Automated control of dialysate temperature to maintain isothermic dialysis (constant body temperature) was superior to thermoneutral dialysis (using lower but constant dialysate temperature) in reducing intradialytic hypotension.[182]

Anticoagulation

Blood clotting during dialysis is a source of patient blood loss and interferes with solute clearance by decreasing the dialyzer surface area.[183] To prevent clotting, a dose of heparin, the most commonly used anticoagulant in dialysis, is usually given at the start of dialysis (2000 to 5000 units or 50 units/kg), then continuously infused (1000 to 1500 units/h) into the blood circuit before the dialyzer, until 15 to 60 minutes before the end of dialysis.[184-186] Alternatively, heparin boluses may be given intermittently during dialysis as needed. The bolus method increases nursing time and results in episodes of overanticoagulation and underanticoagulation. If the patient is at risk for bleeding, low-dose heparin (bolus of 500 to 1000 units followed by 500 to 750 units/h) or no anticoagulant may be appropriate.[185,186] For heparin-free dialysis, pre-rinsing the blood circuit with heparinized saline and flushing the dialyzer with 100 mL of 0.9% sodium chloride every 15 to 30 minutes may help to prevent clotting. Avoiding blood or platelet transfusions through the circuit is also required to minimize clotting. Additional options are the use of heparin-coated dialyzers or regional citrate anticoagulation,[186-188] although heparin-coated dialyzers may be inferior to regional citrate anticoagulation in preventing dialyzer clotting.[187]

Alternatives to heparin and regional citrate anticoagulation include low-molecular-weight heparin,[186,189-191] hirudin,[192] prostacyclin,[193,194] dermatan sulfate,[186] and argatroban.[195,196] Except for low-molecular-weight heparin,[186,191] none is in wide use because of complexity, expense, lack of sufficient clinical experience, or equivalency to heparin. Citrate anticoagulation, in particular, may cause hypocalcemia and death if calcium replacement is inadequate and significant metabolic alkalosis if the dialysate bicarbonate concentration is not decreased,[186] although a simplified treatment protocol may render it safer.[187] In the rare case of confirmed heparin-induced thrombocytopenia, hirudin, argatroban, and citrate anticoagulation have been used with varying success.[186,196] Finally, substituting citric acid for acetic acid in the dialysate with concomitant heparin use during dialysis improves clearance and increases dialyzer reuse, presumably because of decreased clotting.[197,198]

Online Monitoring of Clearance, Hematocrit, and Access Flow

Urea concentration, hematocrit, and access blood flow may be measured online (i.e., during the dialysis). Although the equipment and effort are expensive at present, they may prove cost effective in the long run by improving patient care. Monitoring can minimize the amount of blood drawn and allow more sensitive and frequent assessment of adequacy, control of ultrafiltration, and detection of vascular access stenosis.

Monitoring Clearance

Online monitoring of urea kinetics may provide the best assessment of urea removal and dialysis adequacy.[199-201] Available monitors include those that sample dialysate continuously or periodically to measure urea concentration[106,107,178,202,203] and those that monitor dialyzer sodium clearance by pulsing the dialysate sodium concentration and measuring conductivity.[178,204] The online methods for monitoring urea kinetics provide Kt/V_{urea} based on whole-body urea clearance, not just dialyzer clearance.

Monitoring Hematocrit

Hematocrit can be measured during dialysis using either a conductivity method[205] or an optical technique.[206,207] These methods may benefit dialysis patients at risk for hypotension and cramping because these symptoms are usually caused by intravascular volume depletion, which is reflected by the degree of hemoconcentration.[207] By monitoring the hematocrit online, the filtration rate can be varied during dialysis to minimize the magnitude of hemoconcentration and the occurrence of symptoms during dialysis.[206,208]

Monitoring Access Flow

Vascular access failure is a major problem, costing millions of healthcare dollars each year and diminishing patients' quality of life, prompting the National Kidney Foundation to issue management guidelines.[209] Observational studies[210-213] suggest that an absolute vascular access blood flow of less than 600 mL/min and a 25% decrease in access flow is associated with vascular access failure within 3 to 12 months. Angioplasty prompted by a decrease in access flow is effective in prolonging fistula survival and preventing thrombosis, but prospective studies of surveillance and angioplasty in AV grafts have found mixed results.[214-217] However, because preemptive correction of a stenosis before the access clots is shorter and less expensive and decreases the risk for a missed dialysis treatment or a temporary dialysis catheter, access surveillance and intervention is still preferred in the absence of conclusive evidence for improved graft survival.[218,219]

FUTURE CONSIDERATIONS

Several decades of experience have demonstrated that thrice weekly hemodialysis is not completely successful in reversing the syndrome of uremia. Reasons for this are not entirely clear, but they almost certainly include the residual syndrome (see earlier discussion). Failure to eliminate the residual syndrome may be related to inadequate dialysis, failure of dialysis to reproduce one or more functions of the native kidney, or complications derived from the dialysis treatment itself.

The discovery of dialysis amyloidosis and the subsequent identification of β_2-microglobulin as the amyloid precursor represent major advances in the battle to sustain and maintain a reasonable quality of life over many years of hemodialysis. Because β_2-microglobulin is a relatively large molecule that is not removed by cellulose membranes, its discovery prompted an investigation into the more permeable high-flux dialysis membranes. Accumulated evidence indicates increasingly strongly support for the use of synthetic high-flux membranes to prevent clinical progression of dialysis amyloidosis.

The ever-changing landscape of the residual syndrome now encompasses adynamic bone disease and calciphylaxis, both uncovered during efforts to improve the understanding and treatment of hyperparathyroid bone disease. Other battlefronts in the effort to improve quality of life include studies of nutrition; the cause of the acute-phase response in dialysis patients; the complex interaction among the acute-phase response, nutrition, and atherosclerosis; and methods to prevent both protein and calorie malnutrition. Understanding the mechanisms responsible for accelerated atherosclerosis and myocardial dysfunction in dialysis patients may be a key to improving the high mortality from cardiovascular disease.

The HEMO Study suggests that increasing the urea clearance (Kt/V) to greater than 1.3 during thrice weekly dialysis and enhancing clearance of larger molecular molecules do not alleviate the residual syndrome. In contrast, accumulating data from daily home hemodialysis indicate that blood pressure and serum phosphorus are significantly improved, often while reducing medications. Cardiac hypertrophy, heart failure, sleep patterns, and other quality-of-life markers also present signs of improvement, further correcting the residual syndrome.[220-225] Because the goals for future deployment of hemodialysis include reducing the need for travel to and from the dialysis center and shortening the time required for preparation and administration of hemodialysis, home hemodialysis, especially at night or during sleep, has obvious advantages. Newer developments, including the wearable artificial kidney and the implanted bioartificial kidney, are eagerly awaited.

A full list of references is available at www.expertconsult.com.

23

Vascular Access

Monnie Wasse, MD, MPH, FASN, and Gerald A. Beathard, MD, PhD, FASN

OUTLINE

Vascular access is the *sine qua non* of hemodialysis; it is also the Achilles heel. The process of cleansing the blood of the toxic products of chronic renal failure requires, as its first step, access to the circulation. The importance of the vascular access in the long-term provision of hemodialysis has been apparent from the beginning of the dialysis era. In 1944 Willem Kolff reported, after his first patient had received 12 dialysis treatments over a 26-day period, that all of the veins were "ruined."[1] A surgical cutdown of the radial artery followed but caused severe bleeding during heparinization. Kolff concluded that "we believe to be able to keep patients suffering from uremia and anuria alive so long as blood vessels for puncture are available."[1] It is interesting that more than six decades later we are still in the same position.

Fortunately, today we have better alternatives to provide access to the circulation; yet, it is unfortunate that none of these are ideally suited for the purpose. The ideal vascular access should have the basic characteristics listed in Box 23.1.

Unfortunately, the ideal vascular access does not exist. There are several choices, which are classified as arteriovenous fistula (AVF), arteriovenous graft (AVG), or central vein catheter. Although each of these has its own set of problems, the characteristics of the AVF make it the preferred choice for most patients.

ARTERIOVENOUS FISTULA

There are a number of benefits associated with an AVF. This type of access is associated with the best primary patency rate, the best cumulative patency rate, and the lowest rate of thrombosis and requires the fewest interventions over the duration of its life cycle.[2] Cost of implantation and maintenance of an AVF is the lowest of the three types of access, and AVFs are associated with lower hospitalization rates than are seen in patients with AVGs (relative risk [RR] = 1.47) or catheters (RR = 2.3).[3] Because patients with an AVF have fewer access-related problems, especially infection,[4] they have a lower mortality and morbidity compared with patients with either an AVG or a central venous catheter.[3]

With the exception of transposed fistulas, an AVF can be created with very little patient morbidity associated with the procedure compared with the insertion of a synthetic AVG, and the surgical procedure is relatively simple and is generally quickly accomplished.

TYPES OF ARTERIOVENOUS FISTULAS

Classification of Fistulas

AVF nomenclature incorporates its anatomical location, inflow artery, and outflow vein,[5] such as radial-cephalic (the radial artery and the cephalic vein). Although there are standard AVF configurations, an AVF can be created anywhere there is a cannulatable vein (which may require transposition)

BOX 23.1 Characteristics of Ideal Dialysis Vascular Access

- Easy repetitive access to the circulation
- Ability to reliably provide blood flow > 500 mL/min
- Hemostasis at the end of dialysis accomplished easily and quickly
- Function for the life of the patient
- Freedom from complication
- Cosmetically acceptable

of sufficient diameter to be attached to an adequate inflow artery. AVF types can be classified into three different categories: simple direct, vein transposition, and vein translocation (Table 23.1).

Bioengineered veins have been developed and are currently in phase III clinical trials. The use of these vessels presents a model very similar to a transposition AVF.[6]

Fistula Types Based on Anatomy

Although a variety of different anatomical types of AVF can be surgically created, most AVF creations fall within three basic configurations (Fig. 23.1). There is a separate category of AVFs sometimes referred to as *middle-arm* or *bidirectional fistulas* that have been created when neither of the three basic configurations are possible. These are created using the proximal radial artery with either the median antebrachial vein or the median cubital vein.[7] The suitability of the median antebrachial vein may be contributed to in part by the fact that the venipuncturist does not commonly access it.

According to accepted guidelines,[8,9] the order of preference for the creation of permanent vascular access should start distally in the upper extremity and progress proximally to preserve venous anatomy. According to this approach, the radial-cephalic AVF would be considered primary and the brachial-cephalic and brachial-basilic would be considered secondary choices. Some have advocated that the middle-arm AVFs should be considered tertiary.[10] If it is not possible to create one of the basic configurations of AVF, then reasonable attempts at creating a transposed AVF should be made before consideration is given to the insertion of AVG; however, it is important to consider patient-specific factors (e.g., comorbid conditions, anticipated longevity) at the time a surgical plan is devised. In the event that an AVG is placed, it should ideally be done with the plan that it will be used for the dual purposes of providing dialysis access during its problem-free life and for the development of the upper arm veins for the later creation of a secondary AVF once its use becomes problematic.

TABLE 23.1 Categories of Arteriovenous Fistulas

Simple direct	Easiest of the AVFs to create. Vein and the artery are used in their normal positions. Distal end of the vein is freed and connected to the adjacent artery.
Vein transposition	Most difficult to create. Created using vein that is not easily assessable for dialysis use. Proximal end of the vein is left intact. Distal portion of the vein is transposed to an assessable position. Requires creation of a tunnel or pocket for the newly positioned vein.
Vein translocation	Vessel is removed from one anatomical location and moved to a new site. Requires the creation of both a venous and an arterial anastomosis. Requires the creation of a tunnel for its new location.

Life Cycle of the Arteriovenous Fistula

The life cycle of an AVF can be divided into five distinct clinical phases (Fig. 23.2). The first three phases can be characterized as developmental stages (Fig. 23.3) of the AVF, eventually leading to a clinically functional dialysis access. Although in most successful cases, an AVF progresses through these developmental stages over a period of 4 to 6 weeks, time is

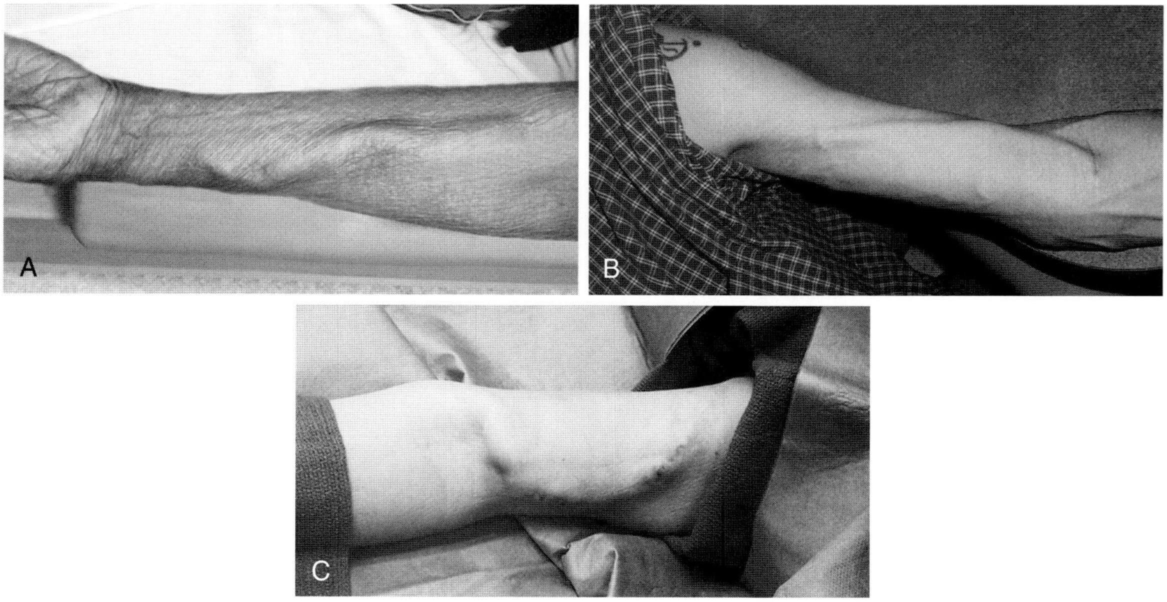

FIG. 23.1 Fistula types based on anatomy. (A) Radial-cephalic fistula (radial artery and the cephalic vein); (B) brachial-cephalic fistula (brachial artery and cephalic vein); (C) brachial-basilic fistula (brachial artery and basilic vein).

not considered an element of these definitions because it does not exert an influence on whether the defined outcome has been achieved.[11]

Phase 1: Creation

Phase 1 of the AVF's life cycle corresponds to the first developmental stage of the access—that is, creating an arteriovenous communication. If this is successful, as demonstrated by the presence of blood flow after creation, a patent AVF has been achieved.

Phase 2: Maturation

The maturation phase corresponds to the second developmental stage of the AVF and is characterized by evolution from AVF patency to a physiologically mature AVF, considered to have the potential for being used as a hemodialysis access. As stated earlier, AVF maturation is characterized by a continuous, progressive, and relatively rapid increase in blood flow and vessel diameter sufficient to permit reproducible clinical usability for hemodialysis. Studies have found that blood flow alone, or a combination of blood flow and vessel diameter, are reliable indirect indicators for predicting the successful use of an AVF for hemodialysis.[12-19] Using these metrics, the physiologically mature AVF is defined as having an internal diameter >0.5 cm (measured without a tourniquet)[12,18,19] and a blood flow >500 mL/min.[11] A blood flow of 400 to 500 mL/min (measured from the brachial artery) has been found to have an accuracy of 53% to 93%,[14-17] sensitivity of 67% to 96%,[14,16-19] and specificity of 65% to 90%[14,16,17,19] for predicting clinical AVF maturation. The combination of both AVF blood flow and internal vessel diameter of the vessel (500 mL/min, 0.5 cm) has been found to have a sensitivity of 84% and a specificity of 93%.[19] It has been reported that most AVFs that mature will do so in 4 to 8 weeks.[12-19]

Phase 3: Clinical Use, Initial

This third phase requires that successful clinical use of the AVF be demonstrated. This is the third and final stage of AVF development, referred to as a *clinically functional AVF*. This definition is necessary to separate from the second stage, AVF

Phase of Life Cycle	Creation	Maturation	Initial Clinical Use	Sustained Clinical Use	Dysfunction
Duration	Immediate	Weeks	Weeks	Unlimited	Immediate
Direction of Movement	→	→	→	←	→
Endpoint	Patent AV Access	Physiologically Mature AV Access	Clinically Functional AV Access	Uninterrupted Clinical Use	Restoration and Preservation of Clinical Use

FIG. 23.2 Five phases of life cycle of an arteriovenous fistula.

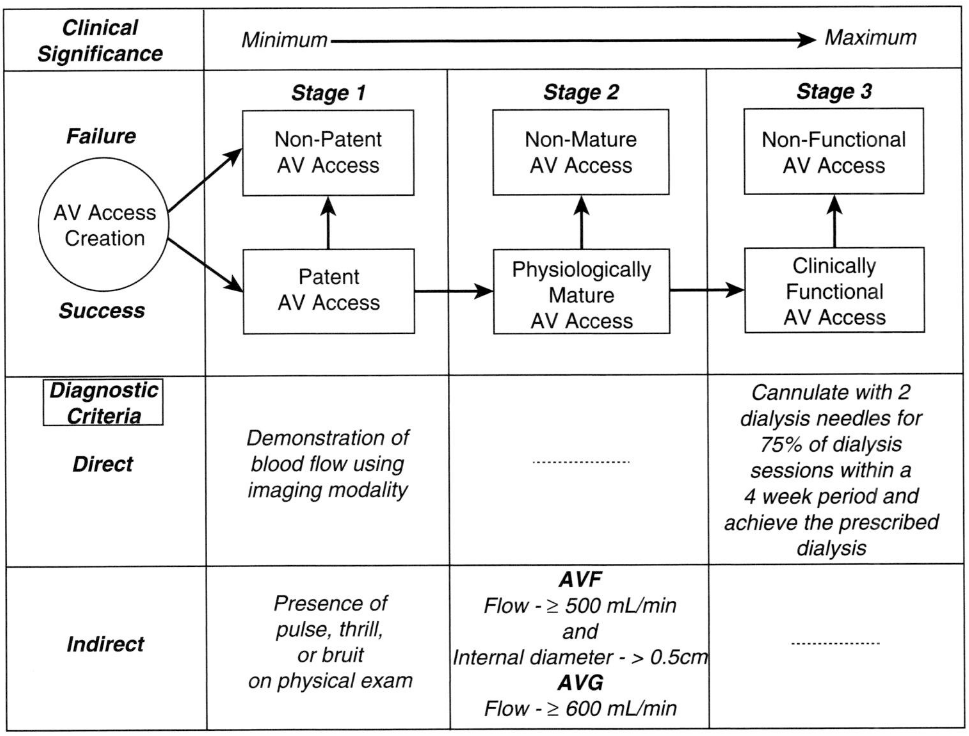

FIG. 23.3 Three stages of arteriovenous fistula development.

maturation, because clinical functionality is dependent on individual patient characteristics in addition to physiological changes that occur within the target vessel. It is possible for an AVF to be physiologically mature and have the capacity to provide adequate dialysis access but be unusable because of its location or depth. In addition, predialysis placement of the access will predictably result in a fully mature (physiologically) AVF not being used for a prolonged period and in some cases never being used.[20,21] In these cases, proof of functionality is never obtained, or at least is delayed, even though optimal physiological changes may have occurred.

A clinically functional AVF is defined as one that can be cannulated with two dialysis needles for at least 75% of dialysis sessions within a 4-week period and achieves the prescribed dialysis.[6] This definition, based on less than 100% success at cannulation, takes into account the fact that many patients with newly created AVFs have cannulation-related complications, although the access is destined to have long-term successful use.[22]

Phase 4: Clinical Use, Sustained

Once the clinical functionality of an AVF has been proven, it enters the fourth phase of its life cycle, characterized by continuous, effective, problem-free use for hemodialysis. This is the ultimate criterion for judging success. Unfortunately, most cases will alternate between this phase and phase 5, characterized as dysfunction. The duration of this phase is indeterminate and is limited by the occurrence of problems and complications.

Phase 5: Dysfunction

This phase is characterized by the occurrence of a problem that interferes with the routine use of the AV access, threatens patency or results in a loss of patency, presents a significant risk for medical complication, or adversely affects the patient's sense of well-being. Intervention is often required to resolve the problem. If this is successful, the AVF returns to phase 4.

COMPLICATIONS ASSOCIATED WITH ARTERIOVENOUS FISTULAS

Although the AVF is associated with fewer complications than are seen with other types of vascular access, they do occur and they should be dealt with effectively. The major complications that occur in conjunction with arteriovenous AVFs can be categorized under the headings of early failure, late failure, excessive flow, ischemia, aneurysm formation, and infection. Both early and late failures have multiple causes.

Failure to Mature

As stated earlier, an AVF is superior to an AVG; however, data on which AVFs' superiority has been established are based on AVFs that successfully mature and become clinically functional and generally exclude AVFs that failed to mature. Were data from all AVFs (nonmaturing and maturing) to be considered, more than a year would elapse before the superiority of the AVF became apparent.[23] This difference is due primarily to early failure. Failure to mature, also referred to as *early* or *primary failure*, is defined as an AVF that is never usable for dialysis or that fails within 3 months of use, and failure rates ranging from 20% to 60% have been reported.[14,24-27] According to US Renal Data System data, 36% of AVFs created in 2014 failed and the average time between AVF creation and first use was 133 days.[28] Although many AVFs can be salvaged,[29,30] those that are often require more than one procedure to become clinically usable[31] and have a shortened primary patency rate, making repetitive interventions necessary for continued clinical use.[32,33]

Reasons for the high incidence of early AVF failure are not totally clear. However, one must realize that the dialysis practice and population at risk for end-stage renal disease (ESRD) have changed over time. When the radial-cephalic AVF first was described in 1966 by Brescia et al.,[34] nearly all patients had chronic glomerulonephritis, the average patient age was 43 years, and blood flows used for dialysis were 250 to 300 mL/min. The early AVF failure rate was 11%. Today's dialysis patients are different—they are much older (many >70 years), and three-quarters of them have five or more comorbidities, with 90% having cardiovascular disease and 50% having diabetes.[35,36] In addition, the average blood pump speed is much higher: 350 to 450 mL/min. Therefore it is not surprising that achieving functional AVFs in today's ESRD population is often a challenge.

Additional risk factors for poorer AVF development include female sex, African American race, older age, greater body mass index (>35 kg/m^2),[37] and history of diabetes, peripheral vascular disease, or coronary artery disease.[26,27]

The three most commonly created AVFs, the radial-cephalic, the brachial-cephalic, and the brachial-basilic transposition, have differing rates of early failure. The early failure rate for the brachial-basilic transposed AVF is reported to be the lowest, followed by the brachial-cephalic and then the radial cephalic, which has the highest failure rate.[38-40] The early failure rate for brachial-basilic transposition AVFs it is reported to be between 0% to 21% in various series.[38-40] Compared with brachial-cephalic AVFs in the same series, brachial-basilic transpositions have an early failure rate of 0% versus 27%, 21% versus 32%, and 18% versus 38%.[39,41] Radial-cephalic AVF failure rates of more than 60% have been reported.[42]

Most investigators agree that nonmaturing AVFs have an associated anatomical problem.[30,43,44] With the exception of thrombosed AVFs, three important principles have been established related to early failure: (1) A distinct lesion or lesions can generally be identified as the underlying cause of failure; (2) the problem can generally be identified by physical examination and confirmed by imaging; and (3) the lesions can be corrected with a high expectation of success (except for certain preexisting lesions, which should have been avoided by quality vascular mapping).

Although several problems commonly exist when an AVF fails to mature,[30,43] the most common lesion observed in these cases is juxta-anastomotic stenosis.[45] This is defined

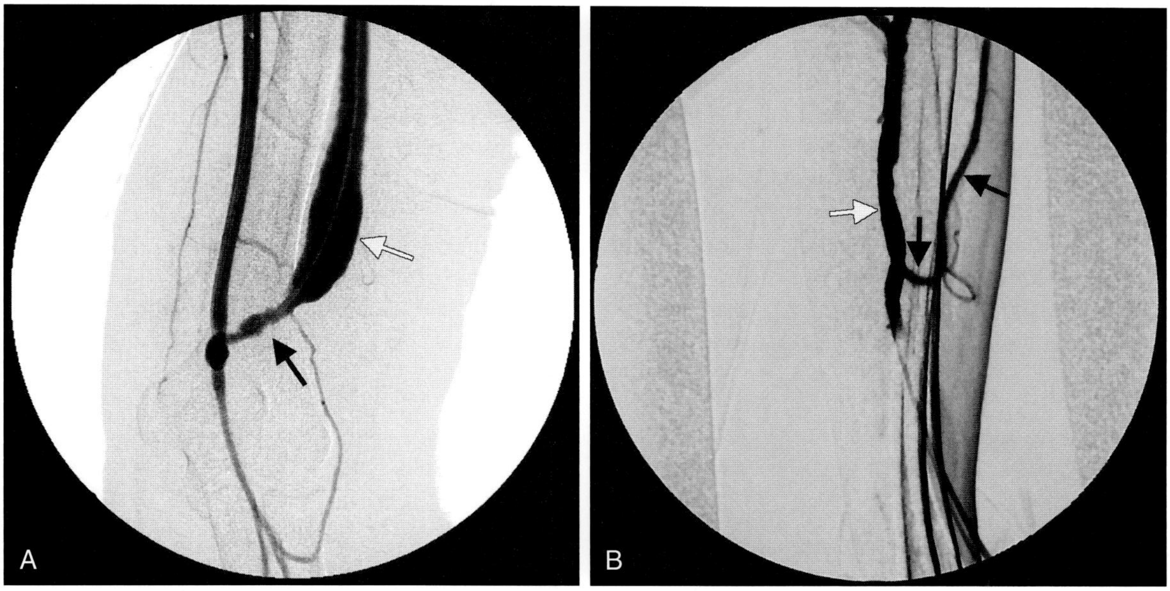

FIG. 23.4 Lesions associated with AVF nonmaturation. (A) Juxta-anastomotic stenosis in radial-cephalic fistula (*black arrow*, lesion; *white arrow*, fistula); (B) accessory vein (*black arrows*, accessory vein; *white arrow*, fistula).

as stenosis occurring within the first 3 to 4 cm of the AVF, immediately adjacent to the arterial anastomosis (Fig. 23.4A). The anastomosis may also be involved, resulting in luminal narrowing, decreased AVF blood flow leading to problems of maturation, and early thrombosis.

In some instances, the problem is poor preoperative vessel selection. The cause of failure to mature may be related to lesions that should have been recognized before the creation of the access. In reported cases, preexisting proximal venous stenosis has been documented as present in 4% to 59% of cases and central venous stenosis in 2.6% to 9% of cases.[30,31,43,46-49] Small arteries or arteries with stenotic lesions may be present and contribute to AVF nonmaturation with an incidence ranging between 4% to 6%.[46,48] When an AVF is created, the inflow artery generally dilates in parallel with dilatation and increasing blood flow in the AVF. If this fails to occur, the AVF will likely not mature.

Another type of preexisting problem that can affect AVF development and maturation is the presence of accessory veins.[30,31,43,47,50-52] These are side branches of the forearm veins used for the construction of an AVF (Fig. 23.4B). Most accessory veins are not problematic; however, because AVF maturation is dependent on blood flow, a large accessory vein that diverts a major portion of the flow away from the target vessel can result in failure of maturation.

Late Arteriovenous Fistula Failure

Late AVF failure is defined as failure that occurs after a period of normal use. The primary causes of late failure are venous stenosis and acquired arterial lesions (Fig. 23.5). These lesions are manifest as a pathophysiological change in the AVF resulting from increasing resistance, leading to a decline in blood flow, followed by inadequate dialysis and eventually thrombosis. The same types of lesions that are seen in association with early failure may be also seen here. Whether present initially and clinically unimportant or whether they developed (or progressed) over time during AVF use is not clear.[52]

The most common cause of late AVF failure is venous stenosis.[46,53] The site of the relevant lesion varies with the site of the AVF arteriovenous anastomosis. In distal radial-cephalic AVFs, virtually all stenoses are found in the inflow region (anastomotic and juxta-anastomotic), whereas outflow lesions are found almost exclusively in midforearm and elbow/upper arm AVF.[54-56] Venous stenosis associated with an AVF generally develops at areas of vein bifurcation, at swing points, and in association with venous valves.[45,52,57] The development of collateral veins is common, often extensive, and tends to preserve flow in the access (Fig. 23.6).

Stenosis of the inflow artery has been reported as a cause of late AVF failure in 6% to 18% of cases.[46,53] These lesions can also lead to decreased blood flow in the access, resulting in inadequate dialysis and eventually thrombosis. In general, 100% of all thrombosed AVFs have either venous or arterial-associated pathological anatomy.[46] Thrombosis is the endpoint of late AVF failure, and it occurs at a rate that is approximately one-sixth of that for an AVG.[58]

Excessive Flow

After the early, rapid increase in dialysis access blood flow (Qa) after AVF creation, there is a tendency for Qa to continue to slowly, yet progressively increase for the life of the access. Although this is generally tolerated and in some cases enhances the dialysis functionality of the AVF, it can also lead to problems, the most clinically relevant of which is high-output heart failure (HOHF). HOHF is a particularly serious problem considering the fact that cardiovascular disease is the leading cause of death in the ESRD population.[59] Currently, there is no generally accepted definition of excess

Qa. It has been suggested that the ratio of Qa to cardiac output (Qa/CO), referred to as *cardiopulmonary recirculation* (CPR), be used as a gauge. Normal values for this ratio are generally considered to be in the range of 20% to 25%. Patients with levels greater than this, or with Qa in excess of 2 L/min (Fig. 23.7), should be considered at higher risk for the development of HOHF.[60]

The risk for HOHF is directly proportional to the Qa and inversely proportional to the patient's preexisting cardiac status.[61] Many patients can tolerate a high Qa associated with an elevated CPR; however, even levels considered to be within the normal range can be excessive for the impaired heart because compromised cardiac function may limit the increase in CO that is required. For this reason, it has been suggested that the cardiac index may be a better gauge for the establishment of HOHF because it is more individualized. Moreover, it has been suggested that patients with symptoms of heart failure (dyspnea either at rest or with varying degrees of exertion; orthopnea; paroxysmal dyspnea; and edema, pulmonary and/or peripheral) that are resistant to medical management and occur in association with a cardiac index >4.0 L/min/m^2 should be considered as having HOHF.[62]

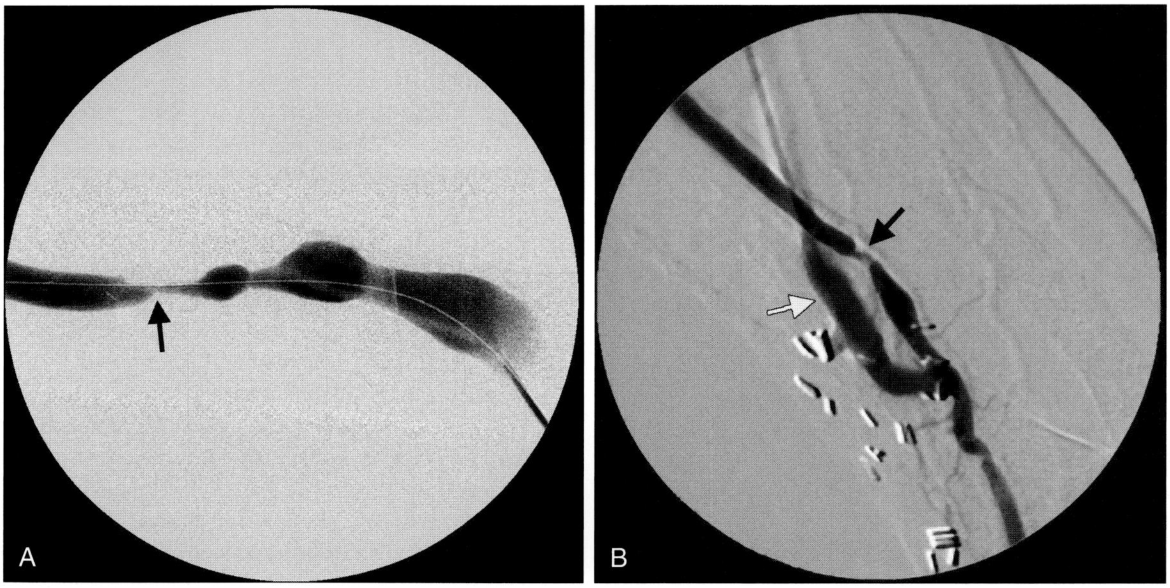

FIG. 23.5 Lesions associated with the late AVF failure. (A) Venous stenosis with pseudoaneurysms upstream from the lesion (*black arrow,* the lesion); (B) arterial stenosis (*black arrow,* lesion; *white arrow,* fistula).

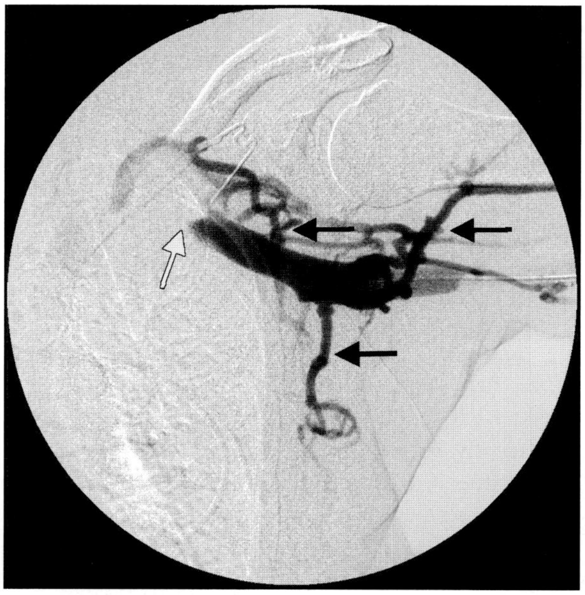

FIG. 23.6 Collateral veins upstream from the stenotic lesion (*black arrows,* collateral veins; *white arrow,* site of stenosis).

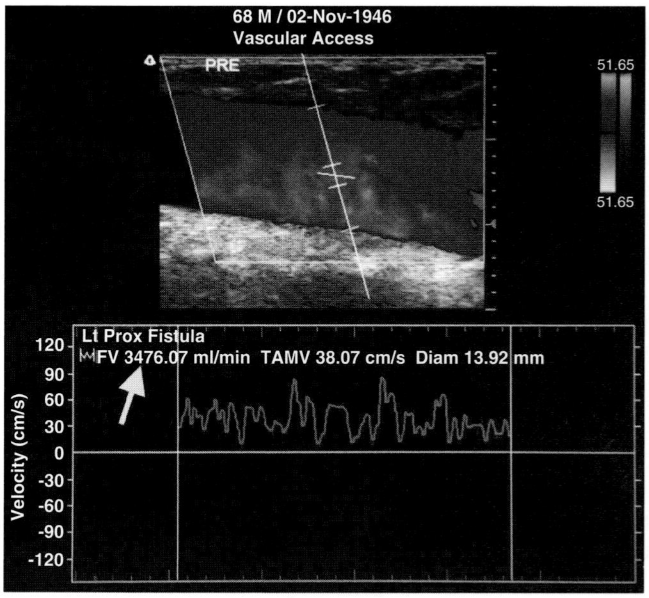

FIG. 23.7 AVF blood flow measured from the radial artery (flow value is indicated by *arrow*).

Hand Ischemia: Dialysis Access Steal Syndrome

When an arteriovenous access is placed in an extremity, a unique physiological state is established, because blood flow to the hand must now also supply the access. This hand/vascular access complex consists of a proximal artery feeding into two competing circuits connected in series—the arteriovenous access and the peripheral vascular bed on which perfusion of the hand is dependent. The former is a low-resistance pathway and is located proximally. The latter is downstream and is characterized by high resistance. Collateral arteries that bypass the access circuit to feed the periphery directly also contribute to this complex.

Most patients tolerate this abnormal physiological state because of compensatory mechanisms. However, in some instances, there is a failure of these mechanisms and hand ischemia, referred to as *dialysis access steal syndrome* (DASS), occurs. DASS can occur with either an AVG or an AVF; however, it is more common with the latter. Two distinct clinical variants of hand ischemia are recognized as associated with the placement of a dialysis access: ischemic monomelic neuropathy (IMN), where changes are confined to the nerves of the hand, and DASS, in which ischemic changes affect all tissues of the hand to a varying degree of severity.[63]

DASS is reported to occur in 1.6% to 8% of cases with an arteriovenous access.[64-69] Major predisposing risk factors include the use of the brachial artery as the inflow, diabetes, female sex, age >60 years, peripheral artery disease, and multiple previous access procedures.[68,70-72] Of these, the use of the brachial artery appears to create the greatest risk for this condition. In addition, DASS is reported to occur more readily in patients with AVFs with large anastomoses and Qa.[69]

BOX 23.2 Stages of Dialysis Access Steal Syndrome

Stage I: Pale/livid hand and/or cool hand without pain
Stage II: Pain during exercise and/or during dialysis
Stage III: Rest pain or loss of motor function
Stage IV: Tissue loss

Based on patient-specific clinical signs and symptoms, DASS is categorized into four stages reflecting increasing clinical severity (Box 23.2, Fig. 23.8). These four stages guide treatment choices for DASS. DASS varies in its time of onset and may be acute, subacute, or chronic.[73,74] Acute DASS is defined as the onset of signs and symptoms that appear immediately or within hours of the time of the surgical procedure. Acute DASS is most commonly associated with the placement of an AVG. DASS that occurs later, but within 1 month of access placement, is defined as subacute. Those cases occurring after this period are classified as chronic. These latter two groups are more commonly seen in association with AVFs and more specifically with brachial artery–based AVFs, although either an AVF or an AVG can be involved at any the three periods.

It is important to differentiate DASS from IMN. IMN is a distinct clinical entity associated with interference of a major limb artery resulting in multiple distal, axonal-loss mononeuropathies.[75] The attributable causal factor is believed to be occlusion of the brachial artery during the AV access surgical procedure. The syndrome develops quickly, typically within minutes to hours of AVF creation. The pathognomic feature is the presence of diffuse neurological dysfunction, usually in the absence of significant ischemic changes in the tissues of the hand and fingers, which differentiates it from DASS. Attributable neuropathic symptoms include pain, paresthesias, and numbness in the distribution of all three forearm nerves along with diffuse motor weakness or paralysis. Involvement of fewer than all three forearm nerves should bring the diagnosis into serious question.[76] Typically the hand is warm, capillary refill is preserved,

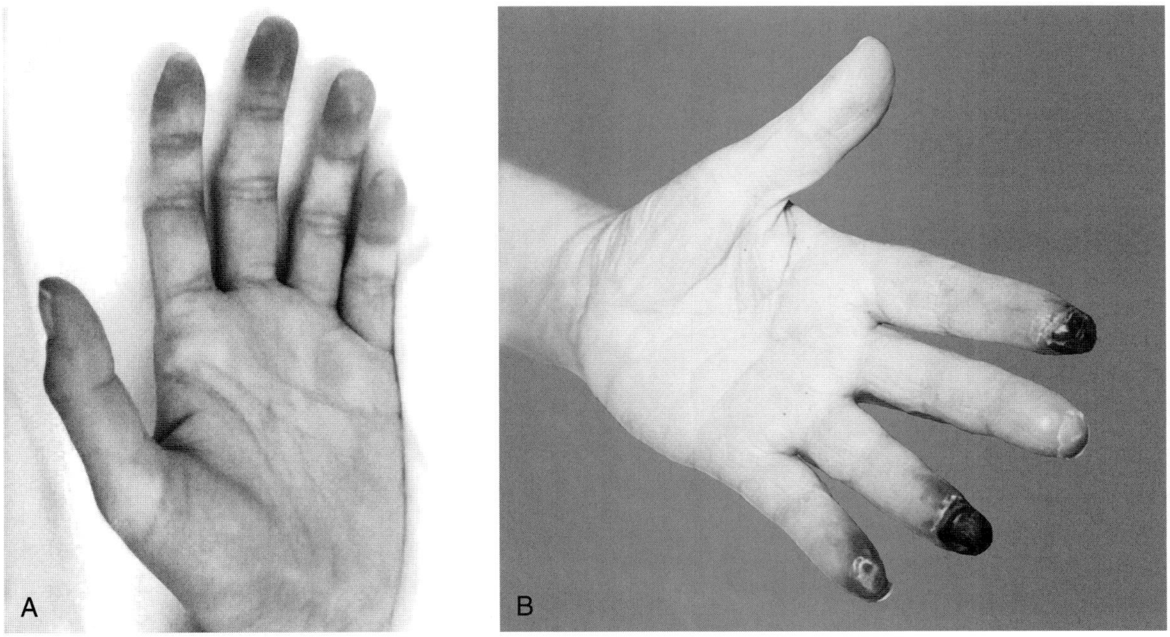

FIG. 23.8 Stages of DASS. (A) Early DASS with no tissue loss; (B) stage IV DASS with tissue loss at the fingertips.

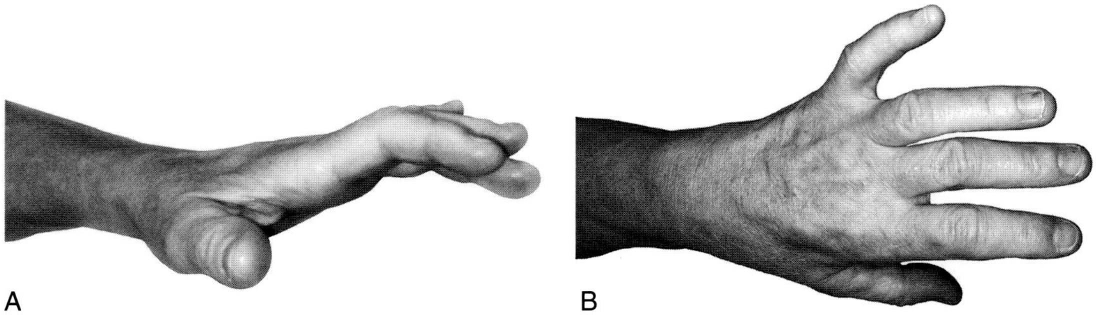

FIG. 23.9 Ischemic monomelic neuropathy with hand deformity and primary median nerve palsy; however, all three forearm nerves were involved. (A) Lateral view; (B) dorsal view.

and a palpable radial or ulnar pulse or audible Doppler signal is present.[76] The motor deficits resulting from the IMN nerve damage cause severe disability to the involved hand (Fig. 23.9).

The exact incidence of IMN is not known, because most of the literature is based on case reports, but it is not believed to be a common occurrence. IMN occurs exclusively in association with an arteriovenous access that is brachial artery based.[76] There are no reports of IMN precipitated by a distal forearm procedure. Although there are case reports to the contrary,[77] the condition occurs almost exclusively in diabetic hemodialysis patients.[78,79]

Aneurysm Formation

Most of the bulges that are noted in association with an AVF are true aneurysms; that is, they contain all layers of the vessel wall. Although there is no universally accepted definition for an aneurysmal AVF, it is commonly defined as an AVF that is three times the diameter of the adjacent normal vein or a minimum of 2 cm.[80] These pathological lesions represent degenerative changes in the vein wall and are relatively common.[81] The features that characterize an aneurysm typically result from the combination of repeated dialysis needle punctures and hemodynamic factors, such as downstream peripheral or central venous stenosis.[82,83] As an aneurysm develops and expands, it can lead to complications such as pain, objectionable cosmetic appearance, difficult cannulation, risk for bleeding, and problems with access blood flow.[82]

Aneurysms can be fusiform, ectatic, or spherical (Fig. 23.10). The fusiform type of aneurysm is commonly seen in association with segmental overuse—that is, repetitive cannulation in a localized area leading to weakening of the vessel wall. With increased pressure, progressive ballooning of the vessel wall develops, generally at the arterial and venous cannulation sites, and have a fusiform appearance. The ectatic type of aneurysm represents a relatively diffuse enlargement of the entire AVF related to downstream stenosis. If allowed to progress, it eventually achieves an appearance that has been referred to as a *megafistula*. The spherical aneurysm is related to a localized defect in the wall of the AVF. At times, this anomaly appears acutely in association with a problematic cannulation and may be a pseudoaneurysm, rather than a true aneurysm.

Infection

Infections in AVF are uncommon and are reported to occur in less than 0.4% of cases in the postoperative period and 0.2% per year thereafter.[84] This is considerably less than that of AVGs and catheters.[4,76] AVF-associated infection can take the form of cellulitis, an abscess, bacteremia, septic emboli, and sepsis.[71,85,86] AVF infections occurring during the immediate postoperative period are generally related to a problem with aseptic technique during surgery, whereas those occurring later are most often related to contamination during cannulation. Late AVF infection has been attributed to the buttonhole cannulation technique.[87]

Secondary Arteriovenous Fistulas

Secondary AVFs (SAVF) are important to the hemodialysis vascular access strategy of all nephrologists. A SAVF is defined as an AVF that is created after an AV access, usually an AVG, using the outflow veins of that access. In general, this is a forearm access and the AVF is created using an upper arm draining vein. Because of the forearm access, the veins of the upper arm undergo the same process of maturation as is seen with AVF development and for the same reasons.[88-92] In most cases this involves the creation of either a brachial-cephalic or a brachial-basilic AVF. Even when one of these veins is not suitable, there may be an adequate vein in the forearm that can be used as a bidirectional, middle-arm SAVF.[93]

When an AV graft is placed in a patient, it should be done with a dual purpose in mind—first, to provide an access for hemodialysis, and second, as a means of maturing veins in the upper arm for a SAVF. The National Vascular Access Improvement Initiative (Fistula First)[94] recommended that every patient receiving dialysis via an AVG be viewed as a potential candidate for a SAVF. To identify a suitable patient for an SAVF, visualizing the veins of the upper arm is necessary and is most easily accomplished by simply having patients roll up their sleeve (Fig. 23.11). With any type of procedure to treat AVG dysfunction, the angiographic studies that are performed can be used to identify optimal candidates for a SAVF if the operator is alert to the issue. In a study of the angiograms that were performed as part of either an angioplasty or a thrombectomy procedure, 75% of the patients with lower-arm grafts were found to have one or both upper-arm superficial veins that were optimal for SAVF conversion.[89]

The success with SAVF creation has been very good, particularly considering that many of these patients were not initially suitable for AVF creation, and they often have a history of prior procedures. The 1-year primary and cumulative

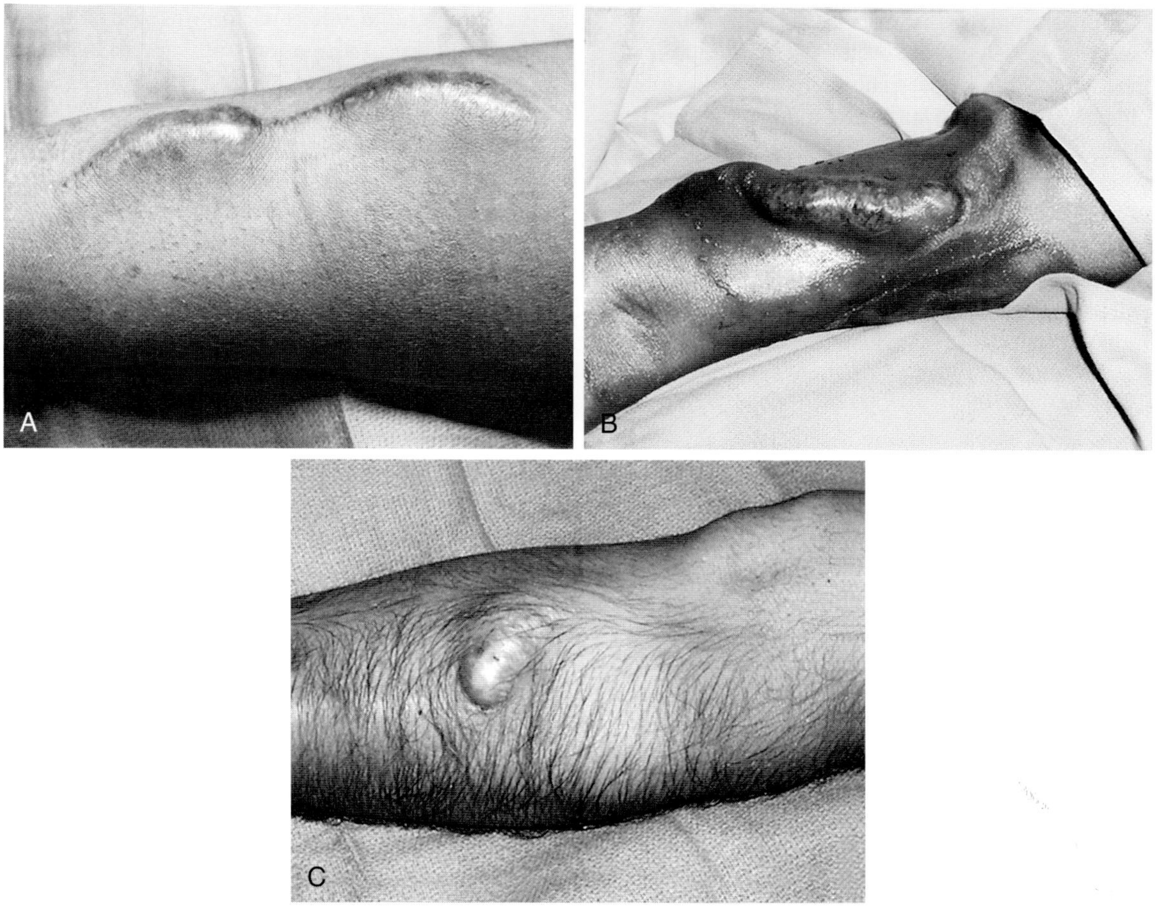

FIG. 23.10 AVF aneurysms. (A) Fusiform aneurysm. (B) Ectatic aneurysm. (C) Spherical aneurysm.

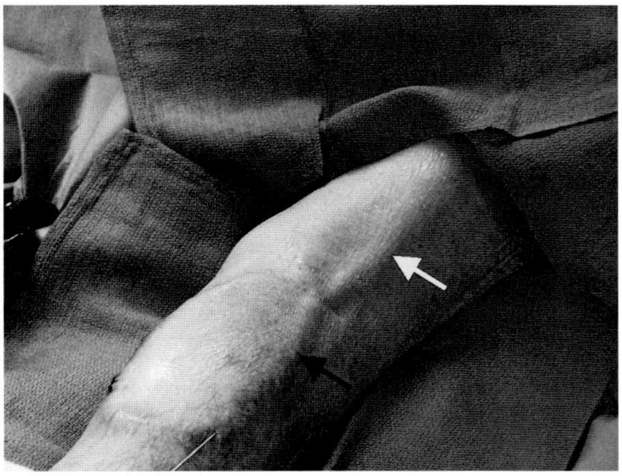

FIG. 23.11 Good candidate for secondary fistula (forearm loop AVG; *black arrow,* upper arm cephalic vein is an excellent candidate for secondary fistula [*white arrow*]).

patency rates for SAVFs have been reported in the range of 71% to 82.5% and 92.5% to 100%, respectively.[95,96]

ARTERIOVENOUS GRAFT

Although the AVF was introduced by Brescia and coworkers in 1966,[34] an AVF was not possible in many patients. After that innovation, vascular access evolved through the use of saphenous vein translocation,[97,98] bovine carotid artery graft,[99] and the Dacron velour vascular graft,[100] but still there were major short-term and chronic problems with these access types. In 1976 the problem of vascular access was solved, or so it was thought, through the use of expanded polytetrafluoroethylene (ePTFE).[101] The AVG was initially considered only as a substitute access in patients in whom an AVF was not possible; however, this philosophy soon became lost and it became the access of choice in the United States, a practice that led to major problems and one that has been very difficult to reverse.

In 1997, the first iteration of National Kidney Foundation Kidney Disease Outcomes Quality Initiative (NKF KDOQI) Clinical Practice Guidelines for Vascular Access was published and stressed the need to decrease the reliance on AVGs.[102] However, in 1998, 58% of patients on dialysis for 2 or more years were still using an AVG.[103] The National Vascular Access Improvement Initiative, which came to be referred to as Fistula First, was launched in January 2003.[94] This was a Medicare initiative designed to decrease AVG reliance and increase AVF use in the United States. Since that time there has been a slow but progressive decline in the prevalence of AVG use, declining to a level of 18.3% in 2014.[104]

It is important to note that there remains a population of patients for whom an AVG represents the best choice for a dialysis vascular access. In general, these patients fall into two categories: (1) patients with vascular anatomy that is not favorable for the creation of an AVF as determined by vascular mapping;

(2) patients with comorbidities that increase the risk for short life expectancy and the time required for an AVF maturation and for whom the high risk for primary failure makes AVF creation imprudent. Elderly patients also fall within this latter group. In a study using Medicare-derived data,[105] dialysis survival was tabulated and four age groups were evaluated: 65 to 79, 80 to 84, 85 to 89, and >90. At 6 months after dialysis initiation, the mortality was 20%, 30%, 40%, and 45%, respectively; in accordance with these results,[106] it was found that an AVF was not associated with better survival compared with an AVG used as the first predialysis access among patients older than 80 years.

Advantages of Arteriovenous Graft

Although considered more problematic than AVFs, AVGs have several advantages. They are comparatively easy to insert and repair, can be used at multiple anatomical sites, can be created in a variety of shapes and configurations, have a short maturation time, are technically easy to cannulate, and offer a large area for cannulation. Although there is a higher infection rate compared with an AVF, their primary disadvantage relates to the development of stenosis from neointimal hyperplasia, which tends to shorten their patency. Reported primary patency rates for AVGs range from 40% to 60% at 1 year,[107] yet with aggressive management of thrombosis, secondary patency rates as high as 90% at 1 year can be achieved.[108]

Types of Arteriovenous Grafts

Unfortunately, a large proportion of patients start dialysis with a central venous catheter, which creates an inordinate risk to the patient. Using the standard ePTFE graft shortens the time required to develop a clinically functional AVF; however, traditional dialysis programs wait 2 to 3 weeks before the use of a newly placed AVG, so a central venous catheter is still required for dialysis access. Data from the Dialysis Outcomes and Practice Patterns Study (DOPPS) was used to examine the average time of AVG cannulation.[109] Investigators found that the relative risk for graft failure (reference group = first cannulation at 2 to 3 weeks) was 0.84 with first cannulation at <2 weeks ($P = 0.11$), 0.94 with first cannulation at 3 to 4 weeks ($P = 0.48$), and 0.93 with first cannulation at >4 weeks ($P = 0.48$), suggesting that earlier cannulation was not associated with AVG failure. Moreover, multilayered early cannulation grafts have been developed that can be cannulated within 24 hours of placement and have no increase in complication rates compared with traditional ePTFE.[110]

An AVG can be placed in a number of different sites and configurations, as long as the cannulation segment is accessible and there is blood return to the right atrium. However, the most common AVG sites are the forearm, the upper arm, and the thigh. Although it is distinctly unusual to see anything other than a loop graft in the thigh, either straight, curved, or loop grafts may be placed in the upper extremity locations.

COMPLICATIONS OF ARTERIOVENOUS GRAFTS

Complications occur much more commonly with AVGs than with AVFs. The major complications are venous stenosis (including the venous anastomosis), arterial stenosis (including the arterial anastomosis) thrombosis, infection, pseudoaneurysm formation, and hand ischemia.[111]

Venous Stenosis

The most common complications associated with an AVG are venous stenosis, arterial stenosis, and thrombosis. In most cases the problems of stenosis and thrombosis share the relationship of disease and symptom. The histological characteristics of venous and arterial stenosis are well characterized as aggressive neointimal hyperplasia.[112] The net result of this process is a progressively expanding lesion that encroaches on the lumen of the vessel, causing a progressive increase in resistance and a decrease in flow, often resulting in eventual thrombosis.

Venous stenosis occurs most often at the venous anastomosis but may occur anywhere within the access conduit, composed of the arterial anastomosis, AVG, the venous anastomosis, and its peripheral and central draining veins. In a review of 2300 cases of venous stenosis,[113] the following distribution of lesions was found: venous anastomosis 60%, peripheral vein 37%, within the graft 38%, central veins 3.2%, and multiple locations 31% (Fig. 23.12).

Percutaneous angioplasty is the treatment of choice for venous stenosis. Among a pooled cohort of 2166 cases from 15 published studies, AVG-related peripheral vein stenosis treated with angioplasty was associated with a primary patency of 62% and a cumulative patency of 85% at 6 months.[114-117] In metaanalysis based on 34 relevant studies, the primary and cumulative patency rate for AVGs at 6 and 18 months was 58% and 33% and 76% and 55%, respectively.[118]

The dialysis vascular access should be thought of as a complete circuit starting and ending with the heart. The venous side represents only one-half of the circuit, whereas the other half is arterial. Arterial lesions adversely affect access inflow, and a hemodynamically significant lesion can develop anywhere in the arterial tree from the ascending aorta to the arterial anastomosis. Reports of inflow stenosis in dysfunctional AVGs range between 14% to 42%.[44,54] These lesions are generally treatable with angioplasty.[54]

Over time, progressive stenosis can result in thrombosis. The frequency of AVG thrombosis is approximately 1 to 1.5 per patient per year.[119] Approximately 85% to 90% of all cases of graft thrombosis are associated with an underlying anatomical lesion.[119]

Infection

Infection (Fig. 23.13) is a common cause of AVG loss[120,121] and a prominent cause of patient mortality.[122,123] In one report, infection was reported to occur at a frequency of 1.3 episodes per 100 dialysis months and was associated with bacteremia at a rate of 0.7 cases per 100 dialysis months.[124] In a prospective Canadian study in which surveillance for hemodialysis-related bloodstream infections was performed in 11 centers during a 6-month period, it was found that the relative risk for bloodstream infection with an AVG access was 2.5 per 1000 dialysis procedures. This was compared with a rate of 0.2 in patients receiving dialysis via an AVF.[125]

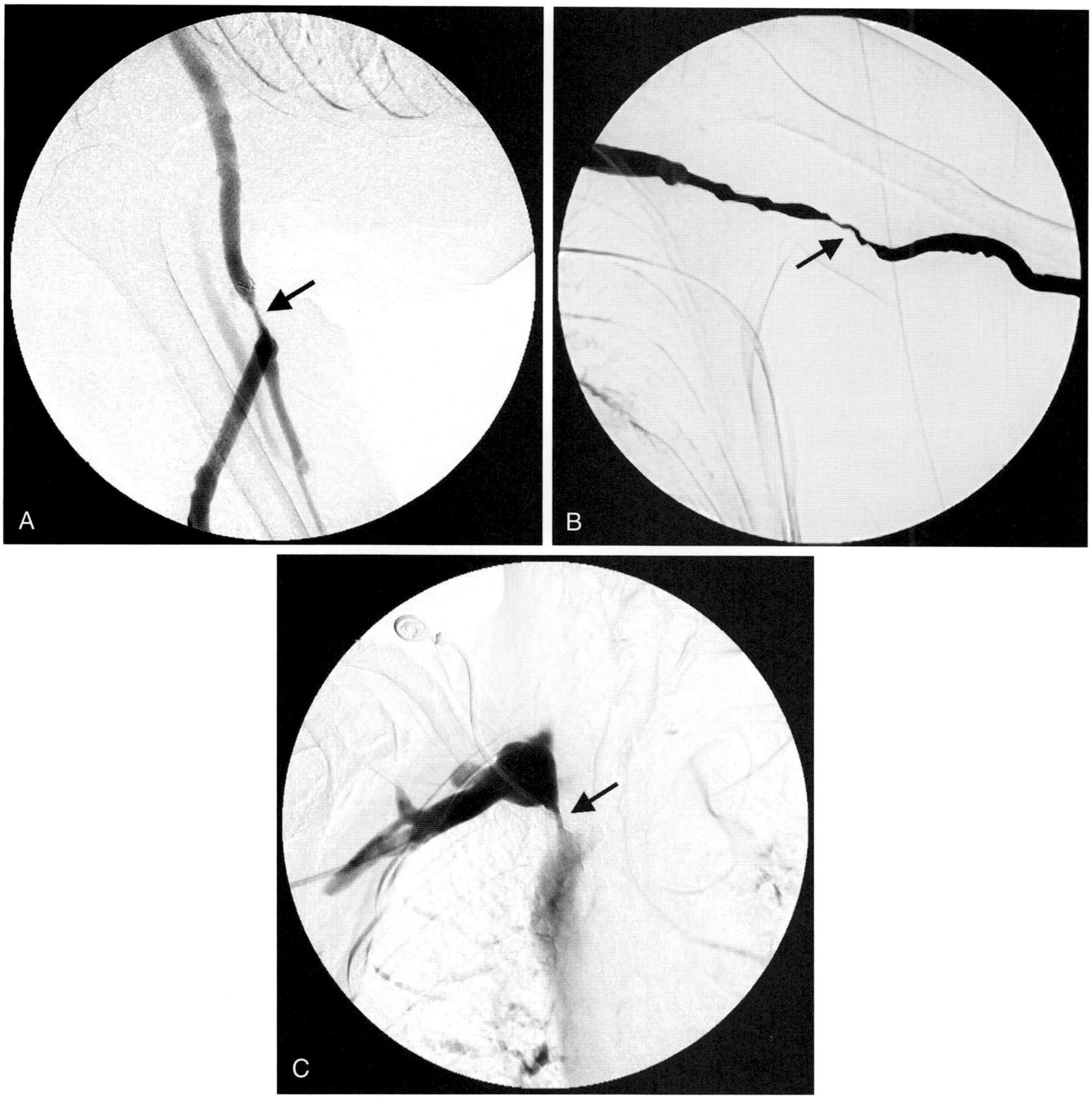

FIG. 23.12 Venous stenosis in AVG. (A) Venous anastomosis stenosis *(arrow)*; (B) draining vein stenosis *(arrow)*; (C) central vein (brachiocephalic vein) stenosis *(arrow)*.

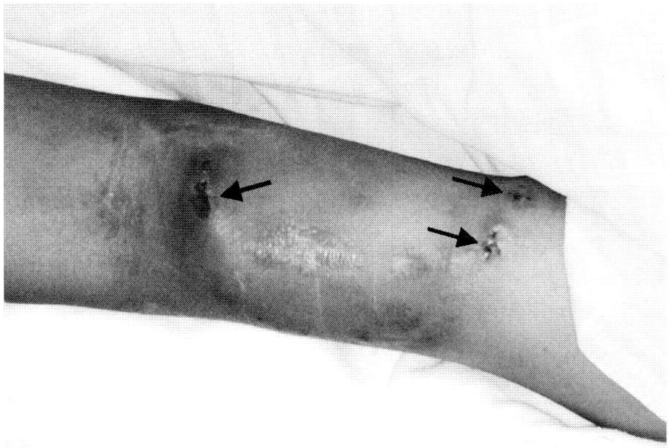

FIG. 23.13 AVG infection at multiple sites *(arrows)*.

The hospitalization rate for dialysis patients is double that of the general population, and infection is the attributable cause in 20% of cases.[56] The development of dialysis access sepsis is associated with a higher incidence of myocardial infarction, congestive heart failure, cerebral stroke, and peripheral artery ischemic disease in the subsequent years.[126] Not only does AVG infection result in significant morbidity, it results in AVG loss in a proportion of affected patients.[127]

A number of risk factors for AVG infection have been recognized, including cannulation technique, AVG location, and duration of use. Patient personal hygiene appears to be the most important risk factor for the development of access-related infection[128]; however, episodes of infection have been traced to individual dialysis facility staff and can be related to poor needle insertion technique.[129,130] This underscores the importance of staff training in infection control measures.

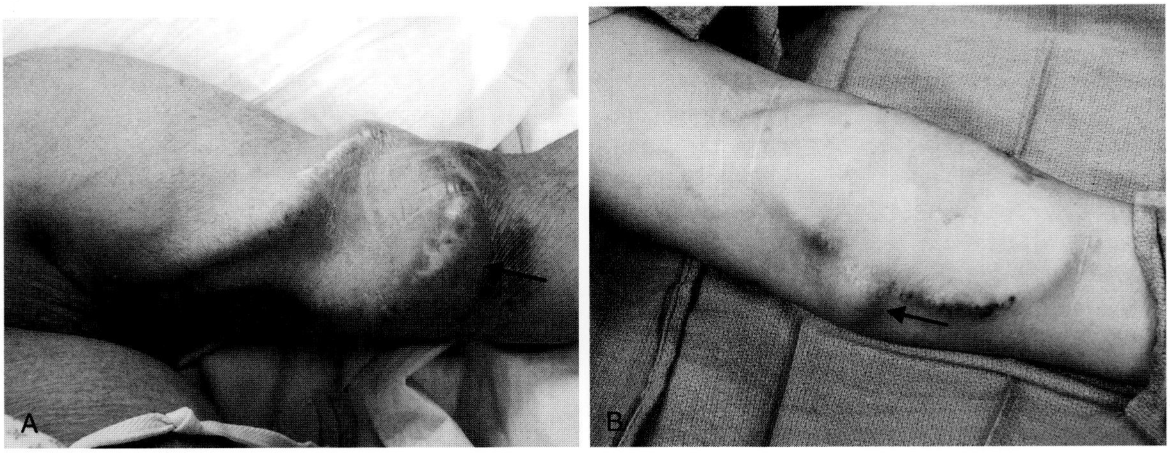

FIG. 23.14 AVG pseudoaneurysms. (A) Ectatic pseudoaneurysm *(arrow)*; (B) spherical pseudoaneurysm *(arrow)*.

Femoral AVGs are often placed when all upper limb access sites have been used. These AVGs are at higher risk for infection.[131] The incidence of graft infection increases with the duration of AVG use,[64,132,133] suggesting another reason to evaluate AVG patients for a SAVF.

AVG infections are generally attributable to common skin microorganisms represented by gram-positive bacteria. In most cases, the causative organism of the AVG infection is *Staphylococcus aureus* or other gram-positive pathogens, such as coagulase-negative staphylococci. *S. aureus* is identified in nearly 68% cases of AVG infection,[128] followed by *Staphylococcus epidermitis.*[134] Gram-negative bacteria are less commonly the cause of infection, and some episodes are polymicrobial.[135]

Pseudoaneurysm Formation

A pseudoaneurysm ("false aneurysm") is characterized by actual disruption of the layers of the AVG leading to a bulging anatomical defect (Fig. 23.14).

Pseudoaneurysm deformities are common and have been reported to have an incidence as high as 60%.[81] Two concurrent events are typically required for the appearance of the dilatation characterizing a pseudoaneurysm. First, the dialysis needle has a thin wall and is very sharp. When it punctures the wall of the AVG, it acts like a cookie cutter, either removing a small plug or creating a flap. Other types of needles, even those of large gauge, make a slit when they puncture the graft. Repetitive cannulation in a localized area eventually results in a defect. Second, increased pressure within the AVG develops as a result of downstream venous stenosis. With the increased pressure, bulging occurs and tends to be progressive. This occurs earlier and is more accentuated if puncture sites are not rotated.[136,137] However, even with site rotation, structural damage to the AVG over a prolonged period will result in a defect. With long-term AVG use, this defect can be quite extensive.

The seriousness of a pseudoaneurysm lies in its associated complications. In addition to the objectionable cosmetic appearance and difficulty with cannulation of the access, pseudoaneurysms can result in pain and an increased risk for thrombosis and infection. The most serious complication, however, is thinning of the skin overlying the defect in the graft. Histological study of the pseudoaneurysm has shown that it consists of only a perigraft fibrous tissue capsule directly overlying the area of the defect.[136] As the enlargement progresses, the skin over the AVG can become scarred, thinned, and avascular. In some cases, this can lead to ulceration and spontaneous bleeding, which can be life threatening.

Hand Ischemia: Dialysis Access Steal Syndrome

DASS is primarily a problem with AVFs; however, it can also occur with an AVG. DASS varies in its time of onset and may be acute, subacute, or chronic. As stated earlier, an AVG patient may develop hand ischemia at any of these times; however, they are primarily acute—that is, immediately after or within hours of the time of the surgical procedure.[73,74]

HEMODIALYSIS RELIABLE OUTFLOW VASCULAR ACCESS DEVICE

Over the years, the average life expectancy of a patient on hemodialysis has improved. Yet an unfortunate consequence of this increased longevity is the potential for recurrent vascular access problems and exhaustion of arteriovenous access options. In the past, there were only two available alternatives that would allow for continuing dialysis treatment in patients with no upper-extremity option—a central venous catheter or a lower-extremity arteriovenous access. Unfortunately, both expose the patient to an increased risk for infection. The development of a hybrid device, the Hemodialysis Reliable Outflow (HeRO) has provided a third alternative in these cases, as long as central venous patency is established for the insertion of a central venous catheter.

The HeRO is a long-term, fully subcutaneous dialysis access that, instead of a venous anastomosis, uses an outflow catheter that is placed percutaneously into the right atrium through the subclavian or internal jugular vein and into the superior vena cava. This outflow component bypasses central vein stenosis by positioning the tip of the outflow component beyond it, in the right atrium.[138] This device, classified as an AVG, consists of two parts—the arterial limb and the venous limb. The arterial limb consists of a 6-mm (internal diameter) AVG that is attached to a peripheral artery at one end and a titanium connector at the other end (Fig. 23.15). This arterial anastomosis and its orientation within the patient's upper arm is like that of a traditional AVG. The titanium connector attaches to the venous limb, a 19F silicone catheter that is reinforced with a nitinol braid that prevents kinking. As with the traditional ePTFE grafts, the HeRO is cannulated by inserting dialysis needles once the graft is tissue incorporated.[139] Relative contraindications to implantation of the HeRO device include a cardiac ejection fraction <20%, systolic blood pressure <100 mmHg, and the presence of infection.[138]

In a systematic review of the literature,[140] the 1-year primary and cumulative pooled patency rates for 409 patients were found to be 21.9% (9.6% to 37.2%) and 59.4% (39.4% to 78%). The range of HeRO-related bacteremia was 0.13 to 0.7 events per 1000 days, and the rate of DASS was 6.3% (1.0 to 14.7%).

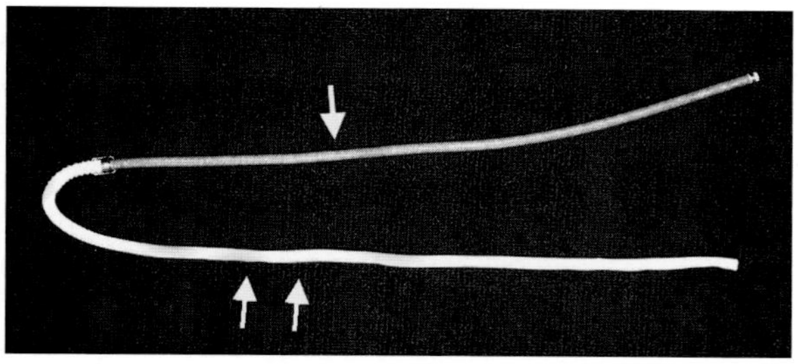

FIG. 23.15 HeRO graft. AVG segment *(double arrow)* connected by titanium connector to outflow catheter *(single arrow)*.

Compared with an AVF or AVG, the HeRO graft patency rate is not as good; however, the patient using this device has already had multiple arteriovenous accesses fail. Moreover, the rate of infection is comparable to that of an AVG. When comparing rates of patency and infection of the upper-extremity HeRO with lower-extremity AVG, results vary most likely because of cohort differences. However, one study concluded that lower-extremity AVGs are preferable because they have better patency rates compared with the HeRO device in the upper extremity.[141] Conversely, compared with a catheter, the infection rate associated with the HeRO was much lower[140] and a cost analysis revealed it to be considerably more economical.[142,143]

The average number of interventions required to maintain HeRO patency ranges from 1.5 to 3 procedures per year. The great majority of these are for the treatment of stenosis commonly associated with thrombosis. In general, the outcomes of these procedures are the same as the treatment of an AVG.[144]

DIALYSIS CATHETERS

The development of a dual-lumen catheter for removing and returning blood has played and continues to play an important role in hemodialysis.[145] Unfortunately, its vantages have been mirrored by serious disadvantages. Catheter use is associated with significant morbidity and mortality risk to the hemodialysis patient, in large part because of their abuse. According to the US Renal Data System, 18.9% of all new hemodialysis patients started dialysis with a catheter in 1996.[146] In 2014 that number was in excess of 80%.[147] Even in patients who had seen a nephrologist before the initiation of dialysis, the majority initiated dialysis with a catheter.

There are two types of dialysis catheter—the acute dialysis catheter (ADC) and the tunneled dialysis catheter (TDC). As the name suggests, the TDC is placed into a central vein through a subcutaneous tunnel (Fig. 23.16). The TDC plays

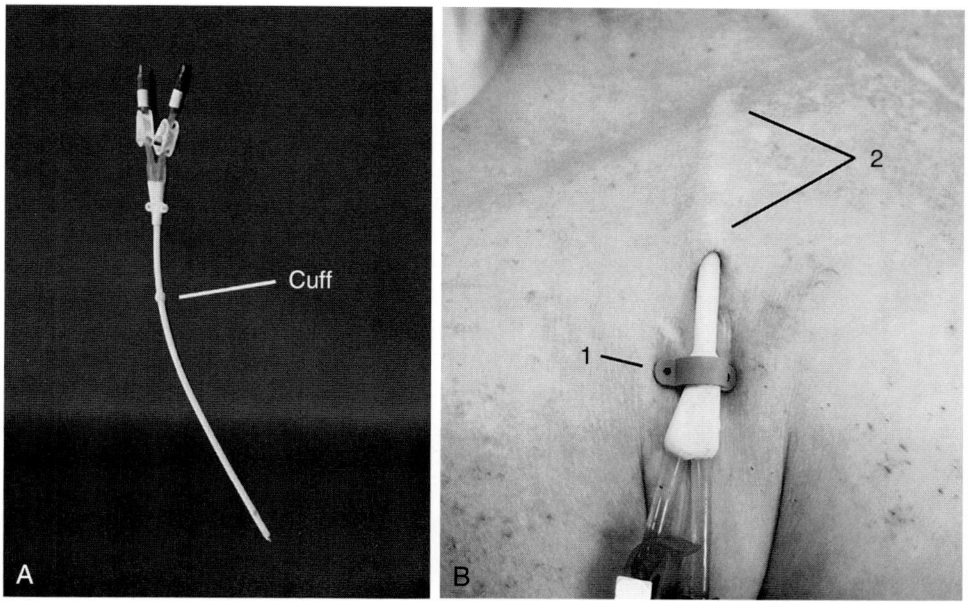

FIG. 23.16 Tunneled dialysis catheter. (A) Appearance of catheter; (B) catheter in place (*1*, wings of catheter to be secured with suture; *2*, catheter in subcutaneous tunnel).

BOX 23.3 Advantages and Disadvantages of Tunneled Dialysis Catheter

Advantages
Universally applicable
Ability to insert into multiple sites
Maturation time not required
Venipuncture not required for dialysis
No hemodynamic consequences
No cardiopulmonary recirculation
Ease and low cost of placement and replacement
Ability to provide access over a period of months
Ease of correcting thrombotic complications

Disadvantages
High morbidity as a result of:
- Thrombosis
- Infection
- Inflammation

Risk of permanent central venous stenosis or occlusion
Discomfort and cosmetic disadvantage of external appliance
Shorter expected life span than other access types

an important role in the management of the hemodialysis patient, being used for a variety of purposes. Although the AVF is the best solution for hemodialysis access, for some patients with comorbidities, a fistula is impractical because of the short life expectancy of the patient. In addition, they are used for emergent dialysis, for short-term treatment, and as a bridge backup for a dysfunctional arteriovenous access.

TDCs have many advantages as a hemodialysis access. Unfortunately, they also have many disadvantages (Box 23.3). Although their advantages are important, they are outweighed by their disadvantages, especially those that create a risk for morbidity and mortality from catheter-associated infection and central venous stenosis and occlusion.

The cardiac effects of an arteriovenous access are not found with a TDC. This makes it the preferred vascular access for the ESRD patient with severe cardiac insufficiency. In addition, CPR observed with an arteriovenous access does not occur with the TDC, resulting in an improved dialysis efficiency.[148]

Catheter Design

In the 1980s the TDC concept was introduced via two different types of catheters: the Quinton PermCath (Quinton Instrument Co., Seattle, Washington) and the Canaud catheter, produced in France. The Quinton PermCath was a single oval-shaped catheter with two circular lumens constructed of silicone rubber. It came in 28-, 33-, 36-, and 40-cm lengths and had a Dacron cuff to anchor the catheter in the subcutaneous tissue. The external end was split into a Y configuration that had external connectors with Luer locks and permanently attached clamps. The catheter-tipped lumen for blood outflow (referred to as the *arterial lumen*) terminated 2.5 cm proximal to the inflow lumen (referred to as the *venous lumen*). It was thought that the Dacron cuff would limit the incidence of infection by presenting a barrier to bacterial migration from the exit site down the catheter tunnel once it was incorporated.

Initially, these TDCs were placed (and removed) surgically in the operating room. Today placement using a peel-away sheath or simply over a guidewire is routine.

Most TDCs are produced with side holes at the tip. The original intent of these holes was to preserve catheter flow if the arterial lumen became occluded by being pressed against the vessel wall; however, this design has the disadvantage of allowing the anticoagulant lock to leak from the tip of the catheter.

Since the TDC was first introduced, there have been numerous modifications, especially to the catheter tip design,[149] that are intended to reduce potential problems that can occur with use of the TDC. There have been tip designs to improve catheter blood flow, minimize recirculation, and inhibit the formation of a fibrin sheath that affects all central venous catheters and is the major cause of dysfunction. The catheters that we have today are generally classified as twin catheters, step-tipped, split-tipped, symmetrical-tipped, and self-centering catheters (Fig. 23.17).

Catheter-Associated Problems

Problems associated with the use of a TDC can be grouped under four headings: (1) adequacy of dialysis, (2) problems associated with placement, (3) catheter dysfunction, and (4) catheter-related infection.

Adequacy of Dialysis

A number of factors influence the adequacy of dialysis; however, the vascular access contribution is generally related to inadequate blood flow. NKF KDOQI defines sufficient blood flow through a catheter as 300 mL/min[32]; however, this should be regarded as the minimum criterion, not the ideal level.[150] Optimally, if a tunneled catheter is to be used for hemodialysis therapy of more than 2 to 3 weeks, it should be capable of delivering no less than the prescribed pump speed blood flow, generally 400 mL/min or greater.

The primary determinant of catheter blood flow is its dimensions. As with the flow of any fluid through any tubular structure, blood flow in a catheter follows Poiseuille's law. Interpolation of this law to apply to a dialysis catheter results in a more practical formula, which states that flow = pressure/resistance.[148] Pressure is applied by the blood pump and resistance is determined by catheter dimensions, the major determinant for resistance being diameter. Resistance decreases in proportion to an increase in radius raised to the fourth power (r^4). This relationship dictates that relatively small increases in catheter diameter will result in major changes in resistance and the potential for flow. Going from a 10F catheter to a 12F (3F = 1 mm), a change of only 26% in diameter, will result in a 60% drop in resistance. Conversely, there is only a direct relationship between resistance and catheter length, making it less important as a determinant to blood flow than the catheter radius. In fact, increasing the catheter radius by only 19% can compensate for a doubling of length.[148]

The higher the resistance, the greater the pressure required to achieve a desired level of blood flow. When a graph is created by plotting pressure against flow in a group of patients, as shown in Fig. 23.18, the slope of the line represents hydraulic

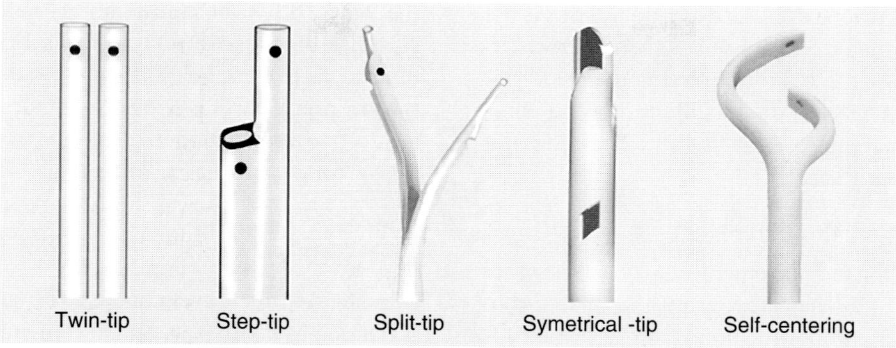

FIG. 23.17 Variations in tunneled dialysis catheter tips.

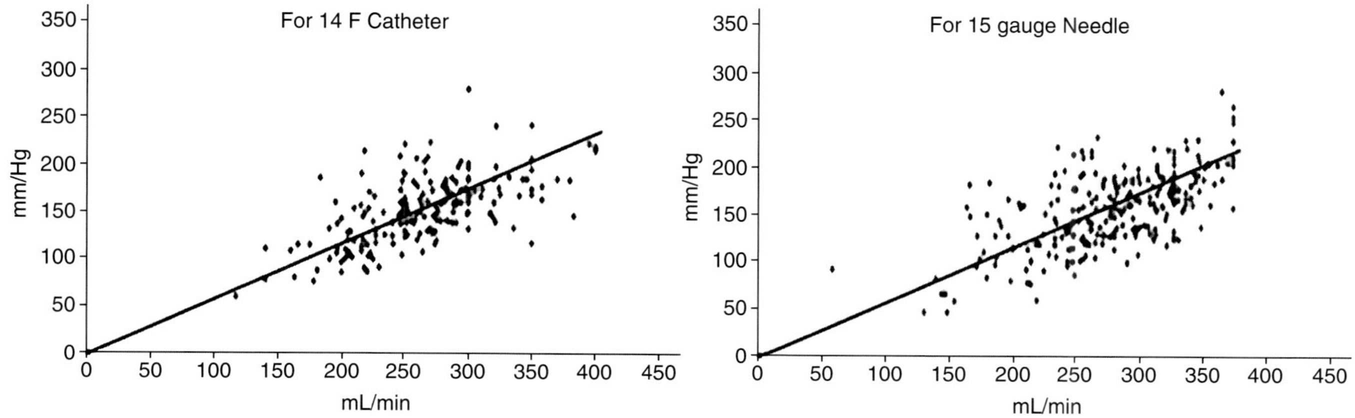

FIG. 23.18 Hydraulic resistance of 14F tunneled dialysis catheter versus 15-gauge dialysis needle. The slope of the line represents hydraulic resistance.

resistance. For a dialysis catheter, hydraulic resistance is a measure of the ease (or difficulty) of passing blood through the catheter or needle. The venous pressure recorded by the dialysis machine is essentially the pressure drop of the catheter lumen and is a reflection of hydraulic resistance—that is, the pressure required to achieve the indicated blood flow. The same is true for the arterial pressure, except that the numbers will be negative. It has been reported that a TDC has approximately the same hydraulic resistance as a standard 15-gauge dialysis needle at comparable flow rates.[151] Comparison of comparably sized split catheters, step-tipped catheters, and twin catheters have found no significant difference in hydraulic resistance.[152]

The roller pump flow meter on the dialysis machine blood pump is not truly volumetric; it is a revolutions-per-minute (rpm) meter. The displayed volume flow is an interpolated value that is based on the assumption that each revolution of the roller pump delivers a constant, known volume of blood (i.e., the volume of the pump segment of the blood tubing). However, if the pump segment volume varies, then actual blood flow will also vary to a proportional degree. This variance often happens and it does so under two circumstances. First, the pump relies on the elasticity of the pump segment to expand and refill as the rollers turn. However, because of elastic hysteresis (failure to return to original size on the rebound), there is some flattening of the pump segment during dialysis as the tubing warms. This results in a slight decrease in blood flow late in the dialysis treatment.[153] Second, the pump segment can be partially collapsed if the prepump pressure is excessive. Because there is a potential for prepump pressure to become more negative with increasing flow demands, problems can occur at high blood flow rate settings, because refilling of the pump segment of the dialysis tubing is less complete as prepump pressure becomes more negative. As the blood pump rpm meter progressively increases, its reflection of true volumetric flow becomes progressively more inaccurate.[154] To prevent errors caused by excessive negative pressure, it is recommended that the prepump pressure be monitored and that alarms be set to detect when it drops to less than −240 to −260 mmHg.[148]

Another issue related to TDCs and dialysis adequacy is that of recirculation. Recirculation occurs when blood returning from the dialyzer returns to the dialyzer rather than mixing with the systemic blood, resulting in a decrease in the efficiency of the dialysis treatment. This is of greater concern with a catheter than with an arteriovenous access. A common strategy for dealing with catheter dysfunction is to reverse the dialysis bloodlines and withdraw blood from the distal venous port and return blood from the proximal arterial port, yet this can increase recirculation. None of the commonly used TDCs have significant recirculation when connected correctly, but recirculation increases as much as

30% when the lines are reversed.[155] An exception to this is the symmetrical-tipped catheter, which has less than 1% recirculation regardless of how the bloodlines are connected.[103] It has been found that increasing dialysis blood flow to compensate for problems and improve dialysis efficiency does not increase recirculation significantly.[104]

Problems Related to Catheter Placement

When choosing a site for the placement of a TDC, there are two issues to consider: (1) The catheter must be placed into a location capable of providing the blood flow necessary for hemodialysis, and (2) care must be taken to minimize the chances of inducing central vein stenosis.

To achieve the blood flow levels demanded by the dialysis prescription, the tip of the TDC must be placed in a location that is capable of delivering a large volume of blood. This requires that it be placed in the vena cava or atrium. If the catheter is in the brachiocephalic vein, blood flow levels are often inadequate.

The primary contributor of central venous occlusive disease (CVO) in the dialysis patient is the central venous catheter. Preservation of the central veins is critical to vascular access selection and outcomes; therefore CVO is a very serious problem. Vein selection for catheter insertion plays an important role in central vein preservation. CVO results from chronic mechanical irritation to the endothelium of the vessel.[156] Although this injury occurs regardless of the target vessel, the degree to which it occurs appears to be related to the anatomy of the vessel—that is, whether the catheter has a straight path to the vena cava and atrium or whether there are curves. When the catheter is in place, there is constant motion because of the movement of the mediastinal structures created by respiration and the beating of the heart. Mechanical irritation is augmented if the catheter follows a curved pathway to its target location. A catheter placed in the right internal jugular vein with its straight descending course to the atrium permits the least amount of contact between the catheter and the vessel wall and therefore the least amount of irritation. Although the incidence of central venous stenosis is in the range of 10%[145,157-160] when the right internal jugular is used, it is by far the best choice for TDC placement. The number of patients with limited venous access options has increased as the dialysis population has grown and patients on dialysis experience greater longevity, creating a need for alternate sites for TDC placement.

Although the incidence of CVO is significantly higher with the left compared with the right internal jugular vein,[145,157-159] it represents the second choice for TDC placement if the right internal jugular is not available. The incidence of CVO resulting from TDC placement in the subclavian vein is reported to be in the range of 30% to 50%.[160-162] Because of this, it has been suggested that this vein never be used for TDC placement unless it is known with certainty that the patient will never need a peripheral arteriovenous dialysis access.[37,163] With loss of the internal jugular veins, other central veins are often enlarged, such as the external and anterior jugular veins, and have been used successfully for the placement of the TDC.[164-167] The transfemoral route to the inferior vena cava has been used[163,168]; however, this site should be used only in cases in which the status of the central veins of the thorax precludes TDC placement or the patient has been reduced to a single upper-extremity vein that needs to be preserved for a future arteriovenous access.

Catheter Dysfunction

The most common complication associated with a TDC is catheter dysfunction secondary to poor blood flow.[169] This is defined as failure to attain and maintain an extracorporeal blood flow sufficient to perform hemodialysis without significantly lengthening the hemodialysis treatment. In general, this is considered to be a blood flow less than 300 mL/min (at a negative pressure ≤–250).[170]

Catheter dysfunction may be classified as early or late.[171] Early catheter failure is defined as that which occurs immediately after placement, whereas late dysfunction is defined as a catheter that initially functioned in an optimal fashion but then became dysfunctional. In general, the problems that result in early dysfunction are related to catheter position or technical problems with placement. Under the heading of improper positioning are catheter tip malorientation, tip malposition, and placement into the wrong vessel. Technical problems that can result in early failure include a kinked catheter and sutures that are constrictive. All these problems should be recognized and corrected at the time of catheter placement.

Late catheter dysfunction is generally the result of either partial or total thrombosis and is classified as either extrinsic or intrinsic.[171] An extrinsic thrombus is one that forms outside of the catheter and is not attached to it. Examples of extrinsic thrombosis include (1) thrombosis of the vessel in which the catheter has been placed; (2) mural thrombus, in which thrombus forms and is attached to the wall of the vein or the atrium at the point of contact with the catheter; and (3) catheter-related atrial thrombus, in which the thrombus presents as a mass within the right atrium and is attached to the catheter. An intrinsic thrombus is one that either forms within the catheter or surrounds it as a sleeve or sheath. Although thrombus may form within the lumen of the catheter, often attached to side holes, the most common cause of delayed catheter dysfunction is a fibrin sheath.

Fibrin sheath formation has been identified in up to 76% of dialysis catheters by pull-back venography.[172-174] Sheathing of the catheter starts as early as 24 hours after catheter insertion and eventually extends to the catheter tip.[175,176] Animal studies have found that the structural components of the fibrin sheath evolve over time as the fibrin sheath becomes organized and is eventually converted into fibroepithelial tissue.[176,177] When the sheath covers the arterial port of the catheter, it acts as a flap valve, often resulting in an inability to aspirate blood from the port, resulting in limited blood flow and abnormal arterial pressures. The reported incidence of catheter dysfunction secondary to this problem ranges between 13% to 57%.[178] In addition to catheter dysfunction, the fibrin sheath has been reported to be associated with additional thrombus formation and subsequent infection.[179,180]

Catheter-Related Infection

Infection associated with TDCs can be classified into three categories: exit site infection, tunnel infection, and catheter-related bloodstream infection (CRBSI). An exit site infection is defined as culture-positive inflammation external to the cuff, localized to the exit site, and not extending above the cuff.[181] A tunnel infection is defined as culture-positive inflammation within the catheter tunnel internal to the Dacron cuff with a negative blood culture.[181] Isolated tunnel infections (negative blood culture) are not a common occurrence but when present are generally associated with CRBSI and should be treated in accordance with the more serious CRBSI classification.

CRBSI is defined as bacteremia in a patient with a catheter and no other explanation for the positive blood culture. Much of the morbidity and mortality related to these infections is due to metastatic infection, which has been reported to range in frequency from 3.2% to 50%, depending somewhat on the type of organism involved,[182-185] with the risk increased in the setting of *S. aureus* infection.[184] Metastatic complications such as septic arthritis, osteomyelitis, endocarditis, and epidural abscess can occur, and although the incidence of these complications is relatively low,[186] they have significant gravity because of their dire consequences.

CRBSI is a biofilm infection. This means that more than 99.9% of bacteria grow as aggregated "sessile" communities attached to the surface of the catheter, rather than as "planktonic" or free-floating cells in the circulation.[187] The biofilm develops when the attached cells excrete polymers that facilitate adhesion, matrix formation, and alteration of the organism's phenotype with respect to growth rate and gene transcription.[94,188] The hallmark of biofilm-related infections is marked resistance to antimicrobials and to host defenses, necessitating infected TDC removal or catheter exchange for optimal eradication of the infection.

ACUTE DIALYSIS CATHETERS

An ADC, also referred to as a *noncuffed dialysis catheter* (Fig. 23.19), is defined as a catheter designed for short-term use as a vascular access in the dialysis patient. Its use should be restricted to acute dialysis and for limited duration in hospitalized patients. Noncuffed femoral catheters should only be used in bedbound patients.[170] The ADCs differ from the TDC in several ways: (1) They are more rigid and are designed to be placed over a guidewire without the use of dilators; (2) most designs are somewhat pointed at the tip; (3) they do not possess a cuff; and (4) they are not placed using a tunnel but rather by a direct insertion into the target vein.

A comparison of ADC and TDC usage is difficult because they are generally used in different patients and for different conditions. One study[189] analyzed the outcome of 37 TDCs and 235 ADCs (149 patients, 11,612 catheter-days) during a 3-year period in an attempt to compare the two. Infection rates were 2.9 per 1000 catheter-days for TDCs, 15.6 for acute catheters (internal jugular), and 20.2 for acute catheters (femoral). They found that within 2 weeks both actuarial and infection-free survival were superior for TDCs ($P < 0.05$ vs. all separate groups).

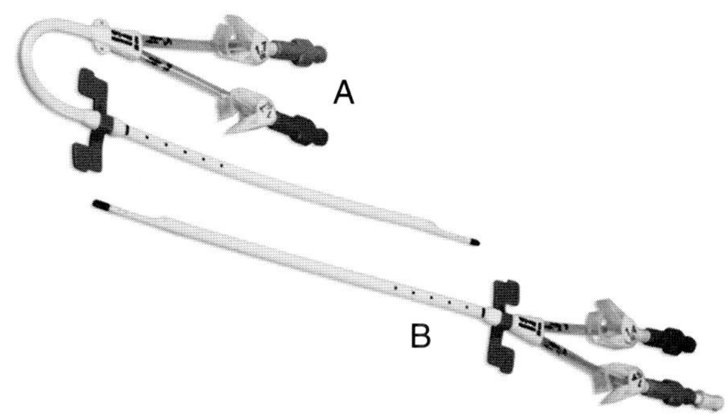

FIG. 23.19 Acute dialysis catheters. (A) Precurved catheter; (B) straight catheter.

From a practical viewpoint, the ADC represents a device that has utility; however, when the choice is between an ADC and a TDC, the decision should always favor the latter. Although the ADC is often inserted at the bedside and often believed to be more easily placed than a TDC, when one considers the risk for placement, time required, and skill necessary for catheter insertion, the ADC has no attribute to recommend it over the use of a TDC.

Adequate dialysis can be achieved using an ADC because most of ADCs are capable of delivering 400 mL/min or greater blood flow. If the catheter is placed properly and is of the appropriate length, recirculation rates are generally within acceptable limits. It is important to note that catheter length is critical because an ADC greater than 15 cm increases the risk for atrial perforation when inserted through the right internal jugular vein. The tips of catheters placed in the neck should reside in the superior vena cava, and those inserted through the groin should be reach the inferior vena cava. Tip placement in a smaller vein increases the risk for significant recirculation. In general, 15-cm catheters should be used in the right internal jugular, 20-cm catheters in the left internal jugular, and 20-cm or 24-cm catheters in the femoral vein.[190] One study[191] looked at recirculation rates for ADCs that were of different links and placed in different veins. Recirculation rates for ADCs have been examined based on catheter length and vessel insertion site. Reported rates were 4%, 5%, and 10% for the 12.5 cm in the internal jugular vein, the 20 cm in the subclavian, and 24 cm in the femoral vein, respectively.

Complications from ADCs include thrombosis, infection, central vein stenosis, and vessel and cardiac perforation. Thrombosis leading to catheter dysfunction is a common problem with all catheters, and although the incidence of dysfunction with the ADC is approximately the same as with the TDC, the risk for infection is considerably higher.[192] The risk for CRBSI from an ADC increases over time in an exponential fashion at both the femoral and internal jugular site; however, the risk for infection at the femoral site is greater. In addition, if an exit site infection occurs and the ADC is left in place, the risk for bacteremia rises dramatically.[193]

Central venous catheters, particularly subclavian catheters, are the major cause of central venous stenosis in the hemodialysis patient.[194-197] The incidence of subclavian stenosis after ADC placement has been reported to be in the range of 42%

to 50%. In contrast, the rate of brachiocephalic stenosis after use of the internal jugular vein has been reported to be 0% to 10%.[160,161] For this reason, subclavian ADCs should be avoided if at all possible. Some nephrologists feel that acute catheter use is better reserved for the femoral vein only.

When an acute catheter is left in place for a prolonged period, progressive vascular erosion can occur and lead to perforation. This is related to the length and relative rigidity of these devices. Improper catheter positioning or migration of the tip out of the proximal superior vena cava increases the risk for this occurrence. This can result in a hemothorax or atrial perforation and pericardial tamponade.[198]

A full list of references is available at www.expertconsult.com.

24

Hemodialysis Adequacy

Scott D. Bieber, DO

OUTLINE

Adequacy, the quality or state of being adequate, is defined as that which is sufficient for a specific need or purpose, a quantity that is acceptable but not better than acceptable.[1]

Since the early days of dialysis, providers and patients have wrestled with the question of the proper amount needed to treat end-stage kidney failure. Currently accepted measures of dialysis dose for hemodialysis often are referred to as *measures of dialysis adequacy*. Dialysis can perform many functions to partially correct kidney failure such as improve balance of fluid volume, correct metabolic acidosis and electrolyte abnormalities, and clear toxins or solutes that are retained in the setting of kidney failure. This chapter is limited to discussion of the removal of solutes that are retained in the setting of advanced kidney failure, known as *uremic retention solutes*, and how best to measure their removal with widely available techniques. The practicing clinician and patients with kidney failure often understand that although dialysis treatments may be described as being adequate, in reality, they fall far short of adequate replacement of native kidney function.

UREMIC RETENTION SOLUTES

When renal function declines, the excretory capacity of the kidney fails and the body accumulates substances that normally would be excreted in the urine. Numerous compounds of varying sizes and origins are retained with decline in kidney function.[2] Some of the solutes that are retained in the course of kidney failure are known to be toxic. Historically, the first solute recognized to be retained in individuals with kidney failure was urea, hence the use of the term *uremia* to describe the clinical condition that patients with advanced kidney failure display. Urea, measureable as blood urea nitrogen (BUN), is generated predominantly by the liver as a product of the urea cycle. The generation of urea is a method by which ammonia can be detoxified. Ammonia generation is a result of protein metabolism and its accumulation can lead to encephalopathy if not properly handled by the liver. Although urea itself is not particularly toxic, except at high concentrations, it is believed that the majority of uremic retention solutes are generated during the course of normal protein metabolism or formed by modifications of amino acids in the gastrointestinal tract by microbial flora.[3,4] Therefore, because urea also is formed as a result of protein metabolism and is easily measureable, it represents an acceptable surrogate marker for the uremic condition. However, it should be recognized that many of the solutes retained in kidney failure have size, shape, charge, and protein-binding characteristics that are very different from that of urea. Therefore it stands to reason that many uremic retention solutes would not behave in the same manner as urea.

Classically, uremic retention solutes have been categorized based on molecular weight (Table 24.1). Size comparison has utility in evaluating expected clearance during dialysis. As is discussed in detail here, the removal of a solute from the body during dialysis depends on many modifiable factors such as membrane characteristics, dialysis technique, and those that are patient specific. Clearance also is affected by the unique characteristics of the solute itself and its resident environment such as molecular weight, solubility, shape, charge, protein binding, Gibbs–Donnan equilibrium, and volume of distribution. Many uremic retention solutes, particularly middle, large, and protein-bound molecules, do not behave in the same manner as urea during dialysis.[5-7] Reliance on urea-based measures of dialysis dose therefore can lead to the misconception that dialysis is adequate for the removal of all toxins retained during the course of kidney failure when in reality the actual clearance may be quite different for larger or protein-bound solutes than what is measured for urea.

TABLE 24.1 Categories of Uremic Retention Solutes

Solute Type	Size (Da)	Examples	Most Effective Means of Removal
Small molecules	<500	Urea, creatinine, sodium, potassium, uric acid, oxalate, asymmetrical dimethylarginine	Diffusive clearance (dialysis) Increase the speed of dialysis: faster blood flow (Qb) and/or dialysate flow (Qd)
Middle molecules Large molecules	500–60,000	3-deoxyglucose, β_2-microglobulin, advanced glycation end products, oxidation products, cytokines, Interleukins, cystatin C, atrial natriuretic peptide, tumor necrosis factor, κ and λ light chains, parathyroid hormone, FGF23, dinucleoside polyphosphates	Increase dialysis time Increase dialyzer surface area, pore size, pore density (high-flux dialyser) Convective clearance (hemofiltration)
Protein bound	Variable	Fructoselysine, hippuric acid, homocysteine, indoxyl sulfate, retinol-binding protein, *p*-cresol	Increase dialysis time Increase dialysate flow Sorbent technology Albumin dialysis
Gut derived	Variable	Phenylacetyl-L-glutamine, 5-hydroxyindole, indoxyl glucuronide, *p*-cresol, indoxyl sulfate, urea	Nutritional modifications Maintenance of gastrointestinal motility Potential in the future: oral sorbents, absorbents Antibiotics or probiotics

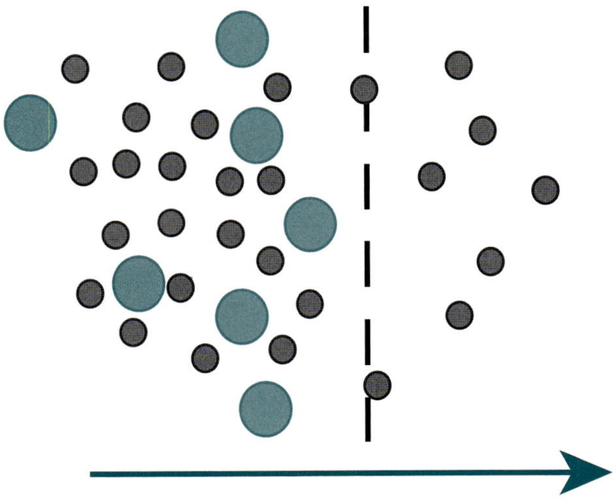

FIG. 24.1 Diffusion. During diffusion, if two compartments are separated by a semipermeable membrane solute that is small enough to pass through the membrane pores, they will move from an area of higher solute concentration to an area of lower solute concentration. *Arrow* represents the direction of molecular movement. Clearance of solute during hemodialysis is predominantly achieved through diffusion of solute from the blood into the dialysate.

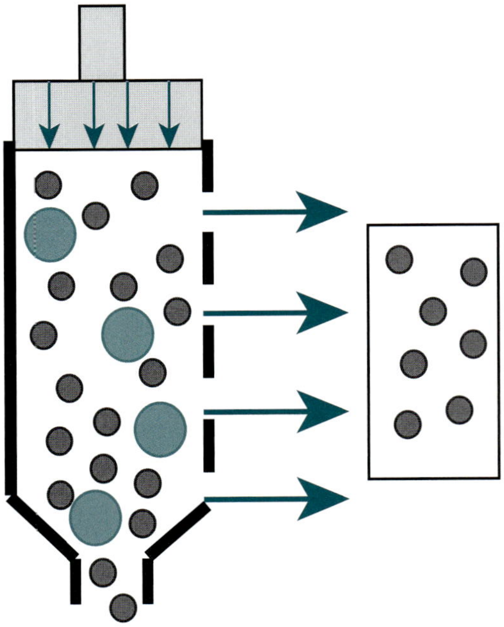

FIG. 24.2 Convection. Convection during dialysis describes the molecular movement that occurs along a pressure gradient. In the image, a compartment is subjected to the pressure applied by a piston, which squeezes fluid through a semipermeable membrane. Solute that is small enough to pass through the membrane pores is cleared from the blood through solute drag. Clearance of solute during hemofiltration or ultrafiltration happens via a convective process driven by transmembrane pressure.

MECHANISMS OF MOLECULAR MOVEMENT DURING DIALYSIS

During contemporary extracorporeal techniques to replace the function of the kidneys, solutes are removed via three mechanisms: diffusion, convection, and absorption.

Diffusion (Fig. 24.1) describes movement of solutes across a semipermeable membrane from an area of higher solute concentration to one of lower solute concentration. Diffusion of solute across the dialyzer and into the dialysate is the predominant method of solute clearance that occurs during standard hemodialysis. Diffusion is bidirectional and limited by the concentration of solute in a solution and membrane characteristics.

Convection (Fig. 24.2) describes the movement of solute suspended in solvent down a pressure gradient from an area of higher pressure to one of lower pressure. This method of solute removal is also termed *solute drag*. During convection, a given amount of solute that is dissolved in a given volume of solvent is cleared after a pressure gradient forces the solvent through the pores of a semipermeable membrane. If the solute is smaller than the pore size of the membrane, it will be dragged along with the solvent into the effluent. Convective clearance is at play during routine ultra- or hemofiltration, the latter example usually representing a larger volume of clearance necessitating replacement fluid administration compared with the relatively minimal convective clearance seen with routine ultrafiltration for volume management.

Absorption refers to the binding of solutes in the blood to parts of the extracorporeal circuit. Given the large surface area and porous nature of most dialysis filters, there is some entrapment of solute that occurs within the membrane. This method of solute removal is comparatively small with contemporary dialysis devices. Historically, sorbent-based systems used for water-efficient dialysis and regeneration of dialysate were quite effective in removal of solute via absorption to sorbent and resin columns and there is some interest in reviving this technology currently.[8-10]

Properties of the membrane can have an effect on the removal of solute during dialysis. During both diffusion and convection, movement of molecules depends on membrane pore size with molecules that are larger than the pore not passing the membrane. One way to describe the porosity of the membrane to an individual solute is by using the sieving coefficient. The sieving coefficient describes the membrane passage of a certain solute and is determined by dividing the solute concentration in the filter effluent by the solute concentration in the blood. Solute with a sieving coefficient of 1 easily passes the dialysis membrane, whereas a sieving coefficient of 0 indicates no movement across the membrane. Differing dialyzers can vary in their efficiency of removal of uremic retention solutes. When discussing dialyzers, the term *efficiency* refers to a dialyzer's ability to facilitate removal of uremic retention solutes. High-efficiency dialyzers have membrane properties that allow them to be more effective at removal of solute compared with low-efficiency dialyzers. The expected clearance of a dialyzer can be determined by in vitro studies and is usually provided on the manufacturer's dialyzer specification sheets in the form of calculated clearances of various solutes (urea, creatinine, phosphorus, vitamin B_{12}) at various blood flow rates (Qb 200, 300, 400, 500 mL/min) and a preset dialysate flow rate (usually 500 to 800 mL/min). Another method for comparison of the performance of different dialyzers is provided by the dialyzer mass transfer-area coefficient (KoA) urea. This is a theoretical clearance of urea provided at infinite blood and dialysate flows. In other words, the KoA urea provides an idea of the maximum ability of the dialyzer to clear small molecule urea when not limited by blood and dialysate flow rates. In this way, it is a reflection of clearance provided by membrane properties alone such as surface area and pore size. A higher value for KoA indicates a more efficient membrane. Manufacturers of hemodialyzers usually will provide KoA urea values as well. These clearance values can be useful for selecting a particular dialyzer from among other dialyzers by allowing the comparison of the expected clearances provided by different dialyzers with urea (MW 60 Da) representing small molecule clearance and vitamin B_{12} (MW 1355 Da) representing middle molecule clearance. However, they are not reliable for calculating expected clearances for individual patients and are not widely used clinically. Methods to directly measure urea removal in the individual patient without comparing expected clearances have gained clinical acceptance and are described in detail here.

USING UREA TO QUANTIFY DIALYSIS DOSE

Over the years, various mathematical constructs have been developed to help describe the drop of urea between the pre- and postdialysis periods as a form of a dialysis index to measure the adequacy of the delivered treatments. This section highlights the more commonly used urea-based measures of dialysis adequacy.

Collection of Blood Samples Before and After Hemodialysis

Accurate measurement of pre- and postdialysis BUN levels is important to ensure proper interpretation of dialysis adequacy. The predialysis urea sample should be drawn before the patient is placed on dialysis and without any influence of dilution from heparin or saline. This is easily accomplished immediately after placement of the dialysis needles if the patient has an arteriovenous access. If the patient has a central venous catheter, care should be taken to discard the lumen dwell content. The postdialysis sample should be drawn at the end of the dialysis procedure. In the postdialysis period, equilibration of urea occurs between various body compartments. The first and shortest period of equilibration is known as *access recirculation*. Access recirculation occurs over a matter of seconds when previously dialyzed blood, which has returned to the venous portion of the dialysis access, is taken up by the arterial needle and sent back through the extracorporeal circuit, decreasing the efficiency of the dialysis procedure. This phenomenon takes place in the dialysis access itself and is more predominant in the setting of a dysfunctional dialysis access and high blood flow through the dialysis circuit. Keeping the possibility of access recirculation in mind, methods have been developed to help ameliorate falsely low BUN levels due to access recirculation. One such method is the "slow-blood-flow" method.[11] At the completion of dialysis, dialysate flow and ultrafiltration are turned off (or if unable to turn off ultrafiltration completely, the ultrafiltration rate can be reduced to 50 mL/h), and the blood pump is slowed to 100 mL/min for 15 to 30 seconds. The sample is subsequently obtained. Alternatively, the "stop-dialysate-flow" method can be used.[12] With this method dialysate flow and ultrafiltration are turned off, 3 minutes are allowed to pass without any changes in the blood flow rate, and blood is subsequently sampled. The idea behind this method is that by stopping the dialysate for the 3-minute period, the dialysate compartment will equilibrate with the blood compartment yielding identical dialyzer blood inlet and outlet concentration. Both methods have been found to be equally effective in eliminating access recirculation. The stop-dialysate-flow method may yield slightly lower indices of dialysis adequacy if a significant amount of tissue equilibration of urea occurs in the 3-minute period when dialysate flow is stopped.

Urea Reduction Ratio

The amount of urea removed during a dialysis session can be described as a fractional reduction of urea:

$$URR = [BUN]_{pre} - [BUN]_{post} / [BUN]_{pre} \quad (1)$$

where $[BUN]_{pre}$ is the BUN concentration before dialysis and $[BUN]_{post}$ is the BUN concentration at the end of dialysis.[13] The result multiplied by 100 will yield a percentage of urea reduction. The urea reduction ratio (URR) is simple, intuitive, and has been embraced as a measure of dialysis dose adequacy. Although appropriate for the measurement of intermittent clearances as seen in standard hemodialytic therapy, it is not applicable to continuous clearances such as peritoneal dialysis, and comparison between hemodialysis strategies of differing frequency and duration would be limited. This is because when the level of kidney replacement increases and predialysis urea levels drop, or continuous clearance is provided, the URR trends toward zero. As can be seen in the equation, there is no accounting for residual renal function, ultrafiltration, or urea generation during dialysis. In contrast to other indices of dialysis adequacy, the URR is not normalized to body size.

Retrospective analyses have been able to demonstrate an inverse relationship between URR and the risk for death.[14] However, this inverse relationship does not always hold up in patients with high URRs as there seems to be a paradoxical relationship between high URR (>75%) and higher risk for death. This has been demonstrated in a reverse J-shape curve between mortality and URR.[15] The paradoxical relationship may be explained by nutritional factors and patient body size. Mortality in dialysis patients is strongly correlated with body weight, with larger patients demonstrating better survival. Patients with lower body weight more frequently have higher URR.[16,17] There also seems to be differences in the relationship between URR and mortality among different demographic groups.[18] These observations draw into question the utility of the URR as a measure of outcome in a population. However, similar to other indices of adequacy, the URR can be useful in trending the adequacy of treatments over time in an individual patient.

Single-Pool Kt/V

The single-pool Kt/V (spKtV) is a mathematical construct that has been proposed as a method by which clinicians can understand the adequacy of dialysis treatments.[19] Although widely used clinically and ever present in clinical practice guidelines, it should be noted that higher Kt/V is not associated with better patient outcomes in clinical trials.[20] To understand the concept of the spKt/V, one must understand the concept of clearance. *Clearance* is defined as the volume from which a substance has been completely removed and usually is expressed per unit time (e.g., mL/min). Clearance does not describe the amount of a substance, or mass removed; rather it describes a volume that has been cleared of a particular substance. Urea resides in the body water and is freely distributed among the body water both in the intracellular and extracellular space. It often is referred to as an *ineffective osmole* due to its relative ease of diffusion across cellular membranes and relatively rapid equilibration between the intracellular and extracellular space compared with other solutes such as sodium. During a typical hemodialysis treatment session, around 120 to 190 L of urea-free dialysate is brought into the dialyzer in contact with the blood, resulting in a net diffusion of urea from the plasma into the dialysate. This volume of dialysate is not routinely collected and is not available for measurement of volume or concentration. Therefore, unlike clearance calculations that may be performed to describe residual renal function, where volume of urine output is known and can be collected for measurement of concentration of urea, or clearance calculations that can be performed in peritoneal dialysis, where volume of peritoneal dialysate effluent is known and can be collected, in hemodialysis we rely on blood side measurements of solute and describe the drop in solute from pre- to postdialysis.

Urea concentration in the blood does not decline in a linear fashion during a dialysis treatment. To express the fractional reduction of urea with a dialysis treatment, a kinetic equation can be proposed that describes the exponential curve of urea disappearance during dialysis.[19,21]

$$C = C_0 e^{-Kt/V}$$

$$Kt/V = -\ln(C/C_0) \quad (2)$$

In this equation, C is the postdialysis urea concentration, C_0 is the predialysis urea concentration, K is clearance, t is time, V is volume of distribution of urea, *e* is a mathematical constant, the base of the natural logarithm. This equation effectively models the removal of a substance from the body where that substance decreases in an exponential fashion. It also can be thought of as the disappearance curve of urea during a dialysis session. The equation yields a result that is unit-less. If we consider the total body water of a patient over a defined period of time to be completely cleared of urea (K = V), this would yield a Kt/V of 1.

The concept of spKt/V urea relies on the assumption that urea is evenly distributed in a single pool of body water that has equal access to the dialyzer. Although urea is an "ineffective osmole" and moves relatively rapidly among the various compartments in the body, due to the extremely efficient and nonphysiological nature of a modern dialysis treatment session where urea is removed from the plasma space at a rate that exceeds equilibration from outside the plasma space, this assumption does not hold true. In contrast to the assumption of the single-pool model, urea is actually distributed in varying concentration throughout the body during dialysis, evidenced by the rebound phenomenon of equilibration at the end of dialysis when urea moves from tissue areas of lower perfusion back into the vascular space. This is sometimes referred to as *two-compartment distribution* or the *double-pool model* where one compartment is considered the vascular space and the other is everything outside of the vascular space.[22] The original logarithmic equations of spKt/V are further flawed in that they do not take into account any fluid removed during the dialysis procedure, which would have an effect on the volume of distribution and alter the concentration of the urea, which in turn affects the clearance. A small amount of urea also is removed via convection or solute drag during ultrafiltration. Furthermore, the simplified single-pool model does not account for urea generation, which would occur during the dialysis session. More advanced formulas have attempted to account for fluid removed with dialysis and estimate urea generation during dialysis. An example follows of a commonly used formula for spKt/V, often referred to as a *second-generation equation* or the *Daugirdas II equation* (not to be confused with the double-pool model, discussed under equilibrated Kt/V [eKt/V]):[23]

$$spKt/V = -\ln(R - 0.008 * t) + (4 - 3.5 * R) * UF/W \quad (3)$$

In this equation, R is the postdialysis BUN divided by predialysis BUN, t is the dialysis session length in hours, UF is the ultrafiltration volume in L, and W is the postdialysis weight in kg. In general, a spKt/V of 1.2 is equivalent to a 65% urea reduction. Some clinical guidelines recommend targeting a minimum spKt/V urea of 1.4.[11] Again, this recommendation has not been shown to improve outcome in any randomized controlled trial completed at the time of this publication.

One disadvantage of using simplified single-pool equations for calculation of dialysis dose is that unlike formal urea kinetic modeling, it does not generate useful information about protein catabolic rate (PCR). Information regarding discrepancy between delivered and prescribed dose may not be appreciated in the way they would with urea kinetic modeling. The equation also is prone to error if used outside standard thrice-weekly 4-hour dialysis in regimens of short, long, or frequent dialysis. To accurately measure the spKt/V using the equation, the decrease in BUN during the dialysis treatment must be significant otherwise error is introduced due to mathematical variance. This inherent property makes the spKt/V models presented here inappropriate for frequent hemodialysis regimens such as daily or nocturnal dialysis. Furthermore, these equations would not be appropriate to calculate continuous clearances such as delivered with peritoneal dialysis where the urea concentration remains at a relative steady state. Fortunately, in such steady-state situations, simple and more direct clearance calculations can be undertaken because the volume of effluent dialysate is known and can be easily sampled. In addition, the calculation or estimation of V by Watson's method or otherwise is likely to be fraught with error and particularly inaccurate at extremes of body size or in women. Finally, there is no adjustment for urea equilibration, or the rebound elevation of urea that occurs after dialysis if the postdialysis BUN level is drawn at the conclusion of the treatment session compared with waiting a period of 30 to 60 minutes for urea to equilibrate.

Equilibrated Kt/V

As already mentioned, one limitation of the spKt/V concept during contemporary dialysis is that urea removal from the plasma space occurs at a rate that exceeds the rate of equilibration from outside the plasma space. To address this problem, dialysis samples could be drawn 1 hour after dialysis to allow adequate time for urea to equilibrate equally between all body compartments. This approach is not practical for the typical dialysis provider nor is it acceptable to the dialysis patient who already has a large amount of time obligated to complete dialysis treatments. The eKt/V, occasionally referred to as the *double-pool Kt/V*, was developed to estimate and adjust the spKt/V for post-urea rebound in lieu of the more time-consuming alternative.

Postdialysis urea rebound is largely believed to have three phases: access recirculation, cardiopulmonary recirculation, and urea redistribution from less accessible body compartments. The phenomenon of disparate urea content in various body compartments is particularly evident with the use of an arteriovenous dialysis access. The first phase, access recirculation, usually resolves in a period of 10 to 15 seconds after the blood pump is stopped or slowed to 50 to 100 mL/min.[24] Cardiopulmonary recirculation refers to the distribution of dialyzed blood to the heart and quickly back to the dialysis access through the cardiopulmonary circuit, bypassing slower areas of circulation that would allow for more even distribution of urea. The effect of cardiopulmonary recirculation lasts only for about a minute after dialysis.[25] The third component, the slow movement of urea from areas of lower perfusion and cellular spaces and can take up to 30 to 60 minutes after the completion of dialysis.[26,27]

Urea rebound is variable between patients. Dialysis-related factors such as blood flow, dialysate flow, volume of ultrafiltration, and patient-related factors such as age, heart function, muscle mass, and blood pressure can affect the amount of urea rebound.[28,29] For example, muscle is thought to contain about 60% of the total body water, yet blood flow to the muscle during dialysis is relatively low contributing to a rebound in urea level after dialysis.[21] In contrast, organs receive a large amount of cardiac output but relatively less body water. This situation is somewhat mitigated by the fact that urea concentration in organ compartments that receive higher amounts of systemic blood flow is likely to be higher than in muscle, which is less perfused during dialysis.[30] Due to these gradients established during dialysis, in the postdialysis period when organ blood combines with muscle blood, one would expect a urea rebound. Furthermore, the rate of dialysis can affect the amount of urea rebound. The following equations were developed through studies of urea equilibration and linear regression analysis with time of dialysis and the value of the spKt/V used as inputs for an equation that converts the spKt/V to an adjusted, eKt/V.[21]

$$eKt/V = spKtV - 0.6\,(spKtV/T) + 0.03\ \text{(arteriovenous access)}$$

$$eKt/V = spKtv - 0.47\,(spKtv/T) + 0.02\ \text{(venous catheter access)} \quad (4)$$

In these equations, spKtV is the result of the spKt/V as calculated from the aforementioned equations and T is equal to dialysis time in hours. The difference in urea distribution during cardiopulmonary recirculation between different dialysis access types necessitates two equations. The first equation should be used in patients with an arteriovenous access and the second equation is for patients where there is no arterial mixing of blood and measurements of urea are strictly venous, such as patients with a typical venous dialysis catheter. Alternative methods to calculate eKt/V are discussed elsewhere.[27,31]

The key advantage of the eKt/V is the avoidance of the error with single-pool methods that overestimate dialysis dose due to urea rebound. This advantage is particularly evidenced when the treatment time is short and the dialysis technique efficient (short, fast dialysis). It should be recognized that the equation provides an approximation based on population data and the coefficients involved are not always accurate for every patient. For example, if blood flow to the muscle is lower in a particular patient then the coefficient of 0.6 is likely to be lower. Limitations of the single-pool model described here are still applicable to the eKt/V and should be kept in mind during interpretation of the results.

Standard Kt/V

The methods just described have utility in describing the kinetics of urea removal during an intermittent dialysis session and are predominantly designed for thrice-weekly intermittent dialysis. More frequent methods of dialysis require a different approach where the dose of dialysis is expressed independently of the frequency of dialysis as a continuous clearance. This concept relies on the steady-state assumption where if one was to maintain a steady plasma concentration then clearance of a solute is equal to the amount that is generated divided by the solute concentration. Thus clearance is inversely proportional to solute concentration and directly affected by the solute generation rate. Furthermore, under a steady-state assumption, urea generation and time-averaged urea concentration can be used to calculate a continuous clearance.

$$K = G/C_{urea} \quad (5)$$

This expression has been termed the *equivalent renal urea clearance* (EKR).[32] Alternatively, if one believes that the peak concentration of urea is more correlated with the toxicity seen in the uremic condition, the average peak or predialysis urea could be input in lieu of the time averaged urea concentration.[33] Using the average predialysis or peak urea concentration results in a lower clearance than if the time averaged urea concentration is used, is more comparable to peritoneal dialysis methods and has been termed the *standard* clearance (K).[34]

$$\text{Standard } K = G/C_m \quad (6)$$

C_m is the mean predialysis urea concentration. Adding the parameter of time (minutes) and normalizing to volume of distribution of urea (mL) yields the dimensionless standard weekly Kt/V (stdKt/V), with the time interval set at 1 week (10,080 minutes):

$$stdKt/V = G/C_m * 10080/V \quad (7)$$

The stdKt/V can be calculated from pre- and postdialysis urea levels with urea kinetic modeling to calculate urea generation (G) or can be approximated with one of the equations below.[11,35] The first equation uses the eKt/V and therefore attempts to adjust for post-urea rebound. Residual renal function is neglected and the equation assumes that the dialysis schedule is symmetrical within the week.

$$stdKt/V = \frac{10,080\,\frac{1 - e^{-eKt/V}}{t}}{\frac{1 - e^{-eKt/V}}{eKt/V} + \frac{10,080}{Ft} - 1} \quad (8)$$

F is the number of treatments in the week, *t* is time of treatment in minutes in the first equation and hours in the second equation and spKt/V or eKt/V is the spKt/V or eKt/V as calculated in the equations presented earlier in this chapter. This method of calculation underestimates the true clearance (K) during dialysis because of fixed volume assumptions. It does not account for ultrafiltration and the convective clearance of solute that happens during ultrafiltration is not appreciated. The change in concentration of urea due to fluid accumulation between dialysis diluting the urea concentration is not appreciated. Furthermore, residual renal function, which can contribute significantly to the patient's overall clearance of uremic retention solute, is ignored. Alternative equations are described elsewhere to adjust for some of these shortcomings.[36]

The utility of standardizing the Kt/V to a continuous weekly clearance can be appreciated mostly when comparing patients on different dialysis regimens. Urea kinetic modeling and the logarithmic equations described above for spKt/V or eKt/V work well for thrice-weekly dialysis but are not designed for use with more frequent dialysis sessions. For example, a patient dialyzing three times a week may achieve an Kt/V of 1.2. If the dialysis regimen was increased to four times weekly, it would not be surprising to see the Kt/V drop to 0.9, despite a greater dose of dialysis delivered over the week on account of the extra day of dialysis. Superficial analysis of the difference between these two values for Kt/V could lead one to erroneously suspect that a lower Kt/V indicates less dialysis delivered. Alternatively, inputting the numbers into the stdKt/V equation just presented would yield a higher stdKt/V for the four-times-a-week regimen. In other words, to compare dialysis adequacy between different dialysis modalities of differing treatment duration, the stdKt/V or the equivalent renal urea clearance is the preferable method. Clinical practice guidelines recommend achieving an stdKt/V of at least 2.[11] Similar to spKt/V, achieving this threshold has not been convincingly tied to a meaningful improvement in patient outcome.[37]

Urea Kinetic Modeling

One of the limitations of taking the simplistic approach to describe the decrease in urea concentration in the blood over a dialysis treatment session as the negative natural logarithm of the final urea postdialysis concentration over the predialysis concentration is that this method does not account for the changes in urea generation and volume of distribution that occur over time. One way to refine the accuracy of the mathematics of the Kt/V to more closely reflect what occurs in real life is to develop more sophisticated Kt/V equations mentioned previously such as the Daugirdas II equation, which use logistic regression modeling of large populations of patients to come up with an equation that can describe the Kt/V. Another method is to use computer programs to perform iterative mathematics that attempt to describe urea kinetic behavior during dialysis. This method is known as *formal urea kinetic modeling*.[38]

$$C = C_o\left[\frac{V - B.t}{V}\right]^{\left(\frac{K_r + K_d + B}{B}\right)} + \frac{G}{K_r + K_d + B}\left[1 - \left[\frac{V - B.t}{V}\right]^{\left(\frac{K_r + K_d + B}{B}\right)}\right] \quad \textbf{(9)}$$

This equation describes a method of urea kinetic modeling where V is postdialysis urea distribution volume, G is urea generation, K_r is native kidney urea clearance, B is the change in V during dialysis, and K_d is dialyser urea clearance.[11,39] Iterative computer programs based on this equation, and others, can be used to predict the urea concentrations that would be expected using in vitro clearance data which provides dialyzer K (from manufacturer specifications or KoA), estimated V (based on total body water estimations from anthropometric nomograms or roughly 50% to 60% of body weight) and dialysis time. If three urea values are known, pre(C_o) dialysis urea concentration for two subsequent treatments and post(C) dialysis urea concentration of the second treatment, rates of urea generation (G) can be calculated. Input variables of pre- and postdialysis urea, dialyzer K, and time allows calculation of a modeled V, which can then be compared with the estimated V. From model output variables of G and V, Kt/V and PCR can be calculated. Modeled values obtained compared with expected values obtained yield insight into discrepancy between prescribed and delivered dose of dialysis. Modeling kinetics with two urea measurements (pre- and postdialysis BUN for a single session) is possible and more frequently used in clinical practice as it does not require an extra blood draw. The two-draw method requires an iterative process over the period of a week rather than over one dialysis session and is limited by the often erroneous assumption that predialysis urea level is consistently the same.[40]

Normalized Protein Catabolic Ratio

Serum urea level is dependent on mass balance relationships with input of urea into the system described as urea generation, G, mg/min. Because urea generation, under steady-state conditions when the patient is neither catabolic nor anabolic, is dependent on dietary protein intake, measurement of urea generation can be used as a marker of nutrition. Due to the close relationship of urea level with dietary protein intake, assessment of dialysis adequacy could be considered to be incomplete without an assessment of nutritional intake. As an example, consider the dialysis patient with subclinical uremia, which is limiting nutritional intake due to nausea. Often in this setting, predialysis urea levels will be low due to decreased protein intake. Low predialysis urea could represent optimal dialysis or, if the uremic condition is present, it is more likely to reflect low dietary protein intake. Indices of adequacy such as Kt/V urea or URR may appear abnormal and serve as a cue to the clinician that more dialysis is necessary; however, this is not universally the case. In certain settings, limited protein intake also can yield indices of dialysis adequacy that are within goal range. In such cases, analysis of nutritional parameters such as the normalized protein catabolic rate (nPCR) along with subjective clinical assessment of the patient are key to the proper interpretation of adequacy indexes. Nutritional status of dialysis patients is likely to have a significant effect on clinical outcome. Low dietary protein intake has been associated with higher mortality in dialysis patients.[41,42] In particular, trends of declining PCR over time in a dialysis patient portend a poor prognosis whereas increasing PCR over time is associated with better survival.[43] The recommended daily protein intake for patients on maintenance hemodialysis is 1.2 g/kg with ≥50% of the protein being of high biological value; meaning that the protein has amino acid composition similar to human protein.[44]

Use of the term *protein catabolic rate* is considered to be a misnomer by some because not all protein in dialysis patients is lost to catabolism. Some of it is lost in dialysate and urine. Subsequently, the total amount of protein breakdown is believed to be larger than what is apparent through urea generation. The term *protein equivalent of total nitrogen appearance* (TNA) or *protein nitrogen appearance* (PNA) has been suggested as more appropriate.[44] For purposes here, PCR and PNA should be considered synonymous. Recall that urea often is measured in the laboratory as BUN, which is a measure of urea nitrogen not urea level. TNA is dependent on losses from residual renal function, stool, skin, and dialysate, as well as urea generation during the interdialytic period. Urea generation (G, mg/min) during the interdialytic period can be calculated by quantifying the rise in urea between dialysis sessions:

$$G = \Delta C * V/\theta \quad \textbf{(10)}$$

ΔC is the difference between the urea concentration at the end of the dialysis session and the beginning of the next session, V is the volume of distribution of urea, and θ is the interdialytic time interval in minutes.[19] This expression assumes a steady state of urea generation with no other outputs in the interdialytic period. Equations have been developed based on this simple relationship to calculate the nPCR using linear regression data of predialysis urea level and Kt/V.[45] The following equations adjust for differences in interdialytic time interval and are most accurate in anuric patients.

Thrice-weekly dialysis:

$$\text{Beginning of week}: C_0/[36.3+5.48KTV+53.5/KTV]+0.168$$

$$\text{Midweek}: C_0/[25.8+1.15KTV+56.4/KTV]+0.168$$

$$\text{End of week}: C_0/[16.3+4.30KTV+56.6/KTV]+0.168 \quad (11)$$

Twice-weekly dialysis:

$$\text{Beginning of week}: C_0/[48+5.14KTV+79/KTV]+0.168$$

$$\text{End of week}: C_0/[33+3.6KTV+83.2/KTV]+0.168 \quad (12)$$

C_o is the predialysis BUN in mg/dL and KTV is the Kt/V that can be calculated by urea kinetic modeling or as a result of the simpler equations described previously. eKt/V would be the most appropriate input for KTV because if single-pool methods for input of KTV are utilized then postdialysis urea rebound will be neglected and nPCR will appear falsely high. For patients with significant residual renal function, the following equations should be used to adjust the C_o upward, accounting for the clearance of urea through the kidneys. The result C_o' (adjusted BUN, mg/dL) can then be input into the appropriate equation.[45]

Thrice weekly dialysis:

$$C_o' = C_o/[1+(0.7+3.08/KTV)\,K_r/V]$$

Twice weekly dialysis:

$$C_o' = C_o/[1+(1.15+4.56/KTV)\,K_r/V] \quad (13)$$

Kr is the residual renal urea clearance in mL/min and V is volume of distribution in L. Goal nPCR should be >1 g/kg/day. nPCR <0.8 should raise suspicion for protein-calorie malnutrition and has been associated with poor outcome.[34,46]

The results of calculations of the PCR as described previously should always be interpreted with an understanding of their inherent limitations in mind. Perhaps the most relevant limitation is the requirement for the patient to be in a steady state of nitrogen balance. This is not always the case, for example, in acutely ill patients where muscle stores are catabolized to meet metabolic demands and conversely in the illness recovery stage when anabolism leads to increased protein storage in the muscle. Also, urine urea nitrogen levels are not consistent and vary with dietary intake. For accurate analysis of the PCR, measurement of the contribution of urea loss in the urine should be performed concurrently, a process that requires cumbersome urine collections. Unmeasured pathways of nitrogen excretion such as skin and respiration also are not accounted for. Finallly, there is some controversy as to the method of normalizing the PCR to body weight, a process that can be misleading in obese, edematous, or malnourished patients.[1]

LIMITATIONS OF UREA-BASED MEASURES OF DIALYSIS ADEQUACY

There are notable caveats that should be kept in mind when interpreting urea-based measures of dialysis adequacy. The uremic condition is complicated and poorly understood. Urea serves as a surrogate marker of the uremic condition but it does not describe the totality of the uremic condition. Notably missing from urea-based measures of dialysis adequacy is assessment of middle molecule solutes, large solutes, protein-bound, and gut-derived uremic retention compounds. These myriad compounds are becoming increasingly recognized as pathological in the uremic condition.[47-57] Urea indices provide information only about small molecular solute clearance. The main limitation of urea kinetic modeling revolves around the assumption that urea is a valid marker for the wide range of biologically relevant toxins. Despite extensive efforts in the past, the clinical significance of urea-based measures of dialysis adequacy has yet to be validated by outcome studies.[20,37,58]

The majority of urea-based measures of dialysis adequacy are based on the premise that V is simply a solvent for urea and does not have any other clinical meaning. This premise is probably not true. V correlates with mortality with larger patients generally enjoying a better survival.[17,59-61] In other words, Kt/V and V may be independently and significantly associated with survival. Patients with smaller body size may require higher Kt/V to achieve the same outcome.[62] Dividing Kt by V fails to normalize results across all body sizes as an index is supposed to do; the expected relationships do not seem to hold up at the extremes of body size. This has been shown to be significant in women with a smaller V as well as big men, particularly when residual renal function drops off.[63,64] Furthermore, there is an implicit assumption that generation of uremic toxins is a function of the volume of distribution (V) and urea is freely and equally distributed within the total body water. In reality, generation of urea is more closely tied to dietary protein intake and there are significant compartmental differences in the distribution of urea that is more pronounced during the dialysis treatment procedure.[65,66]

Relying on laboratory data obtained from a single treatment session assumes that hemodialysis treatments delivered throughout the month are similar to the treatment that was delivered on the day that the laboratory studies were drawn. In reality, dose of dialysis delivered during nonlaboratory draw sessions is less.[67,68] Shortened dialysis time due to treatment interruptions can lower the delivered dose of dialysis but is not accounted for in many of the methods. The sampling procedure of BUN pre- and postdialysis session can be variable and prone to error if not performed correctly. There is no adjustment for hematocrit, recirculation, or loss of dialyzer surface area and volume due to clotting. Modeling of urea disappearance is only feasible in the setting of intermittent dialysis sessions where the drop of BUN between the pre- and postdialysis session is significant. Mathematically, accuracy is lost as treatment sessions become more frequent and many of the methods described earlier in this text would not be appropriate to evaluate a continuous therapy.

KEY STUDIES OF OPTIMAL DIALYSIS DOSE

Finding the answer to the question of the optimal amount of hemodialysis necessary to improve patient outcome has eluded researchers to date. This is not due to lack of effort. The following section summarizes efforts that have attempted to quantify the dose of dialysis and describe an adequate amount necessary to improve patient outcome.

In 1981 the National Cooperative Dialysis Study (NCDS) was a seminal early study seeking to provide a means for quantitative measurement of the optimal dose for thrice-weekly dialysis.[58] Investigators compared time-averaged urea clearances (TAC_{urea}) with long (4.5 to 5 h) or short (2.5 to 3.5 h) treatment durations and TAC_{urea} concentrations that were high (100 mg/dL) versus low (50 mg/dL) using a factorial randomized study design. TAC_{urea} provides a value for the mean concentration of urea over a dialysis cycle. Investigators found that the patients in groups with higher TAC_{urea} had more frequent hospitalizations, most commonly due to nausea, anorexia, and other uremic symptoms. As a result, more patients were withdrawn from the high TAC_{urea} groups for medical reasons likely related to uremia and underdialysis. Regarding the length of therapy, in the high TAC_{urea} patients, the short-duration dialysis group was hospitalized more frequently than the long-duration dialysis group. The benefit of longer dialysis was not seen to reach statistical significance in the two groups with low TAC_{urea}, although there was a trend toward improvement in the long-duration treatment group. The NCDS findings were widely interpreted as suggesting that to prevent morbidity, clearance of urea is more important than dialysis treatment time. This led to the assumption by many clinicians that dialysis time could be shortened as long as urea clearance remained adequate. Notable caveats of the NCDS study include relatively low urea clearances across all groups, a patient population that was healthier compared with the dialysis population in more recent times, and the small size of the study ($n = 151$), which was underpowered to make mortality comparisons.

Following the NCDS study, numerous large observational studies, most of them performed in the 1990s, suggested that higher Kt/V urea values and higher flux dialysis is associated with better outcome.[14,69-75] Subsequently, there was a trend toward lengthening dialysis time and the use of high-flux membranes.

The HEMO (Hemodialysis) study, published in 2002, sought to evaluate the effect of dialysis dose and membrane flux on death from any cause.[20] In a schedule of thrice-weekly dialysis, investigators used a 2 × 2 factorial design to randomize patients to high- or low-dose groups and high- or low-flux groups. To account for urea rebound effects postdialysis, eKt/V was used to measure dialysis adequacy. Investigators achieved an eKt/V in the low-dose group of 1.16 and 1.53 in the high-dose group. The low- and high-flux groups had similar mean eKt/V at 1.34. No significant improvement in survival or hospitalization was seen between standard or high-dose, low- or high-flux dialysis groups. Health-related quality of life, nutritional parameters, and functional status also did not differ between the groups.[76,77] The results of the HEMO study were surprisingly negative in contrast to the earlier observational data of the 1990s. Even so, it is notable that on secondary analysis of the HEMO study, high-flux dialysis was associated with improved cardiovascular and cerebrovascular outcomes.[78,79]

The MPO (Membrane Permeability Outcome) study also was undertaken with a goal of evaluating the effect of membrane permeability (flux) on outcomes.[80] Patients were randomized to dialysis with low- or high-flux membranes and stratified according to their serum albumin level (albumin <4 or >4 g/dL). Both groups were treated with a minimum spKt/V of 1.2. Findings revealed that patients in the low-albumin group (<4 g/dL) had significantly higher survival rates when treated with a high-flux dialyzer. Furthermore, high-flux dialyzers in secondary analysis seemed to improve survival of diabetics regardless of serum albumin. This survival benefit was not seen in patients with higher serum albumin levels or across the group as a whole.

Effect of extended duration of dialysis therapy on patient outcome was not assessed in the aforementioned randomized clinical trials. In 2010 data from the FHN (Frequent Hemodialysis Network) trial were released to help address the issue of the appropriate frequency and duration of dialysis.[37] The rationale for the currently used frequency of dialysis (thrice weekly) is based on limited studies, logistic practicality, cost, and patient acceptance rather than on sound science. The FHN Daily study sought to evaluate the effect of increased frequency of dialysis on outcome with the hypothesis that more frequent dialysis would be found to be more beneficial. Participants were randomized to in-center hemodialysis six times a week compared with standard thrice-weekly dialysis. As expected, solute clearance was higher in the frequent dialysis group (weekly stdKt/V 3.54 vs. 2.49). Results revealed that more short and frequent dialysis was associated with improvement in left ventricular mass, physical composite health score, hypertension, and phosphorus control. The study was conducted for a relatively short period of 12 months and was underpowered to detect any differences in mortality. There was no difference in the rates of hospitalization with more frequent dialysis.

Extended-duration dialysis also can be provided through nocturnal dialysis programs. Numerous observational studies and small prospective studies have suggested benefit in nocturnal patients with regard to improvement in left ventricular mass, superior hypertension control, greater phosphorus clearance, enhanced nutritional parameters, and improved quality of life. These results have been reproduced in two small randomized trials.[81,82] Consistently in nocturnal studies, blood pressure control is superior and mineral metabolism parameters also are easier to control, leading to an overall lower medication burden for the patient.[81,83-91]

The FHN nocturnal trial is the largest randomized clinical trial of nocturnal dialysis to date. This study was underpowered to meet statistical significance for outcomes of death, hospitalization, left ventricular mass, or composite physical health score. However, nocturnal dialysis did improve systolic blood pressure control and phosphorus control. Similar to the results found during the FHN short-daily trials, access complications were more common in the nocturnal hemodialysis group. Unfortunately, this study does not appear to be useful in proving or disproving the utility of increased delivery of dialysis through nocturnal dialysis. As can been inferred from the two prospective studies illustrated here, the study of frequent and nocturnal hemodialysis has been hampered by difficulty in recruitment of patients for these extended therapies.

A full list of references is available at www.expertconsult.com.

25

Hemodialysis-Associated Infections*

Duc B. Nguyen, MD, Matthew J. Arduino, MS, DrPH, and Priti R. Patel, MD, MPH

OUTLINE

INTRODUCTION

Of the patients with end-stage renal disease (ESRD) treated by maintenance dialysis in the United States, approximately 90% are on maintenance hemodialysis and 10% are on peritoneal dialysis.[1] Maintenance hemodialysis patients are at higher risk for infection, because uremia is known to make patients with ESRD more susceptible to infectious agents through defects in cellular immunity, neutrophil function, and complement activation.[2,3] In addition, because the process requires vascular access for long periods in an environment where multiple patients receive hemodialysis concurrently, repeated opportunities exist for transmission of infectious agents. Patient-to-patient transmission of infectious agents, directly or indirectly through contaminated devices, equipment, supplies, injectable medications, environmental surfaces, or hands of healthcare personnel have all been demonstrated. Furthermore, hemodialysis patients require frequent hospitalizations and surgery, which increases their opportunities for exposure and risk for developing healthcare-associated infections. This chapter describes (1) the major infectious diseases that can be acquired in the dialysis center setting, (2) important epidemiological and environmental microbiological considerations, and (3) infection control strategies.

FACTORS CONTRIBUTING TO INFECTIONS AMONG HEMODIALYSIS PATIENTS

Technical development and clinical use of hemodialysis delivery systems improved dramatically in the late 1960s and early 1970s. However, a number of microbiological parameters were not accounted for in the design of many hemodialysis machines and their respective water supply systems. There are many situations where certain types of gram-negative water bacteria can persist and actively multiply in hemodialysis water supplies and aqueous environments associated with hemodialysis equipment. This can result in massive numbers of gram-negative bacteria, which can directly or indirectly lead to septicemia or endotoxemia.[4-17] These bacteria can adhere to surfaces and form biofilms (glycocalyces), which are virtually impossible to eradicate.[6,18-20] Control strategies are designed not to eradicate bacteria but to reduce their concentration to relatively low levels and to prevent their regrowth.

Although certain genera of gram-negative water bacteria (e.g., *Burkholderia, Flavobacterium, Pseudomonas, Ralstonia, Serratia, Stenotrophomonas maltophilia*, and *Sphingomonas*) are most commonly encountered, virtually any bacterium

*The findings and conclusions in this chapter are those of the authors and do not necessarily represent the official position of the Centers for Disease Control and Prevention. The use of trade names and commercial sources in this chapter is for identification only and does not imply endorsement by the Centers for Disease Control and Prevention.

TABLE 25.1 Factors Influencing Microbial Contamination in Hemodialysis Systems

Factors	Comments
Water Supply (Water Source)	
Groundwater	Contains endotoxin and bacteria
Surface water	Contains high levels of endotoxin, bacteria, and other organisms
Water Treatment at the Dialysis Center	
None	Not Recommended
Filtration	
Prefilter	Particulate filter to protect equipment; does not remove microorganisms
Absolute filter (depth or membrane)	Removes bacteria but unless changed frequently or disinfected, bacteria will accumulate and grow through the filter; acts as a significant reservoir of bacteria and endotoxin
Granular activated carbon (GAC)	Removes organics and available chlorine or chloramine; significant reservoir of water bacteria and endotoxin
Water Treatment Devices	
Ion exchange (softener, deionization)	Softeners and deionizers remove cations and anions, contaminants from source water; significant reservoir for bacteria and endotoxin
Reverse osmosis (RO)	Removes bacteria, endotoxin, chemicals, and must be cleaned and disinfected; most systems employed for dialysis applications operate under high pressure
Ultraviolet (UV) germicidal irradiator	Kills most bacteria, but there is no residual; some UV-resistant bacteria can develop
Ultrafilter	Removes bacteria and endotoxin; operates on normal line pressure; can be positioned distal to storage tank and deionizer; must be disinfected or changed
Water and Dialysate Distribution System	
Distribution pipes	
Size	Oversized diameters and length decrease fluic flow and increases bacterial reservoir in the form of biofilms for both treated water and central delivery systems (bicarbonate concentrate or bicarbonate dialysate)
Materials	Pipe materials influence bacterial colonization and biofilm formation, as well as what types of chemical disinfectants can be used
Construction	Rough joints, dead ends, and unused branches can act as bacterial reservoirs
Elevation	Outlet taps should be located at highest elevation to prevent loss of disinfectant
Storage tanks	Generally undesirable because of large surface area and can act as a reservoir for water bacteria; a properly designed tank can minimize this risk
Dialysis Machines	
Single pass	Disinfectant should have contact time with all parts of the machine that are in contact with treated water or dialysate
Recirculating single pass, or recirculating batch	Recirculating pumps and machine design allow for massive contamination levels if not properly disinfected; overnight disinfection recommended

that can grow in water can be a problem in a hemodialysis unit. Several species of nontuberculous mycobacteria may also contaminate water treatment systems, including *Mycobacterium chelonae, M. abscessus, M. fortuitum, M. gordonae, M. mucogenicum, M. scrofulaceum, M. kansasii, M. avium*, and *M. intracellulare*; these microorganisms do not contain bacterial endotoxin but are comparatively resistant to chemical germicides.[21-26]

Gram-negative water bacteria can multiply even in water containing relatively small amounts of organic matter, such as water treated by distillation, softening, deionization, or reverse osmosis, reaching levels of 10^5 to 10^7 microorganisms/mL[6]; these levels are not associated with visible turbidity. When treated water is mixed with dialysis concentrate, the resulting dialysis fluid is a balanced salt solution and growth medium almost as rich in nutrients as conventional nutrient broth.[6,27] Gram-negative water bacteria growing in dialysis fluids can reach levels of 10^8 to 10^9 microorganisms/mL, producing visible turbidity.

Bacterial growth in water used for hemodialysis depends on the types of water treatment system used, dialysate distribution systems, dialysis machine type, and method of disinfection (Table 25.1).[6,18,21,28,29] Each component is discussed separately next.

Microbial Contamination of Water

Water used for the production of dialysis fluid must be treated to remove chemical and microbial contaminants. The Association for the Advancement of Medical Instrumentation (AAMI) published guidelines and recommended practices for the chemical and microbial quality of water used to prepare dialysis fluid and reprocess hemodialyzers (Table 25.2).[30-33] The Centers for Medicare and Medicaid Services (CMS) has incorporated into their ESRD facility conditions for coverage infection control requirements that dialysis facilities need to follow, including water quality standards.[34] Some components of the water treatment system may allow for amplification of water bacteria. For example, ion exchangers such

TABLE 25.2 **AAMI Microbial Quality Standards for Dialysis Fluids**[31,33]

	MICROBIAL BIOBURDEN		ENDOTOXIN	
Type of Fluid	**Maximum Contaminant Level**	**Action Level**	**Maximum Contaminant Level**	**Action Level**
Water for all purposes	100 CFU/mL	50 CFU/mL	0.25 EU/mL	0.125 EU/mL
Conventional dialysate	100 CFU/mL	50 CFU/mL	0.5 EU/mL	0.25 EU/mL
Ultrapure dialysate	1 CFU/10 mL		0.03 EU/mL	
Dialysate for infusion*	This online process shall be validated by the manufacturer to produce fluid that is sterile and nonpyrogenic.			

*Compliance with a maximum bacterial level of 10^{-6} CFU/mL cannot be demonstrated by culturing, but by processes developed by the machine manufacturers.

as water softeners and deionizers do not remove endotoxin or microorganisms and provide many sites for significant bacterial multiplication.[35] Granular activated carbon adsorption media (i.e., carbon filters) are used primarily to remove certain organic compounds and available chlorine (free and combined) from water, but they also significantly increase the level of water bacteria, yeast, fungi, and endotoxins.

A variety of filters are marketed to control bacterial contamination of water and dialysis fluids. Most are inadequate, especially if they are not routinely disinfected or frequently changed. Particulate filters, commonly called *prefilters*, operate by depth filtration and do not remove bacteria or endotoxin. These filters can become colonized with gram-negative water bacteria, resulting in higher levels of bacteria and endotoxin in the filter effluent. Absolute filters, including membrane types, temporarily remove bacteria from passing water. However, some of these filters tend to clog, and gram-negative water bacteria can "grow through" the filter matrix and colonize downstream surfaces of the filters within a few days. Further, absolute filters do not reduce levels of endotoxin in the effluent water. These filters should be changed regularly in accordance with the manufacturer's directions and disinfected in the same manner and at the same time as the rest of the water distribution system.

Ultraviolet germicidal irradiation (UVGI) is sometimes used to reduce microbial contamination in water, but the use of UVGI has some special considerations. The lamp should be appropriately sized for the flow rate of water passing through the device, and the energy output should be monitored to ensure effectiveness of the lamp. Manufacturers of the lamp may require routine replacement schedule. Some bacterial populations may develop resistance to UVGI. In recirculating dialysis distribution systems, repeated exposure to UVGI are used to ensure adequate disinfection; however, this approach allows for progressive removal of sensitive microorganisms and selection of UVGI-resistant organisms. In addition, bacterial endotoxins are not affected.

Reverse osmosis (RO) is an effective water treatment modality that is used in more than 97% of US hemodialysis centers. RO possesses the singular advantage of being able to remove a variety of substances, including microorganisms and endotoxins, from supply water based primarily on particle size and adsorption to the membrane. However, low numbers of gram-negative and acid-fast organisms may penetrate the membrane or by other means (leaks around seals), and colonize downstream portions of the water distribution system. Consequently, the RO unit must be disinfected routinely.

We recommend a water treatment system that produces chemically adequate water while avoiding high levels of microbial contamination. The components in a typical water system should include (1) prefilters, (2) a water softener, (3) carbon adsorption tanks (at least two in series), (4) a particulate filter (to protect the reverse osmosis membrane), and (5) an RO unit. If one includes a deionization unit as a polisher (post–reverse osmosis unit) and a storage tank, the final component should be an ultrafilter to remove microorganisms and endotoxin. As the incoming tap water passes through the system components, it becomes more chemically pure, but the level of microbial contamination increases, which is why ultrafiltration and RO are important. Additional components or processes may be included in the pretreatment chain (see Table 25.1) depending on the pH, potable water disinfectant, and chemical quality of the incoming municipal water. If the system is adequately disinfected and properly maintained, the microbial content of water should be well within the recommended limits.

Distribution Systems

Water that has passed through the water distribution system (product water) is then distributed to individual dialysis machines where it is combined with dialysate concentrates and to a reprocessing area if a facility reprocesses hemodialyzers. It may also be combined with concentrates at a central location where the resulting dialysis fluid is supplied to the individual machines. Plastic pipe (most often polyvinyl chloride) is then used to distribute water, or dialysis fluids to the dialysis machines. Distribution systems should include the use of a loop-based system and no dead-ended pipes. Outlets to dialysis machines should have a relatively short path with the least amount of fittings and the use of valves with minimal dead space. Voids, dead ends, and large surface areas serve as sites for microbial colonization. Also large diameter pipes decrease fluid velocity and increase the wetted surface area available for microbial colonization. In addition, long pipe runs also increase the available surface area for colonization.

Gram-negative water bacteria in fluids remaining in pipes overnight can rapidly multiply and colonize wetted surfaces of the distribution system, producing microbial populations and endotoxin in quantities proportional to the total volume of the surface area. Such colonization results in the formation of protective biofilm, which is difficult to remove and protects the bacteria and other organisms from disinfection.[36] Continuous circulation of water slows down this process.[37]

Disinfection of the water or dialysate distribution system should be performed on a regular basis so that the microbial quality of the fluids is within the acceptable standards range. The frequency of disinfection should be validated by each facility and should be performed after any changes or modifications to the system.[27,38] AAMI standards and recommended practices are community consensus standards, and do not specify a schedule for disinfection other than to suggest that routine disinfection be conducted. In many instances, microbiological monitoring can be used to determine the frequency of testing of disinfection of the distribution system.[38,39] In some circumstances, repeat disinfection of the system cannot adequately control microbial growth because of established biofilm and replacement of the system is the only option.

To prevent disinfectant from draining from pipes by gravity before adequate contact time, distribution systems should be designed with all taps at equal elevation and at the highest point of the system. Furthermore, the system should be free of rough joints and dead-end pipes. Fluid trapped in such stagnant areas can serve as reservoirs for bacteria and fungi that later contaminate the rest of the distribution system.[40]

Storage tanks greatly increase the volume of fluid and surface area of the distribution system. If used, these should be designed with a conical bottom so that water exits the storage tank at its lowest point (and allows the tank to be drained), be fitted with a tight-sealing lid, be equipped with a spray head, and possess an air vent containing a bacteriological filter. If used, the storage tanks should be routinely cleaned, disinfected, and drained. To remove biofilm, use of strong oxidizers may aid in stripping biofilm from surfaces; however, physical scrubbing of the inner surfaces of the tank may be necessary. When using a storage tank, an ultrafilter should be incorporated before water is pumped into the distribution system.

Hemodialysis Machines, Effluent, and Environmental Surfaces

In the 1970s, most dialysis machines were of the recirculating or recirculating single-pass type; their design contributed to relatively high levels of gram-negative bacterial contamination in dialysis fluid. Virtually all dialysis machines in the United States now are single-pass machines (i.e., the dialysate flows through the machine once). Single-pass machines tend to respond to adequate cleaning and disinfection procedures and, in general, have lower levels of bacterial contamination than do recirculating machines. Levels of contamination in single-pass machines depend primarily on the microbiological quality of the incoming water and the method of machine disinfection.[6,38] Earlier dialysis machines had a port (waste-handling option) that allowed disposal of the extracorporeal circuit priming fluids. If one-way check valves in the waste-handling option are not maintained, checked for competency, or disinfected as recommended, it allows backflow from the effluent dialysate path into and contamination of the port and the attached bloodline. This led to outbreaks of infections among hemodialysis patients.[41-43] The waste-handling option is much less commonly used now.

The external surfaces of dialysis machines and components are also likely sources for contamination. These include frequently touched surfaces (e.g., the control panel, dialysis chairs, keyboard, shared charting computers), attached priming buckets used during the priming of the dialyzers, blood tubing draped or clipped to waste containers, or other equipment brought into the station. For example, among nine outbreaks of bacteremia, fungemia, and pyrogenic reactions not related to dialyzer reuse investigated by the Centers for Disease Control and Prevention (CDC), inadequate disinfection of the water distribution system or dialysis machines was implicated in seven (Table 25.3).[4,9,40-45] Surface contamination has been described as a potential contributor to transmission of bloodborne pathogens in the context of other poor practices.[46] A novel source of transmission has been identified: dialysis wall boxes, which contain several connections that allow the dialysis machine to hook up to the water supply and drain effluent. A large outbreak of bloodstream infections caused by *Serratia marcescens, Pseudomonas aeruginosa, Enterobacter cloacae*, and other gram-negative bacteria was identified and wall boxes were determined to be the source.[47] More work is needed to understand the role of wall boxes and other surfaces and related infection control aspects in transmission of pathogens.

Hemodialyzer Reuse

Reuse of disposable hollow-fiber dialyzers in the United States increased between 1976 and 1982, from 18% to 43% of facilities reporting reuse; the highest percentage was 82% in 1997.[48] By 2002 the percentage of facilities reporting reusing dialyzers had declined to 63%.[49] Recent data from the CDC's National Healthcare Safety Network indicated that only 1.8% of facilities reported reuse in 2017 (CDC, unpublished data). This decline coincides with decisions made by several large dialysis organizations to discontinue the practice of reuse and to only use single-use dialyzers. Although dialyzer reuse is still common in developing countries, it has become less popular in developed countries and some have plans to phase out this practice.[50,51] After a series of outbreaks of bacterial infections associated with reuse and reprocessing of dialyzers, CDC recommended that single use of dialyzers be the preferred practice and stated that it should be used whenever possible.[52]

In 1986, AAMI standards for reprocessing hemodialyzers[53] were adopted by the United States Public Health Service and was incorporated into regulation by CMS. In the United States, dialyzer reuse has not been associated with the transmission of bloodborne pathogens such as hepatitis B (HBV), hepatitis C (HCV), or human immunodeficiency

TABLE 25.3 Outbreaks of Dialysis-Associated Illnesses Investigated by the Centers for Disease Control and Prevention, 1975–2016

Description	Cause(s) of Outbreak	Corrective Measure(s) Recommended	Reference
Bacteremia, Fungemia, or Pyrogenic Reactions Not Related to Dialyzer Reuse			
Pyrogenic reactions in 49 patients	Untreated city water contained high levels of endotoxin	Install a reverse osmosis system	4
Pyrogenic reactions in 45 patients	Inadequate disinfection of the fluid distribution system	Increase disinfection frequency and contact time	40
Pyrogenic reactions in 14 patients; 2 cases of bacteremia; 1 death	Reverse osmosis water storage tank contaminated with bacteria	Remove or properly maintain and disinfect the storage tank	28
Pyrogenic reactions in 6 patients; 7 cases of bacteremia	Inadequate disinfection of water distribution system and dialysis machines; improper microbial assay procedure	Use correct microbial assay procedures; disinfect water treatment system and dialysis machines following manufacturer's recommended procedures	302
Bacteremia in 35 patients with central venous catheters (CVCs)	CVCs used as facilities' primary vascular access; median duration of infected catheters was 311 days; improper aseptic techniques	Uses CVCs when only absolutely necessary for vascular access; use appropriate aseptic technique when inserting and performing routine catheter care	303
Three pyrogenic reactions and 10 cases of bacteremia in patients treated on machines with a port for disposal of dialyzer priming fluid (waste handling option [WHO] port)	Incompetent check valves allowing backflow of fluid from the waste side of the machine into attached blood tubing; bacterial contamination of the WHO	Routine disinfection and maintenance of the dialysis machine including the WHO; check competency of WHO before patient treatment	41
Bacteremia in 10 patients treated on machines with WHO port	Incompetent backflow to allow backflow from dialysate effluent side of the machine in the WHO port and attached bloodlines	Routine maintenance, disinfection, and check for check valve competence of the WHO port	42
Outbreak of pyrogenic reactions and gram-negative bacteremia in 11 patients	Water distribution system and machines were not routinely disinfected according to manufacturer's recommendations Water and dialysate samples were cultured using a calibrated loop and blood agar plates—results always indicated no growth	Disinfect machines according to manufacturer's recommendations; include reverse osmosis water distribution system in the weekly disinfection schedule; microbiological assay should be performed via membrane filtration or spread plate using Trypticase soy agar	9
Phialemonium curvatum access infections in four dialysis patients; two of these patients died of systemic disease	Observations at the facility noted some irregularities in site preparation for needle insertion All affected patients had synthetic grafts One environmental sample was positive for *P. curvatum* (condensate pan of HVAC serving the unit)	Review infection control practices clean and disinfect HVAC system where water accumulated; perform surveillance on all patients	304
P. curvatum bloodstream infection (BSI) in two patients	Water system and dialysis machines with WHO ports not routinely maintained; water system contained dead legs and laboratory used wrong assays	Conduct routine maintenance and disinfection of machines and WHO ports; redesign water system to eliminate dead legs; have a routine schedule for disinfection of the water system	43
Outbreak of gram-negative BSI in 58 patients	Poor infection control practices, contamination from dialysis wall boxes	Improve infection control practices, cleaning and disinfection of wall boxes	47
Bacteremia/Pyrogenic Reactions Related to Dialyzer Reprocessing			
Mycobacterial infections in 27 patients	Inadequate concentration of dialyzer disinfectant	Increase formaldehyde concentration used to disinfect dialyzers to 4%	22
Mycobacterial infections in five high-flux dialysis patients; two deaths	Inadequate concentration of dialyzer disinfectant and inadequate disinfection of water treatment system	Use higher concentration of peracetic acid for reprocessing dialyzers and follow manufacturer's labeled recommendations; increase frequency of disinfecting the water treatment system	26
Bacteremia in six patients	Inadequate concentration of dialyzer disinfectant; water used to reprocess dialyzers did not meet AAMI standards	Use AAMI-quality water; ensure proper germicide concentration in the dialyzer	CDC unpublished data

Continued

TABLE 25.3 Outbreaks of Dialysis-Associated Illnesses Investigated by the Centers for Disease Control and Prevention, 1975–2016—cont'd

Description	Cause(s) of Outbreak	Corrective Measure(s) Recommended	Reference
Bacteremia and pyrogenic reactions in six patients	Dialyzer disinfectant diluted to improper concentration	Use disinfectant at the manufacturer's recommended dilution and verify concentration	60
Bacteremia and pyrogenic reactions in six patients	Inadequate mixing of dialyzer disinfectant	Thoroughly mix disinfectant and verify proper concentration	10
Bacteremia in 33 patients at 2 dialysis centers	Dialyzer disinfectant created holes in the dialyzer membrane	Change disinfectant (product was withdrawn from the market by the manufacturer)	305, 306
Bacteremia in six patients; all blood isolates had similar plasmid profiles	Dialyzers were contaminated during removal and cleaning of headers with gauze; staff not routinely changing gloves; dialyzers not reprocessed for several hours after disassembly and cleaning	Do not use gauze or similar material to remove clots from header; change gloves frequently; process dialyzers after rinsing and cleaning	59
Pyrogenic reactions in three high-flux dialysis patients	Dialyzer reprocessed with two disinfectants; water for reuse did not meet AAMI standards	Do not disinfect dialyzers with multiple germicides; more frequent disinfection of water treatment system and conduct routine environmental monitoring of water for reuse	307
Pyrogenic reactions in 14 high-flux dialysis patients; 1 death	Dialyzers rinsed with city (tap) water containing high levels of endotoxin; water used to reprocess dialyzers did not meet AAMI standards	Do not rinse or reprocess dialyzers with tap water; use AAMI-quality water for rinsing and preparing dialyzer disinfectant	308
Pyrogenic reactions in 18 patients	Dialyzers rinsed with city (tap) water containing high levels of endotoxin; water used to reprocess dialyzers did not meet AAMI standards	Do not rinse or reprocess dialyzers with tap water; use AAMI-quality water for rinsing and preparing dialyzer disinfectant	11
Pyrogenic reactions in 22 patients	Water for reuse did not meet AAMI standards; improper microbiological technique was used on samples collected for monthly monitoring	Use the recommended assay procedure for water analysis of water and dialysate; disinfect water distribution system	8
Bacteremia and candidemia among patients in seven dialysis units (in Minnesota and California)	Dialyzers were not reprocessed in a timely manner; some dialyzer refrigerated for extended periods before reprocessing; company made changes to header cleaning protocol	Reprocess dialyzers as soon as possible; follow joint CDC and dialyzer reprocessing equipment and disinfectant manufacturer guidance for cleaning and disinfecting headers of dialyzer	CDC unpublished Data
Outbreak of gram-negative BSI, including *Burkholderia cepacia* and *Stenotrophomonas maltophilia* in 17 patients	*B. cepacia* was isolated from header cleaning machine matched patient isolates Contamination likely was due to incomplete disinfection during reprocessing	Reuse was stopped	52
Transmission of Viral Agents			
26 patients seroconverted to HBsAg+ during a 10-month period	Leakage of coil dialyzer membranes and use of recirculating bath dialysis machines	Separation of HBsAg+ patients and equipment from all other patients	262
19 patients and 1 staff member seroconverted to HBsAg+ during a 14- month period	No specific cause determined; false-positive HBsAg results caused some susceptible patients to be dialyzed with infected patients	Laboratory confirmation of HBsAg+ results; strict adherence to glove use and use of separate equipment for HBsAg+ patients	309
24 patients and 6 staff seroconverted to HBsAg+ during a 10-month period	Staff not wearing gloves; surfaces not properly disinfected; improper handling of needles/sharps resulting in many staff needlestick injuries	Separation of HBsAg+ patients and equipment from susceptible patients; proper precautions by staff (e.g., gloves; handling of needles and sharps)	262
13 patients and 1 staff member seroconverted to HBsAg+ during a 1-month period	Extrinsic contamination of intravenous medication being prepared adjacent to an area where blood samples were handled	Separate medication preparation area from area where blood processing for diagnostic tests is performed	267
Eight patients seroconverted to HBsAg+ during a 5-month period	Extrinsic contamination of multidose medication vial shared by HBsAg+ and HBsAg-susceptible patients	No sharing of supplies, equipment, and medications between patients	(CDC, unpublished data)

TABLE 25.3 Outbreaks of Dialysis-Associated Illnesses Investigated by the Centers for Disease Control and Prevention, 1975–2016—cont'd

Description	Cause(s) of Outbreak	Corrective Measure(s) Recommended	Reference
Seven patients seroconverted to HBsAg+ during a 3-month period	Same staff caring for HBsAg+ and HBsAg-susceptible patients	Separation of HBsAg+ patients from other patients; same staff should not care for HBsAg+ and HBsAg– patients	264
Eight patients seroconverted to HBsAg+ during a 1-month period	Not consistently using external pressure transducer protectors; same staff members cared for both HBsAg+ patients and susceptible patients	Use external pressure transducer protectors and replace after each use; same staff members should not care for HBV-infected and -susceptible patients on the same shift	310
14 patients seroconverted to HBsAg+ during a 6-week period	Failure to review results of admission and monthly HBsAg testing; inconsistent handwashing and use of gloves; adjacent clean and contaminated areas; <20% of patients vaccinated	Proper infection control precautions for dialysis facilities; routine review of serological testing; hepatitis B vaccination of all patients	265
Seven patients on the same shift seroconverted to HBsAg+ during a 2-month period	Same staff members cared for HBsAg+ and HBsAg– patients on the same shift; common medication and supply carts were moved between stations, and multidose vials were shared	Dedicated staff for HBsAg+ patients; no sharing of equipment or supplies between any patients; centralized medication and supply areas; hepatitis B vaccination of all patients	265
Four patients seroconverted HBsAg+ during a 3-month period	Transmission appeared to occur during hospitalization at an acute care facility	Hepatitis B vaccination of all patients	265
11 patients seroconverted to HBsAg+ during a 3-month period	Staff, equipment, and supplies were shared between HBsAg+ and HBs– patients; no patients were vaccinated	Dedicated staff for HBsAg+; no sharing of medication or supplies between any patients; hepatitis B vaccination of all patients	265
Two patients converted to HBsAg+ during a 4-month period	Transmission appeared to occur during hospitalization at an acute care facility; Same staff cared for HBsAg+ and HBs– patients; no patients vaccinated	Hepatitis B vaccination of all patients; dedicate staff for the care of HBsAg+ patients; no sharing of supplies or medication between patients	268
One patient converted to HBsAg+	Transmission from a patient with history of resolved HBV infection, but the infection reactivated as a result of immunosuppression; multiple infection control breaches observed	Awareness of the reactivation/reserve seroconversion situation	271
36 patients with liver enzyme elevations consistent with non-A, non-B hepatitis	Environmental contamination with blood	Use proper precautions (e.g., gloving of staff; environmental cleaning); monthly liver function tests (e.g., ALT)	311
35 patients developed elevated liver enzymes consistent with non-A, non-B hepatitis during a 22-month period; 82% of probable cases were anti-HCV+	Inconsistent use of infection control precautions, especially hand washing	Strict compliance to aseptic technique and dialysis center precautions	312
HCV infection developed in 7 out of 40 (17.5%) HCV-susceptible patients; shift specific attack rates of 29%–36%	Multidose vials left on top of machine and used by multiple patients; routine cleaning and disinfection of surfaces and equipment between patients not routinely done; arterial line for draining prime draped into a bucket that was not routinely cleaned or disinfected between patients	Strict compliance with infection control precautions for all dialysis patients; routine HCV testing	239, 241
HCV infection developed in 5 out of 61 (8%) HCV-susceptible patients	Sharing of equipment and supplies between chronically infected and susceptible patients; gloves not routinely used; clean and contaminated areas not separated	Strict compliance with infection control precautions for all dialysis patients; CDC does not recommend separation of equipment/supplies between HCV-infected and -susceptible patients	239, 241

Continued

TABLE 25.3 Outbreaks of Dialysis-Associated Illnesses Investigated by the Centers for Disease Control and Prevention, 1975–2016—cont'd

Description	Cause(s) of Outbreak	Corrective Measure(s) Recommended	Reference
HCV infection developed in 3 out of 23 (13%) HCV-susceptible patients	Supply carts moved between stations and contained both clean and blood-contaminated items; medications prepared in the same area used for disposal of used injection equipment	Strict compliance with infection control precautions for all dialysis patients	241
HCV infection developed in 7 out of 52 (13%) HCV-susceptible patients; shift-specific attack rates 4%–21%	Medication cart moved between stations and contained both clean and blood-contaminated items; single-dose medication vials used for multiple patients; cleaning and disinfection of surfaces and equipment between patients not routinely done	Strict compliance with infection control precautions for all dialysis patients	241
HCV infection developed in 9 out of 119 (7.6%) patients; attack rate 10%	Cleaning and disinfection of surfaces and equipment between patients not routinely done; gloves not routinely used; medications not stored in separate clean area	Strict compliance with infection control precautions for all dialysis patients; perform routine HCV testing	227
HCV infections developed in 6 out of 66 (9%) patients	Clean and contaminated areas not well delineated; clean supplies accessed with contaminated gloves; medication preparation in proximity to blood specimen processing; reuse of single-dose vial	Strict compliance with infection control precautions for all dialysis patients	CDC unpublished data
HCV infections developed in 8 out of 149 (5.4%) patients; attack rate 8.6%	Multidose heparin vials taken to individual dialysis stations; poor hand hygiene and glove use; poor cleaning and disinfection practices	Strict compliance with infection control precautions for all dialysis patients	244
HCV infections developed in 18 patients; attack rate 16.7%	Poor hand hygiene and glove use; poor cleaning and disinfection practices; blood stains found on machine surfaces after cleaning	Strict compliance with infection control precautions for all dialysis patients	46
HCV infections developed in 16 patients at 9 facilities between 2013 and 2015	Multiple infection control breaches identified	Strict compliance with infection control precautions for all dialysis patients	313

ALT, Alanine aminotransferase; *HBsAg,* hepatitis B surface antigen; *HVAC,* heating, ventilation, and air conditioning.
Updates on HBV and HCV outbreaks among dialysis patients reported to CDC are available at https://www.cdc.gov/hepatitis/outbreaks/healthcarehepoutbreaktable.htm.

virus (HIV).[54,55] However, the reprocessing of dialyzers has been associated with pyrogenic reactions and bacterial infections.[54] These adverse events may be the result of the use of incorrect concentrations of chemical germicides, the failure to maintain appropriate water quality, breaks in reprocessing procedures, or practical challenges to achieving complete disinfection of reused dialyzers. Manual reprocessing of dialyzers, which is allowed in the United States, does not include testing for membrane integrity, such as a pressure-leak test, may fail to detect membrane defects, and relies on disinfection processes that are particularly difficult to standardize.[54,55]

Dialyzer reprocessing can be performed in myriad ways with few quality control checks.[52] Procedures used to reprocess hemodialyzers generally constitute high-level disinfection rather than sterilization.[20,56] Several liquid chemical germicides have been used for high-level disinfection of dialyzers. There are commercially available chemical germicides specifically formulated for this purpose (e.g., peroxyacetic acid, chlorine-based, and glutaraldehyde-based products that are approved by the US Food and Drug Administration [FDA] as sterilants or high-level disinfectants for reprocessing hemodialyzers). During the period between 1983 and 2002, the percentage of centers using formaldehyde for reprocessing dialyzers decreased from 94% to 20%, whereas the percentage using peroxyacetic acid increased from 5% to 72%. Only a minority of facilities (4%) reported used either glutaraldehyde or heat disinfection.[49]

Using a suboptimal disinfectant may lead to outbreaks of infection, such as nontuberculous mycobacteria.[20,22,54,56] An outbreak of systemic mycobacterial infections in five hemodialysis patients, resulting in two deaths, occurred when high-flux dialyzers were contaminated with *Mycobacterium abscessus* during manual reprocessing and disinfected with a commercial disinfectant prepared at a concentration that did not ensure complete inactivation of mycobacteria.[26] These and other outbreaks of infections in dialysis patients emphasize the need to reconsider the safety and necessity of dialyzer reuse.

Outbreaks of pyrogenic reactions (defined as fever or chills in a patient who was afebrile and had no signs or symptoms of an infection before the start of the dialysis treatment session) have often resulted from reprocessing hemodialyzers with water that did not meet AAMI standards (see Table 25.3). In most instances the water used to rinse dialyzers or to prepare the dialyzer disinfectants exceeded the allowable AAMI microbial or endotoxin standards, because the water distribution system was not disinfected frequently, the disinfectant was improperly prepared, or routine microbial assays were improperly performed. Several outbreaks associated with dialyzer reuse have been reported. Breaches in disinfection of dialyzer components (such as an O-ring) and contamination caused by poor infection control practices during reprocessing steps have been identified as major contributors to those outbreaks.[52,57-59] In at least one outbreak, no major breaches in reprocessing were identified. Rather, it was determined that dialyzers are difficult to reprocess safely and completely under typical conditions. This is due to poorly trained staff (often in low-paying jobs), variability in procedures, and few quality control standards.[52]

As described in the most recent investigation of a reuse associated outbreak that resulted in 17 cases, "In practice, reuse and reprocessing of dialyzers poses an increased risk for infection to patients."[52] In this investigation, each additional use of a dialyzer was associated with higher odds of bloodstream infection. In the era of affordable single-use dialyzers, dialysis providers have discontinued reuse in the interest of patient safety.[52] For facilities or regions where reuse and reprocessing continues to be performed, improved standardization of processes and rigorous quality assurance programs are needed.

High-Flux Dialysis and Bicarbonate Dialysate

High-flux dialysis uses dialyzer membranes and hydraulic permeability that are 5 to 10 times greater than conventional dialyzer membranes. There has been concern that bacteria or more likely endotoxin in the dialysate may penetrate these highly permeable membranes.

High-flux membranes require the use of bicarbonate rather than acetate dialysate. Bicarbonate dialysate must be prepared from two concentrates, an acid concentrate (acetic acid or citric acid) with a pH of 2.8 that is not conducive to microbial growth and a bicarbonate concentrate with a relatively neutral pH and a salt molarity of 1.2 M. Because the bicarbonate concentrate will support rapid growth,[60] its use can increase microbial and endotoxin concentrations in the dialysate and theoretically may contribute to an increase in pyrogenic reactions, especially when used during high-flux dialysis.

Some of the concern appeared justified by results of surveillance data during the 1990s showing a significant association between use of high-flux dialysis and reporting of pyrogenic reactions among patients during dialysis.[61] However, a prospective study of pyrogenic reactions in patients receiving more than 27,000 conventional, high-efficiency, or high-flux dialysis with bicarbonate dialysate containing high concentrations of bacteria and endotoxin found no association between pyrogenic reactions and the type of dialysis treatment.[5] Although there seems to be conflicting data on the relationship between high-flux dialysis and pyrogenic reactions, centers providing high-flux dialysis should ensure that dialysate meets AAMI microbial standards (see Table 25.2).

Disinfection of Hemodialysis Systems

Routine disinfection of isolated components of the dialysis system often produces inadequate results. Consequently, the total dialysis system (water treatment system, distribution system, and dialysis machine) should be included in the disinfection procedure.

Disinfection of dialysis systems usually employs sodium hypochlorite solutions, hydrogen peroxide solutions, commercially available peracetic acid disinfectants, ozone, and, in some systems, hot water pasteurization. Sodium hypochlorite solutions are convenient and effective in most parts of the dialysis system when used at the manufacturer's recommended concentrations. Also, the test for residual available chlorine to confirm adequate rinsing is simple and sensitive. However, because chlorine is corrosive, it is usually rinsed from the system after a relatively short dwell time of 20 to 30 minutes. The rinse water invariably contains organisms that can multiply to significant levels if the system is permitted to stand overnight.[27] Therefore disinfection with chlorine-based disinfectants are best used before the start of the first patient treatment session rather than at the end of the day. However, for models of machines that most dialysis facilities are using, options for disinfection include heat at the end of the day and use of other disinfectants with longer contact time that also require overnight dwell. There is no need to disinfect the fluid pathway between patients.

Aqueous formaldehyde, peroxyacetic acid, hydrogen peroxide, or glutaraldehyde solutions can produce good disinfection results.[18,62,63] These products are not as corrosive as hypochlorite solutions and can be allowed to dwell in the system for long periods of time when the system is not in operation. However, formaldehyde, which has good penetrating power, is considered an environmental hazard and potential carcinogen and has irritating qualities that may be objectionable to staff.[64] The US Environmental Protection Agency has also limited the amount of formaldehyde that can be discharged into the wastewater stream, which has drastically reduced the use of this chemical in the dialysis community as a disinfectant. Peroxyacetic acid and glutaraldehyde are commercially available and are designed for use with dialysis machines when used according to the manufacturers labeled instructions. Glutaraldehyde use is also limited because it is considered a sensitizer and may pose a risk to healthcare workers.

Some dialysis systems (both water treatment and distribution systems, some hemodialysis machines) use hot-water disinfection (pasteurization) for control of microbial contamination. In this type of system water heated to >80°C (176°F) is passed through the water distribution system and hemodialysis machine or just the hemodialysis machine at the end of the day. These systems are excellent for controlling microbial contamination. However, it should be noted that heat disinfection of the hemodialysis machine would not

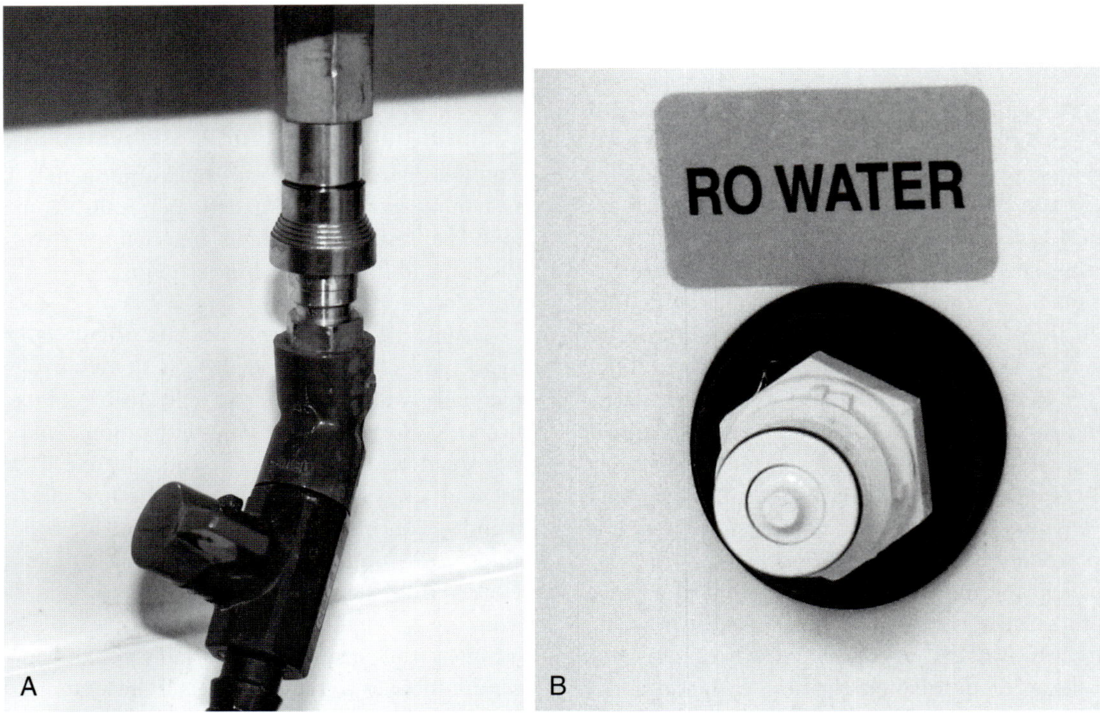

FIG. 25.1 Example of sources to sample water. (A) Connection on water distribution loop, with added adapter to facilitate water sampling. (B) Water connection inside wall box, where water sample can be taken. (Photos courtesy Stephanie Booth.)

control microbial contamination of the waste lines and effluent drains. Additional processes may be needed to disinfect waste lines, drains, and wall boxes.

Monitoring of Water and Dialysis Fluid

Microbiological and endotoxin standards for water and dialysis fluids (see Table 25.2)[30,39,65-67] were originally based on the results of culture assays performed during outbreak investigations. There is increasing evidence that the microbial quality of hemodialysis fluids plays a role in the chronic inflammatory response syndrome, affects anemia management, accelerates loss of residual renal function, and affects serum albumin levels in dialysis patients.[68-82] Increasing data suggest that use of ultrapure water and dialysate would benefit maintenance hemodialysis patients and potentially save costs.[83,84] A large cohort study from Japan found a lower all-cause mortality in facilities using ultrapure water.[85] However, there have been no randomized controlled studies to evaluate and confirm these studies, so regulatory agencies have not yet mandated these higher water standards.[83]

Water samples for routine testing should be collected from a source as close as possible to where water enters the dialysate proportioning unit. In most cases this is the tap (not from that hose connecting the tap to the dialysis machine) at the dialysis station (Fig. 25.1). Water samples should be collected at least monthly from several locations within the dialysis unit, including samples at different dialysis stations. Samples should also be collected using a similar approach after any modifications or maintenance have been made to the water treatment system water distribution system. Dialysate samples should be collected during or at the end of the dialysis treatment from a source close to where the dialysis fluid either enters or leaves the dialyzer (Fig. 25.2). Dialysate samples should be collected at least monthly from a representative number of dialysis machines. Samples of water and dialysate should also be collected when a pyrogenic reaction is suspected. If centers reprocess hemodialyzers for reuse, water used to prepare disinfectant and rinse dialyzers should also be assayed monthly.[30,66] The maximum contaminant levels for water are 100 CFU/mL and 0.25 EU/mL (see Table 25.2).[30,31,33] Methods for microbiological and endotoxin testing are available elsewhere.[86]

In an outbreak investigation, the assay methods may need to be both qualitative and quantitative; also detection of nontuberculous mycobacteria and in some cases fungi in water or dialysate may be desirable. In such instances, plates should be incubated for 5 to 14 days at both 36°C and 28° to 30°C. Laboratories should be notified of special testing requests outside of routine water testing, such as if the facilities would like to look for specific pathogens.

DIALYSIS-ASSOCIATED PYROGENIC REACTIONS

Gram-negative bacterial contamination of dialysis water or components of the dialysis system (water, dialysate, water used for reprocessing) can cause pyrogenic reactions. A pyrogenic reaction is defined as objective chills (visible rigors) or fever (oral temperature ≥ 37.8°C [100°F]) or both in a patient who was afebrile (oral temperature up to 37°C [98.6°F]) and

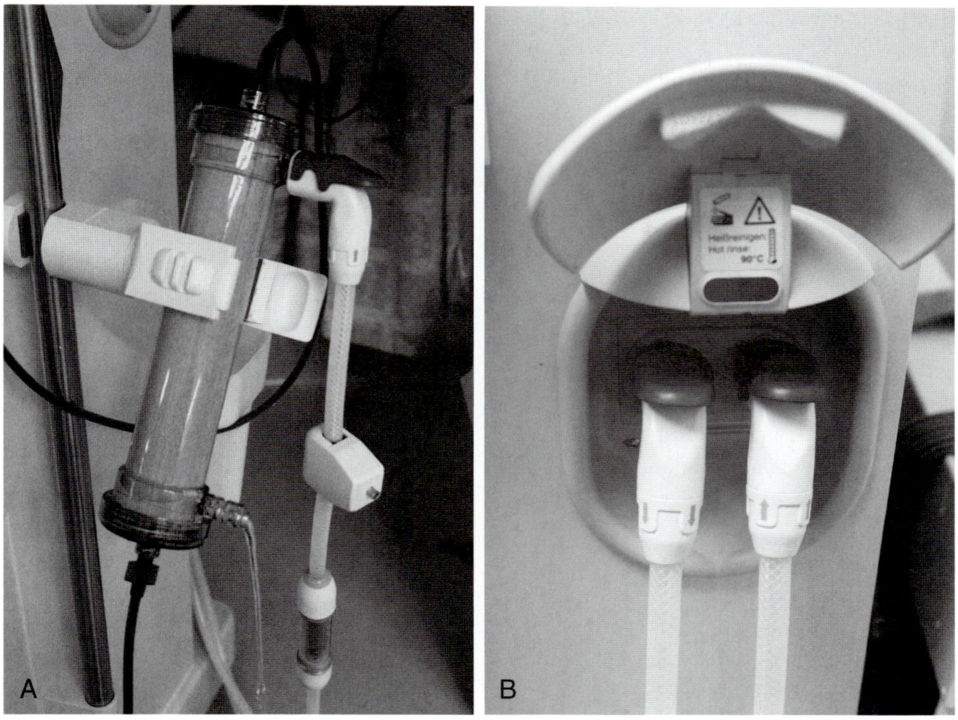

FIG. 25.2 Examples of sources to sample dialysate. (A) Dialyzer port. (B) Hansen connector ports. (Photos courtesy Stephanie Booth.)

had no signs or symptoms of an infection before the start of the dialysis treatment session.[87,88] Depending on the type of dialysis system and the level of contamination, fever and chills may start 1 to 5 hours after dialysis has been initiated. Other symptoms may include hypotension, headache, myalgia, nausea, and vomiting. Pyrogenic reactions can occur without bacteria; because presenting signs and symptoms cannot differentiate bacteremia from pyrogenic reactions, blood cultures are necessary.

During 1990–2002 an annual average of 20% to 24% of the hemodialysis centers in the United States reported at least one pyrogenic reaction in the absence of septicemia in their patients undergoing maintenance hemodialysis.[48,49,89-97] Pyrogenic reactions can result from passage of bacterial endotoxin (lipopolysaccharide) or other substances in the dialysate across the dialyzer membrane[98-102] or from the transmembrane stimulation of cytokine production in the patient's blood by endotoxin in the dialysate.[99,103-105] In other instances, endotoxin can enter directly into the bloodstream with fluids that are contaminated with gram-negative bacteria.[106] The signs and symptoms of pyrogenic reactions without bacteremia generally abate within a few hours after the dialysis has been stopped. If gram-negative sepsis is associated, fever and chills may persist and hypotension is more refractory to therapy.[4,106]

When a patient develops a pyrogenic reaction (i.e., onset of fever or chills) while being dialyzed, the following steps are recommended: (1) careful physical examination of the patient to identify signs and symptoms and evaluate other possible causes of chills and fever (e.g., pneumonia, vascular access site infection); (2) blood cultures, other diagnostic tests (e.g., chest radiograph), and other cultures as clinically indicated; (3) collection of dialysate from the dialyzer (i.e., postdialyzer effluent sample) for quantitative and qualitative microbiological culture; and (4) recording of the incident in a log or other permanent record. In addition, empiric antibiotic treatment should be administered to the patient. Determining the cause of such episodes is important because they may be the first indication of a remediable problem that can affect a potentially large number of patients.

The higher the level of bacteria and endotoxin in dialysis fluid, the higher the probability that the bacteria or their products will pass through the dialyzer membrane to produce bacteremia or stimulate cytokine production. In an outbreak of febrile reactions among patients undergoing hemodialysis, the attack rates were directly proportional to the level of microbial contamination in the dialysis fluid.[6] Prospective studies also reported a lower pyrogenic reaction rate among patients when they underwent dialysis with dialysis fluid from which most bacteria had been removed by filtration, compared with patients who underwent dialysis fluid that was highly contaminated (mean 19,000 CFU/mL).[5,87,107]

DISINFECTION, STERILIZATION, AND ENVIRONMENTAL CLEANING IN DIALYSIS FACILITIES

Good cleaning, disinfection, and sterilization procedures are important components of the infection control program in the hemodialysis center. The procedures do not differ from those recommended for other healthcare settings,[108,109] but the high potential for blood contamination makes the hemodialysis setting unique. In addition, the need for routine aseptic access of the patient's vascular system makes the hemodialysis unit more akin to a surgical suite than to a standard hospital room. Medical items are categorized as critical (e.g., needles and catheters), which are introduced directly into the bloodstream or normally sterile areas of the body; semicritical (e.g., fiberoptic endoscopes), which come in contact with intact mucous membranes; and noncritical (e.g., blood pressure cuffs), which touch only intact skin.[109,110]

Cleaning and housekeeping in the dialysis center have two goals: to remove soil and waste on a regular basis, thereby preventing the accumulation of potentially infectious material, and to maintain an environment that is conducive to good patient care.[110] Crowding of patients and patient stations, as well as overtaxing of staff members, may increase the likelihood of microbial transmission. Adequate cleaning may be difficult if there are multiple wires, tubes, and hoses in a small area. There should be enough space to move completely around each patient's dialysis station without interfering with the neighboring stations. According to the Facility Guidelines Institute, each dialysis station should be at least 80 square feet and allow at least 4 feet distance between stations to avoid contamination.[111] However, most of dialysis facilities do not have space to meet that guideline. To avoid contamination, cleaning should only start when patients have left the station and staff should not allow new patients into chairs until cleaning and disinfection is complete. Creating unit-wide patient-free intervals between treatment shifts is likely to improve the adequacy of station cleaning and disinfection between patients.

Where space is limited, elimination of unneeded items, orderly arrangement of required items and removal of excess lengths of tubes, hoses, and wires from the floor can improve accessibility for cleaning. Because of the special requirements for cleaning in the dialysis center, staff should be specially trained in this task.

After each patient treatment, frequently touched environmental surfaces, including external surfaces of the dialysis machine, should be properly disinfected; some surfaces may also require precleaning (with a detergent) before disinfection. A study in the Netherlands and an investigation of a large HCV outbreak in the United States where the investigators used chemiluminescent agents to detect nonvisible blood contamination have demonstrated the importance of environmental cleaning.[46,112] Antiseptics, such as formulations with povidone-iodine, hexachlorophene, or chlorhexidine, should not be used for surface disinfection because these are formulated for use on skin and are not designed for use on hard surfaces. Given the role of environmental surfaces of components adjacent to the machine (e.g., wall boxes) in transmission of pathogens, as illustrated in recent outbreak,[47] attention should be paid to cleaning and disinfection of those surfaces as well.

BLOODSTREAM INFECTIONS AND OTHER INFECTIONS

The annual adjusted mortality rate among hemodialysis patients is 169 per thousand patient-years at risk. Infection is the second leading cause of mortality in this patient population, accounting for 8% of all deaths.[1] In a number of published studies that have evaluated bacterial infections in outpatient hemodialysis, bacteremia occurred in 0.6% to 1.7% of patients per month and vascular access infections (VAIs; with or without bacteremia) in 1.3% to 7.2% of patients per month.[113-123] A review of four studies published during 2002 estimated that 1.8% of hemodialysis patients have vascular access associated bacteremia each month, amounting to 50,000 episodes nationally per year.[124] In a study of 27 French hemodialysis centers, 28% of 230 infections in hemodialysis patients involved the vascular access, whereas 25% involved the lung, 23% the urinary tract, 9% the skin and soft tissues, and 15% other or unknown sites.[119]

Because of the importance of bacterial infections in hemodialysis patients, the CDC initiated a voluntary ongoing surveillance system in the United States called the Dialysis Surveillance Network (DSN) in 1999.[122] At the time, only bacterial infections associated with hospital admission or intravenous antimicrobial receipt were counted; as a result, this system likely only detected more severe infections. During 1999–2001, 109 dialysis centers reported data. Rates per 100 patient-months were 3.2 for all VAIs (including access infections both with and without bacteremia), 1.8 for vascular access associated bacteremia, 1.3 for wound infection not related to the vascular access, 0.8 for pneumonia, and 0.3 for urinary tract infection. Among patients with fistulas or grafts, wounds were the most common site for infection. Among patients with hemodialysis catheters, infections of the vascular access site were the most common site for infection.[122] The surveillance project expanded and evolved into National Healthcare Safety Network (NHSN), of which Dialysis Event Surveillance is a component (https://www.cdc.gov/nhsn/dialysis/index.html). The NHSN is an Internet-based surveillance system that enables facilities to report healthcare-associated infection data to the CDC. VAIs in dialysis patients and related events are reported to NHSN's Dialysis Event Surveillance. Outpatient hemodialysis facilities in the United States eligible to participate in the surveillance are instructed to follow a standard protocol,[125] by which all outpatients who receive hemodialysis at the facility are monitored for three NHSN-defined dialysis events. The three types of dialysis events (positive blood culture; intravenous antimicrobial start; and pus, redness, or increased swelling at the vascular access site) are reported using a standard data collection form. During 2007–2011, 193 facilities reported to NHSN; the rate of bloodstream infection (BSI) and access-related BSI was 1.27 and 0.88 per 100 patient-months, respectively.[126] Data reported to NHSN have been used by CMS as part of the ESRD Quality Incentive Program since 2012; as a result, almost all outpatient hemodialysis facilities now report to NHSN. In 2014 more than 6000 facilities now reported 160,971 events, including 29,516 BSIs and 22,576 access-related BSIs; the rate of BSI was 0.64 per 100 patient-months. The rate of BSI was much higher among patients with a central venous catheter (2.16 per 100 patient-months) compared with other vascular access types.[127]

Vascular Access Infections

Access site infections are particularly important because they can cause disseminated bacteremia or loss of the vascular access. Local signs of VAI include erythema, warmth, induration, swelling, tenderness, breakdown of skin, loculated fluid, or purulent exudates.[116,117,122,128] Based on data from DSN collected during 1995–2005, the overall VAI rate was 3.1 per 100 patient-months and varied from 0.6 for fistulas to 10.1 for temporary catheters.[129] In the 2014 NHSN surveillance data report, the VAI rate was 1.21 per 100 patient-months.[127] The access-related BSI rate was 0.49 per 100 patient-months, which varied by access type: 0.16 for fistulas, 0.27 for grafts, and 1.83 for central venous catheters (tunneled and nontunneled).

VAIs are caused (in descending order of frequency) by *Staphylococcus aureus* (32% to 53% of cases), coagulase negative staphylococci (20% to 32% of cases), gram-negative bacilli (10% to 18%), other gram-positive cocci (including enterococci; 10% to 12%), and fungi (<1%).[122,129,130] Among BSIs, *S. aureus* remained the most commonly reported pathogen in 2014 NHSN data (31% of BSI and 32% of access-related BSI), and 40% of cases of *S. aureus* were resistant to methicillin.[127]

The primary risk factor for vascular access–related infection is access type, with catheters having highest risk for infection; grafts intermediate; and native arteriovenous (AV) fistulas the lowest.[115,116,120,127,129,130] Other potential risk factors for VAI include (1) location of the access in the lower extremity; (2) recent vascular access surgery; (3) trauma, hematoma, dermatitis, or scratching over the access site; (4) poor patient hygiene; (5) poor needle insertion technique; (6) older age; (7) diabetes; (8) immunosuppression; (9) iron overload; (10) intravenous drug use; and (11) chronic inflammatory state.[116,117,131-136]

Based on the relative risk for both infectious and noninfectious complications, native AV fistulas are considered the preferred vascular access type; a goal of no more than 10% of patients maintained with permanent catheter–based hemodialysis treatment is recommended.[137-141] To minimize infectious complications, patients should be referred early for creation of an arteriovenous access, thereby decreasing the time dialyzed through a temporary catheter. During the period between 1995 and 2002, the percentage of patients dialyzed through fistulas increased from 22% to 33%, with most of the increase occurring after 1999.[49] Data from Dialysis Outcomes and Practice Patterns Study indicated that from August 2010 to August 2013, AV fistula use increased from 63% to 68%, whereas catheter use declined from 19% to 15%.[142] However, the majority of incident patients still initiated dialysis with a catheter. The US Renal Data System (USRDS) annual data report for 2016 indicated that whereas 18.8% of prevalent hemodialysis patients used a catheter, 80.3% of incident patients started dialysis with a catheter.[1]

Etiology and Prevention of Bloodstream Infection

Bacterial pathogens causing infection can either be exogenous (i.e., acquired from contaminated dialysis fluids or equipment) or endogenous (i.e., caused by invasion of bacteria present in or on the patient). Catheter-related infections are most often caused by bacteria from the patient's skin colonizing the outside of the catheter or from direct contact (e.g., touch contamination by healthcare personnel) with the catheter hub, leading to contamination of the inner surface of the catheter. Surveillance data indicate that *S. aureus* and other coagulase-negative staphylococci were the most common pathogens for BSI and access-related BSI.[127,130] Endogenous sources may also be more likely causes of VAI among fistula and graft patients. Contaminated infusates and hematogenous spread are thought to be less common causes of BSI in this patient population, regardless of vascular access type.

Exogenous pathogens have caused numerous outbreaks, most of which resulted from inadequate dialyzer reprocessing procedures (e.g., contaminated water or inadequate disinfectant concentration) or inadequate disinfection and maintenance of the water treatment and distribution system. During 1995–2006, five outbreaks were traced to contamination of the waste handling option on one type of dialysis machine.[41-43,143-145] Recommendations to prevent such outbreaks have been published elsewhere.[146]

Contaminated medication vials are also a source of bacterial infection for patients. In 1999, an outbreak of *Serratia liquefaciens* bloodstream infections and pyrogenic reactions among hemodialysis patients was traced to contamination of vials of erythropoietin. These vials, which were intended for single use, were contaminated by repeated puncture to obtain additional doses and by pooling of residual medication into a common vial.[147]

Recommendations for preventing VAIs have been developed by the CDC[148] and the Healthcare Infection Control Practices Advisory Committee[149] and the National Kidney Foundation.[137-141] The CDC has developed a recommended "Approach to BSI Prevention in Dialysis Facilities" that includes core interventions to prevent BSI among hemodialysis patients (Table 25.4). Facilities that implemented this set of interventions were able to reduce their access-related BSI rates and sustained these lowered rates for at least 4 years.[150] The core interventions include (1) BSI surveillance using NHSN and feedback to clinical staff; (2) hand hygiene observations with feedback to staff; (3) catheter/vascular access care observations to ensure clinical staff adherence to aseptic technique and good infection control practices (with staff feedback); (4) development of staff infection prevention skills, demonstrated through competency assessments; (5) patient education and engagement in infection control processes; (6) decrease catheter prevalence; (7) catheter hub disinfection; and (8) bacitracin zinc/polymyxin B sulfate (Polysporin) triple ointment or povidone-iodine ointment applied to catheter exit sites. The CDC has also developed tools, protocol, and guidance to assist in the implementation of the interventions (https://www.cdc.gov/dialysis/prevention-tools/index.html).

Other strategies that might assist in implementation of recommended interventions include staff engagement and safety culture. Use of a behavioral change strategy ("Positive Deviance"), in which positive BSI prevention practices by certain staff were encouraged among all staff, was found to contribute to the reduction of BSI in one dialysis facility.[151]

TABLE 25.4 Core Interventions for Dialysis Bloodstream Infection Prevention

Surveillance and feedback using NHSN	Conduct monthly surveillance for BSIs and other dialysis events using NHSN, and actively share results with frontline clinical staff.
Hand hygiene observations	Perform observations of hand hygiene opportunities monthly and share results with clinical staff.
Catheter/vascular access care observations	Perform observations of vascular access care and catheter accessing quarterly. Assess staff adherence to aseptic technique when connecting and disconnecting catheters and during dressing changes. Share results with clinical staff.
Staff education and competency	Train staff on infection control topics, including access care and aseptic technique. Perform competency evaluation for skills such as catheter care and accessing every 6–12 months and on hire.
Patient education/ engagement	Provide standardized education to all patients on infection prevention topics.
Catheter reduction	Incorporate efforts (e.g., through patient education, vascular access coordinator) to reduce catheters by identifying and addressing barriers to permanent vascular access placement and catheter removal.
Chlorhexidine for skin antisepsis	Use an alcohol-based chlorhexidine (>0.5%) solution as the first-line skin antiseptic agent for central line insertion and during dressing changes.
Catheter hub disinfection	Scrub catheter hubs with an appropriate antiseptic after cap is removed and before accessing.
Antimicrobial ointment	Apply triple antibiotic ointment or povidone-iodine ointment to catheter exit sites during dressing change.

Additional recommendations for preventing hemodialysis-catheter–associated infections include (1) using sterile technique and maximal sterile barrier precautions (cap, mask, sterile gown, large sterile drapes, and gloves) during catheter insertion; (2) limiting use of noncuffed catheters to 3 to 4 weeks; (3) restricting catheter manipulation and dressing changes to trained personnel; (4) replacing catheter site dressing if damp, loosened, or soiled.[148,152]

A number of studies have looked at the use of various antimicrobial locks to prevent catheter-related BSI among hemodialysis patients. Two meta-analyses of these studies concluded that (1) antimicrobial catheter lock solutions reduce catheter-related bloodstream infections and the (2) use of these lock solutions should be considered in routine clinical practice in conjunction with other prevention modalities.[153,154] However, the long-term consequence of using antibiotics routinely in catheter locking solutions is unknown. CDC and the Healthcare Infection Control Practices Advisory Committee guidelines recommend lock solutions in patients with multiple BSIs despite optimal adherence to aseptic technique.[149] Routine prophylactic use of antimicrobial lock solutions for hemodialysis catheter–related BSI is not recommended at this time.[148,155]

In hemodialysis patients, the Infectious Diseases Society of America has recommended treatment with nasal mupirocin in documented *S. aureus* carriers who have catheter-related BSI with *S. aureus* and continue to need a hemodialysis catheter.[156,157] Otherwise the routine use of nasal mupirocin in patients with hemodialysis catheters is not recommended by either the CDC or the National Kidney Foundation.[137,138,148] The CDC also updated the Guidelines for the Prevention of Intravascular Catheter-Related Infections and included the recommendation of using chlorhexidine-impregnated dressings to protect the insertion site of short-term, nontunneled central venous catheters in patients aged 18 years and older (https://www.cdc.gov/infectioncontrol/guidelines/bsi/c-i-dressings/recommendations.html). However, no recommendations were made for patients with long-term, tunneled catheters, and the effect of chlorhexidine-impregnated dressings on reducing catheter-related bloodstream infections among hemodialysis patients remains unclear.[158,159]

A recently developed chlorhexidine-impregnated catheter cap (ClearGuard®) has been reported in a cluster randomized trial to reduce catheter-related BSIs and hospital admissions for BSI.[160] A needle-free connector (TEGO® needle-free hemodialysis connector [ICU Medical, Inc., San Clemente, Calif.]) was found to be significantly associated with less intravenous antibiotic use among hemodialysis patients; however, the risk for catheter-related BSI among patients who used the connector was not statistically significantly decreased.[161]

Poor injection safety practices have led to BSI among dialysis patients, and thus improving injection practices should be considered as a strategy to reduce the spread of both bloodborne viruses (e.g., hepatitis B and C) and BSIs.[147] To reduce the risk for infection, the CDC recommends (a) preparing medications in a clean room or, if a clean room is not available, in an area separated from the patient treatment area and designated for medications; (b) performing hand hygiene and using aseptic technique when preparing medication; (c) disinfecting the rubber septum of vials with alcohol and using a new needle and a new syringe to withdraw medication; (d) discarding single-dose vials and storing multidose vials appropriately; (e) not handling or storing used supplies, equipment, blood samples, or biohazard containers in or adjacent to areas where medications and clean (i.e., unused) equipment and supplies are handled; (f) delivering medications separately to each patient and not using common carts within the patient treatment area to prepare or distribute medications; and (g) performing hand hygiene, putting on new, clean gloves, scrubbing the injection port with antiseptic, and using aseptic technique when administering medications.[162] Intravenous medication vials labeled for single use, including erythropoietin, should not be punctured more than once. Multidose medication vials should be assigned to a single patient whenever possible.[163]

Respiratory Infections

Hospital admissions for pneumonia have been declining overall for dialysis patients; however, pneumonia rates for hemodialysis patients are 1.8 to 2.0 times that of renal transplant recipients or peritoneal dialysis patients. Hospital admissions for pneumonia are also 102% higher among hemodialysis patients compared with the general population.[164] In one study of a group of 433 dialysis patients over a 9-year period, pneumonia was the third most common cause of infection (after vascular access and infections below the knee) and accounted for 13% of all infections.[165] One- and five-year survival probabilities are 0.55 and 0.17, respectively. Pneumonia is common among hemodialysis patients, carries a poor prognosis, and is often the antecedent to cardiovascular death.[166,167] A recent analysis of incident hemodialysis patients found pneumonia to be associated with chronic obstructive pulmonary disease, inability to transfer or ambulate, hemodialysis as initial therapy, advanced age (≥75 years), and body mass index ≥ 30 kg/m^2.[167] According to the Advisory Committee on Immunization Practices, patients with chronic renal failure should be vaccinated with the pneumococcal polysaccharide vaccine.[168] Both 13-valent pneumococcal conjugate vaccine and 23-valent pneumococcal polysaccharide vaccine can be used; the schedule depends on the vaccination status of patients and is available on the CDC website (https://www.cdc.gov-/dialysis/pdfs/vaccinating_dialysis_patients_and_patients_dec2012.pdf).

Patients with chronic kidney diseases, including hemodialysis patients, are at high risk for developing complications of seasonal influenza,[169] which can be effectively prevented by vaccination. Influenza vaccination is associated with lower risk for hospitalization and death in ESRD patients.[170] Although transmission of influenza, even during pandemics, in US dialysis clinics is not evident through the published literature, anecdotal reports of transmission exist. Because of their higher risk for complications, it is important to maintain influenza vaccination coverage among hemodialysis patients. In addition to influenza vaccination for patients, vaccination for dialysis providers (clinicians, nurses, technicians) is also important. Vaccination for healthcare personnel has been found to decrease absenteeism and healthcare-facility acquired influenza.[171-173] However, coverage among dialysis healthcare personnel was still suboptimal: data indicated that only 73% of healthcare personnel in dialysis clinics received influenza vaccination in the 2011–2012 season.[174] Annual vaccination is therefore recommended for both dialysis patients and healthcare personnel.[169]

ESRD patients with latent tuberculosis (TB) infection are at higher risk for developing TB disease. For this reason, the CDC recommends that all dialysis patients be tested at least once on admission for latent TB infection or TB disease using a tuberculin skin test or TB blood test.[175] Patients who test positive should be evaluated for treatment and for the presence of TB disease. TB transmission in US dialysis facilities has been very rare. The most recently reported instance occurred in 2003 when an infected healthcare worker transmitted the bacteria to patients and other healthcare workers at a dialysis facility.[176] Another episode in 1998 involved a patient with smear-positive pulmonary TB, but no transmission to other patients at the dialysis facility was identified.[177] Suspected or confirmed TB exposure occurring within a dialysis facility should be reported to the appropriate state or local public health authority.

A new emerging respiratory infection, Middle East respiratory syndrome (MERS) caused by a corona virus, was first reported in 2012.[178] No MERS infections or transmissions have been reported in the United States, but because of their significance and transmissibility, healthcare facilities, including dialysis clinics, should remain vigilant for MERS and other respiratory pathogens.

To prevent the transmission of respiratory infections (e.g., influenza) in dialysis facilities, staff should have systems in place to detect patients with respiratory symptoms on presentation to the facilities and implement interventions to decrease transmission. Facilities should educate patients about respiratory hygiene and provide necessary supplies such as tissues, mask, and hand hygiene materials. Patients should be encouraged to notify facility staff of any respiratory symptoms when they arrive. Facilities should also have policies that encourage dialysis healthcare personnel to not work while sick with respiratory infection.[179] For new and emerging pathogens, dialysis providers should maintain awareness of current issues and recommendations from state and local public health departments and the CDC. Any possible instances of transmission of one of these new and emerging pathogens in a dialysis facility should be reported to public health authorities.

Antimicrobial-Resistant Bacteria

Hemodialysis patients have been in the forefront of the epidemic of antimicrobial resistance, especially vancomycin resistance. One of the earliest reports of vancomycin-resistant enterococci (VRE) was from a renal unit in London in 1988.[180] The prevalence of VRE stool colonization among dialysis patients has varied from 1.5% among pediatric dialysis patients in the United Kingdom[181] and 2.4% of adult dialysis patients at three dialysis centers in Indianapolis, Indiana,[182] to 9.5% at a university hospital in Baltimore, Maryland.[183] In one center the prevalence of rectal carriage of VRE was 9%, and 2% of noncarriers developed VRE infections in 1 year.[184] A meta-analysis of studies from 100 facilities and 4800 patients worldwide reported a pooled VRE colonization prevalence of 6.2%.[185] It appears that hospital acquisition of VRE contributes substantially to the increasing prevalence of VRE in the maintenance hemodialysis patient population.[186] Among enterococci causing bloodstream infections in hemodialysis patients, up to 11.4% have been reported to be resistant to vancomycin.[122,127,187,188]

Vancomycin resistance in *S. aureus* has also been reported in dialysis patients. Five of the first six US patients with infections associated with vancomycin-intermediate *S. aureus* were receiving either peritoneal dialysis or hemodialysis.[189,190] In addition, the first US patient found to be infected with a vancomycin-resistant *S. aureus* (VRSA) strain was a maintenance hemodialysis patient; the VRSA was isolated from a diabetic foot wound and from a temporary central venous catheter exit site.[191] In the period between 2002 and 2009 there were nine cases of VRSA in the United States; three of these patients had chronic renal failure and two were hemodialysis patients.[192, 193] Five of those VRSA cases occurred in southeastern Michigan and contained a plasmid carrying the vanA gene, which had been donated from a VRE donor.[194] To date, 14 cases of VRSA have been reported to the CDC, of which the most recent case was in a dialysis patient.[195] A guide to investigation and control of VRSA is available from the CDC[196] and includes suggested strategies for VRSA control in dialysis centers.

The percentage of hemodialysis facilities reporting methicillin-resistant *S. aureus* (MRSA) infection or colonization has increased from 40% in 1995[96] to 76% in 2002.[49] In a 2005 CDC study assessing the incidence of invasive MRSA infection among dialysis patients, the incidence of invasive MRSA infection was found to be 42.5 cases per 1000 dialysis patient population.[197] This is approximately 100-fold higher than the general population, in which rates for invasive MRSA infection are 0.2 to 0.4 cases per 1000 population. The rate of invasive MRSA infections among hemodialysis patients appears to be decreasing.[198] In 2015, invasive MRSA incidence had decreased to 14.8 cases per 1000 population, still much higher than the incidence among general population.[199] A study in the United Kingdom of VAIs found that MRSA was responsible for 30% of *S. aureus* catheter-related infections in hemodialysis patients.[200] In the United States, 30.6% of BSIs in hemodialysis patients were caused by *S. aureus* and 39.5% of the *S. aureus* BSI isolates were methicillin-resistant strains.[127]

Patients with chronic kidney disease, including end-stage renal disease, are at high risk for *Clostridium difficile* infection (CDI).[201] Limited data are available on CDI among dialysis patients in the United States. In a review of USRDS (Medicare claims) data between 2005 and 2008, 4.25% of dialysis patients were diagnosed with first episode of CDI.[202] In a cohort of dialysis patients followed from 1999 to 2007, 14.3% of hemodialysis patients developed CDI (a rate of 8.3 cases per 100 patient-years).[203] The UK Renal Registry reported an incidence of 1.09 CDI per 100 patient-years among hemodialysis patients in 2013–2014.[204] An outbreak of CDI in a hemodialysis facility has been reported. The outbreak investigation revealed several challenges in prevention and control of CDI among dialysis patients (e.g., shared patient environment and equipment, lack of physical barriers between patient treatment stations, and adequacy of typical cleaning and disinfection procedures).[205] CDI control strategies that were employed during this outbreak included designation of select dialysis stations as CDI contact isolation stations, use of dedicated, disposable gown and gloves by staff while caring for a patient in contact isolation, handwashing with soap and water after caring for CDI patients, use of 1:10 dilution of bleach to disinfect environmental surfaces in stations after treatment of CDI patients, and heightened diligence to ensure adequate wet contact time of bleach on surfaces.

To combat emerging antimicrobial resistance in dialysis patients, one must understand the transmission kinetics involved with each organism. For certain patients, including those infected with MRSA or VRE, contact precautions are used in the hospital setting.[162] The CDC has not recommended routine use of contact precautions in hemodialysis centers for patients infected or colonized with multidrug-resistant organisms (MDROs). Transmission of pathogenic bacteria is well documented in hospitals. At least one study has suggested that the majority of transmission and acquisition of resistant pathogens among dialysis patients occurs when these patients are admitted to the acute care setting.[186] However, studies have demonstrated MDRO spread in dialysis centers.[205,206] The CDC recommends additional precautions be used during treatment of patients who might be at higher risk for transmitting pathogenic bacteria (i.e., those with an infected skin wound with drainage that is not contained by dressings or fecal incontinence or uncontrolled diarrhea). These interventions include the following: (1) Staff members treating the patient should wear a separate gown over their usual clothing and remove the gown when finished caring for the patient; (2) patients should be dialyzed at a station away from the main flow of traffic and with as few adjacent stations as possible (e.g., at the end or corner of the unit).[162] However, preventing transmission of resistant pathogens depends primarily on adherence to basic infection control practices and these additional practices. More work is needed to understand the transmission of targeted MDROs in dialysis settings and the effectiveness of interventions to reduce transmission.

One major contributor to the development of antimicrobial-resistant bacteria is inappropriate use of antimicrobial drugs. Antibiotics are commonly used in dialysis patients, especially vancomycin, cefazolin, and third- and fourth-generation cephalosporins. In a small study, as many as 30% of antibiotic indications were found to be inappropriate.[207] Reasons for those inappropriate uses and possible strategies for improved antibiotic stewardship in dialysis facilities have been proposed.[208] More data are needed to understand the relationship between antibiotic prescribing patterns in dialysis centers and antibiotic resistance to better target potential stewardship activities.[209]

HEPATITIS C VIRUS

HCV is a single-stranded RNA virus that belongs to the family *Flaviviridae*.[210] HCV was first recognized as non-A, non-B hepatitis virus in 1974 until cloning of the etiological agent in 1989.[211-213] HCV is a relatively efficiently transmitted bloodborne viral pathogen in the dialysis setting. It is not as efficiently transmitted as HBV in this setting, and generally, recommended infection control practices do prevent transmission among hemodialysis patients (without need for isolation).[162,214-216] However, new acquisition of hepatitis C infection continues to occur among maintenance hemodialysis patients and outbreaks of hepatitis C are far more common than outbreaks of hepatitis B in the dialysis setting.

Epidemiology

In 2002, 63% of dialysis centers tested patients for antibodies against HCV (anti-HCV). In the facilities that performed screening, the incidence rate in 2002 was 0.34%, and among these centers, the prevalence of anti-HCV among patients was 7.8%, a decrease of 25.7% since 1995.[49] Only 11.5% of dialysis facilities reported newly acquired HCV infection among their patients. Higher incidence rates have been reported from cohort studies of dialysis patients in the United States (<1% to 3%), Japan (<2%), and Europe (3% to 15%).[217-224] Higher prevalence rates (10% to >85%) also have been reported in individual facilities and in other countries.[220,224-229]

HCV is moderately stable in the environment and can survive drying and environmental exposure to room temperature for at least 16 hours.[230] Longer survival, up to several weeks, has been reported.[231] HCV is most efficiently transmitted by direct percutaneous exposure to blood, and like HBV, the chronically infected patient is central to the epidemiology of HCV transmission. Risk factors associated with HCV infection among hemodialysis patients include blood transfusions from unscreened donors, injection drug use, low staff-to-patient ratios, dialysis in a facility with high HCV prevalence, and number of years on dialysis.[217,223,232-236] The number of years on dialysis is a risk factor that is independently associated with higher rates of HCV infection. Multiple studies found that as the time patients spent on dialysis increased, their prevalence of HCV infection increased.[217,236-238]

These studies, as well as investigations of dialysis-associated outbreaks of hepatitis C infection, indicate that HCV transmission most likely occurs because of inadequate infection control practices.[239] The practices that have been found to be associated with higher prevalence of HCV in dialysis facilities include handling blood specimens near medication preparation area or other clean areas, use of a mobile cart to distribute medications, poor disinfection of priming buckets, and inconsistent cleaning of dialysis machines.[240] The CDC tracks HCV outbreaks in dialysis settings (https://www.cdc.gov/hepatitis/outbreaks/healthcarehepoutbreaktable.htm); during 1998–2008, the CDC helped investigate five outbreaks of HCV infection among patients in hemodialysis centers.[241,242] From 2008 to 2015, 18 outbreaks involving at least 98 newly infected patients were reported to the CDC.[243] In those outbreaks a common finding was that seroconversions were associated with receiving dialysis immediately after or at a machine adjacent to a chronically infected patient.[46,244] Multiple opportunities for cross-contamination were observed in the involved facilities, including (a) equipment and supplies that were not disinfected between patient use; (b) use of common medication carts to prepare and distribute medications at patient stations; (c) sharing of multiple dose vials, which were used at patients' stations (e.g., observed to be placed on the top of the hemodialysis machine); (d) contaminated priming buckets that were not routinely changed or cleaned and disinfected between patients; (e) machine surfaces that were not routinely cleaned and disinfected between patients; and (f) blood spills that were not cleaned up promptly. Investigation of an outbreak involving four different clusters found multiple lapses in infection control and blood contamination of environmental surfaces as a result of poor cleaning and disinfection practice.[46] In these outbreaks, a single common exposure event is rarely identified, and many outbreaks involve separate chains of transmission occurring over time. Moreover, it has been noted that station turnover procedures are rushed and disinfection of machine surfaces is initiated before the patient has left the treatment station. These common practices are challenges to proper cleaning and disinfection and prevention of cross-transmission of bloodborne pathogens such as HCV.

Other traditional risk factors for acquiring HCV include injection drug use, exposure to an HCV-infected sexual partner or household contact, multiple sexual partners, and perinatal exposure.[245,246] The efficiency of transmission in settings involving sexual or household exposure to infected contacts is low, and the magnitude of risk and the circumstances under which these exposures result in transmission are not well defined. When a new HCV infection (includes acute, symptomatic infection or HCV seroconversion) occurs in a dialysis facility, it should be assumed that the infection was healthcare related and investigated as such. State and local health departments to whom these infections should be reported have extensive expertise in evaluating traditional risk factors that the patient might have in addition to healthcare exposures.

Treatment for HCV infection has gained significant achievements in the past several years, and recent data have indicated that ESRD patients infected with HCV can be treated successfully.[247,248] All dialysis patients with HCV infection should be referred to care and assessment. Because dialysis in a facility with high HCV prevalence is a risk factor for HCV infection, HCV treatment may reduce the number of infected patients and therefore help decrease the number of new infections. However, the effect of HCV treatment on transmission of HCV in dialysis facilities is unknown.

Screening and Diagnostic Tests

FDA-licensed or approved tests to screen for HCV antibodies (anti-HCV) in the United States comprise immunoassays, immunoblot assays, and immunochromatography-based rapid tests. None discriminate between active and resolved HCV infection, and confirmatory recombinant immunoblot tests have been discontinued.[249] All individuals who test anti-HCV positive should be further tested for HCV RNA by an FDA-approved nucleic acid test to determine current infection status.[250]

Routine testing of hemodialysis patients for anti-HCV on admission and every 6 months has been recommended since 2001.[162] For routine HCV screening of hemodialysis patients, the anti-HCV screening immunoassay (either rapid test or laboratory-based assay) is recommended, and if positive, this should be confirmed with HCV RNA testing (Box 25.1).[250]

Prevention of Hepatitis C Virus Transmission

Lessons from investigations of HCV outbreaks in dialysis indicate that breaches in infection control practices are the

BOX 25.1 Interpretation of Test Results for Hepatitis C Virus Infection

Anti-HCV Positive

An anti-HCV positive result is consistent with current HCV infection, past HCV infection that has resolved, or biological false positivity for HCV antibody. Test for HCV RNA to identify current infection.

HCV RNA Positive

An HCV RNA–positive result indicates current (active) infection.

All HCV RNA–positive persons should receive counseling, undergo medical evaluation, and be considered for treatment.

Anti-HCV Negative

Anti-HCV negative result is defined as an anti-HCV screening test negative.

An anti-HCV–negative individual is considered uninfected. However, patients with exposure within the previous 6 months should be tested for HCV RNA or have a follow-up anti-HCV test ≥6 months after last exposure.

Anti-HCV, Antibody to hepatitis C virus.

major contributors to HCV transmission. The following recommendations can be applied to prevent transmission of HCV in dialysis facilities (https://emergency.cdc.gov/han/han00386.asp): (1) Evaluate infection control practices in each facility and ensure adherence to infection control standards. CDC audit tools can be used to help assess practices such as injection medication preparation and administration, hand hygiene, and routine environmental surface cleaning and disinfection; (2) promptly address any gaps in infection control identified; (3) ensure dialysis staff are aware of and trained to implement infection control guidelines[162]; (4) follow CDC recommendations for HCV screening of hemodialysis patients and management of patients who test positive; (5) immediately report any case of new HCV infection among patients undergoing hemodialysis to the state or local health department. Any new HCV infections among hemodialysis patients should be investigated.[251]

HCV-positive patients do not have to be isolated from other patients or dialyzed separately on dedicated machines and can participate in dialyzer reuse programs.[252] They should be referred for evaluation and treatment according to current medical practice guidelines.

HEPATITIS B VIRUS

HBV is the most highly efficiently transmitted pathogen in the dialysis setting. Recommendations for control of hepatitis B in hemodialysis setting were first published in 1977,[253] and by 1980 their widespread implementation was associated with a sharp decrease in the incidence of HBV infection among both patients and staff members.[254, 255] In 1982 the hepatitis B vaccine was recommended for all susceptible patients and staff members.[256] Hepatitis B vaccination is currently the standard of care and is recommended to all susceptible hemodialysis patients. The vaccine series should ideally be administered before starting dialysis for ESRD.[162]

Epidemiology

During the early 1970s, HBV infection was endemic in maintenance hemodialysis units and outbreaks were common. Subsequently, the incidence and prevalence of HBV infection among maintenance hemodialysis patients in the United States has declined dramatically and by 2002 was 0.12% and 1%, respectively.[49] Data from 2002 indicated that newly acquired HBV infections were reported by 2.8% of US hemodialysis centers, and 27.3% of centers reported one or more chronically infected patients.[49] New hepatitis B infections in hemodialysis patients are now rarely reported.

The chronically infected patient is central to the epidemiology of HBV transmission. HBV is transmitted by percutaneous (i.e., puncture through the skin) or mucosal (direct contact with mucous membranes) exposure to infectious blood or body fluids that contain blood. All hepatitis B surface antigen (HBsAg)–positive persons who are also positive for hepatitis Be antigen (HBeAg) have an extraordinary level of HBV circulating in their blood, approximately 10^8 to 10^9 virions per milliliter.[257, 258] With virus titers this high in blood, body fluids containing serum or blood may also contain high levels of HBV and are potentially infectious. Furthermore, HBV at titers of 10^2 to 10^3 virions/mL can be present on environmental surfaces in the absence of any visible blood and still cause infection.[257, 259-261]

HBV is relatively stable in the environment and has been found to remain viable for at least 7 days on environmental surfaces at room temperature.[257,259,261] HBsAg has been detected in dialysis facilities on hemostats, scissors, dialysis machine control panels, and door knobs.[261] Thus blood-contaminated surfaces that are not routinely cleaned and disinfected represent a reservoir for HBV transmission. Dialysis staff members can transfer virus to susceptible patients through contamination in the environment.[257,259,261]

Most HBV outbreaks among hemodialysis patients (see Table 25.3) were caused by cross-contamination to patients via (1) environmental surfaces, supplies (e.g., hemostats, clamps, etc.), or equipment that were not routinely clean and disinfected after each use; (2) multiple-dose vials or intravenous solutions that were not used exclusively for one patient; (3) medications for injections that were prepared adjacent to areas where blood samples were handled; and (4) staff members who simultaneously provided care for both infected (HBsAg-positive) patients and susceptible patients.[106,262-268] Once the factors that promote HBV transmission among hemodialysis patients were identified, recommendations for control were published.[253]

The segregation of HBsAg-positive patients and their equipment from HBV-susceptible patients resulted in 70% to 80% reduction in the incidence of HBV infections among hemodialysis patients.[255,269,270] The success of isolation practices in preventing transmission of HBV infection is linked to other infection control practices, including routine serological surveillance and routine cleaning and disinfection. Frequent serological testing for HBsAg detects patients recently infected with HBV so that isolation procedures can be implemented before cross-contamination can occur. Environmental control by routine cleaning and disinfection procedures reduces the opportunity for cross contamination, either directly from environmental surfaces or indirectly by hands of personnel.

In past studies, independent risk factors among maintenance hemodialysis patients for acquiring HBV infection included the presence of ≥1 HBV-infected patient in the hemodialysis facility who was not isolated, as well as a vaccination rate <50% among patients.[89] However, transmission has been rarely reported in the United States in the past 20 years because of high rates of vaccination, screening, and isolation. The most recent documented transmission in a dialysis clinic in the United States was due to reactivation of hepatitis B infection that occurred in a patient with previous infection who became antigen positive as a result of immunosuppression.[271] The CDC has received anecdotal reports of atypical hepatitis B serological test results among dialysis patients that may represent reactivation of HBV infection or HBV mutant strains; however, no further cases of dialysis-related transmission have been identified.

Other risk factors for acquiring HBV infection include injection drug use, sexual and household exposure to HBV-infected contacts, exposure to multiple sexual partners, male homosexual activity, and perinatal exposure. Dialysis patients should be educated about these and other risks and, for those patients with active HBV infection (HBsAg positive), informed that their sexual partners and household contacts should be vaccinated.[272-274] HBV-infected patients should be evaluated for HBV treatment.

Screening and Diagnostic Tests

Several well-defined antigen-antibody systems are associated with HBV infection, including HBsAg and antibody to HBsAg (anti-HBs); hepatitis B core antigen (HBcAg) and antibody to HBcAg (anti-HBc); and HBeAg and antibody to HBeAg (anti-HBe). Serological assays are commercially available for all of these except for HBcAg because no free HBcAg circulates in the blood. One or more of these serological markers are present during different phases of HBV infection (Table 25.5).[275] HBV infection can also be detected using qualitative or quantitative tests for HBV DNA.[276,277] These tests are most commonly used for HBV-infected patients being managed with antiviral therapy.[278-282]

In some individuals the only HBV serological marker detected is total anti-HBc (i.e., isolated anti-HBc). Among most asymptomatic persons in the United States tested for HBV infection, an average of 2% (range: <0.1% to 6%) test positive for anti-HBc[283]; among injecting drug users, however, the rate is 24% to 28%.[284,285] This pattern can occur after HBV infection among individuals who have recovered but whose anti-HBs have waned or among individuals who have low-level chronic HBV infection and failed to develop anti-HBs. It may also represent a false positive total anti-HBc result or someone in the window of infection. HBV DNA has been detected in <10% of individuals with isolated anti-HBc, and these individuals are unlikely to be infectious to others except under unusual circumstances involving direct percutaneous exposures to large quantities of blood (e.g., transfusion).[286-288] In most persons with isolated anti-HBc, the result appears to be false positive. Data from several studies have indicated that a primary anti-HBs response develops in most of these individuals after a three-dose series of hepatitis B vaccinations.[289,290] No data exist on response to vaccination among hemodialysis patients with this serological pattern. Testing and follow-up recommendations for hemodialysis patients with isolated anti-HBc are available.[162]

TABLE 25.5 Interpretation of Serological Test Results for Hepatitis B Virus Infection

SEROLOGIC MARKERS				
HBsAg	Total Anti-HBc	IgM Anti-HBc	Anti-HBs	Interpretation
–	–	–	–	Susceptible, never infected
+	–	–	–	Acute infection, early incubation
+	+	+	–	Acute infection
–	+	+	–	Acute resolving infection
–	+	–	+	Past infection, recovered and immune
+	+	–	–	Chronic infection
–	+	–	–	False positive (i.e., susceptible), past infection, or low-level chronic infection
–	–	–	+	Immune if titer ≥ 10 mIU/mL

Anti-HBc, Antibody to hepatitis B core antigen; *Anti-HBs,* antibody to hepatitis B surface antigen; *HBsAg,* hepatitis B surface antigen; *IgM,* *Immunoglobulin M.*

Prevention of Hepatitis B Virus Transmission

The following recommendations can be applied to prevent transmission of HBV in hemodialysis facilities: (1) serological screening of patients (and staff members) for HBV infection, including monthly testing of all susceptible patients for HBsAg; (2) HBV vaccination of susceptible patients (and patient care staff); (3) isolation of all HBsAg-positive patients in a separate room; (4) assignment of staff members to HBsAg-positive patients and not to HBV-susceptible patients during the same or overlapping shifts; (5) assignment of dedicated dialysis equipment to HBsAg-positive patients; (6) cleaning and disinfection of nondisposable items (e.g., hemostats, clamps, scissors) before use on another patient; (7) glove use whenever patient or hemodialysis equipment is touched and glove changes and hand hygiene between each

TABLE 25.6 Schedule for Routine Testing for Hepatitis B Virus and Hepatitis C Virus Infections

Patient Status	On Admission*	Monthly	Semi-Annual	Annual
All patients	HBsAg, Anti-HBc (total), Anti-HBs, Anti-HCV, ALT			
HBV susceptible, including vaccine nonresponders		HBsAg		
Anti-HBs positive (≥10 mIU/mL), anti-HBc negative				Anti-HBs
Anti-HBs and Anti-HBc positive		No additional testing is needed		
Anti-HCV negative		ALT	Anti-HCV	

ALT, Alanine aminotransferase.
*Results of HBV testing should be known before patient begins dialysis.

patient (and station); and (8) routine cleaning and disinfection of equipment and environmental surfaces.[162,253] Because dialysis patients can have waning immunity to hepatitis B vaccine, patients who require one or more booster doses of vaccine should not be cared for by the same staff as infected patients.

HEPATITIS DELTA VIRUS

Delta hepatitis is caused by the hepatitis delta (HDV), a relatively small defective virus that causes infection only in persons with active HBV infection. The prevalence of HDV infection is extremely low in the United States, with rates <1% among HBsAg-positive persons in the general population and >10% among HBsAg-positive persons with repeated percutaneous exposures (e.g., intravenous drug users, persons with hemophilia).[291]

Only one transmission of HDV among dialysis patients has been reported in the United States.[292] In this episode, transmission occurred from a patient who was chronically infected with HBV and HDV to an HBsAg-positive patient after a massive bleeding incident; both patients received dialysis at the same station. Therefore, in dialysis settings, HDV-infected patients should be isolated from other HBV-infected patients.

HUMAN IMMUNODEFICIENCY VIRUS INFECTION

During 1985–2002, the percentage of US hemodialysis centers that reported providing maintenance hemodialysis for patients with HIV infection increased from 11% to 39% and the proportion of patients with known HIV infection increased from 0.3% to 1.5%.[49] Although the proportion of patients with HIV infection has remained stable during the past decade, the number of infected patients has increased, as has the number of centers treating patients with HIV infection. HIV is transmitted by blood and other body fluids that contain blood. No patient-to-patient transmission of HIV has been reported in a US hemodialysis center. However, there have been reports of transmission of HIV among patients in other countries. All these outbreaks have been attributed to several breaks in infection control: (a) reuse of access needles and inadequately disinfected equipment, (b) sharing of syringes among patients, and (c) and sharing of dialyzers among different patients.[293-297] The most recent reported outbreak involved three new HIV infections and was associated with sharing of multidose heparin vials, inadequately disinfected hemodialysis equipment, and dialysis staff who used blood-contaminated gloves to manipulate vascular access for multiple patients.[298] Adherence to recommended infection control practices is adequate to prevent HIV transmission in dialysis facilities.[162]

OTHER EMERGING INFECTIONS

In 2014 the largest outbreak of Ebola in history occurred in West Africa. Healthcare personnel caring for Ebola patients are at high risk for becoming infected, and during this outbreak, a significant number of healthcare personnel acquired the virus.[299] Other high-consequence pathogens have continued to be identified, including *Candida auris*, a yeast that is resistant to multiple antifungals.[300] Dialysis center staff and management should prepare for the possible introduction of highly virulent pathogens into their communities and dialysis centers by developing contingency plans, improving baseline adherence to recommended infection prevention practices, and strengthening communication channels with public health departments. The CDC has released on its website recommendations for infection control to prevent transmission of *C. auris* (https://www.cdc.gov/fungal/diseases/candidiasis/c-auris-infection-control.html), including dialysis-specific recommendations.

SUMMARY OF RECOMMENDATIONS AND FUTURE DIRECTIONS

Preventing transmission of pathogens and reducing healthcare-associated infections among maintenance hemodialysis patients requires implementation of a comprehensive infection control program that can support consistent adherence to infection control recommendations (Table 25.6; Boxes 25.2 to Box 25.4) among all staff members. Adherence to core prevention practices (see Table 25.4) has been found to sustainably reduce highly morbid bloodstream infections among dialysis patients with central venous catheters. An active infection control program is the foundation of these efforts. The components of such a program include routine

BOX 25.2 Recommended Infection Control Practices for Hemodialysis Units

Infection Control Precautions for All Patients

- Hand hygiene should be performed:
  - Before and after having direct contact with a patient's intact skin
  - After contact with blood, body fluids or excretions, mucous membranes, non-intact skin, or wound dressings
  - After contact with inanimate objects (including medical equipment) in the immediate vicinity of the patient
  - If hands will be moving from a contaminated-body site to a clean-body site during patient care
  - After glove removal
- Wear disposable gloves when caring for the patient or touching the patient's equipment at the dialysis station; remove gloves and perform hand hygiene (if hands are visibly soiled wash with soap and water) between each patient or station.
- Items taken into the dialysis station should be disposed of or cleaned and disinfected before taken to a common clean area or used on another patient.
  - Nondisposable items taken to the patient treatment station that cannot be cleaned or disinfected (e.g., adhesive tape) should be discarded after use.
  - Unused medications (including multi-dose vials) or supplies (syringes, alcohol swabs, etc.) taken to the patient's station should be used only for that patient and should not be returned to a common clean area or used on other patients.
- When multidose medication vials are used (including vials containing diluents), prepare individual patient doses in a clean (centralized) area away from dialysis stations and deliver separately to each patient. Do not carry multidose medication vials from station to station.
- Do not use common medication carts to deliver medications to patients. Do not carry medication vials, syringes, alcohol swabs, or supplies in pockets. If trays are used to deliver medication to individual patients, they must be cleaned between patients.
- Clean areas should be clearly designated for the preparation, handling, and storage of medications and unused supplies and equipment. Clean areas should be clearly separated from contaminated areas where used supplies and equipment are handled. Do not handle and store medications or clean supplies in the same or adjacent area to where used equipment or blood samples are handled.
- Use external transducer protectors (venous or arterial) for each patient treatment to prevent blood contamination of the dialysis machine's pressure monitoring equipment. Change these external transducer protectors between each patient treatment and when they become wet, and do not reuse them. The redundant internal transducer protectors do not need to be changed routinely between patients. If the external transducer protectors are contaminated with blood the internal transducer protector should be assessed for contamination before dialyzing another patient with the same machine.
- Clean and disinfect the dialysis station (chairs, beds, tables, machines, etc.) between patients.
  - Start cleaning only when patient has left the station and only admit new patient after cleaning and disinfection are complete
  - Give special attention to cleaning control panels on the dialysis machine and other surfaces that are frequently touched and potentially contaminated with patient's blood.
  - Discard all fluid, and clean and disinfect all surfaces and containers associated with the prime waste (including buckets attached to the machines).
- For dialyzers and blood tubing that will be reprocessed, cap dialyzer ports and clamp tubing. Place all used dialyzers and tubing in a leak-proof containers for transport from station to reprocessing or disposal area.

Modified from Centers for Disease Control and Prevention, *Recommendations for preventing transmission of infections among chronic hemodialysis patients.* MMWR Recomm Rep, 2001. 50(RR-5): pp. 1-43.

BOX 25.3 Hepatitis B Vaccination

- Vaccinate all susceptible patients against hepatitis B
- Test for anti-HBs 1–2 months after the last dose
  - If anti-HBs is <10 mIU/mL, consider patient susceptible, revaccinate with an additional three doses, and retest for anti-HBs
  - If anti-HBs is >10 mIU/mL, consider immune and retest annually
- Give booster dose of vaccine if anti-HBs declines to <10 mIU/mL and continue to retest annually

BOX 25.4 Management of HBsAg-Positive Patients

- Follow infection control practices for hemodialysis units for all patients.
- Dialyze HBsAg-positive patients in a separate room using separate machines, equipment, instruments, and supplies.
- Staff members caring for HBsAg-positive patients should not care for HBV-susceptible patients at the same time (e.g., during same shift or during patient change over).

FDA Safety Alert. Modified from Centers for Disease Control and Prevention, *Recommendations for preventing transmission of infections among chronic hemodialysis patients.* MMWR Recomm Rep, 2001. 50(RR-5): pp. 1-43.

implementation of infection prevention and control practices specifically designed for the hemodialysis setting: (1) each dialysis facility should have at least one staff member with basic infection control knowledge and experience in addition to being able to access personnel with advanced infection control expertise; (2) infection prevention training and education should be provided to both staff and patients; (3) regular auditing of infection prevention practices should be conducted (audit and assessment tools are available at https://www.cdc.gov/dialysis/prevention-tools/index.html); (4) a culture of safety should be developed, including engaged leadership and involvement of frontline staff in infection prevention efforts; (5) routine serological testing and immunization of patients and staff should be performed; (6) infection surveillance should be conducted and the data used for continuous quality improvement; and (7) systems should be in place for public health reporting. An excellent review of those essential components of an infection prevention program is available elsewhere.[301] The CDC has also published recommendations describing these components in detail.[162]

Future Directions

Infection control strategies that prevent HBV infection among hemodialysis patients have been well established; however, some questions remain. More work is needed to determine the ideal hepatitis B vaccine dosage regimen for pre- and postdialysis pediatric patients and for predialysis adult patients, as well as the optimal timing for follow-up testing and administration of booster doses among vaccine responders. Also, reports of patients with mutant HBV, patients with reverse seroconversion, and patients with atypical HBV serological test results highlight the need for more research to evaluate their significance in dialysis population. Further work is needed to clarify the specific factors responsible for transmission of HCV among hemodialysis patients and to evaluate the effect of current prevention recommendations, HCV treatment, and other strategies on prevention and control of HCV infection in this setting.

VAIs continue to be a devastating complication among patient receiving maintenance hemodialysis; additional interventions are needed to further reduce rates of these infections. Finally, other important questions about the role dialysis centers play in the spread of MDROs and the effectiveness of interventions designed to prevent MDRO transmission require further investigation.

Acknowledgments

We would like to thank Dr. Saleem Kamili and Ms. Anne Moorman from Division of Viral Hepatitis, Centers for Disease Control and Prevention, for their thoughtful comments. We would like to thank Ms. Stephanie Booth for her contribution to the chapter.

A full list of references is available at www.expertconsult.com.

26

Acute Complications of Hemodialysis

Brendan Bowman, MD, and Mitchell H. Rosner, MD

OUTLINE

Hemodialysis (HD) was first performed in 1945, and since then, millions of patients have undergone this lifesaving and life-sustaining therapy. Technological advances in dialyzer, dialysate, and dialysis machine designs have occurred over the past 70 years, and these have been supplemented with enhanced patient monitoring and the development of safety rules and regulations that govern the operation of HD units.[1] Furthermore, nursing and technical staff at dialysis units are highly trained and certified in their ability to care for patients undergoing HD. In combination, all these factors have increased safety for patients undergoing HD. However, acute complications and safety risks still occur in the HD unit, and the clinician must be aware of these possibilities and ready to intervene to keep patients safe.

HD units are highly complex sites for care where many care providers interact with advanced technology to care for patients with numerous comorbid health conditions. With this complexity comes a risk to patient safety and possible complications associated with the dialysis procedure. A survey by Holley[2] identified an adverse event and error rate of 1 out of every 733 treatments, with dialysis access events, medical errors, circuit clotting, and patient falls as the most common events. Another survey from the National End-Stage Renal Disease (ESRD) Patient Safety Initiative[3] ranked the top five safety issues for HD units as (1) patient falls; (2) medication errors (including deviation from dialysis prescription, allergic reactions, and medication omissions); (3) access-related events (clotting, infiltrates, poor blood flow, difficult cannulation); (4) dialyzer errors (incorrect dialyzer or dialysate and equipment-related sepsis); and (5) excess blood loss or prolonged bleeding. This chapter will focus on acute complications that occur in the HD patient as well as discuss other issues that affect provision of the safest possible HD treatment to patients.

INVESTIGATING AN ADVERSE EVENT ON HEMODIALYSIS

All adverse events that occur during a dialysis session require thorough, stepwise, and multidisciplinary investigation. The process whereby adverse events are investigated is termed a *root cause analysis* (RCA). RCAs seek to identify the origin of a problem using a specific set of steps and tools that aim to determine what happened, why it happened, and what to do to reduce the likelihood that it will happen again. In general, RCA identifies issues in one or more of three broad categories: (1) physical causes, in which a material or machine failed in some way; (2) human causes, in which people did not follow procedures or did something wrong; and (3) organizational causes, in which systems, processes, or policies are faulty. In many cases, issues in several domains may coexist.

Some general principles should follow any dialysis-related incident. Once the patient is stabilized, a complete incident report should be filed and reviewed with the medical director and unit supervisor. If there is any concern regarding the dialysis machine, tubing, dialyzer, or other equipment, these components should be sequestered and inspected by biomedical engineers. The medical director and unit supervisor should also be on alert for clustering of cases that could represent larger issues. Each dialysis unit should have an RCA team that will review the incident report, patient's chart, dialysis log, and unit maintenance reports (including water cultures, conductivity, water system quality reports, and others). The results of the RCA process should lead to improvement plans that are communicated to all parties.

ACUTE REACTIONS OCCURRING DURING HEMODIALYSIS

Adverse reactions occurring during HD may be caused by the exposure of patient blood to surface components of the extracorporeal circuit, including the dialyzer, tubing, and other compounds used in the manufacturing and sterilization processes. This interaction between the patient's blood and the extracorporeal system can lead to various adverse reactions that can range in severity from mild to life-threatening anaphylactic/anaphylactoid reactions.[4]

Anaphylaxis and Anaphylactoid Reactions

Anaphylaxis is a life-threatening allergic reaction that is rapid in onset and typified by symptoms such as hives, pruritus, angioedema, shortness of breath, wheezing, stridor, hypotension, shock, and cardiovascular collapse. Typically, the reaction is due to the release of inflammatory mediators and cytokines from mast cells and basophils that are usually triggered by immunoglobulin E (IgE) binding to an antigen in a sensitized host. Occasionally, nonimmunological mechanisms that lead to direct degranulation of mast cells and basophils (such as that seen with exposure to contrast media) can be operative, and these are termed *anaphylactoid* or *nonimmune anaphylaxis*.[5] The World Health Organization defines anaphylaxis as when any one of the following three events occurs within minutes or, rarely, hours after exposure to a potential antigen: (1) involvement of the skin or mucosal tissue plus either respiratory difficulty or a low blood pressure causing symptoms; (2) two or more of the following symptoms after likely contact with an allergen: (a) involvement of the skin or mucosa, (b) respiratory difficulties, (c) low blood pressure, or (d) gastrointestinal (GI) symptoms; or (3) low blood pressure after exposure to a known antigen.[6]

Dialysis patients are exposed to numerous antigens that could trigger a reaction, and symptoms may develop at any time during the treatment, although characteristic patterns may give clues as to the inciting agent. For example, symptoms that occur within the first 5 minutes after starting treatment point toward issues with the dialyzer, tubing, or dialysate. Symptoms may also be somewhat atypical in ESRD patients, and they include burning or heat sensation throughout the body or at the access site; dyspnea; chest pressure or tightness; angioedema/laryngeal edema; acral or oral paresthesia; rhinorrhea; lacrimation; sneezing or coughing; flushing; pruritus; and nausea/vomiting, abdominal cramps, and diarrhea. Any of these symptoms should prompt consideration that the patient may be having a reaction that requires prompt attention.

Reactions Associated With the Dialysis Circuit

Although reactions to the components of the dialysis circuit are uncommon, it is important to understand the risks associated with exposure of the patient's blood to these components (including the blood tubing, dialysis membranes, sterilizing reagents, and dialysate solutions). In the recent past, acute reactions in patients undergoing HD were more common and were related to the use of bioincompatible, complement-activating dialysis membranes and acetate-containing dialysate solutions; exposure to polyacrylonitrile (PAN) dialysis membranes that stimulated the production of bradykinin; and ethylene oxide sterilization of dialyzers.[7] Studies in the 1980s reported a frequency of approximately 1 reaction in every 12,000 HD episodes; more contemporary data are not available, but reactions are thought to be less frequent.[8]

Allergic reactions occurring during dialysis can be classified by timing and severity: Type A reactions occur within the first 5 to 20 minutes of the HD session and patients develop typical anaphylaxis-type symptoms, whereas type B reactions occur later in the session and symptoms are milder.[9] It has been thought that type A reactions are IgE mediated, whereas type B reactions are anaphylactoid and may be more related to activation of the complement cascade.[9] Given that patients undergoing dialysis are exposed to numerous stimuli (dialysis membrane, dialysate, blood tubing lines, and medications), a careful and thorough assessment of these exposures must be undertaken in any patients who suffer a reaction.

Previously, ethylene oxide was routinely used as a gas sterilizer for dialysis membranes and could lead to IgE-mediated type A reactions. However, the use of ethylene oxide has dramatically decreased and most dialyzers are now sterilized with steam, electron beam, or γ radiation. Likewise, reactions to dialysis membranes were common when cellulose components were used.[10] The cellulose fiber could activate the complement cascade, leading to type B reactions. However, most United States dialysis centers now use synthetic membranes (composed of polymethylmethacrylate, polyether sulfone, polysulfone, or PAN), which are biocompatible and have a much lower risk of reactions.[11] Another source of reactions was seen when dialysis membranes underwent processing for reuse, and in these cases, patients may have been exposed germicides (formaldehyde, glutaraldehyde, and peracetic acid/hydrogen peroxide) that can elicit life-threatening reactions.[12] The near abandonment of reuse in the United States makes these reactions rare.

Despite these changes to alternative sterilization methods and biocompatible dialysis membranes, reactions still occur and, in some cases, may be related to the dialysis membrane. PAN is a negatively charged synthetic membrane, which is composed of a copolymer of acrylonitrile and an aryl sulfonate.[13] In the 1990s, severe anaphylactoid reactions were reported in patients dialyzed with PAN membranes who were also taking angiotensin-converting enzyme (ACE) inhibitors.[14] Binding of Hageman factor XII to a negatively charged membrane leads to formation of kallikrein from prekallikrein and the subsequent release of kinins (i.e., bradykinin) from kininogen. Although cuprophane and polymethylmethacrylate membranes display an ability to activate factor XII, PAN activates it to a greater extent.[15] Bradykinin, a molecule with a very short half-life, in turn activates production of prostaglandin and histamine release, with subsequent vasodilatation and increased vascular permeability.[16] ACE inactivates bradykinin, and therefore ACE inhibitors can prolong the biological activities of bradykinin, which are highly calcium dependent. PAN membranes pretreated with positively charged polyethyleneimine are associated with markedly reduced bradykinin activation, although it is safer to simply use another dialysis membrane for these patients.[17]

Several anaphylactoid reactions have also been reported in patients dialyzed with bleach reprocessed polysulfone membranes and treated with ACE inhibitors.[18] These reactions ceased once the use of bleach was discontinued. Furthermore, a cluster of anaphylactoid reactions was reported in patients dialyzed with different membranes (acrylonitrile 69) who were also taking ACE inhibitors.[19] Hydrogen peroxide/peracetic acid was the reprocessing agent used, and the reactions abated once reprocessing was discontinued, despite continued use of ACE inhibitors.[20]

Recently case series of patients developing acute reactions to dialysis membranes of the polyarylsulfone family (polysulfone, polyethersulfone) have been reported.[21] Typically, patients developed symptoms within the first 30 minutes of dialysis (dyspnea, hypotension, hypoxia, bronchospasm, chest pain, urticaria, and pruritus). Reactions in half of the patients occurred in the first week after starting dialysis with the membrane and in many cases after the first contact. However, another half of patients developed reactions at variable times after exposure (range 1 to 36 months). A careful analysis of these reactions could not isolate the sterilization method, housing materials, or potting materials as causes. Instead, the reactions appeared to be isolated to the type of membrane material. Importantly, 85% of these patients also reacted to other dialysis membranes of the same chemical family, and thus the use of alternative membranes (PAN, substituted cellulose, or polymethylmethacrylate) is needed for these patients. These cases highlight the continued vigilance that is needed for patients undergoing HD and that despite changes in technology, reactions to dialysis membranes still occur.

Although reuse and reprocessing of dialysis membranes has decreased substantially, it is important to realize that disinfectants such as hypochlorite (bleach) and formaldehyde can lead to serious reactions.[7,12] These reactions generally abate when the dialyzer is thoroughly rinsed before use.

Reactions Associated With Drugs and Other Exposures

During a dialysis session, patients may receive numerous medications that include drugs given with each dialysis treatment (heparin, erythropoietin, iron compounds) as well as drugs given on a more sporadic nature for specific indications (antibiotics). Clinicians must be aware that patients can develop reactions to these medications and should carefully review medication administration records in any patient developing a reaction.

Patients undergoing HD are exposed to repeated heparin doses, which have been associated with several forms of allergic reactions.[22] Heparin-induced thrombocytopenia (HIT) is a well-described entity and discussed later in this chapter. However, it is important to note several reports of HIT-associated anaphylactoid reactions in HD patients that occur 5 to 30 minutes after intravenous or subcutaneous administration of either unfractionated heparin (UFH) or low-molecular-weight heparins (LMWH).[23] Clinical features include abrupt falls in platelet counts (consistent with HIT), hypotension or hypertension, wheezing, dyspnea, and cardiovascular collapse associated with the presence of anti-platelet factor (PF) 4/heparin antibodies. In addition, both UFH and LMWH have been linked to episodes of typical anaphylaxis during HD.[24,25] An outbreak of UFH-associated anaphylactic episodes occurred in 2007–2008 and was traced to a lot of heparin produced in China that was contaminated with oversulfated chondroitin sulfate (OSCS).[26] It is not clear if low-level contamination with OSCS is associated with other anaphylactic reactions to heparin seen outside of these cases. A further complicating issue is that heparin "allergy" in an HD patient can also be caused by preservatives in the heparin preparation such as paraoxybenzoic esters.[27]

IgE-mediated allergies to the constituent proteins of natural rubber latex are well known and can occur in HD patients.[28] One study found sensitization to natural rubber latex in 1.1% of nonatopic chronic HD patients.[29] Latex-specific IgE and positive skin testing to latex can help identify these patients, and treatment requires the use of alternative elastomers such as polyvinylchloride, nitrile, or polyurethane. Other potential allergic exposures include washing solutions, chlorhexidine, and other environmental allergens.

The majority of dialysis patients are exposed to repeated doses of intravenous (IV) iron compounds that can be associated with a range of adverse reactions, including severe, life-threatening events. The prevalence of hypersensitivity reactions to IV iron preparations is very low (comparable to the safest radiocontrast agents at 0.01% to 0.1%).[30] There is ongoing debate as to whether certain IV iron preparations are safer than others, and with the exception of higher-molecular-weight iron dextran compounds, which are associated with a higher rate and increased severity of reactions, all other compounds appear similar in their safety profile.[31] Of note, high-molecular-weight iron dextrans are no longer available in the United States. Mechanistically, IV irons reactions do not appear to be IgE mediated and are likely nonimmune in nature.[30] One hypothesis is that IV iron preparations, in susceptible patients, activate the complement system, leading to the formation of anaphylatoxins (C3a, C5a), which can further stimulate mast cells to release vasoactive mediators, leading to the clinical expression of a hypersensitivity reaction.[30] Reactions to IV iron preparations can range from minor symptoms such as pruritus, flushing, arthralgias, and myalgias to more significant symptoms such as chest pain, persistent hypotension, shortness of breath, and cardiovascular collapse.[32] The European Medicines Agency Committee for Medicinal Products for Human Use has issued recommendations for the management of the risk for reactions to IV iron.[33] These recommendations include (1) informing patients of the risk for a reaction; (2) the need for close observation of patients receiving IV iron for any reactions during and for at least 30 minutes after the infusion; and (3) training of staff to recognize and treat reactions, including ready access to resuscitation medications if needed. There is no utility to the practice of using a test dose of IV iron to predict the likelihood of a reaction, and this practice has been largely abandoned. Instead, caution is warranted with all IV iron dosages even if previous dosages have been well tolerated.[33]

Treatment options to manage reactions to IV iron preparations depend on the severity of the reaction. Mild reactions (itching, back/joint pains, flushing) can be managed by stopping the infusion and monitoring the patient. If the symptoms improve, the infusion can be restarted with caution.[34] Moderate reactions (cough, chest tightness, shortness of breath, hypotension) are treated with immediate cessation of the infusion as well as administration of IV fluids and corticosteroids. Severe and life-threatening reactions (wheezing, stridor, cyanosis, persistent hypotension) are treated with a combination of IV epinephrine, fluids, and corticosteroids. In patients who have had life-threatening reactions to IV iron compounds, it is safest to avoid all further IV iron infusions.[34] For patients who may be at higher risk for drug reactions, such as highly atopic individuals, premedication with IV corticosteroids can be considered.[35]

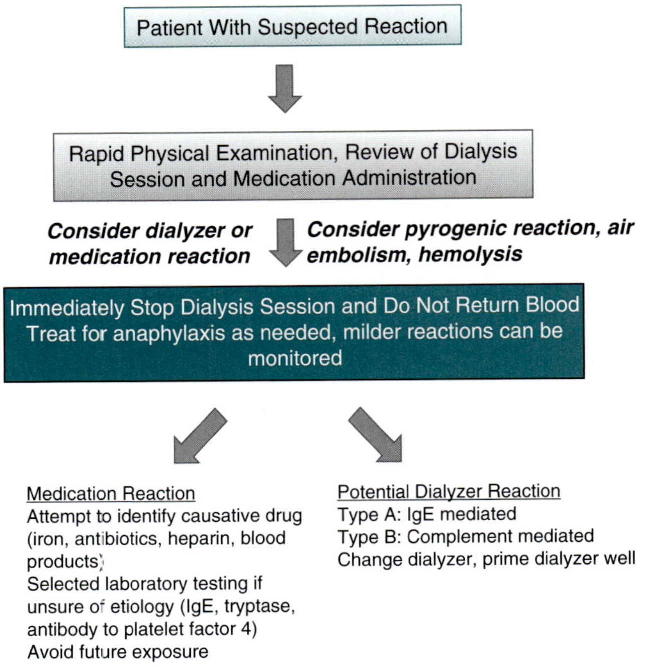

FIG. 26.1 Approach to the patient with a reaction while undergoing hemodialysis.

Approach to the Dialysis Patient With a Reaction

All patients suspected of having a reaction during a HD session should be approached as having a potentially life-threatening event (Fig. 26.1). Given the complexity of the dialysis procedure, a rapid assessment of the patient as well as a review of the dialysis session and any medication administered must occur as a first step. Because the symptoms of a reaction are nonspecific and include cardiovascular collapse, a rapid determination of possible dialysis-related factors such as hemolysis, air embolism, or a pyrogenic reaction (PR) should be assessed (see later) before determining that the patient may be suffering from either a dialyzer- or medication-related event. Furthermore, the dialysis procedure should be halted immediately and blood should not be returned to the patient. For those patients with signs and symptoms of anaphylaxis, rapid administration of subcutaneous epinephrine, IV corticosteroids, and antihistamines (H_1 and H_2 antagonists) should occur along with respiratory support if needed. The maximum initial dose of epinephrine is 0.2 to 0.5 mg in adults and can be given subcutaneously or intramuscularly. Epinephrine should not be administered intravenously unless there is life-threatening shock. The dose of epinephrine can be repeated after 5 minutes if there is no improvement. An inhaled β2-agonist can be added for those patients with bronchospasm. Milder reactions may be treated with corticosteroids and antihistamines or simply monitored closely.

Identification of the offending agent is critical in secondary prevention but may be difficult given the number of potential exposures. Depending on the mechanism of reaction, diagnostic methods that can aid in the identification of the reactive agent include skin tests, specific serum IgE quantification, serum tryptase levels, lymphocyte transformation, and basophil activation assays and in vivo challenge testing.[24] Consultation with an allergy specialist may be helpful in challenging cases.

Complications Associated With Microbiological Contamination

Naturally occurring water bacteria commonly found in HD water systems include gram-negative bacteria (GNB) such as *Pseudomonas* species and nontuberculous mycobacteria. GNB release endotoxin or lipopolysaccharide (LPS) and other bacterial products, and nontuberculous mycobacteria are highly resistant to germicides.[4] Several factors that are operative during dialysis place patients at risk for exposure to bacteria and/or bacterial products, including contaminated water or bicarbonate dialysate, improperly sterilized dialyzers, and cannulation of infected catheters, grafts, or fistulas. The bacteriological quality of treated water and dialysate remains an important issue, and many units report substandard results.[36] The most widely accepted standards for water purity are those recommended by the Association for the Advancement of Medical Instrumentation (AAMI) and the European Pharmacopeia, which respectively allow bacterial growth of <200 colony forming units (CFU)/mL and <100 CFU/mL and an endotoxin concentration of <2 international units (IU)/mL and <0.25 IU/mL. However, a number of multicenter studies have reported that 7% to 35% of water samples have bacterial growth of >200 CFU/mL and up to 44% have endotoxin levels of >5 IU/mL.[37]

Bicarbonate-containing solutions are highly susceptible to bacterial contamination.[4] If stored for too long, sodium bicarbonate breaks down to sodium carbonate, which, along with glucose contained in the dialysate, constitutes a growth medium for bacteria. When GNB reach excessively high concentrations in the dialysate, serious health risks to patients, including PRs with or without bacteremia, can result. Indeed, outbreaks of clusters of infection in HD patients have been ascribed to bacterial contamination, which can occur at multiple places along the HD circuit, including the dialysate, carbon filters, inadequate disinfection, and other sources. For example, in 2007 several patients in a dialysis unit in San Jose, California, developed bacteremia as a result of an unusual GNB, a *Halomonas* species.[38] Tracing back from the dialysis machine, the investigation determined that contamination of the bicarbonate solution was the root cause.

The passage of endotoxin from the dialysate into the blood can occur by diffusion or convection. The use of high-flux dialyzers increases the risk for passage of endotoxin, particularly lipid A (~2000 Da), the active moiety of LPS, from dialysate into blood. LPS interacts with plasma LPS binding protein and mediates cytokine production by interacting with the monocyte CD14 receptor. The subsequent release of pyrogenic cytokines such as interleukin 1 and tumor necrosis factor produce a transient febrile reaction that may be associated with rigors and hypotension. Of note, another source of endotoxin or bacterial infection is intradialytic hypotension (IDH), which can cause transient mesenteric ischemia that may be sufficient to damage the GI mucosa and lead to bacterial and/or LPS translocation.[39]

PRs should be entertained after septicemia has been ruled out. Careful examination of the dialysis access is warranted, and blood cultures should be obtained. Treatment of PR includes antipyretics, empiric broad-spectrum antibiotics, discontinuation of ultrafiltration whenever hypotension is present, and selective hospitalization. An outbreak of bacteremia among several patients involving a similar organism should prompt thorough search for bacterial contaminants of the dialysis equipment. Similarly, an outbreak of PRs should also prompt investigation of the dialysis circuit and water treatment facilities.

The prevention of PRs starts with strict adherence to the AAMI standards.[40] In addition, the Centers for Disease Control and Prevention Division of Healthcare Quality Promotion and the Healthcare Infection Control Practices Advisory Committee have specific guidelines for environmental infection control that should be meticulously followed.[41] In an era of high-flux dialysis and hemodiafiltration, some experts believe that these recommendations are too liberal and that sterile-pyrogen–free dialysis fluids (ultrapure dialysate) with bacteria < 0.1 CFU/mL and endotoxin < 0.03 EU/mL should be used.[37] However, data to widely support this practice in HD are not yet available, even though many dialysis units have adopted this practice in the hope of decreasing chronic inflammatory stimuli.

NEUROLOGICAL AND MUSCULAR COMPLICATIONS DURING HEMODIALYSIS

Neurological and muscular complications are commonly encountered in patients undergoing HD, and they can range from benign but troublesome muscle cramps to life-threatening changes in mental status.

Muscle Cramps

Muscle cramps are defined as prolonged and painful involuntary skeletal muscle contractions. For patients undergoing chronic HD, they are a common occurrence that has been reported in as many as 33% to 86% of treatments and can lead to shortening of HD treatments, failure to reach target weight, and significant impairments in quality of life.[42] Despite this being a common and debilitating condition, there is little research to guide our understanding of the pathophysiology, optimal therapy, and prevention of muscle cramps. Speculation is that muscle cramps may be related to a combination of significant plasma volume contraction, changes in serum osmolality (progressive hypoosmolality), and contributions from deficiencies in magnesium, L-carnitine, vitamin C, and vitamin E.[43] Muscle cramps typically occur near the end of the HD session and most often involve the muscles of the lower extremity, but any muscle may be affected. In terms of the dialysis prescription, lower dialysate sodium levels and higher ultrafiltration rates appear to be risk factors for the development of muscle cramps.[43]

In the past, acute muscle cramps were managed by increasing the plasma osmolality with the administration of hypertonic saline, mannitol, or concentrated (50%) dextrose solutions given intravenously.[44] These therapies are rarely used today given concerns that they may induce thirst and volume overload and limit the ability to get the patient to their target weight. Acute management often includes transiently slowing or stopping ultrafiltration as well as intradialytic massage and stretching of the affected muscle groups.[45] For those patients who develop hypotension along with muscle cramps, prompt attention to raising blood pressure (slowing or stopping ultrafiltration, slowing blood flow rate (BFR), placing the patient in Trendelenburg position, and even administration of midodrine) should be the first course of action.

Preventing or reducing the frequency of muscle cramps during HD should be attempted in patients with frequent intradialytic symptoms. Several strategies have had variable efficacy. For patients who seem to develop muscle cramps associated with the need for high ultrafiltration rates (such as greater than 10 to 13 mL/kg/h), minimizing interdialytic weight gains is critical but often difficult to achieve. Minimizing episodes of IDH by various strategies such as sequential ultrafiltration/dialysis and the use of sodium modeling (such as starting from a dialysate sodium concentration of 145 to 155 mEq/L and decreasing linearly, exponentially, or stepwise to 135 to 140 mEq/L) may also be effective in some patients.[46] It also may be reasonable to empirically increase the target weight by 0.5 kg to see if this lowers the frequency of muscle cramps. Higher dialysate sodium levels or oral salt loading may also ameliorate the frequency of muscle cramps but come at the expense of increased thirst and risk for higher interdialytic fluid gains. Despite very limited data, quinine has been used for the prevention of muscle cramps, perhaps by decreasing the excitability of the muscle endplate.[47] However, the US Food and Drug Administration (FDA) has warned that the use of quinine for the prevention of dialysis-associated muscle cramps is not justified and is associated with severe adverse reactions, including cardiac arrhythmias, allergic reactions, and thrombotic thrombocytopenic purpura–hemolytic uremic syndrome, and thus should not be used. L-carnitine supplementation (administered intravenously [20 mg/kg] after HD or orally [330 mg two to three times per day]) in those patients with low levels may decrease the frequency of muscle cramps, but the data in support of its use are weak.[48] Vitamin E supplementation has also had variable efficacy in decreasing the frequency of muscle cramps in several small trials.[49,50] In one study the combination of both vitamin E and C was more effective in reducing cramp frequency than either alone.[49] In another study, 400 IU of vitamin E reduced the frequency of muscle cramps by 68%.[50] It is thus reasonable to try vitamin E in those patients with frequent muscle cramps. There are very limited data on a variety of other therapies that have been attempted to decrease the frequency of muscle cramps, including the use of gabapentin, short-acting benzodiazepines, and phenytoin.[43]

Headache

Headache is a common complaint in HD patients, occurring with an incidence ranging from 27% to 73%.[51,52] Dialysis-related headaches are defined as those starting or changing their characteristics (such as worsening) when the dialysis treatment starts.[52] Headaches characteristically begin within 1 to 2 hours after initiating dialysis and are variously described as throbbing in nature, moderate in intensity, and most often in the frontotemporal region.[51,52] Often the headache may worsen when the patient reclines, and when severe, it may be accompanied by nausea and vomiting. The headache often, but not always, resolves within 48 to 72 hours after dialysis.[53] Many of these patients will have a history of preexisting headaches and may also have headaches in the interdialytic period, which can confound the diagnosis and therapy.[51] In fact, one study noted that only 6.7% of headaches in the HD population were purely related to the HD session, highlighting the high prevalence of other headaches in these patients.[54]

Although the pathophysiology of dialysis-related headache is not fully defined, certain risk factors are associated with its development. Patients who develop headache typically have lower magnesium levels both pre- and postdialysis, greater intradialytic decreases in serum urea levels, larger changes in body weight during HD sessions, and higher predialysis systolic and diastolic blood pressures.[52-54] Low magnesium levels may be particularly important because this has been reported to potentiate vasospasm and vasoconstriction as well as modulating inflammation and the N-methyl-D-aspartate glutamate receptor associated with nociceptive transmission.[55] Rapid changes in serum osmolality that occur early in the HD session as blood urea and solute levels decrease lead to translocation of water across the blood–brain (hematoencephalic) barrier (because cerebral concentrations of these solutes are stable over the first part of the HD session and an osmotic gradient favoring water movement into the brain occurs). This movement of water into the brain leads to increases in intracranial pressure along with symptoms of headache. In essence, headache may be a milder form of the dialysis disequilibrium syndrome (DDS) (discussed later).[56] Both hypertension and hypotension during the dialysis procedure may also contribute to the development of headache. One study[57] also reported correlations of dialysis headache with higher levels of calcitonin gene–related peptide and substance P. Some have also hypothesized that increases in nitric oxide and bradykinin during the HD session may be headache inducers.[58] One intriguing but unproven hypothesis is that intradialytic removal of caffeine may precipitate headache.[59] Lastly, headache may also be a somatic complaint in patients with depression, and this should be considered in HD patients, where the prevalence of depression is high.[60]

Little data are available to guide the management of dialysis-related headaches, and general management principles are followed: oral analgesics (acetaminophen), magnesium supplementation for those patients with low levels, avoidance of large blood pressure and weight changes, and avoidance of caffeine overuse. In some patients, a reduction in the BFR early in the HD session may be helpful.

Dialysis Disequilibrium Syndrome (DDS)

DDS is defined as neurological deterioration occurring during HD and more typically occurring in patients during or immediately after their first treatment.[61] DDS can be encountered in both acute and chronic kidney failure, and risk factors include high predialysis blood urea nitrogen levels (>175 mg/dL), a rapid fall in blood urea nitrogen levels with HD, preexisting neurological conditions, hyponatremia, and liver disease.[61] The symptoms are nonspecific and mimic those occurring with increased intracranial pressure (such as with acute severe hyponatremia), such as restlessness, headache, nausea, vomiting, hypertension, mental confusion, obtundation, seizures, and coma.[61] Thus a careful assessment of patients presenting with these symptoms should include other causes, such as subdural hematoma, acute cerebrovascular events including intracranial hemorrhage, hypoglycemia, and hypotension. Brain imaging (either computed tomography or magnetic resonance imaging) may reveal cerebral edema in patients with DDS. Although the syndrome is seen less common now than in the past (in part as a result of starting patients on HD with lower blood urea nitrogen levels and using lower blood and dialysate flow rates for the initial sessions), it is still encountered and needs to be recognized.

Although the pathophysiology is not completely known, it is felt that the primary factor is development of cerebral edema and increased intracranial pressure that is driven by water movement into brain cells and the interstitium by an osmotic gradient as a result of rapid falls in serum urea and other effective osmoles (the reverse urea hypothesis).[61] Supporting this concept is the finding that measurement of urea in the blood and cerebrospinal fluid (CSF) indicated that after HD treatment there was a substantial gradient, with the urea concentration in the CSF being higher than that in the blood, and that this gradient caused water to move into the central nervous system, leading to rises in intracranial pressure.[62] The magnitude of the CSF–to–plasma blood urea nitrogen gradient can be as high as 2 immediately after dialysis.[63] Some have also argued that an increase in intracellular brain solutes (idiogenic osmoles), such as myoinositol, glutamine, and taurine, occurs with rapid HD and may also contribute to the osmotic disequilibrium between the CNS and vascular compartments.[64] More recent data supporting the role of the reverse urea hypothesis are that in a rat model of advanced chronic kidney disease there was a decrease in urea transporters as well as an increase in aquaporin channels in brain cells.[65] The consequence of these molecular changes may be a delayed exit of urea from astrocytes, as well as facilitation of water transport into cells by the increase in aquaporin channels.

Prevention of DDS focuses on minimizing the osmotic gradient that leads to water entering the CNS. Various techniques have been used in this regard. No controlled trials are available to guide therapy, and thus clinical judgment on the rate of urea reduction must factor in individual patient characteristics such as the predialysis blood urea nitrogen level, history of neurological disease, and other risk factors. A reasonable goal for a first dialysis session is a reduction in the blood urea concentration of 40% (urea reduction ratio of 0.4).[66] To achieve this goal, the first HD session should be limited to 2 to 2.5 hours and the blood flow should be 200 to 250 mL/h. In addition, the use of hemofiltration (convective solute removal), as opposed to HD, which does not result in as large a solute gradient, may mitigate the risk for DDS.[67] Similarly, in those at the highest risk for DDS (such as those with acute kidney injury and traumatic brain injury or an intracranial hemorrhage), continuous renal replacement therapy with slow urea removal should be considered. The other strategy used to prevent DDS is to raise the osmolality of the intravascular compartment during HD to decrease the osmotic gradient and lessen the risk for cerebral edema. The easiest way to achieve this is to increase the concentration of sodium in the dialysate and use sodium modeling.[68] Studies with this approach have found that higher dialysate sodium concentrations were associated with amelioration of DDS as well as a decrease in electroencephalogram abnormalities compared with standard sodium dialysate.[68] Other osmotic agents such as mannitol and glucose have also been successfully used in the prevention of DDS.[61]

Treatment of DDS, once established, centers on rapidly reducing intracranial pressure by raising blood osmolality with mannitol or hypertonic saline. Even with these maneuvers, patients may not recover, and this highlights the critical importance of prevention of DDS.[69]

Restless Legs Syndrome

Restless legs syndrome (RLS) is characterized by an uncomfortable and urgent need to move the limbs (usually the lower extremities) and typically begins or worsens during periods of rest or inactivity.[70] The International Restless Legs Syndrome Study Group has developed specific diagnostic and severity criteria, and these include the feature that the symptoms are at least partially relieved by movement or stretching.[71] ESRD patients have a much higher prevalence rate of RLS than the general population, reaching approximately 30%.[70] Although the precise pathophysiology of RLS is not well understood, disturbances in dopaminergic neuronal transmission as well reduction in iron stores in specific brain regions are thought to be important, and these insights inform therapeutic maneuvers.[70,72] Uremic toxicity is also thought to be important because the majority of patients recover from RLS after kidney transplantation.[73] Importantly, RLS may manifest itself during the HD session (likely because of inactivity during these 3 to 4 hours), and up to 20% of patients undergoing HD prematurely terminate a dialysis session secondary to the sensory and motor symptoms of RLS.[74]

Studies have found that RLS negatively affects the quality of life for HD patients, with significant negative effects on sleep quality and quantity and a higher prevalence of depression and anxiety.[75,76] Interestingly, RLS is also associated with a higher risk for cardiovascular disease, and this may, in part, be mediated by augmentation of sympathetic nervous system activity.[77] Thus it is not surprising that RLS in ESRD patients is a marker for higher mortality rates and lower survival.[78]

Treatment of RLS in ESRD patients is challenging, and there are very few clinical trials available to guide practice. The first-line pharmacological therapy for RLS is a dopamine agonist such as ropinirole or pramipexole (Table 26.1). Several small clinical trials have reported that these agents can decrease RLS symptoms by approximately 70%.[79,80] Side effects with these agents can include nausea, vomiting, and nightmares. The anticonvulsant gabapentin has also had efficacy and is approved by the FDA for the treatment of RLS.[81] Iron supplementation has also had variable but transient efficacy for RLS, and patients should be treated with IV iron as per protocols used to treat anemia.[82] Intradialytic exercise training is also effective and has been reported to improve sleep quality and decrease RLS symptoms during the HD session.[83]

Seizures

There are numerous potential causes of seizures in the patient undergoing dialysis (Table 26.2). It is important to know the patient's history and medication use, and details of the dialysis session, because this information will often yield significant clues as to the cause of the seizure. A rapid physical examination looking for any focal neurological deficits should be performed because this may suggest an intracranial process. Patients who are just initiating HD may develop a seizure as a result of DDS or from severe electrolyte disturbances such as hyponatremia or hypocalcemia.[84] Erythropoietin, especially in higher doses, had been associated with the development of hypertensive encephalopathy and seizures in as many as 2% to 17% of patients.[85] However, the contemporary use of much lower doses of erythropoietin, as well as more aggressive control of blood pressure, has made erythropoietin-associated seizures an uncommon occurrence.[84]

TABLE 26.1 Pharmacological Therapies for Restless Legs Syndrome

Drug	Recommended Dosing
Ropinirole	0.25–2.0 mg/d
Pramipexole	0.125–0.75 mg/d
Gabapentin	100 mg at bedtime or 200–300 mg dosed three times a week after dialysis
Intravenous iron	Variable depending on preparation used and iron levels

Changes in blood pressure (either acute lowering or elevations) can be associated with seizures, especially in patients with predisposing conditions.[86] IDH should be avoided in these patients. Hypertensive encephalopathy can manifest as headaches, vomiting, confusion, and seizures and can be encountered when the patient presents for dialysis or even during the dialysis session. Proper treatment focuses on controlled decreases in blood pressure, which should be closely monitored in an intensive care unit (ICU) setting.

Numerous electrolyte abnormalities can be associated with seizures, which are usually of the generalized tonic-clonic type.[84] In most cases, rapid changes in electrolyte levels are more likely to precipitate seizures than chronic changes. These include hypocalcemia, hyponatremia, and hypomagnesemia. Rapid recognition and treatment of these disorders can be lifesaving. For instance, for patients with severe hyponatremia, small increases in the serum sodium of 5 mEq/L can be enough to reduce cerebral edema and halt seizure activity.[87] This can be achieved with 100 mL boluses (up to three times) of 3% saline given intravenously.

Patients with a history of seizures and taking chronic antiepileptic medications may pose special challenges in the HD unit. This is due to the fact that ESRD and dialysis alter the distribution, metabolism, and clearance of many antiepileptic drugs.[88] Some medications, such as levetiracetam, phenobarbital, and primidone, are removed by dialysis and thus require supplementation or careful timing of administration to avoid lowering therapeutic levels and precipitating "breakthrough" seizures.[88] Other drugs, such as phenytoin, carbamazepine, and sodium valproate, are poorly dialyzed and do not require supplementation. In all cases, antiepileptic drug levels should be monitored closely.

Aluminum neurotoxicity is largely of historic interest and seldom seen today.[89] The fall in incidence is due to improved water treatment and the avoidance of aluminum-containing phosphate binders. Those few patients who may manifest symptoms of aluminum neurotoxicity, which includes impaired memory, myoclonic jerks, and other neurological symptoms, have generally been on HD for many years and may have received repeated courses of aluminum-containing phosphate binders. Plasma aluminum levels are elevated in these cases.

TABLE 26.2 Causes of Seizures in the Hemodialysis Patient

Dialysis Related	Medication Related	Metabolic	Neurological
Uremic encephalopathy	Erythropoietin	Hyponatremia	Strokes
Dialysis disequilibrium syndrome	High-dose penicillin and cephalosporins	Hypoglycemia and hyperglycemia	Hypertensive encephalopathy
Sudden changes (usually falls) in blood pressure	Meperidine	Hypocalcemia	Posterior reversible encephalopathy
Aluminum intoxication	Ertapenem/meropenem	Hypomagnesemia	Subdural hematoma
Air embolism	Acyclovir		Intracranial infection
			Alcohol withdrawal

Treatment of established seizures requires cessation of dialysis, maintenance of airway patency, and investigation for metabolic abnormalities. Phenytoin and intravenous diazepam or clonazepam may be required. Intravenous administration of 50% dextrose in water should be administered if hypoglycemia is suspected.

Other Neurological Complications

Visual loss is rare during HD and may be caused by central retinal vein occlusion, precipitation of acute glaucoma (because of changes in osmolality), ischemic optic neuropathy associated with IDH, or Purtscher-like retinopathy caused by leukoembolization.[90] Patients experiencing visual changes during HD should have their treatment stopped immediately and be referred for an emergent ophthalmology examination.

CARDIOVASCULAR COMPLICATIONS DURING HEMODIALYSIS

Intradialytic Hypotension

IDH occurs in an estimated 8% to 20% of dialysis sessions.[91] Complicating the evaluation are the variable definitions of IDH. Various studies use a systolic blood pressure (SBP) or mean arterial pressure cutoff (often <90 mmHg SBP), whereas others include only symptomatic episodes. IDH appears to be due to a complex interplay of factors including total volume and rate of fluid removal, rate of intravascular space "refill," degree of osmolar changes between fluid compartments, and impaired compensatory mechanisms caused by underlying medical conditions and/or medications.[92] Symptomatic episodes may include mental status changes such as syncope or seizure in severe cases, nausea, muscle cramping, and end-organ ischemia-related symptoms, among many other manifestations.[93] Even asymptomatic patients may suffer from silent cardiac stunning and cerebral ischemia.[94]

IDH has been associated with a number of negative clinical outcomes, including increased rates of access thrombosis, cardiac remodeling, and higher 1- and 5-year mortality.[95,96] A number of predisposing risk factors have been studied. These include shorter treatment times, higher ultrafiltration rates, higher dialysis dose, left ventricular hypertrophy, diabetes, longer dialysis vintage, higher dialysate temperatures, and dialysis after the "long break" (longer interdialytic interval), among others.[92,97,98]

Strategies to prevent or ameliorate IDH revolve around reducing intradialytic weight gain through patient education, optimizing and limiting ultrafiltration volume and rates during dialysis sessions, lessening the effect of osmolar changes, and increasing vascular tone and/or venous return. Dietary sodium intake is a significant driver of interdialytic fluid gains.[92] As such, patient counseling should include a focus on reducing sodium intake as possible. Once in-center, reducing ultrafiltration volumes and rates via increased total dialysis time or additional sessions may reduce IDH. Various biofeedback technologies to monitor blood volume or heart rate variability have been trialed to optimize ultrafiltration during treatment with varying degrees of success.[99] A high-sodium bath has been used to decrease osmolar-driven fluid shifts and reduce IDH; however, this may lead to significant sodium transfer and higher interdialytic weight gains.[100] A recent metaanalysis suggested that stepwise sodium profiling reduces IDH compared with conventional dialysis and linear sodium profile methods. Thus a dialysis program that uses stepwise sodium profiling with a neutral net sodium transfer may be preferable. Cooled dialysate has been found to have multiple benefits: reduced left ventricular remodeling, reduced brain white matter disease, and lessened IDH.[101-103] The stabilization of core temperature may reduce the reflexive vasodilation from overheating during later stages of dialysis, yielding stable systemic vascular resistance. Cooling may also be the mechanism of reduced IDH seen in online hemodiafiltration because increased thermal energy loss from the circuit yields an unintended method of cooling.[104] Lastly, the selective α_1 receptor agonist midodrine has been found generally safe but variably effective for treatment of IDH.[105]

Other strategies have shown promise in smaller studies and include arginine vasopressin infusion; hypertonic saline administration; modification of dialysate calcium, bicarbonate, and magnesium; L-carnitine administration, and use of pneumatic compression devices.[106-109]

Intradialytic Hypertension

Hypertension in dialysis patients is generally driven by extracellular volume excess. Patients with intradialytic hypertension however, experience paradoxical increases in blood pressure despite ultrafiltration and presumed adequate volume removal. When defined as an increase in systolic pressures of >10 mmHg over the course of treatment, intradialytic hypertension occurs in 12% to 13% of prevalent patients.[110] The pathophysiology varies by patient but is likely multifactorial, including activation of the renin-angiotensin-aldosterone and sympathetic nervous systems, decreased arterial compliance, and increased endothelin 1 production/endothelial cell dysfunction.[111] Removal of dialyzable antihypertensive medications may also play a role. In addition, subclinical volume overload and increased peripheral resistance may also be causative. A study by Van Buren et al.[112] evaluated the role of extracellular water (ECW) at end treatment and found that patients with IDH completed dialysis with higher ratios of ECW to total body water and with increased total peripheral resistance compared with controls.

In those predisposed to intradialytic hypertension, ambulatory blood pressure monitoring has indicated that elevated blood pressure lasts for hours posttreatment.[113] Poor clinical outcomes have been associated with intradialytic hypertension, specifically higher mortality.[114] Despite the prevalence of intradialytic hypertension and potential mortality risk, agreed-on treatment strategies remain opinion based. Given the possible role of subclinical volume overload, it seems reasonable to perform serial target weight challenges on hypertensive dialysis patients and consider longer or additional sessions more than thrice weekly. The Frequent Hemodialysis Network trial reported improved blood pressure control, with lowered target weights and decreased total number of medications.[115] Carvedilol has shown promise in reducing the number of episodes of intradialytic hypertension, possibly through blockage of endothelin 1.[116] Other suggestions include use of less-dialyzable antihypertensives, reducing use of erythropoietin-stimulating agents (ESAs), and lowering dialysate sodium.[117]

Arrhythmias

Arrhythmias, both atrial and ventricular, are a common occurrence in HD patients. Atrial fibrillation is present in 22% of patients, and ventricular arrhythmias occur in another 8% per US Renal Data System (USRDS) data. Lethal arrhythmias are the leading cause of death among patients with ESRD.[118] Dialysis patients have a high burden of cardiovascular disease that predisposes them to arrhythmias, including valvular heart disease, atherosclerotic heart disease, and congestive heart failure—the last two occurring in about 45% of patients.[118] Dialysis-specific risk factors include rapid electrolyte (especially potassium) shifts during dialysis, increased sympathetic tone during treatment, uremia, and myocardial stunning.[119]

Despite the potential mortality, large prospective studies of arrhythmias have not occurred. Two recent trials of implantable cardiac loop monitors in Australian and Brazilian dialysis patients reported that the vast majority of "stable" dialysis patients experience transient arrhythmias and often more than one type.[120,121] In the Brazilian study, most arrhythmias were clinically silent and supraventricular tachycardia predominated. In the Australian group, atrial fibrillation accounted for 62% of transient arrhythmias. Concerning was that both studies had large numbers of patients with ventricular arrhythmias. A study of US patients with loop recorders is currently underway.[122] Management of atrial fibrillation with anticoagulation remains controversial. Some retrospective studies suggest benefit, although a recent metaanalysis reported no mortality benefit and even potential harm.[123] Novel oral anticoagulants such as apixaban have not been well studied in ESRD.

Strategies to reduce the risk for arrhythmias in dialysis patients are mostly opinion based. Most authors advocate reducing electrolyte shifts during dialysis by slowly correcting derangements and avoiding large changes in electrolyte levels. Other strategies include use of antihypertensives that decrease sympathetic tone, such as beta blockers, ACE inhibitors, and aldosterone receptor blockers, and treating underlying cardiac conditions.[124]

Sudden Cardiac Death

Sudden cardiac death (SCD) is the leading cause of death among dialysis patients, accounting for approximately 29% of all deaths. The period of highest risk is in the second month after initiating dialysis.[118] In the general population, SCD is most often associated with coronary artery disease and ventricular arrhythmias.[124] The mechanism in dialysis patients has been presumed to be lethal ventricular arrhythmias. More recently, devices such as implantable cardiac defibrillators and loop recorders have shown bradycardia terminating in asystole as the most common disturbance implicated in SCD.[125] Several studies have found the highest-risk period for SCD is near the end of the "long break"—the 72-hour span in usual thrice weekly dialysis.[121] An earlier study reported clustering of SCD in the 12 hours after dialysis after the long break and a second peak in the 48- to 60-hour period after the final dialysis session in a week. This has led to speculation that the stress of the procedure itself is a risk factor for SCD, as well as the metabolic derangements seen from >48 hours between sessions.[126] Other characteristics associated with SCD in the dialysis population include use of low potassium, magnesium, and calcium baths; underlying structural heart disease; diabetes; use of high doses of ESA, use of vitamin D analogs, excessive heart rate variability, high ultrafiltration rates, and prolonged QTc interval.[126-128]

There are no large prospective randomized trials indicating benefit of a particular intervention for reducing SCD. The use of implantable cardiac defibrillators remains controversial. A small pilot trial of a wearable defibrillator in dialysis patients has found benefit.[129] A recent retrospective trial compared an ESRD implantable cardioverter defibrillator (ICD) recipient cohort with a propensity-matched ESRD non-ICD cohort and found no benefit.[130] A larger prospective study is underway to determine the utility of wearable cardiac defibrillators in incident patients as primary prevention. Medication therapy also remains uncertain. Carvedilol has been found to reduce mortality in a small trial of dialysis patients with reduced left ventricular function, though the reduction in death from SCD was not statistically significant.[131] Given the characteristics of the dialysis procedure itself associated with SCD, it seems prudent to avoid using very low potassium and calcium baths. Ultrafiltration rates should be minimized by increasing time or additional sessions when necessary. Avoiding the components of the long break that may contribute to increases in SCD, such as high volume fluid intake and electrolyte shifts, should be accomplished through counseling if possible.

Finally, management of a cardiac arrest in the dialysis unit should follow the American Heart Association guidelines emphasizing consistent chest compressions. Automated external defibrillators are recommended by the National Kidney Foundation Kidney Disease Outcomes Quality Initiative and present in most dialysis units but have not yet produced improved outcomes.[132] Procedural causes of SCD, such as massive air embolism, acute hemolysis, or errors in dialysate composition, are specific to dialysis and should be managed accordingly when found.

Myocardial Stunning

Myocardial stunning, defined here as transient development of segmental wall motion abnormalities with ventricular dysfunction, has been estimated to occur in 27% to 64% of patients during dialysis.[133] Although IDH may accompany these episodes, more often they are clinically silent.[134] Myocardial stunning has also been associated with higher 1-year mortality.[133] The pathophysiology is thought

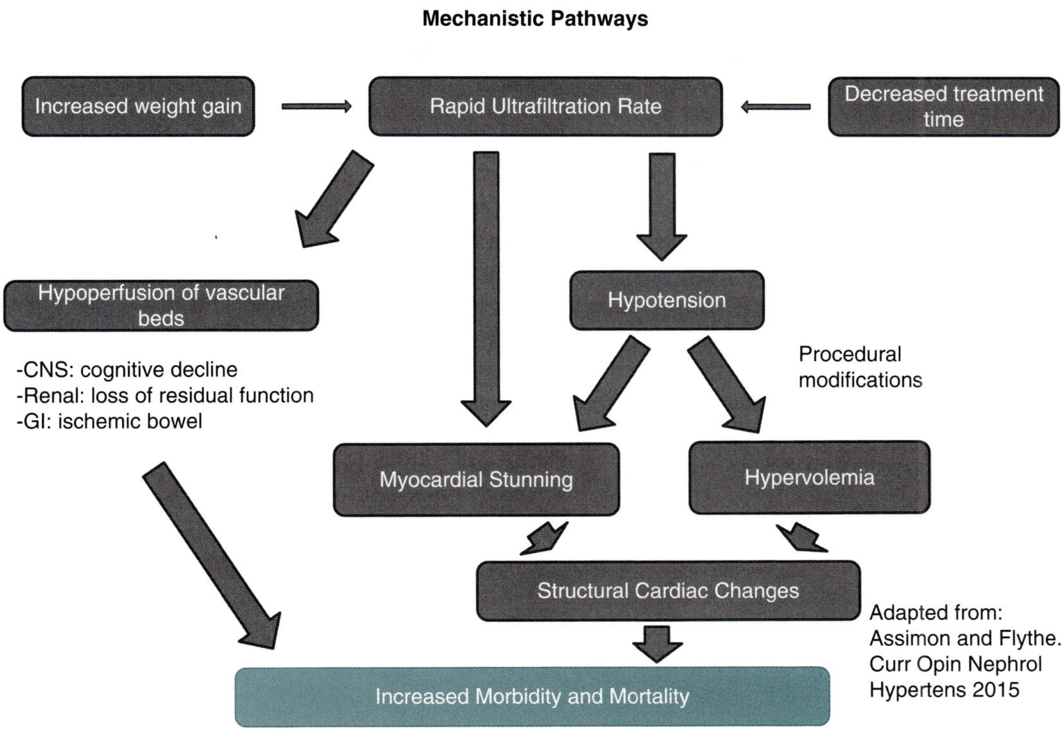

FIG. 26.2 Mechanistic pathway of myocardial stunning–associated morbidity and mortality.

to be decreased coronary artery perfusion, which has been established using various noninvasive imaging modalities, including intradialytic positron emission scans and magnetic resonance imaging.[135] Predisposing factors for myocardial stunning include a history of left ventricular systolic dysfunction, male sex, higher left ventricular mass index, increased age, and higher ultrafiltration rates.[133]

Repetitive myocardial stunning may also predispose to development of permanent segmental abnormalities.[136] This has given rise to the concept of a "vicious cycle" of recurrent ischemia and ensuing cardiac remodeling (Fig. 26.2). The deleterious effects of repetitive myocardial stunning have also been proposed as the potential underlying cause for the higher mortality in patients with high ultrafiltration rates.[137] The mortality link found in patients with ultrafiltration rates >10 mL/kg/h has been significant enough that an ultrafiltration rate quality measure has recently been added to the ESRD Quality Incentive Program (QIP) in the United States.[138]

Strategies to assess and prevent myocardial stunning have not been standardized. Studied interventions have included employing cooled dialysate, lowered ultrafiltration rates, and more frequent dialysis.[139,140] A more recent study compared HD with online hemodiafiltration with an average ultrafiltration rate of ~4 mL/kg/h. Myocardial perfusion was assessed by intradialytic magnetic resonance imaging. In this small crossover trial of 12 patients, no difference was found in the rates of myocardial stunning with equal levels of cooling employed. Implementation of the ultrafiltration rate limit guidelines under the QIP program may also serve to reduce rates of myocardial stunning, but this has not been studied prospectively.

VASCULAR ACCESS–RELATED COMPLICATIONS

This section focuses on those vascular access complications seen specifically during the HD procedure. Other vascular access complications are discussed elsewhere.

Dialysis-Associated Steal Syndrome

The creation of an arteriovenous fistula (AVF) or arteriovenous graft (AVG) results in a variable reduction in blood flow to the distal extremity. Physiological or asymptomatic steal syndrome, with retrograde flow from the distal artery, may occur in up to 90% of accesses.[141] However, clinically severe dialysis-associated steal syndrome (DASS), with limb-threatening ischemia, is relatively rare, occurring in 1% to 10% of upper extremity accesses and in 2% of lower extremity accesses.[142] Mild symptoms, such as transient numbness or coldness, occur less often—in 12% to 50% of patients.[143] The physiology of steal syndrome has been previously described.[144] To summarize, larger fistulas, typically >75% of the diameter of the feeding artery, are favored for dialysis access to support the high required BFRs. Blood then flows preferentially to the lower-pressure vascular bed of the AVF or AVG. Inadequate flow to the distal artery may occur because of retrograde flow after access creation or stenosis of the proximal feeder artery. In addition, arterial collaterals may not develop to sufficiently revascularize the distal arterial supply. In these situations, the signs and symptoms of steal syndrome may occur. Patient-related factors associated with DASS include female gender, age >60, diabetes mellitus, history of atherosclerosis of the coronary arteries, and preexisting peripheral arterial disease.

Access-related associations include use of the brachial artery for inflow and use of a straight graft (as opposed to looped graft) configuration.[145]

Symptoms may be mild, consisting of coolness, numbness, pallor, dialysis-related discomfort; or severe, including cyanosis, severe pain, paresthesias, and even gangrene.[146] The differential diagnosis of steal syndromes includes dialysis- and nondialysis-associated neuropathies, ischemic monomelic mononeuropathy occurring shortly after access creation, and digital eschars/pain associated with calciphylaxis or vasculitis. Diagnosis is generally clinical; however, confirmatory testing may include ultrasound evaluation, angiography, digital blood pressure (DBP) testing, and DBP index (ratio of DBP to contralateral extremity).[147] Nerve conduction studies can be useful to rule out nonischemic-related causes.

Treatment for DASS depends on the underlying cause and the degree of access blood flow. Ischemia has traditionally been treated with ligation of the arteriovenous (AV) access, with the obvious downside of access loss. More recently, distal revascularization with interval ligation (DRIL) has been found to be equally effective for symptom relief and allows preservation of the access.[148] Procedures to reduce blood flow through the AV access such as banding or ligation of venous collaterals are preferred in high-access flow states. When DASS is associated with low or normal flow, treatments that preserve access flow, such as DRIL, proximalization of the arterial inflow, or revision using distal inflow, are favored.[147]

Vascular Access Bleeding

A functional vascular access must sustain a high BFR to ensure adequate dialysis. This high BFR also confers significant risk for morbidity and mortality should access-related hemorrhage occur. The incidence of access-related hemorrhage is difficult to estimate because of limited data. A review of Centers for Medicare and Medicaid Services data from 2000 to 2006 indicated that access hemorrhage was the proximate cause in an estimated 0.4% of dialysis patient deaths.[149] Most fatal hemorrhages occur in the home; however, 1% to 19% may occur in a facility.[141,150] Even nonfatal postdialysis access bleeding, defined as a modest 4 mL of blood loss, has been associated with increased anemia and mortality.[151]

Patient-related risk factors associated with access-related hemorrhage remain unclear. In case series, AVFs and AVGs are more likely to have significant hemorrhage than catheters. One observational study linked later dialysis vintage, diabetes mellitus, use of an AVG, and central venous stenosis with excessive bleeding. A European case series suggested superficial soft tissue infection associated with buttonholes was strongly associated with AVF rupture.[152] The use of antiplatelet agents is presumed to increase hemorrhage risk; however, a large metaanalysis failed to report any major access-related bleeding events.[153] Regarding catheter-related bleeding events, two metaanalyses suggested 4% citrate locks may reduce the risk for bleeding compared with heparin locks.[154] For AV fistulas and especially grafts, recurrent puncture may lead to pseudoaneurysm formation and predispose to access-related hemorrhage.[155] When coupled with increased pressure in the access from a proximal stenosis, this can lead to rupture. A thorough physical examination as part of a vascular access monitoring program can identify signs that suggest possible aneurysm bleed and should prompt emergent vascular surgery involvement and interventional radiology investigation: ulceration or thinning of overlying skin, rapid expansion of the pseudoaneurysm, or unexplained prolonged postdialysis bleeding time.[155]

Treatment of access-related hemorrhage depends on the type of access and nature of bleeding. Some cases of contained bleeding may cause hematoma, leading to a rare presentation of compartment syndrome.[156] For the more typical presentation of access hemorrhage, direct pressure should be applied immediately. Suturing is rarely adequate alone, and vascular surgery supervision is necessary. Usually, an access can be salvaged via either open surgical repair or endovascular repair via stent grafts (where the stent can bridge the pseudoaneurysmal portion of the access), though endovascular repairs often suffer from poorer long-term viability.[157]

Access Thrombosis

Access thrombosis is a common complication of AVFs and AVGs and a leading cause of secondary failure.[158] The details of access monitoring, preemptive intervention, and thrombosis risk factors are reviewed earlier in the text. Although most clinicians encounter thrombosis during the predialysis physical examination, access thrombosis has been known to occur acutely in the setting of HD or may follow as a complication of dialysis treatment. Traditionally, thrombosis has been attributed to intraluminal access narrowing and progressive neointimal hyperplasia.[159] Other factors also play a role, such as increased inflammatory profile, prothrombotic genetic mutations (e.g., factor V mutations), and the presence of a number of thrombophilic biomarkers, such as hyperhomocysteinemia and elevated indoxyl sulfate.[160] Dialysis procedure–related factors may also play a role. Damage of endothelial cells from repetitive needle sticks and reactions to the dialyzer membrane and/or tubing may induce inflammation and thrombosis. Episodes of hypotension from either autonomic instability or excessive ultrafiltration have also been associated with thrombosis. A retrospective study of Hemodialysis (HEMO) trial participants suggested that rates of AVF thrombosis were twice as high for patients with frequent episodes of hypotension compared with those without hypotensive episodes.[161] Lastly, access thrombosis has even been reported to lead to embolic phenomena during dialysis treatment.[162] Medications associated with AV access thrombosis include erythropoietin and thalidomide. A thrombosed AV access in the dialysis unit requires prompt attention and, depending on the patient's need for urgent HD (based on laboratory and physical examination findings), will need to dealt with within 48 hours, with interventional radiologist–performed thrombectomy along with correction of any access-related issue that may have contributed to the thrombosis.

HEMATOLOGIC COMPLICATIONS

Dialysis-Associated Leukopenia

Transient leukopenia is one of the earliest described dialysis-associated phenomena. The first cases reported selective sequestration of granulocytes, particularly in the pulmonary vasculature, which occurs within the first 2 to 15 minutes of treatment.[163] This is followed by rebound where leukocytes return to baseline or greater after about an hour. The underlying pathological condition is thought to be activation of the alternative complement pathway, particularly C3 and C5, with upregulated leukocyte adhesion factors. Transient leukopenia was most often described with cellulose dialyzers, the prevalent type of the day. A lower incidence is reported in other dialyzer types, particularly polysulfone.[164] As bioincompatible dialyzers have been phased out, transient dialysis-associated leukopenia persists but has shifted from a granulocytic predominance to subsets of monocytes ($CD14^+$ and $CD16^+$).[165] The clinical significance of transient leukopenia remains unclear but it is usually self-limited.

Dialysis-Associated Hemolysis

Dialysis-associated hemolysis refers to clinically significant hemolysis occurring either during or as a consequence of the dialysis treatment. Improvements in water treatment and machine safeguards have likely reduced the incidence compared with historical rates. Causes of hemolysis can be broadly categorized into dialysate purity/composition related and machine/procedure related. Subclinical hemolysis occurs during all dialysis sessions from red blood cell (RBC) interaction with the various components of the dialysis circuit—particularly as a result of laminar flow–induced shear stress on RBCs, along with a lesser contribution from blood pump pressure cycling. One estimate suggested 20 mL of blood is lost to hemolysis per session.[166] Other studies have evaluated hematocrit and volume of dysmorphic RBCs in pre- and postdialysis samples and found no meaningful change.[167] Pulsatile, valveless blood pumps have been found to further reduce the risk for hemolysis but are not in common use.

The most important modern-day causes of hemolysis are contaminants altering dialysate composition and mechanical complications (Table 26.3). Regarding contaminants, chloramine compounds—the combination of chlorine and ammonia used to disinfect municipal water supplies—are the most commonly cited cause of hemolysis. Patients may develop fatal hemolysis and methemoglobinemia, along with a constellation of related symptoms.[168] Typically, carbon tank filters remove chloramines early in the water treatment process; however, municipalities may unexpectedly increase levels to respond to changes in bacterial contamination, or breaks in water treatment protocols may lead to chloramine "pass through" to patients.[169] Less common contaminants resulting in hemolysis include trace minerals (zinc, copper from plumbing and fixtures), nitrites and nitrates (from domestic animal waste seepage), and disinfectants such as hydrogen peroxide or formaldehyde, which may be used to sterilize water treatment equipment.[170,171] Incorrect dialysis composition may also cause hemolysis when low-osmolality dialysate is used. One case report cited mistaken use of distilled water in an ICU setting leading to significant hemolysis.[172]

TABLE 26.3 Causes of Hemolysis in Dialysis

Cause	Source
Dialysis Contaminants and Composition Error	
Zinc and copper	Plumbing fixtures, piping
Chloramines and chlorine	Municipal water system additives
	Bleach contamination from inadequate flushing after disinfection of water system
Hydrogen peroxide	Contamination from inadequate flushing after disinfection of water system
Formaldehyde	Contamination from dialyzer reprocessing
Nitrate/nitrites	Well water contamination from domestic animal waste
Hypotonic dialysate	Inappropriate use of distilled water or custom dialysate baths made in pharmacy
Mechanical/Procedural Complications	
Small-gauge needles	When accessing new fistula in conjunction with inappropriately high blood flow rates
Kinked dialysis tubing	Defective tubing sets or improper positioning of blood lines
Blood pump cycling	Pressure variations on red cells inducing shear stress—of modest clinical significance
Defective blood warmer	Mechanical failure

Mechanical and procedural techniques produce high shear stresses on RBCs. Small-gauge needles used in conjunction with high BFRs are an oft-cited cause of hemolysis.[173] Case reports of hemolysis have also been attributed to kinked dialyzer tubing, with occasional severe, near fatal results.[174] Malfunctioning blood warmers were more often reported in the 1970s, and in those cases, temperatures often exceeded 47°C. However, there has only been one reported case in the modern era.[175]

The signs and symptoms of hemolysis may be subtle, such as ESA resistance, but may be fatal. Findings may include hypoxia, nausea, vomiting, abdominal and back pain, hypotension, and cyanosis. Methemoglobinemia may turn blood lines a dark brownish color as haptoglobin is exhausted binding hemoglobin, leaving methemoglobin free. Newer online blood volume monitors used to monitor hematocrit have also been reported to detect major hemolysis events, finding an unexpected drop in hematocrit. Symptom onset may be rapid or delayed—for example, in cases of hyperthermic blood warmers—and last for several days. The sudden onset of unexplained symptoms consistent with hemolysis should prompt an immediate shutoff of dialysis and laboratory evaluation including lysis laboratory values (haptoglobin, hemoglobin), transfusion reaction evaluation, dialysate composition check, and machine removal. Blood should not be returned to the patient.[8]

Dialysis-Associated Thrombocytopenia

Early descriptions of dialysis-associated thrombocytopenia report a similar pattern to leukopenia—transient early drop with rebound to baseline by the end of the dialysis session.[176,177] This phenomenon was originally linked to cuprophane dialyzers with a less severe effect in cellulose-based dialyzers and is also thought to be complement mediated.[178] Polysulfone and PAN dialyzers are less often associated with thrombocytopenia, and occurrence may be related to sterilization technique—electron beam, more so than dialyzer composition, though this is disputed.[179,180] Thrombopoietin levels are actually higher in dialysis patients after treatment, possibly as compensation for treatment-related platelet loss.[181]

HIT is a concerning development in HD patients who are regularly exposed to UFH or LMWH for anticoagulation. Exposure to UFH is considered more likely to cause HIT than LMWH, though the limited data make risk comparisons between the two difficult.[182] HIT has been reported in other dialysis-related scenarios, such as heparin catheter locks and even dialyzers prerinsed with heparinized saline.[183] True incidence in the ESRD population is unclear; however, one Japanese cohort has reported rates of ~4%.[184] Pathophysiology of HIT involves the formation of autoantibodies to PF4 or the heparin-PF4 complex. This leads to platelet activation and increased risk for thrombosis. Findings include rapid platelet drop to <100,000 (within days of exposure), venous and arterial thrombosis, and, less often, bleeding. In dialysis patients, access thrombosis may occur and circuit clotting frequency may increase. Diagnosis is complicated by the high baseline prevalence of heparin antibodies in ESRD patients, and functional tests such as a serotonin release assay, along with clinical scoring systems, may improve diagnosis.[185]

Treatment of HIT should not wait for laboratory confirmation and involves the cessation of heparin and use of alternative anticoagulation agents. The most commonly used alternative anticoagulants include the direct thrombin inhibitor argatroban as well as the factor Xa inhibitor danaparoid. Argatroban is dosed at 250-μg/kg bolus followed by a 2-μg/kg/min infusion to goal 1.5 to 3 times aPTT baseline.[186] Danaparoid, a non-LMWH factor Xa inhibitor, has also been successfully used.[187] A more recent study developed a protocol for use of bivalirudin, another direct thrombin inhibitor, for outpatient dialysis over an average of ~5 months at an initial dose of 0.02 mg/kg/h without bleeding complications.[188] An earlier direct thrombin inhibitor, recombinant lepirudin, has also been shown effective in the treatment of dialysis-associated HIT; however, lepirudin was withdrawn from the market due to manufacturing concerns in 2012 and is no longer available for use.[189,190] Heparin should be avoided in catheter locks, tissue plasminogen activator or other nonheparinoid solutions should be used.

Hemorrhage

Bleeding complications have long been associated with ESRD. The primary defect is decreased platelet function. Castaldi et al.[191] first described the reversible defects of bleeding time and platelet function assays in 19 dialysis patients in 1966. Platelet numbers and thrombopoietin levels are normal in ESRD; however, the ability to activate platelets is reduced.[181] Platelet granules contain lower levels of activating molecules such as adenosine diphosphate and serotonin.[192] Interactions between platelets and vessel walls are also impaired. The glycophosphate IIb/IIIa receptor, which mediates this interaction, is intact but with reduced function.[193] Increased levels of nitric oxide and prostacyclin, which downregulate platelet activity, may also play a role.[194] Additional changes in the clotting cascade include decreases in von Willebrand factor activity, anemia itself, and decreases in various clotting factor activity levels, especially factor VIII.

Medication contributions to bleeding are significant. Antiplatelet agents may increase bleeding risk, especially dual antiplatelet therapy, though single-agent therapy effect is less certain.[195] Oral vitamin K antagonists used to treat complications of atrial fibrillation likely increase rates of bleeding.[196] Novel non-vitamin K–dependent oral anticoagulants, including rivaroxaban, dabigatran, and apixaban, have all recently come to market. Of these three, rivaroxaban and dabigatran have significant renal clearance and are not recommended for use in dialysis patients.[197] Despite this, ESRD patients have been prescribed these drugs with increased bleeding events.[197] Apixaban may not require dosing adjustment; however, a small study recently reported significantly higher blood levels when using typical dosing.[198]

Bleeding time, a measure of platelet–vessel wall interaction, remains the most commonly used test to assess platelets; however, this is a poor predictor of hemorrhage.[199] Other tests, such as the platelet function analyzer and platelet aggregation test, accurately assess platelet function but have not been evaluated to predict hemorrhage.[200]

ESRD patients have high rates of a number of hemorrhagic complications. GI bleeding is common and variable in presentation: AV malformations, gastric antral vascular ectasia, gastroduodenal ulcers, and so on. One analysis of USRDS data found that upper GI bleeds were common—57 per 1000 patient-years—and carried ~10% mortality.[201] Subdural hematomas occur in dialysis patients at roughly four times the rate of non-ESRD patients and at younger ages.[202] Additional bleeding complications include spontaneous retroperitoneal hematomas, spontaneous kidney cyst rupture in acquired cystic kidney disease, retinal hemorrhages, and frequent bruising.

Management of bleeding complications involves stabilizing the patient with fluids and transfusions as needed. Adequate dialysis may treat and prevent platelet dysfunction. Desmopressin, via intravenous or intranasal route, improves bleeding times for several hours with rapid onset. Oral estrogens have been found to improve bleeding times for several days to 2 weeks.[203] Other treatments include recombinant factor VII and cryoprecipitate.[204]

PULMONARY COMPLICATIONS

Dialysis-Associated Hypoxemia

Dialysis-associated hypoxemia occurs in the majority of HD patients, even those without underlying cardiac or pulmonary conditions. The precise etiology is unclear. The typical pattern is a transient hypoxemia occurring within a few minutes of treatment start, nadir at 30 to 60 minutes, followed by gradual return to baseline.[205] Some patients may experience brief periods of hypoxemia in the postdialysis period as well.[206] This pattern coincides with that found in transient leukopenia. Based on this observation, hypoxia was thought to be caused by translocation of leukocytes to the pulmonary vasculature from complement activation as a result of bioincompatible dialyzers.[207] However, a true causal relationship is unclear. Other possible causes include hypoventilation induced secondary to loss of carbon dioxide through the dialyzer occurring with acetate dialysate.[208] High bicarbonate dialysate has also been associated with hypoxemia and hypoventilation, possibly by inducing rapid metabolic alkalosis.[209] Additional contributing factors may be the presence of obstructive sleep apnea and ESRD-related anemia.

Transient hypoxia is generally well tolerated in those without severe underlying cardiopulmonary conditions. However, the long-term implications are not clear. A retrospective cohort study reported higher mortality in a hypoxic group of dialysis patients; however, the hypoxic cohort had a higher burden of comorbidities compared with nonhypoxic patients.[210] Interestingly, ESRD patients residing at high altitude have a better survival versus matched cohorts residing at lower elevations.[211]

Diagnosis of hypoxia can be made with typical monitoring equipment: pulse oximeter or blood volume monitor saturation probe. These detect hemoglobin saturation of oxygen. Access arterial blood line gasses have been found to correlate well with arterial blood gas values for the partial pressure of oxygen.[212] These techniques do not account for the effect of anemia, however. Treatment is usually not necessary. Addressing underlying causes such as anemia and volume overload is important. When necessary, increased fraction of inspired oxygen via nasal cannula can be used to increase hemoglobin saturations when patients are either symptomatic or when oxygen saturations are less than 92%. Lower bicarbonate concentration–based dialysate (29 mmol/L) may cause less hypoxia than high bicarbonate (36 mmol/L).[213]

TECHNICAL ISSUES

Air Embolism

Air embolism is a potentially catastrophic dialysis-associated event. True incidence is unclear. One center reported 7 cases in 14,000 treatments.[214] Air may enter the circulation in several ways: equipment malfunction or loose connections of blood lines; manipulation, placement, or removal of a dialysis catheter; or spontaneous subclinical appearance as microbubbles.[214] The pre–blood pump arterial line is the most common point of entry of air because of high BFRs and strong negative pressures from the blood pump.[215] This can allow a large volume of air to enter the dialysis circuit rapidly. The prepump access port where saline or medication is infused, also under negative pressure, is another point of air entry. Microbubbles may form spontaneously during dialysis and do not trigger machine safety alarms.[216] Central venous catheters (CVCs), through an inadvertent disconnection or catheter crack or even during blood draws, may cause air embolism as a result of negative intrathoracic pressures.[214,217]

In the modern era of dialysis machines, various safeguards prevent air from reaching the patient. Pressure monitors on the venous return line can detect low pressure when a blood line disconnects from a large-caliber CVC, triggering an automatic shutoff of the blood pump. An alarm may not be triggered, however, if the venous pressure results from a small-gauge venous access needle, even when dislodged. More importantly, a venous drip chamber allows air to be captured after the pump. An air detector in the drip chamber can be triggered at a set threshold, leading to pump shutdown, and an additional downstream air detector and clamp rapidly shut off blood flow if air is detected past the chamber. These alarms should not be disabled.

Clinical signs and symptoms depend on the volume of air, speed of the exposure, and patient factors such as position and anatomy. Animal studies suggest a volume of 1 mL/kg can be fatal and 0.5 mL/kg can lead to irreversible brain damage.[218] Smaller volumes can be fatal when exposure is rapid or air enters the arterial circulation. The usual pathophysiological pattern is air trapping in the pulmonary arteries leading to pulmonary hypertension, decreased venous return, and eventual circulatory shock or death. Patients with a patent foramen ovale or large volumes of air in the setting of intrapulmonary shunts are at risk for paradoxical emboli—air crossing into the arterial circulation from venous circulation. For patients in the supine position during exposure, symptoms include dyspnea, palpitations, chest pain, and a sense of "impending doom." Patients in the upright position are more likely to experience retrograde cerebral embolism and display focal neurological defects, syncope, or seizure. Air may also travel to the coronary arteries, leading to acute myocardial infarction, or to the portal venous circulation, causing abdominal pain.[219,220] The clinical significance of long-term exposure to small volumes of air via microbubbles is unclear, though some have suggested a role in dialysis-associated cognitive impairment.[221]

Acute treatment involves arresting any further influx of air—for example, capping an inadvertently disconnected CVC catheter and performing Durant's maneuver—placing the patient in the left lateral decubitus position with head down, or in Trendelenburg position. This traps air in the right side of the heart and prevents retrograde cerebral embolism. Supplemental oxygen should also be applied. Further treatment is supportive and guided by case series and opinion. Direct aspiration of air from the heart with a preexisting CVC or Swan-Ganz catheter may be attempted, and the use of hyperbaric oxygen is warranted, particularly when symptoms are severe or neurological symptoms are present.[222]

Dialysate Composition

The final composition of dialysate results from precise proportioning of purified water, electrolyte concentrates, and buffer. Errors in dialysate concentrations may lead to serious adverse events. Because most buffer is bicarbonate based, the electrolyte concentrate is supplemented with acid (acid concentrate) to prevent magnesium and calcium precipitation. There are two general methods to generate dialysate. Central generation involves mixing a large batch of concentrate and buffer with purified water to service multiple patients using a proportioning machine. Machine-based methods draw concentrate fluid in from a small volume of electrolyte solution located at the machine. Buffer is also added directly at the machine. Bicarbonate buffer may be liquid or powder, and dry acid concentrate is also available.

Monitoring of dialysate composition relies on checking electrical conductivity of the dialysate generated from electrolyte concentrations. These are machine monitors set with strict tolerances. If composition changes and conductivity falls out of range, dialysate flow is stopped. Errors may occur when conductivity monitors fail or, rarely, when an incorrect composition of dialysis yields an appropriate conductivity. For example, severe metabolic acidosis developed in four patients exposed to an overly high ratio of acidic concentrate to bicarbonate solution. All patients developed symptomatic metabolic acidosis with pH <7. Investigation found proper conductivity despite the incorrect proportioning.[223] A pH meter prevents this type of error. In another case series, faulty machine and handheld meters missed rising conductivity leading to symptomatic hypernatremia in two patients.[224] In another case of hypernatremia, excessive bicarbonate triggered a conductivity alarm, which was ignored. This led to seizure during HD after the patient reached a peak sodium concentration of 207 mEq/L.[225] Hypotonic dialysate caused by inadvertent use of distilled water resulting in massive hemolysis has also been reported.[172]

In addition to conductivity and pH monitors, more sophisticated ion-selective monitors are being developed in response to requests for more personalized dialysate solutions.[226] These increasingly complex systems leave additional room for error. Safeguards, both human and machine, must be in place to prevent errors. One group has suggested a dialysis safety checklist with an explicit dialysate check before each treatment.[227]

Blood Loss

Blood loss secondary to access hemorrhage or other nonprocedural causes of bleeding are discussed elsewhere in this chapter. Significant blood loss as a complication of the dialysis procedure is a rare event. The use of anticoagulation for the dialysis procedure and use of oral anticoagulants or antiplatelet agents increases the risk for bleeding. Blood loss may occur in a number of ways. Clotting of the circuit can generally cause the loss of 200 to 300 mL of blood. Inadvertent disconnection of a dialysis access to the machine may lead to large, potentially fatal, hemorrhage. Typically pressure alarms will alert staff and patients of a disconnected catheter because resistance rapidly drops. However, a dislodged arterial or venous needle may not cause a pressure alarm to sound if a small-gauge needle is the source of the resistance. The high BFR through a catheter causes severe and rapid hemorrhage. Another serious cause of blood loss may be dialysis membrane rupture, often preceded by a high transmembrane pressure. A dialysate blood detector will detect hemoglobin in the dialysate and alerts the staff of this. Lastly, hematomas from access infiltration can lead to significant blood loss as well.

Summary

HD is an extremely complex process that owes its safety to a combination of machine and human factors. Each dialysis unit should have processes in place to rapidly investigate complications as well as mechanisms to improve quality. In this manner, the safety of this vulnerable population can be optimized.

A full list of references is available at www.expertconsult.com.

27

Frequent Hemodialysis: Physiological, Epidemiological, and Practical Aspects

Emilie Trinh, MD, and Christopher T. Chan, MD

OUTLINE

End-stage renal disease (ESRD) is associated with poor outcomes including high mortality, significant morbidity, and lower quality of life (QoL).[1-3] Facility-based conventional hemodialysis (HD), performed thrice-weekly for 3 to 5 hours, and peritoneal dialysis (PD) remain the most common forms of renal replacement therapy for the majority of patients worldwide.[1] In recent years, with efforts to improve outcomes for patients with ESRD, there has been resurgence in interest for frequent HD with emerging evidence of benefits. This chapter examines the physiological rationale, established benefits and risks, prescription options, and practical aspects of frequent HD.

DEFINITION OF TERMS

Several terms have been used to describe the various frequent HD regimens, including *short-daily*, *nocturnal*, *quotidian*, *intensive*, *long*, and *alternative*. Conventional HD is typically defined as three to four sessions per week lasting 3 to 5 hours each. As for frequent HD, three predominant regimens are commonly identified: short-daily, long, and long-frequent (Box 27.1).[4] These treatments may be performed either in a dialysis facility or at home. Short-daily HD consists of five or more sessions per week of short duration (2.5 to 3.5 hours). Long HD involves three to four weekly treatments of 6 to 8 hours. On the other hand, long-frequent HD combines both increased frequency (five or more weekly sessions) and longer duration (6 to 8 hours). Both long and long-frequent HD are usually performed at night while patients sleep.[4,5]

HISTORY OF FREQUENT HEMODIALYSIS

HD was first described in 1960, in Seattle, when Scribner and colleagues developed the Teflon arteriovenous shunt.[6] When HD was introduced, treatments were long and infrequent (12 to 18 hours every 10 to 15 days). Since the minimal dose of dialysis required to treat uremic symptoms was unknown, there was no standard session duration or frequency. With time, the frequency of dialysis was increased from every 10 to 15 days to twice then three times a week. Thrice-weekly HD then became the most widely recognized regimen, since it was believed that patients felt better with this schedule. However, as demand for in-center HD began to exceed its availability, home HD became a reality in the 1960s, credited to Shaldon.[7,8] By the 1970s, a large proportion of patients were treated at home, usually at night, twice or three times a week.[6,7,9] Concomitantly, in 1969, DePalma et al. published the first report of daily HD when they changed seven patients from 8 hours thrice-weekly to five times per week for 4 to hours with resulting improvement in blood pressure and urea clearance.[10] In the 1970s, the development of hollow-fiber dialyzers led to a shortening of the length of dialysis sessions to the current 3.5 to 5 hours three times a week. However, the Tassin Center in France continued to perform long intermittent 8-hour thrice-weekly HD until now with excellent reported outcomes of blood pressure and survival.[11-13] During the same period, availability of funding resulted in a rapid expansion of outpatient dialysis units and PD increased in use, thus leading to a rapid decline of home HD.[6]

BOX 27.1 Frequent Hemodialysis: Definition of Terms

Short-Daily
- ≥5 sessions/wk
- 2.5–3.5 h duration
- At home or in-center

Long
- 3–4 sessions/wk
- 6–8 h duration
- Usually performed at night, at home or in-center

Long-Frequent
- ≥5 sessions/wk
- 6–8 h duration
- Usually performed at night, at home

Subsequently, during the 1980s, short-daily HD programs were established in many European centers as rescue therapy after failure of conventional therapy.[14,15] In 1994, slow, frequent nocturnal home HD was first reported by Dr. Robert Uldall in Toronto, Canada. He described results of six patients treated at home during sleep ≥6 nights per week using a central venous catheter (CVC).[16] Ever since, there has been resurgence in the interest for longer and more frequent HD, as well as home HD, with considerable evidence continuing to support the benefits of intensive therapy.

PHYSIOLOGICAL RATIONALE

With progressive renal failure, uremia results from the accumulation of organic waste products normally excreted by healthy kidneys. Since many uremic compounds have yet to be identified, it is still unclear what exactly causes the uremic syndrome. Furthermore, some of these products may not be toxic.[17,18] Nonetheless, three major groups of uremic solutes are described[18,19]:

1) small water-soluble products (molecular weight <500 Da)
2) small protein-bound solutes (molecular weight <500 Da)
3) middle molecules (molecular weight 500 to 60,000 Da)

The differences in molecular weight, availability in the plasma compartment, and water/lipid-solubility of these solutes dictates the efficiency of their removal with dialysis. Plasma availability is, in turn, influenced by the diffusion rate of these molecules across intercompartmental barriers (e.g., cell membrane) and protein-binding capacity.[18,20,21]

Improved "Unphysiology" With Frequent Hemodialysis

Although healthy kidneys continuously excrete uremic compounds, conventional HD is delivered only thrice weekly for 3 to 5 hours. Hence, conventional HD results in wide fluctuations of solutes in a saw-tooth pattern, which has been characterized as the "unphysiology" of dialysis by Dr. Kjellstrand.[22,23] Moreover, conventional HD results in a long 2-day interdialytic interval, a period of higher mortality, and cardiovascular events.[24] Frequent HD results in smaller oscillations with lower time-averaged concentrations of these retention solutes due to longer treatment duration, increased dialysis frequency, and shorter interdialytic intervals.[25] Thus clearance of uremic waste products is potentially increased with frequent HD regimens.

Improved Clearance of Small Water-Soluble Solutes

With small water-soluble solutes, removal rates are highest at the start of HD with subsequent exponentially decreasing rates during conventional HD since the blood-dialysate concentration gradient decreases with time. However, although only solutes in the plasma component are cleared with dialysis, most solutes also are distributed within intracellular and interstitial compartments. In fact, the concentrations of these small uremic compounds begin to rise immediately after conventional dialysis, known as a *rebound*. Even if many of these solutes easily diffuse across cellular membranes, movement from intracellular and interstitial spaces into the plasma compartment may take up to 60 to 120 minutes after a conventional HD session.[25] Increased dialysis treatment time and frequency allow for greater intercompartmental solute diffusion.[21] Thus rebound is decreased and overall solute clearance potentially increased.

Urea is the most widely recognized small water-soluble uremic solute with a molecular weight of 60 Da, and often is used as a measure of dialysis adequacy. Studies have demonstrated that short-daily HD can increase weekly urea clearances by 30% to 50%. By the same token, frequent nocturnal HD has been shown to approximately double weekly urea clearance compared with conventional therapy.[25-27]

Improved Clearance of Small Protein-Bound Solutes

Kinetic patterns of protein-bound molecules differ from that of urea.[20] Shift from intracellular to extracellular compartments are impeded by the degree of protein binding. With longer and/or more frequent treatment, clearance of these molecules is potentially higher with increased time for intercompartmental movement of solutes. However, studies evaluating protein-bound molecules clearance with extended or frequent HD have led to mixed results. In a study of 13 patients who underwent different dialysis regimens, extended HD (8 hours) was associated with a significant increase in removal of protein-bound uremic toxins.[28] Conversely, in a crossover study, Basile et al. demonstrated no significant change in protein-bound solute clearance with prolonged HD, although small and middle molecule clearance was higher.[29] More recently, an analysis of samples from the FHN (Frequent Hemodialysis Network) trial showed no significant reduction in the protein-bound uremic toxins *p*-cresol sulfate or indoxyl sulfate with increased treatment frequency.[30] These conflicting results may be explained by the small sample size of some of these prior studies as well as the varying degree of protein-binding of some of these molecules. It should be noted that other poorly understood factors likely play a role in uremic solute concentration such as nonrenal clearance and changes in solute production.

Improved Clearance of Middle Molecules

Many middle molecules have been shown to be clinically important uremic toxins.[18,31]

Longer dialysis treatment time would potentially allow for more time for middle molecule movement from intracellular to extracellular compartment and thus increase clearance of these molecules. β2-microglobulin (B2M), implicated in the pathogenesis of dialysis amyloidosis, has been the most extensively studied.[32] Higher serum B2M levels have equally been shown to be associated with mortality.[33,34] Several studies have demonstrated that longer dialysis increases B2M removal.[35,36] Similarly, although of small molecular size, phosphate also is considered widely to behave like a middle molecule given its mainly intracellular distribution with slow diffusion across the cell membrane.[37] Increased frequency and dialysis duration have been reported to have a positive impact on dialysis phosphate removal.[26,35,38]

Improved Fluid Status With Lower Ultrafiltration Rates

Fluid overload is common in patients on thrice-weekly HD and is associated with higher mortality and morbidity.[39] To achieve euvolemia, rapid fluid removal with high ultrafiltration (UF) rates often is used in conventional HD. However, this may cause intradialytic hypotension, leading to myocardial, mesenteric, or cerebral ischemia; nausea; cramping; and vascular access complications. Moreover, episodes of intradialytic hypotension may lead to premature discontinuation of dialysis with resulting failure to reach target weight, thus potentially worsening hypertension and left ventricular hypertrophy (LVH). Indeed, it has been shown that UF rates of >10 mL/kg/h are associated with higher mortality and worse cardiovascular outcomes.[40] With increased frequency and/or longer treatment duration, UF rates can be reduced with more time allowed for vascular refill. As such, intradialytic symptoms may be minimized, and this may potentially improve fluid status, and consequently, cardiovascular outcomes. Indeed, frequent HD regimens are associated with lower UF rates in addition to less dialysis-induced myocardial stunning compared with conventional HD.[41]

BENEFITS AND RISKS: REVIEW OF THE CURRENT EVIDENCE

In recent years, there has been growing research investment and continued demonstrated advantages with intensive HD, both short-daily and long nocturnal. In this section, we review the evidence surrounding the clinical benefits with frequent HD and also elaborate on the potential risks with this therapy.

Clinical Benefits

Survival

To our knowledge, there has been no adequately powered randomized controlled trial (RCT) comparing survival between intensive and conventional HD. Although several observational studies have demonstrated excellent patient survival with frequent HD, interpretation of results is limited by potential selection bias, residual confounding, different definitions of frequent HD, and varying practice patterns.

Many studies have shown better outcomes with longer treatment length. In a study that included HD patients from seven countries in the DOPPS (Dialysis Outcomes and Practice Patterns Study), treatment duration >240 minutes was associated with a significant 19% lower risk for mortality after adjustment.[42] Similarly, in a recent retrospective study of a large multicenter US cohort, Rivara et al. demonstrated a 33% lower adjusted mortality risk with extended-hours HD compared with conventional regimens.[43]

There also have been excellent survival reports with intensive nocturnal HD. In a cohort of 247 Canadian nocturnal HD patients, patient survival was 95% and 80% at 1 and 5 years, respectively.[44] Comparably, in an Australian cohort of 286 home nocturnal patients, overall survival was 98% and 83% at 1 and 5 years.[45] For better comparison with conventional HD, Nesrallah et al. matched intensive home HD patients in the International Quotidian Dialysis Registry to conventional HD patients in the DOPPS and demonstrated a 45% better patient survival with intensive HD (hazard ratio [HR], 0.55; 95% confidence interval [CI], 0.34 to 0.87).[46]

Comparatively, in patients on short-daily HD, survival rates have been reported at 92% at 1 year and 73% at 3 years in a cohort of 262 patients from the United States and Europe.[47] Moreover, lower risk for mortality also has been reported with short-daily HD compared with conventional HD. In fact, when daily home HD patients were matched to in-center HD patients using the US Renal Data System (USRDS) database, daily home HD was associated with a 13% lower mortality risk (HR, 0.87; 95% CI, 0.78 to 0.97).[48]

Although most studies have compared intensive to conventional HD, a more recent cohort study from the Australia and New Zealand Dialysis and Transplantation Registry also compared survival with intensive home HD compared with PD. This study showed better patient survival with home HD (HR of mortality 0.47; 95% CI, 0.38 to 0.59) compared with PD.[49]

The largest randomized studies comparing frequent HD to conventional thrice-weekly in-center HD are the FHN Daily Trial and Nocturnal Trial, two companion multicenter RCTs that randomized participants to either conventional thrice-weekly HD or frequent (six times per week) HD for 12 months. In the FHN Daily Trial, patients were randomized to either conventional thrice-weekly in-center HD or six times per week, in-center, short-daily HD. Conversely, patients in the FHN Nocturnal were randomized to either conventional or six times per week nocturnal home HD. However, as it was deemed not feasible to recruit sufficient participants to assess the individual outcome of mortality, these studies examined two coprimary composite outcomes: (1) death or change in left ventricular mass (LVM) and (2) death or change in physical-health score. Although frequent HD was associated with favorable coprimary outcomes in the FHN Daily Trial, there was no significant effect of frequent HD for either of the two co-primary composite outcomes in the FHN Nocturnal Trial.[26,50] Recently, a long-term follow-up of these two trials has been published. Over a median follow-up of 3.6 years of the FHN Daily Trial, patients who had initially been randomized to frequent short-daily HD had a significantly lower mortality risk compared with those who underwent conventional HD (HR, 0.56; 95% CI, 0.32 to 0.99).[51] In contrast, in the long-term follow-up of the FHN Nocturnal Trial, with a median follow-up of 3.7 years, the risk for mortality was significantly higher in the frequent group (HR, 3.88; 95% CI, 1.27 to 11.79).[50] However, the results of these long-term studies should be interpreted cautiously as the FHN trials were not designed to detect mortality differences. Moreover, patients were free to modify their dialysis prescription after the initial 12 months and there was an exceedingly low mortality rate in the FHN Nocturnal Trial.

Cardiovascular Benefits

Cardiovascular disease remains the leading cause of mortality and morbidity in the ESRD population.[1] LVH is well identified as an independent risk factor for mortality and cardiovascular events with significant prognostic value in ESRD patients.[52-54] The prevalence of LVH increases as renal function declines and is present in up to 85% of incident dialysis patients.[55,56] Studies in conventional HD and PD have shown that LVH progresses over time in the majority of patients.[57,58] In contrast, reduction of left ventricular mass (LVM) has been well reported with intensive HD.[59]

In a prospective Canadian RCT by Culleton et al., frequent nocturnal HD was associated with a significant mean reduction in LVM of 15.3 g ($P = 0.04$) compared with conventional HD.[60] Furthermore, in the FHN Daily Trial, LVM significantly decreased in the short-daily group compared with conventional HD (difference in change between groups of 13.8 g; 95% CI, 5.8 to 21.8).[26] Conversely, in the smaller FHN Nocturnal Trial, no significant difference in LVM was observed. However, the small sample size and large proportion of patients without LVH at baseline could have explained the lack of apparent benefit in the nocturnal group.[26]

Several observational studies also have demonstrated beneficial effects of frequent HD on LVM. In an observational cohort comparing 28 patients who converted from conventional to nocturnal HD with 13 control patients, Chan et al. reported a significant reduction in LVM with nocturnal HD (22% decrease from 147 to 114 g/m^2). In comparison, LVM increased in the controls (142 to 150 g/m^2).[59,61] Similarly, in a prospective cohort study by Ayus et al. comparing 26 short-daily HD patients to 51 matched conventional HD patients, short-daily HD was associated with a 30% decrease in LVM, whereas no change was seen in conventional HD.[62] A meta-analysis, including 38 single-arm studies, 5 crossover trials, and 3 RCTs, examining the effect of frequent or extended HD (home or in-center) also reported favorable reduction of LVM compared with conventional therapy, as well as improved left ventricular ejection fraction.[63] Reduction of LVM with frequent HD is likely multifactorial in the context of improved clearance of uremic toxins, better blood pressure control, superior fluid management, and improved abnormalities of mineral metabolism. Downregulation of genes involved in cardiomyocyte apoptosis and fibrosis and improved endothelial dysfunction also have been demonstrated.[64,65] In addition to beneficial effects on LVH, increased dialysis frequency also reduces left and right ventricular volumes and increases heart rate variability, which have both been shown to be associated with cardiovascular events and mortality.[66-69]

The effect of intensive HD on LVM reduction appears to be much more important in patients with LVH at baseline, as seen in a post hoc analysis of the FHN trials.[70] Moreover, recent studies also highlighted the important prognostic implication of LVH regression. In a single-center observational study of 144 intensive home HD patients from Toronto, Canada, regression or prevention of LVH was associated with a significantly lower risk for the composite endpoint of all-cause mortality, technique failure, or cardiovascular hospitalization (HR, 0.42; 95% CI, 0.21 to 0.84). Regression was defined as a reduction of >10% in LVM in patients with baseline LVH.[71]

In addition, a lower cardiovascular hospitalization risk has been reported with frequent HD. When Medicare-enrolled daily home HD patients were compared with matched thrice-weekly HD patients by Weinhandl et al., daily HD was associated with a significantly lower risk for cardiovascular-related admission (HR, 0.89; 95% CI, 0.86 to 0.93).[72] Similar beneficial results on cardiovascular-related hospitalization risk also were seen when daily home HD patients were compared with PD patients.[73,74]

Blood Pressure

Improved blood pressure control has been reported consistently with frequent HD in observational, as well as randomized studies.[26,61,75] In a meta-analysis, intensive HD was associated with significantly lower systolic, and diastolic blood pressure and mean number of blood pressure medications.[63] Although improved fluid status plays a role in better blood pressure control, other established mechanisms with intensive HD have included decreased peripheral resistance, decreased plasma norepinephrine concentration, restoration of brachial artery responsiveness to hyperemia and nitrates, and increased baroreceptor sensitivity and compliance.[76,77]

Mineral Metabolism

Improved phosphate control with decreased use of phosphate binders is extensively described with frequent HD regimens. In the FREEDOM trial, a prospective observational study of short-daily HD, frequent HD was associated with a significant decrease in serum phosphorus.[78] Similar findings were described in the FHN trial and the more recent ACTIVE trial, which randomized patients to extended weekly (>24 hours) or standard (12 to 15 hours) HD.[26,38] However, the effects of intensive HD on parathyroid hormone (PTH) levels appear variable. In an RCT by Walsh et al. comparing the effects nocturnal HD with conventional HD on mineral metabolism, beneficial effects on serum phosphorus and phosphate binders use were described, but there were no significant changes in intact PTH levels. Nonetheless, decline in PTH levels were more frequent in the nocturnal group than in the conventional group (61% vs. 20%; $P = 0.003$).[79]

Sleep

Improvement in symptoms of sleep apnea has been demonstrated with intensive HD.[78,80-82] More recently, studies have linked fluid overload to the pathogenesis of sleep apnea in patients with ESRD. Indeed, it has been shown that there is redistribution of extracellular fluid in the supine position, with interstitial fluid accumulation in the neck tissues and in the lungs, thus leading to increased upper airway collapsibility and pulmonary congestion.[83,84] Consequently, reduction in fluid overload with frequent HD may result in improvement in apnea symptoms. Furthermore, the FREEDOM study demonstrated that short-daily HD was associated with better sleep quality, as measured by the Medical Outcome Study sleep survey. In fact, significant increased sleep adequacy with decreased sleep disturbances and nighttime awakening were reported with frequent HD. Similarly, there was significant improvement in symptoms of restless legs syndrome (RLS), assessed by the International Restless Legs Syndrome (IRLS) Study Group rating scale, with frequent HD. This was even more pronounced in patients with moderate to severe RLS at baseline.[82]

Fertility and Pregnancy

ESRD is associated with decreased fertility and low conception rates. Moreover, pregnancy outcomes are poor with higher risk for intrauterine growth retardation, stillbirth, preterm labor, and preeclampsia.[85] Although data are limited, better pregnancy outcomes have been reported with intensive HD. A recent cohort study compared 22 pregnancies on intensive HD in the Toronto Pregnancy and Kidney Disease Clinic and Registry to 70 pregnancies from the American Registry for Pregnancy in Dialysis Patients. Intensive HD was associated with higher gestational age, higher infant birth weight, and superior live birth rates.[86]

In the setting of chronic kidney disease, numerous factors are thought to contribute to decreased fertility.[85,87] Endocrine disturbances are present with abnormal follicular-stimulating hormone and luteinizing hormone levels leading to lower estrogen and progesterone concentrations and increased prolactin levels.[88,89] In addition, dysregulation of the hypothalamic-pituitary-gonadal axis, menstrual irregularities, sexual dysfunction, anemia, and medications play a role.[85,87] With more intensive HD, it is postulated that the increased clearance of uremic toxins may improve hypothalamic–pituitary–gonadal axis dysfunction and endocrine abnormalities. Furthermore, better blood pressure control with intensive HD also may lead to improved pregnancy outcomes. [85]

Quality of Life

Impaired QoL is common in ESRD patients. As frequent HD includes various different treatment regimens that can be performed in-center or at home, the effects of frequent HD on QoL have yielded inconsistent results.[90] In a RCT of frequent home nocturnal HD versus conventional HD by Culleton et al., frequent therapy was associated with improved selected kidney-specific domains of QoL, although there was no significant difference in overall QoL.[60] More recently, the ACTIVE trial randomized patients to extended weekly (>24 hours) or standard HD (12 to 15 hours), either in-center or at home, and evaluated change in QoL using the EuroQol 5 dimension instrument (EQ-5D). At 12 months, change in EQ-5D score did not differ between groups, but the relatively high baseline scores of participants may have limited significant findings.[38] However, in this study, both physical and mental component scores of the 36-Item Short Form Health Survey (SF-36) did significantly improve with intensive HD.[38] Comparatively, in the FHN trial, one of the coprimary composite outcome included a patient-reported physical health score (RAND-36). Whereas participants in the FHN Daily Trial reported a significant higher score after 12 months compared with conventional HD, there was no significant difference in the FHN Nocturnal Trial.[26] Additional analyses from the FHN trial showed that patients in the frequent daily in-center HD group had higher feeling thermometer scores, and that both nocturnal and short-daily groups had shorter dialysis recovery time compared with the conventional group.[91] The feeling thermometer is a single question that asks patients to rate their health on a scale from 0 to 100, with 100 being perfect health. Shorter recovery time after HD also has been reported in observational studies.[78,92]

The effect of frequent HD on depressive symptoms has been variable. In the FHN trials, no significant differences were found in either the Daily Trial or the Nocturnal Trial.[26] Conversely, in the FREEDOM study, short-daily HD was associated with a significant decrease in Beck Depression Inventory (BDI) score and the proportion of patients with depressive symptoms decreased significantly after 12 months.[78,90]

It should be noted that, although there is a physiological basis for escalation of dialysis dose for mineral metabolism, fertility, and cardiovascular benefits, there may not be a clear rationale for improved overall QoL with more intensive HD. It may be more realistic to expect positive changes in kidney-specific domains of QoL. Furthermore, the heterogeneity of patients (home vs. in-center, different treatment schedules) makes the true effect on QoL difficult to evaluate. For home HD patients, there is the added complexity of the dialysis procedure that needs to be considered. Limitations of QoL measurement tools should be taken into account.

Risks and Complications

Noninfectious Vascular Complications

With frequent HD schedules, the number of vascular access cannulations is higher. With increased vascular access use, the risk for vascular access complications, both infectious and noninfectious, is potentially higher.

In the FHN Daily Trial, Suri et al. reported a higher risk for first vascular access event (repair, loss, or hospitalization) in daily HD compared with conventional HD (HR, 1.76; 95% CI, 1.11 to 2.79). The majority of these events were repairs or losses. Among patients with arteriovenous (AV) access, the increased risk was even more pronounced (HR, 1.90; 95% CI,

1.11 to 3.25). In the corresponding Nocturnal Trial, similar trends were observed but these results failed to reach statistical significance.[93] In an observational Australian study by Jun et al. of 286 patients receiving extended-hours HD, the number of weekly dialysis sessions was found to be associated with higher risk for vascular events. In fact, each one-session-per-week increase in dialysis frequency was associated with a HR of 1.56 (95% CI, 1.03 to 2.36) of adverse access-related event.[45]

Infectious Complications

In patients with ESRD, infection is a major cause of mortality and morbidity, accounting for almost 25% of hospitalizations.[1,94,95] In a study with daily home HD patients matched to conventional in-center HD patients using USRDS data, infection-related hospitalization was higher in the daily group (HR 1.18; 95% CI, 1.13 to 1.23).[72] Vascular-access infection-related hospitalization was significantly higher in the daily group (HR, 1.39; 95% CI, 1.28 to 1.50) as well.[72] However, these results may have been confounded by incomplete information regarding vascular access type and dialysis dose. Conversely, in the FHN trials, there was no overall difference in infection-related hospitalization between intensive and conventional HD.[26,50]

Given more frequent vascular access use, recent studies have evaluated whether central venous catheter (CVC) use leads to worse outcomes in intensive HD patients by the same token as it does in conventional thrice-weekly HD patients. Indeed, similar to studies in conventional HD, two recent registry-based observational studies from Canada and the United States demonstrated that CVC use is associated with higher mortality and hospitalization rates compared with AV fistulae (AVF) and AV graft (AVG) use.[96,97]

Nonetheless, an important factor to consider is the heterogeneity of patients on frequent HD. Moreover, multiple confounders exist when examining vascular access risks with frequent HD, namely differences in operator, infection control practices, frequency of treatment, and cannulation technique.[98] In fact, cannulation technique is an important contributor to infection risk and this information is lacking in several observational studies. Although buttonhole cannulation may be possibly easier to perform at home, studies have indicated it leads to worse outcomes. In a systematic review by Wong et al. examining home HD patients, buttonhole cannulation was associated with higher risk for both local and systemic infections compared with rope-ladder technique.[99]

Residual Kidney Function

Residual kidney function (RKF) is a well-known independent predictor of overall survival in patients with ESRD.[100-102] RKF was examined in both the FHN Daily and Nocturnal trials.[103] The difference in RKF was not as significant in the short-daily group, with comparable urine outputs at 4 and 12 months, as patients on conventional HD. On the other hand, in the nocturnal group, 52% of the patients were anuric at 4 months compared with 18% in patients on conventional HD (P = 0.02). After 12 months, this number increased to 67% in the nocturnal group as opposed to 36% in patients on thrice-weekly HD.[103] However, the FHN studies were likely not designed to detect changes in RKF. Moreover, it is unclear why a more pronounced decline of RKF was seen in the nocturnal group, but not seen with the short-daily group as the HD frequency in both groups was the same. Further studies are needed to better understand RKF trajectory with intensified HD schedules.

Technique Failure

Higher dialysis frequency may be challenging for patients and their caregivers, and this may lead to discontinuation of frequent HD and switch to a thrice-weekly regimen. To our knowledge, few studies have examined the association between dialysis frequency and technique failure in home HD. In a multicenter registry-based Canadian study by Tennankore et al. examining differences in technique survival between different home HD modalities, both short-daily and nocturnal home HD were associated with similar treatment survival when compared with conventional home HD.[104]

There is scarce data examining technique survival in the setting of in-center frequent HD. In a multicenter cohort in the International Quotidian Dialysis Registry, technique failure occurred in 30% of patients receiving facility-based daily HD after a median of 10 months.[94,105]

With increasing efforts to encourage frequent dialysis modalities, it is imperative to better understand technique survival and find strategies to help maintain patients on these therapies. Are there any facility-specific features that predict failure? Are technique failure rates changing with time? It is possible that expanding patient selection criteria may lead to higher discontinuation rates.

CLINICAL INDICATIONS

Frequent HD, particularly home HD, may be beneficial to several patient populations. Box 27.2 outlines situations in which frequent HD and home HD are appropriate as well as contraindications.[4,106]

PRESCRIPTIONS FOR FREQUENT HEMODIALYSIS

Different prescription options exist for frequent HD and can be performed either at home or in a dialysis facility. These prescriptions should be tailored according to clinical status as well as patient preferences. Typical prescriptions for short-daily, long, and long-frequent HD are provided in Table 27.1.

Dialysis Machines

Standard traditional dialysate machines are the same machines used for facility-based conventional HD. Conversely, low-flow dialysate machines (NxStage System One) are designed for short-daily and also long nocturnal home HD. They are used mainly in the United States.[5] As opposed to standard machines, the NxStage System One is portable, giving patients freedom to travel. Moreover, it operates with simple plumbing connections and standard electric current, thus minimizing utility cost and need for modifications to the patient's home. Dialysate is delivered through premixed solution bags, and obviates the need of a water treatment system.[107] A dialysate volume of 15 to 60 L can be delivered at each HD session. As such, clearances with low-flow dialysate systems are lower compared with traditional options, which deliver ≤200 L dialysate per treatment, hence the need for increased dialysis frequency with this system.[5]

BOX 27.2 Clinical Indications and Contraindications for Home Hemodialysis'

Indications for frequent hemodialysis
- Severe obstructive sleep apnea
- Resistant hyperphosphatemia with or without symptoms
- Persistent uremic symptoms
- Uncontrolled hypertension
- Refractory fluid overload
- Right heart failure
- Uncontrolled ascites
- Symptomatic intradialytic hypotension on conventional hemodialysis
- Excessive recovery time after conventional hemodialysis
- Women who are pregnant or planning to conceive

Potential candidates for home hemodialysis
- Employed patients
- Patients attending school
- Patients who have failed peritoneal dialysis and wish to remain on a home modality
- Motivated patients wishing to perform therapy at home

Contraindications to home hemodialysis
- Unstable medical conditions
- Lack of suitable vascular access
- Uncontrolled behavioral or psychological issues
- Contraindication to anticoagulation use
- Uncontrolled seizures
- Significant hemodynamic instability on hemodialysis
- Planned transplant within 6–12 mo

Data from Tennankore K, Nadeau-Fredette AC, Chan CT. Intensified home hemodialysis: clinical benefits, risks and target populations. *Nephrol Dial Transplant.* 2014;29:1342-1349; Rioux JP, Marshall MR, Faratro R, Hakim R, Simmonds R, Chan CT. Patient selection and training for home hemodialysis. *Hemodial Int.* 2015;19(suppl 1):S71-79.

Target Weight

Patients should be educated to adjust their target weights based on clinical symptoms and blood pressure with frequent reassessments.

Phosphate Additives

With intensive nocturnal HD, greater phosphate removal occurs and thus, serum phosphate should be monitored closely as hypophosphatemia is not uncommon. If hypophosphatemia occurs, dietary phosphorus should be increased. If hypophosphatemia persists despite dietary modifications, a phosphate additive, in the form of a phosphate-containing enema (e.g., Fleet), can be added to the dialysate. For every 30 mL of Fleet additive, the dialysate phosphate concentration is raised by approximately 0.2 mmol/L.[108,109]

Anticoagulation

Unfractionated heparin is the most common anticoagulation option used with frequent HD. It is typically delivered as a bolus (50 U/kg) with or without a subsequent infusion of 500 to 1500 U/hour by heparin pump depending on the length of the session. Heparin should be stopped 1 hour before the end of the treatment if the patient has an AVF or AVG and at the end of treatment if the patient has a CVC.[5] Low-molecular-weight heparin also can be effective, with a single dose administered at the start of dialysis.[5,110,111] However, since the duration of anticoagulation effect may be variable depending on the type of low-molecular-weight heparin used, these agents may be less ideal for longer sessions of >6 to 8 hours.[5,110]

Vascular Access

Arteriovenous Fistula. Cannulation of an AVF can be a difficult process and if done improperly, may lead to pain, bleeding, needle infiltration, and hematoma formation. Moreover, with repeated cannulation, aneurysm formation may result due to damage to blood vessel walls.[25] The in-

TABLE 27.1 Frequent Hemodialysis Prescriptions

	Conventional	Short-Daily (NxStage)	Short-Daily (Traditional)	Long (Alternate-Night Nocturnal)	Long-Frequent (Nocturnal)
Frequency	3 d/wk	5–6 d/wk	5–6 d/wk	3–4 nights/wk	5–6 nights/wk
Duration (h)	3–5	2.5–4	2.5–3.5	6–8	6–8
Q_b (mL/min)	300–400	300–400	350–400	250–350	250–350
Q_d (mL/min)	500–800	90–300	350–600	300–500	300
Base (mmol/L)	HCO_3, 32–36	Lactate, 40–45	HCO_3, 32–36	HCO_3, 28–35	HCO_3, 28–35
K^+ (mmolL)	2	2	2	2-3	2-3
Ca^{2+} (mmol/L)	1.25	1.5	1.25	1.25–1.5	1.5–1.75
PO_4 additive	None	None	None	Rare	20%–30% of the time

Ca^{2+}, Calcium; *K^+*, potassium; *PO_4*, phosphate, *Qb*, blood flow rate; *Qd*, dialysate flow rate.
(Adapted from Tennankore K, Nadeau-Fredette AC, Chan CT. Intensified home hemodialysis: clinical benefits, risks and target populations. *Nephrol Dial Transplant.* 2014;29:1342-1349; Lockridge R, Cornelis T, Van Eps C. Prescriptions for home hemodialysis. *Hemodial Int.* 2015;19(suppl 1):S112-127.)

creased frequency of AV access use with intensive HD makes adequate cannulation technique even more critical, especially for patients dialyzing at home.

Two methods of cannulation are used: rope ladder and buttonhole techniques. With the rope ladder technique, needling sites are distributed along the entire length of the AVF.[112] If properly performed, scar tissue formation may be minimized because different puncture sites are used. However, certain needling sites may be preferred, and this technique may weaken the blood vessel wall, thus promoting dilation and aneurysm formation. Conversely, the buttonhole technique involves repeated cannulation of the same site using the same angle and length with blunt needles. To create a buttonhole, a sharp needle is used over 6 to 12 HD sessions to form a scar tissue tract into the fistula.[112,113]

It is hypothesized that the buttonhole cannulation with a blunt needle may be easier to perform at home and cause less vascular damage with reduced cannulation time, fewer needling attempts, decreased risk for needle infiltrations and hematomas, less potential for aneurysm formation and possibly, and decreased pain.[113] However, few studies have demonstrated any significant benefit of buttonhole cannulation compared with the rope ladder technique. In fact, in a systematic review comparing the buttonhole to the rope ladder technique, no demonstrable difference in cannulation pain was found among randomized studies.[99] Similarly, randomized studies have also found no difference in bleeding risk.[114-118] Furthermore, risk for hematoma formation has been inconsistent.[116] Regarding aneurysm formation, beneficial effects were reported with buttonhole cannulation in observational studies, but these studies were limited by small sample size.[116,119,120]

Nevertheless, the infectious risk, both local and systemic, has been well documented with buttonhole cannulation compared with the rope ladder technique. In fact, in a recent metaanalysis, Muir et al. reported significant higher rates of AVF infections with use of buttonhole cannulation (incidence rate ratio 3.85; 95% CI, 1.66 to 12.77) and these results were consistent among randomized and observational studies.[121] Given its associated infectious risk, we recommend that buttonhole cannulation should not be routinely employed. If used, topical antibiotic prophylaxis is strongly advised. Options include Polysporin triple ointment, Mupirocin ointment, or Povidone-iodine ointment. For any self-cannulation, patients should adhere to an appropriate aseptic technique with proper handwashing. After cannulation, a secure and stable taping method should be used.[113]

Arteriovenous Graft. With AVG, only the rope ladder technique is recommended for cannulation.

Central Venous Catheter. For CVC use, proper hand hygiene is crucial with use of an antiseptic to clean the catheter hub. Moreover, to reduce the risk for accidental disconnection and air embolism, a closed-connector device is recommended for home HD use and changed weekly. After each HD treatment, it is common to lock the CVC with either citrate 4% or unfractionated heparin (1000 or 5000 units/mL). Tissue plasminogen activator also may be used in case of catheter malfunction. A dressing (either gauze or nonocclusive transparent) is recommended to be placed at the exit site of the catheter. As for exit-site antibiotic prophylaxis, its use is not consistent across different centers.[113]

Measuring Dialysis Adequacy With Frequent Hemodialysis

Kt/V_{urea} has been used as a measure of dialysis adequacy for more than 30 years. Kt/V_{urea} was first proposed by Gotch et al. in the 1980s when HD was performed thrice-weekly with low-flux dialyzer and of short duration in the United States.[122] At that time, it was determined that Kt/V_{urea} <0.8 was associated with poor dialysis outcomes.[122] In the subsequent HEMO (Hemodialysis) study where patients were randomized to standard (single-pool [sp]Kt/V 1.25) or high-dose HD (spKt/V 1.65), no significant difference in survival was observed between interventions.[123] It should be noted that HD has evolved significantly in the last few years with large-pore high-flux dialysis membranes, more intensive HD regimens and convective strategies.[20]

Treatment duration may deceptively modify Kt/V_{urea}. In fact, shorter sessions may lead to a deflated postdialysis urea value, due to inadequate time for urea rebound, and Kt/V urea may be overestimated. By the same token, urea generation may be increased in extended-hours HD. In fact, an improved equation for spKt/V was recommended by Daugirdas et al. incorporating a urea generation factor adjusted based on length and frequency of treatment.[124]

Nonetheless, for frequent or extended HD regimens, urea clearance can be expressed as weekly standardized Kt/V, as proposed by Gotch et al. (Fig. 27.1).[125] The National Kidney Foundation Kidney's Disease Outcomes Quality Initiative has suggested a target weekly standard Kt/V of 2.3 with a minimum dose of 2.1.[126]

However, although studies have examined the effect of frequent HD regimens on urea clearance, there have been no studies, to our knowledge, examining the association of Kt/V with clinical outcomes in intensive HD. Although urea is still considered by many as a measure of dialysis adequacy, there is little data on its toxicity. Moreover, it should be emphasized that urea kinetics may not be representative of other uremic solutes.[18,20]

More recently, the need for a multidimensional measure to quantify dialysis dose has been highlighted. Ideally, this multidimensional measure would incorporate small solute removal, middle molecule clearance, mineral metabolism control, fluid status, cardiovascular parameters, RKF, and most importantly, patient-reported outcomes.[127]

IMPLEMENTING A FREQUENT HEMODIALYSIS PROGRAM

Frequent Home Hemodialysis program

Implementation of a home HD program requires a specialized infrastructure involving competent personnel, adequate facility space, and appropriate equipment and supplies. An experienced multidisciplinary team is crucial for the success of a home HD program.

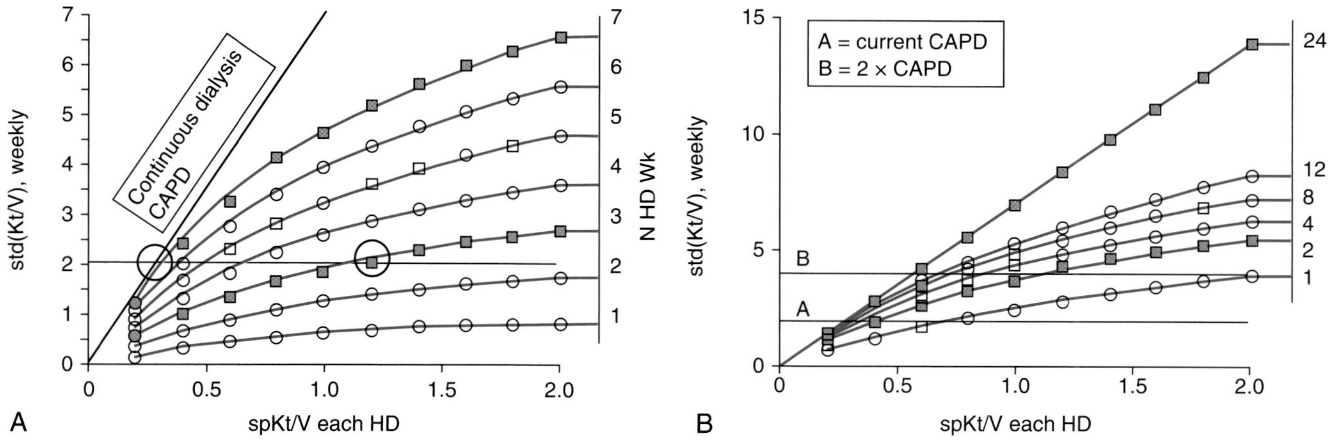

FIG. 27.1 Relationship between weekly standard Kt/V and per-dialysis single-pool Kt/V. (A) The effect of various session frequency with constant dialysis time (3.5 h). (B) The effect of varying treatment time with dialysis frequency of 7 days per week. (From Gotch FA. The current place of urea kinetic modelling with respect to different dialysis modalities. *Nephrol Dial Transplant.* 1998;13(suppl 6):10-14.[125])

There should be arrangements made for adequate and timely delivery of supplies to the patient. This includes dialyzers, dialysate concentrate, blood lines, needles, dressings, tape, gauze, masks, and blood test collection tubes. Typically, delivery is contracted out to a medical supply delivery company.[25]

In-center Daily Hemodialysis Program

Patients who are not suitable candidates for home treatment may benefit from more frequent dialysis. As such, an in-center daily HD program offering short-daily HD could be advantageous for certain patient populations. However, the implementation of an in-center short-daily HD program poses some logistic issues. To start, for most facilities, one HD station will allow six patients to be dialyzed each week on a conventional thrice-weekly schedule. Although treatment duration is reduced with short-daily HD, time is still required for dialysis machine preparation and cleaning. Therefore fewer patients may be able to be accommodated. Moreover, nursing workload is increased and cost for supplies and equipment is raised. To accommodate short-daily HD, facilities may need to stay open longer or to create new HD stations; this would have a much higher financial impact.[25] To overcome some of these constraints, it has been suggested that that the treatment duration for daily patients be about half of a conventional session such that two short-daily HD patients share one conventional HD time slot.[129]

In-center Nocturnal Hemodialysis Program

Analogously, many patients who are not suitable for home therapy may benefit from extended-hours HD through in-center nocturnal HD. Similar to in-center daily HD, implementation of an in-center nocturnal HD program also poses some challenges. It requires additional nursing staff and technicians to work overnight, and adequate infrastructure for patients to be able to sleep while receiving dialysis. However, the numerous benefits with intensive HD potentially outweigh the cost burden.

ECONOMIC CONSIDERATIONS

Although the implementation of a new home HD program may incur high upfront cost, studies have consistently reported financial benefits with home HD compared with conventional HD.[131-134] Cost savings are likely associated with decreased labor costs, lower medication use, and fewer hospitalizations.[9,135] In fact, in a Canadian study by McFarlane et al., home nocturnal HD was reported to provide three times more dialysis treatment time at a one-fifth lower cost.[133] Similarly, in an Australian cohort, Agar et al. also demonstrated significant cost savings of 11% when home nocturnal HD was compared with conventional satellite HD.[131]

As opposed to home HD programs, in-center daily or nocturnal HD programs have a higher financial burden with increased staffing requirements and possible infrastructure changes. However, this must be weighed against the numerous clinical benefits as well as potential for decreased hospital admissions in these patients.

MEDICATION DOSING CONSIDERATIONS

With more intensive HD regimens, clearance of medications during HD may be more difficult to predict. The clearance of a drug during HD depends on numerous factors: the characteristics of the molecule, the type of dialysis membrane, the blood and dialysate flow rates, length of dialysis treatment, and UF rates.[136] Very few studies have examined changes in pharmacokinetics with frequent HD. Manley et al. examined the removal of gentamicin in eight patients on slow-daily home HD. They demonstrated that clearance of the medication was higher compared with conventional HD, but with high variability, and recommended doses of 2 to 2.5 mg/kg post-HD.[137] Likewise, Law et al. studied optimal dosing of cefazolin in a Canadian cohort of nocturnal home HD patients. Although the hourly drug clearance was lower compared with conventional dialyzers, the longer treatment duration resulted in overall increased clearance. After a 6-hour nocturnal treatment, 63% to 76% of drug removal occurred compared with previous reports of clearance up to 60% with high-flux dialyzers during a 4-hour session. Nonetheless, despite increased cefazolin clearance, the same dose of cefazolin as for conventional HD (2 g load then 1 g after each HD) was able to achieve sufficient blood concentrations.[138]

There is paucity of data evaluating dosing strategies in intensive HD. For medications where plasma levels cannot be monitored, it is reasonable to dose medications based on an approximate creatinine clearance of 20 to 30 mL/min.[108] Appropriate clinical follow-up is essential. Nonetheless, further studies are needed to better understand pharmacokinetics with frequent therapy.

INTERNATIONAL TRENDS AND VARIATION

The use of frequent HD continues to increase internationally, but its use varies considerably between and within countries.[1,139] Types of frequent HD also differ around the world. Regarding home HD, short-daily HD predominates in the United States with the NxStage system, whereas long nocturnal regimens of 4 to 7 nights per week are more common elsewhere.[9,140] In the latest USRDS report, the highest rates of home HD use were reported in New Zealand and Australia at 18% and 9% of dialysis patients, respectively. Lower rates of 3% to 6% are seen in Canada, Denmark, Finland, the Netherlands, Sweden, the United Kingdom, and Scotland. In the rest of the world, home HD is either not provided or used in <3% of dialysis patients.[1]

As for facility-based frequent HD, successful in-center nocturnal HD programs have been reported all over the world: Canada, the United States, the United Kingdom, Germany, Italy, Portugal, Slovenia, and China.[130]

OVERCOMING BARRIERS IN UPTAKE OF FREQUENT HEMODIALYSIS

Despite continuing reports of benefits with frequent and home HD, barriers still persist and need to be overcome to increase uptake of these modalities. Barriers exist from the perspectives of patients, healthcare professionals, and governing agencies.[9,135]

As previously discussed, from a patient standpoint, many of the perceived barriers to home HD can be overcome with early comprehensive predialysis education. Home dialysis modalities should be properly presented to all patients with chronic kidney disease as feasible and efficient treatment options. Education should begin early, ideally once estimated glomerular filtration is <30 mL/min/1.73 m^2 and should involve the patient, their family members, and a competent multidisciplinary team. Inadequate or lack of predialysis education typically leads to in-center HD as a renal replacement modality, especially for patients who are referred late. In a randomized trial by McLaughlin et al., a multifaceted education intervention led to a higher likelihood of patients perceiving advantages to home dialysis than standard predialysis education.[141] Moreover, even in the setting of suboptimal dialysis initiation, comprehensive education should be promoted and has been shown to lead to a successful transition to a home modality for a significant proportion of patients.[142]

To provide comprehensive and proper education, it is imperative that all renal healthcare providers be interested and adequately informed on the advantages and disadvantages of intensive HD. This includes physicians, nurses, dietitians, and social workers. Still, physician interest in advocating for home HD remains a challenge. In fact, in an international survey of 439 healthcare professionals, more than half had no home HD patients in their units. The lack of trained staff members and insufficient funding were identified as major challenges in promoting home HD.[143] Furthermore, to ensure competent knowledge, it is imperative that all nephrology trainees be adequately exposed to home HD during their training.

To increase uptake of frequent HD, funding and reimbursement policies also should be adequate. Changes in reimbursement should be implemented so that in-center and home therapy are at least equally remunerated. Furthermore, adequate funding for proper pre-ESRD education is essential to promote uptake of home HD. This also applies for in-center frequent or nocturnal HD programs.

Lastly, another important barrier to home HD use is the complexity of dialysis machines and water treatment system. Development of more user-friendly equipment should be encouraged with smaller, portable machines with simple commands and easier setup. Possible integration of water treatment would be useful to simplify the process.

FREQUENT HEMODIALYSIS IN CHILDREN

Although conventional HD regimens still predominate in children, reports of more intensified regimens are increasing.[144,145] A recent RCT demonstrated feasibility of frequent in-center HD in children, which also led to improved blood pressure control.[146] Home HD has been increasingly described in children.[145] However, the time constraints, disruption of daily life, and potential for increased parental/caregiver burden must be considered in the pediatric population.

FUTURE DIRECTIONS

In recent years, frequent and extended-hours HD have gained in popularity due to numerous established benefits, whether performed in-center or at home. However, many barriers still need to be overcome to increase uptake of these modalities. These include patient reluctance and inadequate education, lack of physician interest and expertise, complexity of dialysis machines, and most importantly, absence of adequate reimbursement and funding policies. Further research is needed to elucidate strategies to reduce technique failure to maintain patients on intensive HD. More quality assurance studies are required to properly quantify and find ways to minimize the potential risks with frequent HD.

A full list of references is available at www.expertconsult.com.

28

Home Hemodialysis

Michael A. Kraus, MD, and Eric Weinhandl, PhD, MS

OUTLINE

INTRODUCTION

Therapy for end-stage renal disease (ESRD) in the United States is dominated by in-center hemodialysis, with less than 2% of the population using home hemodialysis for renal replacement therapy (RRT). However, since 2004 there has been a resurgence of interest in home hemodialysis, with an increase in utilization.[1] This increase can be related to newer devices with less burden and more convenience, as well as the growing interest in increased frequency of hemodialysis. What percentage of patients in the United States could use home hemodialysis? At its peak in 1973, 40% of US patients were treated with home hemodialysis.[2] Patient characteristics have changed over the past 40 years, with an older and sicker population receiving RRT. Certainly, home hemodialysis is not for every patient. However, most would agree that the therapy is underutilized. Moran and Kraus postulated a reasonable estimate of 25%, realizing this growth would take many years to achieve.[3] The benefits of home hemodialysis include flexibility and convenience of home therapies, emphasis on patient-centered care with increased independence, and the simplicity and relatively low cost of providing increased frequency of dialysis, if desired.

BURDEN OF CONVENTIONAL HEMODIALYSIS

Conventional hemodialysis (HD), as it is typically prescribed in the United States, is truly burdensome to the daily lives of patients. Overwhelmingly, conventional HD involves three sessions per week, each 3 to 4.5 hours in duration.[4] Cumulatively, such time "on the machine" consumes 9 to 14 hours per week, typically during the day. Moreover, because patients typically undergo HD in a healthcare facility, there is requisite travel before and after each session. In the DOPPS (Dialysis Outcomes and Practice Patterns Study), more than 2100 US patients responded to the survey question, "How long does it take you to get to your dialysis unit or center (one way)?" Among respondents, 47% reported 15 minutes or less, 33% reported 16 to 30 minutes, 17% reported 31 to 60 minutes, and 3% reported longer than 60 minutes.[5] By this distribution, each dialysis session reasonably necessitates 45 minutes of travel, thus increasing the time that is devoted directly to dialysis therapy to 11 to 16 hours per week. Not surprisingly, the employment rate among dialysis patients between the ages of 18 and 54 years remains low.[6]

Arguably as important as time on the machine is time that is consumed by recovering from a dialysis session. During recovery time, which is highly variable but may tend to range from 6 to 8 hours, physical and mental function may be impaired.[7] With 18 hours per week devoted to recovery, cumulative time either directly or indirectly devoted to dialysis therapy is 29 to 34 hours per week. In tandem with receipt of any additional health care, including hospital admissions, clinic appointments, and pharmacy visits, conventional HD therapy is essentially a (permanent) full-time occupation. Plausibly, patients would appreciate interventions that can ease treatment itself or return some normalcy to the interdialytic interval.

HOME HEMODIALYSIS: BENEFITS AND POTENTIAL RISKS

Home hemodialysis (HHD) represents a strategy to relieve the burden of conventional HD. HHD obviously shifts treatment from a healthcare facility to the home, thereby obviating peri-session travel. More importantly, HHD removes the constraint that shift-based scheduling on Monday–Wednesday–Friday and Tuesday–Thursday–Saturday cycles imposes on

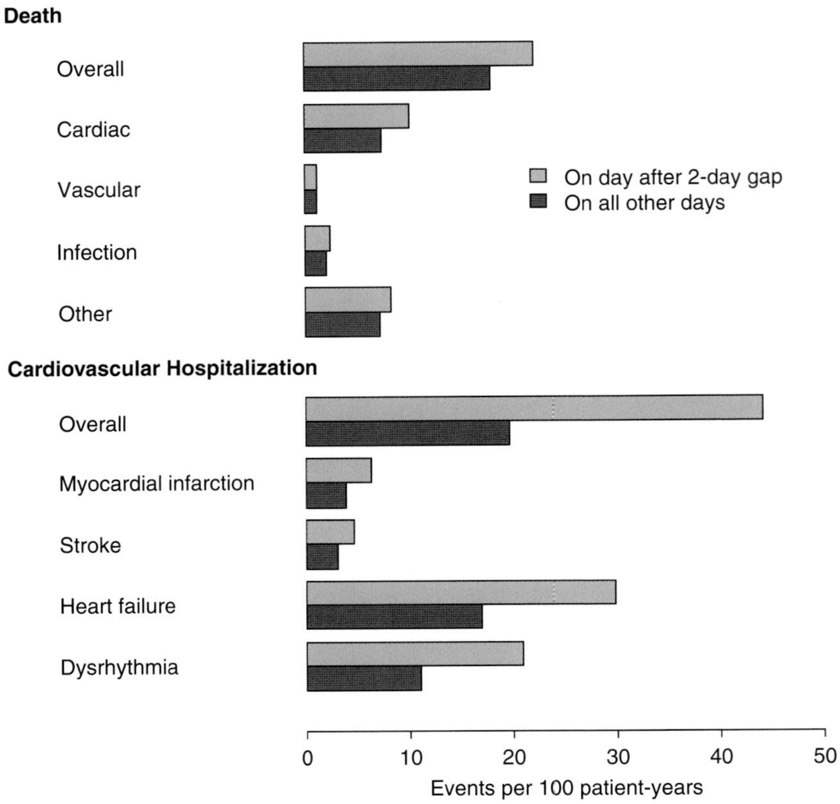

FIG. 28.1 Rates of death and cardiovascular hospitalization on the day after the 2-day gap in dialysis treatment and on all other days. (Reproduced with permission from McCullough P, Chan C, Weinhandl E, et al. Intensive Hemodialysis, Left Ventricular Hypertrophy, and Cardiovascular Disease. *Am J Kidney Dis.* (2016);68(5S1):S5-S14, Fig 1.)

conventional HD. In other words, the cardinal feature of HHD is arguably not the setting of therapy, but rather the intensity of therapy. HHD facilitates intensive therapy (i.e., relative to conventional HD, any schedule that increases the number of treatment sessions per week, the number of hours per session, or both). HHD also readily permits treatment at any time of day or night, thus allowing the patient to dialyze during sleeping hours. The application of intensive HD in the home setting presents several benefits and potential risks, which are described in the following sections.

Left Ventricular Hypertrophy and Cardiovascular Complications

The conventional HD schedule includes a nearly 72-hour interval between consecutive sessions on Friday and Monday or Saturday and Tuesday. Numerous studies have suggested that this interval is associated with higher risks for mortality and morbidity. In a retrospective study of over 32,000 patients, Foley et al. found that the death rate on the day after the long interval was 23% higher than on other days and that the cardiovascular (CV)-related hospital admission rate was 124% higher (Fig. 28.1).[8] These findings have been corroborated by CV-related death patterns in the DOPPS, the United Kingdom, and Australia and New Zealand.[9-11] The long interval at the end of each dialytic week simply allows "unphysiological" fluid and solute accumulation, which puts substantial stress on the heart and the peripheral vasculature. Indeed, CV disease (CVD) is the leading cause of death among dialysis patients.[1]

Left ventricular hypertrophy (LVH) is defined by an increase in LV mass (LVM), due to increased wall thickness. In dialysis patients, LVH itself and serial increases in LVM index are both associated with poor clinical outcomes.[12-15] Two randomized clinical trials (RCTs) have assessed changes in LVM on nocturnal HHD. In the Frequent Hemodialysis Network (FHN) Nocturnal Trial, 87 patients were randomly assigned to receive 12 months of HHD for either six nocturnal sessions per week or three conventional sessions per week. HD was delivered with conventional equipment. Mean LVM decreased significantly with intensive HD, from 141 to 132 g, but remained unchanged with conventional HD, increasing from 132 to only 133 g. The difference in change between groups was almost 11 g, in favor of intensive HD, but lacked statistical significance.[16] The earlier and smaller Alberta trial of nocturnal versus conventional HHD, which also used conventional equipment, generated qualitatively similar results: The effect of intensive versus conventional HD on LVM was over 15 g and statistically significant (Fig. 28.2).[17]

In post hoc analysis of the FHN trials, Raimann et al. examined concurrent influences of interdialytic weight gain and time-integrated estimate of fluid load (TIFL) on change in LVM.[18] TIFL is a metric that estimates the total burden of extracellular fluid volume, with accounting for interdialytic weight gain and urine output. In both the FHN Daily and

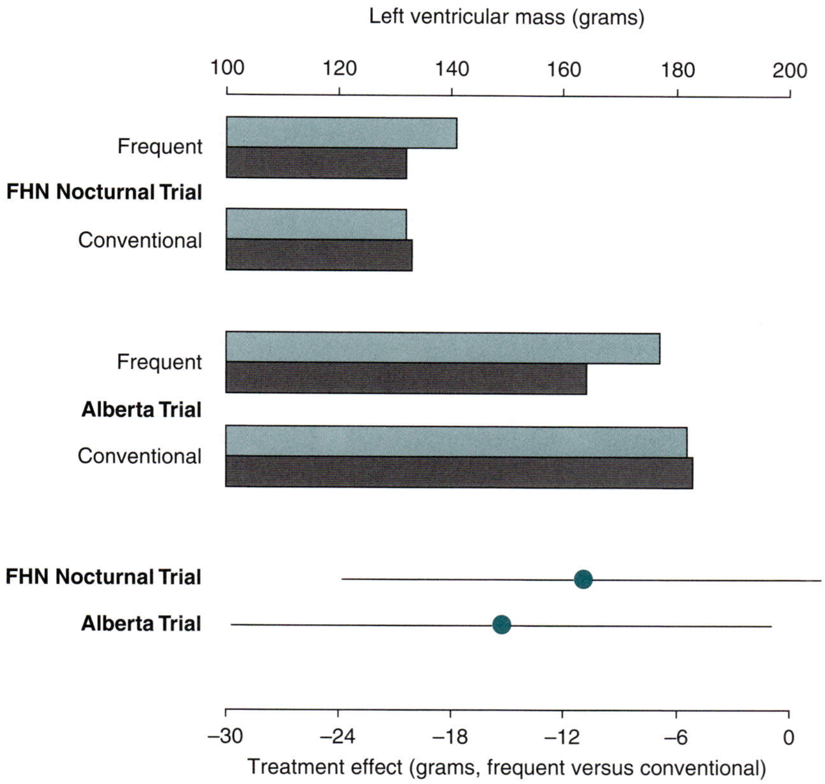

FIG. 28.2 Effects of intensive versus conventional hemodialysis on left ventricular mass in the Frequent Hemodialysis Network Nocturnal Trial and Alberta Trial of nocturnal home hemodialysis. Estimated treatment effects *(solid dots)* and associated 95% confidence intervals *(solid lines)* are displayed at the bottom. (From McCullough P, Chan C, Weinhandl E, et al. Intensive Hemodialysis, Left Ventricular Hypertrophy, and Cardiovascular Disease. *Am J Kidney Dis.* (2016);68(5S1):S5-S14, Fig 3.)

Nocturnal trials, 12-month changes in interdialytic weight gain and TIFL were positively correlated with 12-month change in LVM, albeit with a weaker association between TIFL and LVM in the Nocturnal Trial, possibly due to the lower prevalence of anuria at baseline in that trial.

Whether reduction of LVH portends improvement in clinical outcomes is not entirely certain. Data from the HOPE (Heart Outcomes Prevention Evaluation) trial of ramipril versus placebo strongly suggested such a relationship in the general population.[19] The RCTs of intensive HD offer little guidance, as sample sizes were uniformly too low to evaluate risks for death and hospitalization. However, observational studies of data from the United States Renal Data System (USRDS) support the hypothesis of beneficial effects of intensive HD in the home setting on CV outcomes. Weinhandl et al. compared risks of hospitalization with daily HHD and conventional in-center HD in Medicare beneficiaries. With 3480 daily HHD patients on the NxStage System One, a device that delivers a low volume of dialysate per session, and 17,400 conventional in-center HD patients who were matched according to demographics and comorbid conditions, the hazard ratio (HR) of CV-related admission for daily HHD versus conventional in-center HD was 0.89 (95% confidence interval [CI], 0.86 to 0.93) in intention-to-treat analysis.[20] Regarding types of CV-related admission, daily HHD patients had 25% lower risk for cerebrovascular disease; 41% lower risk for heart failure, fluid overload, and cardiomyopathy; and 16% lower risk for hypertensive disease in on-treatment analysis (Fig. 28.3). In an earlier study, Weinhandl et al. compared risks for CV death with daily HHD on the NxStage System One and conventional in-center HD. In intention-to-treat and on-treatment analyses, the HRs of CV death for daily HHD versus conventional in-center HD were 0.92 (0.78 to 1.09) and 0.83 (0.67 to 1.01), respectively.[21]

Considering the totality of evidence, including the compatibility of randomized studies that have evaluated LVM metrics and observational studies that have examined CV hospitalization, patients with either LVH after an initial trial of conventional HD and patients with overt heart failure, particularly due to diastolic dysfunction, may benefit from intensive HD in the home setting.

Blood Pressure and Antihypertensive Medication Use

Hypertension is very common in patients with ESRD. Hypertensive kidney disease is the primary cause of ESRD for nearly 30% of US patients and the prevalence of hypertension is 85% in incident ESRD patients. In prevalent hemodialysis patients in the United States, as of December 2016, mean predialysis systolic blood pressure (SBP) was 147 mmHg, with 75th and 90th percentiles of 163 and 178 mmHg, respectively.[22] From a different viewpoint, 33%, 21%, and 9% had

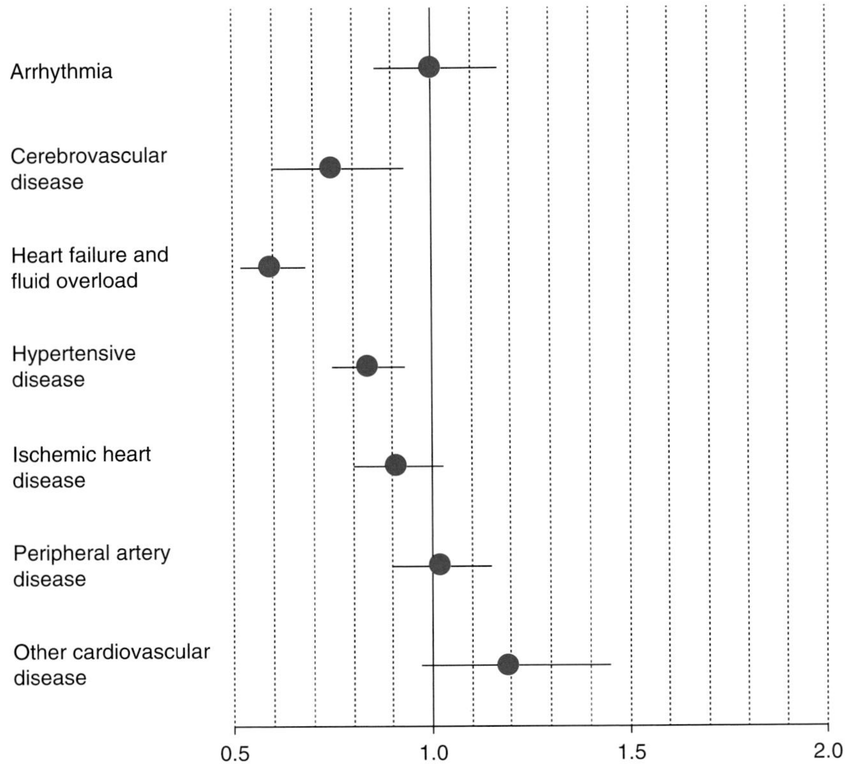

FIG. 28.3 Relative hazards of cause-specific cardiovascular hospitalization for daily home hemodialysis with the NxStage System One versus conventional in-center hemodialysis. *Solid lines* represent 95% confidence intervals around estimated hazard ratios *(solid dots)*. (Adapted from McCullough P, Chan C, Weinhandl E, et al. Intensive Hemodialysis, Left Ventricular Hypertrophy, and Cardiovascular Disease. *Am J Kidney Dis*. (2016);68(5S1):S5-S14, Fig 4.)

predialysis SBP of 140 to 159, 160 to 179, and ≥180 mmHg, respectively. The burden of hypertension cannot be readily attributed to sporadic application of antihypertensive medications, as use of β-blockers, calcium channel blockers, and renin–angiotensin system inhibitors in hemodialysis patients is approximately 70%, 50%, and 40%, respectively.[22] Although observational studies are mixed and many suggest a U-shaped association between either predialysis or postdialysis blood pressure (BP) measurements and clinical outcomes, both ambulatory and home measurements of SBP are strongly associated with mortality risk, with increasing risk along a linear gradient beginning at 120 mmHg.[23-25] Thus lowering BP is likely an effective strategy for improving CV outcomes.[26]

Multiple RCTs have shown that intensive HHD significantly reduces BP.[27] In the FHN Nocturnal Trial, predialysis SBP decreased with intensive HD, from 145 to 142 mmHg at month 2, and steadily declined to 137 mmHg during months 10 to 12.[27] Concurrently, predialysis SBP decreased only slightly with conventional HD, from 153 mmHg at baseline to 151 mmHg at the end of the study. The treatment effect of intensive HD on predialysis SBP was 8 mmHg, in favor of intensive HD, and statistically significant. The Alberta trial of nocturnal versus conventional HD generated similar findings, but without statistical significance (Fig. 28.4).[17] Therefore in patients with uncontrolled hypertension, especially with use of multiple antihypertensive medications, intensive HD in the home setting may be useful. What remains uncertain is whether intensive HHD in the home setting lowers ambulatory SBP, which is a stronger predictor of CV risk than predialysis SBP.

In tandem with lowering BP, intensive HHD also appears to reduce the use of antihypertensive medications. In the FHN Nocturnal Trial, the mean number of antihypertensive medications per patient decreased from 1.9 to 1.1 with intensive HD, whereas the corresponding number of medications with conventional HD remained at 1.6 during follow-up.[27] In the Alberta trial of nocturnal versus conventional HD, antihypertensive medication use was either reduced or discontinued in 62% of patients who underwent nocturnal HD and only 12% of patients who underwent conventional HD ($P < 0.001$). Similar patterns have been seen in observational studies. In the prospective FREEDOM (Following Rehabilitation, Economics and Everyday-Dialysis Outcome Measurements) study, in which patients underwent daily HHD with the NxStage System One, the mean number of antihypertensive medications per patient decreased from 1.7 to 1.0 after 12 months of follow-up ($P < 0.0001$).[28]

Mineral and Bone Disorder and Phosphate Binder Use

Mineral and bone disease (MBD) is another common complication of ESRD. Only one in three hemodialysis patients

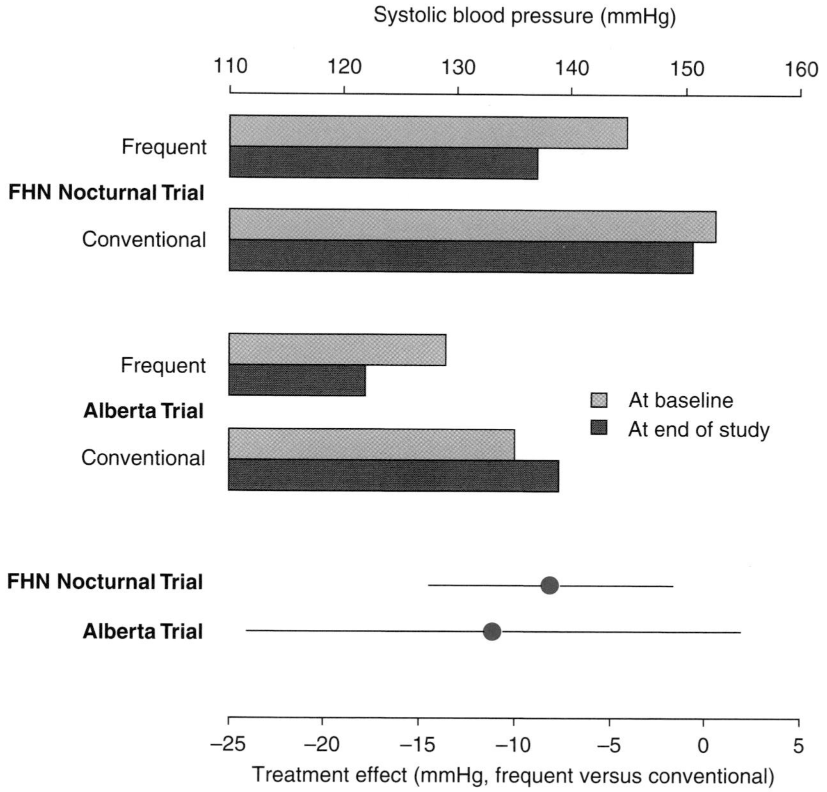

FIG. 28.4 Effects of intensive versus conventional hemodialysis on predialysis systolic blood pressure in the Frequent Hemodialysis Network Nocturnal Trial and Alberta Trial of nocturnal home hemodialysis. Estimated treatment effects *(solid dots)* and associated 95% confidence intervals *(solid lines)* are displayed at the bottom. (Adapted from Bakris G, Burkart J, Weinhandl E, et al. Intensive Hemodialysis, Blood Pressure, and Antihypertensive Medication Use. *Am J Kidney Dis.* (2016);68(5S1):S15-S23, Fig 2.)

have serum calcium, phosphorus, and parathyroid hormone concentrations in target ranges of 8.4 to 10.2 mg/dL, 3.5 to 5.5 mg/dL, and 150 to 600 pg/mL, respectively.[29] There are many pharmacological interventions for MBD, including vitamin D sterols, calcium- and noncalcium-based phosphate binders, and calcimimetics. At least in the United States, these interventions are incredibly costly. In dialysis patients with Medicare Part D coverage during 2014, cumulative spending on phosphate binders exceeded $840 million, whereas cumulative spending on cinacalcet hydrochloride was nearly $480 million; in other words, over 58 cents of every dollar of Part D spending in dialysis patients was devoted to the treatment of MBD.[1] This allocation of resources is problematic, in no small part because of poor adherence.

Although the pathophysiology of MBD is complex, the mechanics of phosphorus intake and excretion merit special attention. Phosphorus is excreted through the kidneys; in the absence of residual renal function, the only exit route for phosphorus is dialysis itself. On the intake side, Noori et al. found that most patients consume between 500 and 1500 mg of phosphorus each day, according to data collected from a food frequency questionnaire.[30] Between 60% and 70% of this intake is absorbed in the gastrointestinal tract. Thus the typical HD patient absorbs around 4500 mg of phosphorus each week. By the way of comparison, a 4-hour HD session clears approximately 1000 mg of phosphorus; the rate of clearance is initially high, but decreases later. Thus there is a significant gap between phosphorus absorption and clearance. With poor adherence to binders, phosphorus accumulates, thus contributing to vascular calcification.

Intensive HD usually increases the cumulative number of treatment hours per week, thus necessarily facilitating increased dialytic clearance of phosphorus. Multiple RCTs have shown that intensive HHD reduces serum phosphorus.[31] In the FHN Nocturnal Trial, mean serum phosphorus declined with intensive HD, from 5.74 mg/dL at baseline to 4.38 and 4.72 mg/dL after 3 to 5 and 10 to 12 months of follow-up, respectively. The adjusted change in serum phosphorus from baseline to end of study was −1.11 mg/dL with intensive HD versus 0.12 mg/dL with conventional HD, thus resulting in a treatment effect of −1.24 (−1.79 to 0.68) mg/dL.[31] In the Alberta trial of nocturnal versus conventional HD, the treatment effect of intensive versus conventional HD was −1.5 mg/dL (Fig. 28.5).[17] In patients with persistent hyperphosphatemia, especially in light of poor adherence to phosphate binders, intensive HD in the home setting, particularly at night, may be a highly effective strategy for controlling serum phosphorus.

Use of phosphate binders also appears to decrease with intensive HHD. In the FHN Nocturnal Trial, the percentage

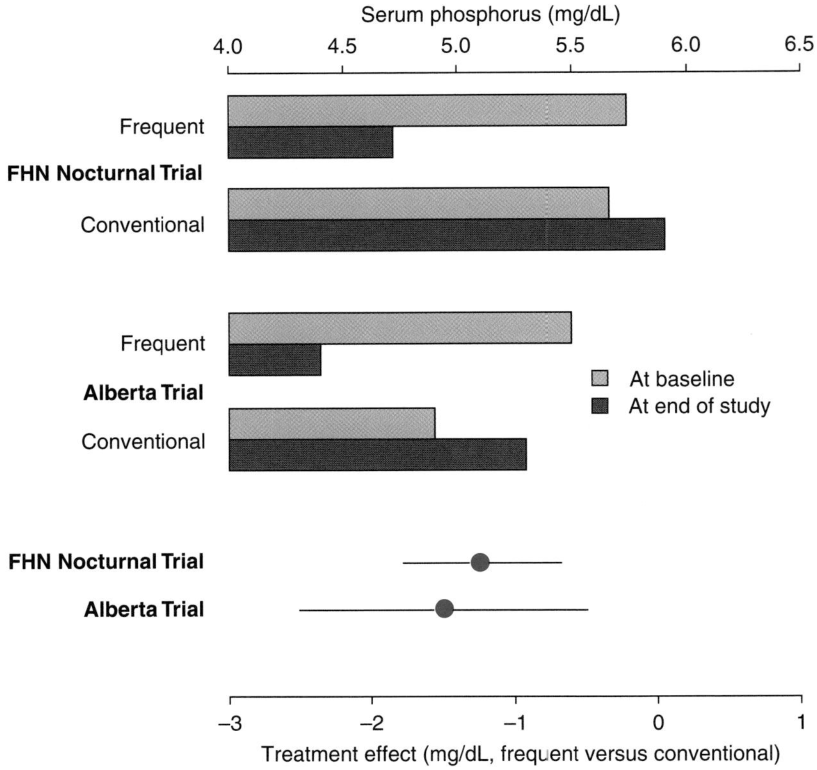

FIG. 28.5 Effects of intensive versus conventional hemodialysis on serum phosphorus in the Frequent Hemodialysis Network Nocturnal Trial and Alberta Trial of nocturnal home hemodialysis. Estimated treatment effects *(solid dots)* and associated 95% confidence intervals *(solid lines)* are displayed at the bottom. (Adapted from Copland M, Komenda P, Weinhandl E, et al. Intensive Hemodialysis, Mineral and Bone Disorder, and Phosphate Binder Use. *Am J Kidney Dis.* (2016);68(5S1):S24-S32, Fig 3.)

of patients who used any phosphate binders decreased from 97% at baseline to only 27% at months 10 to 12 on intensive HD, whereas no such decrease was observed on conventional HD. At the end of the trial, 42% of patients on intensive HD actually required phosphorus supplementation in the dialysate to avoid development of hypophosphatemia.[31]

In contrast to these data, there is little evidence that intensive HHD meaningfully alters either serum calcium or parathyroid hormone, although results about the latter biochemical are limited by the brief follow-up of studies. Of course, serum calcium also reflects the choice of dialysate calcium concentration. Many patients who have performed nocturnal HD have required dialysate calcium ≥3.0 mEq/L.[31]

Health-Related Quality of Life

There is increasing recognition that dialysis patients value quality of life (QoL) more highly than traditional clinical outcomes, including risks for death and hospitalization. In a survey of over 4500 German dialysis patients, safety of treatment, satisfaction with care, and health-related quality of life (HRQoL) were the only outcomes that were rated by greater than 90% of patients as "very important."[32]

HRQoL is typically separated into physical and mental components. In dialysis patients, the prevalence of low physical HRQoL is especially high. In a sample of prevalent HD patients in 2016, 38% of patients had a physical composite summary (PCS) score between 35 and 44 points and another 19% of patients had a PCS score less than 35, according to the 12-item Short-Form Survey, for which the mean and standard deviation are 50 and 10 points, respectively, among US adults. On the other hand, 28% of patients had a mental composite summary (MCS) score less than 45.[33]

In RCTs, intensive HHD appears to exert a positive effect on physical HRQoL, although direct comparisons of effects on intensive and conventional HD suggest cautious interpretation.[15] In the FHN Nocturnal Trial, mean PCS score increased with intensive HD, from 37 at baseline to 40.3 at 12 months, but also increased with conventional HD. Accordingly, the treatment effect of 0.6 points, in favor of intensive HD, lacked statistical significance.[16] In the Alberta trial of conventional versus nocturnal HD, the effect of intensive HD on PCS score was 1.5 points, in favor of intensive HD, despite only 6 months of follow-up, but the effect lacked statistical significance (Fig. 28.6).[34] In an interim analysis of the FREEDOM study of daily HHD with the NxStage System One, but without a comparator group, mean PCS score increased significantly between baseline and at both 4 and 12 months. The percentage of participants with PCS score ≥50 increased between baseline and 12 months in the intention-to-treat (from 8% to 24%) and the per-protocol (from 9% to

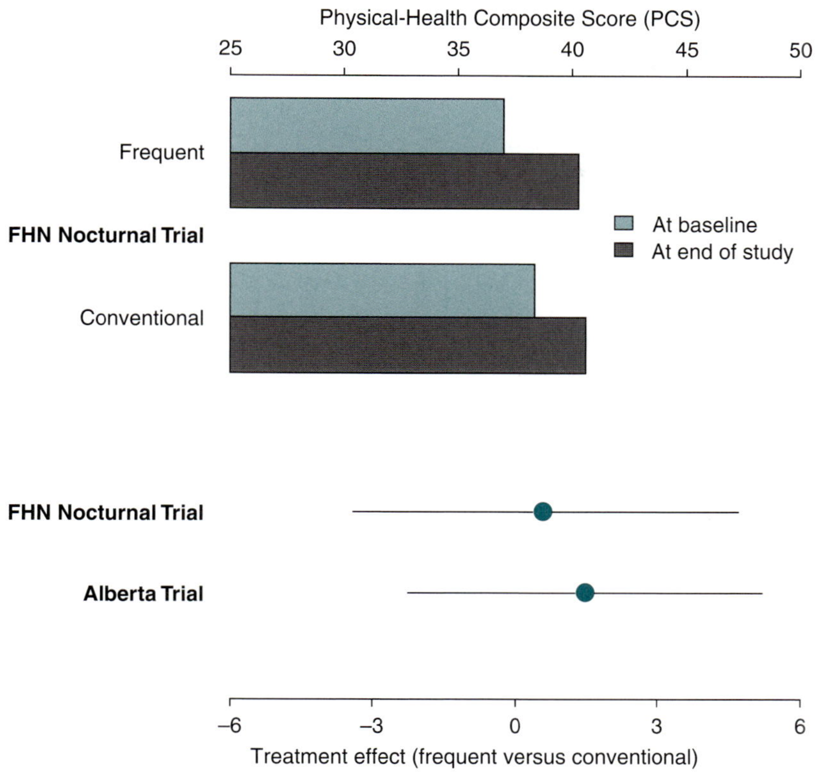

FIG. 28.6 Effects of intensive versus conventional hemodialysis on the physical composite summary score in the Frequent Hemodialysis Network Nocturnal Trial and Alberta Trial of nocturnal home hemodialysis. Estimated treatment effects *(solid dots)* and associated 95% confidence intervals *(solid lines)* are displayed at the bottom. (Adapted from Kraus M, Fluck R, Weinhandl E, et al. Intensive Hemodialysis and Health-Related Quality of Life. *Am J Kidney Dis.* (2016);68(5S1):S33-S42, Fig 1.)

21%) cohorts. [35] Interestingly, in the FHN Daily Trial, which was conducted in a facility, the effect of intensive versus conventional HD on PCS score was larger and statistically significant. One possibility is that although intensive HD improves physical HRQoL, the home setting adds a physical burden to patients' lives, thus resulting in an attenuated effect of intensive HHD on physical HRQoL.

One mechanism that may underlie the modest improvement in physical HRQoL on intensive HHD is improved sleep quality. Hyperphosphatemia, sleep apnea, and symptoms of restless legs syndrome are all associated with poor sleep quality. As described previously, intensive HHD, especially at night, lowers serum phosphorus. Regarding sleep apnea, a study of 14 patients who converted from conventional HD (three sessions per week and 4 hours per session) to nocturnal HD (six or seven sessions per week and 8 hours per session) showed that apnea and hypopnea episodes fell from an average of 25 episodes per hour with conventional HD to 8 episodes per hour with nocturnal HD, whereas oxygen saturation increased after conversion to nocturnal HD.[36] Improvements in sleep quality were similarly observed in the FREEDOM study; improved sleep may partly reflect the observation of fewer symptoms of restless legs syndrome in the FREEDOM study.[37] Nevertheless, some patients on nocturnal HHD fail to sleep well; this observation may explain why the effects of intensive HHD on physical HRQoL in both the FHN Nocturnal and Alberta trials were smaller than the corresponding effect in the FHN Daily Trial, which was conducted in dialysis facilities.

Intensive HHD appears to exert a beneficial effect on mental health.[38] In the FHN Nocturnal Trial, mean PCS score increased with intensive HD, from 45.6 points at baseline to 48.2 at 12 months, but decreased with conventional HD, from 45.9 to 45.6 points. However, the treatment effect of 3.7 points, in favor of intensive HD, was nonsignificant. [38] In the Alberta trial of nocturnal versus conventional HD, intensive HD increased the mean MCS score by 2.5 points, but the result was clearly nonsignificant (Fig. 28.7).[34] Depressive symptoms, as measured by the Beck Depression Inventory (BDI) instrument, have been assessed in multiple studies. In the FHN trials, intensive versus conventional HD lowered the mean BDI score, but neither trial generated a statistically significant finding.[38] In the FREEDOM study, mean BDI score significantly declined between baseline and both 4 and 12 months, with absolute changes that were larger in magnitude than the treatment effects in the FHN trials.[39]

Treatment Complications and Tolerability

Two important complications that are observed on conventional HD are intradialytic hypotension (IDH) and long

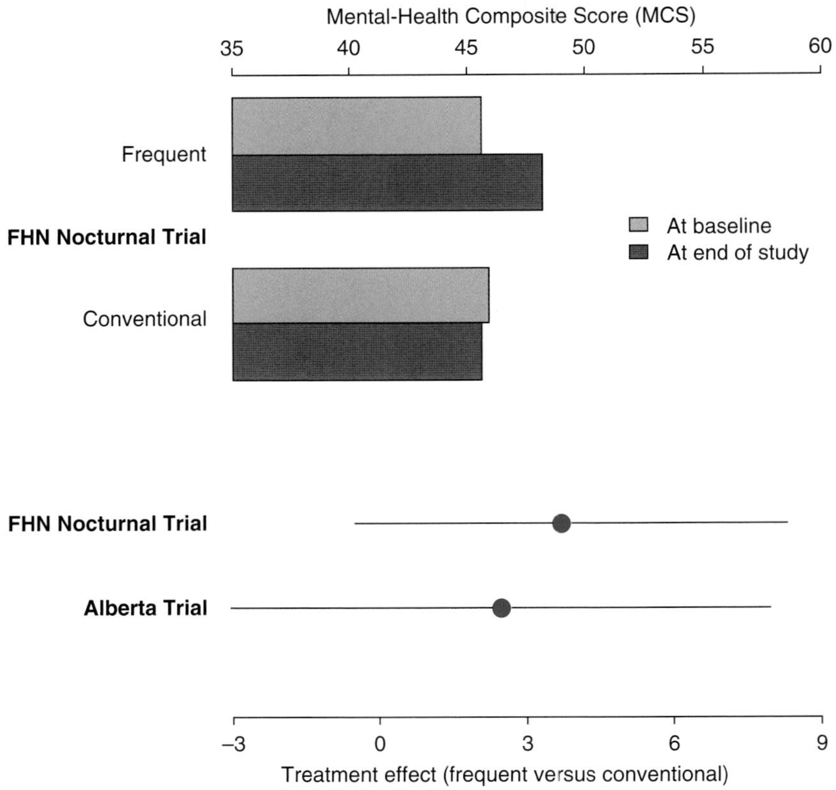

FIG. 28.7 Effects of intensive versus conventional hemodialysis on the mental composite summary score in the Frequent Hemodialysis Network Nocturnal Trial and Alberta Trial of nocturnal home hemodialysis. Estimated treatment effects *(solid dots)* and associated 95% confidence intervals *(solid lines)* are displayed at the bottom. (Adapted from Kraus M, Fluck R, Weinhandl E, et al. Intensive Hemodialysis and Health-Related Quality of Life. *Am J Kidney Dis.* (2016);68(5S1):S33-S42, Fig 2.)

postdialysis recovery time. Regarding the former, treatment-level data about BP dynamics indicate that the incidence of IDH is between 7.5% and 9.7% of conventional HD sessions.[40] The occurrence of IDH is associated with higher risk for death. From a pathophysiological perspective, IDH reflects an inadequate response to decreased intravascular volume when a large amount of fluid is quickly removed. Consequently, aggressive ultrafiltration may be an iatrogenic factor in the pathogenesis of IDH. Lowering the ultrafiltration rate (UFR) is thus a logical strategy to reduce the per-session risk for IDH. Of course, lowering the UFR requires either reducing interdialytic weight gain, including shortening the duration of the interdialytic gap, or increasing session length.

In the FHN trials, symptoms of IDH were classified into three categories: those that led to lowering the UFR or reduced blood flow (level I); those that led to the administration of saline solution, but not to lowering the UFR (level II); and those that led to both the administration of saline solution and lowering the UFR (level III).[27] In the FHN Nocturnal Trial, where UFR was lower with intensive HD, incidences of level I, II, and III IDH were 1.7%, 0.5%, and 0.9%, respectively, with intensive HD (cumulative incidence, 3.1%), whereas incidences of level I, II, and III IDH were 3.1%, 3.7%, and 2.7%, respectively, with conventional HD (cumulative incidence, 9.4%). Both the per-session risk for IDH and the relative number of sessions with level II or III IDH were lower with intensive HD.[27] On the other hand, there is a paucity of data about the incidence of IDH on short daily HD in the home setting.

Long postdialysis recovery time is another complication of conventional HD. In the DOPPS, over 6000 patients were asked how long it takes them to recover from a dialysis session.[7] Recovery times were reported as 2 to 6 hours by 41% of patients, 7 to 12 hours by 17% of patients, and longer than 12 hours by 10% of patients. Each 1-hour increment in recovery time was associated with 5% higher risk for death and 3% higher risk for hospitalization, after adjustment for demographic and clinical factors. Long recovery time is also associated with poor HRQoL. The exact causes of long recovery time are uncertain. A recent study of almost 2700 conventional HD patients in a US dialysis organization linked UFR ≥13 versus <10 mL/h/kg with 28% higher risk for longer recovery time. Moreover, IDH was associated with longer recovery time.[41] Thus ultrafiltration intensity, intradialytic hypotension, and recovery time may be closely connected.

One of the most striking effects of conversion from conventional to intensive HD is the rapid and dramatic decline in recovery time. In an interim analysis of the FREEDOM study, mean recovery time decreased from 7.9 hours (95% CI, 6.4 to 9.4) at baseline to 4 hours (2.9 to 5.1) after 4 months

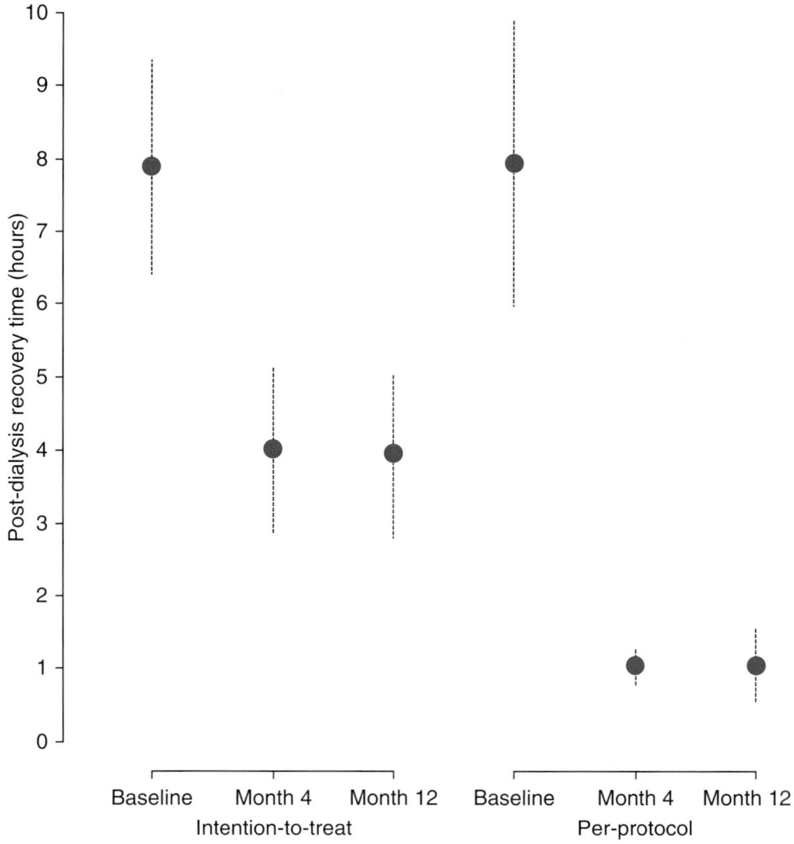

FIG. 28.8 Mean postdialysis recovery time in intention-to-treat and per-protocol cohorts of the FREEDOM study. Dashed bars span 1 SD above and below the mean. (From Morfin J, Fluck R, Weinhandl E, et al. Intensive Hemodialysis and Treatment Complications and Tolerability. *Am J Kidney Dis.* (2016);68(5S1):S43-S50, Fig 4.)

and 4 hours (2.8 to 5.1) after 12 months, by intention-to-treat analysis. By per-protocol analysis, mean recovery time decreased from 7.9 hours (6 to 9.9) at baseline to 1 hour (0.8 to 1.3) after 4 months and 1.1 hour (0.5 to 1.6) at 12 months (Fig. 28.8).[39] These patterns have been recently corroborated by significant treatment effects on recovery time in both of the FHN trials.[42]

Potential Risks of Intensive Hemodialysis

Despite the apparent benefits of intensive HD related to CV outcomes, QoL, and treatment tolerability, intensive HD in the home setting may confer risks for adverse events, including vascular access complications, infection, mortality, accelerated loss of residual kidney function, solute balance, and patient and care partner burden.

Vascular access complications appear to occur more often with intensive HD in trials, although observational studies have not always supported this conclusion. In the FHN trials, the primary vascular access outcome was time to first access repair, access loss, or access-related hospitalization; repair was defined as any access procedure that resulted in continued use of the access, whereas loss was defined as abandonment or removal of the access. In the FHN Nocturnal Trial, primary outcome rates were 58 and 32 events per 100 patient-years with intensive and conventional HD, respectively. Excess risks were driven primarily by repairs, as the risk for access loss was not significantly associated with treatment intensity in either of the FHN trials.[43]

Infection is another potential risk, although it is one that probably reflects the inherent setting (home) of HHD, rather than treatment intensity. Weinhandl et al. evaluated infection-related hospitalization risk in Medicare beneficiaries on daily HHD with the NxStage System One and conventional in-center HD. The HR of first infection-related admission was 1.35 (95% CI, 1.27 to 1.42) for daily HHD versus conventional in-center HD, but the HR of all subsequent infection-related admissions was 1.03 (0.97 to 1.09). In detailed analysis of types of infection-related admission, hazards were statistically significantly greater for daily HHD in cases of bacteremia and sepsis, cardiac infection, osteomyelitis, and vascular access infection (Fig. 28.9).[21] In contrast, the HR of infection-related admission for daily HHD with the NxStage System One versus peritoneal dialysis (PD) appears to favor daily HHD, as the risk for vascular access infections on HHD is lower than the risk for peritonitis on PD.[44] Excess risk with daily HHD versus conventional in-center HD is likely attributable to poor adherence to infection control practices and may be accentuated by use of buttonhole cannulation.[45,46] Use of mupirocin at the buttonhole site after each HD session may sharply reduce the risk for infection-related complications.[47]

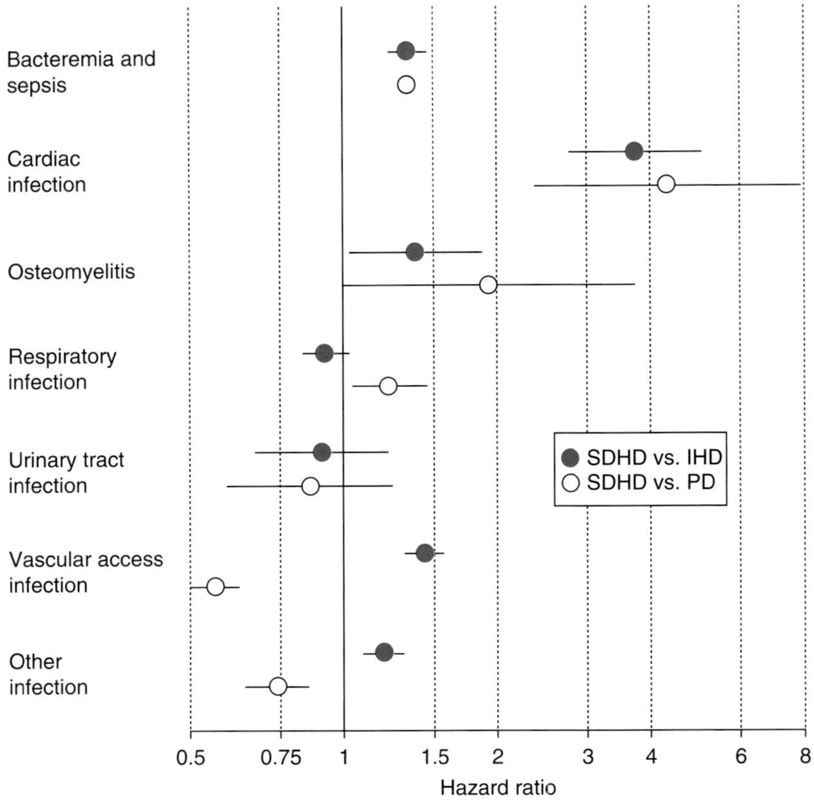

FIG. 28.9 Relative hazards of cause-specific infection-related hospitalization for short daily hemodialysis with the NxStage System One versus conventional in-center hemodialysis and versus peritoneal dialysis. (From Kraus M, Kansal S, Copland M, et al. Intensive Hemodialysis and Potential Risks With Increasing Treatment. *Am J Kidney Dis.* (2016);68(5S1):S51-S58, Fig 1.)

Mortality remains a controversial topic because inference is dependent on observational studies. Many observational studies have suggested that HHD is associated with lower risk for death, relative to conventional in-center HD. However, the home setting may involve selection bias, thus introducing confounding by indication. The FHN trials contribute to the uncertainty. Both trials included extended follow-up periods during which patients may have remained on their randomly assigned treatment schedules or may have switched to alternative schedules.[48] In the FHN Nocturnal Trial, patients who were originally assigned to intensive HD had 288% higher risk for death than those originally assigned to conventional HD.[49] This finding is difficult to interpret, given the high percentages of patients who changed treatment schedules after the protocol-specified 12-month follow-up interval. The role of chance also cannot be excluded. In the Nocturnal Trial, the mortality rate among patients who were originally assigned to conventional HD was only 3.2 deaths per 100 patient-years during the extended follow-up interval; this rate is far below the background rate in the US dialysis patient population. Given the accumulated evidence, it is reasonable to inform patients that intensive HHD simply does not assure longer life expectancy. In fact, in a recent study of HHD patients in Canada, patients undergoing either short daily or nocturnal HD had similar survival as patients undergoing conventional HD.[50]

Residual renal function has long been associated with better survival in patients on PD, but its role in HD patients has garnered less attention, notwithstanding recent interest in incremental HD. In the FHN Nocturnal Trial, a substantial share of participants had relatively low vintage and thus had preserved residual function, with mean daily urine output of 750 mL. (Even this is well below what is often observed in incident dialysis patients who are prescribed PD.) After 4 months, the prevalence of anuria was 52% in patients on intensive HD, but only 18% in patients on conventional HD; this difference persisted after 12 months, although it narrowly lost its statistical significance.[51] Given these results, prescription of intensive HHD in incident ESRD patients with clinically significant urinary output should be carefully considered.

As discussed previously, solute balance may be negatively disrupted by intensive HHD. In patients on nocturnal HD, phosphorus supplementation in the dialysate may be necessary to prevent the development of hypophosphatemia. Higher dialysate calcium concentration may be necessary to prevent the development of hypocalcemia. Loss of carnitine, which occurs even on conventional HD, may be accentuated on intensive HHD.

Patient and caregiver burden almost surely increase when HD is performed in the home setting. Increased burden may lead to feelings of burnout, thus resulting in technique failure. Seshasai et al. reported that the cumulative incidence of HHD technique failure was 25% and 35% at 1 and 2 years after completing HHD training, respectively.[52] However, the risk for

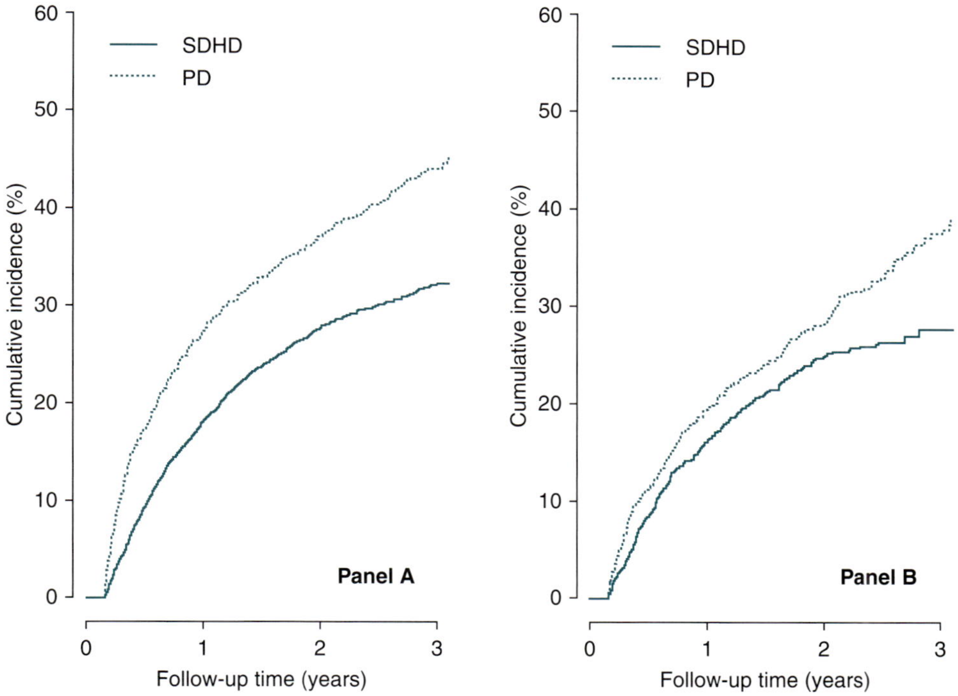

FIG. 28.10 Cumulative incidence of technique failure for short daily hemodialysis with the NxStage System One versus peritoneal dialysis, overall *(panel A)* and in the subset of patients who initiated home dialysis within 6 months of the diagnosis of end stage renal disease *(panel B)*.

HHD technique failure may nonetheless be lower than the risk for PD technique failure, both overall (Fig. 28.10, panel A) and in the subset of incident ESRD patients (Fig. 28.10, panel B).[44] In the FHN Nocturnal Trial, caregiver burden increased significantly with intensive versus conventional HD.[53] Careful and persistent monitoring of HHD patients and their caregivers is necessary to identify increased burden appreciably before it manifests as the decision to revert from home to in-center HD. Use of telehealth monitoring tools may improve HHD patient retention.[54]

PROVIDING HOME DIALYSIS: CLINICAL IMPLICATIONS

Patient Selection

Although patient selection assumes that the provider is choosing patients, it is equally important to set an environment where the patient chooses home dialysis. Many units, especially when first beginning, search for the "ideal patient." The ideal patient may be one who is committed, young, healthy and without significant comorbidity. However, the true question is who is "suitable"? The definition of the suitable patient varies from center to center, but is dependent on the degree of support available. That degree of support is not only support at home, but also support from the dialysis provider. A home unit with greater social work, dietary, physician, and nursing support will be more capable of taking care and evaluating more marginal patients. The availability of appropriate education, re-education, home visits, and respite care should allow for increased care of patients with less social support. Improving connectivity and telemedicine use in the home likely will improve the ability to provide care to more patients in the near future.

Most centers require a partner present for in-home treatments. However, the degree of support provided by partners is variable, extending from total care of a patient to availability only during emergencies. Most partners perform somewhere in the middle of these extremes, although partner responsibility is quite variable. In mid-2017, the FDA cleared the NxStage System One for solo HHD, without a care partner, during waking hours. However, it is known that many patients do perform solo therapies and have done so for many years. Individual units will need to set policies and processes for evaluating and training solo dialysis if desired.

Suitable patients may have greater comorbidity. As noted previously in this chapter, increased frequency dialysis is ideal for CV risks, severe hypertension, fluid control, and when extended hyperphosphatemia and sleep apnea are present. An important note is that the sicker the patient, the greater the perceived benefit. The FREEDOM study of daily HHD with the NxStage System One revealed that patients with the lowest baseline PCS scores experienced the greatest gains in PCS scores at 4 and 12 months.[35]

Another consideration for home dialysis might be patients previously deemed as nonadherent in-center patients. These patients have historically been considered poor home therapy patients. However, the rigid and inflexible schedule of the in-center environment may be the source of this label. Consideration of home therapy may be appropriate after careful evaluation of the reasons for the nonadherent behavior. Active drug abuse, alcoholism, and untreated psychiatric illness are examples of behaviors that should be

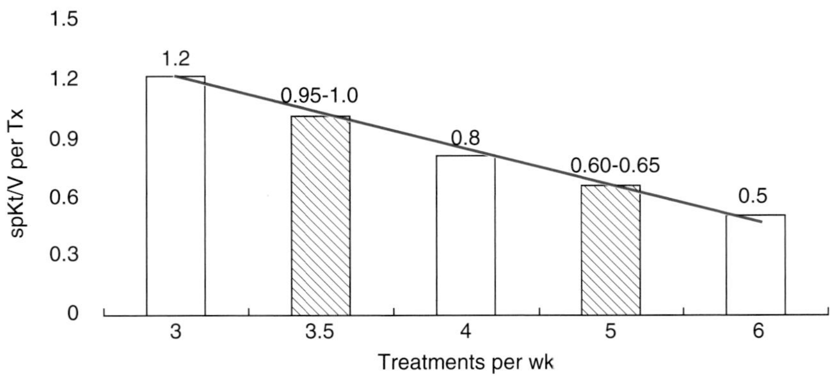

FIG. 28.11 Single-pool Kt/V required to achieve weekly standardized Kt/V >2. Shaded bars represent extrapolation not in KDOQI Clinical Practice Guidelines. (From KDOQI Clinical Practice Guidelines 2006 Updates, page 73.)

avoided in the home. However, a label of nonadherent behavior should be evaluated and considered appropriate in many circumstances.

Patients are more likely to choose home hemodialysis with appropriate education, professional staff, and the assurance of appropriate support around the clock. There should be adequate social work, dietitian support, and nursing. Successful programs generally have a physician and nursing champion. The unit should be attractive and open. Respite care should be available to allow patients and their caregivers necessary respite when needed. Respite may be necessary just for a break from the work of dialysis or may be necessary for medical reasons such as an acute illness or surgery in the care partner.

Patient "selection" is variable among units, but should not be limited to perfect patients. Instead, selection should be widened to provide the best therapy for each individual patient. The dialysis unit should provide support to both patients and caregivers and should be available for around-the-clock support. The unit must be designed to allow patient comfort and trust.

Training and Clinics

The goal of training is to educate patients on how to perform safe dialysis at home, proper antiseptic and cannulation techniques, manage other medical issues, collect appropriate samples for labs, and adjust and manage medications. In addition, the training period is the appropriate time to begin social support and to educate on how to manage and cope with social issues and dialysis-related issues and fears. Training generally takes 4 to 6 weeks but no proscribed time is mandated. Training must be individualized for the patient and care partner and time to complete training should be adjusted. Training generally occurs in a home dialysis unit setting, but may occur in many venues including hospital, extended care facility, or the patient's home. Training is usually a one-on-one session, making certain to understand the patient's and care team's learning ability and styles and ensuring that understanding occurs. When the patient and/or partner is nearing the end of training, they should do several dialyses in the training center without assistance to confirm their independence and ability to do the treatment at home. A formal exit test should be given to the patient or partner to document their understanding and competency. For some patients, it may be helpful for the training nurse to be present (but not assisting unless required) while the patient performs the first dialysis at home.[3] Clinic visits are expected to be monthly and are likely best if multidisciplinary in nature. Successful long-term dialysis and retention depends on the entire team meeting the medical, educational, nutritional, and social support needs of the patient and their care team.

Dialysis Prescription

Home dialysis can be performed with a conventional dialysis machine and water treatment or with a low-flow dialysis device with its own water treatment or bagged dialysate. Whichever technology is used, urea clearance is used as a marker of quality. Kt/V is the accepted marker for urea clearance throughout the world. A standard Kt/V of greater than 2.0 has been defined as the minimum required. A standard Kt/V of >2 is equivalent to single-pool (sp) Kt/V of >1.2 with thrice-weekly hemodialysis. Sp Kt/V of 0.5 can be used with a weekly treatment frequency of 6 days [KDOQI 2016], and sp Kt/V of 0.60 to 0.65 with a frequency of 5 days (Fig. 28.11).

One of the advantages of home dialysis is its ability to meet the needs of the patient with increased frequency, duration of dialysis, or both. Increased frequency above 3 days a week has the advantage of improved BP control and reduction in BP medications, decreased postdialysis fatigue, improved subjective sleep, improved QoL markers, improved restless legs, reduced LVH, and even decreased hospitalization for CV events. In addition, increasing duration can add improved phosphorus removal and control further. Increased duration up to nocturnal therapies can normalize phosphorus without the need of binders and improve sleep apnea. Nocturnal dialysis can potentially decrease the burden of dialysis by increasing the dialysis-free time during daylight hours. Increased frequency and increased duration dialysis can facilitate reduction of the UFR <10 mL/h/kg.

Increased frequency dialysis is defined as a dialysis frequency of more than 3 days per week, ranging form every other day to as many as 7 days. As the frequency is varied, prescription is adjusted to ensure adequate urea clearance. One of the simplest arguments in favor of increased frequency dialysis is to avoid the increased death and hospitalization associated with the 2-day gap seen in the United States. Therefore, when prescribing, training and treating dialysis patients at home on increased frequency, the 2-day gap should be avoided and this must be reinforced regularly. The frequency needs to be individualized for the patient and their care team. Increasing frequency decreases the Kt/V needs, improves ultrafiltration required per dialysis session, and increases phosphorus removal, among other benefits. This must be balanced by the burdens of additional dialysis days on the patient and care partner(s).

Extending therapies to 6 to 8 hours, frequently performed overnight or nocturnal dialysis, is a way to increase middle molecule and phosphorus clearance. Appropriately prescribed, nocturnal dialysis should allow for a normal diet with respect to phosphorus and diminish or completely remove the need for phosphorus binders. Extended therapy combined with increased frequency naturally markedly diminishes UFRs, improves phosphorus control, and improves sleep apnea.

Minimum adequacy of urea clearance can be obtained with appropriate adjustments with conventional dialysis machines and low-flow dialysis. Volume/ultrafiltration control improves with increasing frequency and duration. Phosphorus control improves with frequency and is controlled with increased frequency combined with increased duration of therapies. LVH improves with increased frequency regardless of duration. The improvements associated with home dialysis and increasing frequency need to balance with the burdens of therapy. Improvement in utilization of these therapies can be achieved by improving the education of caregivers and patients.

Barrier to Home Dialysis

When queried, nephrology professionals overwhelmingly prefer home dialysis to in-center dialysis for themselves or family.[55] However, in the United States, only 12% are on any home therapy and just above 2% are estimated to be on HHD.[1] This contradiction between care of oneself and others must be discussed. To decrease these differences, it seems rational that appropriate education must occur, after all, nephrology professionals are well-educated potential patients.

Education to physicians and nurses must occur to help them understand the benefits of home therapies as outlined. Physicians and healthcare professionals must understand their own limitations and explore the possibility of implicit or unintentional bias when deciding which patients are not candidates for HHD. Care must be taken to avoid decisions based on financial status, race, sex, or education.

Patient education should occur often and should include physician input. Patients do not learn easily with one-time exposure or during periods of acute illness. Education should occur early in chronic kidney disease and should be discussed at regular intervals. Care must be taken to match patient learning techniques with education provided. Didactic lectures, clinic discussions, written materials, web-based learning, and DVDs should be made available to patients and their care partners. Time and timing are essential components to adequate education. Risks and benefits to home dialysis, PD, transplant, and especially in-center dialysis need to be discussed frankly.

TABLE 28.1 Educational Barriers and Action Plans

Educational Barrier	Action Plan
Patient Education	Create an easily navigated and organized resource center that recognizes unique needs.
Physician Education	Delineate and adhere to adequate training guidelines. Institute local, regional, and national education seminars with support for fellows. Support visits to centers of excellence for fellows and nephrologists for hands-on home dialysis experience.
Dialysis Staff Education	Designate time and allocate resources toward education. Institute local, regional, and national seminars. Support visits to centers of excellence.

Physician and staff education remain inadequate in the United States. Only a small number of fellowship programs have adequate exposure or time spent on training HHD. Efforts are ongoing to improve education of dialysis staff, but many still have less-than-ideal education and incorrect preconceived biases as to the risks associated with HHD for patients. To correct these limitations, Golper et al. suggested action plans for improvement (Table 28.1).[56]

Preconceived barriers to patient access should be addressed. Many issues such as language, education, age, and IQ are not barriers to therapy but should be clues to proper education and support. Other patient barriers such as fear, adherence, needle phobia, and therapy burden on family can be addressed and potentially overcome with development of support systems, proper education, and peer groups and mentors,

HHD has distinct advantages for many patients. Certain inherent risks exist. The therapy may add additional burden as well. Balancing these issues, individualizing therapies and appropriately educating patients is necessary to provide comprehensive care to all patients with ESRD. It seems reasonable to assume that a greater number of patients could benefit from this therapy. The ability to increase frequency and duration gives HHD an advantage over the in-center unit. Home dialysis therapies are patient-centered modalities that require a distinct partnership between the patient, care partners, dialysis team, and even dialysis device manufacturers. The growth of dialysis may depend on timely and appropriate education, true informed consent, peer support groups and mentorship, excellent training by professional nurses, increased education of nephrology personnel, and true patient advocacy.

29

Peritoneal Physiology

Olof Heimbürger, MD, PhD

OUTLINE

In patients with chronic renal failure, waste products, which normally are excreted in the urine, accumulate in the blood, resulting in uremic intoxication, and the obvious goal of dialysis treatment is to remove uremic toxins (including water) from the patient. Peritoneal dialysis (PD) uses dialysis fluid infused into the peritoneal cavity and a system of biological membranes—the peritoneal barrier—for this purpose. Whereas the artificial hemodialysis membrane has well-characterized, reproducible, solute, and fluid transport characteristics, the peritoneum is not really a membrane but rather a complex structure of living tissues with different transport characteristics, which, furthermore, will differ between patients, a fact that will affect the fluid and solute transport kinetics of PD and dialysis efficiency in PD patients. In addition, the transport characteristics of the peritoneal membrane may not be constant in an individual patient, but may be altered with time because of effects of the dialysis procedure or the dialysis fluids in response to various physiological reactions or pharmacological effects of different drugs.

PERITONEAL ANATOMY

The peritoneal cavity is the largest serosal cavity in the body, with a surface area of approximately 1 to 2 m^2. Although the peritoneal area is commonly suggested to be similar to the body surface area, recent studies suggest that the anatomical surface area of the peritoneum may be only about 50% of the body surface area in adults.[1] *Peritoneum* etymologically means *wrapped tightly around,* which is a good description of the arrangement of this serous membrane that consists of two parts: the parietal peritoneum that covers the abdominal wall, and the diaphragm and the visceral peritoneum that covers the intraabdominal viscera.[2] The parietal peritoneum represents a smaller portion (approximately 10% to 20%) of the total peritoneal surface area[1] and receives its blood supply from the vasculature of the abdominal wall. The visceral peritoneum represents the larger part (approximately 80% to 90%) of the total peritoneal surface area[1] and receives its blood supply through the mesenteric vessels.

However, it should be pointed out that it is the functional peritoneal surface area that is important and not the anatomical surface area.[3] The functional area will be related to the surface area of the capillaries in the peritoneal interstitium, the capillary density, and the spatial arrangement of these capillaries.[1,3] In addition, the peritoneal cavity is only a potential space under normal conditions, and the functional contact area between the peritoneum and the dialysis fluid in the peritoneal cavity during PD will be lower than the anatomical area.[4] In particular, the functional area of the visceral peritoneum is reduced because of the incomplete contact and poor mixing in small fluid compartments within pockets of the visceral peritoneum. In mice, less than half of the peritoneal surface is in contact with a large volume of solution in the peritoneal cavity, but the contact area could be improved by shaking the animal and, particularly, by adding dioctyl sodium sulfosuccinate (a surface tension–lowering agent).[4]

HISTOLOGY

Mesothelium

The surface of the peritoneal cavity is lined by a single layer of mesothelial cells fixed to a continuous basement membrane that, under normal physiological conditions, are covered with a thin (5 μm) film of peritoneal fluid that is kept in place by numerous microvilli.[2] The microvilli and the peritoneal fluid have a lubricating function to prevent formation of adhesions and to allow the free movement of the visceral organs during respiration, peristalsis, and body movement.[2] The peritoneal fluid contains protein, electrolytes, and cells (mainly macrophages, lymphocytes, and desquamated mesothelial cells) and has a high content of phospholipids that are secreted in from the mesothelium by the formation of lamellar bodies, similar to the production of surfactant from type II pneumocytes.[5]

The mesothelial cells may modulate the peritoneal microcirculation by secretion of vasodilators like PGE_2 and nitric oxide (NO) and vasoconstrictors, such as endothelin,[6] and, furthermore, the mesothelial cells have an important role in the initiation of the local immune response regulating leukocyte infiltration through the secretion of chemokines and expression of adhesion molecules.[7] Mesothelial cells have a capacity to produce tissue plasminogen activator (tPA), and the mesothelium normally expresses high fibrinolytic activity.[6] However, the mesothelium also has antifibrinolytic capacity by synthesis of fibrinolytic inhibitors like plasminogen activator inhibitor 1 (PAI-1) and PAI-2, and the balance between the synthesis of fibrinolytic activity and agents in mesothelial cells will determine their capacity to promote fibrin degradation. Under normal conditions the fibrinolytic activity strongly dominates, but the balance may change completely during inflammation, when the antifibrinolytic activity of the mesothelium will dominate, and furthermore, the mesothelium may also exhibit procoagulant activity with expression of tissue factor (which is markedly upregulated in mesothelial cells during inflammation).[6] Thus the mesothelium plays an important role in regulating the balance between fibrinolytic and procoagulant activity in the peritoneal cavity that makes it possible to form adhesions and physically limiting the spread of intraperitoneal infections under normal conditions.

The underlying basement membrane is a very thin laminar network containing collagen type IV, proteoglycans, and glycoproteins such as laminin, and allows macrophages and lymphocytes to pass through it, whereas fibroblasts cannot pass this basement membrane.[6] The thin mesothelial cell layer and their basement membrane seem to offer very little resistance to the transport of small and large solutes, either in vitro or in vivo.[1,8] Thus the mesothelium does not seem to have any major impact on the transport across the peritoneal barrier under normal conditions.

The greater omentum is a large fold of visceral peritoneum that hangs down from the greater curvature of the stomach. It serves as a fat deposit and may, under normal conditions, physically limit the spread of intraperitoneal infections. In addition, the omentum contains "milky spots"—accumulations of mononuclear cells comprising B cells, T cells, macrophages, and mast cells. The milky spots function as secondary lymphoid organs that promote immunity to peritoneal antigens[9] and orchestrate peritoneal cell recruitment.[10] The number of milky spots increases markedly with PD catheter insertion,[11] as well as with start of PD in animal experiments.[11] They are important for the immune response during peritonitis, but their exact role is not completely clear.

Interstitium

Beneath the mesothelium lies the interstitial tissue, comprising an amorphous ground substance or gel-like extracellular matrix interlaced with collagenous, reticular, and elastic fibers; adipocytes, fibroblasts, and granular material; and containing blood capillaries, nerves, and lymphatic vessels.[12-15] The collagen fibers constitute the largest component of the space between the cells in the peritoneum and form a fibrous skeleton in the interstitium.[13] The collagen fibers bind through β_1-integrins to fibroblasts and other cells in the tissue.[14] The interstitial ground substance may be subdivided into a colloid-rich and a water-rich phase, with the two phases being in equilibrium with each other.[1,8,12] The colloid-rich phase contains several different glycosaminoglycans (GAGs), including hyaluronan (HA, which is the major component). All GAGs except HA are covalently bound to a protein backbone forming proteoglycans (the combination of a GAG and a protein), for example, chondroitin sulfate, dermatan sulfate, keratan sulfate, and heparan sulfate. The GAGs are polyanionic and have low isoelectric points, and, consequently, the interstitial ground substance has a high density of negative colloidal charge at physiological pH.[12] Water and small solutes can easily enter the colloid-rich phase, whereas macromolecules are excluded from large parts of this phase. In a complex manner, the interstitium may act as a mucopolysaccharide hydrogel, penetrated with more or less continuous channels of free fluid.[1] Whereas small solutes may pass through interstitial matrix hydrogels without much hindrance, the diffusion of macromolecules may be markedly slowed.[3,13] However, it is important to remember that the capillary wall determines the amount of solutes that are transported from blood to interstitium, and both the interstitium and the capillary wall need to be taken into account when describing the peritoneal transport process.

In general, changes in aggregation and hydration of the ground substance in interstitial tissues affect the physicochemical properties and the functional characteristics of the interstitium,[12] but it is at present not established exactly how PD may affect the functional characteristics of the peritoneal interstitial tissues.[8] However, thickening of the submesothelial interstitial tissue and fibrosis is common in patients on long-term PD[15,16] and may contribute to the observed long-term changes in peritoneal transport by causing uncoupling between increased small solute transport and decreased ultrafiltration coefficient, on one hand, and unchanged or slowed protein transport, on the other hand.[17,18]

Capillary Wall

The microvascular exchange vessels in the peritoneal membrane consist of both true capillaries (diameter 5 to 6 μm) and postcapillary venules (diameter 7 to 20 μm),[3] and the capillary wall is considered to be the major transport barrier for transperitoneal exchange of fluid and solutes during PD. The peritoneal capillaries belong to the continuous type (in which endothelial cells form a continuous layer enwrapped in a negatively charged glycocalyx),[3,19] which functionally restrict solute exchange to less than 0.1% of the total capillary surface area (= the small pores, see later).[1] However, the exact role of the glycocalyx is controversial.[20] The peritoneal capillaries behave functionally as having a heteroporous structure, with a small number of large pores (radius 200 to 400 Å) through which macromolecules are filtered because of convective flow and a large number of "small pores" (radius 40 to 65 Å), which are impermeable for macromolecules larger than albumin (molecular weight 69,000 daltons) but do not restrict the passage of small solutes.[19,20] In addition, "ultrasmall" pores (radius 4 to 6 Å) were postulated to be involved in the water flow induced by the osmotic effect of low-molecular-weight osmotic agents, for example, glucose (Fig. 29.1).[19,21] The anatomical correlate of the water channels was later demonstrated to be aquaporin-1, a protein 28 KDa intramembrane protein shown to be one of the water channels in human proximal tubular cells in the kidney and in various nonfenestrated epithelia.[22] Aquaporin-1 has been demonstrated in peritoneal endothelial cells, at mRNA protein, and at functional levels.[23,24] The anatomical correlates to the small pores are possibly the interendothelial clefts.[3,19,21] The three-dimensional structure of the interendothelial clefts has been described in detail.[25] However, the morphological counterpart to the large pores is not established, although it most likely corresponds to larger interendothelial gaps.[3,19,21] Though there has been considerable controversy about the mechanism of macromolecular transport through the endothelium and the potential role of vesicular transport (transcytosis), it is now established that the quantitative role of transcytosis is negligible.[26]

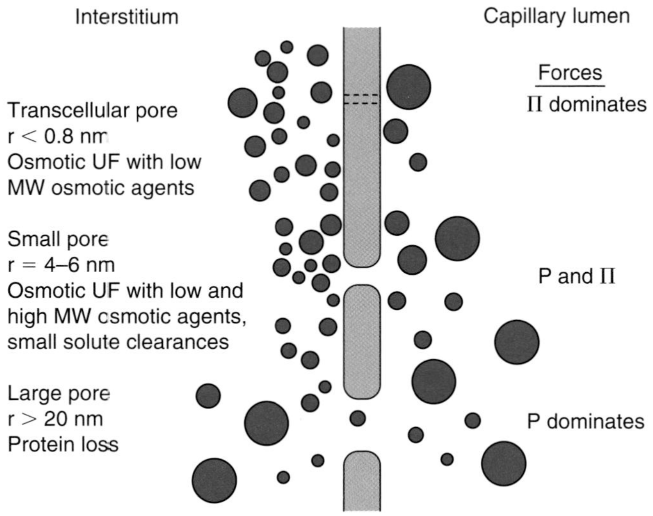

FIG. 29.1 The three-pore model of peritoneal capillary permselectivity, including the transcellular pore (aquaporin-1), the small pores (the interendothelial clefts), and the large pores (possibly large interendothelial clefts). Small circles represent small solutes, and large circles represent proteins. The forces are Π (osmotic pressure) and P (hydrostatic pressure). Crystalloid osmotic pressure induced by glucose is very efficient through the transcellular pores, and about 50% of the ultrafiltered fluid will pass through the aquaporins when glucose is used as an osmotic agent in PD. (From Flessner MF: Peritoneal transport physiology: insights from basic research. *J Am Soc Nephrol* 1991; 2:122–135, with permission.)

The three-pore concept of transcapillary exchange has been successfully applied by Rippe and colleagues[19,27-29] to model the peritoneal transport of small solutes and macromolecules and the peritoneal fluid transport, supporting the view that the capillary wall is the main resistance for transperitoneal fluid and solute transport.

PERITONEAL BLOOD FLOW

The mesenteric blood flow is generally supposed to be about 10% of cardiac output.[30] The effective peritoneal blood flow, that is, the blood flow to the capillaries that are directly involved in peritoneal transport, cannot be directly measured.[30] Indirect estimations suggest that the effective peritoneal blood flow may vary from 20 to 40 mL/min (using estimations of the maximal possible ultrafiltration rate) to more than 100 mL/min (based on the measurements of the clearance of gases).[31] The effective peritoneal blood flow is generally not believed to limit the clearance of small solutes during PD,[32] because the diffusive mass transport coefficient for urea is approximately 20 mL/min. Also, tracer disappearance from small plastic chambers glued to the serosa was not reduced with a 30% decrease in blood flow and only to a minor degree with no blood flow (in dead rats).[33] However, this issue is still controversial, and there are some observations indicating that peritoneal urea clearance may be blood flow limited.[8,30] Rosengren and Rippe[34] reported that a reduction of blood flow by 40% (caused by bleeding of rats) resulted in a decreased transport of glucose and Cr-EDTA by 13% and 24%, respectively. They concluded that there is to some extent a blood flow limitation of peritoneal transport, but that the level of blood flow limitation is much smaller than in other organs. Note that the diffusion rate of small solutes theoretically will not be proportional to the blood flow, but to the square root of the perfusion rate, which to a large extent may explain the small change in transport with marked alterations in blood flow.[35] Vasodilators have been shown to increase peritoneal clearances because of a possible increase in the capillary surface area as a result of vasodilatation and recruitment of capillaries.[30] Furthermore, changes in the distribution of the blood flow may also affect the peritoneal transport rate.

PERITONEAL LYMPHATICS

The Anatomy of Peritoneal Lymphatics

About 4% of the mesothelial surface area is reported to be covered by lymphatic vessels,[36] but the major part of the lymphatic drainage is considered to occur through the lymphatic stomata in the diaphragmatic part of the peritoneum.[37] The diaphragmatic lymphatic stomata, which were first described by von Recklinghausen[38] in 1862, are small openings (diameter 4 to 12 μm) that are formed by intercellular junctions between both mesothelial cells and lymphatic endothelial cells and open directly into underlying lymphatic lacunae.[36] It is through these specific openings that large particles like erythrocytes and bacteria can directly leave the peritoneal cavity. The underlying lymphatic plexuses (which in humans are situated mainly on the muscular portion of the diaphragm) intercommunicate directly with the plexuses on the pleural surface through intercommunicating vessels.[37] After leaving the diaphragm, the lymph is drained through the large collecting ducts associated with the internal thoracic vessels to reach the venous circulation through the right lymphatic duct.[37] The lymphatic drainage of the peritoneal cavity is to a large extent dependent on the periodic compression and release of the lymphatic vessels caused by the movements of the diaphragm during respiration.[37,39]

In addition to the lymphatic vessels in the diaphragmatic part of the peritoneum, subserosal lymphatic vessels can be found in other parts of the peritoneal cavity, including the omentum,[37] and, furthermore, local lymphatic vessels are present in the tissues surrounding the peritoneal cavity, although their role in peritoneal transport seems to be negligible under normal conditions.[37]

Importance of Lymphatic Flow for Peritoneal Fluid Absorption

The disappearance of a macromolecular marker from the peritoneal cavity has often wrongly been used to estimate lymph flow from the peritoneal cavity during PD. It is now well established that the peritoneal absorptive flow of fluid and solutes is composed of two different pathways[8,40]: (1) direct lymphatic absorption (mainly through the lymphatic stomata in the diaphragm, and, to a lesser extent, through visceral lymphatic pathways[40]; and (2) fluid absorption into tissues where the fluid is absorbed through the Starling forces.[19,41] Studies using tracer appearance in plasma have demonstrated that the direct lymphatic flow represents about 20% of the fluid absorptive flow from the peritoneal cavity in clinically stable peritoneal dialysis (PD) patients.[42] (See the later discussion on fluid absorption.)

PERITONEAL LOCAL REACTION TO INFECTION

The peritoneal host defense reaction to infection is a complex network of interactions among mesothelial cells, peritoneal macrophages (PMø), dendritic cells, infiltrating neutrophils, monocytes, and other inflammatory cells and orchestrated by the secretion of vasoactive substances, cytokines, chemokines, growth factors, and components of extracellular matrix.[6] The initiation, resolution, and repair process of inflammation in the peritoneal cavity are very complex processes, which presently are under intense study, and the regulation of these processes is starting to be understood.[6,7,43-47]

The initial inflammatory activation by bacteria entering the peritoneal cavity is likely to occur on the mesothelial surface, where mesothelial cells, together with dendritic cells and PMø, have an important role in the initiation of the local immune response.[46,47] The characteristics of the antigen-presenting cells are starting to be understood.[47] The mesothelial cells are able to contribute to the massive neutrophil influx by generation of chemokines like CXCL8 (previously called *interleukin-8*), a process that is amplified by the PMø-derived cytokines tumor necrosis factor-α (TNF-α) and interleukin (IL)-1β; and the mesothelial cells are also capable of expressing adhesion molecules like ICAM-1, VCAM-1, PECAM-1 and integrins, which may promote leukocyte attachment to the mesothelial cells.[6] The PMø–produced TNF-α and IL-1β are thought to be key mediators in the activation of mesothelial cells.[6] The mesothelial cells are the principal source of IL-6 in the peritoneal cavity and synthesize large amounts of IL-6 upon inflammatory challenge.[48] However, mesothelial cells do not express the cognate IL-6 receptor, and therefore they initially are unresponsive to IL-6. There is a rapid accumulation of neutrophils within the peritoneal cavity during the first 12 to 24 hours. The proinflammatory cytokines will also lead to differentiation and activation of dendritic cell precursors in the peritoneum into mature dendritic cells that migrate to the lymphoid tissue to active adaptive immunity.[46] The activated Th1 cells and resident natural killer cells will produce interferon-γ, which upregulates the bactericidal activity of the peritoneal macrophages and is also involved in the recruitment and clearance of neutrophils.[46] Early upregulation of the receptor-interacting protein-2 (RIP2) in peritoneal macrophages is required for the rapid resolution of peritonitis, and RIP2 expression likely is required for the decrease of intracellular infection and regulation of migration of antigen-presenting cells.[45] RIP2 has been suggested as a biomarker for resolution of peritonitis to be used in the clinic.[45]

After a few days the neutrophils are replaced by a more sustained population of monocytes and lymphocytes.[7] In fact, this temporal switch in the recruitment of leucocytes (which is under complex regulation) determines whether or not the infection is cleared.[49] Liberation of the soluble IL-6 receptor (SIL-6R) from the initial neutrophils allows for the formation of the IL-6 and SIL-6R complex that allows IL-6 responsiveness in cell types (including mesothelial cells) lacking the cognate IL-6 receptor.[49] The IL-6 and SIL-6R complex will downregulate the expression of CXCL8 and other neutrophil-activating chemokines, and the SIL-6R may also directly promote MCP-1 expression, resulting in the more sustained mononuclear leukocyte infiltration.[7] In addition, the release of oncostatin M from the infiltrating neutrophils will have a synergistic effect with the SIL-6R for the temporal switch from neutrophil influx to mononuclear cell recruitment as oncostatin M suppresses IL-1β–mediated expression of CXCL8.[43] Interferon-γ also has an important role in this process by controlling both the initial neutrophil recruitment independently of IL-6 (through regulation of chemokine expression) and the neutrophil clearance phase by regulating local IL-6 levels.[44,50] The neutrophils will, to a large extent, undergo apoptosis and then be phagocytized by mononuclear cells.[50] This transition from the recruitment of neutrophils (typically associated with innate immunity) to the leukocytes typically associated with acquired immunity is considered to facilitate the successful resolution of the inflammatory reaction.[7,46]

PERITONEAL TRANSPORT PHYSIOLOGY

Barriers to Transperitoneal Exchange

The peritoneum is a complex structure of at least five different resistance barriers coupled in a series: (1) the unstirred fluid layer in the capillaries, (2) the capillary wall (endothelium and basement membrane), (3) the interstitial space, (4) the mesothelium and its basement membrane, and (5) the unstirred fluid layers in the peritoneal cavity.[51] Each of these barriers has its specific transport properties. The capillary wall is considered to represent the major transport barrier for transperitoneal exchange,[19,21] but the interstitium is also important, particularly in long-term PD patients with markedly increased thickness of the submesothelial tissue.[17] The mesothelium, on the other hand, is highly permeable and is not a significant transport barrier.[19,21] The mucopolysaccharide hydrogel of the interstitium will exclude solutes from part of the interstitial water volume and force solutes to follow a tortuous path,[8] and furthermore, the negative charge of the interstitial ground substance may markedly slow the transport of charged molecules through the interstitium.[12] Unstirred fluid layers in the peritoneal cavity may represent transport resistances for the diffusion of small solutes,[8] but are likely of much less importance than the interstitium because the diffusibility is much less in the interstitium compared with the stagnant fluid layers.[1,52]

Modeling of Peritoneal Transport

To completely model the peritoneal transport process, all transport barriers and their specific transport characteristics should be taken into account, including the distribution of the capillaries within the peritoneal interstitium. This will result in very complex models that are difficult to apply in the clinical situation, and, at present, even complex models fail to predict ultrafiltration with better accuracy than simpler models.

Single-membrane models have been used to estimate transport parameters in clinical PD.[53-57] In the single-membrane models, the peritoneal barrier is regarded as a single membrane separating the well-mixed blood and dialysate compartments. The single-membrane models will work very well to describe the transport of small solutes (up to the size of small proteins like β_2-microglobulin) from plasma to dialysate, but they will not work as well for the description of dialysate to plasma transport, and in particular, they cannot correctly describe the osmotic fluid transport when a high-molecular solute (e.g., icodextrin) is used as an osmotic agent.[3,58] The distributed model by Flessner et al.[59] takes into account the distribution of capillaries in the interstitium and should be preferred from a theoretical point of view. However, the simpler three-pore model by Rippe and colleagues,[27-28] which takes into account the three pore systems in the capillary wall (see earlier text), is still as accurate in predicting both fluid and solute transport during clinical PD, using both small-molecular-weight and macromolecular osmotic agents (Fig. 29.2).[27,28,58] Also, a model describing the peritoneum as two heteroporous membranes in series (presumably the capillary wall and the interstitium) has been developed.[60] This model was further developed based on the current understanding of the long-term changes in peritoneal membrane, combining the concept of the capillary three-pore model with an interstitial fiber-matrix barrier, and has been successful in describing the long-term changes in peritoneal transport of fluid (with uncoupling of small solute transport from the peritoneal ultrafiltration coefficient) and of small and large solutes.[17] A detailed description of the different models lies outside the scope of this chapter.

Fluid Transport

Ultrafiltration

The intraperitoneal dialysate volume over time curves during a PD exchange are characterized by three phases: (1) initial net ultrafiltration (rate and duration depend on the osmotic pressure of the solution); (2) dialysate isovolemia (during which ultrafiltration is counterbalanced by fluid absorption); and (3) net fluid absorption (independent of the osmolality of the solution) (Fig. 29.3).[61]

Ultrafiltration in PD is achieved by the application of a high concentration of an osmotic agent (usually glucose) in the dialysate, resulting in a high osmotic pressure gradient across the peritoneal barrier.[8,23] However, the osmotic pressure gradient across the peritoneal barrier decreases rapidly because of the absorption of the osmotic agent when small

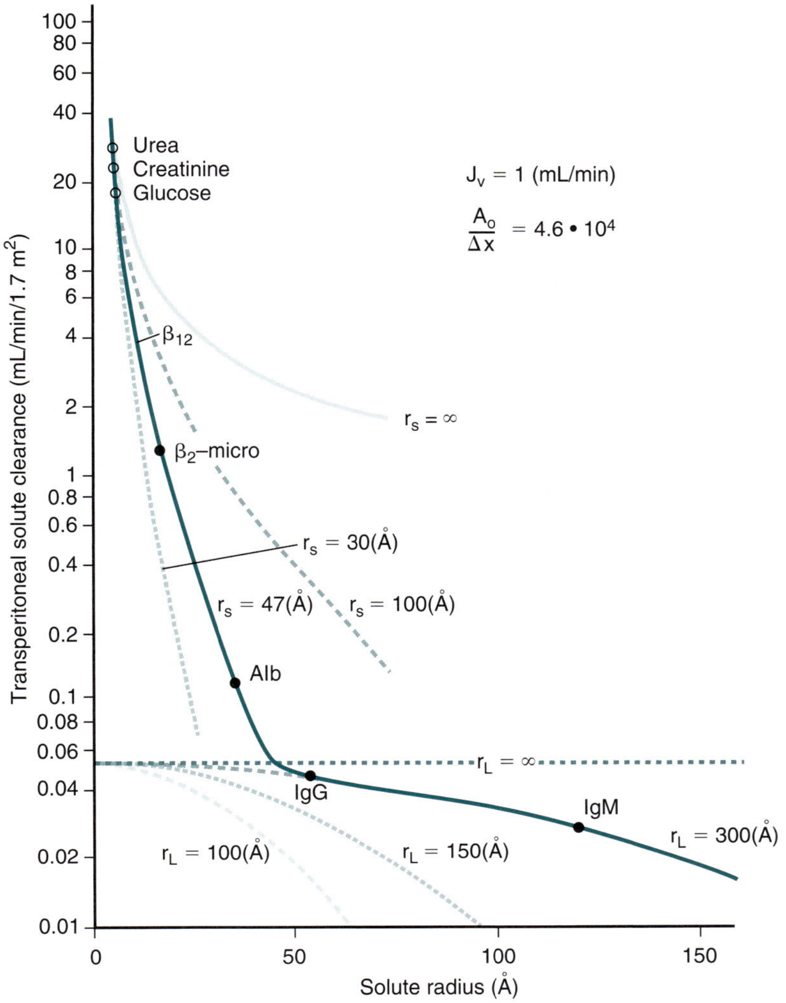

FIG. 29.2 Semilogarithmic plot of transperitoneal unidirectional clearances versus molecular radius. The solid line represents the theoretic clearances simulated for a small pore radius of 47 Å, a large pore radius of 300 Å, a pore area over unit diffusion distance ($A_0/\Delta x$) of 45,000, and a total blood to peritoneal cavity filtration rate at 1 mL/min/1.73 m² body surface area. (From Rippe B, Krediet RT: Peritoneal physiology-transport of solutes. In: R. Gokal, K.D. Nolph, eds., *The textbook of peritoneal dialysis*. 1994. Dordrecht, Kluwer Academic Publishers, pp. 69–113, with permission.)

solutes like glucose, amino acids, or glycerol are used as osmotic agents. When a large molecular solute—for example, icodextrin—is used as an osmotic agent, the absorption of the osmotic agent is much slower, resulting in a much longer-lasting osmotic gradient and positive net ultrafiltration.

Applying the thermodynamic theory of volume transport through selective membranes to the peritoneal membrane, the ultrafiltration rate (Q_U) is directly proportional to the ultrafiltration coefficient (L_PA), which, in turn, represents the product of the hydraulic conductance (L_P) and the effective surface area (A).[61,62] The ultrafiltration rate is therefore described as:

$$Q_U = L_PA\left(\Delta P - \sigma_{prot}\Delta\pi_{prot} - \sum_{i=1}^{n}\sigma_i\Delta\pi_i\right) \quad \textbf{(1)}$$

where ΔP is the hydrostatic pressure gradient, σ_{prot} is the reflection coefficient for total protein, $\Delta\pi_{prot}$ is the colloid osmotic pressure difference caused by the plasma proteins, and the third term within the parentheses represents the sum of all effective crystalloid osmotic pressure gradients across the peritoneal barrier.[62] Note that this equation is a simplification that applies to the capillary wall and, for the full description of the total process, local effects in peritoneal tissue (e.g., the distribution capillaries in the interstitium, interstitial tissue pressure gradients) also will have an impact on the ultrafiltration rate. Thus the ultrafiltration induced when glucose is used as an osmotic agent in PD is dependent on the osmotic pressure difference for glucose, the hydraulic conductance (L_P), the surface area (A), and the reflection coefficient for glucose (σ_g).[62] A wide range of values for the ultrafiltration coefficient (L_PA) has been reported in the literature because markedly different values of σ_g have been estimated.[54] The reason for these discrepancies is that σ_g in several studies has been calculated as $\sigma_g = 1 - S_g$ (where S_g is the "lumped" glucose sieving coefficient for the whole peritoneal membrane), which is true for homogeneous membranes. However, as

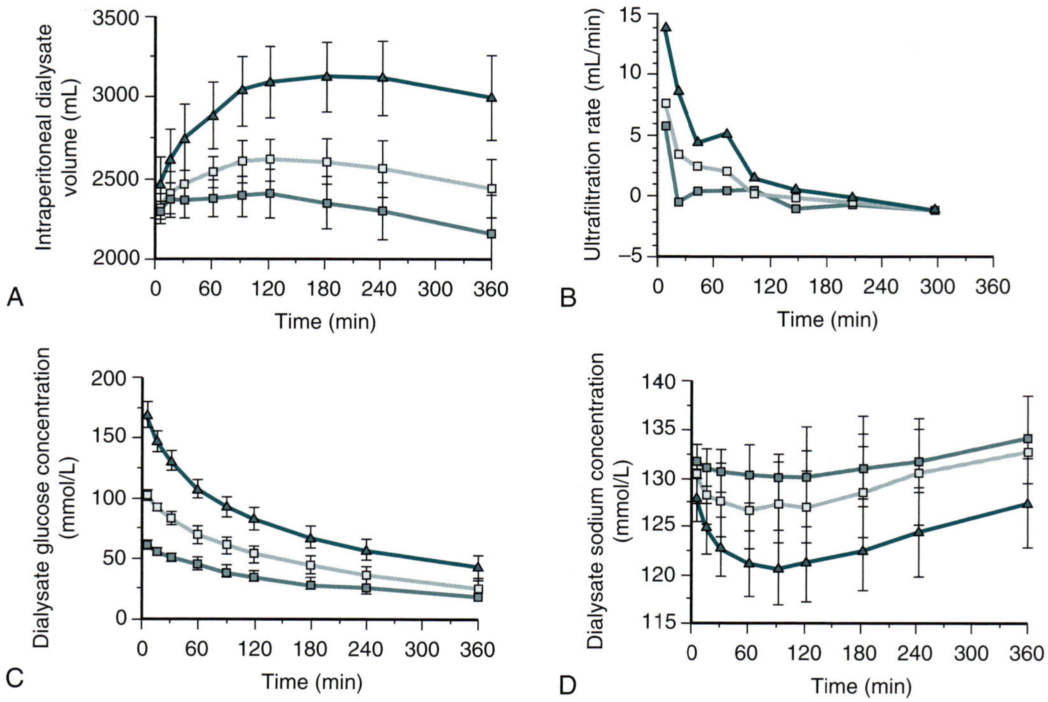

FIG. 29.3 Intraperitoneal dialysate volume (A), net ultrafiltration rate (B), dialysate glucose concentration (C), and dialysate sodium concentration (D) versus time during a 6-hour dwell study with an exchange of 2 L of 1.36% (■), 2.27% (□), and 3.86% (▲) glucose solution (mean ± SD). The intraperitoneal dialysate volumes were assessed from the dilution of the tracer (radioiodinated human serum albumin) with a correction applied for the elimination of the tracer. Note that when hypertonic 3.86% glucose dialysis solution is used, there is a marked dip in dialysate sodium concentration because of the dilution of the dialysate by the ultrafiltrate. The sodium concentration in the ultrafiltrate is much less than the sodium concentration in plasma because sodium sieving as about half of the ultrafiltered fluid will pass through the aquaporins. (From Heimbürger O, Waniewski J, Werynski A et al.: A quantitative description of solute and fluid transport during peritoneal dialysis. *Kidney Int.* 1992;41:1320-1332, with permission.)

the peritoneal membrane is a heteroporous membrane, the relationship between σ_g and S_g may vary. In fact, one of the most convincing arguments for the heteroporous character of the peritoneal membrane is that the direct determinations of L_pA for the peritoneal membrane (assuming $\sigma_{albumin} = 0.9$) in cats and rats (scaled to humans using the scaling factor body weight $(BW)^{0.7}$) yielded an L_pA value of approximately 0.1 mL/min/mmHg, which, in turn, yielded a σ_g of approximately 0.02.[58] These values are well in agreement with the reported initial ultrafiltration rate of 10 to 20 mL/min with 3.86% glucose solution (4.25% dextrose).[54,61,63]

For the peritoneal barrier, the total σ of a solute is equal to the sum of the product of σ and the fractional hydraulic conductivity α for each set of pores. Thus when applying the three-pore model for the peritoneal membrane, the total σ for a solute will be given by the equation:

$$\sigma = \alpha_A \cdot \sigma_A + \alpha_S \cdot \sigma_S + \alpha_L \cdot \sigma_L \quad (2)$$

where subscripts A, S, and L denote aquaporins, small pores, and large pores, respectively. Because the aquaporins are impermeable for glucose, $\sigma_A = 1$ for glucose across the aquaporins, whereas the relative osmotic efficiency of glucose is much less across the small pores ($\sigma S = 0.03$) and negligible across the large pores (σL approximately 0).[28] During normal conditions, the aquaporins account only for a small fraction (approximately 2%) of the LpA, and they will play a minor role in fluid transport, whereas the small pores account for about 90% of LpA. However, when applying a high crystalloid osmotic pressure over the membrane by using a small-molecular osmotic agent, the importance of the aquaporins for fluid transport markedly increases. As $\alpha \cdot \sigma$ will be quite similar for the aquaporins ($0.02 \cdot 1 = 0.02$) and the small pores, ($0.90 \cdot 0.03 = 0.027$) about half of the ultrafiltration will pass through the aquaporins, resulting in marked sieving of solutes (for the large pores, $\alpha \cdot \sigma$ will approximately be zero, as σ_L is approximately 0).[28]

Fluid Absorption

During PD, ultrafiltration is partly counterbalanced by the peritoneal fluid absorption (Q_A).[64] Thus the net change in dialysate volume (V_D) is equal to:

$$\frac{dV_D}{dt} = Q_U - Q_A \quad (3)$$

Because Q_A is considered to be bulk flow, it can be estimated by the disappearance rate (K_E) of a macromolecular marker applied in the dialysate (see Ref. 99 for a detailed discussion).

Pathways for Peritoneal Absorptive Flow

The peritoneal absorptive flow consists of two different pathways[8,19,40-41]: (1) direct lymphatic absorption (through the lymphatic stomata mainly in the diaphragm and, to a lesser extent, through visceral lymphatic pathways)[40]; and (2) fluid absorption into tissues (where the fluid is absorbed into the capillaries because of the Starling forces, whereas the macromolecules are absorbed slowly through local lymphatics).[19,41] Sieving of macromolecules is assumed to be negligible with the direct lymphatic absorption, and with the second pathway (fluid absorption into tissues), sieving of macromolecules at the site of the mesothelium is considered to be negligible from a practical point of view. Thus the macromolecular disappearance rate from the peritoneal cavity may be used as an estimate of the peritoneal bulk absorptive flow[64] because it is mainly dependent on the two components of peritoneal absorption, which both are considered to be bulk flows.[41,64] When the fluid, which has entered the peritoneal interstitial tissue compartment, is absorbed across the capillary wall (because of the Starling forces), sieving of macromolecules should occur at the site of the capillary wall. It is generally agreed that almost no protein may enter the plasma compartment directly through the capillary wall (although direct capillary uptake of radioiodinated human serum albumin [RISA] has been demonstrated under certain conditions). The macromolecules that have entered the interstitial tissue compartment may thus accumulate in the interstitial tissue compartment before they are slowly absorbed by local lymphatics.[41]

The peritoneal absorptive flow is independent of the intraperitoneal osmotic pressure[64] and thus not influenced by ultrafiltration induced by the osmotic agent in the dialysate (i.e., osmotic pressure–driven convective flow). On the other hand, the peritoneal fluid and protein absorption rate in animal experiments has been shown to be directly proportional to the intraperitoneal hydrostatic pressure.[65] Studies by Flessner[41] of tissue concentration profiles of RISA and labeled immunoglobulin G (IgG) (absorbed from the peritoneal cavity in rats) strongly support the notion that hydrostatic pressure–driven convection is the most likely mechanism driving the fluid and protein transport into adjacent tissues. It may seem puzzling that osmotic pressure–driven convection during dialysis and hydrostatic pressure–driven convection are considered to go simultaneously in different directions through the peritoneal barrier without any major interaction. However, this apparent paradox may be explained by the nonhomogenous nature of the peritoneal barrier, where different parts have different vascularization, hydrostatic pressure gradients, and so forth.[3,41] Furthermore, osmotic pressure–driven convection will take place close to the capillaries only, whereas the major part of the peritoneal surface area will allow hydrostatic pressure–driven convection in the opposite direction.[41]

Relative Importance of Lymphatic Absorption and Absorption into Adjacent Tissues

The relative contribution of the two different components of peritoneal absorptive flow (lymphatic absorption and absorption into tissues) has been controversial.[8,19,41] In fact, the disappearance rate of a macromolecular marker has previously been assumed to provide an estimate of the lymphatic absorption rate in PD patients. However, several studies have shown that the plasma appearance rate of a macromolecular marker is, on average, only about 10% to 20% of its disappearance rate from the peritoneal dialysate (in clinically stable PD patients[42] and in animals).[66-67] Furthermore, studies in animals have demonstrated that a major part of the lost marker accumulates inside the tissues adjacent to the peritoneal cavity, mainly in the liver, diaphragm, and anterior abdominal wall.[52,66] Thus the interstitial adjacent tissues may serve as a reservoir for RISA, from which it is slowly absorbed into local lymphatic vessels.[8,41]

Theoretically, it is also possible that RISA transport is delayed in lymph nodes compared with the fluid accompanying RISA in the lymphatic vessels. However, trapping in lymph nodes has not been found to be of major importance,[68] and furthermore, this would not explain the high tissue concentrations of macromolecular tracers reported by Flessner[41] from studies in the rat.

Solute Transport

During PD, solutes are transported bidirectionally through the peritoneal barrier mainly by diffusion (as a result of the concentration gradient between blood and dialysate) and, to a lesser extent, by convection into the peritoneal cavity (as a result of hydrostatic pressure differences and the osmotic disequilibrium caused by the osmotic agent).[61] Also, the solute transport accompanying the convective fluid absorption from the peritoneal cavity into the surrounding tissues and to blood through the lymphatics (see earlier mention) needs to be taken into account.[59,66]

Diffusive Transport

Diffusive transport through a membrane is driven by the concentration gradient over the membrane. If diffusion is unrestricted, the solute transfer rate (J_S) is proportional to the concentration gradient between dialysate and plasma (ΔC), the solute's diffusion constant (D, which is inversely proportional to the solute's radius), the surface area available for diffusion (A), and inversely proportional to the diffusion distance (Δx)[1]:

$$J_S = \frac{D}{\Delta x} A \Delta C \tag{4}$$

The ratio of the solute's diffusion constant to the diffusion distance ($D/\Delta x$) is called *permeability* (P), and the product of P and surface area is usually denoted *permeability surface area product* (PS), which in PD has also been denoted as *diffusive mass transport coefficient* (K_{BD}), *mass transfer coefficient* (MTC), or *mass transfer area coefficient* (MTAC). Thus

PS = K_{BD} = MTC = MTAC. Inserting PS into Eq. 4 yields the following description of diffusive solute transfer rate for a solute across the peritoneal barrier:

$$J_S = PS\ \Delta C \quad (5)$$

However, because the peritoneal barrier behaves as a porous structure, the diffusion of a solute may be restricted by the pore passage; the solute has to hit the pore entrance area and may also be restricted by interaction because of friction with the pore wall.[1] The diffusion through the peritoneal barrier will therefore be restricted, and a restriction factor (A/A_0) needs to be introduced (where A is equal to the apparent pore surface area and A_0 the total cross-sectional pore surface area), and inserting this into Eq. 4 yields:

$$J_S = \frac{DA}{\Delta x}\Delta C = \frac{DA_0}{\Delta x}\frac{A}{A_0}\Delta C \quad (6)$$

From this it follows that the diffusion rate over the peritoneal membrane for a solute will be governed by the solute's diffusion constant (D), the restriction factor (A/A_0), the concentration gradient (ΔC), and the term $A_0/\Delta x$, which represents the unrestricted pore area over unit diffusion distance.[1] Because A_0 and Δx cannot usually be determined, $A_0/\Delta x$ will be the central term describing the membrane's diffusive properties. Knowing $A_0/\Delta x$, the PS can be calculated for different solutes using their diffusion constants (based on the solute radius).[3] Also, when PS is known for one solute, $A_0/\Delta x$ can be estimated and used to estimate PS for other solutes.

Permeability Surface Area Product Under Standard Conditions

Several authors have estimated PS for various small solutes and proteins under standard conditions. The PS values for different solutes decrease with increasing molecular weight, and there seems to be a good agreement between the results from different studies, with reported PS for urea about 18 mL/min, creatinine 10 mL/min, glucose 11 mL/min, inulin 4 mL/min, β_2-microglobulin 1.2 mL/min, albumin 0.12 mL/min, IgG 0.06 mL/min, and α_2-macroglobulin 0.02 mL/min.[1,69,70] The variation in PS from different studies seems to be largest for urea, which is not surprising because dialysate urea concentration is close to equilibration with plasma concentration after 4 hours; the estimated value of PS for urea will be highly dependent on the estimation procedure, in particular, the model applied for PS estimation,[55] and whether or not urea concentrations in plasma are corrected for plasma protein content.[71]

Convective Transport

The magnitude of convective transport is determined by the ultrafiltration rate (J_V) through the peritoneal membrane, the average solute concentration within the membrane (C_M, which for low flow rates is equal to the average of dialysate and plasma concentration), and the sieving coefficient (S, describing the fraction of the solute, which passes through the membrane with the water flow; $0 \le S \le 1$). The rate of solute flow through the membrane, J_S, as a result of diffusion and osmotic pressure–induced convection, can be described as:

$$J_S = PS\Delta C + SJ_VC_M \quad (7)$$

Note that solutes are also transported from the peritoneal cavity because of the peritoneal fluid absorption (J_A, vide supra), which is considered to be a bulk flow.[41,64] Thus the intraperitoneal solute mass will decrease with a term proportional to J_A and C_D. The net solute flow to the peritoneal cavity (Q_S) is equal to[72]:

$$Q_S = PS\Delta C + SJ_VC_M - J_AC_D \quad (8)$$

For the peritoneal barrier, the sieving coefficient for small solutes will be dependent on the fraction of ultrafiltration that passes through small and large pores in relation to the total ultrafiltration flow (through aquaporins, small pores, and large pores), because no solutes will pass through the aquaporins and the convective passage of small solutes through the other pores will not be subject to any sieving.

Importance of Different Parts of the Peritoneum for Peritoneal Transport

Different parts of the peritoneal barrier may have different transport characteristics. These differences will influence the relative importance of different parts of the peritoneum on the total solute and fluid transport through the peritoneal barrier. In particular, the permeability, distribution, and surface area of the capillaries within different parts of the peritoneal membrane may have an impact on the relative importance of different parts of the peritoneal membrane for the overall fluid and solute transport.[8] Furthermore, the mixing of dialysate may be different in different parts of the peritoneal cavity, with particularly poor mixing in pockets of the visceral peritoneum, which may decrease solute transport in regions of the peritoneal cavity where mixing is poor.[4] This is likely one reason why studies of peritoneal transport after evisceration suggests that the hollow viscera may play only a minor role in the overall peritoneal transport because evisceration was found to reduce absorption of urea, creatinine, glucose, and inulin only by about 10% to 20% despite removal of approximately 60% of the peritoneal surface area during experimental PD in rats.[73] After evisceration the contact between dialysate and the membrane is likely to be improved in some areas because of redistribution of fluid to areas not accessible to the dialysate before evisceration.

The parietal peritoneum seems to have only a minor role in peritoneal solute transport, because shielding of the parietal wall with plastic patches did not affect the overall peritoneal transport of urea, creatinine, glucose, or inulin.[73]

The role of different parts of the peritoneal membrane for lymphatic absorption has been studied by Rippe and colleagues[74] by measuring the peritoneal to plasma clearance of I^{125}-RISA in rats after evisceration, or after sealing the diaphragm or the anterior abdominal wall with histoacrylate glue, compared with control rats. They concluded that lymphatic absorption mainly occurs (60%) through diaphragmatic pathways, whereas about 30% occurs through visceral lymphatic pathways, and just a small fraction passes through parietal tissue pathways. On the other hand, the total bulk fluid absorption from the peritoneal cavity (as assessed by the disappearance of RISA) decreased markedly after sealing the anterior abdominal wall, indicating that the anterior abdominal wall plays an important role in peritoneal fluid absorption.[74] This is in agreement with the studies in rats by Flessner and colleagues[66] demonstrating that a significant portion (28%) of the tracer leaving the peritoneal cavity is absorbed into the anterior abdominal wall, resulting in local tracer accumulation within the tissues of the anterior abdominal wall.

Tests to Assess Peritoneal Transport

Several tests are available for the assessment of peritoneal transport characteristics. Commercial computer programs are available to assess basic peritoneal transport parameters and to predict effects of various treatment schedules on peritoneal small solute clearances and ultrafiltration.[29,75,76] In general, the results will be closely dependent on the quality of data used for calculations or put into the computer. In particular, if only long dwells are used and the solutes are close to equilibration, it will be impossible to calculate transport characteristics (see later text). The laboratory methods may also be very important for the results, and, in particular, creatinine levels in dialysate measured with the Jaffé method must be corrected for the interference with high concentrations of glucose in dialysate.[77] Sodium levels should preferably be measured with flame photometry or indirect ion-selective electrodes, because measurements with direct ion-selective electrodes may give different results.[78]

Diffusive Mass Transport Coefficients

For small solutes, the diffusive mass transport coefficient PS (= K_{BD} = MTC = MTAC, see previous text) can be assessed with high accuracy using Eq. 8, if the sieving coefficients and the volume flow are known. If there are no large volume changes, PS can easily be determined using the solute concentrations in dialysate at the beginning (C_{D1}) and in the end of a dwell (C_{D2}), the solute concentration in plasma (C_P)[1,79]:

$$PS = \frac{\overline{V}}{t_2 - t_1} \ln \frac{C_P - C_{D1}}{C_P - C_{D2}} \quad (9)$$

Where t_1 and t_2 are start and end of the exchange, respectively, and $\overline{V}$ is the average volume during the exchange. This equation has been widely used for the estimation of PS, but should be used only when there is a low ultrafiltration rate. Also, it is important to note that the result is closely dependent on the difference between solute concentration in dialysate and plasma at the end of the dwell. Therefore when using this method, solute concentration in plasma (C_P) should be preferably recalculated to achieve the concentration in plasma water (C_{PW}) by correcting for plasma protein and lipid content to avoid overestimation of PS.[79] This can be done using the equation[71]:

$$C_{PW} = C_P \frac{1}{1 - V_{Lip} - 0.000718 \cdot C_{prot}} \quad (10)$$

where V_{lip} is the fractional volume for lipids (often approximated to 0.016) and C_{prot} is the concentration of total protein (often approximated to 65 g/L) in plasma. However, for solutes that are almost equilibrated at the end of an exchange, this method should still not be used, because small random errors in solute concentration will result in large variations in PS. Instead, a shorter dwell time (when the solute concentrations are not equilibrated between dialysate and plasma) should be used for estimation of PS.

There are also much more sophisticated methods to estimate PS for small solutes, but results agree quite well, bearing the limitations of different methods in mind. Presently, computer software is available for the calculation of PS.[29,75,76]

Peritoneal Equilibration Test

The most widely used approach to evaluate peritoneal transport characteristics in individual patients is to measure the dialysate to plasma solute concentration ratio (D/P) for particular solutes during an exchange with conventional PD fluid (Fig. 29.4).[61] This procedure (which was first proposed by Verger and colleagues)[80] has been standardized in the peritoneal equilibration test (PET) by Twardowski and colleagues[77] and has won wide acceptance as a routine method to assess clinically important alterations in peritoneal transport characteristics. The PET procedure is standardized with regard to sampling procedures, duration of dwell, evaluation of the results, and so forth.[77,81] Briefly, the overnight dialysate is drained and 2 L of 2.27% glucose (2.5% dextrose) dialysis fluid are infused. The original PET description included several dialysate samples,[77] but usually, the procedure is simplified and dialysate samples are taken after infusion and then after 2 and 4 hours, at which time the dialysate is drained and the volume recorded. A blood sample is drawn at 2 hours dwell time. Usually, the dialysate drainage volume (used as a measure of ultrafiltration capacity [UFC]), D/P for creatinine, and D/D_0 (dialysate concentration/initial dialysate concentration) for glucose, are compared with standard values. The D/P for creatinine and D/D_0 for glucose from the PET will be closely related to the diffusive mass transport coefficient for these solutes.[82] The patients are usually classified according to D/P creatinine at 4 hours using Twardowski's initial classification into different transport groups (Table 29.1).[69,75,77,81,83-86]

It has been suggested to use 3.86% glucose (4.25% dextrose) solution instead of 2.27% glucose (2.5% dextrose) solution for the PET because it will give a better estimate of UFC because the ultrafiltration rate is higher and the discrimination between patients better. Thus the net ultrafiltration will be less dependent on variations in residual volume between the start and end of the dwell, and the common definition of decreased UFC is a net ultrafiltration <400 mL after 4 hours with use of 4.25% dextrose/3.86% glucose solution.[87] The use of a more hypertonic solution also makes it possible to use decrease in dialysate sodium as an additional parameter to

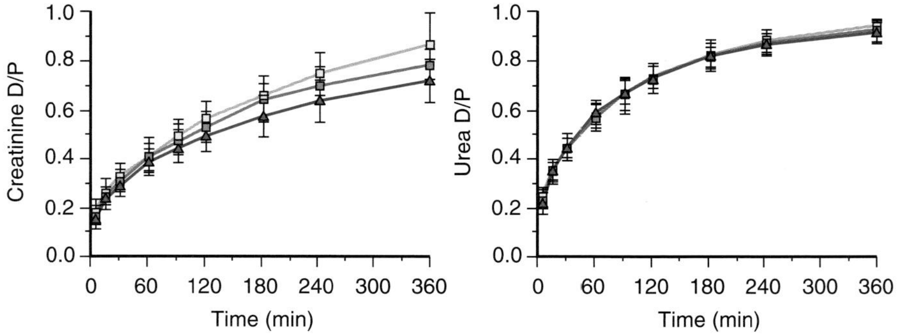

FIG. 29.4 Dialysate to plasma equilibration curves (mean ± SD) for creatinine and urea during a 6-hour dwell study with an exchange of 2 liters of 1.36% (□), 2.27% (■), and 3.86% (▲) glucose solution. (From Heimbürger O, Waniewski, J Werynski A, et al.: Dialysate to plasma solute concentrations [D/P] versus peritoneal transport parameters in PD. *Nephrol Dial Transplant* 1994;9:47–59, with permission.)

TABLE 29.1 Characteristics of the Four Different Peritoneal Solute Transport Groups as Classified by D/P Creatinine After 4 Hours of a Peritoneal Equilibration Test, According to Twardowski's Initial Classification.[77]

Transport Category[a]	4-h PET D/P Creatinine[77,81]	Mini-PET With 3.86% Glucose[81]	$A_0/\Delta x$[75] (cm/1.73 BSA)	UF[81]	Standard PD-2 L × 4/24-h[69] Kt/V Creatinine Clearance		APD Compared With PD[84] Kt/V[a] Creatinine Clearance[b]	
Fast	>0.81	>0.52	>30,000	⇊	=	⇈	⇈	⇈
Fast Average	0.65–0.81	0.43–0.52	23,600–30,000	↓	=	↑	⇈	⇈
Slow Average	0.5–0.65	0.34–0.43	17,200–23,600	↑	=	↓	⇈=-↑	
Slow	<0.5	<0.34	<17,200	⇈	=	⇊	↑	= -↓

[a]The transport categories have previously been denoted high, high average, low, and low average, but it is now recommended to use fast, fast average, slow average, and slow peritoneal transport instead.
[b]The resulting clearances from APD will be strongly dependent on the APD prescription. The table is based on an APD prescription with a total dialysis fluid volume of about 15–20 L for APD and a wet day with an additional daytime exchange.
APD, Automated peritoneal dialysis; *PD*, peritoneal dialysis; *PET*, peritoneal equilibration test; *UF*, ultrafiltration.

identify patients with poor ultrafiltration.[87,88] When hypertonic 3.86% glucose (4.25% dextrose) dialysis solution is used, there is a marked dip in dialysate sodium concentration because of sieving of sodium and about half of the ultrafiltered fluid will pass through the aquaporins (see earlier text) (see Fig. 29.3). In patients with normal transport characteristics, the decrease in dialysate sodium is marked during the first 60 minutes, then it decreases slightly to reach its lowest value after approximately 90 minutes, and thereafter the dialysate sodium concentration increases because of sodium diffusion from plasma.[61]

PET is a simple procedure and easy to perform, the standard values are well established, and it does not require any complicated calculations. On the other hand, the D/P and D/D_0 results are rather sensitive to laboratory errors (only three samples are used), and the net ultrafiltration (measured as drained minus infused volume) is sensitive to variation in the intraperitoneal residual dialysate volume because of incomplete drainage. Furthermore, PET does not provide any details of the peritoneal transport process. However, a commercial computer software program (PD-Adequest) has been developed using results from the PET and the preceding overnight exchange to allow for calculation of basic transport parameters and to simulate the effects of changes in treatment schedules in individual patients.[29,76] The PET has also been modified by using more frequent sampling and adding a tracer to the dialysate to allow for more detailed analysis of changes in intraperitoneal volume.[89]

The D/P values generated by the PET procedure show an excellent correlation with the diffusive mass transport coefficient PS for small solutes, and PS and D/P for creatinine and PS and D/D_0 for glucose can be used to identify patients with loss of UFC because of increased diffusive transport.[88,89] When using 2 L of 4.25% dextrose/3.86% dextrose/glucose solution for the PET, it was suggested to define loss of UFC as a net ultrafiltration below 400 mL after 4 hours. This definition has won wide acceptance, and the use of hypertonic solution for the PET is strongly recommended for the evaluation of UFC.

Mini-PET and double mini-PET. Recently, a short 1-hour "mini-PET" with hypertonic 3.86% glucose (4.25% dextrose) solution was suggested for the evaluation of ultrafiltration and free water transport.[86] It was also found to give estimates of solute transport (D/P creatinine) and classification of patients into different transport groups in good agreement with a 4-hour PET. In addition, free water transport could be estimated from the net ultrafiltration and sodium removal.[86] A further improvement of this test was done by combining two consecutive 1-hour mini-PETs (with 1.36% and 3.86% glucose or 1.5% and 4.25% dextrose solutions, respectively) in the double mini-PET. This approach gives the possibility to calculate an estimate of the free water transport, the osmotic conductance for glucose, and the ultrafiltration through the small pores. The double mini-PET seems to be a simple, fast, and useful test, in particular, for the evaluation of patients with reduced UFC.[90]

Personal Dialysis Capacity Test

The personal dialysis capacity (PDC) test involves urine, blood, and dialysate sampling. The patient collects urine and dialysate during a standardized PD day using a special exchange schedule, with two short (2 to 3 hours) and two medium-length exchanges (4 to 6 hours), each with two different glucose solutions, and one long overnight exchange. A sample is taken from each bag, and the volume of each bag is measured to give the variation in net ultrafiltration and solute equilibration with time and with the two glucose-based dialysis fluids.[75,91] The data are put into a special software program, Personal Dialysis Capacity, based on the three-pore model of peritoneal transport, and calculates the following transport parameters (in addition to adequacy parameters and residual renal function): (1) area parameter ($A_0/\Delta x$), determining the diffusion capacity of small solutes, and indirectly, the hydraulic conductance of the membrane (LpA); (2) reabsorption rate of fluid from the peritoneal cavity to the blood after peak time, when the glucose gradient has dissipated; and (3) large-pore fluid flow, which determines the loss of proteins to the PD fluid. The $A_0/\Delta x$ is a more general parameter than PS for a specific solute and can be also used to classify the patients into similar transport groups as the PET (see Table 29.1). Because the PDC is based on five different determinations of dialysate concentration, it should have better and more reliable classification of an individual patient's transport rate, if a correct sampling procedure has been carried out.[91]

Peritoneal Transport Groups

PD patients are usually classified according to D/P creatinine at 4 hours of the PET using Twardowski's initial classification into high transporters (above mean + 1 SD), high average transporters (between mean and mean + 1 SD), low average transporters (between mean and mean − 1 SD), and low transporters (below mean − 1 SD), but this classification may also be done using the PDC "area" parameter (see Table 29.1).[92] However, preferably fast and slow transport should be used instead of high and low because the net removal of very small solutes (e.g., urea) is often low in "high" transporters as a result of poor ultrafiltration and lower drained volume. Fast and fast average transporters have more rapid equilibration of creatinine and poorer net ultrafiltration because of more rapid glucose absorption, whereas slow average and slow transporters will have lower solute transport, resulting in slow glucose absorption and high net ultrafiltration but low peritoneal clearances for creatinine and larger solutes. Usually, Twardowski's initial limits[77,81] are used to define transport groups, although most studies show an average creatinine D/P equilibration rate that is more rapid than in the study of Twardowski.[83,93,94] It is also likely that there are different types of fast transporters.[83,95] (See later discussion.)

Effluent Soluble Markers of the Peritoneal Membrane

In addition to solutes originating from the circulation, the drained peritoneal dialysate contains substances that are locally produced or released from the surrounding tissues or from cells released into the dialysate. These substances include lubricants and surface tension–lowering substances, such as phospholipids, various cytokines, growth factors, chemokines, prostanoids, and constituents of the extracellular matrix (e.g., GAGs and procollagen peptides), and also coagulation, fibrinolytic, and antithrombogenic substances.[96] Some of these substances have been measured in effluent dialysate to better understand the local intraperitoneal immune system and the local reaction to complications like peritonitis, and the concentrations of some of these substances have also been used as markers of the peritoneal membrane status in apparently stable PD patients.[97,98] However, it should be noted that the interindividual variation is very large, even in clinically stable patients without overt complications, and surprisingly little data are available on the long-term evolution of these markers in patients treated with PD. It should also be stressed that appearance rate (i.e., the amount of solute in the drained bag multiplied by the drained volume and divided by time) should be used when comparing patients, and not the concentration, if there is a marked interpatient variation in drained volume or dwell time. Otherwise, the marker concentration may vary because of differences in dilution as a result of differences in infused volume or in net ultrafiltration, for example.

The most widely used marker of membrane status in clinical studies has been the dialysate effluent concentration of cancer antigen 125 (CA125).[97,98] CA125 is a 220 kD glycoprotein produced by mesothelial cells, and the CA125 level in dialysate increases linearly with dwell time and correlates with the number of mesothelial cells in the effluent. Patients on long-term PD and patients with peritoneal sclerosis have low levels of dialysate CA125.[99] Based on these observations, CA125 has been suggested to be a marker of the mesothelial cell mass or turnover in stable PD patients.[98] Increased levels of dialysate CA125 have widely been used as a marker of improved biocompatibility of new PD solutions, and effluent levels of CA125 consistently increase with the use of more biocompatible dialysis solutions in clinical studies.[100,101] However, the interpatient variation in dialysate CA125 is large, and it is not completely clear exactly what it represents. Therefore the CA125 levels in dialysate effluent need to be interpreted with some caution.

Other potentially important markers are the central proinflammatory cytokine IL-6 and its soluble receptor (sIL-6R) because of their central role in the regulation of intraperitoneal inflammation.[7,102] In particular, IL-6 has gained more and more interest as a marker of local intraperitoneal inflammation. Increase in effluent IL-6 has been reported to relate to more rapid peritoneal transport rate for small solutes as well as for changes with time.[102-104] This is strongly supported by finding that a functionally relevant genetic polymorphism of the IL-6 gene was shown to be related to the initial interpatient variability in small solute transport rate at the start of PD.[105]

Several other effluent candidate markers of peritoneal membrane health status during long-term PD have been used, including HA, which is an important constituent of the interstitial tissue and is produced by mesothelial cells and fibroblasts. HA is involved in several physiological processes, such as tissue repair and wound healing. The fraction of HA that is produced by mesothelial cells forms a coat on the mesothelial cells, together with other GAGs and phospholipids. HA concentration increases with intraperitoneal inflammation and decreases with use of more biocompatible PD solutions.[101,102] The procollagen peptides, procollagen-1-C-terminal peptide and procollagen-3-N-terminal peptide, are produced locally by fibroblasts and mesothelial cells during the synthesis of collagen 1 and 3, respectively, and have also been measured in dialysate as potential markers of local collagen synthesis,[100,101] but it is not completely clear what the levels represent.

Vascular endothelial growth factor (VEGF) is also a potentially interesting marker, because it enhances vascular permeability and angiogenesis, and it is upregulated in peritoneal capillary endothelium in long-term PD patients.[106] Interestingly, both IL-6 and VEGF have been reported to decrease with the use of more biocompatible solutions,[107] though no difference was seen in dialysate IL-6 levels in the randomized balANZ study.[103]

Recent studies have also focused on potential peritoneal tissue injury biomarkers. In particular matrix metalloproteinase-2 (MMP-2) and the tissue inhibitor of metalloproteinase-1 (TIMP-1) have been studied. Both of these markers increase with the duration of PD, and higher effluent levels of MMP-2 were reported to be associated with faster peritoneal transport rate, as well as the risk for future peritonitis.[108] However, the effluent levels of these biomarkers were not influenced by use of biocompatible PD solution.

Factors Affecting Peritoneal Transport

A number of factors have been shown to influence peritoneal transport, possibly by altering the underlying physiological conditions that govern the exchange rate between blood plasma and dialysate. In particular, vasodilatory factors have been shown to increase peritoneal clearances as a result of a possible increase in capillary surface area available for transperitoneal exchange.[30]

Temperature

Klapp[108] reported that heating the anterior abdominal wall resulted in increased fluid absorption from the peritoneal cavity, whereas the opposite effect was noted with cooling of the abdominal wall. The effect of increased temperature was possibly mediated through local vasodilation because local hyperemia could be observed at the serosal and parietal peritoneum.[109] An increase in dialysate temperature will result in an increased solute transport, in addition to the increased fluid absorption.[110]

Intraperitoneal Hydrostatic Pressure

The intraperitoneal hydrostatic pressure is the driving force for convective movement of fluid and solutes into the adjacent tissues.[41] The hydrostatic pressure increases with increasing intraperitoneal dialysate volume[111,112] and varies with body position; the pressure is higher in sitting and standing than in the supine position.[111] The intraperitoneal hydrostatic pressure seems to increase in an almost linear fashion with increased and infused dialysis volume in PD patients,[111] but a study in rats using a larger variation in infused dialysate volume shows that this relationship, in fact, seems to be exponential.[112]

The increased intraperitoneal pressure results in increased fluid absorption,[113] mainly because of increased fluid absorption into adjacent tissues and not increased lymphatic absorption, because the peritoneum to plasma clearance of a radioactive tracer was unchanged when the intraperitoneal pressure was increased in a study in rats.[114] In agreement with these findings, Durand and colleagues[114] reported on a negative correlation between net ultrafiltration and intraperitoneal pressure at the end of a 2-hour dwell in stable PD patients.

Dialysate Volume

In a systematic study of infused dialysate volumes between 0.5 and 3 liters in 10 stable PD patients, Keshaviah and colleagues[115] found that PS for urea, creatinine, and glucose increased in an almost linear fashion between 0.5 and 2 L infused volume, with its values almost doubling over this range. Between 2 and 3 L infused dialysate volume, there was only a small increase in PS values. However, infused volumes yielding maximum urea PS were found to increase with increasing body surface area. The authors attributed the increase in PS to a more effective contact between dialysate and the peritoneal surface area.[116] Krediet and colleagues[116] studied the effect of a 3-L exchange compared with a 2-L exchange with 1.36% glucose (1.5% dextrose) solution and reported significantly higher PS for creatinine, kanamycin, and inulin with the larger volume, but no difference in PS for urea, lactate, glucose, β_2-microglobulin, albumin, or IgG was found. However, the net ultrafiltration relative to the volume at 5 minutes was lower at almost all occasions because of a markedly increased fluid absorption rate with the 3-L exchange volume, possibly related to an increased intraperitoneal hydrostatic pressure.[117]

Effect of Body Posture on Peritoneal Transport

The effect of upright body position has been addressed in a few studies showing a slightly slower D/P equilibration and a decreased net ultrafiltration rate in sitting or standing compared with recumbent position.[118,119] The slightly slower transport rates are likely due to a decreased contact between dialysate and the peritoneal membrane in sitting position, as ultrasound investigation revealed that the bulk of the dialysate was found in the subumbilical region of the peritoneal cavity,[118] and the reduced net ultrafiltration is due to an increased peritoneal fluid absorption as a result of an increased hydrostatic pressure in the upright position compared with supine position.[119] Upright position will also increase the hydrostatic pressure gradient over the anterior abdominal wall, where a large part of the convectively induced peritoneal absorption takes place.[41]

Effect of Dialysate Composition on Peritoneal Transport

Several factors related to the PD solutions per se may also affect peritoneal transport, for example, hyperosmolality, type and concentration of osmotic agent applied, pH, type of buffer, buffer concentration, glucose degradation products (GDPs), and other contaminants.

Glucose Concentration and Osmolality

Because hyperosmolality is a known vasodilatory factor,[120] it is reasonable to expect that hyperosmolality may induce changes in peritoneal transport rates. The use of a 7% glucose solution for PD in uremic patients was associated with an increased solute clearance (compared with 1.5% dextrose solution), which exceeded the possible contribution of convective transport,[121] and similar effects have been found in animal studies. In contrast, the clinical use of the presently available hypertonic 3.86% (anhydrous glucose, corresponding to 4.25% of hydrous glucose or dextrose) dialysis solutions does not seem to affect the peritoneal diffusive transport characteristics in PD patients.[61]

In addition, during heat sterilization and storage of glucose-containing PD solutions, several toxic GDPs are formed, for example, formaldehyde, 3-deoxyglucosone, 3,4-dideoxyglucosone-3-ene, and several other low-molecular-weight aldehydes.[122,123] Although GDPs do not seem to have any major acute effect on peritoneal transport in the concentration found in currently used PD solutions, these pollutants are likely involved in the evolution of changes in peritoneal structure and function observed in long-term PD patients.[123]

Alternative Osmotic Agents

In general, osmotic agents with a lower molecular weight compared with glucose, for example, amino acids and glycerol, will be absorbed more rapidly than glucose, resulting in a shorter period of positive net ultrafiltration than with glucose solutions of the same osmolality.[124,125] However, the presently available amino acid solution will induce similar, or slightly better, ultrafiltration compared with 1.36% glucose (1.5% dextrose) solution because of the slightly increased osmolality of the amino acid solution.[125] Although the use of the presently available 1.1% amino acid solution does not seem to affect peritoneal transport using the PET,[126] they seem to slightly increase peritoneal solute transport and blood flow in one study,[127] and hypertonic 2.7% amino acid solution has also been reported to be associated with slightly increased peritoneal transport rates.[124,128]

Several large-molecular-weight osmotic agents, such as starch, glucose polymers, dextran, gelatin, albumin, and polypeptides, have been used in experimental studies.[129] Because the capillary wall is easily permeable to water and small solutes but restricts the passage of large-molecular-weight solutes, the osmotic effect of colloid during PD is much more prolonged than the osmotic effect of small solutes. Therefore even with a relatively low osmolality, the colloid osmotic pressure may ensure the sustained osmotic transport of water.[130] Note that the main osmotic effect of the polymers will occur over the small pores, and sodium sieving will thus not be observed.[58]

Icodextrin, which is the only commercially available large-molecular-weight osmotic agent in clinical practice, is a specific fraction of dextrin isolated by fractionation of hydrolyzed cornstarch.[131] Icodextrin is a polydispersed mixture of polymers with varying chain lengths, with the majority of icodextrin polymers (>85%) having a molecular weight between 1680 and 45,000 daltons. The osmotic pressure from icodextrin will be relatively high over the small-pore system because icodextrin cannot pass through the small pores, whereas the water flow through the aquaporins will be small because of the low difference in osmolarity and the small total area of the aquaporins. As the ultrafiltration with icodextrin solution will occur almost entirely through the small pores, no sieving of small solutes will be observed with this solution.

The presently used 7.5% icodextrin solution is, in fact, hypoosmolar compared with plasma but will result in a sustained net ultrafiltration for more than 14 hours because of the sustained colloid osmotic gradient.[58] The icodextrin-based solution does not affect peritoneal solute transport characteristics,[132,133] but the large osmotic fluid flow through the small pores will result in increased clearance of sodium and of low molecular proteins like β_2-microglobulin and leptin.[58,133]

Absorption of icodextrin occurs primarily because of the relatively slow convective fluid movement out of the peritoneal cavity.[132,133] As a result the absorption of the osmotic agent is much slower, resulting in a longer duration of the osmotic gradient and a positive net ultrafiltration. Thus the osmotic pressure created by icodextrin will be relatively constant during the dwell and ultrafiltration is sustained throughout the long dwell.[58,130,132,133] Only about 20% to 40% of the administered icodextrin is absorbed from the peritoneal cavity during a long dwell.[134]

Because of the slow absorption of icodextrin and the sustained ultrafiltration with icodextrin solution, it is theoretically well suited for patients with poor ultrafiltration because of rapid glucose absorption. Several clinical studies also demonstrate that this is the case in the clinical situation[134-136] where icodextrin solution can provide good ultrafiltration in these patients. In contrast to the decline in ultrafiltration with glucose-based solutions during peritonitis episodes, icodextrin solution will preserve its UFC during peritonitis.

Effect of pH and Different Buffers on Peritoneal Transport

Conventional glucose-based dialysis solutions were reported to be vasoactive when applied directly to capillaries, with an initial transient vasoconstriction (for less than 2 minutes) followed by a maximal vasodilatation sustained during the whole study period.[137] The high osmolality or high concentration of buffers, acetate, or lactate was indicated as a possible factor.[137] The unphysiologically low pH in traditional dialysis fluids is also considered to be vasoactive and may thus theoretically influence the vascular responses in the peritoneum during dialysis. A few studies have been conducted to assess the effect of pH per se on peritoneal transport. However, the low pH in dialysis fluids was not found to induce distinguishable vasoactive responses in the peritoneum[138] or to affect the peritoneal solute transport characteristics in rats[139] or humans.[140]

Acetate, lactate, and bicarbonate have been used as buffers in PD solutions. As pH and other factors may also differ between solutions with different buffers, it is difficult to assess the possibly independent effects of pH and buffer on peritoneal transport. Furthermore, the long-term effects of the dialysis solution on peritoneal transport seem to differ between similar solutions produced by different manufacturers,[141] and it is possible that differences in their production processes may have resulted in differences between the solutions, for example, in different content of GDPs.

Acetate was previously used as a buffer in dialysis fluids. However, although acetate buffered solutions seem to have no effect on peritoneal UFC in short-term studies,[141] long-term use of acetate was associated with high frequency of UFC failure[140,142] and has furthermore been suggested to be implicated in the etiology of encapsulating peritoneal sclerosis (EPS, previously called *sclerosing encapsulating peritonitis*).[141] However, use of acetate-based solutions from different manufacturers was associated with markedly different risks for EPS, suggesting that other factors were different between the solutions.

Because of the side effects of acetate solutions, lactate was for many years the almost exclusively used buffer in commercially available PD solutions. At present, different bicarbonate solutions are available, and the transport does not seem to differ to a major extent in clinical studies among lactate, bicarbonate/lactate, or pure bicarbonate solutions.[138]

Effect of Biocompatible Solutions on Peritoneal Transport

During the last decade, several new, more biocompatible PD solutions have been introduced. These solutions are characterized by more physiological characteristics with neutral pH, by markedly reduced content of GDPs, and in some cases by use of bicarbonate as buffer (either in combination with lactate or pure bicarbonate).[142] These solutions have got widespread use in some areas of the world in the hope that they will be beneficial in the long-term preservation of the structure and function of the peritoneal membrane. However, so far this is not established. Early studies of bioincompatible PD solutions were relatively small with medium-term follow-up (up to 24 months). Most of these short-term studies show either no effects or small effects on peritoneal transport with a slight increase in small solute transport and a slightly reduced ultrafiltration in some of the studies.[100,143-149] These effects seem to be rapid and disappear relatively shortly after switching back to traditional bioincompatible solutions.[143,145] In the largest randomized study so far, the 2-year balANZ study,[149-150] 167 patients had peritoneal membrane function evaluated. Whereas the initial 4-hour D/P creatinine ratios were significantly higher in the group using biocompatible PD solution, mean D/P creatinine at 4 hours remained stable in this group, whereas they increased significantly in controls. Similarly, peritoneal net ultrafiltration increased significantly in the biocompatible solution group but remained stable in controls.[149] These results suggest a beneficial long-term effect of biocompatible PD solution.

In addition, use of biocompatible PD solutions is associated with increased effluent levels of CA125, suggesting increased mesothelial cell turnover or cell mass.[100, 143,148] Though mechanisms behind the changes in peritoneal transport with biocompatible solutions remain elusive, it is possible that the effect of the solutions on the mesothelial cell may in turn affect the peritoneal capillaries and, in turn, the effective peritoneal surface area. However, use of biocompatible PD solutions does not seem affect the effluent levels of IL-6.[102,103]

Pharmacological Effects on Peritoneal Transport

Several drugs and hormones have been reported to alter peritoneal transport rates.[30,151] The results of many of these studies must, however, be interpreted with caution because the experimental conditions are not always standardized, and several other factors may also have been altered by the experimental conditions. In addition, accurate determinations of dialysate volume are often lacking.

Vasoactive Drugs

Intravenous administration of norepinephrine significantly decreases peritoneal clearances, whereas dopamine increases the peritoneal solute transport rate, possibly because of vasodilation caused by stimulation of mesenteric dopamine receptors.[30,151] In general, vasodilatory drugs have been reported to increase peritoneal transport[30,152,153]; for example, theophylline, furosemide, hydralazine, and sodium nitroprusside (an NO donor) have all been reported to augment peritoneal clearances—an effect that is possibly related to an increased peritoneal capillary surface area. On the other hand, splanchnic vasoconstrictors, like norepinephrine,[151] generally tend to decrease peritoneal clearances.[30]

Changes in Peritoneal Transport During Peritonitis

Peritonitis is associated with several changes in peritoneal transport. A fall in UFC is often noted during peritonitis,[154,155] but this alteration is transient, and UFC usually returns to normal within less than 1 month.[154]

The decreased UFC is most commonly associated with increased small solute transport and rapid glucose absorption and consequently loss of the osmotic driving force.[154] In addition, the peritoneal fluid absorption is markedly increased.[75] Detailed studies of peritoneal fluid absorption have not been performed, but it is likely that the increase in fluid absorption is due to both increased lymphatic flow and increased convective fluid transport into adjacent tissues.[69]

The increased small solute transport seems to be related to an increased peritoneal capillary surface area, probably as the result of inflammatory recruitment of microvessels.[28,75] This effect is likely, to a large extent, mediated by NO and both endothelial nitric oxide synthase (eNOS) and inducible nitric oxide synthase (iNOS), which have been demonstrated to be markedly upregulated in a rat model of acute peritonitis with poor ultrafiltration and increased small solute transport.[156] Also, the structural changes, the increased solute transport, and the poor ultrafiltration were much less pronounced in eNOS knockout mice.[251]

Furthermore, peritonitis is associated with markedly increased protein losses in dialysate,[75,154,155] indicating an increase in the number or size of the large pores.[75] The intraperitoneal production of prostaglandins (e.g., PGE_2 and PGI_2) is increased during peritonitis.[155] Since the increased peritoneal protein loss during peritonitis correlates with the increased dialysate concentration of prostanoids, and, furthermore, the increased protein loss partly may be inhibited by indometacin,[155] it may be suggested that the increased peritoneal protein loss during peritonitis is mediated, at least partly, by the vasoactive prostaglandins.

Changes in Water and Solute Transport With Time on Peritoneal Dialysis

Changes in peritoneal solute transport are common after initiation of PD. Several studies using the PET have reported on a significant increase in 4-hour D/P creatinine from the PET after 6 months of PD compared with initial results obtained during the first 2 weeks of PD, whereas ultrafiltration was rather stable.[158,159] It has also been reported that in patients with initially high solute transport, transport rate may, in fact, decrease.[158]

Changes in Peritoneal Transport With Long-Term Peritoneal Dialysis

In the majority of patients treated with PD for up to 3 years, the peritoneal UFC and small solute transport characteristics seem to be relatively stable,[158,160] although several studies demonstrate a tendency toward increasing diffusive mass transport coefficients for small solutes and a tendency toward decreasing net UF.[158-161] However, individual patients may behave markedly different; some patients demonstrate increased diffusive solute transport and decreased ultrafiltration, whereas other patients show opposite patterns.

In patients treated with PD for 4 years or more, the tendency toward decreasing ultrafiltration and increasing small solute transport is evident in almost all prospective studies.[158,161] In contrast, macromolecule transport (as assessed by protein clearances) has been reported to be stable or to decrease with time on PD,[85,162] indicating a stable or decreased peritoneal permeability for macromolecules.

However, the interpretation of most studies (and in particular the cross-sectional studies) of peritoneal transport with time may suffer from methodological fallacy in that patients with "inadequate" peritoneal transport will drop out, so that both fast transporters (insufficient fluid removal) and slow transporters (insufficient small solute clearances) may drop out, resulting in selection bias.

Loss of Ultrafiltration Capacity

With time on PD there is an increasing risk for developing loss of UFC. Using the standard lactate-based solutions, the risk for developing permanent loss of UFC (using a clinical definition) increases markedly with time on PD, being 9% after 48 months and 35% after 72 months of PD.[85] There is hope that the use of biocompatible PD solutions and less use of hypertonic PD solution will decrease this risk, and the results of the balANZ trial give some hope for this.[149,150]

There are several pathophysiological mechanisms behind ineffective fluid removal as a result of permanent loss of UFC (Box 29.1). Increased transport of small solutes with rapid glucose absorption is the most common mechanism observed in PD patients with impaired UFC.[85,158,160-162] The rapid glucose absorption results in rapid loss of the osmotic driving force (glucose gradient) and, consequently, a rapid decline in ultrafiltration rate. However, detailed kinetic analyses of patients with UFC as a result of rapid diffusive transport also show that the remaining osmotic gradient cannot induce water flow as effectively as in patients with normal UFC, indicating a decreased osmotic conductance of the peritoneal membrane.[56,163]

A selective decrease in ultrafiltration in patients with normal diffusive glucose transport has also been reported in some PD patients (with loss of UFC), who also had a minor decline of dialysis sodium concentration when using hypertonic glucose solution.[88,164] This may imply a decreased hydraulic conductivity of the peritoneal membrane, and it was suggested

BOX 29.1 Suggested Causes of Ineffective Fluid Removal in PD

A. Obstructed outflow and increased residual dialysate volume
B. Loss of residual renal function
C. Subcutaneous or retroperitoneal leakage
D. Loss of ultrafiltration capacity as a result of:
   1. Increased solute transport (most common mechanism)
   2. Reduced osmotic conductance (impaired transcellular water transport or reduced UF coefficient; not uncommon, often combined with 1. in long-term PD patients)
   3. "Hypopermeable peritoneum" with decreased water transport or decreased surface area (extremely rare)
   4. Increased peritoneal fluid absorption (probably rare)

that these alterations may be the result of decreased transcellular water transport (deficient aquaporin-mediated ultrafiltration) and that this may be an additional cause of UFC failure. However, this finding needs to be interpreted with caution because when the ultrafiltration rate is low, a reduction of dialysate sodium caused by the dilution of dialysate by ultrafiltrate will not occur to the same degree. Sodium sieving will always be markedly reduced when ultrafiltration is poor, even when the aquaporin function is normal.[165] An alternative explanation to the normal glucose transport without decline of dialysate sodium could be a combination of selective changes in the peritoneal ultrafiltration coefficient in combination with increased surface area.[17] This would result in unchanged diffusive solute transport in combination with reduced ultrafiltration coefficient across both transcellular water pores (aquaporins) and small pores.[87]

Loss of peritoneal surface area with slow solute transport as a result of fibrosis and the formation of adhesions has been reported during the late stage of EPS in a few cases. However, detailed studies in four patients developing EPS showed increasing PS in three of the patients,[166] suggesting that loss of UFC associated with increased solute transport in these patients was an early sign that preceded the development of more overt signs of EPS. A recent report suggests that a decreased sodium dip with hypertonic solution was seen in EPS patients before the onset of EPS.[167] Thus initially EPS seems to be associated with increased peritoneal solute transport, which later is followed by formation of adhesions and finally encapsulation of the intestinal loops, resulting in slow peritoneal solute transfer caused by loss of the surface area. However, slow solute transport seems to be an extremely rare cause of UFC loss, and only a few cases have been reported.

Increased peritoneal fluid absorption has also been reported as the cause of UFC loss.[85] The increase in peritoneal fluid absorption in these patients is not due to increased lymphatic absorption, but to increased fluid absorption into the peritoneal interstitial tissue, indicating changes in the interstitial tissue fluid hydraulic conductivity.[42] The mechanisms behind these changes are not clear. Increased fluid absorption may also be caused by subcutaneous or retroperitoneal leakage of the dialysate.[168] Because retroperitoneal dialysate leakage can be diagnosed with only computed tomography, magnetic resonance imaging (MRI) scan, or scintigraphy, it is possible that some cases of increased fluid absorption in fact are due to undiagnosed retroperitoneal leakage.[168]

Relation Between Peritoneal Transport Characteristics and Clinical Outcome

Peritoneal transport characteristics have a major impact on the clinical management and outcome in PD patients. The patient's peritoneal small solute transport characteristics will have a major impact on the optimal dialysis prescription with regard to ultrafiltration and small solute clearances. Furthermore, a high/fast peritoneal transport rate has been identified as an important risk factor for both PD technique failure and mortality.[83,92,169,170]

Although the reasons for this are not established, several different mechanisms may contribute. At first, there is an association between a fast peritoneal transport rate and comorbidity, including diabetes, cardiovascular disease, and chronic inflammation (with elevated plasma levels of C-reactive protein [CRP] and IL-6).[94,103,171,172] Second, high transporters have a more rapid glucose absorption and thus an impaired fluid and sodium removal, and have a high risk to chronic fluid overload,[173] which in itself is associated with left ventricular hypertrophy (LVH) and left ventricular (LV) dysfunction in PD patients[174] and may cause immune activation because of bacterial or endotoxin translocation in patients with severe gut edema as a result of severe volume overload.[175] In contrast, although a low fluid removal may result in low urea clearance, peritoneal clearances for larger solutes than urea are usually not lower in fast transporters. During standard PD, the Kt/V_{urea} is not different between transport groups, and creatinine clearance is usually higher in high/fast transporters (see Table 29.1).[69]

The role of overhydration[176] as a cause of poor clinical outcome in PD patients with fast peritoneal transport is supported by the fact that the clinical outcome has improved markedly with the more frequent use of icodextrin solution and automated PD (APD) and that there is no increased mortality in fast transporters treated with APD.[170,177]

Because there is a close relationship between the peritoneal transport characteristics of solutes of different molecular weights up to the size of albumin (see Fig. 29.2),[27,69] it is not surprising that many patients with fast peritoneal transport also exhibit increased protein losses and that these patients have more severe hypoalbuminemia than patients with lower D/P ratios.[178] It is interesting to note that the low serum albumin levels are already present in high transporters before the initiation of PD,[178] indicating that another mechanism, such as inflammation, may also contribute. Furthermore, a large influx of glucose absorbed from the dialysate may suppress appetite, although Davies and colleagues[179] reported that calories derived from the dialysate in PD patients did not seem to reduce appetite in PD patients. The low albumin levels and increased glucose absorption in high transporters lead to the hypothesis that a fast transport state will lead to protein-energy wasting, which, in turn, may affect clinical outcome. However, except from low serum albumin levels, high transporters do not seem to have more severe protein-energy wasting with regard to other nutritional parameters.[92] Furthermore, there were no signs of change in any nutritional parameters in fast transporters in a longitudinal study of nutritional parameters.[162,297]

It is striking that the relation between peritoneal transport rate and serum albumin[92] and some other nutritional markers was seen already at the start of PD.[180] Therefore it is likely that the relation between peritoneal transport and some nutritional parameters seen in some studies, in fact, are due to a relation between peritoneal transport and the malnutrition, inflammation, and atherosclerosis (MIA) syndrome.[181] Fast peritoneal transport characteristics may thus be another feature of the MIA syndrome.[181]

Moreover, it is important to note that the etiology and clinical features of fast transporters may be different. It has recently been suggested that there may be different types of fast transporters[182] and that the prognosis may depend on the type of fast transporter.[156] Type I is an early inherent type that is associated with higher mortality, mainly because it is associated with comorbidity, low residual renal function, and inflammation; these patients would also have a poor prognosis if they were treated by hemodialysis. Type II is an early inherent type with a large peritoneal surface area, and type III is a late acquired type with transport changes that develop with time on PD; the latter two types do not necessarily have higher prevalence of inflammation or comorbidities, such as diabetes mellitus and cardiovascular disease. These patients will have a good prognosis if fluid balance is controlled using APD and icodextrin-based PD solution.[177,183] In addition, other patients may perhaps exhibit an increase in transport rate over time on PD because of the development of clinical complications, resulting in increasing inflammation. The relative importance of the different types of fast transporters and their contribution to the poor clinical outcome of high/fast transport patients is not known.

In addition, an increased peritoneal albumin clearance (or large pore flux from the PDC test) has recently been reported as an independent predictor of poor clinical outcome.[184] It may, to some extent, be related to inflammation and cardiovascular disease and has furthermore been suggested as a marker of endothelial dysfunction.[185]

Changes in Peritoneal Morphology With Time on Peritoneal Dialysis

During the last 20 years, several small studies have demonstrated marked changes in peritoneal morphology in patients treated with PD, including mesothelial denudation, submesothelial thickening and fibrosis, and vascular changes with vascular basement membrane reduplications.[304-307] More recently, myofibroblasts suggested to be transdifferentiated from mesothelial cells that have undergone epithelial to mesenchymal transition (EMT),[15,187] vascular changes with subendothelial hyalinization and neoangiogenesis,[188,189] and accumulation of advanced glycation end-products (AGEs) in the peritoneum[188,190] have been reported, factors that also were related to functional changes with increasing peritoneal solute transport.

The Peritoneal Biopsy Registry reported the analysis of biopsies from the parietal peritoneum in 130 PD patients and compared them with peritoneal biopsies from normal individuals and uremic subjects not treated with PD.[16] The most dramatic changes were the marked increase in the submesothelial compact zone (which approximately equals the interstitium), which was 50 μm in normal subjects, 150 μm in hemodialysis patients, and 270 μm in PD patients. The thickness increased markedly with time on PD from 180 μm in patients treated with PD for less than 2 years to a median value of 700 μm in patients treated for more than 97 months (Fig. 29.5).[16] Vascular changes with progressive subendothelial hyalinization and luminal narrowing or obliteration were seen in 56% of the PD patients and increased with time on PD. Patients with membrane failure had higher submesothelial thickness and a higher density of blood vessels, which correlated with the degree of fibrosis.[16]

In a few patients who had been treated with PD for several years, progressive peritoneal fibrosis with development of EPS has also been reported. This is a frightening complication with fibrotic thickening of the peritoneal membrane, formation of adhesions, and in the last phase encapsulation of the intestinal loops and formation of an intestinal cocoon.[141] Research has recently focused on finding predictors of EPS like free water transport[167] and effluent biomarkers.[191,192]

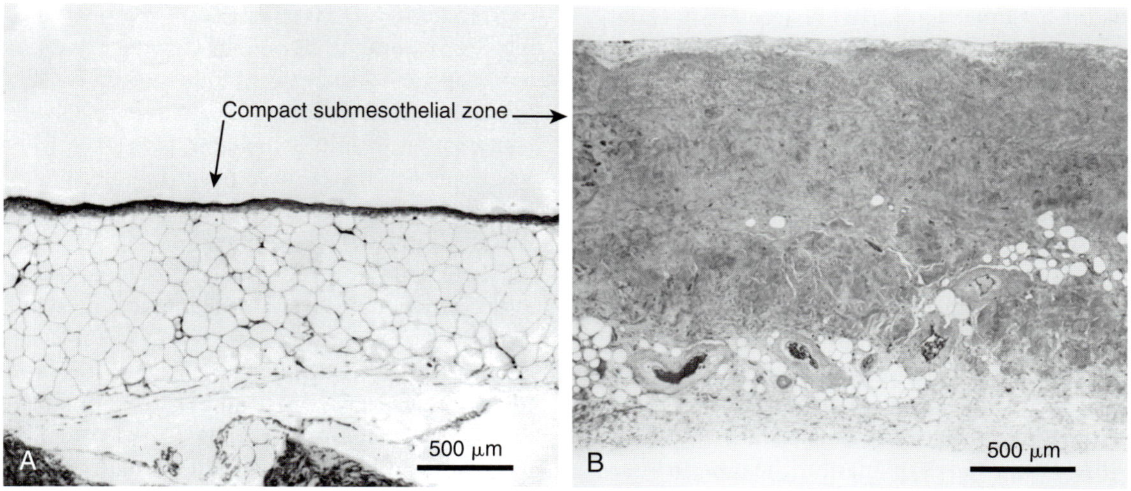

FIG. 29.5 Parietal peritoneal biopsies from a normal individual (A) and from a patient who had been treated with PD for 9 years (B). Note the marked expansion of the submesothelial compact zone in B. (From Williams JD, Craig KD, Topley N et al.: Morphological changes in the peritoneal membrane of patients with renal disease. *J Am Soc Nephrol* 2002;13:470-479.)

Pathophysiological Considerations

Potentially Causative Factors

The pathogenetic mechanisms behind the structural and functional alterations in the peritoneal membrane are not clear, but both bioincompatibility of the PD solutions and the effect of peritonitis have been discussed. Davies and colleagues[159] reported that recurrences or clusters of peritonitis and the cumulative dialysate leukocyte count were related to increased D/P creatinine and reduced UFC, whereas D/P creatinine and UFC were stable in patients with no or single isolated peritonitis episodes. However, the relationship between peritonitis and high solute peritoneal transport rate is not evident in studies of patients with loss of UFC, where most studies have failed to demonstrate any relation between the number of peritonitis episodes and loss of UFC.[85] Although numerous studies have demonstrated the bioincompatibility of the presently used PD solutions in vitro, and bioincompatibility has been extensively discussed as a cause of changes in peritoneal solute transport,[193] there have been limited clinical data demonstrating such a relationship, except from the relation between loss of UFC and the use of acetate as a buffer. However, it should be noted that until recently, almost all standard PD solutions have had similar composition and biocompatibility. The results of the 2-year balANZ study (see earlier) suggest a beneficial long-term effect of biocompatible PD solution, but the study was limited in time.[149,150] Much attention has focused on the relatively high content of reactive carbonyls in the conventional PD solutions.[122,194] These reactive carbonyls are particularly of interest because they are more potent promoters of formation of AGEs than glucose itself.[194] The potential pathogenetic role of carbonyls and AGEs in the changes of peritoneal function are supported by the facts that increased AGE content has been found in the peritoneum of long-term PD patients and was furthermore associated with increased peritoneal small solute transport.[188,190] In addition, AGEs may stimulate the transdifferentiation of mesothelial cells to undergo EMT.[15] Also, it has been reported that patients with increasing small solute transport (as assessed from the PET) with time on PD had a higher glucose exposure compared with patients with stable peritoneal membrane transport.[195]

Physiological Mechanisms

The mechanism(s) by which small solute transport increases in patients with poor ultrafiltration and increased small solute transport is not yet understood. It has been suggested that the cause of the increased small solute transport rate is an increase in peritoneal vascular surface area as a result of neoangiogenesis, which has been demonstrated in the peritoneal membrane.[16,105,188,189] However, if this was the only explanation, the protein losses should also be increased among these patients because of the larger vascular surface area. However, the markedly expanded interstitium (submesothelial compact zone) will slow macromolecular transport more than small solute transport, resulting in an increased small solute transport and normal macromolecular transport.[17,18]

In reduced osmotic conductance (reduced osmotic efficiency of glucose) observed in many patients, it has been suggested that this is due to decreased transcellular water transport (deficient aquaporin-mediated ultrafiltration).[88,164] However, this is still not established, and the aquaporin expression was, in fact, reported to be normal in a long-term PD patient with poor ultrafiltration attributed to impaired transcellular water transport.[196] Furthermore, computer simulations have demonstrated that sodium sieving will always be markedly reduced when ultrafiltration is poor, even when the aquaporin function is normal.[165] Also, an expanded matrix of fibers coupled in series with the three-pore membrane can simulate these changes with reduced osmotic conductance (uncoupling of small solute transport from the peritoneal ultrafiltration coefficient, LpA).[17,18] Therefore further research is needed to establish the pathophysiological mechanisms behind the reduced osmotic conductance in many PD patients with poor ultrafiltration.

Devuyst[197] has suggested a model where the increased reactive carbonyls (caused by uremia and the carbonyls in the PD fluid) will amplify the AGE formation in the peritoneal membrane. The carbonyls and AGEs will have several effects, including stimulation of peritoneal cells to produce VEGF. AGEs will also stimulate mesothelial cells to undergo EMT, and transdifferentiated mesothelial cells are an important source of VEGF.[198] However, the origin of the submesothelial myofibroblasts in long-term PD patients is not well established. The origin of the myofibroblasts from EMT has been questioned, and there are other potential sources, including resident progenitor cells in the peritoneum, endothelial cells, and circulating fibrocytes.[199,200]

The local peritoneal inflammation caused by peritonitis or cellular stress and tissue injury due to the dialysis process or the PD solution may trigger Toll-like receptors on mesothelial cells, resulting in release of proinflammatory as well as fibrotic mediators (e.g., IL-6, tumor growth factor-β [TGF-β], TNF-α, and IL-8).[201,202] Treatment with soluble Toll-like receptor-2, a negative modulator of Toll-like receptors, markedly reduced bacteria-induced fibrosis in vivo.[201] IL-6 in combination with its soluble receptor (sIL-6R) will promote VEGF expression of mesothelial cells through a transcriptional mechanism.[203] The sIL-6 is needed, as mesothelial cells lack the cognate IL-6 receptor.[203]

The inflammatory response to bacterial peritonitis results in upregulation of several cytokines and growth factors (e.g., TGF-β, IL-1, IL-6, fibroblast growth factor-2, and angiotensin II) that further stimulate EMT.[198] sIL-6R can be delivered to mesothelial cells by shedding from infiltrating neutrophils and forming the IL-6 and sIL-6R complex stimulating mesothelial cells to VEGF production.[203] VEGF will stimulate neoangiogenesis and interact with endothelial cells to produce eNOS, which is markedly increased in long-term PD patients[105] and will cause vasodilation and further stimulate neoangiogenesis. NO is a crucial regulator of vascular tone and permeability, and the finding that eNOS knockout mice, to a large extent, were protected against the structural and functional changes induced by acute peritonitis[157] underscores the importance of NO in the pathophysiology of peritoneal membrane dysfunction. The correlation seen between submesothelial fibrosis and neoangiogenesis suggests that these two processes are related,[16,189] and it is likely that transdifferentiated mesothelial cells that have undergone EMT are not only an important source of VEGF,[198] but also play an essential role in the initiation of fibrosis and in the synthesis of matrix components such as collagen I and fibronectin.[15] It is in this context of interest that uremia per se and the binding of VEGF to the extracellular matrix will induce the release of basic fibroblast growth factor (bFGF), which has fibrotic and angiogenetic effects.[197]

However, even if much progress has been made during the last few years, our knowledge is still insufficient about which factors will be most important in causing the long-term changes in the peritoneal membrane structure and function, and about the pathogenetic mechanisms involved in the evolution of these alterations. Much further research is clearly needed in this area.

A full list of references is available at www.expertconsult.com.

30

The Use and Outcomes of Peritoneal Dialysis

Matthew J. Oliver, MD, MHS, and Robert R. Quinn, MD, PhD

OUTLINE

Peritoneal dialysis (PD) is associated with equivalent outcomes to hemodialysis but can be provided in most countries at significantly lower costs. Individuals receiving PD generally report good quality of life and high satisfaction with their care and can live a more independent lifestyle. Given the current pressures on healthcare budgets, PD is actively promoted in many countries. The stated justification for these policies is "to increase patient access to care, control costs through lower infrastructure and capital investments, empower patients, and optimize treatment provision".[1]

However, the use of PD varies widely among regions, suggesting that optimization of PD use is a complex and variable process. It is important to understand the variance in use among regions, recent changes in PD use, and what factors may explain the observed variance. It is also relevant to understand how the outcomes of patients on PD compare with those on hemodialysis, given that PD is promoted in many countries.

Peritoneal Dialysis Use

Jain et al.[2] conducted a comprehensive review of PD use between 1997 and 2008 by contacting a representative from the national dialysis registries for each country. PD use was reported as number of patients on PD, PD incidence, PD prevalence per million population, and PD prevalence as a percentage of dialysis patients. Focusing on the latter statistic, countries can be classified into high use (50% of greater), moderate use (10% to 50% use) and low use (less than 10%) (Table 30.1).

This study, although comprehensive in its methods, does not reflect the most recent PD use statistics, and some countries have implemented policies to increase PD use since 2008. For example, in the United States, the Center for Medicare and Medicaid Services (CMS) implemented an expanded prospective payment system that bundled most of the services provided to dialysis patients starting January 1, 2011[3,4] to promote PD use. Prevalent PD use, according to the US Renal Data System (USRDS) renal report, has increased from 7.2% to 9.8% from 2010 to 2014.[5]

In Thailand a PD-first policy was implemented in 2008 that dramatically increased prevalent PD use from 9.5% in 2008 to 30.0% in 2014, according to the Thailand Renal Replacement 2014 report.[6] In Ontario, Canada, the Ministry of Health and Long-Term Care began actively promoting PD in 2005.[7] The policy was followed by the formation of a renal agency called the Ontario Renal Network in 2011, which has a strategic goal to increase home dialysis. Prevalent PD use has grown modestly from 18% in 2005 to 19.4% in 2015.[8]

Framework for Understanding Peritoneal Dialysis Use

The use of PD can be explained by a variety of frameworks. For example, Liu et al. identifies the importance of government policies, economic factors, and provider and patient education.[1] Other explanations focus on system, provider, and patient factors. Our preferred framework is to focus on the process of care that requires patients to pass through six steps to successfully start PD therapy. At each step, the impact of policies, education, and provider and patient factors can be considered.[9]

Identification of Potential Peritoneal Dialysis Patients

PD use will be increased in programs that have a robust intake and accounting process to identify all potential PD candidates. The majority of patients are followed in predialysis clinics by nephrologists or interdisciplinary teams. The receipt of predialysis care is strongly associated with PD use. For example, a predialysis education program implemented by Fresenius Medical Care in the United States was associated with an adjusted odds ratio (OR) of 5.13 (95% confidence interval [CI], 3.58 to 7.35) for selecting PD.[10]

In our quality improvement system (DMAR system) we have found that interdisciplinary meetings conducted every 2 weeks to identify and review all new patients starting dialysis can greatly improve the identification of potential PD patients.[9] These meetings are particularly important for patients who start dialysis acutely in the hospital. Hughes et al. found that 46% of the patients starting dialysis in Canada began as an inpatient, despite 62% having received at least 4 months of predialysis care.[11]

TABLE 30.1 Peritoneal Dialysis Prevalence in Selected Countries

Country	Prevalent Use of PD (%)
Use >50%	
Hong Kong	79.4
Mexico	65.8
Use between 10% and 50%	
New Zealand	36.3
Sweden	23.8
Australia	22.6
Canada	18.3
United Kingdom	17.0
China	14.0
Brazil	10.6
Use <10%	
United States	7.0
Thailand	5.5
Germany	5.3
Japan	3.3

Modified from data reported in Jain AK, Blake P, Cordy P, Garg AX. Global trends in rates of peritoneal dialysis. *J Am Soc Nephrol* 23:533-544, 2012.

Prevalence is extracted from annual reports from national registries from 1997 to 2008, but the prevalences cited were primarily from 2008 (personal communication, Arsh Jain).

Patients starting dialysis urgently in the hospital are normally treated with hemodialysis using a central venous catheter. The advent of urgent start PD programs, usually defined as PD catheter use within 2 weeks of insertion, allows these patients to consider PD as their initial dialysis modality rather than receive hemodialysis (HD) as a default.[12] Urgent-start PD studies indicate that this strategy can be successful, with acceptable rates of complications, although catheter dysfunction was increased in some studies because patients were acutely ill and could not undergo the same level of preparation before PD catheter insertion as those with elective PD starts. The impact on PD use is less clear, but urgent-start PD should increase PD incidence use by offering acute patients the option to start on PD rather than hemodialysis. Studies are generally small, with sample sizes of fewer than 100 patients, and some patients used their catheter for PD within 48 hours of insertion.[13,14]

Identification of PD candidates among patients starting dialysis acutely may also be facilitated by use of nurse navigators. Rioux et al., in a study from Toronto, Canada, found that 21.5% of patients starting dialysis urgently without prior modality education chose PD when targeted by an advanced nephrology practice nurse.[15] Similarly, use of a nurse navigator for urgent starts was found to increase the likelihood of transitioning from in-center hemodialysis to independent forms of dialysis (OR 3.75; 95% CI, 1.08 to 13.05) in a single-center study from Vancouver, Canada.[16]

Assessment of Peritoneal Dialysis Eligibility

All end-stage renal disease (ESRD) patients who are likely to initiate or have initiated chronic dialysis therapy should be assessed for PD eligibility. The average rate of eligibility among multiple dialysis programs in Ontario was 65%, although experienced programs have considered up to 80% of their patients eligible for PD.[17] Eligibility is generally determined by either a nephrologist or interdisciplinary team based on the presence of contraindications to PD, barriers to self-care PD, and the availability of support.

Contraindications to PD are not completely objective, and providers in programs may have different levels of comfort treating patients with different medical conditions (Fig. 30.1). Some programs may also use extended PD

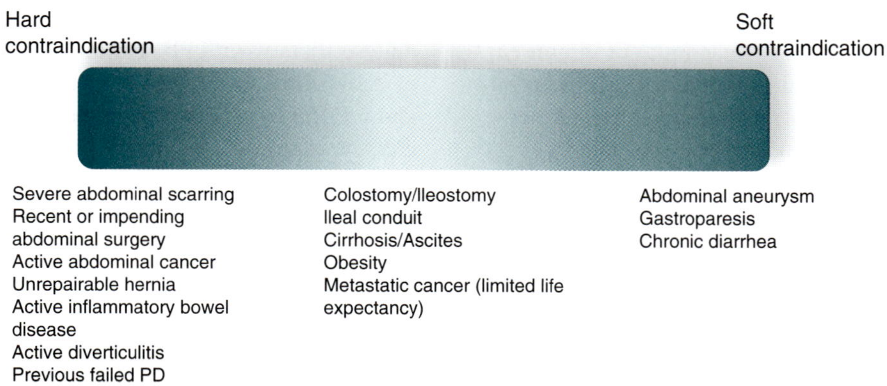

FIG. 30.1 Contraindications to peritoneal dialysis *(PD).*

catheters or presternal PD catheters, which allow patients with a large pannus or a colostomy/ileostomy to receive peritoneal dialysis.[19] Some programs may also have access to surgeons who can perform PD catheter insertion using advanced techniques such as adhesiolysis and hernia repair, which expands eligibility for PD.[19] With these considerations in mind, our prospective study found that 22% of patients were considered by their nephrology team to have a contraindication to PD.[20]

Studies also indicate physical, cognitive, and social barriers to self-care PD are common. Our prospective study found that 53% of patients assessed for PD (excluding those with contraindications) had at least one physical barrier to PD, such as decreased strength, dexterity, vision or hearing.[20] At least one cognitive barrier to PD was present in up to 15% of patients and included language barriers, dementia, a history of nonadherence, and active psychiatric conditions.[22] When PD patients are screened for cognitive dysfunction using a battery of validated tests, up to 45% of PD patients have evidence of cognitive decline.[21] Social barriers may be present when patients are primary caregivers for others (children or elderly parents), have employment issues, or live in residences such as small apartments or retirement homes that make PD more difficult. Although these physical, cognitive, and social barriers are common in PD patients, it is not known if they explain variance in PD use among programs within or between countries.

In contrast, the availability of support likely influences PD use at the program or regional level. We previously reported that the availability of home care support for PD increased eligibility from 65% to 80% in an elderly dialysis population in a single-center study.[22] In France, assisted PD was chosen by 1232 out of 1613 (76%) of PD patients older than 75 years.[23] We also reported that the availability of family support increased PD eligibility from 18% to 46% depending on the presence of barriers to self-care PD. The availability of home care assistance varies from country to country, but this model of PD delivery has been reported in studies from Canada, United Kingdom, France, Denmark, Switzerland, Spain, Brazil, Taiwan, and China.[24,25,26]

Offer and Choice

Once a patient is deemed potentially eligible for PD, he or she is provided modality education. Modality education takes many forms and can be provided by physicians, nurses, or specialized educators. The format of educational programs can include one-to-one sessions, group education, printed materials, videos, or websites. Patients may also now access material directly from the Internet or benefit from peer-to-peer education. Given these many options, it is not surprising that education varies widely among dialysis programs. Regardless of the format of modality education, it is necessary to increase PD use. For example, Mehrotra et al. reported that only 34% of patients in the ESRD Network 18 reported being offered any form of PD when they started renal replacement therapy.[27] This may partly explain the low penetration of PD in the United States because receipt of education is consistently associated with choosing PD. A recent review of educational studies we conducted found that modality education increased PD choice by a factor of 4.6 in a randomized study and a factor of 2.2 in prospective observational studies.[28] Decision aids for patients, such as the Yorkshire Dialysis Decision Aid,[29] "My Kidneys, My Choice Decision Aid",[30] and "My Life, My Dialysis Choice"[31] may also allow patients to make better choices. A prospective study by Winterbottom et al. found their Yorkshire dialysis decision aid was associated with higher information scores, higher decision clarity and feelings of control, and higher levels of shared decision making among patients' families. These are all positive results, but they did not evaluate the impact on actual home dialysis use.

Patient choice, or whether patients are given a choice at all, is a relatively easy factor to modify and likely explains much of variance in PD among programs. In prospective studies, approximately 50% of patients chose PD when they were offered it in a systematic fashion.[20,32,33] However, the choice rate will vary widely from program to program depending on their philosophy. Some programs employ a neutral approach where patients are provided fact-based education with little promotion, similar to consent for a clinical trial. For example, France has a legal requirement to offer patients modality choice.[23] However, most programs likely encourage patients to consider home-based therapies and actively promote them by strongly emphasizing the benefits of home dialysis. Other countries, like Hong Kong, Thailand, and Mexico, employ PD-first policies where choice is explicitly restricted.[1] Other countries such as New Zealand may not explicitly restrict choice but make it challenging for some patients to receive in-center hemodialysis, resulting in high home dialysis rates.

PD-first policies may conflict with the patient-centered care and the principle of shared decision making. Shared decision making is defined as "an approach where clinicians and patients share the best available evidence when faced with the task of making decisions, and where patients are supported to consider options, to achieve informed preferences".[34] Other research suggests shared decision models, when employed thoughtfully, can increase home dialysis without restricting patient choice.[35]

It is important to note that expressed choice before the initiation of dialysis does not always translate into actual receipt of PD therapy. For example, Leibmen et al. found of 124 patients who chose PD at the time of education, 59 started dialysis therapy with PD, and 65 started with HD.[36] On day 91 of dialysis therapy, a total of 60 patients were on PD therapy and 55 were on HD therapy. Proponents of buried PD catheters have argued this technique can "lock in" patient choice and is one of the advantages of placing buried PD catheters at higher levels of GFR.[37] Buried catheters are inserted so the external limb of the catheter is buried under the skin, permitting healing and tissue ingrowth of the cuffs in a sterile environment. Buried catheters cannot be flushed and must be externalized before use.[18]

The availability of support can also increase PD choice. Family or home care support was associated with increased likelihood of choosing PD,[20] and the impact of support was more pronounced in patients with barriers to self-care.

Insertion of the Peritoneal Dialysis Catheter

Patients who chose PD must undergo PD catheter insertion to receive PD. PD catheter insertion among eligible patients is an objective measure of choice and can be used to compare choice rates among programs in epidemiological studies.[17] Methods of insertion include percutaneous techniques, generally performed by nephrologists and radiologists, and surgical techniques, including laparoscopic and open insertion, performed by surgeons. Randomized trials have not consistently found significant differences in complication rates between the different methods, and the most recent guidelines of the International Society for Peritoneal Dialysis (ISPD) recommend using local expertise and availability to guide the method of insertion.[38,39,40,41] Some advocates of laparoscopic placement with advanced techniques report outstanding results with very low complications rates,[18,19,42] but it is not known whether these results are generalizable to all programs.

A study we conducted in Ontario, Canada found patients who had PD catheters inserted by nephrologists were more likely to receive at least 4 weeks of PD use.[43] However, it was not known if this result was due to be better timing of insertion, patient selection, or reduce complication rates. Higher-risk patients with previous abdominal surgeries and scarring may be selected for surgical placement of PD catheters. In this study, 17% of PD catheters did not provide at least 4 weeks of PD therapy during follow-up, but the reasons could not be determined from the administrative data. Asif et al. reported an increase in the prevalent use of PD at three centers from 16% to 18% to 22% to 32% when nephrologist-based insertion of PD catheters was introduced.[44]

In summary, methods of insertion vary widely and it is not clear the impact the method of insertion has on PD use. Laparoscopic insertion with advanced techniques could provide superior technical results, but its impact on use is unknown. In contrast, nephrologist-based insertion may also improve use, but the mechanism is not known. Regardless of technique, high rates of insertion-related complications, particularly ones causing early technique failure, will negatively affect PD use.

Receipt of Peritoneal Dialysis

Once the catheter is in place, PD can be initiated. ISPD guidelines recommend at least 2 weeks of healing before using PD catheter. However, urgent-start PD programs have used PD catheters 24 to 48 hours after insertion.[12] In contrast, buried catheter studies are often exteriorized months or years after initial placement (Table 30.2).

TABLE 30.2 Summary of Factors Potentially Influencing Peritoneal Dialysis (PD) Use

Steps in Process of Care	Factors Potentially Increasing PD Use
Identify PD candidates	Predialysis care Urgent-start PD programs Nurse (modality) navigators Interdisciplinary meetings to review new patients
Assess for PD eligibility	Predialysis care Nurse (modality) navigators Interdisciplinary meetings to review new patients
Determine patient is eligible	Availability of family support Availability of home care support
Offer PD	Modality education Peer support programs
Patient chooses PD	PD-first policies Shared decision-making models Decision aids Availability of family support Availability of home care support
Patient receives PD	Method of PD insertion Operator inserting PD catheter Timing of PD catheter insertion

Outcomes of Peritoneal Dialysis Therapy

Kidney transplantation is felt to provide the best patient outcomes and quality of life and is the most cost-effective form of renal replacement therapy available[45,46,47,48] in settings that have the necessary health system infrastructure to support transplant programs. However, donor organs are a scarce resource and not all patients are eligible for a transplant. As a consequence, the vast majority will receive dialysis as the first form of treatment for end-stage kidney failure.[5,49]

In an ideal world, information about patient outcomes from several, well-designed randomized controlled trials comparing different dialysis treatments would be available to guide shared decision making and help patients and providers choose between the different options. Unfortunately, attempts at randomized comparisons have been unsuccessful.[50] Although there are numerous potential comparators (e.g., transplantation, home hemodialysis, or conservative management), we focus our discussion on studies that have compared the outcomes of patients treated with PD and HD.

Attempts at Randomized Comparisons of Peritoneal Dialysis and Hemodialysis

Investigators in the Netherlands attempted to conduct a randomized trial of incident dialysis patients at 38 participating sites.[50] Although 63% of screened patients were deemed eligible for the trial, only 38 of 773 eligible patients consented to participate and it was stopped because of poor accrual. This study was nonetheless informative because it demonstrated the fact that patients appeared to form strong preferences for one modality or another when educated about their treatment options and were unwilling to subject themselves to randomization. This is an important consideration, particularly in environments where PD-first policies are being contemplated.

A subsequent feasibility study was conducted in China to determine whether patients would be willing to be randomly assigned to either PD or HD (clinicaltrials.gov NCT00510549). The investigators had planned to enroll 50 patients to determine whether a larger trial looking at the impact of treatment modality on mortality, morbidity, quality of life, and cost effectiveness was feasible. According to clinicaltrials.gov, recruitment was completed in August 2008 and a protocol for the larger trial was registered in 2011 (clinicaltrials.gov NCT01413074). Recruitment was terminated in 2013 after 416 patients were enrolled, and final data collection for the primary outcome measure was to be completed in December of that year. The results of the pilot and larger trial have not been published to our knowledge.

In the absence of data from randomized controlled trials, we must rely on outcomes of observational studies. Although there is a general feeling among experts that the outcomes of patients treated with PD and HD are equivalent, much of the existing literature is based on registry studies with unclear data quality, which have included patients who might not be eligible for both therapies and patients who are acutely ill, have a poor prognosis, and are treated almost exclusively with HD. These and other issues may introduce bias into nonrandomized comparisons. Given that many jurisdictions are actively promoting PD and some have implemented PD-first policies, it is important to be aware of the methodological challenges inherent in such comparisons and the level of confidence we should have in prior comparative studies.

Data Validity

It is important that data regarding baseline patient characteristics, changes in treatment modality, and patient-level outcomes are valid to ensure a fair and unbiased comparison of PD and HD. If differential reporting of patient characteristics or outcomes occurs, this can lead to systematic bias. Ideally, data collected as part of a well-designed prospective cohort study [61,68] or data from a validated source [67] would be used for PD versus HD comparisons. However, the majority of studies comparing outcomes in individuals treated with PD and HD have been based on data from regional or national dialysis registries, particularly in recent years.

Registries can be an important source of information and are often used for comparative studies of PD and HD. It is generally assumed that data from dialysis registries are valid, but very little work has been done in this area to confirm the validity of the data sets and the available information raises some important concerns. Longenecker et al.[52] compared comorbidity information collected using Form 2728 (Medical Evidence Report for end-stage renal disease in the US Renal Data System Registry) to data from the prospective Choice for Healthy Outcomes in Caring for ESRD (CHOICE) study. The authors found that comorbidities were "significantly underreported on Form 2728" and found that performance of the registry data were systematically different among those treated with PD compared with HD. In fact, they cautioned, "bias may be introduced if Form 2728 data are used to study associations between comorbid conditions, treatment, and mortality or other outcomes." Subsequent studies examining the validity of Form 2728 for identifying glomerular diseases have shown poor agreement with kidney biopsy results.[53]

Validation studies of other national registries, such as the Canadian Organ Replacement Register [49] and the Australia and New Zealand Dialysis and Transplant Registry (ANZDATA), have been conducted. Moist et al. found that there was underreporting of comorbidities in CORR, similar to the USRDS.[54] However, when hazard ratios were calculated for individual comorbidities using CORR data and compared with those obtained using information taken from chart review, there was good agreement between the two sources. Although this is somewhat reassuring, the authors didn't specifically look to see if there were systematic differences between the coding of comorbidities in PD and HD patients or determine the validity of other important variables required to conduct an unbiased comparison of these two modalities (e.g., changes in treatment status or the occurrence of important patient outcomes). Similar findings were reported in a retrospective audit of 175 HD patients registered in the ANZDATA registry.[73] Gray et al. found that primary renal disease was correct in 86% of cases; date of first dialysis was correct in 94% of cases, but there was significant underreporting of most comorbidities (low sensitivity and relatively high specificity). No information was available for PD patients or for important patient outcomes.

Valid data are necessary foundation for robust, unbiased comparisons of PD to HD. However, several other methodological considerations can influence the observed results. It follows that it is important to ensure that studies are well designed, in an attempt to minimize bias and avoid misleading results and conclusions.[67] These issues will be explored further in the context of the relevant outcomes discussed next.

Comparing the Outcomes of Patients Treated With Peritoneal Dialysis and Hemodialysis: Survival

Studies examining the impact of dialysis treatment modality on patient survival have been inconclusive, but most experts believe that PD and HD are associated with similar survival. Some studies have found a benefit with PD,[55,56,57] whereas others have reported a survival advantage of HD[58,59,60,61,62,63] or little or no difference between modalities.[64,65,66,67]

Eligibility for Peritoneal Dialysis and Hemodialysis

It is important to note that not all individuals with kidney failure are candidates for PD or other home dialysis therapies. Some patients have medical and social conditions that are considered contraindications to treatment.[33,69] These include morbid obesity, massive polycystic kidneys, diverticulitis, other disease states that make the peritoneal cavity unsuitable for PD, and living in a nursing or retirement home that does not permit PD. Many patients without an absolute contraindication to therapy still have barriers to home dialysis that must be overcome to perform it safely. Examples of barriers include decreased physical strength and manual dexterity, poor vision, cognitive impairment, and a fear of social isolation.[33] After taking barriers and contraindications into consideration, two-thirds of patients are candidates for both PD and HD and must choose between them with the help of their healthcare providers.[50,17]

In the setting of a randomized controlled trial, all participants would be screened to ensure that they are eligible for the two strategies being compared. The choice of dialysis treatment modality is only relevant to those who are eligible for both therapies because this is the only group that is faced with the decision in clinical practice. Ideally, observational studies comparing PD with HD would include only those eligible for both therapies and therefore faced with a choice between the two in clinical practice. However, eligibility for PD and HD is not routinely recorded in national dialysis registries and has not generally been accounted for, even in prospective studies.[61] This is relevant because approximately one-third of patients are deemed ineligible for PD, either because of medical or social contraindications or their constellation of barriers to doing home therapies.[50,17] Including ineligible patients in comparisons of PD and HD means that patients who are generally older and sicker are included in the PD group, and this may bias analyses against PD. Several studies have conducted comparisons of outcomes in patients who are judged to be eligible for both therapies according to the local multidisciplinary team and based on a structured assessment.[70,71,72] However, the majority of studies have not addressed this issue. Some authors have attempted to overcome the lack of information about PD eligibility by using propensity scores.[61,82] In this approach, statistical methods (e.g., matching on propensity score or adjustment for propensity score) are used to make groups more similar with respect to the likelihood of receiving PD. This approach attempts to level the playing field but is not the same as comparing eligible patients.

Cohort Formation

In addition to restricting analyses to patients who are eligible for both PD and HD, the definition of a "chronic" dialysis patient varies. Many registries follow patients for 90 days from the time of dialysis initiation before calling them a chronic dialysis patient. Although the impact of cohort selection on the results of PD versus HD comparisons has not been studied extensively, a Canadian study by Quinn et al.[51] explored the impact of several different cohort definitions and reported that results differed significantly according to the definition employed.[67] Restricting the analysis to elective, outpatient dialysis starts that had received at least 4 months of predialysis care identified no difference in mortality in those treated with PD compared with HD. When the results were compared with those obtained using traditional definitions of chronic dialysis, they differed in important ways. The interaction between diabetes status and treatment modality was no longer present and the change in the relative hazard of death over time that has been described in prior studies was no longer present, suggesting it is related to the inclusion of urgent dialysis starts, rather than an effect of dialysis modality.

The Impact of Urgent Starts

There are several potential trajectories for patients who develop end-stage kidney failure: slowly progressive kidney disease, acute kidney injury superimposed on chronic kidney disease, and acute kidney injury in an individual with no known history of kidney disease. Patients who have an acute component to their kidney failure may not have been adequately prepared to start dialysis, may have a poorer prognosis, and are preferentially treated with HD in most centers.[75,76] It is important to note that the increased mortality observed in this population persists for up to 6 months, so analyses based on traditional definitions of chronic dialysis may not overcome this inherent selection bias by restricting the cohort to "chronic, stable" patients.

Incident Versus Prevalent Patients

It is generally well accepted that comparisons of HD and PD should be conducted in incident patients, rather than prevalent patients. Outcomes in the incident patient population are more relevant to clinical decision making because decisions about modality choice are generally made before the start of dialysis or soon thereafter in patients who start dialysis in an unplanned manner (Quinn J Nephrol 2007). Comparisons among prevalent patients are difficult to interpret given the heterogeneous patient population, variable time on therapy, and influence of other interventions and complications that have occurred since the initiation of renal replacement therapy.[51]

Changes in Treatment Modality

The method used to account for switches between treatment modalities must also be considered. The two main approaches have been described as intention to treat (ITT), in which patients are classified according to their initial treatment modality, or as treated (AT), in which modality is treated as a time-varying exposure and outcomes are attributed to the current dialysis modality. In ITT approaches, patients can be censored when they switch to a different modality or modality switches can be ignored. In AT approaches, it is possible to introduce a lag period where outcomes that occur during a prespecified time after a change in modality are attributed to the prior treatment. This is done because patients may suffer a complication that leads to a change in modality (e.g., fungal peritonitis) but that also adversely affects prognosis or the likelihood of other complications. Although it is generally recommended that both approaches should be performed, ITT analyses are likely the most clinically relevant to inform decision making.

Setting

It is important to consider the setting in which a study is conducted. Differences in the way that care is structured and the proportion of patients treated with PD and HD may influence the results of observational comparisons. As a result comparisons of HD to PD in one country may not be generalizable to another because of different outcomes by country, center experience with a given modality, cost considerations that are unique to that jurisdiction, or patient factors that influence quality-of-life measures.[77,78] Finally, the outcomes of patients treated with PD appear to have improved over time in the United States and many other parts of the world, whereas the outcomes of patients treated with HD have not.[79,80]

Statistical Considerations

Case-mix severity refers to an individual's risk for experiencing adverse outcomes based on measured clinical characteristics and is important to account for when comparing outcomes in two or more groups.[81] Groups may differ on the likelihood of experiencing a particular event because important risk factors are unevenly distributed between them. As a result, they confound the observed relationship between group assignment and the risk of the outcome. Failing to account for differences in case mix between groups may lead to biased or inaccurate results. The drivers of case-mix severity vary depending on the population being studied, as well as the exposure and outcome being examined. In comparison of PD and HD, demographic information, comorbidity data, laboratory variables, measures of functional status, genetic makeup, and treatment-related factors, such as those related to dialysis therapy, are all potentially relevant.[76]

In addition to accounting for case-mix severity, it is important to screen for important effect modifiers and account for them when present. In mortality comparisons, age, race, ischemic heart disease, congestive heart failure, diabetes, and the presence or absence of comorbidities have all been found to be effect modifiers.[83] This means, for example, that the impact of treatment modality on survival may be different for patients with diabetes mellitus than it is for those without diabetes. In situations where effect modification is present, results should be presented for all subgroups separately.

The important considerations when modeling mortality data in this patient population are reviewed by Vonesh et al.[84] They concluded that Cox and Poisson survival models appeared to produce consistent results and the choice of model should depend on the nature of the available data and the preference of the investigator. Since the publication the report by Vonesh et al., other approaches, including marginal structural models, the use of propensity score techniques, and methods to account for competing risks (e.g., transplantation), have been employed. Although an in-depth review of the relative advantages and disadvantages of each approach is beyond the scope of this chapter, choice of statistical approach does not appear to have a significant impact on the observed results.

The relative benefit of PD and HD has been found to change over time in a number of studies. Most reported that the benefit of PD was greatest in the first 2 years of therapy and then declined.[55,56,61,85] It has been suggested that PD is associated with a better preservation of residual renal function compared with HD and that this may explain the change in the relative hazard of death over time.[86,87,88] Residual renal function tends to decrease with time on therapy and is a potent predictor of survival on both PD and HD.[89,90,91] The loss of residual renal function is slower in PD patients, and some feel that this is the reason that there is an initial survival advantage that gradually disappears. Alternatively, it may be explained by a tendency to start PD patients while they have a higher residual renal function than their HD counterparts.

Another potential explanation for the initial survival advantage noted with PD is that patients who start dialysis urgently on HD require a temporary form of dialysis access. This typically means that the patients have a central venous catheter placed to access the bloodstream for dialysis. Catheters are associated with a risk for bacteremia and sepsis that is present soon after the catheter is placed, particularly in the acutely ill patient.[92] In this situation, it is possible that treatment with HD is associated with higher short-term mortality as a result of the prevalence of central venous catheters in this population, rather than simply being a surrogate for a higher risk patient.[93] Perl et al. found that the initial survival advantage of PD disappeared when PD patients were compared with HD patients who initiated dialysis with a functioning arteriovenous fistula or graft for vascular access. HD patients who started dialysis with a central venous catheter for vascular access had an 80% higher mortality in the first year of therapy (adjusted hazard ratio [HR] 1.8; 95% CI, 1.6 to 1.9).

However, it is likely that the observed initial survival advantage with PD is related to selection bias rather than an effect of treatment modality or choice of vascular access. The mortality rate on HD has been found to initially be quite high, fall to a nadir at 12 to 18 months, and then rise in a relatively linear fashion thereafter.[55] In contrast, the mortality rate on PD has been found to rise in a linear fashion from baseline and meet the HD curve between 30 and 36 months. After that time, the mortality rates were fairly consistent. If HD is the default option in a higher proportion of urgent starts, it might explain why patients treated with HD have elevated mortality rates shortly after the start of therapy. In studies that include urgent starts, the vast majority would be included in the HD group rather than the PD group, and given that they have a worse prognosis, this would tend to artificially inflate the mortality rate on HD at the start of therapy. A study by Quinn et al. supports this hypothesis. When traditional definitions of chronic dialysis were used, the relative risk of death on PD compared with HD increased over time, consistent with prior studies. However, the association disappeared when the authors excluded patients who started dialysis therapy urgently, suggesting that the apparent increase in the relative risk of death over time on PD compared with HD is due to bias rather than a specific effect of dialysis modality or vascular access.[67]

Some have suggested that it may be worth testing a strategy of switching patients from PD to HD after a specified period to optimize survival in ESRD patients, based on the fact that the relative hazard of death on PD increases with time.[56,94] In the absence of a controlled trial suggesting that elective switch at a particular point in a PD patient's treatment history is beneficial, it is our opinion that this approach should not be recommended based on the existing evidence.

Comparing the Outcomes of Patients Treated With Peritoneal Dialysis and Hemodialysis: Hospitalization

Rates of hospitalization are very similar among those treated with PD and HD. The most recent data from the USRDS suggest that rates of hospitalization, measured as hospital days per patient-year of follow-up, were 11.1 and 10.9 for PD and HD in 2014, respectively.[5] The same data suggest that rates have decreased over time from 14.7 days spent in hospital per year for dialysis patients in 2005 to 10.9 for all patients in 2014.

Although the absolute rates of hospitalization have varied, studies that have compared them between patients treated with PD and HD have found similar rates of hospitalization between PD and HD.[5,65,72,74,95–102,104] Much of the information regarding cause of admission comes from administrative data, which generally track the most responsible diagnosis for each admission rather than the reason for admission. The most responsible diagnosis is the condition that led to the most resource consumption during a hospital stay. For example, if a patient is admitted with catheter-related bacteremia and suffers an acute myocardial infarction that leads to an extended stay in the cardiovascular intensive care, the myocardial infarction would be coded as the most responsible diagnosis, even though the reason for admission was catheter-related bacteremia. This is relevant when one considers hospitalization through the lens of quality improvement. If the intent is to prevent hospitalization, it is important to understand the factors that led to admission to hospital and to be able to distinguish them from complications that occur during a hospital stay. In a study by Murphy et al., the authors reported that dialysis-related hospitalizations were responsible for 10 hospital days per 1000 patient-days of follow-up, or 23% of the total duration of time spent in hospital.[74] Metcalfe et al. reported that 46% of hospitalizations in the first year of dialysis were for dialysis-related reasons, based on data from the Scottish Renal Registry.[105] However, creation of a vascular access for dialysis and PD training made up 17% of the admissions. These procedures and events tend to occur on an outpatient basis in North American programs, and if they were omitted from the analysis, 29% of admissions were for dialysis-related reasons. Quinn et al. found that dialysis-related complications were responsible for 19% of admissions and complications of kidney disease, such as volume overload and hyperkalemia, were responsible for an additional 4%, taking the total to 23%.[72] The proportion of hospitalizations for dialysis-related reasons therefore appears to be relatively consistent across studies. This is important to note because the majority of hospital days incurred are the consequence of comorbid illness, rather than complications of dialysis therapy or complications directly related to kidney disease.

There are several methodological and design issues that deserve mention that may influence the observed absolute and relative rates of hospitalization. Many of the limitations of the literature highlighted earlier in the discussion of survival outcomes apply to the hospitalization literature, such as the lack of randomized comparisons of PD and HD. The inclusion of prevalent patients who have been treated with dialysis for a longer period likely inflates estimates of hospitalization rates compared with studies done in incident populations, because the burden of comorbid illness increases with time. If hospital days are counted from the start of dialysis therapy, urgent starts that occur in the context of an admission to hospital will tend to inflate hospitalization rates and bias against HD, because the vast majority of these patients are treated with HD. Only one small study to date has restricted the comparison of PD and HD to patients who were eligible for both therapies and found no difference between the two therapies in rates of hospitalizations.[72,104] Finally, there are considerations when choosing the appropriate modeling strategy for adjusted hospitalization rates. Although Poisson regression models are traditionally used, they may not be appropriate in situations where a large proportion of patients are not hospitalized during the period examined.[106] It is important to test the assumptions underlying these models when applying them to hospitalization data, because negative binomial or zero-inflated models may be more appropriate in certain settings. Inappropriate model selection may lead to biased or misleading conclusions.[106]

Comparing the Outcomes of Patients Treated With Peritoneal Dialysis and Hemodialysis: Cost

In general, PD has been found to be less expensive to provide than other forms of dialysis, particularly in middle- and high-income countries.[106a] Some of the most robust data come from microcosting studies of different dialysis therapies in Canada that found the total annual healthcare costs associated with treating PD patients were approximately $56,000 compared with $95,000 to $107,000 for in-center HD and $71,000 to $90,000 for home HD.[107] A more recent review of costing data from 46 developed countries found a similar trend among 17 of 20 developed countries. In these countries, the cost of HD was 1.25 to 2.35 times higher than PD.[110]

The relative costs of PD and HD do vary somewhat in less developed nations. In 26 countries with low- or middle-income status, PD was less expensive than HD in 5, similar in cost in 13, and more costly than HD in the remaining 8 nations.[110] Another review of data from 2004 to 2012 by Liu et al. reported that three countries (Chile, India, and Turkey) had similar costs for providing PD and HD, whereas HD was more expensive than PD in the remaining five lower- to middle-income nations.[112] Discrepancies between countries may relate to economic differences (e.g., wages of healthcare workers), the frequency with which HD is provided, the ability to manufacture supplies required for PD locally versus the need to import supplies from elsewhere, economies of scale (e.g., higher PD prevalence tends to lower PD costs), and the presence of geographical barriers or a lack of developed health system infrastructure to support HD therapy.[110,112]

This finding appears to be consistent, even in patients who experience technique failure.[108,109] If one looks separately at PD submodalities, CAPD appears to be slightly less expensive than CCPD, although the differences are small and not significantly different.[111]

Costing studies comparing PD and HD are at risk for bias because they are typically nonrandomized. Although well-conducted observational studies can include large sample sizes, offer more prolonged follow-up of patients, and capture costs and resource use accurately, the nonrandom allocation of patients to their treatments means that the costs associated with medication use, emergency or hospital visits, and other events that may be affected by selection bias could skew the results. Patient-borne costs typically have not been included in studies and are another important consideration when taking a societal perspective. Klarenbach et al. have conducted a thorough review of the issues pertaining to the conduct and interpretation of economic evaluations of different forms of renal replacement therapy.[106a]

Comparing the Outcomes of Patients Treated With Peritoneal Dialysis and Hemodialysis: Quality of Life

The cost savings associated with PD and the fact that PD and HD are associated with equivalent clinical outcomes have led many jurisdictions to actively promote it as the preferred form of dialysis therapy. It has also led many to suggest that choice of dialysis therapy should be guided by quality-of-life considerations and the form of treatment that aligns most closely with patient preferences.[113]

The quality of life of patients treated with dialysis therapy is generally poor, and little progress has been made in recent decades to improve it.[117] Patients on dialysis therapies have a significant symptom burden, and many of the symptoms that cause patients the most distress in their day-to-day lives do not have good treatments and are poorly studied. In recent years there has been a shift in focus toward patient-centered care, and increasing attention is being paid to issues that are important to patients and caregivers. Manns et al. engaged adult patients on or nearing dialysis, their caregivers, and the healthcare professionals who care for them in research priority-setting exercise.[118] A national survey was undertaken, followed by an in-person meeting to identify the top 10 research uncertainties from their perspective. They identified communication between patients and providers, information about dialysis modality options, itching, access to transplantation, heart health, dietary restrictions, depression, and vascular access as the most important areas of focus for future research. There has also been increasing interest in the patient–caregiver dynamic and the impact of caring for a patient on dialysis therapy at home.[119]

With that in mind, in studies that have compared PD and HD, PD has been found to be associated with comparable or slightly improved overall quality of life.[114,115,116,120,121,122,123] In the absence of randomized comparisons of quality of life between the two therapies, we look to observational studies for guidance. Many of the studies done have been small, single-center, cross-sectional studies with their attendant limitations, and many have not used instruments for measuring health-related quality of life that have been validated for use in this patient population. A lack of longitudinal follow-up and examination of how measures change over time on therapy as well as inadequate control for differences in baseline patient characteristics are further limitations.

In the prospective CHOICE study, conducted at 81 clinics in the United States between 1995 and 1998, participants were asked to complete the Choice Health Experiences Questionnaire (CHEQ) at baseline, 3 months, 6 months, and 1 year. CHEQ is a tool that includes the generic Short Form 36 (SF-36) Health Survey as well as dialysis-specific domains. In a well-conducted study, Wu et al. reported on internal consistency and test-retest reliability for CHEQ and reported baseline and 1-year results, as well as change in various domains over the first year of therapy.[123] They concluded that nearly all patients had some improvement in overall well-being and general functioning. When they compared modalities, there were differences in scores for certain domains, but after adjustment for important patient characteristics, there were no significant differences in change in general or dialysis-related quality of life over the first year of therapy.

Summary

In summary, PD use varies greatly across regions, and to understand that variation, it is helpful to have a conceptual framework. We have presented a standardized approach that includes six steps that drive incident PD use: identification of all potential candidates, assessment for PD eligibility, determination of eligibility, offer of PD, choice of PD, and receipt of PD. This framework can be used to categorize interventions that are designed to increased PD use. More importantly, it lends itself to quality improvement initiatives that target increased PD use because it provides a framework for understanding the process of care that drives incident PD use and the collection of data to measure performance at each step. This allows for the identification of specific areas in the process of care that require further attention to increase PD use and focuses efforts on potential interventions. In our opinion, this approach to optimizing the safe and effective use of home therapies is preferred in an era of patient-centered care and shared decision making.

Given the interest worldwide in expanding the use of PD, it is also important to critically examine the outcomes of PD compared with other forms of renal replacement therapy. Although transplant is generally the preferred treatment where it is available for eligible patients, the majority of patients with kidney failure will receive some form of dialysis. We critically examined the literature comparing in-center HD to PD. In general, PD and HD are felt to be equivalent with respect to clinical outcomes and quality of life and PD is cost saving compared with HD. However, there are no randomized comparisons of these two therapies to guide decision making, and the existing observational literature has important limitations that should be considered.

With increasing focus on patient-centered care and patient-centered decision making, it is worth noting that attempts at randomized trials have highlighted the fact that patients develop strong preferences for one therapy or another when educated about their treatment options. These considerations are relevant to areas that have adopted or are contemplating PD-first policies because patients no longer have a choice of treatment modality, which may affect patient satisfaction with care and health-related quality of life and ultimately could influence clinical outcomes and costs.

A full list of references is available at www.expertsonsult.com.

31

Peritoneal Dialysis Solutions, Prescription and Adequacy

Angela Yee-Moon Wang, MD, PhD

OUTLINE

The use of a novel portable or wearable equilibrium peritoneal dialysis (PD) technique was first described by Moncrief et al.[1] in 1976 and named as continuous ambulatory peritoneal dialysis (CAPD) 2 years later. In the last 40 years, significant advances have been made in the understanding of peritoneal membrane function, residual kidney function (RKF), and dialysis adequacy and in the development of PD technology, solutions, and prescription. A significant growth in PD use has been reported worldwide, with some countries, such as Hong Kong and Thailand, adopting a "PD first policy." A more thorough understanding of PD solutions, adequacy, and prescription is therefore essential for successful delivery of PD programs worldwide.

This chapter covers three major issues in relation to PD:

1. *PD solutions.* This includes conventional standard glucose PD solutions, more biocompatible PD solutions, and solutions using alternative osmotic agents as well as other novel solutions that are under development. Various other constituents of PD solutions are also reviewed and their importance discussed in light of more recent studies.
2. *PD adequacy and prescription.* This section defines standard indices of dialysis adequacy, peritoneal membrane function and their measurements. Prescription strategies used to increase PD dose are reviewed. Specific discussions will be made on ultrafiltration failure (UFF) and management of volume overload.
3. *Residual kidney function.* This section reviews the importance of RKF in its contribution to the overall clearance and clinical outcomes in PD patients. Potential strategies in retarding loss or decline of RKF are discussed.

PERITONEAL DIALYSIS SOLUTIONS

Constituents of Peritoneal Dialysis Solutions

Conventional commercially available PD solutions contain sodium (132 to 135 mmol/L), calcium (1.25 to 1.75 mmol/L), magnesium (0.5 mmol/L), chloride (95 to 103.5 mmol/L), and lactate (35 to 40 mmol/L) and varying concentrations of glucose/dextrose ranging from 1.36%/1.5% to 2.27%/2.5% and 3.86%/4.25%. This results in an overall osmolality of 344 to 347, 395 to 398, and 483 to 486 mOsmol/L, respectively (Table 31.1). The concentrations of various components of PD solutions were designed to facilitate ultrafiltration and removal of water-soluble uremic toxins while maintaining electrolyte and acid–base balance of PD patients. The various glucose concentrations of PD solutions provide an osmotic gradient of different degrees that allows ultrafiltration to take place across the peritoneum. However, standard glucose-based PD solutions are acidic in pH (5.0 to 5.8) to prevent dextrose caramelization during the sterilization procedure. As a result of their high lactate, high glucose concentration, high osmolality, and high levels of glucose degradation products (GDPs), long-standing use of these standard glucose PD solutions has been associated with progressive peritoneal membrane injury, neovascularization, peritoneal sclerosis, and fibrosis.[2] Furthermore, the low pH, high osmolarity, and glucose content of standard glucose PD solutions inhibit phagocytic functions of peritoneal leukocytes and impair host immune defense mechanisms.[3,4] Instillation of these solutions may also be associated with inflow pain in some patients.[5]

TABLE 31.1 **Composition of Various Current Commercially Available Peritoneal Dialysis (PD) Solutions**

	Dianeal Standard Glucose PD Solutions	Physioneal	Icodextrin or Extraneal or 7.5% Solution	Amino acid or Nutrineal or 1.1% Solution	StaySafe Standard Glucose PD Solutions	StaySafe Balance	Bica Vera
Sodium (mmol/L)	132	132	133	132	134	134	134
Calcium (mmol/L)							
Low	1.25 (PD-2)	1.25	—	1.25	1.25	1.25	—
Standard	1.75 (PD-4)	1.75	1.75	—	1.75	1.75	1.75
Ultralow	1.00 (PD-1)	—	—	—	—	—	—
Magnesium (mmol/L)	0.25	0.25	0.25	0.25	0.5	0.5	0.5
Chloride (mmol/L)	96	95 (Physioneal-40) 101 (Physioneal-35)	96	105	103.5	100.5 for 1.25 mmol Ca 101.5 for 1.75 mmol Ca	104.5
Lactate (mmol/L)	40	15 (Physioneal-40) 10 (Physioneal-35)	40	40	35	2	0
Bicarbonate (mmol/L)	—	25	0	0	0	35	35
Glucose (mmol/L)	1.36%, 76 2.27%, 126 3.86%, 214	1.36%, 75.5 2.27%, 126 3.86%, 214	0	0	1.5%, 83.2 2.3%, 126.1 4.25%, 235.8	1.5%, 83.2 2.3%, 126.1 4.25%, 235.8	1.5%, 83.25
Icodextrin (g/L)	0	0	75	0	0	0	0
Amino acids (mmol/L)	0	0	0	87[a]	0	0	0
Overall pH	5.5	7.4	5.2	6.6	7	7	7.4
Approximate osmolality	PD-2 1.36%, 346 mOsm 2.27%, 396 mOsm 3.86%, 485 mOsm PD-4 1.36%, 345 mOsm 2.27%, 395 mOsm 3.86%, 483 mOsm PD-1 1.36%, 344 mOsm 2.27%, 394 mOsm 3.86%, 484 mOsm	1.36%, 344 mOsm 2.27%, 395 mOsm 3.86%, 483 mOsm	284 mOsm	365 mOsm	1.25 mmol/L Ca solution 1.5%, 356 mOsm 2.3%, 399 mOsm 4.25%, 509 mOsm 1.75 mmol/L Ca solution 1.5%, 358 mOsm 2.3%, 401 mOsm 4.25%, 511 mOsm	1.25 mmol/L Ca solution 1.5%, 356 mOsm 2.3%, 399 mOsm 4.25%, 509 mOsm 1.75 mmol/L Ca solution 1.5%, 358 mOsm 2.3%, 401 mOsm 4.25%, 511 mOsm	358 mOsm

[a]The 1.1% solutions consist of a combination of amino acids, including histidine, valine, isoleucine, alanine, leucine, arginine, lysine, glycine, methionine, proline, phenylalanine, serine, threonine, tyrosine, and tryptophan.

Dialysate Buffer

The buffer present in standard PD solutions is lactate, with concentrations varying between 35 to 40 mmol (see Table 31.1). In patients with normal liver function, lactate is rapidly converted to bicarbonate such that 1 mM lactate absorbed generates 1 mM bicarbonate. The rapid metabolism of lactate to bicarbonate maintains the high dialysate to plasma lactate concentration gradient necessary for continued absorption without accumulation of lactate in the circulation.[6] Absorption may be reduced with hypertonic glucose PD solution, because increased ultrafiltration may dilute the concentration of lactate in the peritoneal cavity, thus decreasing the concentration gradient for diffusion. Lactate in standard PD solution is normally present in a racemic mixture of approximately equimolar concentration of D-lactate and L-lactate isomers. L-Lactate was suggested to be more rapidly absorbed than D-lactate.[6]

Bicarbonate is regarded as the most physiological and biocompatible buffering system. However, calcium and magnesium precipitate in the presence of bicarbonate and with an alkaline pH. Thus magnesium and calcium must be omitted from bicarbonate-containing dialysate. Patients doing PD with these calcium-free and magnesium-free solutions may develop deficits of calcium and magnesium. A dual-chamber dialysate bag in which one chamber contains the bicarbonate buffer of 34 mmol/L and the other contains a solution with calcium and magnesium has therefore been designed. The two solutions are mixed together only before instillation into patients' abdomen, thus preventing calcium and magnesium carbonate precipitation. The neutral pH bicarbonate solution has been found to be well tolerated and effective in ameliorating metabolic acidosis[7] and is currently used in daily clinical practice in some parts of the world. Treatment of metabolic acidosis is well known to be associated with downregulation of muscle ubiquitin–proteasome complex and inhibition of muscle degradation.[8] More details are discussed in the Biocompatible Peritoneal Dialysis Solutions section. Bicarbonate-containing solutions (e.g., 25 mmol/L) may also be available in a mixture form with lactate (15 mmol/L), because solutions with pure supraphysiological concentration of bicarbonate have been associated with more abdominal pain than mixed bicarbonate and lactate solution.[5]

Dialysate Calcium

Patients treated with PD may be in negative, positive, or neutral calcium balance, depending on various factors, including dialysate calcium concentration, dietary calcium intake, dose of calcium-based phosphorus binders used, and use of vitamin D analogs. Hou et al.[9] found that a high dialysate calcium concentration of 1.75 mM may lead to positive calcium balance and increased plasma calcium, whereas a low dialysate calcium concentration of 0.75 mM may lead to negative calcium balance and decreased plasma calcium. A dialysate calcium concentration of 1.25 mM maintained neutral calcium balance with minimal perturbation in plasma calcium[9] (Fig. 31.1). However, plasma calcium does not reflect body calcium balance because 99% of calcium resides in the bone.[10]

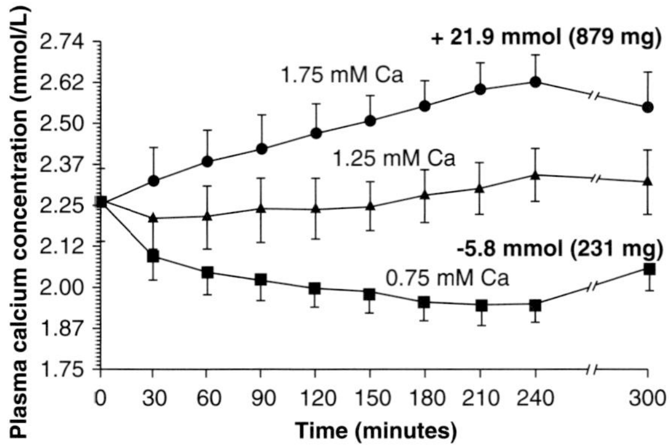

FIG. 31.1 Changes in plasma calcium concentration over a 4-hour dwell of PD fluid with different dialysate calcium concentrat ons, namely 0.75 mM, 1.25 mM, and 1.75 mM. (Reproduced with permission from Hou SH, Zhao J, Ellman CF, Hu J, Griffin Z, Spiegel DM, et al. Calcium and phosphorus fluxes during hemodialysis with low-calcium dialysate. *Am J Kidney Dis.* 1991;18(2):217-224.)

The addition of vitamin D analogs and calcium-based binders may increase extracellular calcium and increase the risk for positive calcium balance even when 1.25 mM calcium dialysate is used.[10]

In fact, it is somewhat of a misnomer that current commercially available high-calcium (1.75 mM) PD solution is termed *standard* calcium solution, whereas 1.25 mM calcium concentration solution is termed *low-calcium* solution but in fact is the more physiological calcium concentration (see Table 31.1). As nicely demonstrated in two calcium balance studies, an elemental calcium intake of 1.5 to 2 g induced positive calcium balance in patients with chronic kidney disease (CKD).[11,12] There are concerns that high-calcium dialysate may induce low parathyroid hormone and has been associated with a higher risk for cardiovascular death in hemodialysis patients.[13] On the other hand, low-calcium dialysate may stimulate an increase of parathyroid hormone and worsen secondary hyperparathyroidism.[14-16] Although an earlier study[17] suggested that low-calcium (1.25 mM) dialysate use may increase parathyroid hormone in the short term, addition of calcium-based phosphorus binders and vitamin D analogs appeared to inhibit parathyroid hormone increase and stabilize its level over time. Furthermore, use of low-calcium (1.25 mM) dialysate may be associated with a lower incidence of hypercalcemia in PD patients.[18,19] A previous small randomized controlled trial[15] (RCT) found no difference in bone histomorphometry for PD patients randomly assigned to receive 1.25 mM or 1.75 mM calcium solution for 1 year. There were some suggestions that PD patients using 1.25 mM calcium dialysate may have less progression in arterial stiffness than those receiving 1.75 mM calcium dialysate.[20,21]

In a 2016 prospective RCT,[22] 425 hemodialysis patients with intact parathyroid hormone ≤ 300 pg/mL were randomly assigned to receive either 1.25 mM or 1.75 mM calcium dialysate; those receiving 1.75 mM calcium dialysate had significantly more progression in coronary artery calcium score over 24 months than those using 1.25 mM calcium dialysate.

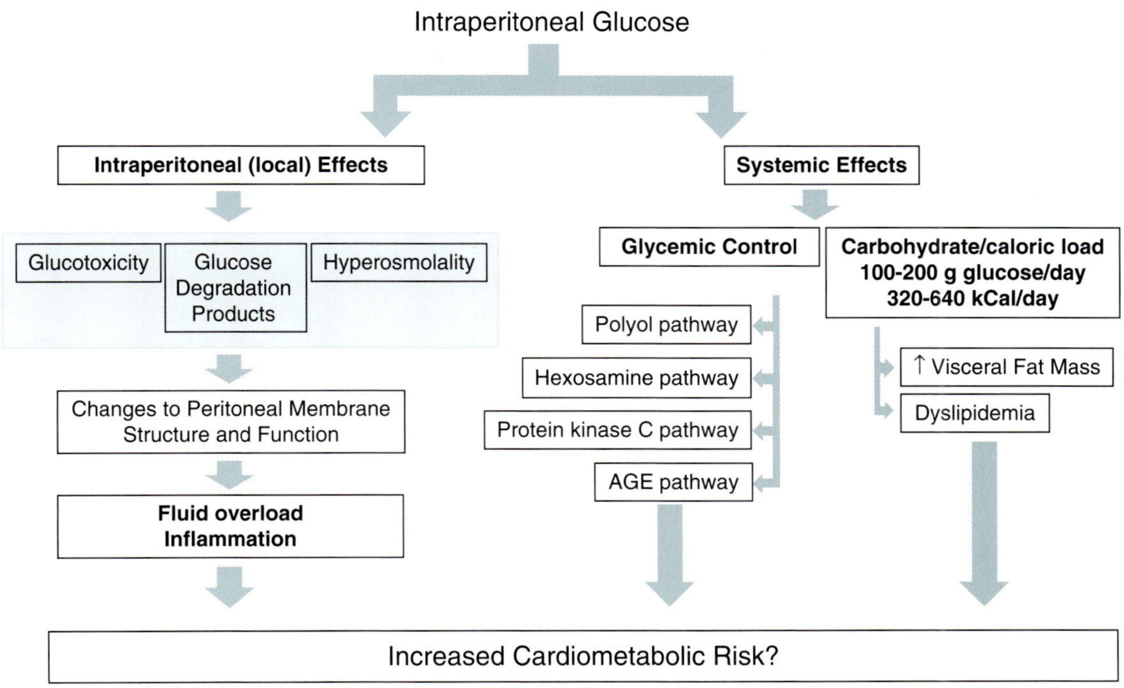

FIG. 31.2 Local and systemic effects of PD glucose solutions. (Reproduced with permission from Holmes CJ. Reducing cardiometabolic risk in peritoneal dialysis patients: role of the dialysis solution. *J Diabetes Sci Technol.* 2009;3(6):1472-1480.)

Subgroup analysis indicated that progression of coronary artery calcification was found mainly in the subgroup with poor phosphorus control, namely serum phosphorus level ≥ 4.7 mg/dL. Furthermore, the 1.25-mM low-calcium dialysate group had a significant decrease in the prevalence of histologically diagnosed low bone turnover, from 85% to 41.8%, whereas the prevalence of low bone turnover did not change over 24 months in the 1.75-mM high-calcium dialysate group. Although a similar study is not available in PD patients, both the Kidney Disease Improving Global Outcomes 2017 CKD-mineral bone disease (MBD) guideline[23] and the International Society of Peritoneal Dialysis (ISPD) Adult Cardiovascular and Metabolic guidelines[24] suggested a 1.25-mM calcium-containing PD solution be used to avoid positive calcium balance or hypercalcemia.

Glucose-Based Solutions

One study[25] found that initial ultrafiltration rate across the peritoneum is directly proportional to the initial glucose osmotic gradient. Generally, 1.36%/1.5% glucose/dextrose solution generates a 100 to 200 mL ultrafiltration, 2.27%/2.5% glucose/dextrose solution generates a 200 to 400 mL ultrafiltration, and 3.86%/4.25% glucose/dextrose solution generates more than 400 mL ultrafiltration. A 4-hour dwell of 2.5% PD dextrose solution has been used as the standard for peritoneal membrane equilibration test (PET).[26] A net ultrafiltration of more than 200 mL from a standard 4-hour dwell of 2.27%/2.5% glucose/dextrose or more than 400 mL from a standard 4-hour dwell of 3.86%/4.25% glucose/dextrose solution is regarded as sufficient ultrafiltration. Values less than this indicate relative UFF.[27] Symptoms of UFF may not manifest overtly until RKF has declined significantly or is completely lost.

Other than serving as an osmotic agent to facilitate ultrafiltration, glucose in the PD solution provides an important source of energy. The amount of glucose absorbed varies proportional to the concentration of glucose in the dialysate. The amount of glucose absorbed per liter of dialysate (y) can be predicted using the equation of Grodstein et al.[28] as $y = 11.3 \times x - 10.9$, $r = 0.96$, in which x denotes the concentration of glucose from the dialysate. With an average peritoneal solute transport rate (PSTR), it is estimated that almost two-thirds of the PD fluid glucose is absorbed during a 4-hour dwell and more than 85% in an 8-hour dwell. This translates to an obligatory absorption of 43 g and 73 g of glucose with an 8-hour dwell of 2.5% and 4.25% solutions, respectively. Patients receiving four PD exchanges with three exchanges of 1.5% dextrose and one exchange of 2.5% were estimated to have absorbed 88 g glucose in a day. Typically glucose absorbed from PD fluids may amount to 100 to 300 g/day and may account for approximately 12% to 34% of total energy input. Thus it may lead to weight gain in some patients,[29] although this has not been reproduced in other studies.[30,31] Hypertonic glucose solutions may also add satiety and reduce appetite in PD patients.

Glucose-based PD solutions have various other local and systemic adverse effects (Fig. 31.2).

Local Effects

Glucose exerts direct cytotoxic effects on peritoneal mesothelial cells and causes diabetiform changes in the postcapillary venules, leading to changes in peritoneal membrane structure and function.[32] The standard heat sterilization of glucose-based PD solutions accelerates the generation of GDPs.[33-35] The formation of GDPs during heat sterilization may be reduced by lowering the pH of the solution.[36] GDPs are locally cytotoxic and glycated local proteins form advanced glycation end-products (AGEs)[37] and contribute to the long-term bioincompatibility of PD solutions. GDP and AGEs exert damaging effects on the peritoneal membrane by causing mesothelial cell loss, inflammation, submesothelial fibrosis, calcification, vasculopathy, and diabetiform neoangiogenesis.[38,39]

Data from the Peritoneal Biopsy Registry indicated a thickening of the submesothelial compact zone and development of a diabetiform occlusive vasculopathy of small arterioles and postcapillary venules with neovascularization with increasing time on PD.[40] Peritoneal biopsy specimens taken from PD patients with low ultrafiltration capacity demonstrated that AGE accumulation in the peritoneal membrane was positively correlated with the development of severe interstitial fibrosis and microvascular sclerosis.[41] All these negative effects on the peritoneum decrease the effectiveness of the peritoneum as a dialysis membrane, resulting in an increased PSTR with time on dialysis and intensifying the need for using hypertonic glucose solutions.[42] This may eventually lead to peritoneal membrane failure (PMF), increased risk for fluid overload, and protein energy wasting (PEW). Several studies[43-47] reported that a high PSTR was associated with worse patient survival, and some studies[43,44] also reported a trend toward worse PD technique survival with high PSTR. A more contemporary analysis based on a nationally representative cohort of PD patients in the United States, of whom 87% were treated with automated peritoneal dialysis (APD), reinforced a similar finding; that is, the dialysate to plasma (D/P) creatinine ratio was associated with survival outcome and linearly associated with mortality. For every 0.1 unit increase in the D/P creatinine ratio, the adjusted mortality risk increased by 7% (95% confidence interval [CI], 1.02 to 1.13), the adjusted hospitalization risk increased by 5% (95% CI, 1.03 to 1.06). On the other hand, ultrafiltration volume was inversely related with hospitalization rate but not with all-cause mortality.[46]

Systemic Effects of Glucose-Based Peritoneal Dialysis Solutions

The cumulative, systemic PD glucose absorption through the peritoneum may aggravate various metabolic disturbances, including insulin resistance, hyperglycemia, accumulation of atherogenic visceral fat, weight gain, and dyslipidemia, and worsen glycemic control in PD patients with diabetes.[48]

Insulin resistance has been found to be associated with a higher cardiovascular mortality and worse clinical outcomes in dialysis patients.[49] New-onset hyperglycemia has been reported in end-stage renal disease (ESRD) patients sometime after commencing PD treatment. Intraperitoneal glucose absorption gives rise to higher plasma glucose levels as well as a more extended period of hyperinsulinemia compared with an equivalent dose of oral glucose.[48] Hyperglycemia not only stimulates hyperinsulinemia but also increases mitochondrial superoxide generation, which activates four key pathways—namely, the polyol pathway, hexosamine pathway, protein kinase C pathway, and AGE pathway—causing hyperglycemic damage.[50,51] Activation of these pathways induces the expression of endothelin 1, vascular epithelial growth factor, transforming growth factor beta, fibronectin, collagen, and leptin genes and at the same time downregulates endothelial nitric oxide synthase and upregulates transcription factor nuclear factor kappa B. Together with an increased oxidative stress, this results in a heightened inflammatory response, insulin resistance, and peritoneal membrane damage as well as a higher risk for accelerated atherosclerosis.[52,53]

Derangements in glucose and insulin metabolism are evident in early CKD.[54] With progression of CKD, peritubular insulin uptake increases, which compensates for the decline in the metabolism of filtered insulin. As kidney function further deteriorates, insulin clearance also decreases. In addition, insulin resistance and tissue insensitivity to insulin increase, resulting in suboptimal insulin secretion in response to a glucose load or hyperglycemia.[55,56] Usually around 60% of the glucose in PD solutions may be reabsorbed during the dwell, thus causing disturbed carbohydrate metabolism even in nondiabetic PD patients, further aggravating insulin resistance. Hyperinsulinemia also contributes to hypertriglyceridemia. Insulin enhances hepatic triglyceride synthesis and indirectly reduces the metabolism of very-low-density lipoprotein cholesterol.

Use of glucose-based PD solutions has been associated with more weight gain and fat mass increase than non–glucose-based PD solutions.[57,58] Increased truncal fat mass and visceral adiposity over time using glucose-based PD solutions has been positively associated with serum leptin and inflammation and negatively associated with serum adiponectin,[59,60], providing indirect evidence of an important link between truncal fat mass and cardiometabolic risk markers. Increased abdominal adiposity has been implicated to contribute significantly to a higher cardiovascular risk in PD patients.[61] An in vitro study[62] found that leptin secretion is directly stimulated in adipocytes being exposed to glucose-based PD solutions via activation of the hexosamine pathway. The degree of leptin secretion correlated directly with the amount of glucose being exposed. Similar stimulation on leptin secretion was not noted with non–glucose-based solutions.[62] In keeping with these experimental data, higher leptin levels were reported in PD patients than in hemodialysis patients.[63]

Several studies have examined whether long-standing exposure to glucose-based PD solutions may be associated with worse clinical outcomes. So far, most available studies were retrospective and results were inconsistent. A retrospective analysis from Taiwan[64] suggested that a higher initial glucose load within the first 6 months of initiation of PD was associated with higher prevalent diabetes mellitus, lower serum albumin, and lower RKF and a higher risk for technique failure but not mortality. Another extended follow-up study[65] using time-dependent covariate analysis reported that long-term glucose exposure was associated with a greater risk for mortality and technique failure. In keeping with these observations, a retrospective analysis from China[66] found that use of PD solutions of higher glucose concentration over the initial 6 months of PD treatment was associated with a greater risk for all-cause and cardiovascular disease mortality. Metabolic syndrome, which consists of a constellation of clinical features including central obesity, hypertension, atherogenic dyslipidemia, hyperglycemia, and insulin resistance, has been found to be associated with adverse cardiovascular outcomes in nondiabetic PD patients.[67]

Hyperglycemia and hyperinsulinemia induced by hypertonic glucose PD solutions may also be associated with short-term adverse hemodynamic changes. A 4.25% dextrose solution has been found to increase blood pressure and cardiac output acutely in the absence of any acute changes in left ventricular diameter, whereas non–glucose-based PD solution was not associated with similar hemodynamic disturbance.[68]

Non–Glucose-Based Peritoneal Dialysis Solutions

Glucose Polymer Solutions

Icodextrin is a starch-derived, branched, water-soluble glucose polymer with an average molecular weight between 13,000 and 19,000 Da. The current commercially available formulation is a 7.5% icodextrin solution with a sodium concentration of 133 mmol/L and a lactate concentration of 40 mmol/L and is isoosmotic (284 mOsmol/L) (see Table 31.1). Icodextrin is not significantly metabolized in the peritoneum. Instead it is slowly absorbed into the bloodstream via the lymph vessels, with around 40% being absorbed after a 12-hour period, and is metabolized into oligosaccharides and maltose by circulating α-amylase. The maltose cannot be metabolized in the circulation of humans because maltase is not in the circulation but is present in the kidney and intracellularly in the body. Nevertheless, there is no evidence to date that maltose accumulates within patients treated with icodextrin. Because icodextrin stays in the peritoneal cavity for a considerable period and very little gets reabsorbed, icodextrin is a superior osmotic agent and has better ultrafiltration capacity compared with conventional glucose, especially with longer dwell hours. Icodextrin was approved for use by the Food and Drug Administration of the United States in 2002 to increase ultrafiltration in PD patients.

Effects on ultrafiltration, volume status, and technique survival. Over the years, considerable clinical data demonstrated the efficacy of icodextrin in increasing ultrafiltration in PD patients compared with standard glucose solutions.[69-72] When used as once-daily overnight long dwell in CAPD or long day dwell in continuous cycler PD (CCPD), icodextrin can achieve a net ultrafiltration equivalent to or even more than that of 2.27% or 3.86% glucose solution, depending on the peritoneal membrane transport characteristics and length of dwell.[71,73,74] Generally the ultrafiltration, relative to glucose, is greater in patients with high PSTR. In patients with high or high-average peritoneal membrane transport, the ultrafiltration volume with icodextrin is significantly larger than that with 2.27% or 3.86% PD solution.[71,75] As a result of better ultrafiltration, more sodium is also removed by convection using icodextrin compared with 2.27% glucose PD solution.[76] Thus it has been used as a salvage therapy in patients with clinically inadequate ultrafiltration or PMF. There is a suggestion that icodextrin may extend the life of PD treatment.[77]

Two earlier short-term RCTs both demonstrated better overall ultrafiltration with icodextrin compared with conventional glucose solution, resulting in better volume status as assessed by bioimpedance.[69,70] Konings et al.[70] also suggested a decrease in left ventricular mass index with icodextrin. Davies et al.[69] reported that an icodextrin group had weight loss, whereas a standard glucose solution group had weight gain. This may be explained by more fluid removal or less fat mass gain with icodextrin. Another prospective RCT found that icodextrin improved technique survival rate in PD patients with background diabetic nephropathy, though a more rapid decline in RKF was found over a 24-month follow-up period.[78]

Several meta-analyses have reviewed the use of icodextrin versus standard glucose PD solutions in relation to peritoneal ultrafiltration and small solute clearance (Table 31.2).[79-82] All studies showed significantly better daily peritoneal ultrafiltration with icodextrin than standard glucose PD solutions. The systemic review by Cho et al.[79,80] additionally found a significantly lower incidence of uncontrolled fluid overload with icodextrin compared with standard glucose PD solutions without compromising RKF. Icodextrin may be a useful salvage therapy in PD patients with refractory fluid overload or UFF and may prolong technique survival.[77,83,84] However, so far there are no prospective trials examining the effects of icodextrin on patients' survival as the primary endpoint. Based on available evidence, the ISPD Adult Cardiovascular and Metabolic Guidelines 2015[24] recommended that once-daily icodextrin be considered as an alternative to hypertonic glucose PD solutions for long dwells in those experiencing difficulties to maintain euvolemia as a result of insufficient peritoneal ultrafiltration, taking into account the PSTR. The level of recommendation for the statement was given a grading of 1B.[24] Similarly, the European Best Practice Working Group (EBPG) recommended icodextrin be used as the long dwell in high transporter patients with a net peritoneal ultrafiltration <400 mL during a PET with a 3.86% glucose solution.[85]

Effects on metabolic profile. Use of icodextrin as the long-dwell solution also minimizes glucose exposure and incurs less metabolic derangement compared with standard glucose PD solutions. Changes in triglycerides level have been suggested to correlate with the amount of peritoneal glucose absorption.[86] Several prospective RCTs found that icodextrin, by minimizing glucose absorption, may improve glucose metabolism, improve insulin sensitivity, and reduce dyslipidemia compared with standard glucose PD solutions. An earlier prospective open-label multicenter study from Japan[87] found that switching PD patients from standard glucose PD solutions to icodextrin reduced triglycerides and mean total and low-density lipoprotein cholesterol levels. Among

TABLE 31.2 Table Summarizing Systemic Reviews on Clinical Trials With Icodextrin

Author, Year	No. of Studies *(N)*	Key Results
He et al., 2011[82]	Total nine trials:	
	Two trials (n = 131), peritoneal creatinine clearance	Significant ↑ in peritoneal efficiency ratio with icodextrin vs. control (MD 6.84, 95% CI, 4.43–9.25)
	Five trials (n = 528), peritoneal creatinine clearance rate	Significant ↑ in peritoneal creatinine clearance rate with icodextrin vs. control (MD 0.51, 95% CI, 0.35–0.67)
	Four trials (n = 508), peritoneal urea clearance rate	Significant ↑ in peritoneal urea clearance rate with icodextrin vs. control (MD 0.43, 95% CI, 0.26–0.61)
Cho et al., 2013[79] and Cho et al., 2014[80] (same findings)	Total 11 trials:	
	Four trials (n = 102), peritoneal ultrafiltration	Significant ↑ in peritoneal ultrafiltration with icodextrin vs. control (MD 448.54, 95% CI, 289.28–607.80 mL/d)
	Two trials (n = 100), fluid overload episodes	Significant ↓ in uncontrolled fluid overload episodes with icodextrin vs. control (RR 0.30, 95% CI 0.15–0.59)
	Four trials (n = 114), RKF Three trials (n = 69), urine volume (n = 69)	Did not compromise RKF (standardized MD 0.12, 95% CI, −0.26 to 0.49) or urine output (three trials; 69 patients; MD −88.88, 95% CI, −356.88 to 179.12 mL/d) with icodextrin use for up to 2 years

MD, Mean difference; *RKF,* residual kidney function; *RR,* relative risk.

those with glycated hemoglobin ≥6.5%, glycemic control also improved with icodextrin.[87] A randomized study from Mexico found that diabetic PD patients using icodextrin as the long dwell had reduced insulin requirement, lower fasting glucose, lower glycated hemoglobin, lower serum triglycerides, and fewer adverse events compared with a standard glucose group.[75] IMPENDIA and EDEN trials evaluated the clinical effects of a glucose-sparing PD regimen, namely icodextrin and amino acid–based PD solutions, in a multicenter study of 251 diabetic PD patients.[88] The study[88] reported an average of 0.5% improvement in glycated hemoglobin (as the primary study outcome) in the intervention group versus standard glucose group at 6 months. The mean glycated hemoglobin reduced from 7.7% to 7.2%. Secondary outcomes included a significant reduction in very-low-density lipoprotein cholesterol, serum triglyceride, and apo-B levels in the intervention group compared with control group. However, a significantly higher incidence of treatment-related adverse events, serious adverse events, hypoglycemia, and volume overload as well as study withdrawal were reported in the intervention group.[88] Icodextrin may also have favorable effects on plasma adipokines.[89]

Another prospective open-label RCT from Japan[78] failed to find a significant benefit of icodextrin on glycemic control or lipid profile in diabetic PD patients, but both glycemic control and lipid profile were secondary study outcomes. A more recent multicenter open-label short-term (90 days) RCT[90] of 60 nondiabetic automated PD patients found that icodextrin use as the long dwell significantly reduced insulin resistance as denoted by homeostatic model assessment (HOMA) index. There are some suggestions that using twice-daily exchanges of icodextrin in place of standard glucose PD solution may reduce peritoneal glucose exposure by up to 50%, thus lowering systemic glucose absorption by 60%.[91] Longer-term studies are needed to evaluate the safety of this approach because icodextrin metabolite levels will be higher than a single daily exchange.

Effects on residual kidney function. Although there were some earlier suggestions that increased ultrafiltration with icodextrin may jeopardize RKF, a systematic review by Cho et al.[79,80] did not find any significant difference between icodextrin and standard glucose PD solution in relation to decline in RKF and urine volume. However, RKF and urine volume were not primary outcomes in these studies. In a prospective multicenter RCT from Korea[92] examining changes in residual glomerular filtration rate (GFR) and urine volume as the primary outcomes, there were some suggestions that icodextrin may be associated with slower residual urine volume loss compared with standard glucose PD solutions over a period of 12 months in both the intention-to-treat analysis and per-protocol analysis.

Potential adverse effects. Use of icodextrin may be associated with potential adverse events such as sterile peritonitis or skin rash as a result of allergy to starch. Sterile peritonitis with icodextrin has been described and was related to contamination of icodextrin by peptidoglycan, which is a constituent of bacterial cell walls.[93,94] Clinically, patients with sterile or chemical peritonitis may remain well despite having cloudy effluent. The differential cell count of PD fluid is associated with leukocytosis with predominantly eosinophilia but not neutrophils.[95] PD effluent usually clears up rapidly on withdrawal of icodextrin. According to the systematic review by Cho et al.,[79,80] the incidence of chemical peritonitis was not increased with icodextrin compared with standard glucose PD solutions. The reported incidence of skin rash with icodextrin use is around 10% but may be up to 18.9%.[96,97] It is usually mild and localized to the palm of hands. Occasionally, a more severe form of exfoliating dermatitis may occur, requiring withdrawal of icodextrin.[98]

The presence of icodextrin and its metabolites in plasma may interfere with some laboratory analytical methods on glucose measurements. For example, certain glucometers that use glucose dehydrogenase–pyrroloquinoline quinone will overestimate blood glucose in patients using icodextrin.[99,100]

Biocompatible Peritoneal Dialysis Solutions

Neutral pH, low-GDP solutions. Epithelial-to-mesenchymal transition (EMT) of peritoneal mesothelial cells is a hallmark feature in the peritoneum of PD patients[101] and was suggested in earlier studies to play an essential role in the initiation of peritoneal fibrosis,[102] leading to peritoneal membrane function decline and failure.[103,104] In vitro experiments found that mesothelial cells culturing in neutral pH, low-GDP solutions had less EMT than in standard glucose solutions.[105] Effluent mesothelial cells grown ex vivo from patients treated with neutral pH, low-GDP solutions also had a trend toward maintaining more of an epitheloid phenotype with less induction of proinflammatory cytokine production, whereas mesothelial cells from patients treated with lactate-buffered standard glucose PD solution invariably transdifferentiated into a nonepithelial phenotype by 24 months.[105] This led to the development and clinical application of more "biocompatible" PD solutions to minimize adverse effects to the peritoneum. However, a later experimental study[106] used inducible genetic fate mapping and demonstrated type I collagen–producing submesothelial fibroblasts as specific progenitors of α-smooth muscle actin–positive myofibroblasts that accumulated progressively in various models of high-glucose solutions or transforming growth factor β_1–induced peritoneal fibrosis. Notably, only submesothelial fibroblasts but not mesothelial cells expressed α-smooth muscle actin after induction of peritoneal fibrosis in mice. Furthermore, pharmacological inhibition of platelet derived growth factor receptor, which is expressed by submesothelial fibroblasts but not mesothelial cells, attenuated peritoneal fibrosis. These data provide important novel evidence that submesothelial fibroblasts may be the key cell source of myofibroblasts driving peritoneal injury and fibrosis.[106]

For the glucose-based PD solutions to be more biocompatible clinically, a dual-chamber bag system was designed to allow heat sterilization and storage to occur at a lower pH in a separate bag to minimize GDP generation. Some of the low-GDP solutions used bicarbonate instead of lactate as the buffering system to minimize exposure to lactate as well. Thus mixing the contents of the two chambers just before use would produce a more physiological and neutral pH of around 7.0 (see Table 31.1). Earlier preclinical studies found that use of neutral pH, low-GDP solutions was associated with better preserved peritoneal membrane morphology and function[40] and better host immune defense.[107] Several subsequent observational studies also suggested similar findings, that use of neutral pH, low-GDP solutions may be associated with more favorable peritoneal membrane morphology,[108] less systemic inflammation,[109] and better patient survival outcomes.[110,111] Numerous RCTs[112-122] were conducted in the last 10 years on neutral pH, low-GDP solutions; these are summarized in Table 31.3.

Effects on residual kidney function and urine volume. The Euro Balance Trial[123] was the first RCT that examined the effects of neutral pH, low-GDP solutions on the peritoneal membrane and RKF in a crossover design. The study found that use of neutral pH, low-GDP solutions is accompanied by a significant improvement in peritoneal membrane integrity as reflected by higher levels of peritoneal cancer antigen 125 (CA125) and procollagen peptide and significantly decreased circulating AGE levels compared with standard glucose solution over a 12-week time frame. Renal urea and creatinine clearance (CrCl) and urine volume also increased after exposure to neutral pH, low-GDP solutions.[123]

To date, the balANZ trial represents the largest RCT with the longest follow-up (2 years) that examined the effect of neutral pH, low-GDP solution on RKF and various other patient outcomes. It was an investigator-initiated, multicenter, multicountry, open-label, parallel-design RCT including 185 incident PD patients. The primary outcome of the study was slope of RKF decline, which did not have a significant difference between the neutral pH, low-GDP solution group and the control group (standard glucose solution) up to 2 years. However, the biocompatible group had significantly longer times to anuria ($P = 0.009$), longer time to first peritonitis episode ($P = 0.01$), and lower rates of peritonitis (0.30 vs. 0.49 episodes per year, $P = 0.01$) compared with the standard glucose solution group. Nevertheless, these were secondary outcomes. No significant difference was reported between the two groups in relation to technique survival and patient survival.[118] In keeping with the findings from the balANZ trial, several other investigators found that neutral pH, low-GDP solutions attenuated decline of RKF in incident PD patients in an RCT setting.[116,117,120,122] However, some other controlled trials did not reproduce similar results,[112,114,115] which may be related to the rather short study durations of up to 12 months and relatively small sample sizes.

The findings from these RCTs were summarized in the systematic review by Cho et al.[80,124-127] Essentially, the use of neutral pH, low-GDP solutions appeared to produce better preservation of RKF and greater urine volumes. In the Cochrane review, the benefit of low-GDP solutions in preserving RKF was found most significantly between 12 to 23 months ($P = 0.0005$) but also from 24 months and beyond, though less significant ($P = 0.04$). Similarly, low-GDP solutions were beneficial in preserving urine volume between 12 to 23 months ($P = 0.0005$) and from 24 months and beyond ($P = 0.04$)[80] (Fig. 31.3). In addition, in 2016 the Trio study[128] involving 67 incident PD patients also reported significantly slower decline in RKF in the lactate-buffered low GDP solution (Gambrosol Trio) group compared with the standard glucose PD solution (see Table 31.3). Based on these data, the 2015 ISPD Adult Cardiovascular and Metabolic Guidelines recommended that neutral pH, low-GDP solutions be considered for better preservation of RKF if used for 12 months or more (grading 2B).[24]

Effects on peritonitis risk. In the balANZ trial, the time to first peritonitis episode was longer and overall peritonitis rates were lower with neutral pH, low-GDP solution compared with standard glucose solutions.[118] A separate analysis on the same trial suggested a broad reduction in peritonitis caused by gram-positive, gram-negative, and specifically non-*Pseudomonas* gram-negative organisms as well as less severe peritonitis in patients using biocompatible solutions.[129]

However, similar findings were not reported in other trials. The Cochrane review did not find any difference in peritonitis rates between neutral pH, low-GDP solutions and standard glucose PD solutions.[80]

Effects on peritoneal solute transport and ultrafiltration volume. The effects of biocompatible solutions on ultrafiltration volume were inconclusive. Several studies suggested lower ultrafiltration volume with neutral pH, low-GDP solutions compared with standard glucose solutions.[118,122] In a separate analysis of the balANZ trial, the mean D/P creatinine ratio at 4 hours remained stable in the neutral pH, low-GDP solutions group but increased significantly in the control group over 2 years.[130] Ultrafiltration volume was lower in the neutral pH, low-GDP solution group compared with the control group up to 6 months. However, over 2 years, ultrafiltration volume increased significantly in the neutral pH, low-GDP solution group but remained stable in the control group.[130] The differential effects of neutral pH, low-GDP solutions on peritoneal solute transport and ultrafiltration over time remain poorly understood.

Another study[115] suggested that neutral pH, low-GDP solution may be associated with a higher ultrafiltration volume. Overall the recent Cochrane and Canadian systematic reviews suggested a trend toward lower ultrafiltration volume with biocompatible PD solutions compared with standard glucose solutions but not reaching statistical significance. No significant difference was found in the peritoneal creatinine clearance.[80,124]

Other clinical outcomes. Earlier studies suggested a potential benefit in reducing inflow pain with more biocompatible PD solutions.[5,131] However, a recent Cochrane review suggested that the trend toward lower incidence of inflow pain with neutral pH, low-GDP solutions did not reach statistical significance. There is no convincing evidence to indicate that use of neutral pH, low-GDP solutions improve patients' survival and technique survival.[80] So far, no studies have been

Comparison: 1 Low-GDP (all buffer types) versus standard glucose dialysate

Outcome: 5 Residual renal function: PD fluid types

Study or subgroup	Neutral pH, low GDP N	Mean (SD)	Standard glucose N	Mean (SD)	Std. Mean Difference IV, Random, 95% CI	Weight	Std. Mean Difference IV, Random, 95% CI
1 Balance							
Bajo 2011	9	4.2 (2.6)	3	4.2 (4)		1.6%	0.0 [−1.31, 1.31]
balANZ Trial 2006	40	3.4 (2.79)	48	3.2 (2.82)		15.8%	0.07 [−0.35, 0.49]
Choi 2008	38	4.7 (10.7)	30	1.86 (6.44)		12.0%	0.31 [−0.17, 0.79]
Kim 2003	16	2.3 (1.2)	10	1.8 (2.2)		4.4%	0.29 [−0.50, 1.09]
Kim 2008	25	3.5 (3.4)	21	1.65 (1.97)		7.9%	0.64 [0.04, 1.24]
Szeto 2007	24	2.72 (2.08)	24	2.81 (2.87)		8.7%	−0.04 [−0.60, 0.53]
Subtotal (95% CI)	**152**		**136**			**50.5%**	**0.22 [−0.02, 0.45]**
Heterogeneity: Tau² = 0.0: Chi² = 3.45, df = 5 (P = 0.63): I² = 0.0%							
Test for overall effect: Z = 1.79 (P = 0.073)							
2 Purely bicarbonate buffered							
Fernandez-Perpen 2012	5	6 (4.4)	3	4.2 (4)		1.3%	0.37 [−1.09, 1.82]
Schmitt 2002	13	2.54 (2.62)	11	2.92 (1.98)		4.3%	−0.16 [−0.96, 0.65]
Weiss 2009	15	4.77 (3.78)	11	4.1 (2.8)		4.6%	0.19 [−0.59, 0.97]
Subtotal (95% CI)	**33**		**25**			**10.2%**	**0.07 [−0.46, 0.59]**
Heterogeneity: Tau² = 0.0: Chi² = 0.55, df = 2 (P = 0.76): I² = 0.0%							
Test for overall effect: Z = 0.25 (P = 0.80)							
3 Multiple fluid types in treatment group							
Fan 2008	44	5.1 (4.08)	49	5.38 (3.75)		16.8%	−0.07 [−0.48, 0.34]
Lai 2012a	58	2.3 (2.74)	67	1.69 (2.29)		22.4%	0.24 [−0.11, 0.59]
Subtotal (95% CI)	**102**		**116**			**39.3%**	**0.10 [−0.20, 0.41]**
Heterogeneity: Tau² = 0.01: Chi² = 1.29, df = 1 (P = 0.26): I² = 23%							
Test for overall effect: Z = 0.66 (P = 0.51)							
Total (95% CI)	**287**		**277**			**100.0%**	**0.16 [−0.01, 0.32]**
Heterogeneity: Tau² = 0.0: Chi² = 5.78, df = 10 (P = 0.83): I² = 0.0%							
Test for overall effect: Z = 1.85 (P = 0.064)							
Test for subgroup differences: Chi² = 0.47, df = 2 (P = 0.79): I² = 0.0%							

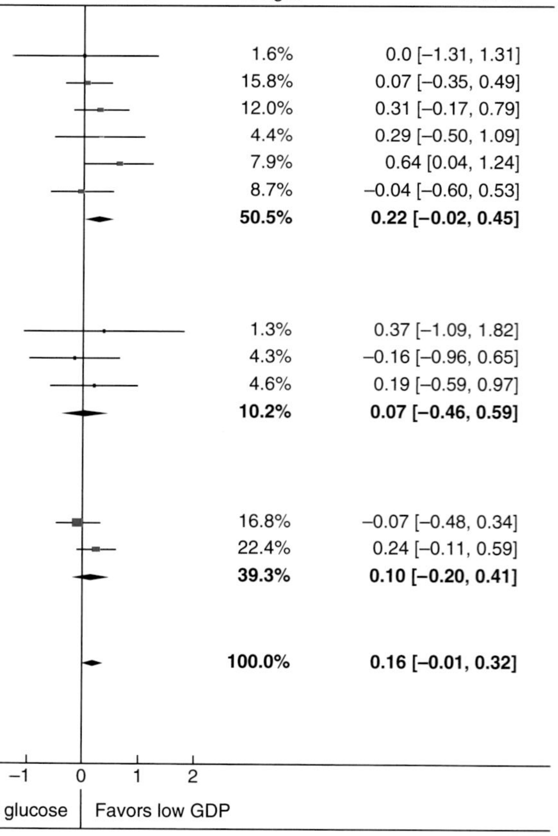

A

FIG. 31.3 Cochrane systematic review on studies comparing low-GDP (all buffer types) solutions versus standard glucose solution in relation to (A) residual kidney function, (B) urine volume, (C) analysis of residual kidney function from 12 to 24 months, and (D) residual kidney function up to 12 months. (Reproduced with permission from Cho Y, Johnson DW, Craig JC, Strippoli GF, Badve SV, Wiggins KJ. Biocompatible dialysis fluids for peritoneal dialysis. *Cochrane Database Syst Rev.* 2014(3):CD007554.)

Review: Biocompatible dialysis fluids for peritoneal dialysis

Comparison: 1 Low-GDP (all buffer types) versus standard glucose dialysate

Outcome: 6 Urine volume

Study or subgroup	Neutral pH, low GDP N	Mean (SD)[mL.AD]	Standard glucose N	Mean (SD)[mL.AD]	Weight	Mean Difference IV, Random 95% CI
1 3 months						
Fan 2008	44	800 (663.3)	49	1000 (700)	109%	−200.00 [−477.1R, 77.18]
Weiss 2009	15	1346.1 (870.8)	12	1000.6 (770)	25%	345.50 [−774.17, 965.17]
Subtotal (95% CI)	**59**		**61**		**13.4%**	**−0.54 [−515.46, 514.38]**
Heterogeneity: Tau^2 = 88804.91: Chi^2 = 2.48, df = 1 (P = 0.12): I^2 = 60%						
Test for overall effect: Z = 0.00 (P = 1.0)						
2 12 months						
Choi 2008	38	290 (236.6	30	143 (172.9)	41.8%	137.00 [39.60, 234.40]
Kim 2008	36	750 (6.79)	33	532 (408)	12.0%	218.00 [−43.87, 479.87]
Szeto 2007	24	800 (600)	24	690 (520)	8.6%	110.00 [−207.65, 427.65]
Subtotal (95% CI)	**98**		**87**		**62.4%**	**144.03 [56.29, 231.77]**
Heterogeneity: Tau^2 = 0.0: Chi^2 = 0.37, df = 2 (P = 0.83): I^2 = 0.0%						
Test for overall effect: Z = 3.22 (P = 0.0013)						
3 24 months						
balANZ Trial 2006	42	814 (624)	48	699 (639)	12.0%	115.00 [−146.33, 376.33]
Subtotal (95% CI)	**42**		**48**		**12.0%**	**115.00 [−146.33, 376.33]**
Heterogeneity: not applicable						
Test for overall effect: Z = 0.86 (P = 0.39)						
4 3 years +						
Lai 2012a	58	745.7 (819.23)	67	475.1 (635.92)	12.1%	220.60 [1053, 530.67]
Subtotal (95% CI)	**58**		**67**		**12.1%**	**270.60 [10.53, 530.67]**
Heterogeneity: not applicable						
Test for overall effect: Z = 2.04 (P = 0.041)						
Total (95% CI)	**257**		**263**		**100.0%**	**126.39 [26.73, 226.05]**
Heterogeneity: Tau^2 = 3711.80: Chi^2 = 7.51, df = 6 (P = 0.28): I^2 = 20%						
Test for overall effect: Z = 2.49 (P = 0.043)						
Test for subgroup difference: Chi^2 = 1.24, df = 3 (P = 0.74), I^2 = 0.0%						

−1000 −500 0 500 1000

Favors standard glucose | Favors low GDP

B

Review: Biocompatible dialysis fluids for peritoneal dialysis

Comparison: 1 Low-GDP (all buffer types) versus standard glucose dialysate

Outcome: 2 Residual renal function: 24 months and beyond

Study or subgroup	Neutral pH, low GDP N	Mean (SD)	Standard glucose N	Mean (SD)	Weight	Std. Mean Difference IV, Random, 95% CI
1 24 months						
Bajo 2011	9	4.2 (2.6)	3	4.2 (4)	3.3%	0.0 [−1.31, 1.31]
balANZ Trial 2006	40	3.4 (2.79)	48	3.2 (2.82)	32.3%	0.07 [−0.35, 0.49]
Fernandez-Perpen 2012	5	6 (4.4)	3	4.2 (4)	2.7%	0.37 [−1.09, 1.82]
Kim 2008	25	3.5 (3.4)	21	1.65 (1.97)	16.0%	0.64 [0.04, 1.24]
Subtotal (95% CI)	**79**		**75**		**54.3%**	**0.25 [−0.07, 0.57]**
Heterogeneity: Tau^2 = 0.0: Chi^2 = 2.51, df = 3 (P = 0.47): I^2 = 0.0%						
Test for overall effect: Z = 1.51 (P = 0.13)						
2 3 years +						
Lai 2012a	58	2.3 (2.74)	67	1.69 (2.29)	45.7%	0.24 [−0.11, 0.59]
Subtotal (95% CI)	**58**		**67**		**45.7%**	**0.24 [−0.11, 0.59]**
Heterogeneity: not applicable						
Test for overall effect: Z = 1.34 (P = 0.18)						
Total (95% CI)	**137**		**142**		**100.0%**	**0.25 [0.01, 0.48]**
Heterogeneity: Tau^2 = 0.0: Chi^2 = 2.51, df = 4 (P = 0.64): I^2 = 0.0%						
Test for overall effect: Z = 2.02 (P = 0.044)						
Test for subgroup differences: Chi^2 = 0.00, df = 1 (P = 0.98), I^2 = 0.0%						

−2 −1 0 1 2

Favors standard glucose | Favors low GDP

C

FIG. 31.3, cont'd.

Continued

Review: Biocompatible dialysis fluids for peritoneal dialysis

Comparison: 1 Low-GDP (all buffer types) versus standard glucose dialysate

Outcome: 2 Residual renal function: 24 months and beyond

Study or subgroup	Neutral pH, low GDP N	Mean (SD)	Standard glucose N	Mean (SD)	Std. Mean Difference IV, Random, 95% CI	Weight	Std. Mean Difference IV, Random, 95% CI
1 24 months							
Bajo 2011	9	4.2 (2.6)	3	4.2 (4)		3.3%	0.0 [−1.31, 1.31]
balANZ Trial 2006	40	3.4 (2.79)	48	3.2 (2.82)		32.3%	0.07 [−0.35, 0.49]
Fernandez-Perpen 2012	5	6 (4.4)	3	4.2 (4)		2.7%	0.37 [−1.09, 1.82]
Kim 2008	25	3.5 (3.4)	21	1.65 (1.97)		16.0%	0.64 [0.04, 1.24]
Subtotal (95% CI)	**79**		**75**			**54.3%**	**0.25 [−0.07, 0.57]**
Heterogeneity: $Tau^2 = 0.0$: $Chi^2 = 2.51$, df = 3 (P = 0.47): $I^2 = 0.0\%$							
Test for overall effect: Z = 1.51 (P = 0.13)							
2 3 years +							
Lai 2012a	58	2.3 (2.74)	67	1.69 (2.29)		45.7%	0.24 [−0.11, 0.59]
Subtotal (95% CI)	**58**		**67**			**45.7%**	**0.24 [−0.11, 0.59]**
Heterogeneity: not applicable							
Test for overall effect: Z = 1.34 (P = 0.18)							
Total (95% CI)	**137**		**142**			**100.0%**	**0.25 [0.01, 0.48]**
Heterogeneity: $Tau^2 = 0.0$: $Chi^2 = 2.51$, df = 4 (P = 0.64): $I^2 = 0.0\%$							
Test for overall effect: Z = 2.02 (P = 0.044)							
Test for subgroup differences: $Chi^2 = 0.00$, df = 1 (P = 0.98), $I^2 = 0.0\%$							

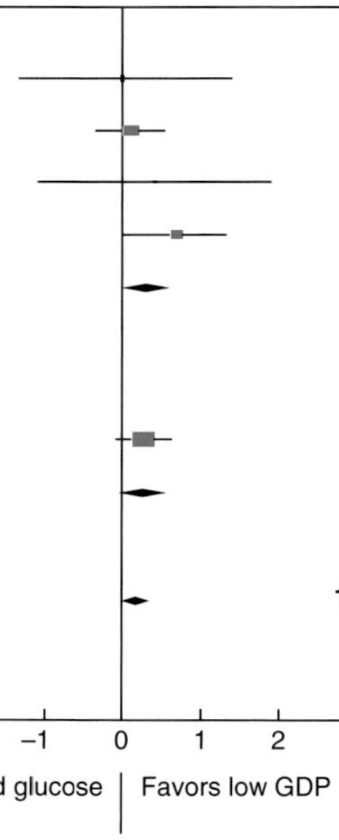

D

FIG. 31.3, con'd.

TABLE 31.3 An Overview of Randomized Controlled Trials of Neutral pH, Low-GDP Solutions in Relation to Residual Kidney Function (RKF) or Urine Volume

Reference	*n*	I/P	Follow-up Duration	Results
Feriani et al., 1998[113]	69	I	24 weeks	No significant difference was found in decline in residual renal clearances between biocompatible, 2.7 ± 2.8–2.8 ± 4.4 mL/min, and standard glucose group, 3.6 ± 4.1–3.0 ± 3.3 mL/min.
Szeto et al., 2007[114]	50	1	12 months	No significant difference was found in the rate of decline of RKF between neutral pH, low-GDP solutions (−1.19 ± 2.23 mL/min/1.73 m²) and control group (−1.02 ± 3.27 mL/min/1.73 m²).
Choi et al., 2008[115]	104	1	12 months	No significant difference was found in the change in renal clearances or urinary volume between neutral-pH, low-GDP solution and standard glucose group.
Fan et al., 2008[112]	93	I	12 months	No significant difference was found in the change in RKF between biocompatible and standard glucose groups.
Kim et al., 2009[116]	91	1	12 months	No significant difference was found in urine volume in the two groups at any time point. Using a mixed-models method and adjusting for baseline differences in kidney function, the residual GFR at 12 months was significantly higher in the neutral pH, low-GDP solution group (*P* = 0.048).
Haag-Weber et al., 2010[117]	69	I	18 months	The rate of decline in RKF was significantly slower with biocompatible PD solution Gambrosol Trio (−1.5%/month [95% CI, −3.07% to 0.03%]) vs. standard glucose solution (−4.3%/month [95% CI, −6.8% to −2.06%, *P* = 0.04]); also, there was a slower decline in 24-hour urine volume (12 vs. 38 mL/month, *P* = 0.02)
Johnson et al., 2012[118]	185	I	2 y	No significant difference was found in the slope of decline in RKF in either year 1 (−0.22 vs. −0.28 mL/min/1.73 m²) or year 2 (−0.09 vs. −0.10 mL/min/1.73 m²). A significantly longer time to anuria was reported in individuals assigned to neutral pH, low-GDP solution (*P* = 0.009).

TABLE 31.3 **An Overview of Randomized Controlled Trials of Neutral pH, Low-GDP Solutions in Relation to Residual Kidney Function (RKF) or Urine Volume—cont'd**

Reference	*n*	I/P	Follow-up Duration	Results
Lai et al., 2012[119]	125	I	Mean, 2.3 years	No significant difference was found in RKF in patients at end of follow-up (2.30 ± 0.36 vs. 1.69 ± 0.28 mL/min/1.73 m^2); urine volume was higher in neutral pH, low-GDP solution group (745.7 ± 107.57 vs. 475.1 ± 77.69 mL/d).
Lui et al., 2012[120]	150	I	12 months	No significant difference was found in the rate of decline in RKF between the group using 1.5%/1.1%/7.5% vs. standard solutions (–0.76 ± 1.77 vs. –0.91 ± 1.92 mL/min/1.73 m^2 per year; $P = 0.60$); patients using the biocompatible PD fluids had better preservation of daily urine volume (959 ± 515 vs. 798 ± 615 mL/d; $P = 0.02$).
Park et al., 2012[121]	146	I	12 months	No significant difference was found in RKF (2.9 ± 2.3 vs. 2.9 ± 3.1 mL/min) or urine volume (625 ± 488 vs. 644 ± 575 mL) in neutral pH, low-GDP solutions vs. standard solutions group.
Cho et al., 2013[122]	60	I	12 months	No significant difference was found in RKF (2.4 ± 1.7 vs. 2.2 ± 2.1 mL/min) or urine volume (714 ± 537 vs. 682 ± 460 mL) in neutral pH, low-GDP solution vs. standard glucose solution group.

GDP, Glucose degradation products; *I,* incident; *P,* prevalent.

adequately powered to examine the impact of neutral pH, low-GDP solutions on clinical hard outcomes such as hospitalizations or cardiovascular events.

Amino Acid Peritoneal Dialysis Solutions

Amino acid PD solution was launched back in the 1990s with an aim to supplement and replace nitrogen losses in PD patients. PD patients may lose up to 3 to 4 g/day of amino acids and 4 to 15 g/day of proteins even in the stable condition. The amount of peritoneal protein and amino acids loss may increase further with peritonitis. The only commercially available amino acid PD solution is 1.1% solution, which contains 87 mmol/L of amino acids, the majority (61%) of which is essential amino acids (see Table 31.1). A 1.1% amino acid solution exerts a similar osmotic force to 1.36% glucose solutions, thus providing an ultrafiltration volume comparable to that achieved with 1.36% glucose solutions. The peak plasma amino acid concentration is usually achieved around an hour. Usually approximately 72% to 82% of amino acids are absorbed in a single daily dwell and this may amount up to 18 g/day, thus providing a good source of protein supplement without adding phosphorus load.[132]

The 1.1% amino acid solution has been found to have a very small vasodilatory effect on peritoneal blood flow and may increase small solute transport.[133] Earlier balance studies suggested that the nitrogen absorbed from a single daily dwell of 1.1% amino acid solution is sufficient to offset the daily losses of amino acids and protein from the peritoneum.[132] Compared with using glucose solution only, combined amino acids and glucose PD solutions have been found to improve protein kinetics and whole-body protein synthesis in PD.[134,135] Nevertheless, this was not accompanied by a parallel increase in serum albumin, suggesting different pathways involved in albumin and skeletal muscle protein synthesis.[136]

Several RCTs have been conducted to evaluate the safety of 1.1% amino acid solution and its efficacy in treating malnutrition, or what is now called *protein-energy wasting*, in PD patients.[137] An earlier 12-week multicenter study[138] reported an increase in circulating insulin growth factor I in PD patients randomly assigned to 1.1% solution compared with controls, suggesting an increase in protein synthesis. A subgroup analysis indicated an increase in plasma prealbumin and transferrin levels, yet no change in midarm muscle circumference levels among those with plasma albumin <35 g/L.[138] Another RCT[139] using 1.1% amino acid solution was conducted in Chinese malnourished PD patients. In the 3-year study, participants who were randomly assigned to use 1.1% solution had an improvement in serum albumin, triglyceride, and total cholesterol level as well as a reported increase in dietary protein intake and an increase in normalized protein equivalent of nitrogen appearance (nPNA). Some anthropometric markers improved, although composite nutrition scores did not differ between treatment and control groups. Interestingly, the nutritional benefits appeared more prominent in women, whose lean body mass and body mass index were well maintained with combined amino acids and glucose PD solution but not with glucose solutions. The study was not powered to detect a difference in survival outcomes because only 60 participants were included. No significant difference was noted in inflammatory profile, mortality rates, and duration of hospitalization.[139] Another 6-month crossover study[140] failed to find any positive benefit on lipid metabolism with 1.1% amino acid solution in PD patients. In relation to peritoneal membrane function, preliminary data suggested that 1.1% amino acid solution may be more biocompatible to the peritoneal membrane and mesothelial cells than standard glucose solutions, as reflected by both in vitro and in vivo response of peritoneal CA125.[141]

In summary, the overall clinical value of 1.1% amino acid solution in PD patients has remained equivocal and uncertain. Generally, 1.1% amino acids PD solution is safe. Potential adverse effects include increased nausea and anorexia. Some patients may develop mild metabolic acidosis.[142] This may be ameliorated by adjusting to use a bicarbonate-based buffer in the remaining PD exchanges. 1.1% amino acids solution may be reserved as a glucose-sparing solution in PD subjects and also for use in subjects at risk or exhibit features of PEW syndrome. Adequately powered randomized studies are needed to better define the outcome benefits of this solution.

Low-Sodium Peritoneal Dialysis Solutions

Sodium removal is largely achieved by convection in PD through ultrafiltration. The concept of using low-sodium dialysate is to enhance sodium removal by diffusion, given the larger concentration gradient between plasma and dialysate sodium. However, low-sodium dialysate is currently not in use in clinical practice. In a 2009 nonrandomized controlled trial by Davies et al.,[143] two novel solutions designed from predictions using the three-pore model were compared. In one group, sodium concentration was 115 mmol/L and glucose concentration was increased to 2.0% to compensate for reduced osmolality. In the other group, sodium concentration was 102 mmol/L and glucose concentration was unchanged (2.5%). Both solutions were substituted for one 3- to 5-hour exchange per day and no change was made to the rest of the PD regimen. The results indicated that use of the compensated low-sodium dialysate increased the diffusive component of sodium removal while maintaining ultrafiltration. This in turn translated to an improvement in blood pressure, thirst, and fluid status. However, uncompensated low-sodium dialysate had no effect at all on blood pressure, thirst, and fluid status, suggesting that these benefits cannot be achieved just by manipulating the dialysate sodium level alone.[143]

In a prospective multicenter double-blind RCT conducted to prove noninferiority of total weekly urea clearance (Kt/V) with low-sodium versus standard-sodium PD solutions, 108 patients were randomly assigned to low-sodium dialysate (sodium concentration 125 mmol/L) versus standard sodium dialysate (sodium concentration 134 mmol/L) for a 12-week treatment. The noninferiority of low-sodium PD solution for total Kt/V could not be confirmed. Although no difference was found in PD Kt/V, renal Kt/V was different between the two groups, being higher in standard-sodium than in low-sodium group. Low-sodium group showed higher mean daily dialysate sodium removal than high-sodium group. Blood pressure also decreased more with the low-sodium group, resulting in less antihypertensive medication use.[144] Freida et al.[145] created their own compensated “bimodal solution” using a combination of icodextrin and glucose solution. The combination solution had a sodium concentration of 121 mmol/L, and a 15-hour dwell was associated with enhanced net ultrafiltration (mean 990 mL) and sodium removal (mean 158 mmol) compared with 7.5% icodextrin (mean net ultrafiltration 462 mL, mean net sodium removal 49 mmol) or 3.86% glucose-based PD solution (mean net ultrafiltration −85 mL, mean net sodium removal 16 mmol). Compared with 7.5% icodextrin, the combination solution was also associated with significantly higher urea and creatinine clearances, by 41% and 26%, respectively.[145]

Another nonrandomized trial from the same group of investigators[146] using the bimodal solution combining colloids and crystalloids solution found that over a 4-month period, net ultrafiltration and peritoneal sodium removal using bimodal solution as the long dwell increased more than twofold compared with baseline. The estimated change (95% CI) from baseline in net daytime ultrafiltration was 150% (106% to 193%) for the bimodal solution versus 18% (−7% to 43%) for icodextrin and was highly significant. The estimated change from baseline in peritoneal sodium removal was 147% (112% to 183%) for the bimodal solution versus 23% (−2% to 48%) for icodextrin ($P < 0.001$). The estimated change from baseline in ultrafiltration efficiency was also significantly higher with bimodal solution than icodextrin (71% vs. −5%).[146] These data suggest that a bimodal solution based on a mixture of glucose (2.6%) and icodextrin (6.8%) significantly improved both ultrafiltration and peritoneal sodium removal and warrants further evaluation.

Future Development in Peritoneal Dialysis Solutions

Hyperbranched polyglycerol (0.5 to 3 kDa) is a nontoxic, nonimmunogenic, water-soluble polyether polymer and has been found to be an efficacious and biocompatible osmotic agent in a rodent model of PD.[147] Preclinical data suggested that hyperbranched polyglycerol functioned as colloids and induced osmosis mainly through capillary small pores and provided superior fluid and waste removal compared with Physioneal solution.[148] More recent animal data indicated that hyperbranched polyglycerol solution may preserve peritoneal membrane function and structure better than standard glucose solution in a rat model of chronic PD.[149] Pyruvate has been suggested as the other alternative buffer. However, all these alternative solutions require further testing and evaluation before clinical application.

CONCLUSIONS

The standard glucose-based PD solutions have adverse effects both locally to the peritoneal membrane and systemically to the metabolic profile of PD patients. There is a need to move to a glucose-sparing regimen for PD patients. Preclinical and observational studies suggested that biocompatible neutral pH, low-GDP solutions may improve peritoneal membrane morphology. However, this was not confirmed in the RCT setting. Data from RCTs indicated that the biocompatible neutral pH, low-GDP solutions preserved RKF and urine volume better than standard glucose solutions without finding any increase in adverse events and thus should be adopted more readily clinically in patients with preserved RKF. The latest evidence from a systematic review of RCTs suggested that glucose polymer solution significantly increased peritoneal ultrafiltration and reduced episodes of uncontrolled

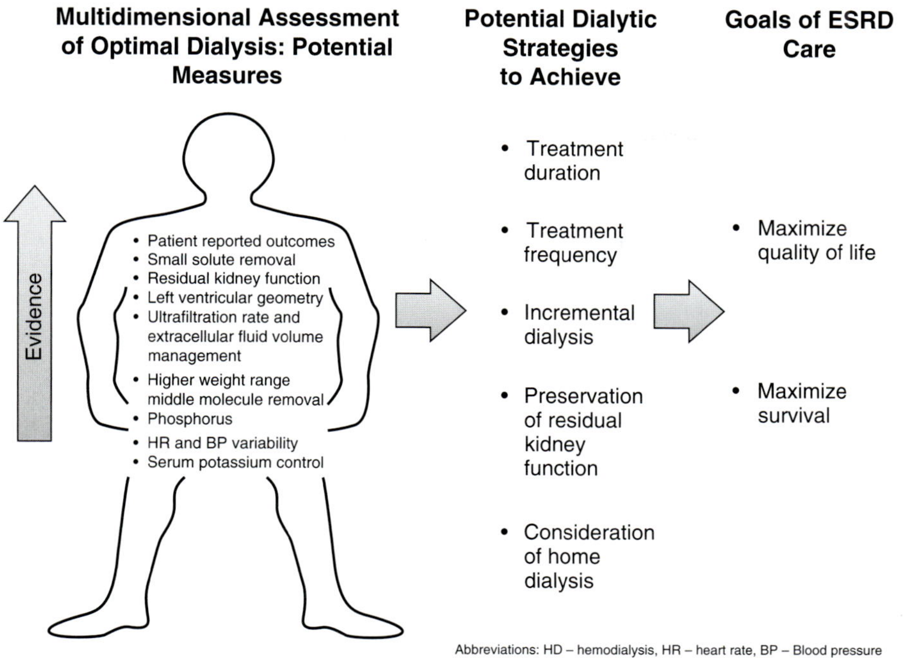

FIG. 31.4 Multidimensional measure of optimal dialysis. (Reproduced with permission from Perl J, Dember LM, Bargman JM, Browne T, Charytan DM, Flythe JE, et al. The use of a multidimensional measure of dialysis adequacy-moving beyond small solute kinetics. *Clin J Am Soc Nephrol.* 2017;12(5):839-847.)

volume overload compared with standard glucose solutions. None of these solutions produced a difference in the peritonitis risk compared with standard glucose solutions.

DIALYSIS ADEQUACY AND PRESCRIPTION

Defining Dialysis Adequacy

Starting in the 1990s, the term *peritoneal dialysis adequacy* was used to denote small solute clearance, namely Kt/V normalized to total body water and CrCl normalized to body surface area.[150] Total weekly Kt/V and CrCl are each composed of two components, namely clearance from RKF and clearance from PD. The dialysis component is modifiable. Thus the term *dialysis prescription* was introduced to denote the prescription of PD therapy to optimize dialysis adequacy to reach adequacy targets.

The United States Centers for Medicare and Medicaid Services ESRD Dialysis Incentive Program included Kt/V as a dialysis adequacy comprehensive clinical measure. However, there is increasing recognition that the term *dialysis adequacy* should encompass more than small solute clearance, Kt/V. Adequacy of dialysis should reflect measures that maximize the sum of survival, cardiovascular outcomes, extracellular volume status, CKD-MBD control, and patient-centered outcomes such as quality of life, appetite, nutrition status, and sleep, in addition to biochemical indices of dialysis adequacy.

The American Society of Nephrology Dialysis Advisory Group recently proposed a multidimensional measure that moves beyond small solute clearance and that aims to quantify dialysis adequacy. This multidimensional measure of optimal dialysis encompasses not only small solute removal, ultrafiltration rate, and extracellular volume overload but also left ventricular geometry, higher weight range middle molecule and phosphate removal, blood pressure variability, serum potassium control, anemia management, and, most importantly, patient-reported outcomes[151] (Fig. 31.4). There are evolutionary changes coming from the concept of *adequacy of dialysis* to *optimal dialysis* in the Standardised Outcomes in Nephrology (SONG)–PD Initiative, which accounts more for patient-centered outcomes such as self-reported quality-of-life measures[152] (Fig. 31.5). Adequacy of dialysis should not just include numerical indices of biochemical or clinical parameters but also, more importantly, how patients themselves feel with the therapy received.

Measuring Biochemical Indices of Dialysis Adequacy

The measurement of biochemical indices of dialysis adequacy requires the simultaneous collection of all PD effluent drained out and all urine output passed within the same 24-hour period together with a blood sample for serum urea and creatinine collected around the same time frame. In practical terms the blood sample is usually collected at the time when patients return both the 24-hour PD effluent and simultaneous 24-hour urine to the dialysis center. The PD component of Kt/V and CrCl is calculated by measuring urea and creatinine quantity in a 24-hour collection of PD fluid, respectively (Table 31.4). These values are divided by serum urea and creatinine levels to give the PD Kt/V and CrCl, respectively. The PD and residual renal component of urea and CrCl are then added to give a total weekly Kt/V and CrCl, respectively. Both

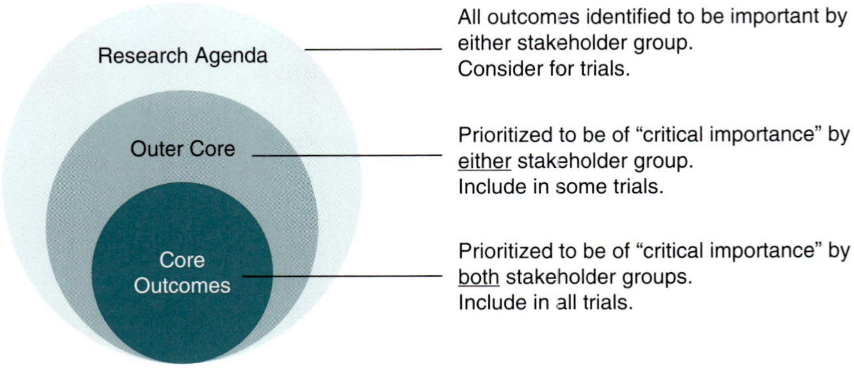

FIG. 31.5 Standardised Outcomes in Nephrology–Peritoneal Dialysis aims to identify outcome measures that are important to patients and caregivers in PD and establish a set of core outcome domains for trials conducted in PD. (Reproduced with permission From Tong A, Manns B. Establishing Core Outcome Domains in Hemodialysis: Report of the Standardized Outcomes in Nephrology -Hemodialysis (SONG-HD) Consensus Workshop. *Am J Kidney Dis*. 2017 Jan;69(1):97-107.)

TABLE 31.4 Formulas for Calculation of Indices of Dialysis Adequacy

Indices of Dialysis Adequacy	Formulas
Total weekly Kt/V	= (Daily PD + renal urea clearance) × 7 and normalized by V
Daily PD Kt/V	= [(24-hour PD volume in L) × (24-hour PD fluid urea concentration in mmol/L) / Plasma urea concentration in mmol/L] and normalized by V
Daily renal Kt/V	= [(24-hour urine volume in L) × (24-hour urine urea concentration in mmol/L) / Plasma urea concentration in mmol/L] and normalized by V
Total weekly CrCl	= (Daily PD + renal creatinine clearance) × 7 and normalized by BSA
Daily PD CrCl	= [(24-hour PD volume in L) × (24-hour PD fluid creatinine concentration in umol/L) / Plasma creatinine concentration in μmol/L] and normalized by BSA
Daily renal CrCl	= [(24-hour urine volume in L) × (average of 24-hour urine urea and creatinine concentration in μmol/L) / Plasma creatinine concentration in μmol/L] and normalized by BSA
nPNA (g/d) equations*	
Bergstrom formula I	= 20.1 + (7.5 × UNA in g/d)
Bergstrom formula II	= 15.1 + (6.95 × UNA in g/d) + (dialysate + urine protein in g/24 h)
Randerson I	= 10.76 × (UNA/1.44 + 1.46) and UNA is in g/d
Randerson II	= 10.76 × (UNA + 1.46) and UNA is in mg/min
Teehan	= 6.25 × (UNA + 1.81 + 0.031*BW) and UNA is in g/d
Blumenkrantz I	= 34.6 + 5.86 × UNA in g/d
Blumenkrantz II	= 22.5 + 6.16 × UNA in g/d
Residual GFR (mL/min/1.73m^2)	= Average of (24-h urine urea clearance + creatinine clearance in mL/min)
Normalization factor	Formulas
V (L)	= 2.447 + (0.3362 × BW in kg) + (0.1074 × BH in cm) – (0.09516 × age in years) for male patients
V (L)	= –2.097 + (0.2466 × BW in kg) + (0.1069 × BH in cm) for female patients
BSA	= 0.007184 × BW in kg$^{0.425}$ × BH in cm$^{0.725}$

BH, Body height; *BSA,* body surface area; *BW,* body weight; *CrCl,* creatinine clearance; *Kt/V,* urea clearance; *PD,* peritoneal dialysis; *UNA,* urea nitrogen appearance; *V,* total body water estimated by Watson method.

*These equations make the assumption that the patient is in steady state, where urea nitrogen output equals urea generation. The Randerson equation also assumes that the average daily protein loss in the dialysate is 7.3 g/day. In PD patients with substantial protein losses in dialysate or urine, these losses must be added to the equation in calculating nPNA.

Kt/V and CrCl values are conventionally expressed as weekly rather than daily to allow comparisons with hemodialysis.

Notably, when 24-hour PD fluid and urine collections are repeated on separate occasions in the same patient receiving the same PD prescription, significant intraindividual variations occur, especially in the renal component of clearance.[154] These variations may be accounted for by inaccuracies in the 24-hour urine and dialysate collection because they are cumbersome to do or by the timing of blood sampling. There could also be genuine day-to-day variation in the amount of dietary protein intake and fluid intake; urine volume, peritoneal ultrafiltration volume, and degree of equilibration of PD fluids; timing of PD exchanges; and concentrations of PD glucose solutions used. In CAPD either the patient is asked to bring all the dialysate drained out over the 24-hour period to clinic and the total 24-hour dialysate volume is measured in the laboratory, or the patient can measure the volumes of all dialysate drained out over a 24-hour period, mix up all the dialysates drained out well, and bring back a representative volume to the dialysis center. In automated PD the dialysate volumes involved are even larger. APD patients are usually trained to record or measure total cycler effluent volumes at home using the machine reading and bring back a representative aliquot of the dialysate to clinic for measurement of urea and creatinine concentrations.

In CAPD the timing of blood sampling for urea and creatinine may not be as critical because generally serum urea and creatinine do not fluctuate significantly during the day. In automated PD, however, there may be a 10% or greater variation in serum urea and creatinine from a trough value after completion of PD cycles in the morning to a peak value before the patient resumes PD cycles in the evening. This may be a problem especially if patients have no PD fluids dwell during daytime. Thus in patients receiving APD with no PD fluids during daytime, serum samples should be taken approximately halfway through the noncycling period, which means mostly in the early afternoon.

The target total weekly Kt/V values achieved in PD are usually around half to two-thirds of those in hemodialysis. This difference may be explained by the fact that, in contrast to hemodialysis, PD provides a continuous removal of small solute clearance and thus is greater than intermittent hemodialysis that delivers a similar quantity of clearance.[155,156] Furthermore, the continuous nature of PD avoids the day-to-day fluctuations in small solute clearance as found in intermittent hemodialysis. The concept of a "peak concentration hypothesis" put forward by Keshaviah et al.[155] suggested that peak levels rather than mean levels of small solutes determined uremic toxicity. Theoretically, continuous modalities may be better, because peak levels of uremic waste solutes should be lower for a given clearance than as in the case of intermittent modalities.[155,156]

Normalization Factor for Urea and Creatinine Clearance

Total weekly Kt/V is normalized to total body water, V, which can be estimated using anthropometric formulas such as Watson[157] or Hume,[158] which are based on age, gender, body weight, and height information. Estimates of V using the Watson formula are on the average slightly lower compared with the gold standard methods for estimating total body water such as deuterium oxide dilution.[159] However, the discrepancy varies substantially in patients with extreme body weight, such as obesity. By far, the Watson formula remains the most commonly adopted equation used to calculate V. Total weekly CrCl is normalized to body surface area (BSA), which is usually estimated by the du Bois formula.[160] In general, edema-free body weight should be used in the formulas to calculate V and BSA[153] (see Table 31.4). If patients have significant weight loss as a result of PEW, the ideal body weight rather than actual body weight has been suggested to be used in the formula. This is because wasted patients would have a misleadingly high normalized clearance value as a result of significant weight loss, whereas obese patients would have a misleadingly low value because of overweight. Ideal body weights provided by the National Health and Nutrition Evaluation Survey tables give the median body weight of North Americans of the same age, sex, height, and frame as the patient and are regularly updated. However, it is uncertain whether these values are also directly applicable to non-white populations.

Estimation of Residual Kidney Function

The renal component of urea and CrCl is calculated in the same way as with a 24-hour urine collection, except that in the case of creatinine clearance, an average of residual renal urea and CrCl is typically used (see Table 31.4). This is because unmodified urine CrCl substantially overestimates the true GFR because of tubular secretion of creatinine, whereas using renal Kt/V underestimates GFR.[164] Both creatinine and urea are freely filtered by the glomeruli. As part of the biochemical indices of dialysis adequacy, residual GFR is estimated using the average of 24-hour urine urea and CrCl and is normalized to BSA[164] (see Table 31.4). It is important to take into account both the peritoneal membrane transport characteristics and RKF of each patient when doing PD prescription and interpreting biochemical indices of dialysis adequacy.

Frequency of Monitoring of Biochemical Indices of Dialysis Adequacy

For all CAPD or APD patients, total weekly Kt/V and RKF should be measured around 4 weeks after initiation of PD therapy. Thereafter, they should ideally be monitored at least once every 6 months to allow for prescription modification if necessary.

Peritoneal Equilibration Test

PET is a simple clinical method that assesses the diffusive transport capacity of urea, creatinine, and other solutes across the semipermeable membrane, as well as ultrafiltration, in different patients.[26]

Patients who are high transporters equilibrate very quickly and have excellent diffusive transport capacity. However, they tend to have a low ultrafiltration volume using standard glucose PD solutions because the osmotic gradient for glucose dissipates relatively quickly (Fig. 31.6). These patients may do better with short dwell times as in APD. However, long hours' day dwell in APD using standard glucose solution may be a problem in high transporters because PD fluids will be largely reabsorbed. Glucose polymer solution or icodextrin would be preferred as the long day dwell solution for high transporters receiving APD.[72] In contrast, low transporters ultrafiltrate well but equilibrate slowly. Thus longer dwell times may be more effective in removing small solutes in low transporters. Generally, Kt/V is much less affected by peritoneal transport characteristics than CrCl in CAPD because more than 90% of Kt/V and equilibration occurs with the long dwell hours of CAPD, regardless of peritoneal transport characteristics. This differs from creatinine clearance, which may have two to three times difference between low and high transporters even after a 4- to 6-hour dwell (see Fig. 31.6). In APD, dwell time is usually shorter than CAPD except for the long day dwell. Thus peritoneal membrane transport characteristics may be considered in the prescription of PD modality and regimen.

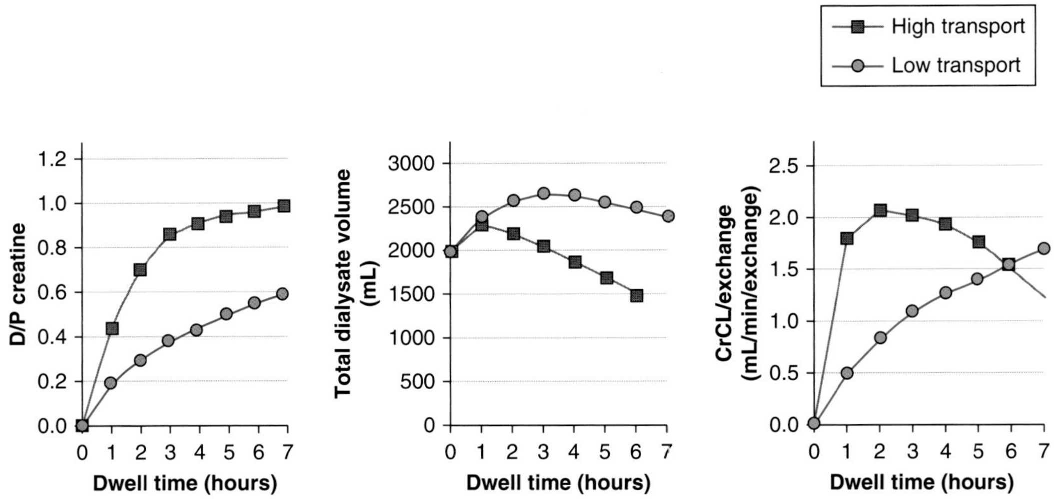

FIG. 31.6 Solute and fluid transport in low transporters versus high transporters in PD. High transporters reach equilibrium for creatinine more quickly than low transporters *(left panel)* and have a gradual reduction in dialysate drain volume after 2 hours or so as a result of glucose absorption and loss of osmotic gradient *(middle panel)*. Creatinine clearance also gradually decreases after 4 hours as a result of continued absorption of creatinine with the glucose and fluid *(right panel)*. This is in contrast to the low transporters, who have a very gradual increase in creatinine clearance, dialysate-to-plasma creatinine ratio, and dialysate drain volume over the 4-hour dwell. (Reproduced with permission from Twardowski ZJ. Nightly peritoneal dialysis. Why, who, how, and when? *ASAIO Trans.* 1990;36(1):8-16.)

In patients with complete loss of RKF, there could be limitations in achieving optimal clearance targets, depending on the peritoneal transport characteristics.

Importance of Dialysis Adequacy and Defining Numerical Targets for Biochemical Indices of Dialysis Adequacy

The CANUSA (Canada-USA) study[43] was a prospective multicenter cohort study of 680 incident CAPD patients from Canada and United States that examined the importance of adequacy. Over a 2-year period of follow-up, a significant positive association was identified between the total weekly Kt/V and CrCl and clinical outcomes including overall survival. For every 0.1 unit higher total weekly Kt/V, the relative risk for mortality was lower by 6%, and for every 5 L higher total weekly CrCl, the relative risk for mortality was lower by 7%. Subsequent to the CANUSA study, Maiorca et al.[168] also reported an association between weekly Kt/V >1.96 and better survival in another prevalent cohort of CAPD patients followed over 3 years.[168] These two important studies formed an important basis for the recommended total weekly Kt/V target of at least 2.0 and a CrCl target of at least 60 L/week/1.73 m^2 for those receiving CAPD with high and high-average transporters and a CrCl target at least 50 L/week/1.73 m^2 for those with low and low-average transporters by the National Kidney Foundation Dialysis Outcome Quality Initiative (K/DOQI) Guidelines in 1997 and 2000.[169] If there is discordance in achieving these targets, Kt/V was recommended to be the immediate determinant of dialysis adequacy because it directly reflects protein metabolism and is less affected by extreme variations in RKF. However, a cause for the discrepancy should be looked for and the patient should be followed closely for signs of underdialysis. One potential explanation for the discrepancy could be patients being underweight, which may result in a small V and overall a higher Kt/V.

Subsequent to these studies, two large prospective RCTs found no significant difference in the mortality risk for PD patients by increasing peritoneal small solute clearance. In the ADEquacy of PD in MEXico (ADEMEX) study,[170] increasing weekly peritoneal Kt/V from 1.62 to 2.13 (weekly CrCl from 46.1 to 56.9 L/week/1.73 m^2) had no significant effect on mortality risk (relative risk 1.00, 95% CI, 0.8 to 1.24). In another randomized trial from Hong Kong,[171] 320 PD patients with baseline renal Kt/V <1.0 were randomly assigned to three groups of different Kt/V targets, namely 1.5 to 1.7, 1.7 to 2.0, and >2.0. Patients in the group with the lowest Kt/V target 1.5 to 1.7 had more clinical problems and were more likely to be withdrawn from the study by their physicians based on clinical ground. The overall 2-year survival was 84.9% with no significant difference reported between the group with a Kt/V target of 1.7 to 2.0 and the group with a Kt/V target >2.0.[171] Another retrospective analysis from an administrative database of anuric PD patients in the United States demonstrated higher mortality rates in patients with a weekly Kt/V <1.7.[172]

With the exception of the study from Hong Kong, all the other studies failed to find a relationship between peritoneal small solute clearance and survival in PD patients. The ADEMEX RCT and the Hong Kong PD RCT formed the key basis for a subsequent revision of the 2006 K/DOQI, 2005 EBPG, and 2006 ISPD guidelines, all recommending a minimum weekly Kt/V target of 1.7 in CAPD patients.[169,173,174] There are no trial data to support benefit of further increasing dialysis to reach a total weekly Kt/V beyond 2.0 or a CrCl of more than 60 L/week/1.73 m^2. Furthermore, there are trial

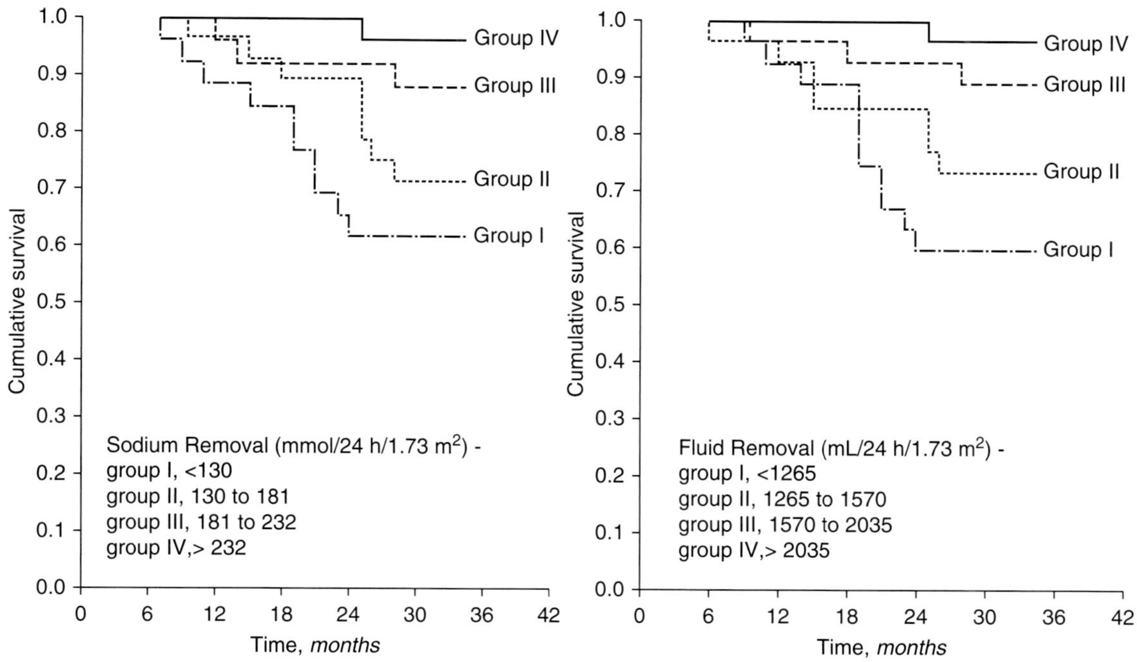

FIG. 31.7 Effects of sodium and fluid removal on survival in PD patients. (Reproduced with permission from Ates K, Nergizoglu G, Keven K, Sen A, Kutlay S, Erturk S, et al. Effect of fluid and sodium removal on mortality in peritoneal dialysis patients. *Kidney Int.* 2001;60(2):767-776.)

data to suggest that a weekly total Kt/V <1.7 was associated with more clinical problems and greater need for erythropoietin.[171] In the Netherlands Cooperative Study on the Adequacy of Dialysis (NECOSAD) study, peritoneal Kt/V <1.5 and CrCl <40 L/week/1.73 m^2 were associated with higher mortality.[175] The 2005 EBPG guideline, 2006 ISPD guideline update, and K/DOQI 2006 guideline suggested a minimum weekly peritoneal Kt/V of 1.7 for anuric PD patients.

In APD a cycler is used to perform multiple overnight exchanges. A minimum weekly Kt/V target of ≥1.7 per week is recommended and is in line with the 2006 K/DOQI guideline.[169,173] In APD patients who are anuric or have minimal urine volume, an additional manual day exchange is suggested to increase PD clearance, because the recommended Kt/V targets for APD patients are based on studies in CAPD patients who underwent continuous PD over a 24-hour period. In the 2006 ISPD guideline, a separate target for CrCl was not suggested for CAPD. In APD, because of more variable relations between Kt/V and CrCl, an additional target of 45 L/week/1.73 m^2 for CrCl was recommended.

Novel concepts in defining dialysis adequacy or optimal dialysis. The minimum target Kt/V defines the minimum but not necessarily the optimal dose of dialysis that should be performed. Optimal dialysis prescription should be personalized, based on an assessment of RKF, peritoneal membrane function, status of clinical and biochemical parameters, acid–base status, uremic symptoms, volume status, nutrition profile, control of mineral metabolism, and patients' self-perceived well-being on dialysis (see Fig. 31.4). In some situations, dialysis dose may need to be increased despite achieving the minimum weekly Kt/V target of 1.7. Examples of these situations are persistent acidosis, persistent uremic symptoms such as nausea and anorexia, clinical manifestations of PEW, and hyperphosphatemia despite dietary restriction and use of phosphorus binders.

Ultrafiltration and Volume Control as a Target for Dialysis Adequacy

Ultrafiltration is an important parameter for assessing adequacy of dialysis, and ultrafiltration has been found to be associated with survival in anuric APD patients; ultrafiltration volume less than 750 mL/day was associated with a higher mortality.[176] However, a numerical target for daily ultrafiltration volume was not formulated or recommended by different guideline bodies. It is because the overall volume status depends also on the residual urine volume as well as salt and fluid intake of patients and there may be substantial intraindividual variation. Both the 2006 ISPD guidelines and the recent 2015 ISPD Cardiovascular and Metabolic guidelines emphasized the importance of maintaining euvolemia in PD patients as one of the treatment goals in PD and recommended that attention be paid to both the urine volumes and PD ultrafiltration volumes.[24,169]

The negative findings from the ADEMEX study that increasing small solute clearance did not improve survival of PD patients[170] suggested the need to look for factors other than small solute clearance that may be important in determining clinical outcomes of PD patients. A reanalysis of data from the CANUSA study indicated that every 250 mL of urine output was associated with a 36% lower mortality risk, suggesting the importance of urine volume in determining the clinical outcome of PD patients.[177] Sodium and fluid removal are associated with survival in PD patients. The lower the sodium and fluid removal from PD, the greater the mortality risk[178] (Fig. 31.7). Extracellular volume overload is a highly prevalent complication in PD patients.

BOX 31.1 Clinical Evaluations and Checklist for Patients With Volume Overload

1. What is the PD outflow pattern lately? Has there been a recent change in PD ultrafiltration or drain volume? Any recent change in PD prescription? What's the outflow volume for each bag of PD exchanges used?
2. What's the daily amount of urine volume lately? Has there been a recent decrease in urine volume?
3. Are there any nonadherence issues related to salt and fluid restriction?
4. Has the patient been dining out often or eating high-salt or -fluid meals?
5. Is there any nonadherence to dialysis prescription? Or missed exchanges by patients?
6. Does the patient have undiagnosed cardiovascular disease or heart failure? Any features to suggest silent myocardial ischemia?
7. What kind of peritoneal transport characteristics does the patient have?
8. Does the patient reach the minimum target for Kt/V and CrCl?
9. If drain volume is low:
   (i) Are there any mechanical issues with PD outflow that may explain low drain volume?
   (ii) Does the patient have constipation?
   (iii) Is outflow position related?
   (iv) Is the catheter positioned correctly?
   (v) Are fibrin clots present that may obstruct outflow?
   (vi) Is there omental wrap?
   (vii) Are there clinical features to suggest peritoneal adhesions or encapsulating peritoneal sclerosis?

CrCl, creatinine clearance; *Kt/V*, urea clearance; *PD*, peritoneal dialysis.

Using bioimpedance spectroscopy, the estimated prevalence of extracellular volume overload was at least more than 50%[179,180] and was even higher when patients completely lost their RKF.[179] Extracellular volume overload is associated with a higher risk for mortality in PD patients.[181] Apart from loss of RKF, UFF with low drain volume is another important cause of volume overload (see Ultrafiltration Failure). Other non–membrane-related causes of volume overload include dietary nonadherence with excess salt and fluid intake, nonadherence to dialysis prescription, and inappropriate choice of PD solution strengths that may affect the PD outflow. Mechanical complications such as dialysate leaks, hernias, catheter malposition, and loculations in the peritoneal cavity may also cause low drain volume. In fact, retroperitoneal dialysate leaks have been suggested to be an important cause of acute UFF and can be diagnosed using computed tomography peritoneogram.[182] Hyperglycemia may also contribute to low drain volume by decreasing the glucose osmotic gradient–driven ultrafiltration.[183]

It is therefore essential to take a thorough history and physical examination and review the PD outflow records and dietary intake pattern in the preceding days before the episode of volume overload to identify the exact cause. Box 31.1 details a checklist of questions to be asked when assessing a patient with volume overload. Fig. 31.8 provides an algorithm on the clinical evaluation of patients who present with volume overload.

Nutrition Status as a Target for Dialysis Adequacy

The importance of nutrition status in clinical outcomes and survival of dialysis patients has long been recognized. A study by Owen et al.[184] found that serum albumin concentration was at least 20-fold more powerful than urea reduction ratios in its association with a higher risk for mortality in dialysis patients.[184] In PD patients, various nutritional indices, including subjective global assessment, serum albumin, handgrip strength, and lean body mass, have been found to be associated with survival and cardiovascular outcomes.[185-187]

In 2008 the International Society of Renal Nutrition and Metabolism (ISRNM) commissioned an expert panel to standardize the definition and terminology used. The term *protein-energy wasting* was recommended to denote loss of body protein mass and fuel reserves. The diagnosis of PEW is made based on the presence of three out of the four characteristics, namely (1) at least one biochemical parameter of the following: low serum levels of either albumin, transthyretin, or cholesterol; (2) reduced body mass (low or reduced body fat mass or weight loss with reduced intake of protein and energy); and (3) reduced muscle mass (muscle wasting or sarcopenia, reduced midarm muscle circumference) (Box 31.2). Unintentional weight loss should lead one to consider the presence of PEW. The panel regarded loss of 5% of nonedematous weight within 3 months or an unintentional loss of 10% of nonedematous weight over the past 6 months as an indicator of PEW, independent of weight-for-height measures. Loss of body fat and muscle mass are considered important criteria for diagnosing PEW. Other potential tools such as a nutrition scoring system (e.g., subjective global assessment, malnutrition-inflammation scoring, appetite assessment, dietary intake assessment) or body composition assessment may also be used, though they are not included as a diagnostic criteria for PEW.[188] In fact, a simple questioning of appetite has been found to be useful in predicting clinical outcome and hospitalization in dialysis patients.[189] Inflammatory markers such as C-reactive protein are usually elevated in the setting of PEW.[188]

Various urea kinetics equations have been used to estimate nPNA, a surrogate for protein intake in PD patients. However, these equations made the assumption that the patient was stable and urea generation, excretion, and other nitrogen losses were proportional and in equilibrium to the amount of protein intake. Among the various equations, the best validated is the Bergstrom formula. Both the Randerson and Bergstrom formulas are often used (see Table 31.4). These formulas are derived using the same variables as Kt/V. In the early 1990s, the cross-sectional association between solute clearance Kt/V

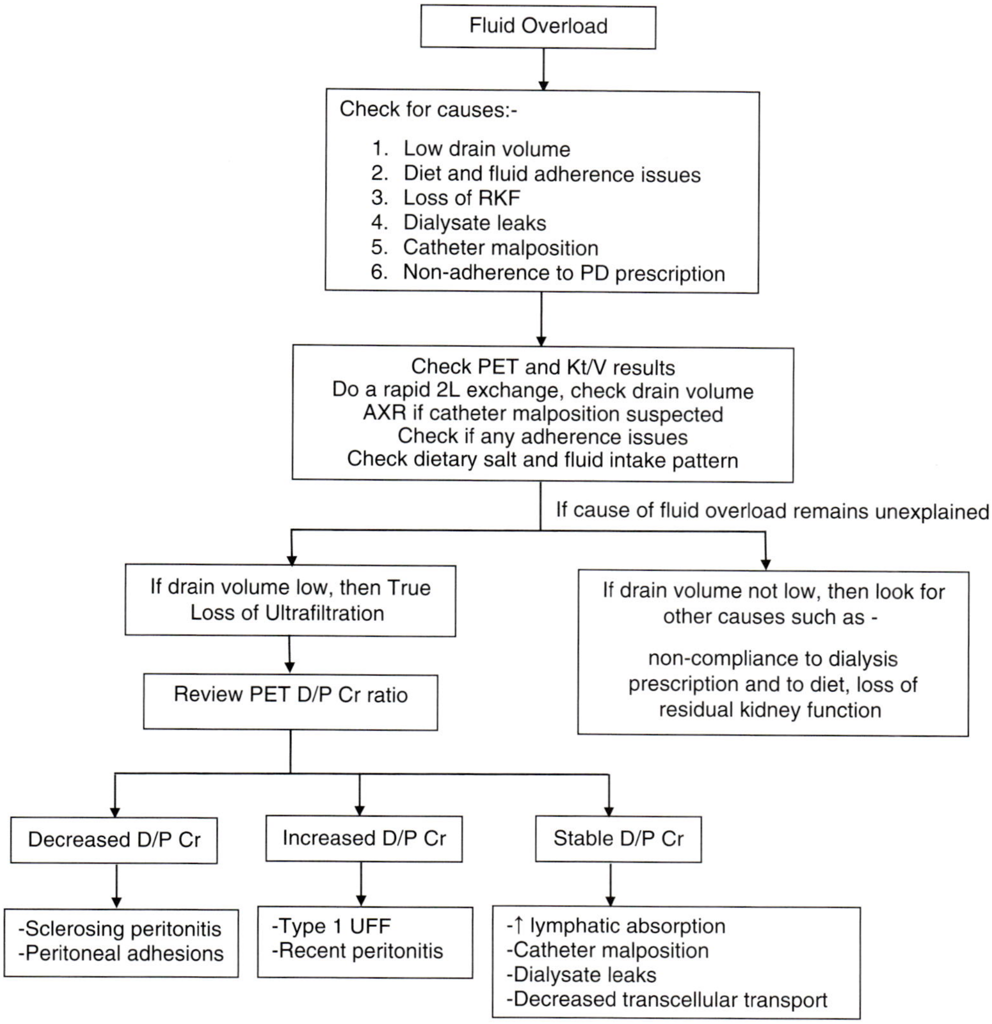

FIG. 31.8 Algorithm of clinical evaluation of patients with volume overload.

BOX 31.2 ISRNM Consensus Statement on Diagnosis of Protein-Energy Wasting (PEW)[188]

A diagnosis of PEW requires that at least three out of the four listed categories be met and at least one test in each of the selected category should be included.

Serum Chemistry

- Serum albumin level (measured using the bromocresol green method) <38 g/L
- Serum prealbumin level (transthyretin) <30 mg/dL
- Serum cholesterol level <2.59 mmol/L (not valid if low concentrations are caused by abnormally high urinary or gastrointestinal protein losses, liver disease, or cholesterol-lowering medicines)

Body Mass

- BMI <22 kg/m^2 ≤65 years, <23 kg/m^2 >65 years (a lower BMI might be desirable for certain Asian populations; weight must be edema-free mass)
- Unintentional weight loss over time: ≥5% over 3 months or ≥10% over 6 months
- Total body fat percentage <10%

Muscle Mass

- Muscle wasting: reduced muscle mass ≥ 5% over 3 months or ≥10% over 6 months
- Reduced MAMC area as measured by a trained anthropometrist (reduction >10% in relation to the 50th percentile of the reference population)
- Creatinine appearance (of note, appearance is influenced by muscle mass and meat intake)

Dietary Intake

- Unintentionally low DPI <0.80 g/kg per day for at least 2 months (which can be assessed by dietary diaries and interviews, or for protein intake by calculation of the normalized protein equivalent of total nitrogen appearance [normalized protein nitrogen appearance or normalized protein catabolic rate] as determined by urea kinetic measurements)
- Unintentional low DEI <25 kcal/kg/d for at least 2 months

BMI, Body mass index; *DEI,* dietary energy intake; *DPI,* dietary protein intake; *MAMC,* midarm muscle circumference.

and dietary protein intake, nPNA, led to the conclusion that dialysis dose was one of the important determinants of dietary protein intake.[187] However, subsequent concerns were raised that the close correlation reported between Kt/V and nPNA may have been due to mathematical coupling because these two parameters contained some common variables.[190] Wang et al. found that total weekly Kt/V and CrCl had important associations with actual intake of dietary protein, energy, macronutrients, and micronutrients, estimated using a 7-day food frequency questionnaire, independent of other confounding clinical and biochemical covariates. The associations with intake of various dietary components including protein and energy were essentially contributed by RKF but not PD clearance.[191,192] These data provided important evidence that the correlations reported between small solute clearance and protein intake were not simply the result of mathematical coupling. RKF but not PD clearance contributed significantly to the overall nutrition status and dietary intake of PD patients. In keeping with this finding, the ADEMEX RCT reported no difference in nutrition status and dietary protein intake with increasing PD clearance to 60 L/week/1.73 m^2 compared with the control group with average PD clearance of 45 L/week/1.73 m^2, suggesting that increasing PD dose to 60 L/week/1.73 m^2 did not further improve nutrition status.[170]

The current recommended protein intake nPNA for stable PD patients is ≥1.2 g/kg body weight per day and energy intake is ≥30 to 35 kcal/kg/day including energy derived from peritoneal glucose absorption.[193] Other than loss of RKF, a multitude of other factors may contribute to lower dietary intake and increased catabolism, causing PEW in PD patients (Box 31.3). Some of these factors included uremic anorexia, inflammation, metabolic acidosis, insulin resistance, resistance to growth hormone/insulin growth factor I, impaired protein anabolism, volume overload, and associated comorbidities. In PD, dialysate protein losses, impaired gastric emptying as a result of diabetes or peritoneal fluids, and infections such as peritonitis may additionally predispose patients to PEW. Fig. 31.9 provides a conceptual model of the etiology and consequences of PEW.

The current estimated prevalence of PEW in PD patients ranges from 18% to 55%.[191,194] Regular monitoring of nutrition status and screening for PEW are therefore essential in PD patients and in particular when complication sets in. Serum albumin alone is not a reliable marker of PEW because systemic inflammatory processes lower serum albumin. Hypoalbuminemia may also be a marker of overhydration.[195] In managing PD patients with PEW, it is essential to identify and treat the underlying cause of PEW. Oral nutrition supplement (ONS) and enteral nutrition supplement should be considered in patients who fail to achieve the recommended level of protein and energy intake and have features of PEW such as unintentional weight loss, low serum albumin, and loss of body fat mass and muscle mass. Trials on ONS have been lacking in the PD population. Nevertheless, in hemodialysis, small RCTs have reported that ONS improved various nutritional parameters.[193] Other potential treatments for PEW, such as growth hormone and anabolic steroids, that may stimulate net muscle protein synthesis or appetite need further evaluation in PD patients. Fig. 31.10 provides an algorithm proposed by ISRNM on nutrition management and support in CKD, including patients receiving PD treatment.[193] Detailed discussion on management of PEW in CKD is provided in another section.

BOX 31.3 Causes of Protein-Energy Wasting in Peritoneal Dialysis Patients

Protein and Nutrient Losses in Dialysate
- Increased loss during peritonitis

Decreased Intake of Dietary Protein, Energy, and Other Nutrients
- Uremic anorexia
- Loss of residual kidney function
- Accumulation of uremic toxins
- Dietary restrictions
- Abdominal distension as a result of peritoneal fluids in situ
- Early satiety as a result of peritoneal glucose
- Encapsulating peritoneal sclerosis
- Peritoneal collections and adhesions
- Diabetes mellitus
- Atherosclerotic vascular disease and peripheral vascular disease
- Heart failure and volume overload
- Infections (e.g., peritonitis, exit site infections, pneumonia)
- Psychological factors such as depression
- Poor dentition or dental caries, periodontitis

Hypermetabolism
- Inflammation relating to comorbidities (such as atherosclerotic vascular disease, peripheral vascular disease, heart failure, volume overload, MIA syndrome)
- Inflammation relating to infections (e.g., peritonitis, exit site infections, pneumonia)
- Loss of residual kidney function
- Insulin resistance
- Increased glucocorticoid activity
- Sympathetic overactivity
- Dialysis-related inflammation
- Dialysis-related hypermetabolism
- Metabolic acidosis
- Inflammation caused by periodontitis

Decreased anabolism
- Resistance to growth hormone/insulin growth factor 1
- Testosterone deficiency
- Low thyroid hormone levels
- Decreased nutrient intake

Initial Peritoneal Dialysis Prescription

The initial CAPD prescription may need to be empirically set based on patients' weight, degree of RKF, and lifestyle constraints even before information on peritoneal transport status is available. Generally, PET is recommended to be conducted at least 4 to 6 weeks after long-term continuous PD initiation. CAPD or APD may be initiated incrementally or as a full therapy, depending on the degree of RKF at the time of dialysis initiation.

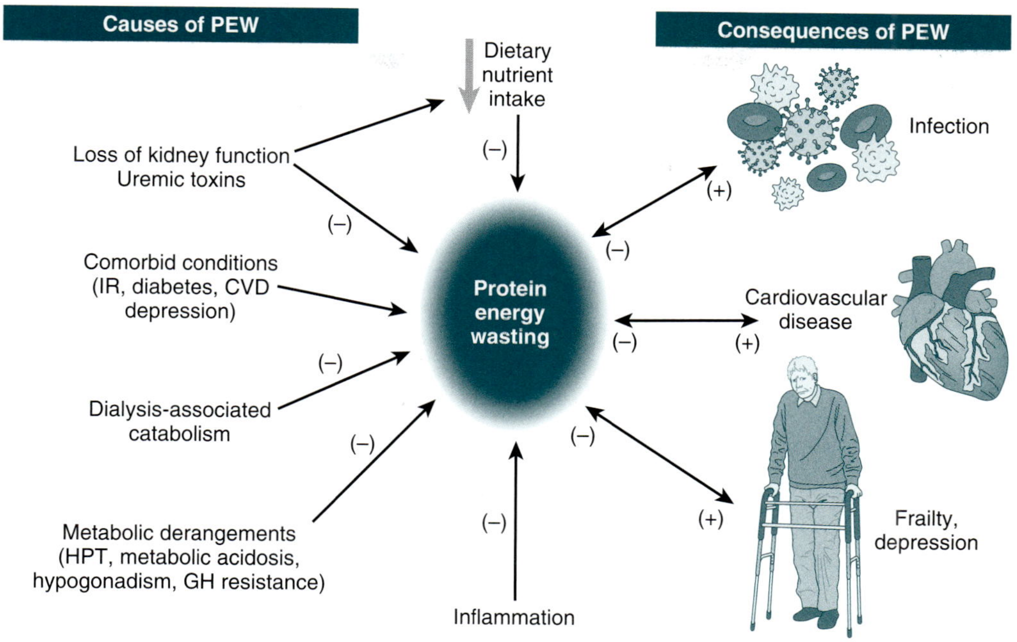

FIG. 31.9 The conceptual model for etiology and consequences of protein energy wasting in chronic kidney disease. *CVD,* Cardiovascular disease; *GH,* growth hormone; *HPT,* hyperparathyroidism; *IR,* insulin resistance. (Reproduced with permission from Ikizler TA, Cano NJ, Franch H, Fouque D, Himmelfarb J, Kalantar-Zadeh K, et al. Prevention and treatment of protein energy wasting in chronic kidney disease patients: a consensus statement by the International Society of Renal Nutrition and Metabolism. *Kidney Int.* 2013;84(6):1096-1107.)

Clinical Evaluation of Patients With Low Delivered Urea Clearance

In PD patients with a low Kt/V, evaluations should include the following potential causes:

1. Check if the dialysis prescription, namely the number of cycles and the concentration of PD solutions, is sufficient for the patient.
2. Check for nonadherence or nonadherence to the dialysis prescription or missed cycles.
3. Check if actual dwell times may differ from that prescribed.
4. Check for loss of RKF.
5. Check for incomplete draining.
6. Check for hypercatabolic conditions in the patient.

Adjusting Peritoneal Dialysis Prescription

If kinetic modeling is not available, dialysis dose may be increased by increasing the instilling volume as tolerated, thereby maximizing mass transfer and dwell time. The other possibility would be to increase the number of daily PD exchanges while maximizing the dwell time. For example, for PD patients who are prescribed three exchanges daily of 2 L × 1.5% and have a low Kt/V because of loss of RKF, one may increase the dialysis dose by increasing to four exchanges daily of 2 L × 1.5% or by increasing the volume per exchange to 2.3 to 2.5 L × 1.5% as required and as tolerated. If there is a need to increase ultrafiltration volume as well, then one may consider replacing 1.5% with 2.5% solution.

If computer-assisted kinetic modeling is available, then the kinetic modeling may be used to tailor PD prescriptions to individual's transport type, RKF, body size, and lifestyle habits and thus enable a more personalized PD treatment to be prescribed. Kinetic modeling is especially important for APD prescription because the dwell times are variable and may not be optimized for many patients. Computer-assisted kinetic modeling accurately and reliably predicts the delivered dose and facilitate the prescription process and achievement of the target delivered PD dose. Actual measurements will still need to be carried out to confirm that an adequate PD dose has indeed been delivered.

In patients performing APD, an initial prescription may consist of three to four daily exchanges of 2 L × 1.5% or 2.5% in various combination, depending on the ultrafiltration volume and urine output of patients. A dry day may be considered in those who still have significant RKF, but this implies that the total daily number of hours of dialysis will be reduced by at least 8 to 10 hours, depending on the hours of the dry day. As patients lose their RKF or in patients who are underdialysed with dry day, usually a wet day or a single day dwell using 2 L exchange of 1.5%, 2.5%, or icodextrin solution will be required to achieve adequate dialysis. The use of icodextrin as the long day dwell has the advantage of achieving a better ultrafiltration volume compared with the standard glucose solutions. In patients who remain underdialysed with a single long day dwell, the prescription can be modified to using two shorter day dwells—for example, 2 × 2 L exchanges of 1.5% or 2.5%—to increase dialysis clearance. Other ways to increase dialysis clearance in APD patients include increasing the number of exchanges overnight to five exchanges or increasing the dwell volume—for example, from 2 L to 2.5 L as tolerated. In patients who are low transporters and in whom clearance critically depends on the dwell time, using cycler therapy shorter than 2-hour dwells may not achieve

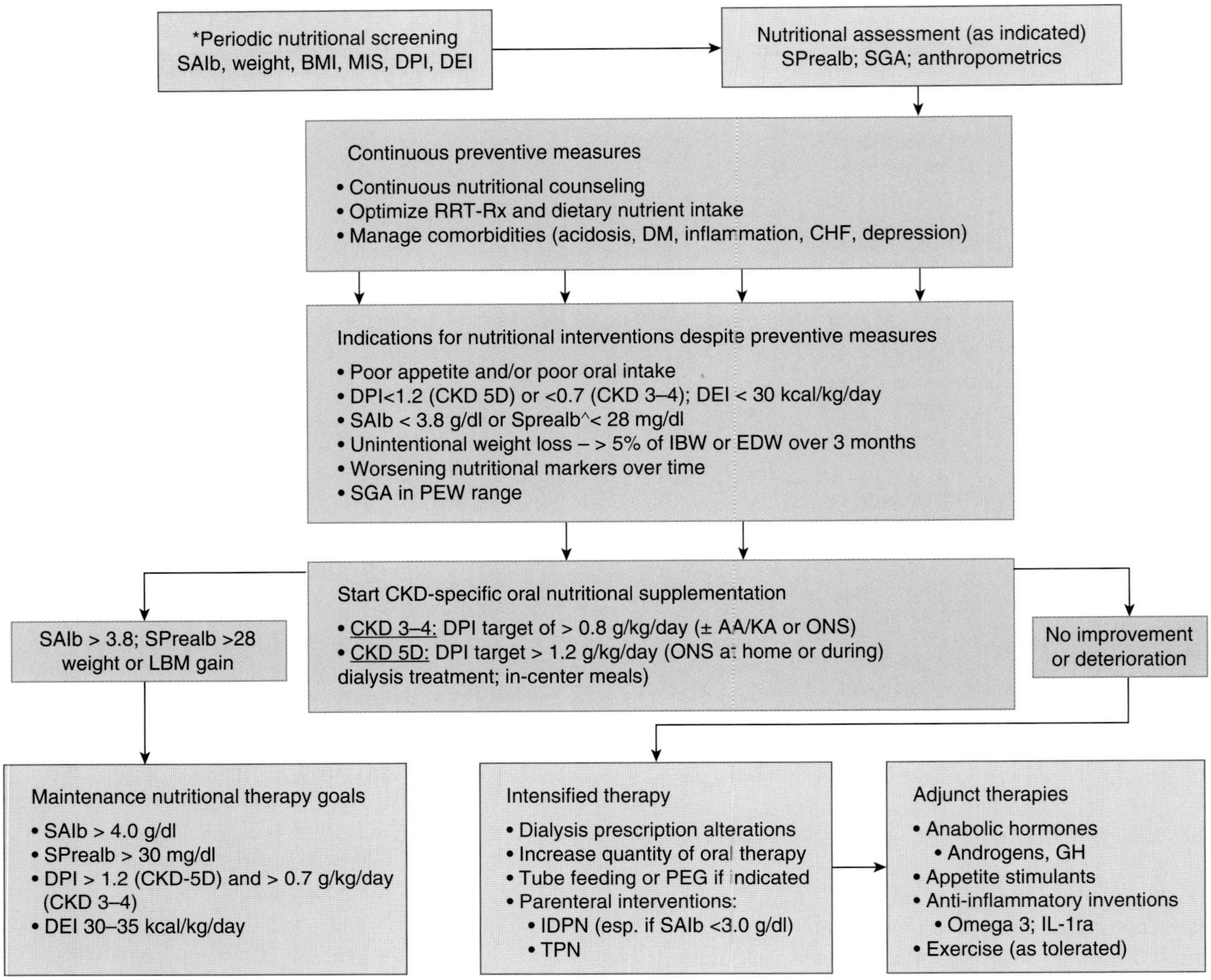

FIG. 31.10 A consensus statement from ISRNM on nutritional management and support in PD patients. *AA,* Amino adics; *BMI,* body mass index; *CHF,* congestive heart failure; *CKD,* chronic kidney disease; *DEI,* dietary energy intake; *DM,* diabetes mellitus; *DPI,* dietary protein intake; *EDW,* expected dry weight; *GH,* growth hormone; *IBW,* ideal body weight; *IDPN,* introdialytic parenteral nutrition; *IL-1ra,* interleukin-1 receptor anatogonist; *KA,* ketoanalog; *LBM,* lean body mass; *MIS,* malnutrition inflammation syndrome; *ONS,* oral nutrition supplement; *PEG,* percutaneous endoscopic gastrostomy; *SAlb,* serum albumin; *SGA,* subjective global assessment; *SPrealb,* serum prealbumin; *RRT-Rx,* renal replacement therapy prescription; *TPN,* total parenteral nutrition. (Reproduced with permission from Ikizler TA, Cano NJ, Franch H, Fouque D, Himmelfarb J, Kalantar-Zadeh K, et al. Prevention and treatment of protein energy wasting in chronic kidney disease patients: a consensus statement by the International Society of Renal Nutrition and Metabolism. *Kidney Int.* 2013;84(6):1096-1107.)

a higher dialysis clearance. Rather, increasing dwell volume without changing dwell time will help increase dialysis clearance.

High Transporters

High transporters have the highest rates of diffusive transport. Small solutes such as glucose, urea, and creatinine are transported quickly in these patients, leading to equilibration between dialysate small solute concentration and that of the blood relatively early in a dwell. As a result of rapid absorption of dialysate glucose, there is early dissipation of the osmotic gradient between dialysate and blood that is required for ultrafiltration to take place and so ultrafiltration ceases. Furthermore, there is a slow but continuous absorption of fluid via the peritoneal lymphatics. Thus a major clinical problem encountered by rapid transporters is suboptimal ultrafiltration, low drain volume, and inadequate solute clearance (see Fig. 31.6).

Some PD patients are high transporters at the start of dialysis, whereas others gradually become high transporters over increasing time on PD. A high peritoneal transport status is associated with a higher mortality in PD patients.[43-45,203-205]

Factors Contributing to More Adverse Outcomes in High Transporters

Several mechanisms have been proposed for the higher risk for mortality reported in high transporters, including fluid overload, chronic inflammation, increased protein loss through the peritoneum, and PEW.[206,207] Some cross-sectional analyses indicated that peritoneal transport characteristics, namely the D/P creatinine ratio, had an inverse relationship with serum albumin, independent of dialysis dose.[208] This may be explained by increased dialysate protein losses that may amount up to 15 g/day (generally, an average of 5 to 6 g of protein is lost in the dialysate per day in CAPD patients). The other possibility may relate to the chronic inflammation that is associated with high peritoneal transport status and that explains the associated hypoalbuminemia.[207] A 2006 meta-analysis included mainly studies of patients receiving CAPD, which is a less favorable modality for high transporters as a result of poor ultrafiltration volume and solute clearances. In a small study comparing CAPD patients who were low transporters with those who were high transporters, patients who were high transporters were more likely to be hypertensive and had more left ventricular hypertrophy.[209]

In theory, high transporters would do best with short dwell times (up to 3 hours per dwell). Thus high transporters fare best with APD or NIPD with 3 hours per dwell overnight when using standard glucose solution and then either have a long day dwell using icodextrin or a day dwell with a midday exchange when using standard glucose solutions. In contrast, low transporters would do best with prolonged dwells such as CAPD or CCPD with fewer overnight exchanges. Patients with low average or low transport may need to use larger PD fluid volumes, which increase clearance by maximizing contact surface area with the peritoneum. In practice, most patients could be prescribed either CAPD or APD. Previous observational studies did not demonstrate any significant difference in the overall survival for patients doing CAPD or APD.[210-212] Another analysis based on the Australia and New Zealand Registry suggested a better survival outcome for high transporters treated with APD versus CAPD.[213] Summarizing current available data, there is no conclusive evidence to suggest one modality is superior to the other and thus modality of PD should be individualized according to patients' need, peritoneal transporter characteristics, and RKF.

Acute Membrane Injury

Patients with acute peritonitis may develop acute peritoneal membrane dysfunction, resulting in reduced ultrafiltration volume and increased solute transport. This is usually the result of an increased effective surface and an increased vascular permeability. Usually, PET will not be conducted during or immediately after peritonitis because the acute membrane dysfunction will largely resolve after peritonitis.[214,215] However, in the acute phase, a short-term adjustment of the PD prescription is usually required to improve ultrafiltration—for example, by using more hypertonic glucose solution or by shortening the dwell time of an exchange.

Ultrafiltration Failure

UFF is classically defined as having a net ultrafiltration volume less than 400 mL with a standard 2 L 3.86% glucose solution during a 4-hour exchange.[27] In fact, any patient who requires three exchanges of 3.86% glucose PD solution to maintain dry weight is considered to have an inadequate ultrafiltration capacity.

UFF is classified into three types (Table 31.5). Type I UFF is the most common, in which equilibration across the membrane is so rapid that the osmotic gradient for glucose dissipates before adequate ultrafiltration has occurred. It is characterized by inadequate ultrafiltration and increased solute transport and generally has a more gradual onset. The prevalence of high transport status may increase with increasing time on PD. In some cases, temporary cessation of PD or resting the peritoneal membrane may allow remesothelialization and may transiently improve ultrafiltration capacity.[216] However, in some cases, encapsulating peritoneal sclerosis (EPS) may develop after switching to hemodialysis.[217]

According to some previous surveys, the cumulative incidence of UFF was 2.6% after 1 year on PD, rising to 9.5% after 2 years and to 30.9% after 6 years.[218] The cumulative increase in the incidence of high peritoneal transport status over time on PD has been suggested to be partly attributed to the long-standing exposure of the peritoneal membrane to glucose-based PD solutions. In particular, exposure to hypertonic glucose solution has been implicated as one of the key culprits. Pathologically, peritoneal membrane of PD patients had increased submesothelial fibrosis, vasculopathic changes, and neovascularization compared with healthy controls and

TABLE 31.5 Classification of Ultrafiltration Failure

Types	Characteristics
I	Inadequate ultrafiltration is caused by rapid solute transport, resulting in early dissipation of the osmotic gradient. Has been attributed to long-standing exposure of peritoneal membrane to glucose-based PD solutions or hypertonic glucose solutions, which resulted in submesothelial fibrosis, vasculopathic changes, and neovascularization of the peritoneum as well as an increase in the effective peritoneal surface area. Classically presents with a low drain volume in patient who has been on PD for some years. PET indicates a high D/P creatinine ratio.
II	Decrease in peritoneal transport of small solutes and water is caused by loss of peritoneal surface area. Characterized by a decrease in the osmotic conductance to glucose and an attenuation of sodium sieving. Usually occurs in the context of peritoneal adhesions secondary to severe peritonitis, encapsulating peritonitis or postoperative complications. Classically presents with a low drain volume and PET indicating a low D/P creatinine ratio.
III	Occurs when there is high lymphatic reabsorption of fluid from the peritoneal cavity that reduces ultrafiltration.

D/P, Dialysate to plasma; *PD*, peritoneal dialysis; *PET*, peritoneal equilibration test.

hemodialysis patients.[2] The neovascularization increases the effective peritoneal surface area, leading to more rapid peritoneal transport. In animal models of PD, glucose and GDPs of glucose solutions induced vascular endothelial growth factor (VEGF) expression, which in turn promoted vasculopathic changes and neovascularization of the peritoneal membrane through induction of nitric oxide. Treatment with neutralizing anti-VEGF monoclonal antibodies largely prevented the hyperglycemia-induced structural and functional microvascular alteration of the peritoneum and prevented deterioration of ultrafiltration in animal models of PD.[219,220]

Similarly, in human studies, patients who develop high peritoneal transport characteristics were noted to have more exposure to hypertonic glucose solutions for some years before its development, compared with other patients who maintained relatively stable transport characteristics. However, glucose exposure may not be the sole factor contributing to an increased peritoneal transport. There are some suggestions that patients who develop high peritoneal transport characteristics also had a faster decline in RKF.[221] However, a causal link cannot be determined based on the cross-sectional study design.

As reported in a longitudinal follow-up study, peritonitis may also partly influence the time course of small solute and solute-free water transport. Patients with previous peritonitis had an earlier and more pronounced increase in the mass transfer area coefficient for creatinine and glucose compared with the group with no peritonitis. A decrease in solute-free water transport and ultrafiltration rate occurred only in the peritonitis group. The decrease in ultrafiltration was evident after 1 year in patients with severe peritonitis. On the other hand, in long-term peritonitis-free PD patients, small solute transport decreased and ultrafiltration increased.[222,223] Systemic inflammation may also be associated with high peritoneal transport in patients receiving PD for more than 6 months.[224]

Type II UFF occurs as decrease a result of loss of peritoneal surface area, resulting in a decrease in peritoneal transport of small solutes and water. This is less common and usually occurs in the context of peritoneal adhesions secondary to severe peritonitis or after surgical complications. As a result of the peritoneal adhesions, the surface area and capacity for peritoneal transport for both solutes and water are substantially reduced. There is some suggestion that type II UFF may be a manifestation of EPS, although in early stages of EPS, a high rather than a low peritoneal transport is usually seen.[225] The diagnosis of EPS may be confirmed by a contrast-enhanced computed tomographic scan of the abdomen.[218]

Type III UFF occurs when lymphatic reabsorption of fluid from the peritoneal cavity is large enough to reduce ultrafiltration. Peritoneal fluid absorption occurs either by direct lymphatic absorption that occurs predominantly through the diaphragmatic stomata or by hydrostatic pressure into the anterior abdominal wall tissues. From there, peritoneal fluid is gradually reabsorbed by the lymphatics or into systemic capillaries. The total amount of fluid reabsorbed is approximated to be 60 to 120 mL/hour. The incidence of type III UFF is not known and is a diagnosis of exclusion, because peritoneal lymphatic flow is not measured in most PD centers. There is some preliminary suggestion that peritoneal lymphatic flow may increase with increasing time on PD.[226]

To best assess UFF, a modified PET using 3.86% glucose solution is preferred over 2.5% dextrose solution to maximize osmotic drive.[227] During the PET, the D/P sodium curve typically shows an initial fall because of the high ultrafiltration rate. Ultrafiltration is initially low in sodium concentration as a result of sodium sieving. Dialysate sodium concentration reduces, resulting in a fall in the D/P sodium ratio. With the cessation of ultrafiltration later in the dwell, dialysate sodium gradually equilibrates with that of plasma and the D/P sodium ratio gradually returns back to baseline. Absence of the initial fall in D/P sodium ratio is a feature of UFF and typically occurs in the early phase of EPS.[228]

CONCLUSIONS

There is an evolving concept to define adequate dialysis, or more preferably *optimal* dialysis, using a multidimensional measure that moves beyond urea and CrCl targets. Optimization of PD prescription also should be based on various other therapeutic targets, including ultrafiltration and volume control, nutrition status, uremic toxins removal, CKD-MBD control, blood pressure, left ventricular hypertrophy, and function as well as patient-centered outcomes. This multitargeted approach may be useful in improving clinical outcomes of PD patients.

RESIDUAL KIDNEY FUNCTION

Importance of Residual Kidney Function in Peritoneal Dialysis

The importance of RKF in clinical outcomes of PD patients was first recognized in the 1990s when Maiorca et al.[168] reported that in a prospective cohort of hemodialysis and PD patients every 1 mL/min higher residual GFR was associated with a 40% lower mortality risk in the overall cohort and a 50% lower mortality risk in the PD patients. Subsequent to this study, several other investigators reported a similar association between residual GFR and overall survival in other prospective PD cohorts. A reanalysis of data from the CANUSA study confirmed notable differences in the contribution of RKF and PD to the overall total small solute clearance in PD patients. The predictive power of total weekly small solute clearance for survival of PD patients was attributed to RKF but not to PD clearance. Every 5 L/week/1.73 m^2 higher residual GFR was associated with a 12% lower risk for mortality. However, no association was reported between the PD component of small solute clearance and survival of PD patients.[177] These data suggest that the contribution of these two components of small solute clearance cannot be considered equivalent.

Extending these observations in relation to hard outcomes, Wang et al.[229] reported an important inverse relationship between the degree of left ventricular hypertrophy and total

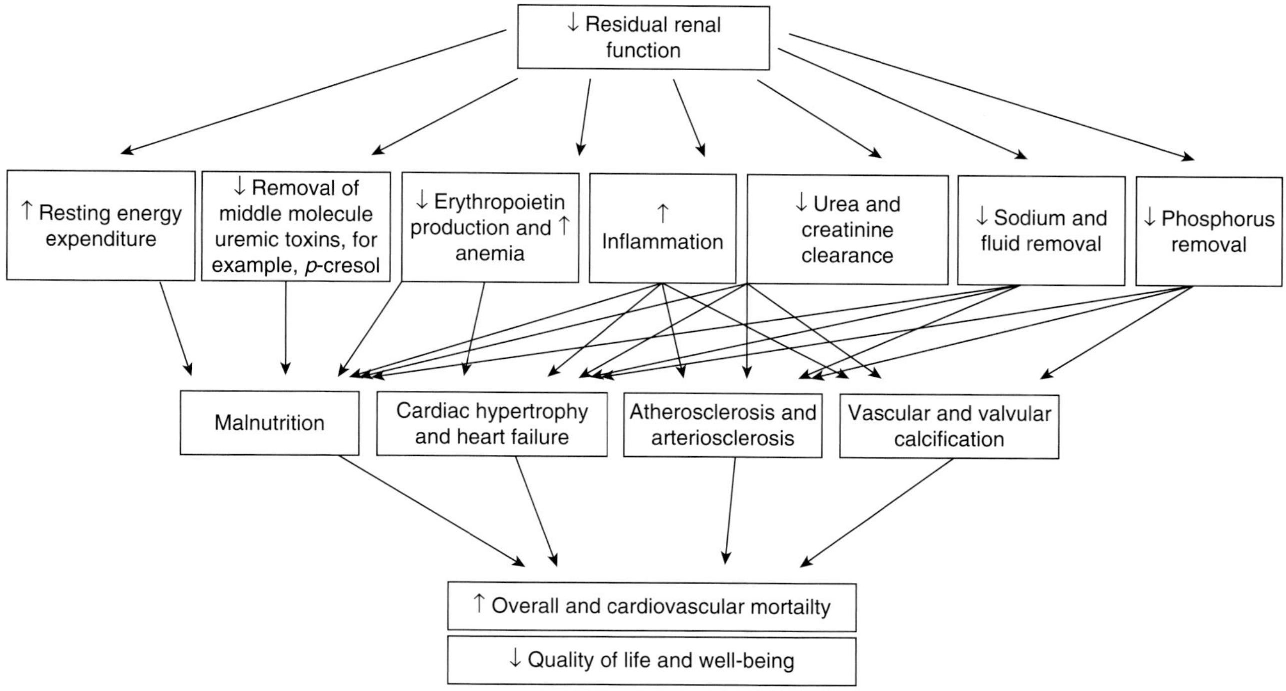

FIG. 31.11 Importance of residual kidney function in PD patients. (Reproduced with permission from Wang AY, Lai KN. The importance of residual renal function in dialysis patients. *Kidney Int.* 2006;69(10):1726-1732.)

small solute clearance and that this association was attributed to residual GFR but not to PD small solute clearance. Several factors have been suggested to explain the association between RKF and clinical outcomes of PD patients[230] (Fig. 31.11), one of which was related to extracellular volume overload. Konings et al.[231] found that loss of residual GFR was associated with extracellular volume overload as determined by bromide dilution in PD patients. In keeping with this early observation, a 2008 study[232] found that left ventricular filling pressure, estimated by echocardiography and tissue Doppler imaging–derived ratio of early diastolic transmitral flow velocity to early diastolic mitral annular velocity (E/Em), was inversely associated with residual GFR, independent of other clinical, biochemical, and echocardiographic factors. A higher left ventricular filling pressure as determined by E/Em ratio was predictive of a greater risk for mortality and cardiovascular events in PD patients.[232]

An increased inflammatory response also contributes to adverse clinical outcomes of PD patients and is in part attributed to the loss of RKF.[233] C-reactive protein and interleukin 6, prototype markers of inflammation, are well-recognized predictors of a higher mortality and cardiovascular events in PD patients.[47,233-236] Previous studies from Wang et al.[233,237] and other investigators found that PD patients with less residual GFR had more inflammation as denoted by different inflammatory parameters, including C-reactive protein, interleukin 6, and soluble vascular cell adhesion molecule 1. The loss of RKF together with more severe cardiac hypertrophy and more inflammation combined additively to increase the mortality and cardiovascular death risk for PD patients. Compared with patients who exhibited none of the risk factors, PD patients having all three risk factors had a nearly sevenfold higher all-cause mortality risk and more than fivefold higher cardiovascular death risk.[238]

Accumulation of protein-bound uremic retention solutes and middle molecules has been suggested as the other key factor linking loss of RKF to more adverse clinical outcomes of PD patients.[239] Higher circulating levels of uremic retention solutes such as free *p*-cresol and β_2 microglobulin were associated with higher risk for mortality in dialysis patients.[239,240] Accumulating evidence suggests that some of these uremic retention solutes, such as *p*-cresol sulfate, indoxyl sulfate, and *p*-cresol glucuronide, activate monocytes, macrophages, and endothelial cells that are pivotally involved in the process of atherosclerosis and mediated vascular injury by stimulating cross-talk between leukocyte and vascular endothelium.[241,242] Furthermore, RKF appears to have a substantially greater contribution compared with PD clearance to the overall clearance of protein-bound uremic retention solutes and middle molecules such as free *p*-cresol and indoxyl sulfate.[239,243,244] (Fig. 31.12). There are similar data from hemodialysis populations indicating that RKF contributes significantly to the clearance of β_2 microglobulin.[240] Thus the decrease in protein-bound uremic retention solutes and middle molecules clearance with decline in RKF may not be equivalently replaced by increasing PD.[243]

RKF also plays an important role in the CKD-MBD axis. Residual GFR was one of the most significant contributing factors to serum phosphorus control among those with preserved RKF, second only to nPNA. Its importance outweighed that contributed by PD clearance. Among anuric PD patients, PD clearance and nPNA were the most significant factor associated with serum phosphorus level.[245] In keeping

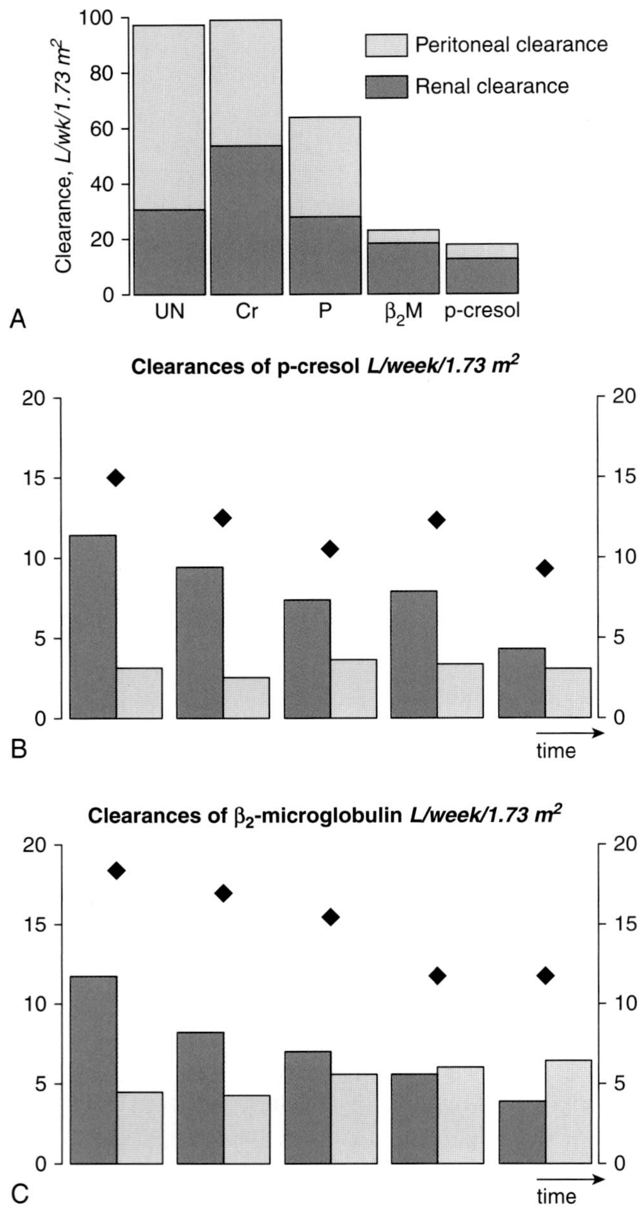

FIG. 31.12 Renal and peritoneal clearance of uremic retention solutes. (A) Important contribution of residual kidney function to middle molecular uremic toxins clearance (e.g., *p*-cresol sulfate and β_2 microglobulin [β_2M]) in PD patients. (B) Time course of renal *(gray bars)*, peritoneal *(white bars)*, and total clearances *(black diamonds)* (in liters per week per 1.73 m^2) of β_2M from visits 1 to 5 (*N* = 24). (C) Time course of renal *(gray bars)*, peritoneal *(white bars)*, and total clearances (in liters per week per 1.73 m^2) of *p*-cresol from visits 1 to 5 (*N* = 24). Median values are shown. (Reproduced with permission from Bammens B, Evenepoel P, Verbeke K, Vanrenterghem Y. Time profiles of peritoneal and renal clearances of different uremic solutes in incident peritoneal dialysis patients. *Am J Kidney Dis*. 2005;46(3):512-519.)

with these observations, a greater prevalence of valvular calcification was reported in anuric PD patients compared with those with preserved RKF and appeared to be contributed to both by an increased inflammatory response and worse calcium phosphorus control.[246] A combination of inflammatory and calcification markers further increased the long-term mortality and cardiovascular event risk in PD patients.[247] Loss of RKF also increased the prevalence of 25-hydroxyvitamin D deficiency in PD.[248] A previous meta-analysis[249] found that having a higher 25-hydroxyvitamin D level was associated with a better survival in patients with CKD. RKF was also associated with other parameters of CKD-MBD, such as fibroblast growth factor 23, which has also been found to be associated with mortality in dialysis patients.

RKF contributes significantly to the nutrition status of dialysis patients.[250] Bammens et al.[251] found that retention of middle molecule uremic solutes may explain uremic symptoms in dialysis patients. In PD patients, better preserved RKF but not PD clearance has been associated with a greater amount of dietary protein, energy, other macronutrient and micronutrients intake, and better nutrition status as determined by subjective global assessment.[191,192] On the other hand, loss of RKF was associated with increased catabolism in PD patients. This is evident by the strong, inverse, novel association between residual GFR and resting energy expenditure independent of other factors, including diabetes, cardiovascular disease, C-reactive protein, and serum albumin in PD patients. Having a better preserved RKF was associated with a lower resting energy expenditure, whereas PD patients who lost their RKF were associated with an increased resting energy expenditure.[252] In keeping with these data, PD patients who lost their RKF were also noted to have more muscle wasting as reflected by less handgrip strength.[186] Having less handgrip strength was associated with higher risk for mortality and cardiovascular death[186] and was found to be predictive of higher risk for heart failure in PD patients.[185]

In conclusion, having a better preserved RKF was associated with better small solute clearance as well as middle molecule uremic retention solute clearance, better extracellular volume control, less inflammation, better control of the CKD-MBD axis, better dietary intake profile, less muscle wasting, and less resting hypercatabolism in PD patients, thus explaining a better survival and cardiovascular outcome (see Fig. 31.9). Having a better preserved RKF was also noted to be associated with a better quality of life in PD patients.[253] Specifically, this included several dimensions of the Kidney Disease Quality of Life scale in PD patients: physical health, kidney disease issues, and patient satisfaction (unpublished observation of Wang et al.).

Decline of Residual Kidney Function

There have been some suggestions that PD may be associated with a slower rate of decline in RKF than hemodialysis.[254-257] The rates of decline in RKF on average may be 24% to 80% faster in hemodialysis than PD patients,[258] although there have also been studies that suggested similar rates of decline of RKF in PD and hemodialysis patients.[259,260] However, it is important to caution that these studies were all observational and not randomized. Notably, there were some suggestions that the rate of decline of RKF matters in dialysis patients. PD patients with faster rates of decline in RKF were associated with worse patient survival and technique survival.[261]

BOX 31.4 Potential Strategies Being Studied for Better Preservation of Residual Kidney Function

Avoid hypotension.
Avoid nephrotoxins and radiocontrast use.
Use low-GDP solutions (randomized trials and data suggest its use may keep RKF and urine volume better up to 24 months).
Use icodextrin (no conclusive data to suggest icodextrin use increases RKF loss).
Use angiotensin-converting enzyme inhibitors or angiotensin receptor blockers (only two very small randomized trials available).
Use oral N-acetylcysteine (only two pilot single-arm small studies available).
Supplement with a low-protein diet (only one small randomized controlled trial available).
Use diuretics (no data to suggest their use preserves RKF better).
Consider PD vs. APD (no randomized studies, only observational studies; no conclusive data to suggest any difference in RKF decline between PD vs. APD).

APD, automated peritoneal dialysis; *GDP*, glucose degradation products; *PD*, peritoneal dialysis; *RKF*, residual kidney function.

According to a marginal structural model analysis from the NECOSAD study group, dialysis patients who completely lost their RKF had a higher mortality risk compared with those who retained some degree of RKF.[262] The importance of RKF and its rate of decline were further confirmed in a recent large nationally representative cohort of incident hemodialysis patients from Obi et al.[263] reporting that the annual change in residual renal Kt/V and urine volume were associated with all-cause mortality. Patients with better preserved residual Kt/V and urine volume at 1 year had significantly lower hazards for mortality.

How Can We Better Preserve Residual Kidney Function in Peritoneal Dialysis Patients?

Box 31.4 summarizes potential therapeutic strategies that may be useful to better preserve RKF in PD patients.

It is generally recognized that avoiding overdehydration and hypotensive episodes may be important in preserving RKF in dialysis patients. As found in the analysis based on the NECOSAD cohort, having hypotensive or dehydration episodes was associated with a more rapid decline in residual GFR at the initial 3-month period of dialysis in both hemodialysis and PD patients, and that was independent of other confounding factors such as age, gender, background kidney disease, comorbidity, and dialysis urea clearance.[259] On the other hand, there are also data to suggest that having extracellular volume overload did not help preserve RKF better in PD patients. In an earlier analysis based on the United States Renal Data System Dialysis Morbidity and Mortality Study Wave 2, factors that were found to hasten the loss of RKF included female gender, nonwhite race, background diabetes, and history of heart failure. Use of converting enzyme inhibitors and calcium channel blockers as well as having a higher baseline residual GFR was associated with a lower risk for losing RKF in PD patients.[264] Another, more observational analysis based on the International Pediatric PD Network found that background glomerulonephritis, use of icodextrin, and the ultrafiltration volume were associated with greater hazards of losing RKF, whereas use of diuretics may be associated with a lower hazard of losing RKF.[265]

Biocompatible low-GDP solutions. The effects of biocompatible low-GDP solution on RKF have been examined in several RCTs (detailed earlier in Biocompatible Peritoneal Dialysis Solutions), the largest of which is the balANZ trial. Although the primary endpoint of this trial, rate of decline in RKF, was negative, the biocompatible group had a significantly longer time to anuria ($P = 0.009$) than the standard glucose solution group.[118] In keeping with the findings from the balANZ trial, several other RCTs also reported that neutral pH, low-GDP solution attenuated the decline of RKF in incident PD patients.[116,117,120,122] Some other controlled trials did not reproduce similar results,[112,114,115] which may be explained by their rather short study durations of only up to 12 months and relatively small sample sizes.

The findings from these randomized trials were summarized in two systematic reviews[80,124-127] (see Fig. 31.2). Essentially, the systematic reviews suggested that use of neutral pH, low-GDP solutions resulted in better preservation of RKF and greater urine volumes. In the Cochrane review, the benefit of low-GDP solutions in preserving RKF was found most significantly between 12 to 23 months ($P = 0.0005$) but also from 24 months and beyond, though less significantly ($P = 0.04$). Similarly, low-GDP solutions also had significant benefit in preserving urine volume between 12 to 23 months ($P = 0.0005$) and from 24 months and beyond ($P = 0.04$).[80] More recently, the Trio study of 67 randomly assigned incident PD patients also found significantly slower decline in RKF in the lactate-buffered low-GDP solution (Gambrosol Trio) group compared with the standard glucose PD solution group.[128] Based on the cumulative evidence, the ISPD Adult Cardiovascular and Metabolic Guidelines made the recommendation that neutral pH, low-GDP solutions be considered for better preservation of RKF if used for 12 months or more. The grading of the recommendation was 2B.[24]

Renin-angiotensin system blockers. The efficacy of angiotensin-converting enzyme inhibitors or angiotensin receptor blockers in preserving RKF were examined in two randomized open-label trials. In the RCT by Li et al.,[266] 60 PD patients were studied. Residual GFR declined by 2.07 ± 1.12 with ramipril 5 mg daily versus 3.00 ± 1.86 mL/min/1.73 m^2 in the control group over a 12-month period ($P = 0.03$). In the study by Suzuki et al.,[267] 34 PD patients were randomly assigned to either valsartan or no valsartan. Valsartan 40 to 80 mg daily was associated with a change in residual GFR from 3.2 ± 0.3 to 4.3 ± 0.7 mL/min/1.73 m^2, whereas the control group had a change in residual GFR from 5.9 ± 0.5 to 2.8 ± 0.4 mL/min/1.73 m^2 ($P < 0.01$) over a treatment period of 24 months. It is important to caution that both studies were small and from a single center. Thus these findings can only be regarded as preliminary and need to be confirmed in larger, adequately powered studies.

Ketoacid-supplemented low-protein diet. There is some preliminary suggestion that a ketoacid-supplemented low-protein diet may be useful in preserving RKF in PD patients. In a small RCT conducted by Jiang et al.,[268] 60 PD patients were randomly assigned to a high-protein diet (1.0 to 1.2 g/kg/day protein diet), low-protein diet (0.6 to 0.8 g/kg/day protein diet), or ketoacid-supplemented low-protein diet (0.6 to 0.8 g/kg/day). Over a treatment period of 12 months, the ketoacid-supplemented low-protein diet group had significantly better preserved residual GFR and urine volume compared with the other two groups.[268] These interesting preliminary findings warrant further confirmation in larger RCTs.

N-acetylcysteine. Two small single-arm pilot studies, one in PD and one in hemodialysis patients, suggested that oral N-acetylcysteine 1200 mg twice daily for 2 to 4 weeks may be useful in increasing urine volume and residual GFR.[269,270] These very preliminary findings need further evaluation in a longer-term RCT.

Diuretics. The role of diuretics is mainly to increase urine volume and sodium excretion and minimize use of hypertonic PD glucose solutions without preserving RKF in PD patients. A previous prospective RCT in 61 PD patients found that patients randomly assigned to receive furosemide 250 mg daily had higher urine volumes at 6 and 12 months than those randomly assigned to no furosemide. However, both urea and CrCl declined at a constant rate in both groups.[271]

Aminoglycosides. Given the nephrotoxicity of aminoglycosides, use of aminoglycosides should be cautioned in PD patients to minimize loss of RKF, although several studies reported no effect of aminoglycosides use on RKF decline.[272] In a small RCT in which 50 PD patients with preserved RKF >1 mL/min/1.73 m^2 were randomly assigned to receive cefazolin and netilmicin versus cefazolin and ceftazidime, residual GFR had transient reduction by day 14 but returned back to baseline by day 42 with no significant difference between the two groups.[273]

Iodinated radiocontrast. Because iodinated radiocontrast agents can cause acute tubular necrosis and acute kidney injury, its use is generally cautioned in PD patients because it may jeopardize RKF. Several observational studies reported no significant loss of RKF after radiocontrast agent administration. However, none of these studies were randomized or controlled.[274,275] Thus one should cautiously weigh the risks versus benefits before subjecting PD patients to any contrast studies.

PD modality. There has been some suggestion that APD might be associated with a more rapid decline in RKF than CAPD.[276,277] However, other studies did not find any significant effect of PD modality on RKF loss in PD patients.[278-280] So far, none of the studies were RCTs and thus it remains inconclusive whether the modality of PD, namely APD versus a continuous form of PD, may influence the decline of RKF differentially. Further confirmatory studies are required to answer this question.

Monitoring of RKF

The 2015 ISPD guideline recommended that monitoring of RKF be performed at least once every 6 months in PD patients with urine output.[24]

CONCLUSION

RKF contributes significantly to uremic toxins clearance and various metabolic and hemodynamic controls in PD patients and is not equivalent to that contributed by PD. Regular interval monitoring of RKF is essential in all patients who still have urine. Use of biocompatible low-GDP solutions may better preserve urine volume and RKF up to 24 months according to a systematic analysis.

A full list of references is available at www.expertconsult.com.

32

Peritoneal Dialysis-Related Infections

Cheuk-Chun Szeto, MD, FRCP, and Philip Kam-Tao Li, MD, FRCP, FACP

OUTLINE

Peritoneal dialysis (PD)-related infection is a broad term that encompasses PD-related peritonitis and catheter-related infections (CRIs), and the latter is used as a collective term to describe exit-site infection (ESI) and tunnel infection. PD-related infections are important complications of PD and could lead to serious consequences, including catheter loss,[1,2] transfer to hemodialysis, hospitalization, and death.[3,4] Peritonitis is the leading cause of technique failure in PD patients.[5,6] Although the mortality of a peritonitis episode is <5%, peritonitis is the major contributing cause of death in >15% of PD patients.[7,8]

Every PD unit should monitor, at least on a yearly basis, the incidence of peritonitis and CRIs.[9,10] The latest guideline published by the International Society for Peritoneal Dialysis (ISPD) suggests that rates of peritonitis and CRIs should be reported as the number of episodes per patient-year[9,10] rather than as number of patient-month per episode, which was commonly used in the past. There is a substantial variation in the peritonitis rate reported by different countries or even different centers within the same country.[11-13] However, the overall peritonitis rate should be no more than 0.5 episodes per year at risk.[9]

PERITONEAL DIALYSIS-RELATED PERITONITIS

Pathogenesis

PD-related peritonitis could be caused by touch contamination, catheter-related problems, bowel pathology, gynecological disease, or systemic bacteremia. The common microbiological causes of PD-related peritonitis are summarized in Table 32.1. Despite the advances in PD system connectology, touch contamination at the time of the PD exchange remains a common cause of peritonitis.[1,14] Organisms that are commonly grown from specimens in contamination-related peritonitis are coagulase-negative staphylococcal species (CNSS) and diphtheroids (*Corynebacterium* species).[15-17] Nasal carriers of *Staphylococcis aureus* often have the same bacteria on their hands and at the exit sites, which can lead to peritonitis through either touch contamination or CRI. Organisms found in the oral cavity, such as *Streptococcus* species, may cause peritonitis by droplet spread or transient bacteremia (e.g., after a dental procedure).

Approximately 15% to 20% of peritonitis episodes, especially those due to *S. aureus* or *Pseudomonas aeruginosa,* are caused by catheter infection.[1,18] ESIs can spread to involve the catheter tunnel and then the peritoneum.[18,19] Such infections often are refractory or relapsing.[20] A warm and humid climate may favor the accumulation of sweat and dirt around the catheter exit site, and therefore the growth and colonization of bacteria, resulting in a seasonal variation in the incidence of PD-related peritonitis that peaks in the months that are hot and humid.[21,22]

Many bacteria can form biofilm on the walls of catheters. Bacteria within the slime layer of biofilm are protected from host defense and antibiotics.[23] Refractory or relapsing peritonitis episodes often are caused by the release of planktonic bacteria from the biofilm.[20,24,25] However, biofilm also can be found in asymptomatic PD patients without peritonitis.[26]

Gram-negative bacteria that cause PD-related peritonitis are generally considered to originate from the bowel.[17] Most of these cases are presumably caused by the transmural movement of bacteria rather than perforation. This phenomenon is similar to the scenario of spontaneous bacterial peritonitis in patients with liver cirrhosis.[27,28] Uremia per se is associated with impaired intestinal barrier function to macromolecules, bacterial fragments,[29,30] and possibly bacteria.[31] Constipation,[32] diarrhea,[33,34] and

TABLE 32.1 Microbiological Causes of Peritonitis

Bacteria, %	80
Gram-positive organisms	40
Gram-negative organisms	30
Polymicrobial	10
Mycobacterium species, %	1
Fungus, %	2.5
Culture negative, %	15

diverticular disease may further increase the risk for such happening. Gastric acid inhibitors have been reported to be associated with gram-negative peritonitis.[35] Surgical diseases of intraabdominal organs also may result in enteric peritonitis.[36,37] Traditionally, polymicrobial peritonitis is believed to be caused by the perforation of internal viscera, and surgical exploration often is recommended.[38,39] Recent reports show that many patients with PD-related polymicrobial peritonitis do not have overt surgical pathology in the abdomen and response to antibiotic therapy alone often is satisfactory.[40,41]

Peritonitis may follow colonoscopy with polypectomy,[37] hysteroscopy,[42] endoscopy with sclerotherapy,[43] and dental procedures.[44] Peritonitis after dental procedures is most likely related to transient bacteremia. Vaginal leak of dialysate,[45] the use of intrauterine devices,[46] and endometrial biopsy[47] are other recognized contributing factors of PD-related peritonitis. Because of the risk for peritonitis related to such procedures, antibiotic prophylaxis administered before any such procedure is necessary. Antibiotic prophylaxis should be given before colonoscopy and invasive gynecological procedures.[9]

Host Defense Mechanisms of the Peritoneal Cavity

Uremia per se causes a wide range of defects in the immunological defense against infection, which is beyond the scope of this chapter. Both humoral and cellular factors participate in the local peritoneal defense processes against peritonitis.[48] Under physiological circumstances, bacteria entering the peritoneal cavity are digested by resident peritoneal macrophages and neutrophils. Individual variation in the phagocyte function may partly account for interindividual variation in the risk for peritonitis.[49]

Humoral Immunity

The concentrations of immunoglobulin G (IgG) and complement in normal peritoneal fluid are similar to serum. In PD effluent, however, these values are reduced by 100- to 1000-fold,[50,51] even after several hours of dwell time. This dilutional effect severely compromises the humoral immunity within the peritoneal cavity. An inverse relationship between the frequency of PD-related peritonitis and peritoneal opsonic activity or IgG concentration has been reported.[52]

For mechanisms that are not entirely clear, the opsonic activity of spent dialysate against gram-negative bacteria is substantially lower than that against gram-positive bacteria.[52] This may partly account for the greater clinical severity of gram-negative peritonitis. In addition to complement, fibronectin has opsonic activity against gram-positive organisms.[53] Low fibronectin concentrations in spent dialysate is a risk factor of PD-related peritonitis.[50]

Cellular Immunity

The leukocyte count in PD effluent is 100- to 1000-fold less than in normal peritoneal fluid.[54] Macrophage is the predominant cell type in noninfected spent dialysate; lymphocyte percentages vary between 2% and 84%, and polymorphonuclear leukocytes (PMNs) are usually 5% to 10%.[55] However, baseline peritoneal leukocyte count is not associated with the risk for PD peritonitis.[55] When there is peritonitis, neutrophils and macrophages quickly migrate from the systemic circulation and interstitial matrix into the peritoneal cavity.

Lymphocytes and cell-mediated cytotoxicity do not play a significant role in the defense against bacterial peritonitis. On the other hand, resident peritoneal macrophages constitute the first line of defense against bacterial invasion. Peritoneal macrophages probably originate from blood monocytes, and their phagocytic and bacteria-killing capacity from PD patients is normal when incubated in culture media.[48] However, the oxidative metabolism of macrophages is reduced in dialysis solution[54] or after repeated peritonitis episodes.[51] PMN from PD patients exhibit decreased binding of C5a, decreased chemotaxis, and impaired opsonic activity.[54]

Mesothelial cells along the peritoneal membrane also play important roles in the local defense against peritonitis.[56] The interaction between mesothelial cells and peritoneal macrophages early in the course of peritonitis occurs via cell–cell interaction and secretion of various inflammatory mediators.[56]

Effects of Peritoneal Dialysis Solutions on Peritoneal Defense

The effects of commercial PD solutions on peritoneal defense are related to dilution, high osmolality, low pH, lactate, and heat sterilization of the dialysate. In addition to the dilutional effects on intraperitoneal (IP) immunoglobulin and complement levels, decreased density of peritoneal macrophages reduces the phagocyte-bacterium encounter and thus bacterial killing.[54] The high osmolality and low pH of dialysis solution suppress peritoneal PMN and macrophage functions.[57] Although dialysate pH rises to physiological levels within 30 minutes of infusion, the period of low pH coincides with that of a high risk for bacterial entry. Lactate in dialysis solution may have independent adverse effects on peritoneal defense.[58] Some studies showed that biocompatible PD solutions with normal pH and bicarbonate-buffer dialysis solution may reduce the risk for peritonitis.[59,60] However, in vitro PMN function after incubation in bicarbonate-based dialysis solution also is impaired.[61] A metaanalysis of six randomized controlled trials (RCTs) concluded that the use of neutral pH or bicarbonate-buffered PD solutions had no definite effect on the rate of peritonitis.[62] The effect of glucose polymer-based or other novel PD solutions on leukocyte function has not been well studied.

Presentation

Patients with peritonitis typically present with cloudy dialysis effluent and abdominal pain.[63] Other common symptoms at presentation include diarrhea, vomiting, chills, and reduction in PD outflow. Although theoretically possible, abdominal pain with clear PD effluent seldom indicates peritonitis. A small but non-negligible group of patients present with cloudy PD effluent but no abdominal pain. The severity of illness varies widely and partly depends on the etiological microorganism.[64] For example, *S. epidermidis* or diphtheroids often cause minimal abdominal pain. On the other hand, virulent organisms such as *S. aureus, P. aeruginosa,* and fungi often cause severe abdominal pain and, not uncommonly, diarrhea. Fever and hypotension indicate systemic sepsis, bacteremia, and severe peritonitis.[64,65]

Diagnosis

Most practicing nephrologists can diagnose PD-related peritonitis on clinical grounds. Nonetheless, a standard set of diagnostic criteria has been designed to facilitate dialysis unit audit and assist in making the diagnosis by nonspecialists. The latest ISPD guideline states that peritonitis should be diagnosed when at least two of the following are present: (1) clinical features consistent with peritonitis (i.e., abdominal pain and/or cloudy dialysis effluent); (2) dialysis effluent white cell count >100/μL or $>0.1 \times 10^9$/L (after a dwell time of ≥2 hours), with >50% PMN; and (3) positive dialysis effluent culture.[9] For patients receiving machine-assisted PD with rapid cycles, the PD effluent white blood cell (WBC) count may be <100/μL during peritonitis. In this circumstance, one should rely on the differential WBC count, and a PMN >50% is indicative of peritonitis.

The differential diagnosis for infectious peritonitis includes chemical peritonitis, peritoneal eosinophilia, hemoperitoneum, pancreatitis, chylous effluent, and malignancy.[66] Peritoneal eosinophilia usually occurs early in the course of PD, resolves spontaneously after 2 to 6 weeks, and is usually not associated with infection.[67] The mechanism is believed to be allergic reaction to the plasticizers on the dialysis tubing. IP administration of amphotericin[68] can cause chemical peritonitis. Sterile chemical peritonitis also has been reported after icodextrin PD solution.[69] The episodes are characterized by mild abdominal discomfort, dialysate leukocytosis with a predominance of macrophages, and the absence of systemic symptoms. PD patients who develop pancreatitis may present with abdominal pain and cloudy dialysis effluent. Typically, culture of the effluent yields no bacterial growth, and the effluent amylase level is >100 U/L.[70] Chylous ascites is a rare cause of sterile cloudy effluent, and the effluent WBC count is normal.[71] Patients with intraabdominal malignancy may have cloudy effluent, and the diagnosis can be established by cytological evaluation.[72]

Treatment of Peritonitis

Initial Evaluation

PD patients presenting with cloudy effluent should be presumed to have peritonitis and should be treated as such until the diagnosis can be confirmed or excluded.[9] In a patient presenting with possible peritonitis, evaluation should include questioning about possible touch contamination, adherence to sterile exchange technique, recent procedures that may lead to peritonitis, and change in bowel habits. A formal root-cause analysis is valuable in preventing further episodes of peritonitis, but it can be performed after the patient improves with treatment. The physician should review any history of recent peritonitis episode so as to determine the possibility of relapsing episode or antibiotic resistance. In addition to the usual physical examination, one must carefully search for coexisting ESI or tunnel infection. PD effluent should be tested for WBC count, differential, and Gram stain and should be cultured whenever peritonitis is suspected.[9] Blood-culture bottle is the preferred technique for bacterial culture of PD effluent.[9] At present, there is insufficient evidence to support the use of novel laboratory and molecular techniques for the diagnosis of peritonitis.[9]

Empirical Therapy

As just emphasized, PD patients presenting with cloudy effluent should be presumed to have peritonitis, and empirical antibiotic therapy should be initiated as soon as possible after appropriate microbiological specimens have been obtained.[9] Many patients with PD-related peritonitis could be managed on an outpatient basis. The decision to hospitalize a patient depends on clinical factors (e.g., severity of signs and symptoms) as well as practical ones (e.g., feasibility of administering IP antibiotics).

The recommended treatment regimen has been described in detail by the latest ISPD guideline.[9] In essence, empirical antibiotic regimens should be center-specific and cover both gram-positive and gram-negative organisms.[9] Gram-positive organisms could be covered by vancomycin or a first-generation cephalosporin, whereas gram-negative organisms could be covered by a third-generation cephalosporin or an aminoglycoside.[9]

For gram-positive coverage, a metaanalysis showed that vancomycin-based regimens result in a higher complete cure rate than first-generation cephalosporin, but there is no difference in the rate of primary treatment failure, relapse, or catheter removal.[73] Theoretical concern of inducing vancomycin resistance would favor the use of first-generation cephalosporin, except for PD units that have a high rate of methicillin-resistant organisms. For the coverage of gram-negative organisms, previous studies showed that aminoglycosides and third- or fourth-generation cephalosporins are equally effective[74,75] Aminoglycosides are inexpensive, and there is no evidence that short courses of aminoglycosides accelerate the loss of residual renal function.[76,77] However, repeated or prolonged aminoglycoside treatment (>3 weeks) is associated with a high incidence of vestibular and oto-toxicity and should be avoided.[78] Table 32.2 summarizes the algorithm

TABLE 32.2 Algorithm of the Initial Assessment and Therapy for Peritoneal Dialysis-Related Peritonitis

Goal	Steps	
Evaluation	Clinical evaluation; examine exit site and catheter tunnel.	
	Collect dialysis effluent for cell count, differential count, Gram stain, and bacterial culture.	
Treatment	Start intraperitoneal antibiotics as soon as possible	
	Allow to dwell for at least 6 h	
	Empirical gram-positive and gram-negative coverage, based on patient history and center sensitivity patterns	
	Gram-positive coverage: first-generation cephalosporin or vancomycin	Gram-negative coverage: third-generation cephalosporin or aminoglycoside
Adjunctive measures	Consider adjuvant treatment: pain control; IP heparin; antifungal prophylaxis.	
	Education and assess IP injection technique.	
	Ensure follow-up arrangements.	

IP, Intraperitoneal.
Adapted from Li PK, Szeto CC, Piraino B, et al. ISPD peritonitis recommendations: 2016 update on prevention and treatment. *Perit Dial Int.* 2016;36:481-508.

BOX 32.1 Empirical Initial Therapy for Peritoneal Dialysis-Related Peritonitis

Gram-positive coverage
- Cefazolin
  - intermittent: 15–20 mg/kg IP daily
  - continuous: 500 mg/L IP loading, 125 mg/L IP maintenance
  - APD: 20 mg/kg IP daily in long day dwell
- Vancomycin
  - intermittent: 15–30 mg/kg IP every 5–7 d
  - APD: as above, in long day dwell

Gram-negative coverage
- Ceftazidime
  - continuous: 500 mg/L IP loading, 125 mg/L IP maintenance
  - APD: 1000–1500 mg IP daily in long day dwell
- Aminoglycoside (gentamicin/netilmicin/tobramycin)
  - intermittent: 0.6 mg/kg IP daily
  - APD: as above, in long day dwell

APD, Automated peritoneal dialysis; *IP*, intraperitoneal.
Adapted from Li PK, Szeto CC, Piraino B, et al. ISPD peritonitis recommendations: 2016 update on prevention and treatment. *Perit Dial Int.* 2016;36:481-508.

for the initial assessment and empirical antibiotic therapy of PD-related peritonitis. Suitable agents and dosages are listed in Box 32.1. In general, IP antibiotics are the preferred route of administration unless the patient has features of systemic sepsis.[9]

Practical Aspects of Antibiotic Therapy

For many antibiotics, IP regimen can be given as continuous (i.e., in each exchange) or intermittent dosing (i.e., once daily to once every few days). Because of its concentration-dependent bactericidal effect, IP aminoglycoside should preferably be administered as daily intermittent dosing.[9] There is no evidence that monitoring aminoglycoside levels mitigates toxicity risk or enhances efficacy.[79] IP vancomycin could be administered intermittently, usually at a dosing interval of every 4 to 5 days.[9] Redosing is probably appropriate to keep serum vancomycin levels >15 μg/mL.[79]

For cephalosporins, basic pharmacological principles would favor continuous dosing because this group of agent kills bacteria in a time-dependent manner. However, there are few data to support that continuous dosing is more efficacious than intermittent dosing. Moreover, intermittent dosing regimens are valuable in some situations. For example, some elderly or debilitated patients would require helpers or healthcare visitors for the administration of IP antibiotics, and intermittent dosage may be the only practical solution when the injection could only be performed once or twice daily and drug stability in PD solution is a concern.

Intermittent dosage is also the only possible means of administering antibiotics for patients treated with machine-assisted PD. In this case, the intermittent IP dosing could be given in the day dwell.[9] Because extrapolation of pharmacokinetic data from continuous ambulatory peritoneal dialysis (CAPD) to machine-assisted PD may result in significant underdosing when antibiotics are given IP intermittently, a higher daily dose often is required.[9] Alternatively, patients on machine-assisted PD who develop peritonitis may temporarily switch to CAPD.[9] However, it is not always practical to switch because patients may not be familiar with the exchange technique, and the supplies for CAPD may not be immediately available.

Adjuvant Therapy

Extensive rapid-cycle peritoneal lavage during the first 24 hours of peritonitis does not affect the clinical outcome and is not advisable for routine clinical use.[80] Patients with cloudy PD effluent may benefit from the addition of IP heparin (e.g., 500 units/L) to prevent occlusion of the catheter by fibrin. Antifungal prophylaxis, preferably by oral nystatin, should be given during antibiotic therapy to prevent secondary fungal peritonitis.[9,81] The benefit of IP urokinase for the treatment of relapsing or refractory peritonitis has not been confirmed.[82,83]

TABLE 32.3 **Treatment Regimen for Gram-Positive Peritonitis**

Enterococcus	*Staphylococcus aureus*	Coagulase-Negative *Staphylococcus*
At 24–48 h		
• Stop cephalosporins • Start IP vancomycin • Consider adding IP aminoglycoside	• Stop ceftazidime or aminoglycoside, continue IP cefazolin • Consider adding oral rifampin 450–600 mg/d for 5–7 d • If methicillin resistant or clinically not responding, change to IP vancomycin	• Stop ceftazidime or aminoglycoside, continue IP cefazolin • If methicillin resistant or clinically not responding, change to IP vancomycin
Duration of Therapy		
• 21 d	• 21 d	• 14 d

IP, Intraperitoneal.
Adapted from Li PK, Szeto CC, Piraino B, et al. ISPD peritonitis recommendations: 2016 update on prevention and treatment. *Perit Dial Int.* 2016;36:481-508.

Because of the systemic inflammatory response and increased peritoneal protein loss, protein-energy wasting develops quickly during PD peritonitis. During peritonitis, ultrafiltration (UF) by PD is usually reduced. Protein-energy wasting should be screened for and appropriate supplement should be considered in patients with prolonged peritoneal inflammation. In patients with diabetes, glycemic control may worsen during peritonitis because of the rapid glucose absorption. Blood glucose monitoring with appropriate adjustments of insulin dosage may be needed. Fluid overload is a frequent complication, and the usual PD regimen may need to be adjusted according to the clinical condition. A recent study suggested that the use of icodextrin solution during acute peritonitis resulted in better UF and fluid control in CAPD patients.[84]

Therapy for Specific Organisms

Gram-Positive Microorganisms. The treatment for gram-positive peritonitis is outlined in Table 32.3. Peritonitis episodes due to CNSS, *S. aureus, Streptococcus,* and *Enterococcus* species are distinctly different in presentation, pathogenesis, and outcome. Treatment must therefore be individualized.

Coagulase-Negative Staphylococcal Species

Peritonitis episodes caused by CNSS should be treated with IP first-generation cephalosporins or vancomycin, according to the antimicrobial susceptibility, for 2 weeks.[9] These episodes often are secondary to touch contamination. Exchange technique of the patient and adherence to aseptic technique should be checked. Nowadays, some centers have very high prevalence of methicillin resistance,[85] and vancomycin may need to be considered as empirical therapy. On the other hand, vancomycin may be slightly less effective than first-generation cephalosporins when the bacteria are methicillin-sensitive. Relapsing coagulase-negative staphylococcus peritonitis suggests colonization of the PD catheter with biofilm, and catheter removal should be considered. The benefit of IP urokinase and oral rifampicin for the prevention of relapsing episode remains controversial.[86]

Staphylococcus aureus

Peritonitis episodes caused by *S. aureus* should be treated with effective antibiotics for 3 weeks.[9] These episodes often are secondary to ESIs or tunnel infections, which should be carefully searched for. Ultrasound study of the catheter tunnel may help to diagnose occult tunnel infections and identify a subgroup of patients who are likely to require catheter removal. Screening for nasal *S. aureus* carrier also should be considered, especially in patients with relapsing or repeated peritonitis episodes caused by *S. aureus.*

Two retrospective studies found that the initial empiric antibiotic choice between vancomycin and cefazolin had similar clinical outcomes.[87,88] One study showed that the use of adjuvant rifampicin for 5 to 7 days may reduce the risk for relapsing or repeat *S. aureus* peritonitis.[87] However, rifampicin is a potent liver enzyme inducer and interaction with other concomitant medications may be problematic. For patients with concomitant *S. aureus* ESI or catheter tunnel infection, catheter removal should be considered.

Streptococcal Species

Streptococci frequently originate from the mouth,[89] although *Streptococcus bovis* typically comes from the colon.[90] Peritonitis episodes caused by streptococci usually respond well to IP cefazolin or vancomycin treatment.[81,89] Patients often are advised to wear a face mask during PD exchange to prevent further episodes of streptococcal peritonitis, but there is no published evidence to support this practice.

Enterococcus Species

Peritonitis episodes caused by *Enterococcus* species are usually severe. In about half of the cases of enterococcal peritonitis, other coexisting organisms could be isolated, and intraabdominal pathology must be considered. Since enterococcal species have intrinsic resistance to cephalosporins, and ampicillin may be unstable in PD solution, enterococcal peritonitis should be treated with IP vancomycin for at least 3 weeks.[9] IP aminoglycoside could be added as adjunct for severe cases.[9] Treatment of peritonitis episodes caused by vancomycin-resistant enterococcus should be individualized. Linezolid, quinupristin/dalfopristin, daptomycin, or teicoplanin are all valid options.

Gram-Negative Organisms. Peritonitis due to gram-negative organisms often is associated with fever, nausea, vomiting, and abdominal pain. The treatment of gram-negative peritonitis is summarized in Table 32.4. Satisfactory therapeutic responses have been reported with either IP aminoglycoside or ceftazidime.[91] Other third- or fourth-generation cephalosporins are

TABLE 32.4 Treatment Regimen for Gram-Negative Peritonitis

Single Gram-Negative Organism	*Pseudomonas* Species	Multiple Gram-Negative or Anaerobes
At 24–48 h		
• Stop cefazolin or vancomycin • Continue IP ceftazidime or aminoglycoside • Adjust antibiotics according to sensitivity	• Continue ceftazidime or aminoglycoside • Treat with both IP ceftazidime and IP aminoglycoside • Adjust antibiotics according to sensitivity	• Stop cefazolin • Continue IP ceftazidime or aminoglycoside • Start IP vancomycin and oral or intravenous metronidazole • Consider surgical evaluation
Duration of Therapy		
• 14–21 d	• 21 d	• 21 d

IP, Intraperitoneal.
Adapted from Li PK, Szeto CC, Piraino B, et al. ISPD peritonitis recommendations: 2016 update on prevention and treatment. *Perit Dial Int.* 2016;36:481-508.

probably equally effective. Alternatively, fluoroquinolones, such as levofloxacin, ciprofloxacin, and moxifloxacin, have the advantage of good oral bioavailability, and can be used with acceptable result.[92]

Pseudomonas Species

Recent antibiotic therapy is the major risk factor of *Pseudomonas* peritonitis.[93] Patients with immunosuppression are also at higher risk for *Pseudomonas* peritonitis.[94] *Pseudomonas* peritonitis should be treated with two antibiotics (e.g., IP gentamicin or oral ciprofloxacin with IP ceftazidime or cefepime) for 3 weeks.[9] When there is concomitant ESI or tunnel infection, catheter removal is usually necessary. In this circumstance, simultaneous removal and reinsertion of a new PD catheter (with a new tunnel and exit site) may avoid the need of temporary hemodialysis and often is successful in preventing further relapsing episodes.

Other Gram-Negative Bacteria

Single-organism gram-negative peritonitis may be secondary to touch contamination, ESI, or transmural migration from constipation or colitis. In general, non-*Pseudomonas* gram-negative peritonitis should be treated with effective antibiotics for at least 3 weeks.[9] A retrospective study suggests that treatment with two antibiotics may reduce the risk for relapse and recurrence compared with treatment by a single agent.[95] In recent years, there has been an increase in incidence and probably recognition of peritonitis episodes caused by gram-negative bacilli with extended-spectrum beta-lactamases and carbapenem-resistant *Enterobacteriaceae*. Their treatment should be individualized. A number of new second-line antibiotics, such as ceftaroline, ceftolozane plus tazobactam, and tigecycline, are potentially effective.[96]

Polymicrobial Peritonitis

When multiple enteric organisms (multiple gram-negative or mixed gram-negative and gram-positive organisms) are grown from the PD effluent, it often indicates the presence of intraabdominal pathology. Treatment should include oral or intravenous metronidazole plus IP vancomycin and either IP aminoglycoside or IP ceftazidime for a minimum period of 3 weeks.[9] Similarly, the presence of anaerobic bacteria or fungus as part of the mixed microbial growth from the PD effluent usually suggests underlying surgical pathology. On the other hand, if multiple gram-positive organisms are grown from PD effluent, intraabdominal pathology is less likely and the prognosis is usually favorable. These patients should be treated with effective antibiotics for 3 weeks.[9] Routine surgical intervention for this group of patients is often not necessary.

Culture-Negative Peritonitis. In approximately 15% of episodes that meet the criteria for peritonitis on the basis of cell count and clinical features, culture of the PD effluent would not yield any pathogenic organisms. Most of the culture-negative peritonitis could be explained by recent antibiotic therapy or technical problems during the collection of PD effluent for culture.[97] Negative PD effluent cultures on day 3 warrant a repeat dialysis effluent WBC count with differential.[9] If the culture-negative peritonitis is resolving at that time, the empirical antibiotic that covers gram-positive organisms (i.e., first-generation cephalosporin or vancomycin) should be continued for 2 weeks, although it remains controversial whether the empirical antibiotic that covers gram-negative organisms should be stopped. In general, IP aminoglycoside should be discontinued to avoid extended or repeated exposure,[9] whereas third-generation cephalosporins may be continued, especially in centers with a high background incidence of gram-negative peritonitis. If the culture-negative peritonitis is not resolving on day 3, special culture techniques should be considered for isolation of unusual organisms.[9] Fungus and mycobacterial species may not be recovered by routine bacterial culture of PD effluent and should also be considered as the causative organisms.

Fungus. Fungal peritonitis occurs in patients undergoing PD at the rate of 0.01 to 0.19 episodes per dialysis-year, accounting for 3% to 6% of episodes.[4,98,99] More than 70% of the episodes of fungal peritonitis are caused by *Candida* species.[99,100] Recent antibiotic therapy, frequent episodes of bacterial peritonitis, and immunosuppression are the major risk factors of fungal peritonitis.[101] Patients often are severely ill with marked abdominal tenderness.[100,102]

Catheter removal is indicated once fungi are identified in PD effluent, and an appropriate antifungal agent should be continued for at least 2 weeks after catheter removal.[9] Traditionally, the therapy for fungal peritonitis is a combination of amphotericin B and flucytosine. However, this regimen has a high incidence of adverse effects, and the response often is less than satisfactory because amphotericin B has poor penetration through the peritoneal membrane. Fluconazole is commonly used for peritonitis episodes caused by many *Candida* species and *Cryptococcus*,[103] but this agent is fungistatic. Echinocandins (especially caspofungin) is now often advocated for the treatment of fungal peritonitis caused by *Aspergillus* species and nonalbicans *Candida* species,[104] whereas posaconazole and voriconazole are reasonable choices for episodes caused by other filamentous fungi.[105] However, it should be noted that intravenous voriconazole is contraindicated in dialysis patients because it contains cyclodextrin in the solvent and may cause neurotoxicity in patients with severe renal impairment.

Mycobacterial Peritonitis

Tuberculous Peritonitis

Tuberculous peritonitis is uncommon in the Western world, but is more common in Asian countries. Contrary to the common belief, the WBCs in the effluent, at least during the early phase of peritonitis, are predominantly PMN cells, and an acid-fast bacilli stain of an effluent specimen is usually negative.[106] Abnormal chest radiograph and ascitic fluid lymphocytosis only identify one-third of the cases.[107] Conventional microbiological diagnostic methods are slow and have a low sensitivity. New fluid medium (e.g., Septi-Chek, BACTEC; Becton Dickinson) could reduce the time to develop and positive culture. Overall diagnostic yield could further be improved by centrifuging 50 to 100 mL effluent, followed by culturing the sediment in both solid and fluid media. Alternatively, mycobacterial DNA polymerase chain reaction can be performed on dialysis effluent, although false-positives are common.[108] Peritoneal biopsy often is recommended for expedite diagnosis of tuberculous peritonitis in clinically suspicious cases, but this strategy is not practical for PD patients.

Regarding the treatment, standard antituberculous chemotherapy is highly effective,[106,107] but it takes at least 12 months to complete the course. Drug interactions between rifampicin and other concomitant medications are common. Removal of PD catheter is usually not necessary, but UF problems may occur as a delayed complication.[109]

Nontuberculous Mycobacterial Peritonitis

In subtropical countries, there is an increase in incidence of peritonitis caused by nontuberculous mycobacteria in the past decade.[110,111] More than half of the cases are caused by rapidly growing species, such as *Mycobacterium fortuitum* and *M. chelonae*.[110] It has been postulated that extensive use of topical antimicrobial ointment (especially gentamicin) for exit-site care may predispose patients to nontuberculous mycobacterial infection of the exit site.[112] The treatment regimen for nontuberculous mycobacterial peritonitis is not well established, but catheter removal is usually necessary.[9]

Reassessment After Therapy

Most patients with PD-related peritonitis show considerable clinical improvement after 2 to 3 days of antibiotic therapy. Antibiotic therapy should be adjusted to narrow spectrum agents, as appropriate, once culture results and sensitivities are known. If the patient has not shown definitive clinical improvement after 3 days of empirical therapy, effluent cell counts, Gram stain, and cultures should be repeated. PD effluent WBC count ≥1090/mm^3 on day 3 predicts treatment failure.[113] Theoretically, catheter removal should be considered if the response to antibiotic therapy is poor after 4 days of antibiotic therapy (see next section), but this recommendation is difficult to follow in practice as it is limited by the availability of surgeon, operating theatre, as well as patients' own preference.

TABLE 32.5 Terminology of Peritonitis

Recurrent	An episode that occurs within 4 wk of completion of therapy of a prior episode but with a different organism.
Relapsing	An episode that occurs within 4 wk of completion of therapy of a prior episode with the same organism or one sterile episode.
Repeat	An episode that occurs >4 wk after completion of therapy of a prior episode with the same organism.
Refractory	Failure of the effluent to clear after 5 d of appropriate antibiotics.

Adapted from Li PK, Szeto CC, Piraino B, et al. ISPD peritonitis recommendations: 2016 update on prevention and treatment. *Perit Dial Int*. 2016;36:481-508.

Catheter Removal

The definitions of refractory, relapsing, recurrent, and repeat peritonitis are summarized in Table 32.5. PD catheter should be removed promptly in refractory peritonitis.[9] Timely catheter removal also should be considered for relapsing peritonitis, refractory ESI and tunnel infection, and fungal peritonitis.[9] In most patients, temporary hemodialysis is needed after catheter removal. However, simultaneous removal and reinsertion of catheters is a safe and effective method for the treatment of refractory ESI[114] as well as for the prevention of relapsing peritonitis after dialysis effluent clears up.[115,116]

Effective systemic antibiotics should be continued for at least 2 weeks after catheter removal for peritonitis.[9] Insertion of a new PD catheter could be attempted at least 2 weeks after catheter removal and complete resolution of peritoneal symptoms.[9] Reinsertion should be done by laparoscopic or minilaparotomy approach so that adhesion can be directly visualized. In about 50% of the patients who have had their catheter removed, PD can be successfully resumed,[117,118] but UF problems are common subsequently.[117] Peritoneal equilibration test should be considered around 1 month after resuming PD for the tailoring of PD regime.

Complications of Peritoneal Dialysis Peritonitis

Peritonitis results in a marked increase in dialysis effluent protein losses, which may aggravate the protein-energy wasting of PD patients.[119] Attention should particularly be paid on the nutritional status of patients with prolonged peritoneal inflammation. Reduction in UF is common during peritonitis episodes because peritoneal permeability is increased.[120] The use of hypertonic exchanges and short dwell times may be needed during this period to maintain adequate fluid removal, but appetite may be further worsened with this approach. Temporary use of icodextrin solution may prevent

TABLE 32.6 Exit-Site Scoring System

	0 Points	1 Point	2 Points
Swelling	No	Exit only; < 0.5 cm	>0.5 cm or involve tunnel
Crust	No	<0.5 cm	>0.5 cm
Redness	No	<0.5 cm	>0.5 cm
Pain	No	Slight	Severe
Drainage	No	Serious	Purulent

Catheter-related infection is diagnosed if score ≥4.
Modified from Schaefer F, Klaus G, Müller-Wiefel DE, Mehls O. Intermittent versus continuous intraperitoneal glycopeptide/ceftazidime treatment in children with peritoneal dialysis-associated peritonitis. *J Am Soc Nephrol.* 1999;10:136-145.

fluid overload in PD patients with acute peritonitis, and the therapeutic response is not affected.[84] Because of rapid glucose absorption, glycemic control may worsen during peritonitis in patients with diabetes. Blood glucose monitoring with appropriate adjustments of insulin dosage may be needed.

The change in the peritoneal permeability during peritonitis is usually transient.[121] However, after multiple peritonitis episodes or an episode of severe peritonitis, permanent increase in solute transport and loss of UF capability may occur.[117,122] The risk is probably proportional to the extent of inflammation and the number of peritonitis episodes.[123] The final stage of this process is peritoneal fibrosis, sometimes referred to as encapsulating peritoneal sclerosis (EPS).[122] EPS is present in approximately 1% of patients undergoing PD and is possibly more common in some countries (e.g., Japan).[124] In addition to UF failure, the EPS patient becomes progressively malnourished because of recurrent partial intestinal obstruction from encasement of the bowel. PD cannot be continued and this complication is frequently lethal despite conversion to long-term hemodialysis.

CATHETER-RELATED INFECTIONS

CRIs are used as the collective term to describe ESI and tunnel infection. These two entities may occur on their own or simultaneously. Bacterial colonization of the PD catheter exit site may lead to infection of the catheter exit site, which may further spread along the subcutaneous tunnel of the catheter to the inner cuff and subsequently to the peritoneum, resulting in tunnel infection and peritonitis, respectively. The reported incidence of CRIs, as well as the prevalence of individual causative organism, varies considerably in the literature,[125,126] but for most PD centers, *S. aureus* and *P. aeruginosa* are the most common causes of CRIs.

Definitions

ESI is defined as the presence of purulent discharge, with or without erythema of the skin at the catheter-epidermal interface.[10] The classification of catheter exit-site appearance is summarized in Table 32.6.[127] Peri-catheter erythema without purulent drainage is sometimes an early indication of infection, but also can be an allergic skin reaction, or in a recently placed catheter or after trauma to the catheter.[128]

Catheter tunnel infection is defined as the presence of clinical or ultrasonographic evidence of inflammation or collection along the catheter tunnel.[10] Tunnel infections are commonly occult, and often only detected by ultrasonography of the subcutaneous catheter tunnel.[19,129] ESI caused by *S. aureus* or *P. aeruginosa* often are associated with concomitant occult tunnel infections.[130]

Risk Factors

The major risk factor in *S. aureus* catheter infections is nasal carriage of *S. aureus*,[131,132] which is present in around 50% of new and prevalent PD patients.[132] Patients who were *S. aureus* carriers had significantly higher incidences of *S. aureus* ESIs, tunnel infections, and peritonitis than noncarriers.[131,132] Only 33% of the *S. aureus* carriers had the same phage type upon repeat culture, and 16% patients are intermittent carriers only.[132]

ESI, especially episodes caused by *S. aureus* and *P. aeruginosa*, is the major risk factor for tunnel infection. In addition, tunnel infections are probably more common in patients with diabetes.[130] Immunosuppressed patients are at increased risk for catheter infections.[133] A downward-directed catheter exit site is associated with easier-to-treat infections, with fewer episodes of catheter-related peritonitis.[1]

Treatment

Clinical Presentation and Assessment

ESI generally presents as purulent drainage from the exit site, with or without surrounding erythema. Tunnel infection, if clinically apparent, usually presents as erythema, edema, induration or tenderness over the subcutaneous pathway, and often occurs in the presence of ESI. Peri-catheter erythema without purulent drainage could be an early sign of ESI but also can be a local skin reaction without infection. Gram stain of exit-site drainage and bacterial culture with aerobic and anaerobic media are valuable to guide the treatment. A review of the previous bacterial culture from exit-site swab often gives valuable information in guiding the choice of antibiotics for patients presenting with ESI or tunnel infection.

Exit-Site Care

During an episode of acute CRI, the exit site should be cleansed at least daily.[10] However, there is no published trial on the efficacy of intensified exit-site care for the treatment (not prevention) of overt CRIs,[50,51] and the choice of the optimal cleansing agent has not been defined. Although commonly used, there are few data on the efficacy of topical antibacterial agents in the treatment of active CRIs.[134]

Antibiotic Therapy

When a clinical diagnosis of ESI or tunnel infection is made, empiric oral antibiotic treatment with appropriate *S. aureus* cover, such as a penicillinase-resistant penicillin (cloxacillin, dicloxacillin, or flucloxacillin) or first-generation cephalosporin, are reasonable choices.[10] If the patient has a history of infection or colonization with methicillin-resistant *S. aureus* (MRSA), empirical therapy with a glycopeptide

TABLE 32.7 Recommended Dosage of Common Oral Antibiotics for Catheter-Related Infections

Amoxicillin	250–500 mg bid
Amoxicillin/clavulanic acid	875 mg/125 mg bid
Ciprofloxacin	250 mg bid or 500 mg/d
Cloxacillin/flucloxacillin	500 mg QID
Levofloxacin	300 mg/d
Trimethoprim/sulfamethoxazole	80 mg/400 mg/d to 160 mg/800 mg bid

bid, Twice a day; *QID*, four times a day.
From R Gokal, Ash SR, GB Helfrich, et al. Peritoneal catheters and exit-site practices: toward optimum peritoneal access. *Perit Dial Int.* 1993;13:29-39; Zimmerman SW, O'Brien M, et al. Randomized controlled trial of prophylactic rifampin for peritoneal dialysis-related infections. *Am J Kidney Dis.* 1991;18:225-231; lowey DL, Warady BA, McFarland KS. The treatment of Staphylococcus aureus nasal carriage in pediatric peritoneal dialysis patients. *Adv Perit Dial.* 1994;10:297-299. Hardy DJ, Guay DR, Jones RN. Clarithromycin, a unique macrolide. A pharmacokinetic, microbiological, and clinical overview. *Diagn Microbiol Infect Dis.* 1992;15:39-53.

or clindamycin should be considered.[10] Similarly, if there is a past history of CRI or peritonitis caused by *Pseudomonas* species, empirical therapy with a fluoroquinolone or third- or fourth-generation cephalosporins may be preferred. Oral antibiotics appear to be as efficacious as parenteral agents.[134] The recommended dosage for commonly used oral antibiotics are summarized in Table 32.7.

When the result of Gram stain or culture becomes available, the oral antibiotic regimen should be tailored according to the specific organism identified. *S. aureus* catheter infections often respond to penicillinase-resistant penicillin, first-generation cephalosporin, or trimethoprim-sulfamethoxazole.[134,135] Rifampin may have activity within bacterial biofilm and can be used as adjunctive therapy, although there is no prospective study to support the benefit of this practice. Potential interaction with other concurrent medications (e.g., antihypertensive agents) also should be considered during rifampicin treatment. ESI caused by *Pseudomonas* species preferably should be treated with two antibiotics.[10]

Patients should be reviewed regularly to determine the clinical response to treatment. Most ESIs should be treated with at least 2 weeks of effective antibiotics.[10] However, tunnel infections and ESI caused by *Pseudomonas* species should be treated with at least 3 weeks of effective antibiotics.[10] Repeating exit-site wound swab for bacterial culture after the discontinuation of antibiotic treatment probably is not necessary. Ultrasonography of the catheter tunnel also has been advocated for evaluating the response to therapy, and may be used to decide on the need for surgical intervention.[135,136]

Catheter Removal

The PD catheter should be removed in patients with ESI that progresses to, or occurs simultaneously with, peritonitis. These patients should receive temporary hemodialysis, and reinsertion of a PD catheter could be considered at least 2 weeks after catheter removal and complete resolution of peritoneal symptoms.[10] On the other hand, simultaneous removal and reinsertion of the dialysis catheter with a new exit site under antibiotic coverage could be considered in patients with refractory ESI or tunnel infection without peritonitis,[10] or, when there is concomitant peritonitis, after the PD effluent has cleared up with IP antibiotics. Refractory ESI or tunnel infections are usually defined as failure to respond after 3 weeks of effective antibiotic therapy.

Other Catheter Interventions

Observational data suggest that partial catheter reimplantation[137] and catheter diversion procedure with exit-site renewal[138,139] could be considered for catheter salvage in refractory CRIs. In selected cases, cuff-shaving under systemic antibiotic cover may be considered as the alternative to catheter replacement for tunnel infection.[140] The unroofing technique, with or without *en bloc* resection of the skin and tissues around the peripheral cuff, has been advocated. However, the procedure is associated with a risk for immediate peritonitis and also should be performed with systemic antibiotic coverage.[141,142]

PREVENTION

CRIs are major predisposing factors to PD-related peritonitis.[89] The primary objective of preventing ESIs and tunnel infections is to prevent peritonitis. Many prevention strategies aim primarily at reducing the incidence of peritonitis, and clinical trials in this area often report the rate of ESIs or CRIs as a secondary outcome.

Catheter Design and Insertion

Detailed description on the recommended practice of PD catheter insertion has been covered in a recent ISPD position paper.[90] RCTs consistently show that prophylactic systemic antibiotics before the placement of PD catheter reduces the risk for early peritonitis and probably CRIs.[81] Although first-generation cephalosporin may be slightly less effective than vancomycin in this regard, the former should be the agent of choice because of the concern of inducing vancomycin resistance.[9]

In addition to prophylactic antibiotics, the design and insertion technique of the PD catheter have little effect on the risk for peritonitis or CRIs. Specifically, there is no consistent difference in peritonitis risk between laparoscopic and mini-laparotomy catheter placement, midline and lateral incisions, single and double cuff, straight and coiled catheter, or downward and lateral facing exit site.[143] Novel designs such as buried catheter or presternal and abdominal swan neck catheters have other practical advantages but do not consistently lead to a lower infection rate.

Connectology and Dialysis Solutions

For CAPD, prospective studies consistently show that disconnect systems with a "flush-before-fill" design result in a lower peritonitis rate than traditional spike systems[144] and should be used whenever available. The use of disconnect systems, however, has become the routine practice and spike systems are no longer available, at least in most developed countries. There is no significant difference between various disconnect systems (e.g., double bag and standard Y systems) in terms of peritonitis rate.[144]

Some data suggest that PD solutions with low glucose degradation product are associated with a lower risk for peritonitis.[60] However, the results of published trials are not consistently positive.[62] The latest ISPD guideline does not have any specific recommendation on the choice of PD solution in relation to the prevention of peritonitis.[9]

Training and Continuous Quality Improvement Programs

The training program of PD patients has an important influence on the risk for peritonitis and catheter infections.[145] High-quality evidence that guides how, where, when, and by whom PD training should be performed, however, is lacking[145] In general, the latest ISPD recommendations for teaching PD patients and their caregivers should be followed.[146] In addition to the initial training, home visits by PD nurses, usually shortly after the patient returns home for regular PD, often are useful in detecting practical problems.[147] Retraining in selected patients may reduce the risk for peritonitis. However, the indication of retraining is not well defined. The latest ISPD guideline recommends retraining after peritonitis or catheter infection; prolonged hospitalization; change in dexterity, vision, or mental acuity; change to another supplier or a different type of connection; or other interruption in PD.[9] It also has been suggested by some experts that regular retraining may be beneficial. However, published evidence in this regard is lacking. The optimal frequency of routine retraining has not been generally agreed on, and the impact on nursing manpower should be considered.

In addition to a formal patient training program, a continuous quality improvement program within a PD unit may help reduce the rate of peritonitis.[148] The latest ISPD guideline recommends that multidisciplinary teams running continuous quality improvement programs in PD centers should meet and review their units' performance metrics regularly.[9]

Exit-Site Care

There is a strong association between ESIs and subsequent peritonitis.[149] Early detection and prompt management of ESIs are logical steps to reduce the risk for subsequent peritonitis. During patient training, education on exit-site care and meticulous hand hygiene should be emphasized. The exit site should be cleansed at least twice weekly and every time after a shower.[10] In countries with a hot and humid weather, daily exit-site cleansing may be necessary. Gauze is commonly used for exit-site dressing and protection, and immobilization of the catheter often is recommended, but there is no published evidence to support this kind of practice.

A number of topical cleansing agents have been tested for the prevention of CRIs, but none has been shown to be superior with respect to preventing them.[10] Antibacterial soap and water are commonly used to clean the exit site but that efficacy has not been proved. Povidone-iodine, chlorhexidine, and electrolytic chloroxidizing solutions also are widely used. However, a systematic review shows that topical povidone-iodine disinfection does not reduce the risk for peritonitis compared with simple soap and water cleansing or no treatment.[150] We believe chlorhexidine solution may be a better choice for exit-site cleansing.

Contrary to exit-site cleansing and dressing, a good body of published evidence shows that daily use of topical mupirocin cream or ointment to the catheter exit site could effectively reduce the incidence of peritonitis.[9,151] Once-weekly topical mupirocin is less effective than more frequent administration.[152] Intranasal mupirocin reduced *S. aureus* ESIs but not peritonitis, and is less well tolerated by patients.[153,154] Daily application of gentamicin cream is an acceptable alternative to mupirocin.[9] Gentamicin cream application to the exit site is effective in reducing the risk for peritonitis, and has the additional advantage of reducing ESI caused by *Pseudomonas* species.[155] The potential risk for resistance to mupirocin and gentamicin has always been a concern but the clinical ramifications remains unclear. The association between gentamicin cream and nontuberculous mycobacterial infection of the exit site has been suspected but never proved. Despite the initial enthusiasm, topical application of antibacterial honey or polysporin triple ointment were not found to be superior to conventional exit-site care.[156,157] Other alternative topical antibacterial agents have been tested but none has gained wide acceptance for routine clinical use.[9]

Management of *S. aureus* Carrier

Nasal carrier of *S. aureus* is an important risk factor of CRIs. Although the evidence to support routine screening of nasal *S. aureus* carriage in PD patients is limited, the efficacy of prophylactic intranasal antibiotics, especially intranasal mupirocin, for the treatment of confirmed cases of nasal carriage of *S. aureus* has been shown to reduce the risk for CRIs.[153] The effect on reducing peritonitis rate, however, is less clear. Cyclical oral rifampicin therapy (typically one 5-day course every 3 months) is effective in reducing the rate of CRIs, presumably by eradicating *S. aureus* carriage.[158] Nonetheless, the routine use of oral rifampicin for the treatment of nasal *S. aureus* carrier or prevention of peritonitis is not recommended because adverse reactions, drug interactions, and rifampicin resistance are all common and important problems.[10]

Other Modifiable Risk Factors

Peritonitis commonly follows invasive interventional procedures (e.g., colonoscopy, hysteroscopy, cholecystectomy) in PD patients. Observational data showed that prophylactic antibiotics before most endoscopic interventions, including colonoscopy, sigmoidoscopy, and invasive gynecological procedures (but not upper gastrointestinal endoscopy) were associated with a lower peritonitis rate.[159] The optimal antibiotic regimen, however, has yet to be defined. A previous systematic review recommended the use of intravenous ampicillin plus an aminoglycoside, with or without metronidazole, for this purpose.[81] In our own experience, a single dose of amoxicillin/clavulanic acid or third-generation cephalosporins (e.g., cefotaxime) are convenient and effective alternatives.

Common clinical sense suggests that prophylactic antibiotics should be used after wet contamination.[9] There is no widely accepted standard regimen, but a 2-day course of fluoroquinolone is a reasonable regimen. Hypokalemia should be treated, partly because it is associated with an increased risk for enteric peritonitis.[160] Pets should not be allowed where the PD procedure is being performed.[161] A number of other modifiable risk factors for PD peritonitis have been described,[162] but it remains unknown whether treating these risk factors would reduce the risk for peritonitis.

Secondary Prevention of Peritonitis

Most fungal peritonitis episodes are preceded by antibiotics treatment.[163] Prophylactic treatment with either oral nystatin or fluconazole during systemic antibiotic therapy, especially when used for the treatment of bacterial peritonitis, significantly reduces the risk for secondary fungal peritonitis.[81,164] Nystatin is generally the agent of choice because it is cheap and has no systemic effect. However, nystatin is not available in some countries. In some centers, nystatin is only available as a mouthwash solution; patients need to be reminded to swallow the solution to ensure the efficacy of prophylaxis. Although fluconazole is effective, interaction with other concomitant medications is common, and the possibility of inducing resistant strains should be considered.

For each peritonitis episode, a root-cause analysis should be performed to determine the etiology and contributing factors. Whenever possible, interventions directed against any reversible risk factor should be made to prevent further peritonitis episodes. The PD exchange technique should be reviewed (especially after an episode of gram-positive peritonitis), and focused retraining may be needed. Replacement of the catheter is more effective than urokinase in preventing further peritonitis episodes due to biofilm or bacterial adherence to the catheter, and should be considered in patients with relapsing or repeat peritonitis.[73] In this scenario, catheter removal and reinsertion can be performed as a single procedure without the need for temporary hemodialysis after PD effluent has cleared up with antibiotic treatment.[165]

A full list of references is available at www.expertsonsult.com.

33

Noninfectious Complications of Peritoneal Dialysis

Clare B. Jones, MB, ChB, Athanasios K. Roumeliotis, MD, and Joanne M. Bargman, MD, FRCPC

OUTLINE

Although peritonitis is regarded as the Achilles heel of peritoneal dialysis (PD), a number of serious noninfectious complications can develop in patients on PD. These complications can lead to significant morbidity and mortality. Some complications, such as catheter malfunction, hernias, and dialysate leaks, are commonly encountered; others, such as encapsulating peritoneal sclerosis, are rare and can be devastating (Table 33.1). This chapter will address these and other noninfectious complications of PD.

COMPLICATIONS RELATED TO INCREASED INTRAABDOMINAL PRESSURE

The instillation of dialysate into the peritoneal cavity leads to an increase in intraabdominal pressure (IAP).[1] Two principal factors govern the magnitude of the rise in IAP: the volume of dialysate instilled and the position the patient assumes during the dwell.[1] A strong positive relationship exists between the amount of dialysate instilled into the peritoneal cavity and IAP. The effect of patient position is also important, with the supine position generating the lowest IAP for a given volume of dialysate.[2] Other factors that may increase IAP include higher body mass index (BMI) and activities such as exercising, coughing, and straining.[1]

Hernia Formation

In accordance with Laplace law, the tension on the abdominal wall increases with instillation of dialysate as a result of the increase in IAP and the larger radius of the abdomen. High abdominal pressure and abdominal wall tension place mechanical stress on the supporting structures of the abdomen and can lead to hernia formation in those with congenital or acquired weakness or defects. The areas of weakness are probably very important in the pathogenesis of hernias.

Incidence, Types of Hernia, and Etiological Factors

The prevalence of hernia in PD patients has been reported to range from 10% to 25%. This is higher than in the general population.[3,4] The true prevalence of this condition may, in fact, be even higher due to the presence of asymptomatic hernias that are not detected until a complication occurs.[4]

Umbilical hernias are the most commonly described hernia occurring in PD patients (Fig. 33.1).[4] However, a multitude of other types of hernia have been reported. These include incisional hernia, hiatal hernia, inguinal hernia, ventral hernia, epigastric hernia, femoral hernia, Spigelian hernia, cystocele, Richter hernia, and herniation through the foramen of Morgagni.[3,5,6]

Numerous risk factors for hernia formation exist, including older age, female sex, multiparity, midline PD catheter insertion, and having undergone a previous hernia repair (Table 33.2).[7] Moreover, some studies have demonstrated a correlation with an increased BMI, whereas others have reported the opposite effect.[1,8,9] Continuous ambulatory peritoneal dialysis (CAPD), rather than night-cycler–based dialysis, has been reported as a risk factor for hernia, possibly as the result of an increased duration of time spent upright leading to sustained increased IAP.[7] In addition, hernias are more common in patients who have previously undergone transplantation. Interestingly, they are generally not associated with the transplant incision and

TABLE 33.1 Summary and Timeline of Noninfectious Peritoneal Dialysis Complications

Early (d, wk)	Late (mo)
Catheter malfunction	
Displacement, kink, omental wrap	
Leak (<30 d)	**Leak (usually within first year)**
Usually at exit site or pericatheter (positive result when glucose test strip dipped in exit-site fluid)	Leak through defect in peritoneum e.g., into an abdominal hernia or through a patent processus vaginalis
Drain pain	
Often worse on cycler	
	Encapsulating peritoneal sclerosis
	Major risk factor = long peritoneal dialysis vintage
Hydrothorax	**Hydrothorax**
Likely congenital diaphragmatic defect	Likely acquired diaphragmatic defect, sometimes presents coincident with peritonitis
Hernia	**Hernia**

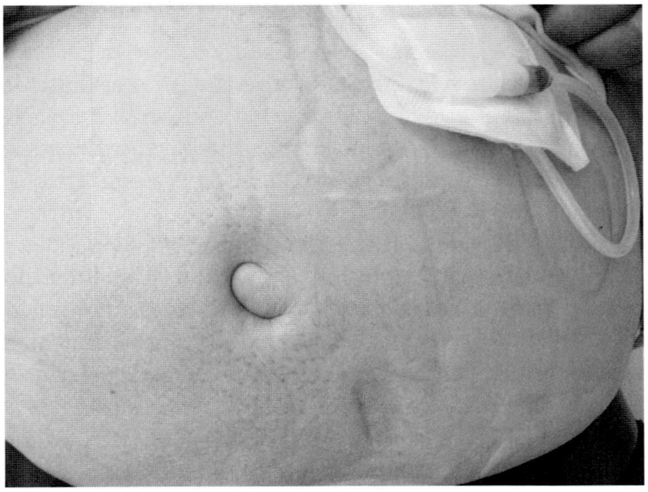

FIG. 33.1 Umbilical hernia. There is a small umbilical hernia leading to leak of dialysis fluid into the abdominal wall soft tissue. The imprint of the catheter and clothing is clearly visualized.

TABLE 33.2 Risk Factors for Hernia Formation

Large dialysate volumes
Sitting position
Raised intraabdominal pressure (during activities, e.g, exercise)
Recent abdominal surgery
Deconditioning
Multiparity
Pericatheter leak
Obesity
Congenital anatomical defects
Polycystic kidney disease

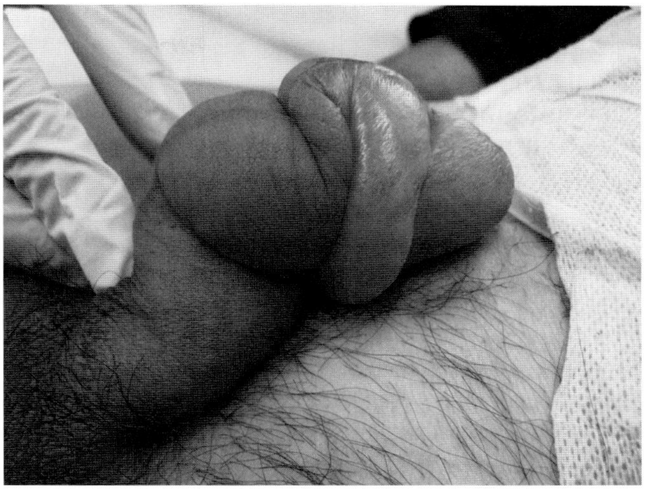

FIG. 33.2 Edema of penis. The long-term transplant patient underwent peritoneal dialysis catheter insertion uneventfully. When a day exchange was added, he developed penile edema. Computed tomography with intraperitoneal contrast demonstrated leak of fluid through a laparoscopic port hole.

it is thought they may be related to chronic steroid use or changes in abdominal musculature.[10]

Finally, polycystic kidney disease can predispose PD patients to hernia development through multiple mechanisms, including higher IAP caused by the enlarged kidneys, a patent processus vaginalis, or as a manifestation of a generalized connective tissue disorder leading to weakening of the abdominal wall.[11,12] However, the theory that increased IAP caused by PD results in increased hernia risk is controversial with studies demonstrating conflicting results.[2,13]

Clinical Presentation and Diagnosis

Typically, hernias present as a painless swelling. This may occur after an antecedent event such as a coughing bout or after physical exertion. Some hernias may be clinically occult and present with diminished effluent return or abdominal edema resulting from dialysate leak through defects in the abdominal wall.[14] The most worrisome complications of hernia are incarceration and strangulation of bowel, which occurs most commonly with umbilical hernias.[15] Patients may present with a tender lump, recurrent episodes of peritonitis with multiple gram-negative organisms, and signs and symptoms of bowel obstruction.[5]

Diagnosing hernia usually is straightforward in the clinical setting. However, other tests may be needed to confirm the diagnosis. Ultrasonography is an excellent modality to distinguish pericatheter hernias from masses caused by hematomas, seromas, or abscesses.[15] With ultrasound, hernias often appear solid, whereas the other conditions are characterized by fluid collections.[16]

Although ultrasound is helpful in detecting pericatheter hernias, computed tomography (CT) is the most sensitive and specific modality to delineate other hernias.[17] The diagnostic utility of the CT is improved by the use of intraperitoneal dye.[17] Typically, 100 mL of dye is added to the dialysate, which is infused into the peritoneal cavity.[18] The patient should remain ambulatory over the next 2 hours to facilitate the entry of peritoneal fluid containing the dye into the hernia sac and any other potential areas of leak. CT is then performed (Fig. 33.2).

Magnetic resonance imaging (MRI) also has been used to diagnose hernias associated with abdominal wall and genital leaks.[19] This modality is beneficial in that dialysate is used as the "dye," thereby making it devoid of ionizing radiation. Furthermore, MRI will detect where dialysate is residing in the soft tissues, whereas CT will only pick up what has leaked following instillation of the dye.

Treatment

The vast majority of patients on PD who develop a hernia should undergo surgical repair. A notable exception is those individuals who are an unacceptably high surgical risk. In these patients, however, the development of a hernia does not necessarily obviate the use of PD.[20] In fact, PD may be continued if the patient uses methods to lower IAP such as dialysis while supine (night-cycler treatment), lower dialysate volumes, and wearing an abdominal binder for external support. Although hernias may be cosmetically unappealing, most should be repaired to prevent the serious complications of bowel incarceration and strangulation and to avoid the development of dialysate leaks. The risk for bowel incarceration and strangulation is particularly important for smaller umbilical hernias.[21] In contrast, ventral hernias carry little risk for strangulation. However, the defect in the abdominal wall integrity associated with these hernias serves as a source of dialysate leak leading to the formation of abdominal edema.[21]

Hernia repair sometimes incorporates a preperitoneal mesh placement. This allows development of an inflammatory state around the mesh, which helps to seal the peritoneal cavity.[22] For a patient who has not yet initiated dialysis, hernia repair can occur at the same time as PD catheter insertion.

Reports have demonstrated that PD patients undergoing hernia repair need not be automatically converted to hemodialysis (HD) around the surgery.[20,23] These patients can continue standard PD therapy until the morning of surgery, drain the PD fluid before surgery, and withhold dialysis for the first 24 to 48 hours after surgery. Dialysis can then be safely reintroduced using the principles of low IAP (low volumes using a night-cycler and day dry) for a 2-week duration particularly in patients who have significant residual kidney function. Temporary transfer to HD should be initiated when the hernia is associated with bowel strangulation, which may compromise the bacterial barrier of the bowel wall and subject the patient to peritonitis. In the patient without renal kidney failure, it may be prudent to consider temporary support with HD. An example of a management strategy for PD before and after hernia surgery is outlined in Table 33.3.

Previously, there was concern regarding the potential for mesh infection in patients on PD, although there is no compelling evidence for this. Generally, mesh infection rates are assumed to be higher in patients treated with intraperitoneal mesh (with exposure of the mesh to the peritoneal cavity) compared with preperitoneal mesh (with minimal breach of the peritoneum).[24] Regardless, numerous published reports of mesh hernia repairs in PD patients report no episodes of mesh infection even in the presence of peritonitis.[25]

TABLE 33.3 Protocol for Peritoneal Dialysis Before and After Hernia Surgery

- Continue on standard PD therapy until the morning of surgery
- Drain the PD fluid before the surgery
- No dialysis for the first 48 h
- Laboratory investigation at start of IPD and weekly
- IPD 3 times per week (1-L exchange × 10 for 10 h) for 2 wk for CAPD patients and for 1 wk for CCPD patients
- CAPD patients resume low volume (1–1.5 L × 5 exchanges for 2 wk)
- CCPD patients to continue on NIPD for an additional 4 wk
- Patients resume preoperative PD prescription after 4–5 wk

CAPD, Continuous ambulatory peritoneal dialysis; *CCPD*, continuous cycling peritoneal dialysis; *IPD*, intermittent peritoneal dialysis; *NIPD*, nocturnal intermittent peritoneal dialysis; *PD*, peritoneal dialysis.
From Shah H, Chu M, Bargman JM. Perioperative management of peritoneal dialysis patients undergoing hernia surgery without the use of interim hemodialysis. *Perit Dial Int.* 2006;26(6):684-687.

Recurrence of surgically repaired hernias in PD patients has been reported to be as high as 27%,[26,18] although a more recent study (primarily using mesh repairs) was around 10%.[10] In the event of recurrence, a long-term option for those on CAPD would be to switch to overnight ambulatory peritoneal dialysis (APD). A 2012 retrospective study evaluated the effect of hernia repair in PD patients over a 10-year period. Repair was done in 49 of 73 hernias (mainly umbilical). There was no significant effect on residual kidney function or technique survival with 86% of patients remaining on PD long-term.[10]

Dialysate Leaks

The loss of dialysate from the peritoneal cavity, either into another compartment or around the PD catheter itself, is known as a peritoneal dialysate leak. This phenomenon often is a consequence of the loss of peritoneal membrane integrity caused by a defect within the membrane. It may manifest with a wide spectrum of presentations: from moisture around the PD catheter exit site to genital and abdominal wall edema. The ramifications of dialysate leaks can be distressing as they may lead to technique failure.[14]

Incidence, Classification of Leaks, and Risk Factors

The incidence of dialysate leaks varies widely in the literature. Conservative reports demonstrate an incidence of 5% in PD patients; however, others have noted rates as high as 10%.[12,27] The variability in incidence may be the result of heterogeneity in the reporting of leaks. Dialysate leaks may be classified as early or late depending on the time course they develop after PD catheter insertion (Table 33.4). Early leaks are those that develop within 30 days of catheter insertion.[12,28] They are usually related to catheter placement and present as dialysate leakage at the exit site or incision. In contrast, late leaks most often are related to a defect in the peritoneal membrane.[12,28] These leaks more often present with hydrothorax and genital and abdominal wall edema, sometimes in association with hernias.

TABLE 33.4 Comparison Between Early and Late Dialysate Leaks in Peritoneal Dialysis Patients

	Early Leaks	Late Leaks
Pathogenesis	• Poor tissue healing • Midline catheter insertion • Use of PD immediately after catheter insertion	• Poor tissue healing/tensile strength • Straining, infections, hernias • Method of catheter insertion may have an effect
Site	• Exit site, incisional site, or subcutaneous	• Subcutaneous
Diagnosis	• Usually by clinical means (leak through exit site or incision)	• Often requires imaging
Management	• PD interruption alone often effective	• Usually requires surgery • Occasionally conservative means (change to other modality of PD, observation) are sufficient
Prevention	• Paramedian surgical insertion with meticulous closure of the peritoneum and obliteration of all potential open tunnel spaces. Waiting period of 10–14 d if feasible • Starting PD with low volumes • Avoiding heavy straining	• Same as early leak prevention. Avoid day dwell in at-risk cycler patients with residual kidney function

PD, Peritoneal dialysis.
From Tzamaloukas AH, Gibel LJ, Eisenberg B, et al. Early and late peritoneal dialysate leaks in patients on CAPD. *Adv Perit Dial.* 1990;6 :64-71.

The risk factors for the development of leaks are similar to those for hernia development. However, early leaks can be the result of not placing a secure purse-string suture around the deep cuff of the catheter. In addition, initiating dialysis too soon after catheter placement may increase the likelihood of a leak. A recent randomized controlled trial analyzed the appropriate time to initiate PD after catheter insertion. The trial randomized 122 patients to one of three groups: commencing PD at 1 week postcatheter insertion, at 2 weeks, or at 4 weeks. Catheter leak was significantly higher in the first group than in the third group (28.2% vs. 2.4%) but not compared with those waiting 2 weeks.[29]

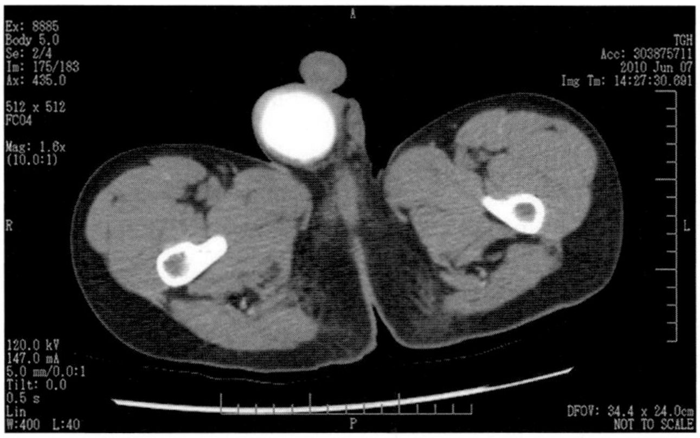

FIG. 33.3 Radiocontrast dye in the scrotal sac. A peritoneal dialysis patient presented with a swollen testicle compatible with hydrocele. Computed tomography with intraperitoneal contrast showed dialysis fluid in the right scrotal sac, as a result of a patent processus vaginalis.

Complications of Dialysate Leaks

Genital Edema. Genital edema occurs in 4% to 10% of PD patients.[30,31] Two mechanisms have been proposed to explain the formation of genital edema.[31] First, dialysate can track through a patent processus vaginalis into the labia or scrotum, leading to a hydrocele composed of dialysis fluid. Along with dialysate, bowel also can migrate along the processus vaginalis into the scrotum, leading to a concurrent and often occult indirect inguinal hernia.[32] The second mechanism leading to genital edema is imparted by defects in the abdominal wall, particularly at the catheter insertion site. These defects allow dialysate to track inferiorly along the abdominal wall, leading to edema of the mons pubis, scrotum, and foreskin (see Fig. 33.2). Women have a lower incidence of genital edema, which has been attributed to the processus vaginalis being patent more often in males due to the spermatic cord.[31]

The diagnosis is usually obvious, but it is important to rule out other processes that may lead to similar presentations such as epididymitis or more generalized fluid overload. CT is the modality of choice to delineate the cause of the genital edema.[22,33] The technique is similar to that used for the detection of hernias with dye being instilled into the peritoneal cavity with the dialysate. The subsequent scan, if positive, will show the movement of dialysate through a patent processus vaginalis or abdominal wall defect into the scrotum or labia (Fig. 33.3). Radionuclide scanning also may be used.[34]

The initial steps in the management of genital edema should address the risk factors leading to fluid accumulation. Specifically, measures aimed at decreasing IAP and minimizing fluid translocation along low-resistance pathways, such as the processus vaginalis, should be undertaken.[30] In this regard, a conservative approach is used, which involves the discontinuation of CAPD, bed rest, scrotal elevation, and the initiation of continuous cyclic peritoneal dialysis (CCPD) or nocturnal intermittent peritoneal dialysis using low volumes with the patient supine.[14,28] This is done for approximately 1 to 3 weeks.[35] The success of this approach is usually dependent on having adequate residual renal function to compensate for the decrease in dose of PD. If the patient does not have adequate residual renal function, they should receive HD temporarily while waiting for the edema to dissipate and

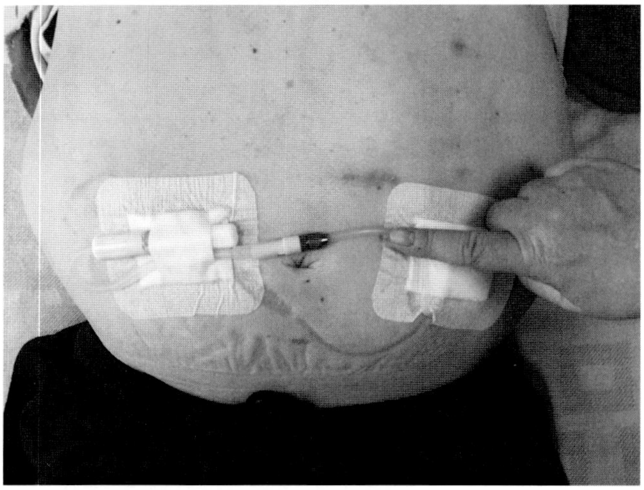

FIG. 33.4 Abdominal wall edema. This patient with polycystic kidney disease presented with leak of dialysis fluid through an occult hernia into the soft tissue. The edema is appreciated in the lower abdomen.

surgical repair of the defect. One center's experience with this approach noted only a 14% rate of recurrence of genital edema.[28]

If conservative treatments fail, surgical repair can be undertaken. In these cases, the same preoperative and postoperative principles as hernia repair apply.

Abdominal Wall Edema. The incidence of abdominal wall edema is not well defined in the literature; however, it is believed to occur less frequently than hernias.[14] The presence of abdominal wall edema suggests that the origin of the peritoneal defect is located within one of the following sites: the incisional site for the insertion of the PD catheter, the catheter tunnel and exit site, from a soft tissue defect within a hernia (Fig. 33.4), or from a peritoneal-fascial defect.

Abdominal wall edema may be difficult to detect clinically because it may present with nonspecific signs and symptoms. These include diminished effluent returns and weight gain due to dialysate accumulating in tissues of the abdominal wall. Other presenting features include abdominal asymmetry or increased abdominal girth. Patients with suspected abdominal wall edema should be examined while standing to better detect any abdominal asymmetry.

CT peritoneography or radionuclide scanning can be used for diagnostic purposes.[17,18,33] MRI scanning also has been used, with one study revealing better delineation of dialysate movement than with CT.[36] This finding is likely because MRI will detect dialysate residing in soft tissue, whereas CT will only detect dialysate that has leaked over the course of the study.

The principles of management of abdominal wall edema are similar to those of genital edema (see previous discussion). In brief, the dialysis regimen is converted to CCPD in the supine position with low volumes and a dry day. The goal is to allow the abdominal wall defect to heal on its own. Should this fail to occur, surgical intervention to close the defect is undertaken. If the leak is from a hernia, the hernia should be repaired.

Pericatheter Leak. Typically, pericatheter leaks are clinically obvious, presenting as wetness around the catheter exit site, or wetness of the exit-site dressing. The diagnosis can be proven using similar CT techniques as for hernias, genital, and abdominal wall edema.[17,18]

The treatment of these leaks differs from that for abdominal wall and genital edema. Here the patient should be drained of dialysate and PD should be discontinued for at least 48 hours.[27] Sometimes this yields enough time for the leak to seal; however, should this not be the case, then the patient should commence HD for a few days if dialysis is needed. If this fails to allow enough time for the leak to seal, then the catheter should be removed and reinserted at a different site. Overall, leaks have required catheter replacement in 37% to 48% of patients.[28,37] Other interventions aimed at sealing the leak, including the placement of purse-string sutures or fibrin glue around the cuff after the fact have not been efficacious.[38] A stitch should never be placed at the exit site. The source of the leak is where the catheter exits the peritoneal cavity, so exit-site stitches will only mask the problem and pose a risk for exit site infection.

Although dialysate leak at the exit site increases the risk for peritonitis or tunnel infection, the use of prophylactic antibiotics is usually not warranted unless there are signs of obvious infection.[37]

Prevention of Dialysate Leaks

As previously discussed, there is evidence that delaying PD initiation for 2 weeks after catheter insertion can reduce the risk of a leak developing.[29,39] It is important to use low volumes of dialysate if PD is to be initiated after a short or no break-in period to reduce the risk for pericatheter leakage.[40,41] Similarly to hernia risk, failed transplant patients are probably at increased risk for leak presumably secondary to a long history of corticosteroid (CCS) use. Steroid use should be minimized where possible and sirolimus discontinued as long as possible before PD catheter insertion.[42]

There is a growing interest in "acute-start" PD wherein a patient needing to start dialysis undergoes PD catheter insertion, avoiding exposure to a tunneled HD venous line. PD is started 1 or 2 days after PD catheter insertion, sooner than is typical for elective PD starts. Despite the increased incidence of leaks with this approach, patients rarely endure significant consequences and the vast majority do not need to transfer to HD.[43]

Hydrothorax

Increased IAP can lead to the translocation of dialysate from the peritoneal cavity across the diaphragm and into the pleural space. The accumulation of dialysis fluid in the pleural space is called hydrothorax (Fig. 33.5).[44] This complication can occur almost immediately or as a late leak.

Pathogenesis

The pathogenesis of hydrothorax formation in PD patients has not been clearly elucidated. It has been speculated that two factors, possibly occurring concurrently, may be involved in hydrothorax development: (1) diaphragmatic defects combined with a large pleuroperitoneal pressure gradient and (2) abnormalities in lymphatic drainage.[45]

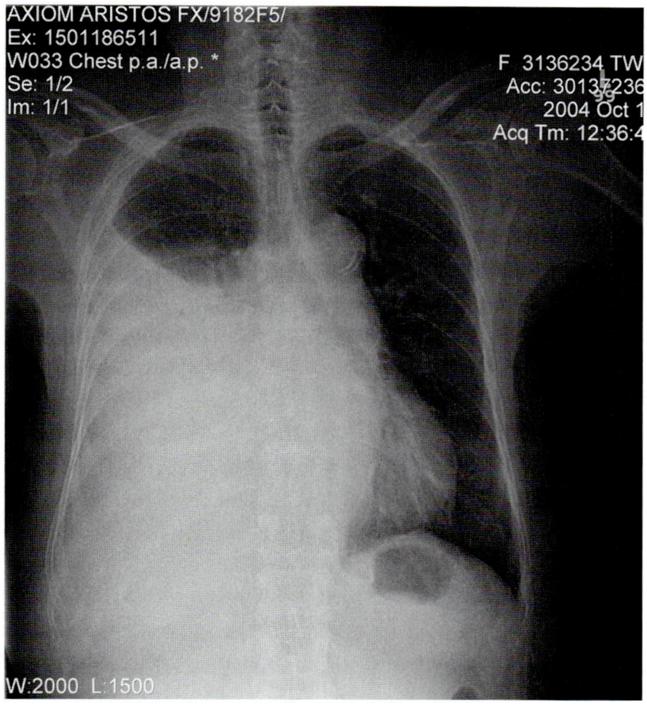

FIG. 33.5 Hydrothorax. This patient presented with shortness of breath soon after starting peritoneal dialysis. Chest x-ray shows a large right-sided pleural effusion as a result of movement of dialysis fluid across the hemidiaphragm.

Diaphragmatic Defects Combined with a Pleuroperitoneal Gradient. To allow the flux of dialysis fluid from the peritoneal cavity into the pleural space, a defect in the diaphragm, acting as a source of communication between the two spaces, must be present. However, it is not enough to have a defect; a pressure gradient also must exist between the two compartments to create a driving force for the movement of fluid. Higher IAP created by the instillation of dialysate combined with the negative pressure in the pleural space leads to a pressure gradient favoring fluid movement from the peritoneum into the pleura. Fluid will continue to move into the pleural space until there is equalization of pressure between the two compartments or there is an impediment to further movement. It has been postulated that a valve-like defect in the diaphragm or the action of the hepatic capsule to tamponade backflow of dialysate from the pleural to peritoneal space may be such impediments.[45]

Other than a peritoneal-pleural gradient, one or multiple defects in the diaphragm must be present to allow hydrothorax formation. These defects may be congenital or acquired. The nature of the underlying defect may explain why some individuals develop hydrothorax with their first-ever infusion of dialysis fluid. Coughing and stretching of the diaphragm are common causes of pleural defects raising IAP to 120 to 150 mmH_2O compared with "normal" baseline pressures of 0.5 to 2.2 mmH_2O. The presence of PD fluid raises IAP to 2 to 10 cmH_2O.[46]

From a pathological point of view, it has been noted that anomalies in the formation of the diaphragm can lead to defects and herniations of this structure. Autopsy studies have revealed localized absence of muscle fibers in the hemidiaphragm, which are replaced with a disordered network of collagen.[47,48] This collagen network is more susceptible to rupture when exposed to high pressures such as those provided by the instillation of dialysate. Moreover, when hydrothorax has been investigated by surgery, "blisters" or "blebs" have sometimes been noted on the pleural surface of the diaphragm.[47] With the instillation of dialysate into the peritoneal cavity, these blebs can be seen to swell and even rupture, thus providing a pathway to the movement of fluid.[47]

Patients presenting with hydrothorax months to years after PD initiation probably have an acquired defect of the diaphragm. Their attenuated diaphragmatic tissue is likely the consequence of ongoing injury from repeated exposure to raised IAP or recurrent episodes of peritonitis.[49,50]

Abnormalities in Lymphatic Drainage or the Lymphatic Transfer Theory. The Lymphatic Transfer Theory was proposed to explain the contribution of impaired lymphatic drainage to the formation of hydrothorax in PD patients.[51] Based on surgical findings, this theory suggests that in susceptible individuals, the instillation of dialysis fluid leads to engorgement of the phrenic lymphatic system resulting in the transudation of fluid into the pleural space. Although plausible, this mechanism cannot explain all cases of hydrothorax formation.

Incidence and Risk Factors

The incidence of hydrothorax in patients receiving PD has been reported to be 2%.[52] Similar to hernias, it has been speculated that this figure is an underrepresentation of the true incidence of hydrothorax as the result of asymptomatic cases.[53]

Multiple risk factors for the development of hydrothorax in PD patients have been described in the literature.[45,47,49,50,52,54,55] However, it is interesting to note that in most cases of hydrothorax, a risk factor is not identified.[11,52]

Polycystic kidney disease (PCKD) has been consistently associated with hydrothorax formation.[54] Two potential explanations for this correlation are (1) the polycystic kidneys compound the rise in IAP when dialysate is infused into the peritoneal cavity, and (2) there is a greater inherent weakness of the diaphragm as a part of a generalized connective tissue defect seen in this condition.[54]

Another important risk factor for hydrothorax is peritonitis.[52,55] Although the link between these two conditions is not clear, it has been postulated that peritonitis may contribute to the further weakening of attenuated diaphragmatic tissue, thereby making it more susceptible to increases in IAP.[55] Women are more likely than men to develop hydrothorax. The reason for this sexual predominance is unknown, although stretching of the hemidiaphragm from previous pregnancy contributing to its weakness has been suggested.[47]

Clinical Presentation

Most commonly, patients with PD-associated hydrothorax present with increasing shortness of breath. Other reported symptoms include pleuritic chest pain, diminished effluent volume, and weight gain as a result of decreased ultrafiltration.

The use of hypertonic solutions often can make the situation worse due to increased ultrafiltration and greater IAP.

Moreover, as previously mentioned, it is not uncommon for hydrothorax to be clinically silent and only discovered incidentally during radiographic procedures done for some other reason.[56]

It is interesting to note that the vast majority of hydrothoraces occur on the right side.[56] One possible explanation for this predisposition has been attributed to cardiac and pericardial surfaces providing a protective effect by covering diaphragmatic defects on the left.[53]

Diagnosis

In the correct clinical setting, the diagnosis of hydrothorax in PD patients may be quite simple to make. Having said that, it is important to consider other causes of dyspnea in PD patients including congestive heart failure, parenchymal lung disease, and pulmonary embolism. Physical findings are consistent with pleural effusion and include absent breath sounds and stony dullness to percussion in the base of the affected lung. Chest x-ray demonstrates a pleural effusion that is usually right-sided and layers out when the patient is placed in the decubitus position. The clinical scenario wherein a patient develops a large right-sided pleural effusion within the first few dialysis exchanges is strongly suggestive of hydrothorax.

Historically, thoracentesis with pleural fluid analysis has been the first step in the diagnosis of PD-associated hydrothorax. As the pleural fluid is composed of dialysate, it should possess the same biochemical characteristics. That is, it should be a transudate, have a low lactic acid dehydragenase, and have a low white blood cell count.[45,52] Because the glucose concentration in the dialysate solution is very high, the pleural glucose concentration in the hydrothorax should similarly be elevated; this diagnostic tool has led to the term *sweet hydrothorax.* Typically, a pleural fluid glucose concentration 50 mg/dL greater than serum glucose concentration is 100% sensitive and specific for diagnosing PD associated hydrothorax.[57] However, cases with borderline glucose values are not uncommon. This may occur if the fluid has been left in the pleural cavity for many hours and is partially reabsorbed by the parietal lymphatics.

Another instance in which the pleural fluid may not have elevated glucose concentration is if the patient is using icodextrin for the long dwell. The presence of icodextrin in a pleural effusion can be demonstrated by the addition of iodine to a pleural fluid sample. This complexes with the starch resulting in a blue/black discoloration.[58]

Instillation of methylene blue into the dialysate has been used in the past with subsequent pleural fluid analysis yielding a blue color. However, this is no longer recommended due to reports of a chemical peritonitis from this agent.[59,60]

Radiological techniques used include scintigraphy, CT peritoneography, and MR peritoneography.[61] Studies comparing techniques have generally had small numbers of patients. Peritoneal scintigraphy uses technetium-99m tagged macroaggregated albumin or sulfur colloid that is instilled into the peritoneal cavity with dialysate. It is a simple, noninvasive technique with low radiation exposure but has sensitivity rates of only 40% to 50%.[62] In addition, although scintigraphy can provide evidence of a leak, the precise location of a defect is not demonstrated. Kang and Kim described the benefits of CT peritoneography, which has the additional benefit of locating the defect. They used 1 mL/kg of nonionic contrast mixed with 30 mL/kg of dialysate. After 30 to 60 minutes of ambulation, CT images can be taken.[63] Sometimes a delayed scan may be warranted, particularly if the defect is small and fluid translocation time is long. MRI also has been used; it provides detailed information but without the radiation risk.[64]

Management

Before commencement of definitive treatment, immediate treatment of hydrothorax must be undertaken if there is respiratory compromise. This involves an emergent thoracentesis, which often dramatically improves the patients' symptoms and provides pleural fluid for analysis.

Subsequent treatment is dictated by whether the patient chooses to continue on PD. If the patient wants to transfer to HD, further management is not required once the effusion has resolved. However, if the patient desires to continue on PD, a multitude of treatment options are available. These include conservative management with temporary interruption of PD, conventional pleurodesis, and surgical thoracotomy or video-assisted thoracoscopic (VATS) repair of the diaphragmatic defect.[53,65] The underlying goal of treatment is simple: prevent recurrence of hydrothorax through the closure of the diaphragmatic defect. It is prudent to consult and discuss management plans with the thoracic surgical team. As no guidelines exist for the management of hydrothorax in PD patients, it is unclear which approach confers the best long-term outcomes.

Temporary Interruption of Peritoneal Dialysis (Conservative Management). There is a clear consensus that interruption of PD should be the initial step in the definitive management of hydrothorax. It is believed that discontinuation of PD acts to reduce the size of the effusion and in some cases promote spontaneous resolution of the pleuroperitoneal communication. It is thought that the acidic hypertonic PD fluid may act as an irritant and hence a sclerosing agent to close small defects in the hemidiaphragm. Discontinuation of PD should occur for a period of 2 to 6 weeks.[53,65] A temporary transfer to HD often is necessary, especially if the patient has limited residual renal function. Using this approach, one case series noted a 53% success rate in the return to long-term PD. However, a high recurrence rate also was noted.[65]

Occasionally, patients who experience hydrothorax on CAPD are able to resume PD by cycler after only being treated with conservative measures (i.e., temporary interruption of PD). As previously mentioned, the main determinants of IAP are volume and position, and therefore a dialysis prescription emphasizing low-volume, supine-based dialysis should be initiated in these patients. Although somewhat counterintuitive, the supine position is not conducive to fluid migration into the pleural cavity. One explanation is that the decrease in IAP afforded by the supine position more than compensates for the movement of fluid into the pleura when supine.[66]

TABLE 33.5 **Causes of Catheter Malfunction**

	Cause	Presentation	Management
One-way obstruction	Constipation—stool extrinsically impinges on catheter	Poor dialysate outflow Evidence of fecal loading on abdominal x-ray	Laxatives, stool softeners, suppositories; omission of constipating agents such as iron, calcium, and opioids peri-insertion
	Catheter tip migration (may be precipitated by constipation; intestinal peristalsis)	Poor dialysate outflow Catheter tip incorrectly positioned on abdominal x-ray	Radiological manipulation Surgical manipulation or replacement, often laparoscopic
	Extraluminal occlusion by omentum, adhesions, or catheter "engulfment" by fallopian tube fimbriae	Poor dialysate outflow Abdominal x-ray may or may not show catheter displacement	Forceful flushing—but risk for mechanical damage Surgical manipulation—omentopexy can be performed. Laparoscopic "salpingopexy" or salpingectomy when obstructed by fallopian tube
Two-way obstruction	Intraluminal catheter occlusion by thrombus/fibrin	Poor dialysate inflow and outflow Adhesions may be visible on CT peritoneography—limited distribution of dialysate is suggestive	Heparin in dialysate: 500 units/L Urokinase: instilled for 1 h Recombinant tPA
	Catheter kinking	Poor dialysate inflow and outflow	Catheter manipulation—radiological vs. surgical At the time of insertion, the operator should check for good inflow and outflow

CT, Computed tomography; *tPA*, tissue plasminogen activator.

Pleurodesis. Pleurodesis is another option for repairing the pleuroperitoneal communication leading to hydrothorax. This method involves the instillation of a sclerosing agent into the pleural cavity, which causes an inflammatory reaction, leading to pleural fibrosis and subsequent obliteration of the diaphragmatic defect. No consensus has emerged regarding the optimal timing for pleurodesis.[65] Some have proposed using it concurrently with conservative measures, whereas others have advocated its use as a second-line measure after conservative treatments have failed.

Several agents have been used successfully for pleurodesis. These include talc, tetracycline, autologous blood, fibrin glue, and hemolytic streptococcal preparation OK-432.[67,68,56] Pleurodesis can be undertaken via the chest tube or now, more commonly as part of a VATS procedure. This enables direct visualization to ensure effective talc poudrage as well as identification of diaphragmatic defects.[69] Tetracycline and talc appear to have similar success rates.[69]

Some authors advocate for the resumption of PD as early as 10 days after pleurodesis.[53] In contrast, others favor a more conservative strategy opting to resume PD after 4 to 6 weeks. Although it is currently unclear which is the best approach, the use of pleurodesis in the management of hydrothorax is associated with good long-term results. In fact, a large systematic review demonstrated 48% of patients treated with pleurodesis were able to resume long-term PD.[65]

Surgical Intervention. VATS has become the preferred modality to obliterate the diaphragmatic defect as the pleuroperitoneal communication can be directly visualized.[70] The "blebs" in the diaphragm often can be seen and then sutured, stapled, or reinforced with Teflon patches.[47] As previously described, VATS is also an effective vehicle for pleurodesis. It is recommended that 2 to 3 L of dialysate be infused intraoperatively at the conclusion of the procedure to ensure that there is no seepage of dialysate indicating an ongoing defect. Surgery utilizing a thoracotomy is significantly invasive and reserved as a last resort. Unsurprisingly, recurrence rate is highest when the communication is not detected at the time of surgery. VATS treatment of hydrothorax has been associated with excellent long-term outcomes. In one study, 88% of patients were able to resume long-term PD without recurrence of hydrothorax.[65]

MALFUNCTION OF THE PERITONEAL CATHETER

Malfunction of the peritoneal dialysis catheter is one of the most common complications of PD occurring in up to 20% of patients, not infrequently necessitating transfer to HD.[71]

Malfunction frequently manifests early in the course of PD and is highlighted by poor drainage from the catheter.

Drainage problems can be broken down into "one-way obstruction," which involves adequate inflow but poor outflow; and "two-way obstruction," which entails both poor inflow and outflow.

The primary causes of catheter malfunction are summarized in Table 33.5.

Poor catheter outflow is usually the result of obstruction around the holes in the intraperitoneal portion of the dialysis catheter.[72] During instillation of dialysate, the increased pressure pushes away the obstruction, so inflow is preserved. However, with the negative Bernoulli force involved in drainage of effluent, the obstructing material comes into contact with the catheter and envelopes it, limiting outflow. A 2006 case series reported that catheter tip migration was the most

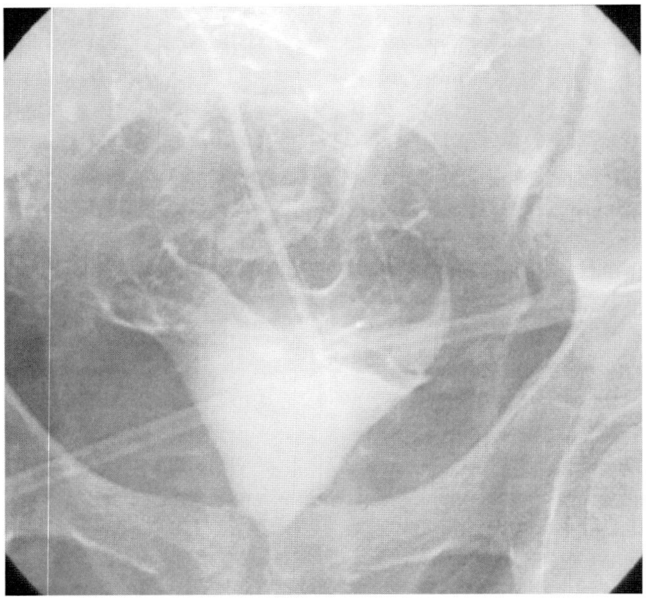

FIG. 33.6 Radiocontrast study of a nonfunctioning catheter. This patient had a history of previous abdominal surgery. A catheter was inserted without direct visualization. There were problems with both inflow and outflow. Injection of dye through the catheter showed that the catheter was in a pocket of the peritoneal cavity defined by adhesions on either side.

common cause of one-way obstruction of the PD catheter.[73] A more recent retrospective pediatric study reviewed 452 access revisions over an 8-year period.[74] Sixty percent of the access revisions were for mechanical obstruction and this doubled the risk for technique failure compared with infectious causes.

Investigating for causes of poor outflow or one-way obstruction should begin with a plain abdominal x-ray. This is a simple technique that allows for easy identification of the common causes, namely, constipation and catheter migration. If the abdominal film does not identify a cause, then a CT can be undertaken with contrast injected through the PD catheter. A catheter dye study can suggest omental wrap or adhesions as causes of outflow obstruction (Fig. 33.6).

An uncommon but nonetheless important cause of catheter malfunction is obstruction by fallopian tube fimbriae. Direct visualization by laparoscopy is thought to be the most efficient diagnostic tool for this complication not least because catheter manipulation along with salpingopexy or salpingectomy can be undertaken if appropriate.[75]

The management of outflow obstruction is dependent on the cause. Constipation usually can be easily treated with judicious laxative use; this may be sufficient to restore catheter function.[76] It is prudent to try this approach even in the absence of radiological evidence of constipation. It is important to ensure that other potentially constipating medications such as iron and calcium are held temporarily before catheter insertion as these medications may contribute to constipation.

For catheter tips that have migrated into the upper abdomen, a guidewire can be inserted through the PD catheter radiologically to enable maneuver back to the pelvis.[77] Although successful repositioning will occur in almost all

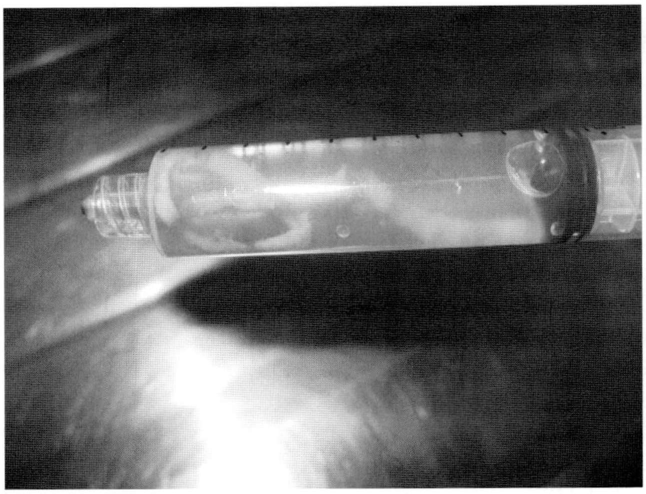

FIG. 33.7 Fibrin strand flushed from the catheter. A recently placed peritoneal dialysis catheter had poor inflow and outflow. Aspiration of the catheter withdrew a large fibrin plug (seen inside the syringe barrel).

patients, the rate of recurrence is high with long-term patency being <50%.[78] Laparoscopic manipulation or catheter replacement is frequently used and can be particularly appropriate for the management of omental wrap.

In recent years, tacking of the omentum to the upper abdomen, or omentopexy, has been performed at the time of laparoscopic PD catheter insertion in an attempt to prophylactically avoid future problems. A retrospective review of PD catheter insertions performed over a 10-year period showed that "advanced" laparoscopic insertion using the creation of a rectus sheath tunnel, selective omentopexy, and adhesiolysis significantly reduced catheter dysfunction rate and increased PD longevity.[79-81]

Problems with both inflow and outflow, or two-way obstruction, are usually the result of intraluminal obstruction or a kink in the PD catheter.[82] There have been multiple case reports highlighting materials that cause intraluminal obstruction. These include blood clots, cryoglobulins, fibrin strands (Fig. 33.7), stones, and fungal balls.[83,84]

Before initiating a diagnostic workup for suspected two-way obstruction flushing the catheter under high pressure with heparinized saline followed by aspiration should be attempted.[85] If this maneuver is unsuccessful, then tissue plasminogen activator (tPA) should be instilled and allowed to dwell for a few hours to lyse old clots or other foreign material.[86,87] The transfer set should be inspected to ensure it is not occluded with fibrin.

If the catheter obstruction persists, then a diagnostic workup similar to that of one-way obstruction should be implemented. If an occlusion or kink in the PD catheter is found, a guidewire or balloon can be inserted via the catheter using a fiberscope.[88] Alternatively, surgical manipulation via a laparoscopic approach can be undertaken and has yielded positive results.[89]

DRAIN PAIN

Drain pain during PD is a commonly encountered problem. It frequently occurs during training and can negatively affect a patient's progress as well as confidence levels. Despite this, there is a paucity of published data regarding the problem. A Canadian survey questioned 293 patients on automated PD and found that 72 were using a tidal modality. Of these, 25% had been started on tidal dialysis in an attempt to alleviate drain pain.[90]

The precise cause of drain pain is unclear. However, it is usually a problem occurring during cycler usage. Postulated explanations have therefore included the application of negative pressure to the sensitive parietal peritoneum during the hydraulic suction of the cycler. Another theory relates to suction on the bowel wall. In addition, it has been suggested that low catheter insertion sites may be contributory as a result of the catheter tip being more likely to be in contact with parietal peritoneum.[41]

Tidal PD was first introduced as a method to increase contact time of dialysis fluid with the peritoneal membrane and so improve solute clearance. In tidal PD, a residual volume is left in the peritoneal cavity. For example, for a patient with a 2 L dwell volume, 85% tidal flow would imply that after the first 2 L infusion, 1.7 L (rather than 2 L) is drained, and the next inflow and outflows are again 1.7 L until the final drain, when all the residual fluid is drained. Therefore during this process a residual volume resides in the peritoneal cavity. Due to its relative complexity, tidal PD is not used often for clearance purposes, but can be very helpful in those with inflow and outflow pain. The tidal volume can be increased even further (e.g., to 50%). In the past, there were some concerns regarding the use of tidal volumes as the rates of increased intraperitoneal volume events or "overfill" were increased.[91] However, newer cyclers guard against this by continuing to suck on an empty peritoneal cavity that can then unfortunately lead to worsening drain pain. If this fails to alleviate symptoms, a switch to CAPD may be needed; drainage is gentler and less likely to incur symptoms.

HEMOPERITONEUM

Bloody dialysate or hemoperitoneum is a complication of PD that can be very distressing to the patient. As little as 2 mL of blood can render a 1 L bag of dialysate visibly blood-tinged.[92] Intraperitoneal bleeding may occur frequently in those not on PD; however, it is clinically silent. On the other hand, in patients on PD, a window to the peritoneum is provided by the PD catheter, and therefore intraperitoneal bleeding is easily detectable.

The incidence of hemoperitoneum in PD patients is quite varied, ranging from 7% to 52% depending on the report.[93-95] The largest review to date demonstrated an incidence of 8.4% of PD patients.[93]

A wide variety of causes has been reported and a categorization as benign and malignant has been proposed.[96] Another approach includes causes due to complications involving the PD catheter, obstetrical and gynecological issues, intraabdominal organs (such as kidneys, liver, spleen, and gastrointestinal [GI] tract), vasculature, endoscopic procedures, coagulopathies, infection, and other more rare causes (Table 33.6). Catheter insertion can lead to hemoperitoneum, especially in the presence of platelet dysfunction and predisposition to bleeding associated with uremia.[97] Bloody dialysate can lead to fibrin and clot formation inside the catheter lumen, leading to inflow and outflow dysfunction.[95] Catheter placement also can traumatize vessels or organs, but direct visualization through laparoscopy minimizes the risk.[92]

TABLE 33.6 Causes of Hemoperitoneum

Catheter-related
Obstetrical and gynecological
Menstruation
Ovulation
Hemorrhagic luteal cyst
Ovarian cyst rupture
Pregnancy (uterine tear)
Intraabdominal
Kidneys
Renal cyst rupture
Acquired cystic kidney disease
Autosomal dominant polycystic kidney disease
Tuberous sclerosis (angiomyolipomas)
Liver
Liver rupture
Hepatic tumors
Hepatocarcinoma
Hepatocellular adenoma
Liver metastasis
Liver cyst rupture
Spleen
Splenic rupture
Splenic infarct
Gastrointestinal tract
Vascular
Erosion of mesenteric vessel by Tenckhoff catheter
Aneurysm rupture
Procedure related
Pericardiocentesis
Radiation
Colonoscopy
Bleeding diatheses
Uremic platelet dysfunction
Anemia
Infection
Cytomegalovirus infection
Peritonitis
Other
Retroperitoneal hematoma
Iliopsoas spontaneous hematoma

From Lew SQ. Hemoperitoneum: bloody peritoneal dialysate in ESRD patients receiving peritoneal dialysis. *Perit Dial Int.* 2007;27(3):226-233.

The majority of hemoperitoneum episodes, however, are the result of menstruation and they occur in more than half of menstruating women on PD.[98] This is why women on PD are twice as likely as men to experience an episode of hemoperitoneum.[93] Two mechanisms have been proposed to explain the occurrence of blood in the peritoneal cavity associated with menstruation. First, uterine blood can be expelled retrograde by uterine contraction into the fallopian tubes that open into the peritoneal cavity. This process is known as *retrograde menstruation*.[99] Second, endometrial deposits in the peritoneal cavity also may cause bloody effluent. This is because this ectopic endometrial tissue is under the same hormonal control as the intrauterine endometrium and therefore sheds at the same time.[100] Both mechanisms lead to a periodic appearance of bloody effluent and may sometimes be mistaken for mild peritonitis related to the presence of blood in the peritoneal cavity.[96]

Although menstruation is the most common cause, hemoperitoneum has been reported in pregnant women receiving PD.[101] More rare causes include intraabdominal pathology of solid organs. These can either be benign such as bleeding of ruptured ovarian or renal cysts or serious such as spleen, liver, renal, or GI malignancies.[92,96,102,103] Disruption of blood vessels, such as during Tenckhoff catheter placement, can lead to hemoperitoneum.[104] Additional causes are rupture of omental artery,[105] abdominal aorta aneurysm rupture,[106] and splenic artery pseudoaneurysm, with the latter being treated via embolization.[107] Intraabdominal trauma, bleeding diatheses, intraperitoneal infections, and conditions such as encapsulating peritoneal sclerosis (EPS) also are possible etiological factors.[92,102,107,109] Some rarer causes of hemoperitoneum have been reported. These include spontaneous rectus sheath hematoma[110] colonoscopy-related[111] and cardiac catheterization-related.[112] As some of the causes—such as ischemic bowel, colon or urological cancer, pancreatitis, encapsulating peritoneal sclerosis—may be serious, it is important to consider them in a patient presenting with bloody effluent.

The presentation of hemoperitoneum should initially trigger the PD patient to undertake several rapid PD exchanges to determine whether the bleeding is persistent or an acute event.[113] These exchanges are carried out using room temperature dialysate, which causes vasoconstriction of the intraperitoneal blood vessels and often abrogates the bleeding.[114] However, patients must be reminded to seek medical attention, especially if the bloody effluent persists or darkens or they develop symptoms of volume depletion, hemodynamic disturbance, and abdominal or back pain.

The diagnostic evaluation of hemoperitoneum should be guided by the clinical setting. As menstruation is most often associated with this condition, an exhaustive workup for potential causes need not be undertaken in a menstruating female who is otherwise well. However, should this not be the case or should the hemoperitoneum persist, investigations must be undertaken to account for the source of the bleeding. At the very least, an abdominal ultrasound should be performed to assess for intraabdominal pathology. If this investigation is negative, then CT of the abdomen and pelvis should be performed. Routine blood work should also be undertaken including a complete blood cell (CBC) and a coagulation profile to assess for a coagulopathy. If the bleeding persists, despite negative radiographic investigations, then an isotope-labeled red blood cell scan can be done to localize the site of bleeding.

The management of hemoperitoneum in PD patients is dependent on the underlying cause. As previously mentioned, a majority of patients will not require any definitive therapy; however, in severe cases of bleeding investigations or even laparoscopy for both diagnostic and therapeutic reasons, flushes with dialysate at room temperature may need to be performed.

In the majority of patients presenting with hemoperitoneum, there are often no long-term deleterious sequelae.[93,115,116] Specifically, studies have demonstrated that hemoperitoneum, be it a single episode or recurrent episodes, imparts no change on peritoneal membrane characteristics, ultrafiltration, or a predisposition of the peritoneum to peritonitis.[93,116]

That being said, the main complication associated with this condition is the coagulation of blood in and around the intraperitoneal portion of the PD catheter leading to its obstruction. Although this complication is uncommon, it is recommended that heparin be instilled intraperitoneally at a dose of 500 to 1000 units/L as long as the dialysate has visible blood or fibrin, to prevent this problem.[87,92] Although administering anticoagulation in a patient having some degree of bleeding may appear counterintuitive, anecdotal accounts have demonstrated it to be efficacious in hemoperitoneum caused by menstrual bleeding.[116] When hemoperitoneum is a manifestation of other causes, the use of heparin needs to be weighed against the risk for increased bleeding.

CHYLOPERITONEUM

Chyloperitoneum, or chylous ascites, is defined as the pathological accumulation of chylomicrons rich in triacyglycerides (TGs) into the peritoneal cavity. It is a rare complication of PD that can be confused with signs of peritonitis. It is important to differentiate between the two, so that appropriate management can be undertaken. This phenomenon arises from the interruption of the lymphatic drainage from the GI tract to the main lymphatic trunks.[117] The etiology is, so far, unclear, but involves a communication between lymphatics and the peritoneal cavity (Table 33.7).

After a fatty meal, long-chain fatty acids are absorbed directly into the lymphatic system and increase the flow of lymph, whereas medium-chain TGs are absorbed into the portal circulation, bypassing the lymphatic system. Hence, chyloperitoneum is an intermittent event occurring after a fatty meal, and it has been treated by following a diet in which long-chain fatty acids are avoided.

For the PD patients, chyloperitoneum presents as a history of painless cloudy peritoneal effluent. The peritoneal fluid has the characteristic milky appearance due to high percentage of TGs, whose concentration in the dialysate is greater than the one in the plasma. Diagnosis is established by analysis of the fluid showing normal peritoneal fluid white cell count, and Sudan III staining that reveals fat globules and high TG content.

Treatment is conservative and the aim is to reduce the flow of lymph into the mesenteric nodes. Therefore temporary cessation of PD, a low-fat medium-chain TG diet, parenteral nutrition and octreotide administration may be helpful until its resolution.[118]

TABLE 33.7 Etiology of Chyloperitoneum

After Intervention/ Operation	Drug Use	Cancer	Other
Catheter insertion	Calcium channel blocker	Lymphoma	Spontaneously
Bilateral nephrectomy (postoperatively)	Renin inhibitor	Intraabdominal malignancies	Tuberculous peritonitis
G-tube insertion	Sirolimus after renal transplantation		Superior vena cava syndrome
			Intravenous administration of high doses of long-chain fatty acids

METABOLIC COMPLICATIONS

Glucose has served well as the first, and for three decades the dominant, osmotic agent in PD. However, the absorption of glucose and its byproducts through the peritoneum causes metabolic complications in patients on PD such as hyperglycemia, insulin resistance (IR), obesity, lipid abnormalities, and hyperleleptinemia.[119] As all of these can potentially increase cardiovascular risk, it is important to recognize, prevent, and manage these complications.

Hyperglycemia

There is a substantial glucose load with traditional solutions in PD patients. Plasma insulin levels rise along with intraperitoneal glucose in a dose-dependent manner.[120] The amount of glucose absorbed from the peritoneal membrane significantly increases in rapid transporters and depends on the dialysis modality.[121] There is a debate as to whether the more glucose the patients absorb, the more prone they are to obesity, dyslipidemia, IR, loss of the osmotic gradient required for sustained ultrafiltration capacity, and development of cardiovascular disease.[122]

The consequences of the glucose burden can be divided into the systemic effects and the local effect on the peritoneal membrane.

Systemic effects can be attributed to a combination of hyperglycemia, excess calorie uptake, and carbohydrate load.[123] Glucose absorption from the peritoneum results in an extended period of hyperglycemia followed by a similar period of hyperinsulinemia, increased oxidative stress, weight gain, and hypertension.[124] New-onset hyperglycemia in nondiabetic patients on PD has been reported to result in lower survival, although it may be a marker for a group of patients with more comorbidities.[120] Yet, another study has reported no influence of glucose solutions on glucose and hemoglobin A_{1c} levels in patients after 1 year on PD.[125] In addition, prolonged peritoneal exposure to hypertonic glucose solutions can induce structural and functional alterations on the peritoneal membrane,[126] although the clinical significance of these changes remains unclear.

Aside from fat restriction and glycemic control, minimizing the need for hypertonic dialysate should be employed via three complementary strategies. The first is to limit dietary salt and fluid intake, the second to maintain residual kidney function and optimize renal salt and water excretion with diuretics, and the third to optimize peritoneal ultrafiltration with minimal glucose use. Glucose-sparing solutions, such as those with amino acids or icodextrin, could potentially benefit both diabetic and nondiabetic PD patients by improving disturbances in carbohydrate metabolism,[127,128] reducing fasting insulin levels, body weight, and fat mass and as well as improving insulin sensitivity.[129,130] However, it is unclear how much these strategies will reduce cardiovascular events in this population.

Lipid Abnormalities

Patients on PD present a more atherogenic lipid profile than HD patients, as they have elevated levels of lipoprotein (a), apolipoprotein (Apo)-B, total cholesterol (C), low-density liporotein-C, very low-density lipoprotein (VLDL)-C, and TGs.[123] Proposed mechanisms for this phenomenon are (1) glucose absorption from the dialysates leading to increased insulin levels and (2) protein loss in the dialysate leading to hyperlipidemia akin to that with nephrotic syndrome. Both of these lead to enhanced hepatic synthesis and secretion of TGs, lipoproteins, and VLDL.[123]

Although dyslipidemia represents a major important risk factor for cardiovascular disease development in the general population, its role in the atherogenesis of PD patients remains controversial.

The treatment of this abnormality is problematic. No prospective study of hypolipidemic drugs has proved their efficiency in cardiovascular morbidity and mortality reduction.[123] However, effective lowering of Apo-B, TGs, and VLDL has been found with a low-glucose PD regimen or icodextrin use compared with a conventional glucose regimen.[131,132]

Insulin Resistance

IR develops simultaneously with deterioration of kidney function in early stages of chronic kidney disease.[133] After PD initiation, partial correction of uremia and metabolic acidosis improves IR, which is once again deranged by glucose-containing PD fluids.[134] As an acknowledged cardiovascular risk factor in PD patients, even in the absence of diabetes, strategies are being investigated to reverse this process.[135] Replacement of dextrose solutions by icodextrin in CAPD and APD, in diabetic and nondiabetic patients, seems to reduce hyperinsulinemia and improve IR according to homeostatic model assessment (HOMA).[128]

Hepatic Subcapsular Steatosis

Hepatic Subcapsular Steatosis (HSS), first described in 1989, is an atypical form of hepatic steatosis and a rare PD complication in CAPD patients receiving intraperitoneal insulin.[136] In one study, HSS was present in 18% of diabetic CAPD patient receiving intraperitoneal insulin.[137] The pathogenesis is thought to result from high insulin concentrations in the subcapsular hepatocytes, which stimulates TG synthesis; high glucose concentration in the dialysate may potentiate this process. HSS does not appear to cause liver dysfunction and is probably clinically insignificant.[138] Imaging features include lack of mass effect and subcapsular distribution of fatty deposits. Ultrasound has good sensitivity for the detection of HSS, whereas in CT it appears as multiple lesions with low attenuation in a subcapsular location and MR may be required to confirm the fatty nature of hepatic steatosis.[61] HSS decreases in severity or even resolves after cessation of intraperitoneal insulin administration.[139]

ELECTROLYTE DISORDERS

Hypokalemia

Hypokalemia is the most common electrolyte abnormality encountered in PD patients. It is found in 10% to 36% of PD patients.[112] Although the role of hypokalemia in producing arrhythmias and muscle weakness is well documented, it recently has been found to be associated with increased peritonitis rate and mortality in Asian PD patients.[140] In a more recent study, the population-attributable risk for all-cause mortality in PD patients for serum potassium <4 mEq/L was twice as high as that in patients with levels >5.5 mEq/L.[141] Moreover, hypokalemia also could induce a kaliopenic nephropathy, which may hasten the loss of residual renal function.[142]

Three processes have been postulated to explain hypokalemia in PD patients: potassium loss through the bowel and dialysate, poor nutritional intake of potassium-rich fruits and vegetables, and intracellular shift of potassium.[140,143]

Previously, hypokalemia was ascribed to be the result of losses of potassium in the dialysate; however, a recent study has discounted this.[144] Although dialysate losses of potassium are important (each 2-L exchange has the potential to remove 8 mEq per dwell), poor nutritional intake, particularly of potassium-rich foods, seems to be more important. This is especially the case for certain ethnic groups who either avoid fruits and vegetables because of ethnocultural preferences or reduce the potassium content of foods substantially through traditional cooking methods.[140] Patients who have poor nutrition may also be catabolic. In this state, there is breakdown of intracellular macromolecular organic phosphates (RNA) into inorganic phosphates that are excreted in the dialysate, along with potassium. The result is hypokalemia, metabolic alkalosis, and hyponatremia.[143] Finally, potassium may be shifted into cells by a wide variety of mechanisms, particularly the stimulation of insulin secretion from the absorption of the dialysate glucose load.[145] It recently has been postulated that perhaps the lactate buffer added to dialysate solutions may promote intracellular shift of potassium through a similar mechanism as insulin, that is, activation of the NHE3 antiporter creating a driving force for potassium to move into the cell. The role of diuretics and residual renal function has been found to have very little impact on the development of hypokalemia.[140]

The management of hypokalemia in PD patients often is straightforward. As hypokalemia is a risk factor for cardiorespiratory dysfunction, potassium supplementation should be commenced to bring the serum potassium into the normal range. Food sources are preferred as first-line therapy and a dietitian should be consulted. If nutritional intake fails to increase serum potassium concentration, then oral potassium supplementation should be attempted. However, close monitoring of serum electrolytes is warranted, particularly in patients with limited renal reserve, as it is not uncommon to find that a small amount of oral potassium supplementation can lead to a surprising increase in serum potassium concentration. Potassium chloride also can be added to the dialysate to diminish the concentration gradient for the diffusion of potassium into the dialysate to abrogate potassium loss, or can be added in high enough concentration to allow potassium to diffuse from the dialysate to the patient.[146] In the acute setting, up to 20 mmol/L can be added to the dialysate, whereas in chronic cases 3 to 4 mEq/L are usually added. The former dose has been reported to increase the plasma potassium concentration by an average of 0.44 mmol/L over 2 to 3 hours.[147] However, given that the toxicity of the high intraperitoneal potassium concentrations is unknown, its use should be reserved for short-term emergency situations.

ENCAPSULATING PERITONEAL SCLEROSIS

EPS is recognized as the most serious and devastating noninfectious complication of PD. The first case in PD patients was reported in 1980 by Gandhi et al.[148] Since then, our knowledge of this rare condition has improved.

Definition and Epidemiology

EPS has been defined by the International Society of Peritoneal Dialysis as "a clinical syndrome continuously, intermittently, or repeatedly presenting with symptoms of intestinal obstruction due to adhesions of a diffusely thickened peritoneum."[149] Its incidence has been reported to be up to 19.4%,[150] but more recent studies report ranges from 0.5% to 4.4%.[151-153] It has been proposed that the use of less bioincompatible PD solutions and improvements in peritonitis rates have accounted for this decrease. Although the overall incidence of EPS in PD patients is low, the mortality associated with this condition remains high. Mortality rates among PD patients with EPS have been reported to range between 38% to 83%,[150,154] but in more recent studies the survival may vary from 6 to 48 months[155] or from 26% to 56%.[153] Furthermore, a large Japanese study has described a direct relationship between mortality, PD duration, and incidence of EPS. Specifically, they noted a 17.2% incidence of EPS and a 100% mortality rate in patients who were on PD for greater than15 years versus a 2.1% incidence and 8.3% mortality rate in those on PD for less than 5 years.[154]

A geographical predilection for EPS also has been reported. Japan has the highest incidence of EPS among its PD population, whereas North America has the lowest.[156] The limited availability of kidney transplantation in Japan making lifelong PD a necessity has been cited as the main reason explaining this trend.

TABLE 33.8 Factors Implicated in the Etiology of Encapsulating Peritoneal Sclerosis

Unrelated to Peritoneal Dialysis	Related to Peritoneal Dialysis
Idiopathic	Duration of PD
Inflammatory conditions	Peritonitis
Systemic lupus erythematosus	Acetate dialysis solutions (historical)
Familial Mediterranean fever	Chlorhexidine plasticizers
Sarcoidosis	Glucose/hypertonic solutions
Exposures	
β-blockers	
Talc	
Asbestos	
Intraperitoneal chemotherapy	
Abdominal lavage disinfectants	
Gastrointestinal diseases	
Hepatic ascites	
Intraabdominal malignancies	
Diseases of reproductive organs	
Luteinizing thecoma of the ovary	
Endometriosis	
Ventriculoperitoneal shunt	

PD, Peritoneal dialysis.
From Kawaguchi Y, Kawanishi H, Mujais S, et al. *Encapsulating peritoneal sclerosis: definition, etiology, diagnosis, and treatment.* International Society for Peritoneal Dialysis Ad Hoc Committee on Ultrafiltration Management in Peritoneal Dialysis. *Perit Dial Int.* 2000;20(suppl 4):S43-S55.

Risk Factors

A number of risk factors are associated with the development of EPS in PD patients. These can be classified as PD-related and non–PD-related (Table 33.8). Common to all these factors is the disruption of normal peritoneal membrane physiology and subsequent membrane damage. Although there are many PD-related risk factors associated with EPS, three seem to be the most important: duration of PD (believed to be the most significant), persistent or frequent episodes of peritonitis, and cessation of PD.

The duration of PD is believed to be the most significant risk factor for EPS. As previously mentioned, Japanese and Australian studies have demonstrated progressive increases in EPS incidence after 8 years on PD.[154,157] It has been speculated that this relationship may be a consequence of the cumulative exposure of the peritoneum to nonphysiological PD solutions, leading to progressive membrane damage. Interestingly, although a severe peritonitis episode can trigger EPS in a long-term PD patient, the overall number of peritonitis episodes is not a very strong predictor of EPS. Perhaps, this is because a patient with frequent episodes may have to give up the method sooner.[158]

Compounding the damage from PD solutions, persistent or recurring episodes of peritonitis have also been considered strong risk factors for EPS development. From a pathophysiological point of view, peritonitis superimposes a large inflammatory response on an already damaged peritoneal membrane leading to further membrane damage. This is especially the case for peritonitis episodes caused by *Staphylococcus aureus*, fungal organisms, and *Pseudomonas*.[149] In fact, a large Japanese study recently reported that PD patients who developed EPS had peritonitis rates three times greater than their non-EPS counterparts.[159] Conversely, some investigators have questioned the significance of peritonitis in the development of EPS given that it is also well documented in patients who have never had an episode of peritonitis.[150,154] Nevertheless, the sheer complexity of EPS development makes it difficult to discount the contribution of peritonitis based on this observation alone.

It has been observed that PD patients are developing EPS at increasing rates upon discontinuation of PD.[160] This was demonstrated by Kawanishi et al.[154] who reported that 93% (37 of 40) of patients developed EPS upon withdrawal from PD for various reasons. Moreover, it was noted that the onset of EPS was quite abrupt, occurring within 4 months of discontinuation. It is tempting to speculate that the withdrawal of PD abrogates the continued removal of cytokines, growth factors, and fibrin from the peritoneal cavity by dialysate. Consequently, these lingering humoral factors propagate ongoing inflammation ultimately leading to the development of EPS.

Another important PD-related risk factor is membrane transport status. Patients who developed EPS have been reported to have higher dialysate-to-plasma-creatinine ratios, signifying rapid transport status, earlier in the course of their PD than those who did not.[161] The early onset of rapid transport status may aid in the exudation of cytokines and other growth factors, thereby promoting damage to the peritoneal membrane. On the other hand, rapid transport status may signify peritoneal membrane inflammation, an early harbinger of EPS.

Other PD-related risk factors such as acetate-based dialysis solutions, chlorhexidine disinfectants, plasticizers, β-blockers, and an acute abdominal event have all previously been implicated in the development of EPS.[162]

Pathophysiology

In PD patients, morphological changes occur in the peritoneal membrane over time. These changes include the loss of mesothelium, epithelial to mesenchymal transition of mesothelial cells, expansion of the submesothelial compact zone (acellular collagen layer and collagen fibroblast layer), fibrosis, angiogenesis, and vascular degeneration.[163] Collectively, this process is called *peritoneal sclerosis* and is the result of ongoing damage to the peritoneum caused by a variety of factors.[163] It is important to realize that peritoneal sclerosis is not EPS. Rather, it is considered by some to be an early change that may or may not be a step in the evolution of the peritoneal membrane toward EPS. Although both conditions share many morphological features, recent studies of patients affected by EPS have demonstrated unique membrane changes. In the advanced stage of EPS, a dense, hard, fibrous tissue rich in microvessels and an encapsulating, thickened membrane cover the bowels. Morphological studies of peritoneal membranes with EPS have informed the stratification of EPS development into two stages: the initial stage, which is characterized by a marked inflammatory state; and the late stage, which is distinguished by the resolution of inflammation and the appearance of peritoneal membrane fibrosis as described previously.

The "Two-hit" Hypothesis. The "two-hit" hypothesis is based on the principle that two events or insults are required for the development of EPS. The first "hit" leads to peritoneal deterioration both in structure and function and is the consequence of ongoing injury to the peritoneal membrane from a variety of factors. Historically, the best described factor is such as the use of bioincompatible dialysis solutions.[164] The second "hit" often is facilitated by factors that cause a marked inflammatory response in the peritoneum such as acute and chronic bacterial peritonitis episodes and PD discontinuation.[164] This results in fibrosis, encapsulation of the peritoneum, and intestinal obstruction.

It has been well established that the ongoing exposure of the peritoneum to high levels of glucose, glucose degradation products from heat sterilization, and an acidic pH is associated with morphological changes in the membrane.[165] Specifically, the mesothelial cells are preferentially targeted by this "toxic" milieu.[163] The role of advanced glycation end-products (AGEs) also have been implicated in the development of peritoneal damage.[166] The binding of AGEs to their receptors on mesothelial and other cells leads to the upregulation and secretion of a variety of humoral factors involved in peritoneal damage.[166] Other factors such as plasticizers from the PD catheter, recurrent episodes of peritonitis, and various medications such as chlorhexidine have been implicated in contributing to peritoneal membrane deterioration.[162]

Proponents of the "two-hit" theory believe that an additive relationship exists between the degree of peritoneal damage (first "hit") and the intensity of the inflammatory response (second "hit").[167] Given that the extent of peritoneal damage increases with the duration of PD, the degree of the inflammatory stimulus ("second hit") need not be as strong over time, which explains why EPS can develop on long-term PD after a seemingly mild inciting events.

Clinical Presentation and Diagnosis. EPS is a slowly progressive disorder that may remain asymptomatic for a prolonged period of time. When symptoms and signs do arise, they often are vague and nonspecific; therefore a high index of suspicion of EPS is required.[168] Abdominal discomfort, nausea, vomiting, changes in bowel habits, fever, and new-onset inflow pain often are the initial inflammatory manifestations of EPS. As peritoneal sclerosis progresses and GI function further declines, these symptoms increase in frequency and intensity. Soon anorexia sets in, leading to weight loss and protein-energy wasting. Other important clinical signs indicating peritoneal damage may be present such as hemorrhagic effluent, recurrent episodes of "culture negative" peritonitis, and acquisition of rapid transporter status

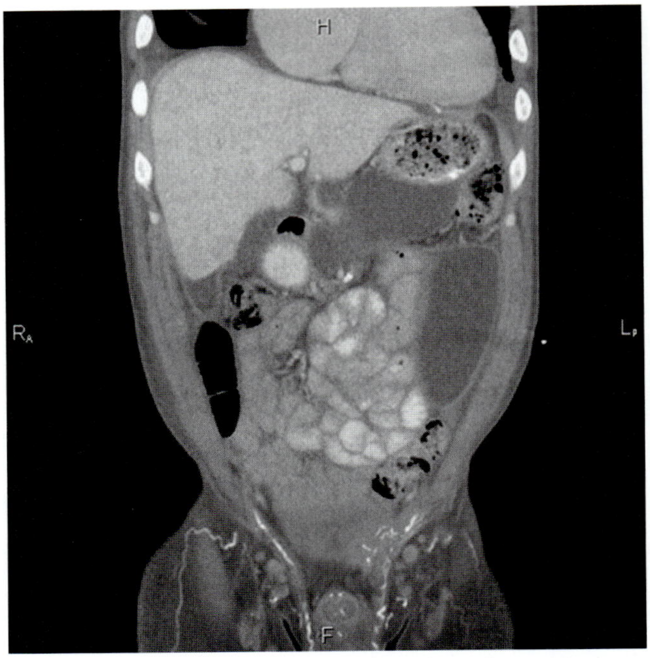

FIG. 33.8 Computed tomography scan of a patient with encapsulating peritoneal sclerosis. A patient on peritoneal dialysis for 12 years developed recurrent small bowel obstruction. The coronal slice on computed tomography shows the bowel (with oral contrast) cocooned in the center of the peritoneal cavity, surrounded by pockets of intraperitoneal fluid.

with a falloff in ultrafiltration. Ultimately, frequent episodes of bowel obstruction occur, which clinically herald a state of peritoneal fibrosis.

Biochemically, EPS may present with aberrations in laboratory findings consistent with systemic inflammation. These include elevated levels of C-reactive protein (CRP), refractory anemia, and hypoalbuminemia.[160]

Given the large variability in the presentation of EPS, further testing is usually warranted. Historically, radiological evaluation of the peritoneum and its structures has been the first step in confirming the diagnosis of EPS and in ruling out other conditions. UK EPS group clinical practice guidelines, as of 2009, proposed two major criteria for EPS diagnosis: (1) symptoms of obstructive ileus with or without systemic inflammation and (2) radiological evidence of peritoneal thickening, encapsulation, or intestinal obstruction (Fig. 33.8). There are four radiological findings that are pertinent to confirmation of the diagnosis of EPS: (1) peritoneal thickening and encapsulation, (2) intestinal obstruction, (3) peritoneal calcification, and (4) cocooning.[149] These findings can be quite variable in a given patient depending on the radiological modality chosen and the stage of EPS.

Plain abdominal films have demonstrated limited utility in diagnosing EPS, whereas abdominal ultrasound is an excellent modality for detecting changes associated with EPS.[61] It can demonstrate multiple abnormalities in the peritoneal cavity including the characteristic trilaminar appearance of the bowel wall.[61] However, it requires the presence of fluid in the peritoneum for optimal sensitivity and is operator dependent.

Although x-rays may detect dilated small bowel loops, air-fluid levels, and peritoneal calcification, they possess limited specificity.[61]

On the other hand, CT is the most sensitive and specific modality for demonstrating findings characteristic for EPS,[61] although these can be subtle and therefore subject to interpretation by the reviewing radiologist. This may be the reason for the "overcalling" of EPS based on CT findings. In an attempt to abrogate such variability, a study has demonstrated that in the correct clinical setting, the diagnosis of EPS can be made if bowel tethering and peritoneal calcifications are found on CT study.[169] Another study concluded that sensitivity reached 100% for EPS diagnosis with increased radiologist experience and a combination of CT findings.[170] When three of the following six parameters are present (or two of the five if no intravenous contrast medium is administered), it results in 100% sensitivity and 94% specificity for EPS diagnosis:

1. Peritoneal enhancement
2. Peritoneal thickening
3. Peritoneal calcification
4. Bowel tethering
5. Bowel dilatation
6. Fluid loculation/septation

Despite CT scanning being a valuable tool in the diagnosis of EPS, it is not useful as a screening tool.[169] Specifically, in a retrospective study of 13 EPS patients with CT scans 4 months before their diagnosis, this modality was unable to detect any abnormal findings in nine patients.[169] This may attest to the notion that EPS may have a fulminant course and early detection through screening may be unwarranted. Obviously, further study is needed to confirm this observation. The role of MRI in diagnosing EPS is still being evaluated; however, data suggest results similar to CT.[61,171]

Follow-through examinations of small and large bowels may be helpful in locating the obstruction site. However, they are invasive, time consuming, and require preparation and thus are rarely used.[178]

The gold standard for diagnosing EPS is direct visualization of the peritoneal membrane. At times, histological examination may be required; however, the diagnosis of EPS is essentially confirmed when gross examination of the peritoneal cavity demonstrates thickening of the peritoneum, encasing some or all of the intestines in a tanned, leathery cocoon.[172]

Pathologically, EPS is characterized by complete loss of the mesothelium, accompanied by gross interstitial thickening within the membrane. The thickened interstitial layer is composed of fibroblasts, collagen, abnormal vasculature, and at times inflammatory mononuclear cells.[167,172] Marked fibrin staining also is found along the membrane indicating extensive fibrin deposition.[167,172]

Biomarkers. A number of biomarkers have been studied in the PD effluent. It has been suggested that potential diagnostic markers included in PD patients are cancer antigen 125 (CA-125) and interleukin (IL)-6. CA-125 appears to be a surrogate marker for mesothelial cell mass, and some studies find that its levels reduce years before EPS. In addition, IL-6 levels were high even 2 years before EPS diagnosis. The combination of low dialysate CA-125 with high IL-6, exhibit 70% sensitivity and 100% specificity for EPS in PD patients appearing with ultrafiltration failure.[173]

Therapeutic Approaches in Encapsulating Peritoneal Sclerosis

The relative paucity of EPS cases imparts substantial difficulty when attempting to study therapeutic interventions. In fact, most studies focusing on EPS therapy are small, anecdotal, or observational accounts, which limits the generalizability of the results.[160,172] Since the original reports of EPS were published, the management of this condition has evolved. Although surgical management was the mainstay of treatment in the past, insights into the pathophysiology of EPS have permitted the introduction of novel medical therapies. Despite being unable to demonstrate a substantial change in the natural history of EPS on a consistent basis, these therapies have helped reinforce the notion that early initiation of treatment is paramount to potentially facilitate some degree of improvement. In this regard, a staging classification of EPS has recently been proposed by Kawanishi.[174] It stratifies EPS into four stages based on clinical and pathological findings at different times in the course of EPS development. This allows for rational therapeutic interventions to be used according to the stage of EPS (Table 33.9).

Conservative Measures. As previously mentioned, GI symptoms are pervasive in EPS. As a result, patients often decrease their oral intake substantially. In addition, patients are frequently highly catabolic. Both factors ultimately lead to protein-energy wasting, which plays an important role in the morbidity and mortality associated with this condition.

In mild cases of EPS, where the GI side effects are tolerable, nutritional support through nasogastric feeds or high caloric beverages combined with antiemetics should be instituted. This is in contrast to more severe cases, particularly those with obstruction, where parenteral feeding and bowel rest may be necessary. Although one small study demonstrated a 51% recovery rate in patients treated with only total parenteral nutrition (TPN) and transfer to HD, other reports demonstrate substantially worse outcomes.[154,175] This disparity may be due to complications related to use of TPN itself, but more importantly, it may relate to the cessation of PD, which may accelerate progression of EPS. Given the small numbers of patients in these studies, it is difficult to fully elucidate the contribution or lack thereof of TPN.

Corticosteroids. CCSs have become paramount in the treatment of EPS, with some studies documenting response rates as high as 100%.[176] Although this rate was demonstrated in a small study, the largest study to date involved 39 patients and showed a 38.5% rate of recovery.[154] CCS are particularly useful in early EPS inflammatory stages,[176] and most patients who have responded to CCS were on PD for shorter duration than their counterparts who did not respond. Failure to respond may lead to fibrosis, capsule formation, and the full-blown manifestations of EPS. This has been suggested in

TABLE 33.9 Proposed Staging of Encapsulating Peritoneal Sclerosis

Stage	Clinical Findings	Therapeutic Approach
Stage 1 (pre-EPS period)	Loss of ultrafiltration capacity Development of a high transport state Hypoproteinemia Bloody dialysate, ascites Calcification of peritoneum	Peritoneal rest Peritoneal lavage Glucocorticoids
Stage 2 (inflammation period)	Increase in C-reactive protein Increase in white blood cells Fever Bloody dialysate Ascites Weight loss Appetite loss Diarrhea	Glucocorticoids
Stage 3 (encapsulating or progressive period)	Disappearance of the signs of inflammation Appearance of symptoms/signs of ileus (nausea, vomiting, abdominal pain, constipation, abdominal mass, ascites)	Glucocorticoids Total parenteral nutrition Tamoxifen
Stage 4 (ileus or complete period)	Anorexia Complete ileus Abdominal mass	Surgical intervention

EPS, Encapsulating peritoneal sclerosis.
From Nakamoto H. Encapsulating peritoneal sclerosis: clinician's approach to diagnosis and medical treatment. *Perit Dial Int.* 2005;25(suppl 4):S30-S38.

both animal models and humans, where the early initiation of steroid therapy minimized the progression to EPS, improved bowel function and survival.[164]

Although there is consensus for early steroid initiation, there is no marker to indicate optimal timing. Furthermore, it is unclear which is the best dosing regimen—pulse or continuous CCS. In the past, markers of inflammation such as CRP, ferritin, and hypoalbuminemia have been used to guide clinical decision making; however, these markers are neither sensitive nor specific for EPS. Both low-dose steroids and pulse-steroid regimens, followed by maintenance therapy, have been used successfully.[154]

Ultimately, clinical judgment must be used to decide the therapy and dose initiation. In this regard, a trial of CCS should be administered fairly quickly in most patients who fail to respond to more conservative therapies after peritonitis or other intraabdominal infection has been ruled out.

Tamoxifen. Tamoxifen is a selective estrogen receptor modulator with antifibrotic properties used in the treatment of various fibrotic disorders and therefore has garnered interest as a therapeutic agent for EPS.[177] In a recent large retrospective Dutch study, significantly lower mortality was demonstrated in EPS patients treated with tamoxifen (45.8%) compared with those not treated with tamoxifen (74.4%).[177] Tamoxifen seems to act through inhibition and modulation of transforming growth factor (TGF)-β. In vitro and in animal models, tamoxifen blocked TGF-beta induced epithelial-to-mesenchymal transition. It also preserved the fibrinolytic activity and reduced the migration capacity of mesothelial cells, leading to reduced fibrosis and decreased vascular endothelin growth factor (VEGF) in PD-effluent and subsequent reduced angiogenesis in the peritoneum.[178] However, tamoxifen has been almost always used in combination with CCS, leaving its use as monotherapy uninvestigated, and further work is warranted. Potential side effects include deep vein thrombosis, endometrial cancer, and calciphylaxis.[179] Obviously, further study into the role of tamoxifen in the management of EPS is warranted.

Surgical Management. Despite the use of steroids and tamoxifen in the management of EPS, approximately 50% of patients do not respond and eventually require surgery in the late stages of EPS.[176] The Japanese have a wealth of experience in the surgical management of EPS and have demonstrated that in experienced hands, surgery can improve symptoms and survival.

The current surgical technique used for EPS involves peritonectomy (peritoneum resection) and enterolysis (resection of fibrous tissue with lysis of intestinal adhesions to release the bowel).[176] Postsurgery mortality ranges from 19% to 34.5%.[176] Surgery is the most successful form of treatment, and recurrence rates after surgery tend to be as high as 25%. However, in Japan, the recent introduction of Noble placation (suturing the intestines to each other to prevent obstruction) along with routine enterolysis has reduced the recurrence rate to 12.3%.[176] CCSs and tamoxifen also may be continued postoperatively, as they may have a role in preventing EPS recurrence.[176]

Surgical intervention should be sought before the appearance of protein-energy wasting, which may increase postoperative morbidity and mortality. According to the UK EPS Clinical Guideline Group, there are four accepted indications for surgery in EPS—persistent bowel obstruction, failing nutritional status, failure to respond to conventional therapy, and recurrent episodes of peritonitis secondary to bowel compromise. Surgery should be performed by a dedicated surgeon familiar with the management of EPS.[176]

Immunotherapy and Other Experimental Agents. There are reports in the literature of immunosuppressants being used to treat EPS.[180] Agents such as azathioprine or mycophenolate mofetil (MMF) combined with prednisolone have been used in the past and have demonstrated some efficacy.[180] Although the results are promising, the number of cases is small and confounded by concurrent steroid use. Other novel therapies, including blockers of the renin-angiotensin system (RAS), VEGF inhibitors, mammalian target of rapamycin (mToR) inhibitors, hepatic growth factor (HGF) inhibitors, colchicine, and gene therapy, have demonstrated benefit in animal models.[181-183] Sirolimus and everolimus (mToR inhibitors) as antiproliferative agents have a basis for EPS treatment but their adverse effects should be kept in mind and further evaluation is needed. [181]

Prevention of Encapsulating Peritoneal Sclerosis

Despite recent advances in determining the pathogenesis of EPS, preventing this condition continues to be extremely difficult. Thus far, the most logical approach to prevent EPS is to implement practices that address risk factors such as (1) effective peritonitis prevention strategies, (2) early and aggressive management of peritonitis, and (3) PD catheter removal in nonresolving peritonitis. The use of more biocompatible, with lower glucose-degradation products, peritoneal solutions is still under debate in terms of preventing EPS. Although it is unclear whether the introduction of these practices is efficacious, they are relatively safe, simple, and inexpensive to initiate. Therefore there is little risk in initiating them.

Similarly, more controversial practices aimed at mitigating the development of EPS also have been attempted with equivocal results. These practices include the preemptive discontinuation of PD, peritoneal lavage upon cessation of PD, and the use of novel antifibrotic medications.[154,157,184]

The practice of preemptive discontinuation of PD with transfer to HD has not demonstrated any merit in a prospective study.[154] In fact, this practice may unintentionally act as a stimulus for the development of EPS. It has been recommended by the UK EPS Clinical Guideline Group that preemptive transfer to HD only be considered in patients with a very high risk for EPS. These patients usually possess many of the risk factors previously discussed. The effect of this management strategy is currently unknown. Obviously close follow-up would be warranted as EPS can develop many years after discontinuation of PD.

Another early intervention aimed at preventing EPS with cessation of PD is peritoneal lavage. It has been proposed as a therapy to remove accumulated fibrin, which is a key player in capsule formation. Although one small study demonstrated improvement in transport state after 6 months of daily lavage, subsequent studies have failed to confirm this trend.[184] In fact, in these studies, EPS developed in 50% and 52% of patients undergoing lavage.[184] Because of this, peritoneal lavage has been abandoned as a prophylactic measure.

ENCAPSULATING PERITONEAL SCLEROSIS AND RENAL TRANSPLANTATION

There has been much speculation about the role transplantation plays in the development of EPS after a report from two Dutch units demonstrating an increase in the number of EPS cases occurring after renal transplantation.[185] These cases presented with an acute onset of EPS that was characterized by severe symptoms of obstruction, which is in contrast to the typical presentation of EPS. Further work by de Freitas et al.[186] reported 23 cases of EPS occurring within 1 year after renal transplant in patients previously on PD. Current data advocates that the prevalence of posttransplantation EPS is reported to be 1% to 3% in PD patients undergoing kidney transplantation and is associated with significant mortality.[185,187] The time from kidney transplantation to development of EPS is typically short, with the vast majority occurring within the first year of transplantation.[187] However, a late-onset EPS has been reported in one patient presenting 33 months after transplantation.[188] In contrast to primary EPS, posttransplantation EPS patients tended to be younger at PD initiation and did not necessarily have a prolonged PD duration.[152,189]

To explain the phenomenon of posttransplant EPS, both termination of PD and transplantation-related factors can be invoked.[154] As mentioned previously, the discontinuation of PD leads to an increase in concentrations of fibrin and proinflammatory mediators, which can give rise to and propagate EPS. Certain immunosuppressant medications have been implicated in the pathogenesis of EPS.[190] This is especially the case for profibrotic agents such as calcineurin inhibitors, which may enhance the inflammatory fibrotic processes already initiated in the visceral peritoneum.[190] Using rat models, it has been demonstrated that the addition of cyclosporine (CSA) in conjunction with ongoing PD leads to angiogenesis and increased peritoneal fibrosis.[190] Moreover, the trend toward use of CCS withdrawal protocols in newer immunosuppressive regimens may reveal an inherent tendency to develop EPS posttransplantation. By withdrawing steroids, the inflammatory response can propagate unabated, leading to the progression of EPS. This has been noted in a case report of EPS developing after steroid tapering in a transplant patient.[191] Increase in steroid dose leads to a regression of EPS. The prognosis of posttransplantation patients seems to be better compared with the nontransplanted ones.[189]

The approach to the diagnosis and management of posttransplantation EPS is similar to that of the nontransplant population. However, the differential diagnosis must include transplant-related causes of GI disturbances including MMF-induced GI dysmotility, lymphomas, and various infections. Consideration could be given to changing a calcineurin inhibitor to sirolimus. Referral of eligible patients to a transplant waiting list early after starting PD may significantly contribute to EPS prevention in clinical practice.

A full list of references is available at www.expertconsult.com.

SECTION IV

Transplantation

34

The Epidemiology, Outcomes, and Costs of Contemporary Kidney Transplantation

Tarek Alhamad, MD, MS, David Axelrod, MD, MBA, Krista L. Lentine, MD, PhD

OUTLINE

INTRODUCTION

Although the successful transplantation of the Herrick twins in 1954 established the feasibility of kidney transplantation, widespread adoption required the introduction of effective immunosuppression medications, the ability to avoid preformed anti-HLA antibodies through crossmatching, and the systematic allocation of donated organs. Over the ensuing 70 years, kidney transplant outcomes have improved, and graft survival rates now routinely exceed 96% at 1 year.[1] Long-term patient survival with kidney transplant significantly exceeds that achieved by hemodialysis at a lower cost to society.[2,3] However, changes in recipient characteristics, donor quality, and treatment strategies have affected the resources required for successful transplantation, increasing the cost of transplant, especially for novel treatment strategies.

KIDNEY TRANSPLANT CANDIDATES: CHARACTERISTICS AND TRENDS

The complexity of candidates on the waiting list has changed markedly over the past 20 years. Once used primarily in young patients with glomerular disease, kidney transplant is now the treatment of choice for patients with long-standing chronic illness. Diabetes is the leading etiology of kidney failure among listed candidates (36%), followed by hypertension (24%), and glomerulonephritis (14%).[1] Successful kidney transplantation is routinely performed in patients previously believed to be too high risk to benefit, including the elderly and patients with significant pretransplant comorbidities. Transplant in patients aged 65 years and older improves survival compared with remaining on dialysis.[4,5] Even transplant recipients aged 70 years and older experience lower mortality risk than waitlisted dialysis patients (age 70 to 74: hazard ratio [HR], 0.59; age ≥75: HR, 0.58).[6] As a result, patients older than age 50 have become the fastest-growing cohort of waitlisted candidates, increasing from 34,871 patients in 2005 (56% of the list) to 64,408 in 2015 (66% of the list).[7] The percentage of candidates aged 65 years or older rose from 14.5% in 2005 to 22% in 2015. Patients previously excluded from transplant due to medical comorbidities can now be successfully treated. Gill and colleagues demonstrated a significant survival benefit from transplant among patients who with existing ischemic heart disease (7.9 years), peripheral vascular disease (7.9 years), and or congestive heart failure (6.7 years) compared with long-term dialysis.[8] These authors also demonstrated a 48% reduction in the risk for death by 1-year posttransplant in patients with body mass index (BMI) >40 kg/m^2 compared with a 66% reduction in patients with BMI <40 kg/m^2.[9] Patients with prior failed allografts in need of retransplantation now comprise 13% of the waiting list, as the outcomes after retransplantation have improved sufficiently to consider this treatment option.

The proportion of candidates on the waiting list with more than 5 years of dialysis dependence increased from 11.4% in 2005 to 15.7% in 2015. Longer pretransplant dialysis contributes to waitlist mortality and is a risk factor for poor outcomes after transplant.[10,11] Although prolonged waiting times contribute to the extended periods of dialysis, delay in timely referral for transplant evaluation also remains a major barrier to transplantation. Almost half of the patients newly listed for transplant have been on dialysis for more than 4 years.[1] Lower socioeconomic status was associated with lower kidney transplant access, and residing farther from a transplant center or in rural regions is associated with lower deceased donor transplant access.[12,13] Members of racial and ethnic minorities, such as African Americans, face barriers to transplant evaluation and delays in listing, exacerbating racial disparities in access to transplant.[14,15] These differences begin at the local level. One recent study examined referral patterns for incident dialysis patients in Georgia and found that although the average rate of referral for evaluation within 1 year of dialysis was only 24%,[16] rates varied from 0% to 75% across dialysis centers. Dialysis facilities with the lowest transplant referral rates were more likely to treat patients living in high poverty neighborhoods, had higher patient-to-social worker ratios, and were more likely nonprofit.

CHANGES IN THE TRANSPLANT WAITING LIST

Unfortunately, the limited supply of deceased and living donor organs has not kept pace with growing demand for kidney transplant. As of May 2017, more than 117,000 patients were waiting for kidney transplantation, compared with 62,166 in 2005.[1] The average national waiting time for a deceased donor organ exceeds 3.5 years.[17] Despite the directive of the "Final Rule" issued by the Department of Health and Human Services for the Organ Procurement and Transplantation Network (OPTN)/United Network for Organ Sharing (UNOS) to reduce disparity in access to transplantation, marked differences in average waiting time and transplant rates persist. Patients in some areas of the United States experience disparities in transplant access, due, in part, to differences between the local supply of organs and demand for transplant. Other factors that contribute to differences in waiting times include the degree of competition between centers and aggressiveness in organ acceptance practices.[18,19] Rates of living donor transplant also vary markedly, and are reduced in areas with low socioeconomic status, high minority populations, and greater obesity.[20]

The wait for transplant for an individual candidate is influenced by biological factors as well as regional variation in waiting list size and organ availability. High levels of allosensitization are associated with reduced access to transplant due to greater difficulty identifying compatible organs. Although the recent revision of the US kidney allocation system (KAS; discussed later) has been effective in increasing decreased donor transplant rates among the most highly sensitized (panel reactive antibody [PRA] level 98% to 100%), from 7% per 100 patient-years in 2013 to almost 30% in 2015,[1] patients with slightly lower levels of sensitization continue to have reduced access to transplantation. The incidence of highly sensitized patients is likely to further increase as patients with prior transplants are considered for retransplantation.

TRANSPLANT RECIPIENTS: CHARACTERISTICS AND TRENDS

In 2015, 18,597 adult and pediatric kidney transplants, including multiorgan transplants, were performed in the United States, an increase from 17,388 in 2005. Living donor transplant constituted 30% of the transplants in 2015, down slightly from its peak in 2004.[1] Recipient demographics mirror that of the waiting list, as older patients now comprise a higher fraction of transplant recipients. Recipients older than 60 years of age increased from 15% in 1995 to 2000 to 31.5% in 2011 to 2016[21] (Fig. 34.1).

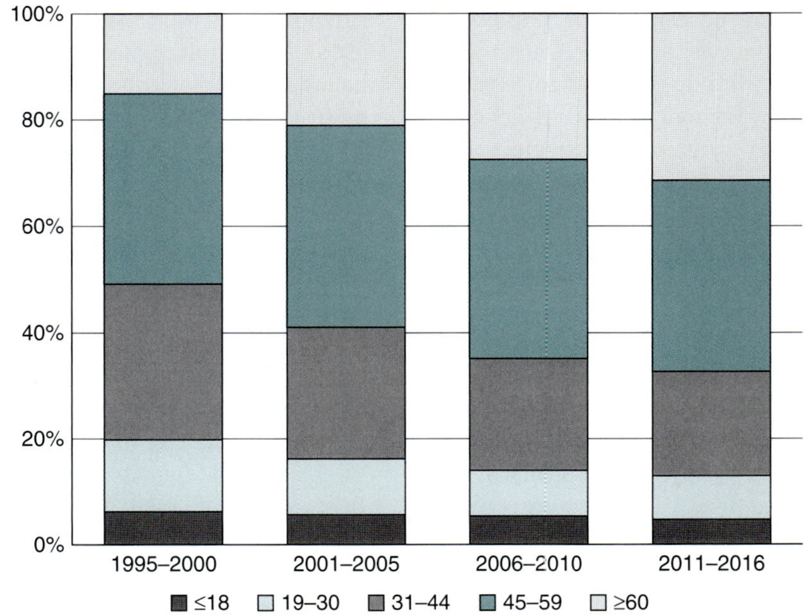

FIG. 34.1 Evolution in the age distribution of US kidney transplant recipients over time. Prepared by the authors from Scientific Registry of Transplant Recipients data through December 2016.

The proportion of non-Caucasian recipients has increased slowly over recent decades: 49% of recipients transplanted from 2010 to 2015 were white compared with 60.8% in 1995 to 2000. Mirroring the obesity epidemic in the general population, obese transplant recipients (BMI >30 kg/m^2) increased from 13.5% between 1995 and 2000 to more than 33% of recipients in 2011 to 2016.[22] Half of the transplants were performed in recipients whose end-stage renal disease (ESRD) was reported to be caused by diabetes and hypertension. Hypertension is also the most commonly reported comorbid condition among transplant recipients (72%), followed by diabetes (32%).[8]

The proportion of deceased donor kidney transplants in recipients with calculated panel reactive antibody (cPRA) 98% to 100% rose from 4.8% in 2014 to 14.6% in 2015,[1] reflecting changes in the KAS to increase access for patients with highest levels of allosensitization. Recipients with cPRA 80% to 89% declined from 6.6% in 2014 to 3.2% in 2015, whereas recipients with a cPRA from 90% to 97% remained the same.[23]

CHANGES IN DECEASED DONOR ORGAN CHARACTERISTICS, ALLOCATION, UTILIZATION, AND ACCESS

The growing organ shortage has led to increased recovery of deceased donor organs with a higher risk of graft failure, delayed graft function (DGF), and primary nonfunction. Factors associated with higher rates of early kidney graft failure include donor age, comorbidities, premortem renal function, and associated medical comorbidities. The use of kidneys from donors older than 50 years of age, and particularly older than 65 years of age, is associated with increased risk for DGF, acute rejection, and graft loss.[24-26] Grafts from older donors have more age-related changes of atherosclerosis and fewer functional nephrons. Therefore they have limited reserve to adapt to new insults in the setting of kidney transplant. It also is proposed that kidneys from older donors are more immunogenic than kidneys from younger donors, and thus have higher risk for rejection.[24] Despite these effects on graft outcomes, the use of donors older than 50 years of age remained stable (approximately 25% of all decreased donors) between 2004 and 2015.[1] The proportion of deceased donors with history of hypertension also remained at approximately 25% during this period. Most organs are recovered after brain death, a mechanism of death that offers the opportunity to sustain organ perfusion with oxygenated blood until the time of actual recovery followed by immediate cooling to minimize ischemic injury. Donors who do not meet the legal definition of brain death for whom organs are recovered after cessation of cardiac activity are known as *donation after cardiac death* (DCD). DCD donors are classified using the Maastricht categorization of controlled and uncontrolled cardiac death.[27] Controlled DCD donors are those who suffer cardiac arrest after planned and witnessed withdrawal of support. Uncontrolled donors are those whose heart has stopped before arrival to the hospital, with or without successful resuscitation. In the United States, the vast majority of DCD donors are controlled donors. DCD has been associated with higher rates of DGF and primary nonfunction.[28] After DGF recovery, however, recipients of DCD kidneys have long-term allograft and survival comparable to those of recipients of kidneys recovered after brain death, especially when organs are procured from donors younger than 50 years of age.[29-31] DCD utilization has increased from 10% in 2005% to 18% in 2015, but varies widely between transplant programs and donation service areas.

In December 2014, the OPTN implemented changes to the US KAS designed to improve the utility of deceased donor kidneys and equity in transplant access. As noted previously, sensitization is a barrier to transplant access because it reduces the likelihood of identifying an organ against which the candidate does not have preformed donor-specific antibodies. For minority race candidates, such as African Americans, who face barriers to transplant evaluation and listing, delays in listing reduces allocation priority and exacerbate racial disparities in access to transplant.[14,15] Important changes incorporated in the revised KAS include defining the start of waiting time at the date of chronic dialysis initiation for patients who were already on dialysis. This change provides better equity for patients who were referred late or had delayed access to transplant services. Candidates receive an allocation point for every year of dialysis before registration. A sliding scale of increasing allocation points was incorporated for the most highly sensitized patients, such that candidates with calculated cPRA scores of 98%, 99%, and 100% receive 24.4, 50.1, and 202.1 points, respectively. This priority is designed to improve access to potentially compatible organs. To improve access for blood type B candidates, they are now being offered blood type A2 and A2B kidneys at transplant programs willing to accept such organs, based on evidence that transplantation care be safely performed without preconditioning treatments as the A2 antigen has a low level of expression on the cell membrane, rendering the A2 kidney similar to a blood group O kidney.[32]

The revised KAS also was designed to increase transplant utility through incorporation of "longevity matching" based on scores for organ quality and expected recipient survival. The previous binary division of deceased donors as standard and expanded criteria donors was replaced with continuous, more granular grading of organ quality using the kidney donor risk index (KDRI) based on 10 donor characteristics: age, height, weight, ethnicity, history of hypertension, history of diabetes, cause of death, serum creatinine, hepatitis C serology (HCV), and DCD.[33] The KDRI provides an estimate of the relative risk for posttransplant kidney graft failure from a particular deceased donor compared with the median donor in the previous calendar year. Kidney donor profile index (KDPI) is estimated from KDRI as a percentage from 0% to 100%, designed to rank the quality of a specific donor organ relative to other kidneys; lower KDPI values are associated with better donor quality and vice versa. Kidneys with KDPI >85% are comparable to previously designated expanded criteria kidneys. A continuous scale also was developed to compute estimated posttransplant survival (EPTS) in transplant candidates based on candidate age, length of dialysis, diabetes, and prior solid organ transplant status.[34] Lower EPTS score (on a scale ranging from 0% to 100%) indicates that the candidate is expected to benefit from more years of graft function compared with candidates with higher scores. To optimize utility, the revised KAS prioritizes candidates with the highest predicted posttransplant benefits (EPTS ≤20%) to receive offers for kidneys from donors with KDPI <20%. Assessment of the effects of the revised KAS over the first year postimplementation demonstrated the following trends:

- Increased transplant rate among highly sensitized candidates (cPRA >98%), from 7 per 100 waitlist years in 2014 to 27 per 100 waitlist years in 2015.[23]
- Increased likelihood of transplantation among candidates aged 18 to 40 years (adjusted hazard ratio [aHR], 1.47; 95% confidence interval [CI], 1.38 to 1.57), but reduced access for candidates aged >50 years (aHR, 0.93; 95% CI, 0.87 to 0.98 for age 51 to 60 and aHR, 0.90; 95% CI, 0.85 to 0.96 for age >70).[35]
- Increases in the proportions of African American and Hispanic transplant recipients.[35] Two-year post-KAS analysis demonstrates that African Americans and Hispanics are now transplanted in proportion to their representation on the waitlist.[36] Importantly, these estimates do not consider disparities in access to transplant services and initial listing.
- Increase in the correlation between donor age and recipient age, from 0.35 to 0.38.[23]
- Greater likelihood of waitlisted candidates with the top 20% of life expectancy (EPTS <20%) to undergo transplant with shorter waiting time: approximately 50% of these candidates underwent transplant by 3.2 years after listing, compared with an average waiting time of 4.5 years under the prior policy.[37]

The use of kidneys from infection risk donors (IRD) also has expanded in light of the ongoing organ shortage and the epidemic in opiate overdose-associated mortality. These are kidneys recovered from donors with behaviors associated with HIV, hepatitis B, and HCV infection, generally intravenous drug use, incarceration, and certain sexual practices. These behaviors were formally defined by the US Public Health Services (US PHS) and must be disclosed to potential recipients.[38] A change from the Centers for Disease Control and Prevention criteria increased the number of organs defined as being recovered from "increased risk" donors. Strikingly, 20% of kidneys are now classified as US PHS increased risk.[39] Notably, the vast majority of organs are screened with nucleic acid testing (NAT) to identify the presence of HIV or HCV, which has dramatically reduced the risk for unintentional disease transmission during the "window period." Risk prediction tools to compare outcomes with dialysis may guide use of IRD organs in patients who can benefit.[40] IRD kidneys often are high-quality organs from young donors with excellent long-term survival. Although not directly factored into the calculator, it is also notable that both HIV and HCV are treatable infections, such that the rare transmission can be managed, which is a consideration compared with the high mortality of dialysis. The UNOS Disease Transmission Advisory Committee (DTAC) recently released an educational resource to help patients and providers understand the risks and benefits associated with these organs.[41] Kidneys from donors with known HCV can benefit HCV-positive recipients by markedly reducing time to transplantation.[42] Patients with HCV who accept an HCV-positive kidney wait an average of 395 days less than those who wait for an HCV-negative kidney. Recent experimental protocols have been introduced to allow transplantation of HCV-positive donor organs into HCV-negative recipients to expand access to organ from these donors, provided that recipients undergo posttransplant antiviral treatment.[43,44]

Other nonstandard organs that may provide benefit to some patients include kidneys procured from donors with high terminal creatinine due to acute tubular necrosis. These organs are frequently discarded. Analysis of the UNOS database from 1995 to 2007 showed that among donors with terminal creatinine >2 mg/dL, neither kidney was recovered in 44%, whereas when terminal creatinine was ≤1.5 mg/dL neither kidney was recovered in only 2%.[45] However, emerging data show these kidneys can be safely used with recognition that a period of posttransplant dialysis will likely be needed. In one single-center experience, transplants from donors with terminal creatinine >2 mg/dL had a higher rate of DGF (66%) and longer DGF (median 10 days) compared with transplants from donors without acute kidney injury (DGF 27%, with median duration 8 days), but similar estimated glomerular filtration rate and graft survival at 1 year posttransplant.[46]

Unfortunately, the discard rate (i.e., the proportion of organs recovered but not used) has remained at approximately 20% despite the organ shortage and the changes in KAS described previously. The discard rate does vary with donor factors and quality measures, increasing with donor age and higher KDPI.[1] Notably, the discard rate begins to rise earlier than risk for adverse outcomes: Whereas graft failure and DGF risk starts to accelerate at KDPI >70, the discard rates rise in a linear manner at KDPI >40 (Fig. 34.2).[47] A caveat to this comparison is that transplant outcomes apply to the selected subset of higher risk organs that are used, but the observation raises that use should be considered. Despite higher rates of graft failure, high KDPI organs provide substantial benefit in appropriate populations. A recent study of national registry data by Massie et al. showed that high-KDPI transplant, defined as KDPI >70, was associated with increased short-term death risk over 6 months, but better long-term survival, compared with waiting for a higher-quality organ among older patients, diabetics, and those living in regions with prolonged waiting times.[48] This study also found that the highest-risk organs (KDPI 91 to 100) benefit patients older than 50 years of age at centers with waiting times longer than 3 years.[49]

LIVING DONOR TRANSPLANTATION

Living kidney donors can be related, unrelated, nondirected, or participants in donor exchange (kidney paired donation [KPD]) programs. Living donor transplantation provides benefits over deceased donor kidney transplantation including faster access to transplant, which reduces time on dialysis and its associated risks, as well as superior long-term patient and allograft survival at the lowest cost.[50] Unfortunately, living donor kidney transplantation in the United States has declined from a peak of 6000 in 2004 to current rates of approximately 5500 per year.[1] Multiple barriers to living

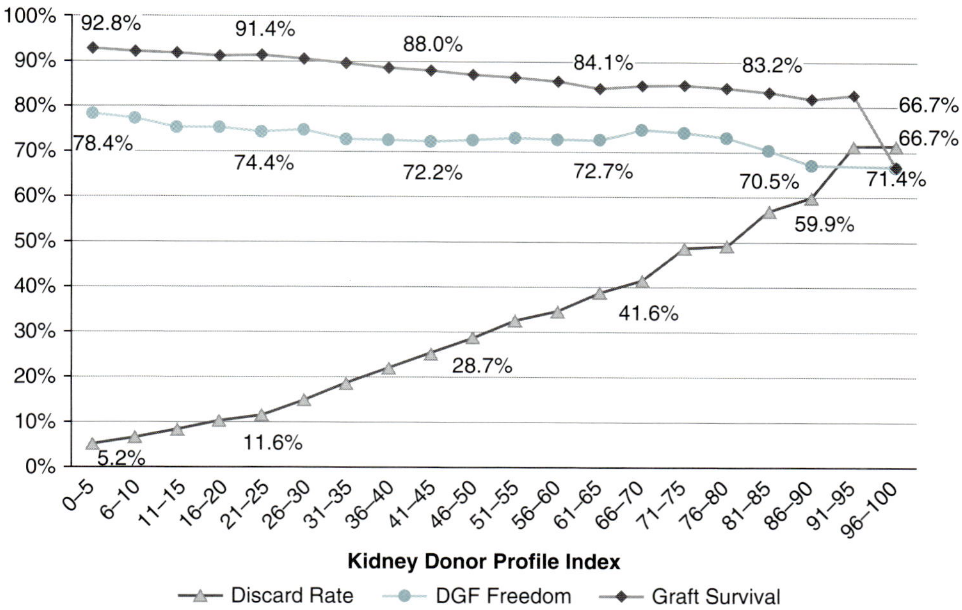

FIG. 34.2 The discard rate rises more rapidly with higher KDPI than graft failure and DGF rates. Prepared by the authors from Scientific Registry of Transplant Recipients data from 2010 to 2016. *DGF*, Delayed graft function; *KDPI*, kidney donor profile index.

donor transplantation exist, including the transplant candidate's ability to identify a willing donor, ensuring donor health and proper selection, and uncompensated costs for the donor.[51] Based on clear evidence of recipient benefit and surveys supporting positive public perceptions of living donation, a number of recent initiatives are underway to increase awareness of living donor transplantation and reduce disincentives, including a 2015 American Society of Transplantation Consensus Statement promoting living donor transplantation as the "best treatment option" for eligible patients with kidney failure.[52]

The pool of potential living donors has been expanded through the widespread access to laparoscopic donor nephrectomy and the development of KPD programs for patients with willing but biologically incompatible donors. Laparoscopic nephrectomy offers reduced surgical risk, pain, and cost. The laparoscopic approach also has enabled expansion of the living donor pool to older patients and has reduced the fear of donation.[53] KPD programs apply algorithms to exchange kidneys among two or more pairs of incompatible donors and recipients so that all candidates receive compatible organs.[54] Paired donation has been the fastest growing living donor transplant modality, and currently comprises approximately 10% of living donor transplants per year.[1] Survey of potential donors supports strong willingness of potential donors to participate in KPD to facilitate transplant access for their intended recipient.[55] However, it is widely believe that KPD is underused: It is estimated that if all centers used paired donation at the rate of high-performing centers, another 1000 transplants could be performed per year.[56] Entry of compatible pairs into KPD has been suggested as an approach to increase the pool of potential matches.[57] Entry of biologically compatible pairs in KPD systems may result in the compatible recipient receiving a better matched organ or organ from a younger donor. Best practices for the living kidney donor selection are out of the scope of this chapter; however, a comprehensive review is found in the 2017 Kidney Disease Improving Global Outcomes (KDIGO) "Guideline on the Evaluation and Care of Living Kidney Donors."[58]

IMMUNOSUPPRESSION: TRENDS AND CURRENT PRACTICE

Induction Immunosuppression

The success of kidney transplantation is largely the result of the advances of immunosuppression including better induction therapy and maintenance regimens. The KDIGO guideline recommends induction therapy in all kidney transplant recipients (1A).[59] This guideline also recommends interleukin-2 receptor antibody (IL2rAb) for first-line induction therapy (1B), while offering a class 2B recommendation for use of cell-depleting agents in patients considered high risk for acute rejection. A higher risk for rejection has been associated with African American heritage, significant allosensitization, history of prior transplantation, longer cold ischemic time, younger recipient age, and DGF. In addition, the choice of maintenance medications influences the need for induction therapy. In 2015, 91% of kidney transplant recipients received induction therapy. Use of IL2rAb fell from 35% in 2004% to 20% in 2015, whereas use of T-cell depleting agents (including thymoglobulin, alemtuzumab) continued to increase, from 39.5% in 2004 to 70% in 2015.[1] The percentage of recipients receiving no induction therapy continued to decline from 22% in 2004 reaching a low of 9.1% in 2015 (Fig. 34.3).[60]

Choice of induction therapy should be determined based on patient and donor characteristics. For instance, black, highly sensitized, or recipients who experience DGF are, appropriately, more likely to be treated with cell-depleting agents (alemtuzumab, thymoglobulin) than IL2rAb (Fig. 34.4).[60] Alemtuzumab is more commonly used with steroid-free

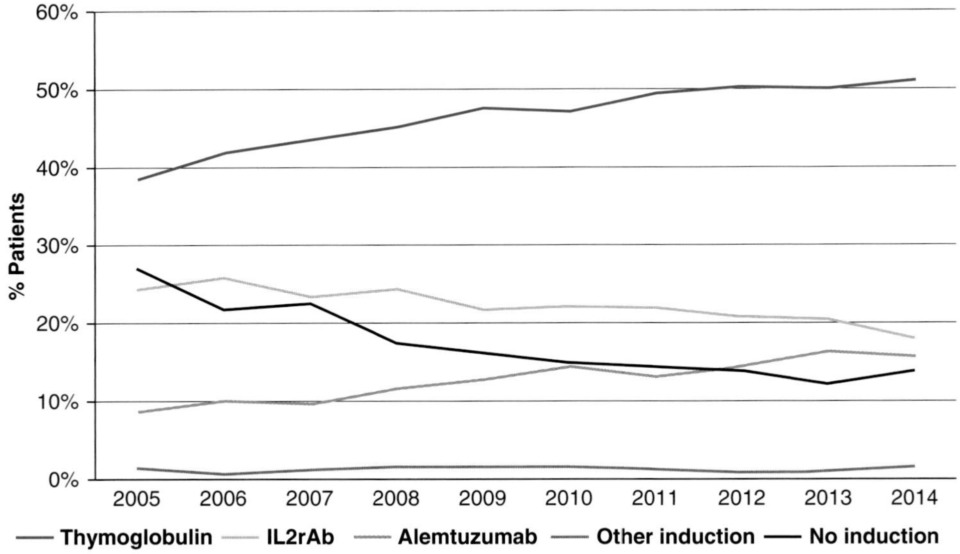

FIG. 34.3 National trends in kidney transplant induction over time. *IL2rAb*, interleukin-2 receptor blocking antibodies. (Reproduced with permission from Dharnidharkaa VR, Naik AS, Axelrod DA, et al. Center practice drives variation in choice of U.S. kidney transplant induction therapy: a retrospective analysis of contemporary practice. *Transpl Int.* 2018;31:198-211.)

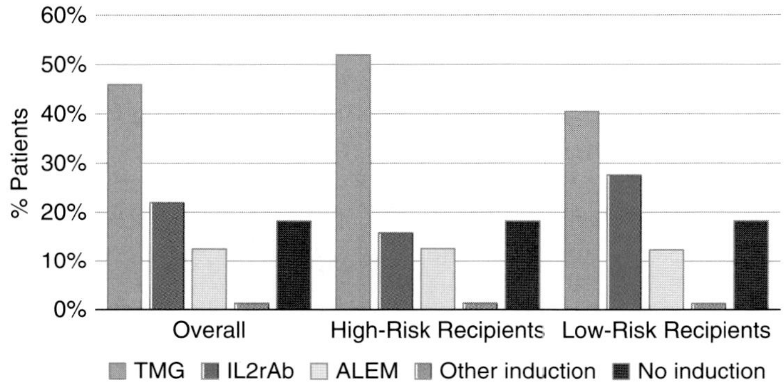

FIG. 34.4 National trends in kidney transplant induction by recipient immunological risk profile. *ALEM*, Alemtuzumab; *IL2rAb*, interleukin-2 receptor blocking antibodies; *TMG*, thymoglobulin. High risk was defined as black race, PRA >20, or retransplantation. (Reproduced with permission from Dharnidharkaa VR, Naik AS, Axelrod DA, et al. Center practice drives variation in choice of U.S. kidney transplant induction therapy: a retrospective analysis of contemporary practice. *Transpl Int.* 2018;31:198-211.)

maintenance regimens (tacrolimus and antimetabolite), whereas induction may not be used in patients on triple maintenance therapy.[61,62] Although low-risk patients, such as 2 haplotype-matched white recipients, may be transplanted safely with no induction, the majority of patients seem to benefit from induction treatment.[63] However, recent evidence suggests that center practice patterns, rather than patient and donor characteristics, dominate the decision about whether or not to use induction agents, and if so, which one.[60]

Maintenance Immunosuppression

Initially, maintenance immunosuppression was relatively standardized (cyclosporine, azathioprine, and corticosteroids) due to limited options available to transplant physicians. The nephrotoxicity of cyclosporine was recognized as a limiting factor in improving the long-term outcomes of kidney transplantation, as was the risk for skin cancer associated with azathioprine. The introduction of tacrolimus, mycophenolate, mammalian target of rapamycin inhibitors (mTORi: sirolimus and everolimus) and belatacept has now given transplant providers a wider variety of choices and the potential for tailoring to optimize individual patient outcomes. However, in reality, the variation of regimens among transplant centers is largely driven by center practice and preference rather than patient demographic and transplant characteristics (Fig. 34.5).[64] In national studies, despite similar patient and donor demographics, there is wide variation in selection of antirejection regimen. This variation emphasizes the need for more evidence-based practice, as well as collaborative clinical trials and secondary data analyses of contemporary practice to optimize posttransplant outcome.[64] Here, we will review the trends of individual agent use and immunosuppression regimen preference among the transplant centers in the United States.

Calcineurin inhibitors (CNIs) continue to form the cornerstone of maintenance immunosuppression medications despite the modest adoption of belatacept at some transplant centers. Among CNIs, tacrolimus has been the dominant medication and its use increased from 75% in 2004 to reach 97% in

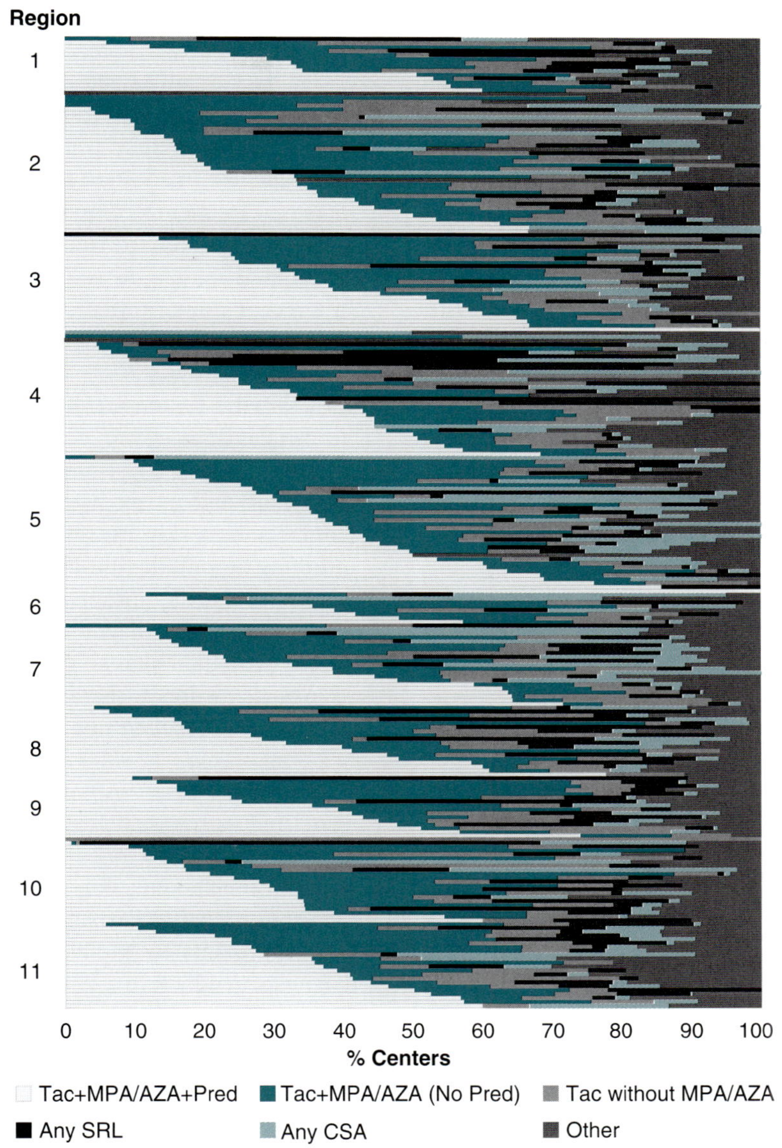

FIG. 34.5 Proportion of US patients receiving one of six mutually exclusive immunosuppression regimens during months 6 to 12 posttransplant. Each horizontal bar represents an individual center within US regions ordered by the proportion of patients who received triple immunosuppression (Tac + MPA/AZA + Pred). Overall percentage of regimen use at patient-level across centers: Tac + MPA/AZA + Pred, 33.8%; Tac + MPA/AZA (No Pred), 25.8%; Tac without MPA/AZA, 11.3%; SRL-based, 9.9%; CSA-based, 7.8%; and other regimens, 11.6%. *AZA*, Azathioprine; *CSA*, cyclosporine; *MPA*, mycophenolate; *Pred*, prednisone; *SRL*, sirolimus; *Tac*, tacrolimus. (Reproduced with permission from Axelrod D, Naik AS, Schnitzler MA, et al. National variation in use of immunosuppression for kidney transplantation: a call for evidence-based regimen selection. *Am J Transplant*. 2016;16:2453-2462.)

2015.[1] Tacrolimus has two new extended-release formulations to allow once-per-day dosing.[65] However, the immediate-release formulation remains the most commonly used, possibly because it is available as a generic option. Mycophenolate has been established as the antimetabolite medication of choice, with one of two formulations (mycophenolate mofetil, mycophenolate sodium) comprising more than 95% of antimetabolite use. Less than 5% of recipients are prescribed azathioprine in current practice.[1] Although the mycophenolate formulations are believed to differ in side-effect profile, clinical outcomes have not been shown to differ significantly.[66]

Modern renal transplant immunosuppression is generally based on a combination of two or more agents. One-third of kidney transplant recipients transplanted from 2004 to 2010 received triple immunosuppression composed of tacrolimus, an antimetabolite, and corticosteroids.[64] The second most commonly prescribed regimen in this period was tacrolimus and antimetabolite (steroid avoidance) in 26% of the recipients, followed by tacrolimus alone or tacrolimus plus prednisone (antimetabolite sparing) in 11.3%, mTORi-based (with or without CNI) in 9.9%, and cyclosporine-based in 7.8%. Although the use of these regimens varies significantly among transplant centers, the use of triple-therapy immunosuppression is more likely among patients with higher immunological risk such as highly sensitized patients, retransplant recipients, and those with a history of glomerulonephritis.[64] The use of mTORi-based regimens is more likely in patients with lower GFR at 6 months posttransplant. Overall, mTORi use in kidney transplant recipients declined from approximately 15% in 2004% to 5% in 2015.[1] This decline is mainly driven by recognition of associations with increased risk for poor wound healing, acute rejection, and proteinuria without realization of substantial benefits in long-term allograft survival.[67]

Despite the wide variety of choices of immunosuppression medications, long-term graft survival remains limited by chronic transplant glomerulopathy, interstitial fibrosis/tubular atrophy, inflammation, and subclinical cellular and antibody medicated rejection.[68,69] Complications of immunosuppression, including infection and malignancy as discussed here, pose challenges for long-term patient survival. Further advances in medications and new strategies for posttransplant monitoring, being explored in the evolving field of biomarkers,[70] are needed to improve the long-term outcomes after kidney transplantation.

COMPLICATIONS OF KIDNEY TRANSPLANTATION

The increased potency of contemporary immunosuppression has yielded substantial reductions in acute rejection rates. In the early 1980s, 50% to 60% of renal allograft recipients experienced at least one acute rejection episode compared with less than 15% today.[71,72] In the ELITE-Symphony study, which simultaneously compared low- or high-dose cyclosporine-based to tacrolimus-based or sirolimus-based regimens, the acute rejection rates and graft failure rates were much higher in the nontacrolimus-based arms, contributing to widespread adoption of tacrolimus-based regimens.[73] However, the benefits of preventing acute rejection are balanced by the risks for overimmunosuppression, including infection and malignancy.[74,75] In this section, we review the epidemiology and effects of clinical complications such as infections, malignancy, and new-onset diabetes after transplant (NODAT).

Urinary tract infections (UTIs), pneumonia, and sepsis occur in 10% to 30% of recipients in the first year after a kidney transplant.[74,76,77] Analysis of infection diagnoses among Medicare-insured US kidney transplant recipients in 2000 to 2011 demonstrated an association with increased mortality in the first-year after transplant, ranging from 41% (aHR, 1.41; 95% CI, 1.25 to 1.56) for UTI alone, 6-fold risk for pneumonia, 12-fold risk for sepsis, and 34-fold risk (aHR, 34.38;, 95% CI, 30.35 to 38.95) for those with all three infections in the first year.[78] Infections also significantly increase the first-year cost of kidney transplant care by $17,691 UTI alone, $40,000 to $50,000 for pneumonia or sepsis alone, and $134,773 for those with UTI, pneumonia. and sepsis in this period. Clinical and economic effects persist in years 2 to 3 posttransplant.[78]

Viral-derived malignancies, such as lymphoma, Kaposi sarcoma, lip cancer, and genitourinary tract cancer, are substantially more common in transplant patients than age-adjusted estimates in the general population or patients with chronic kidney disease and ESRD.[79,80] Cancer has become second only to cardiovascular disease (CVD) as the leading cause of posttransplant mortality, surpassing death from infection.[81] Furthermore, although the risk for death from CVD appears to be stable or even decreasing despite higher comorbidity burdens among transplant recipients, cancer mortality after kidney transplant appears to be increasing over time.[82,83] In addition to viral-linked cancers, there is an increased frequency of nonmelanoma skin cancers and certain solid organ tumors (including kidney, prostate, and colon carcinoma) compared with nontransplant populations.[84,85] In a recent study of Medicare-insured US transplant recipients, the cumulative incidence of cancer diagnosed by 3 years posttransplant was 5.7% for nonmelanoma skin cancers, 1.9% for viral-linked, and 6.3% for almost all other cancers.[86] Viral-linked cancer was associated with more than threefold increased risk in subsequent mortality within 3 years after transplant, and nearly twice the mortality risk after year 3. Nonmelanoma skin cancer was associated with 33% higher mortality beyond the third year posttransplant.

Cancer also significantly increases the costs of posttransplant care. Newly diagnosed viral-linked cancer was associated with incremental costs, after adjustment for other recipient and donor characteristics. A diagnosis of a viral-linked cancer resulted in $22,000 to $27,000 per year higher inpatient costs and $9000 to $11,000 per year higher outpatient costs per case.[86] A newly diagnosed "other" cancer was associated with $14,500 to $18,000 per year higher inpatient expenses and $8000 to $9000 per year higher outpatient costs. Nonmelanoma skin cancers was associated only with increased outpatient expenditures, and the cost impact rose from approximately $1400 to $2000 per year in the year of diagnosis to $2500 to $2800 per year in subsequent years.[86] Overall, cancer accounted for 3% to 5.5% of total inpatient Medicare expenditures and 1.5% to 3.3% of outpatient expenditures in the first 3 years posttransplant (Fig. 34.6).

The risk for NODAT has been increasing with the incidence of obesity and racial minorities in the recipient population. The risk is highest in the first year after transplant, ranging from 15% to 30%.[87-89] Subsequent annual incidence is approximately 5% per year. Risk factors for NODAT include potentially modifiable (e.g., BMI) as well as nonmodifiable factors (e.g., race/ethnicity).[90-92] NODAT has been associated with adverse outcomes after transplantation, including graft failure and death, as well as rejection, infection, and cardiovascular complications including myocardial infarction (MI) and congestive heart failure.[75,93,94] NODAT also increases the cost of posttransplant care.[95] The risk for developing NODAT is associated with African American race, Hispanic ethnicity, obesity, HCV infection, and pretransplant glucose intolerance. Multiple immunosuppressive agents have been implicated, but risk is highest with steroids and tacrolimus, particularly in African Americans.

A population-based analysis of US kidney transplant recipients (2000 to 2011) demonstrated variation in the risk for posttransplant complications over 3 years according to initial immunosuppression regimen (Fig. 34.7).[67] Compared with a regimen of thymoglobulin induction and maintenance tacrolimus, mycophenolate and prednisone, sirolimus-based immunosuppression was associated with increases

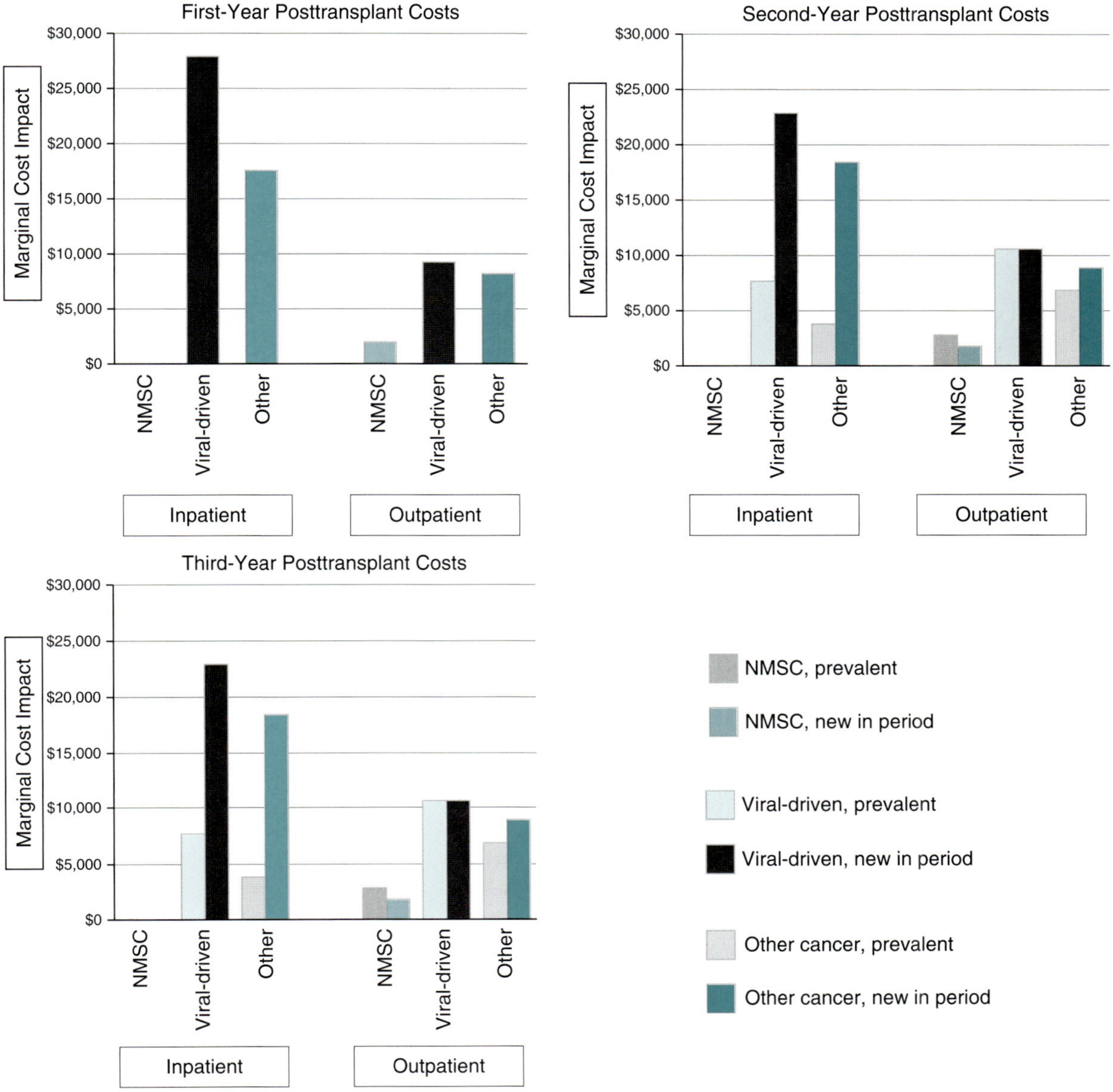

FIG. 34.6 Cost effects of posttransplant cancer. NMSC, nonmelanoma skin cancer. (Reproduced with permission from Dharnidharka VR, Naik AS, Axelrod D, et al. Clinical and economic consequences of early cancer after kidney transplantation in contemporary practice. *Transplantation.* 2017;101:858-866.)

in the 3-year risks for pneumonia (aHR, 1.45), sepsis (aHR, 1.40), diabetes (aHR, 1.20), acute rejection (aHR, 1.33), graft failure (aHR, 1.78), and patient death (aHR, 1.40), but 29% lower risk for skin cancer.[67] Cyclosporine-based immunosuppression was associated with increased risks for pneumonia (aHR, 1.17), sepsis (aHR, 1.16), acute rejection (aHR, 1.43), and graft failure (aHR, 1.39), but 17% less risk for diabetes. Steroid-free immunosuppression was associated with the 11% reduced risk for pneumonia, 20% reduced risk for sepsis, and 33% reduced risk for diabetes, but 35% higher risk for graft failure.[67]

Azathioprine has been associated with nonmelanoma skin cancer.[79] A recent case–control study of kidney and heart transplant recipients reported that azathioprine, but not mycophenolate, was associated with increased risk for nonmelanoma skin cancer, and that the association was independent of CNI choice.[96]

In summary, the choice of immunosuppression medication has an effect on the risk for posttransplant complications, cost, and graft survival. Further study is warranted to better guide the choice of immunosuppression and tailor efficacy and morbidity to the characteristics of the patient and the donor organ.

POSTTRANSPLANT OUTCOMES

Solid organ transplantation is unique among medical specialties in the universal collection of clinical data. Through the mechanism of the OPTN as mandated by the National Organ Transplant Act (NOTA), transplant centers have been required to submit baseline and follow-up clinical data describing all patients listed for and receiving solid organ transplants in the United States since 1986.[97] Posttransplant follow-up information is collected at 6 months after transplant, at the

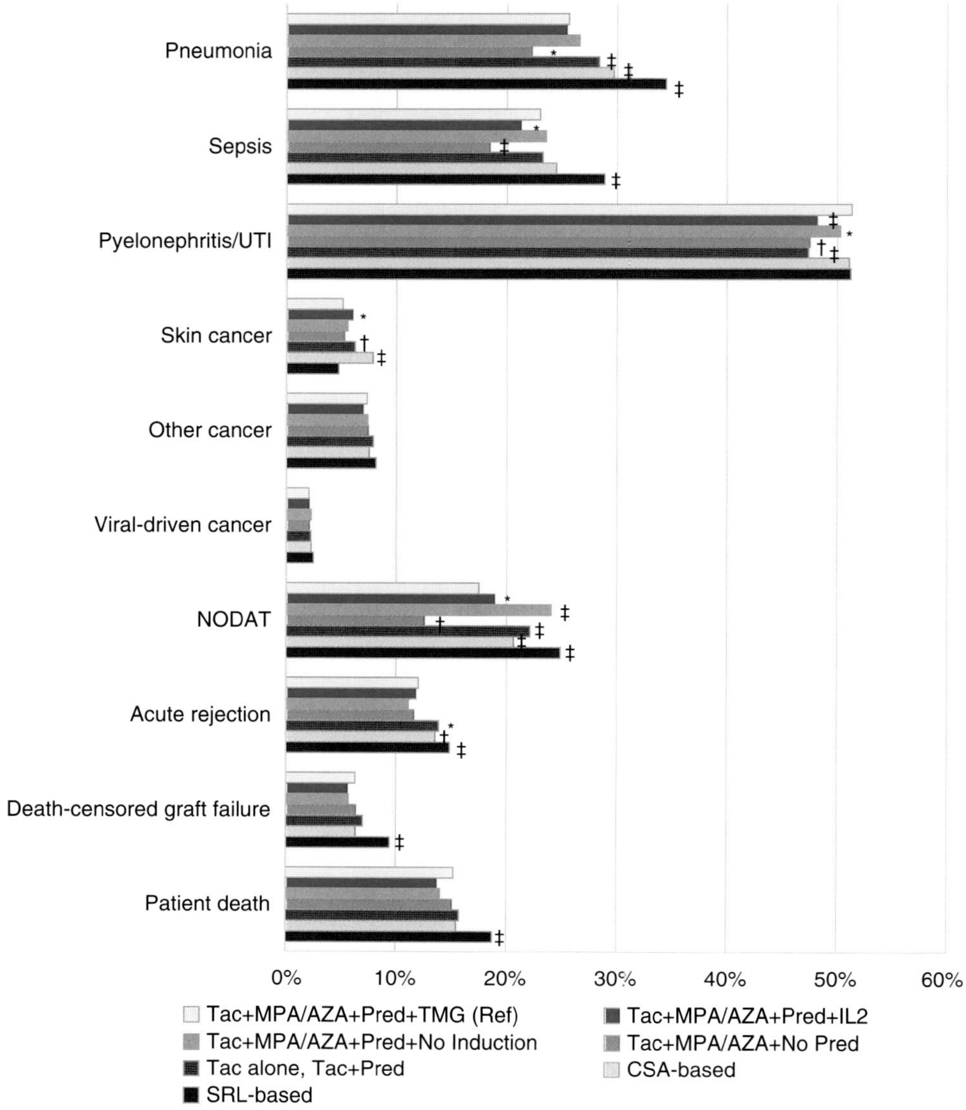

FIG. 34.7 Incidence of clinical events at 3 years posttransplant according to early immunosuppression. *AZA*, Azathioprine; *CSA*, cyclosporine; *MPA*, mycophenolate; *NODAT*, new-onset diabetes after transplant; *Pred*, prednisone; *SRL*, sirolimus; *Tac*, tacrolimus; *UTI*, urinary tract infection. (Reproduced with permission from Dharnidharka VR, Schnitzler MA, Chen J, et al. Differential risks for adverse outcomes 2 years after kidney transplantation based on initial immunosuppression regimen: a national study. *Transpl Int.* 2016;20:1226-1236.)
$^*P < 0.05–0.002$
$^{\dagger}P = 0.001–0.0002$
$^{\ddagger}P < 0.0001$

first transplant anniversary and then annually. The Scientific Registry of Transplant Recipients (SRTR) augments OPTN data with national death and dialysis records. Major events that are applicable for outcomes studies include acute rejection, graft failure (defined by return to dialysis, retransplantation, or patient death), death-censored graft survival (defined by return to dialysis or retransplantation), and patient death.

Acute Rejection

There are two types of acute rejection: T-cell mediated and antibody-mediated. Both types of rejection can occur early or late, individually, simultaneously, or sequentially. The incidence of acute rejection within the first year decreased for both living and deceased donor transplant recipients from 10% in 2009 to 2010 to 7.9% in 2013 to 2014. However, in a greater proportion of acute rejection episodes, renal function did not return to baseline after treatment, which was associated with an incremental increase in the relative hazard for graft survival.[98,99] Acute rejection events recognized later after transplant have more serious graft loss implications, especially within the first 90 days after an acute rejection event.[72] Even when successful, treatment of rejection is expensive. Examination of Medicare-insured US kidney transplant recipients in 2000 to 2007 found that antibody-treated (year 1: \$22,407, year 2: \$18,803, year 3: \$13,909) and nonantibody-treated (year 1: \$14,122, year 2: \$7852, year 3: \$8234) acute rejection events were associated with significant increases in the cost of care.[48] These costs do not include the cost of return to dialysis for patients whose transplant never recovered.

Graft Survival

Graft loss within the first 12 months after transplant are primarily due to technical failures (very early), surgical compilations, primary nonfunction, severe rejection, or severe recurrent glomerulonephritis (such as recurrent focal segmental glomerulosclerosis). Beyond the first-year posttransplant, the main causes of graft loss are patient death and chronic allograft nephrology. Historically, improvements of long-term graft survival have not paralleled the robust improvements in short-term outcomes. However, the SRTR annual report issued in 2017 found that average longer-term graft and patient survival appears to be improving.[1] Overall, 1-year deceased donor graft survival improved from 90% in 2005 to 94% in 2015, and 10-year graft survival improved from 41% in 2005 to 47% in 2015.[1] Five-year graft survival for recipients of DCD organs was identical to recipients of organs from brain dead donors at 75%. One-year graft survival of living donor transplant recipients increased from 95% in 2005 to 98% in 2015, whereas 10-year graft survival improved from 55% in 1995 to 63% in 2005. Interestingly, the results for first deceased donor transplants were largely static, suggesting that these improvements in long-term outcomes were due to better outcomes among retransplant recipients.[100]

Patient Survival

In the first 3 months after kidney transplant, there is an increased risk for mortality compared with waiting on dialysis, reflecting the risk of undergoing surgery and starting immunosuppression. Beyond this period, the relative risk for death is lower in transplant recipients than in candidates on the waitlist, although the benefit varies by patient and donor factors.[2] By 4 years, kidney transplant recipients have an average 70% reduction in mortality. One-year patient survival after deceased donor kidney transplantation has exceeded 95% in the past two decades and reached 97% in 2015.[1] For living donor kidney transplant recipients, 1-year patient survival is now 99%. The most common causes of death with a functioning transplant are CVD, infection, and malignancy.

CENTER PERFORMANCE GRADING

The availability of national, comprehensive data on transplant outcomes has facilitated public reporting of transplant center-specific data. As required under NOTA, the SRTR produces program-specific reports describing outcomes at each transplant program. These data include detailed analyses of waitlist activity, transplant rates, graft survival, and patient survival. Because transplant recipient and donor characteristics vary substantially between centers, the SRTR has developed a complex risk adjustment methodology to attempt to account for differences in case mix. This methodology is used to calculate the center's observed-to-expected (O/E) event ratios in comparison to other transplant programs. The current risk adjustment equation for kidney recipient outcomes uses 33 variables and 125 different coefficients (for different variable ranges, known as *spline* terms). In addition to public reporting, these data are provided to two regulatory bodies, the OPTN/UNOS Membership and Professional Standards Committee (MPSC) and the Centers for Medicare & Medicaid Services (CMS). The MPSC oversees the compliance of the transplant programs with federal regulations and OPTN policies. The MPSC uses the SRTR program-specific reports to identify programs that do not meet performance standards and should be considered for further review, probation, or, if egregious, be declared as a "Member Not in Good Standing," which results in exclusion from deceased donor allocation.[101,102] The MPSC uses a set of established criteria to "flag" programs for performance (Box 34.1).

BOX 34.1 OPTN/UNOS Membership and Professional Standards Flagging Criteria

For large programs (≥10 transplants in a 2.5-year period), the MPSC will review a transplant program if it has a higher hazard ratio (HR) of mortality or graft failure than expected for that transplant program. The criteria used to identify programs with a hazard ratio that is higher than expected include either of the following:

1. The probability is >75% that the HR is >1.2.
2. The probability is >10% that the HR is >2.5.

For small programs (<10 transplants in a 2.5-year period), the MPSC will review a transplant program if the program has one or more events.[68]

MPSC, Membership and Professional Standards; *OPTN/UNOS*, Organ Procurement and Transplantation Network/United Network for Organ Sharing.

BOX 34.2 Centers for Medicare & Medicaid Services Performance Criteria

1) Observed/Expected >1.85
2) Observed/Expected >3
3) The probability that an observed excess (rather than difference) of observed events compared with expected events is likely due to random chance with a one-sided $P < 0.05$.

Centers for Medicare & Medicaid Services

The CMS oversees transplant programs that receive Medicare reimbursement, which includes most of the kidney transplant centers in the United States. In 2007 the CMS began periodic reviews of all Medicare-approved transplant programs.[103] The SRTR provides analyses to CMS with separate models that use frequentist (rather than Bayesian) methods. Centers that meet all three of the following criteria (Box 34.2), in two out of five semiannual reports, are considered to be in violation of CMS's conditions of participation (CoP). These centers are at risk for removal from the Medicare program and, most likely, being closed.

Effect of Performance Monitoring

The current posttransplant outcome review process creates disincentives for programs to transplant higher-risk recipients or nonstandard organs, due to concern that early graft failures or patient deaths will cause the program to be reviewed. Schold et al. examined center behavior after a poor performance evaluation, and found a striking increase in the frequency of waitlist removals, a reduction in total size of the waiting list, and reduced numbers of transplants.[104] These practices were associated with reduced access to transplant. In other words, more conservative patient and organ selection is a common response to poor prior performance, which may, or may not, be justified by critical review of the program's data. A recent analysis prepared by the SRTR demonstrated that the use of higher-risk organs was not associated with a higher risk for regulatory citation by the MPSC.[105] However, this analysis did not consider other outcomes of high-risk transplants, including the effects of public reporting of less-than-expected outcomes on private payer Center of Excellence network membership. To address these issues, the UNOS Board of Directors approved a new policy directing the MPSC to only review programs with poor outcomes for all kidney transplants performed if they remained a poor performing center after excluding "higher-risk" transplants, wherein a higher-risk transplant is defined by recipient EPTS score >80, or donor KDPI >85. In other words, the MPSC will not review kidney programs for outcomes if the only reason they did not meet the expected threshold for performance was the outcomes of higher-risk transplants. This proposal is designed to further protect centers that chose to use higher-risk organs in patients most likely to benefit compared with dialysis. Further study is needed to determine whether the perception of using higher-risk kidneys remains after starting these review criteria. It is important to recognize that without corresponding changes in CMS review criteria, the potential consequences of worse-than-expected performance remain severe as centers may still find themselves out of compliance with the CoP. CMS has indicated a willingness to consider the use of high-risk organs as a potential mitigating factor, which will result in the program escaping citation for less-than-expected outcomes; however, this has not been tested.

UNMEASURED AND NOVEL RISK FACTORS

The pool of potential risk adjustment factors in the SRTR graft and patient survival models is constrained by data collected in the OPTN/UNOS registry. These data elements include only limited measures of comorbid conditions and no measures of medical or pharmaceutical care. An evolving body of literature suggests that supplementing the national transplant registry with additional data elements, such as pharmaceutical and medical billing claims, may provide novels measures of posttransplant risk.

Symptomatic hypotension is a common complication in patients with ESRD, especially among those with prolonged dialysis dependence, which is not currently captured using UNOS data.[106,107] Symptomatic hypotension has been estimated to complicate approximately 25% of hemodialysis treatments and may result in dialysis session interruptions and prevent delivery of adequate clearance and fluid removal.[108] When standard interventions (such as dialysate sodium modeling, low-temperature fialysate) fail to prevent intradialytic hypotension, pharmacological treatment with midodrine may be used.[109] Midodrine was recently examined as a marker for symptomatic hypotension before kidney transplant and was shown to be associated with graft failure and posttransplant death. Based on integrated national transplant registry data, outpatient pharmacy fill records from a pharmaceutical claims clearinghouse, and Medicare billing claims, patients who filled midodrine before transplant were found to have twice the risk of developing DGF and 3.5 times the risk for death at 3 months posttransplant than nonusers.[110] Similar patterns of graft failure and death occurred at 12 months posttransplantation. Pretransplant midodrine exposure also was associated with other medical complications after transplant including hypotension, acute MI, ventricular arrhythmia, and cardiac arrest. The effects of midodrine use before transplant was augmented in the recipients of nonstandard organs (ECD, DCD, and high KDPI >85%) compared with standard-criteria donor allografts.[110]

CVD remains poorly characterized in the UNOS data despite the high prevalence of significant disease in kidney transplant candidates. The OPTN/UNOS registry collects only limited measures of baseline CVD and no measures of posttransplant CVD, which significantly affects posttransplant survival. The incidence of death-censored graft failure after a posttransplant MI is 8.7% at 1 year and 12.9% at 2 years after infarction, whereas all-cause graft loss after posttransplant MI is 30.7% at 1 year and 38.8% at 2 years.[75] Clopidogrel is a medication indicated for MI, stroke, or refractory ischemia in patients with non-ST-segment elevation acute coronary syndrome as well as unstable angina, including those who are managed medically and those with coronary revascularization. According to the drug monograph, it is also indicated to reduce the rate of death from any of the above causes and reduce the rate of combined endpoints of death, reinfarction, or stroke in patients with ST-elevation MI, as well as to reduce the rate of combined endpoint of new ischemic stroke or MI, and other vascular deaths in patients with history of recent MI or stroke, or established peripheral vascular disease.[111] A recent study of integrated national registry and pharmacy fill data found that clopidogrel use within 90 days of transplant was associated with a 61% increased risk for mortality and 23% increased risk for graft failure.[113] Risks were higher with clopidogrel use >90 days before transplantation (111% for death, 59% for graft loss).

The use of prescription opioids is emerging as another novel risk factor in transplant patients. Although opioid analgesics serve an important role in management of both acute and chronic pain, patients with chronic kidney disease are prone to more complications related to the misuse, abuse, and inherent potential toxicity of prescription opioids due to altered drug protein binding, metabolism, and excretion, leading to accumulation of parent agents and potentially toxic metabolites.[114,115] Recent studies based on integration of US transplant registry with pharmacy fill records showed that 29% of the kidney transplant recipients filled an opioid prescription in the year before transplant. The highest quartile of opioid use before kidney transplantation was associated with increased posttransplant death (aHR, 2.3; 95% CI, 1.7 to 3.1) and graft loss (aHR, 1.7; 95% CI, 1.4 to 2.3).[116] Pretransplant opioid use was associated with posttransplant ventricular arrhythmias, hypotension, hypercapnia, mental status changes, drug abuse and dependence, alcohol abuse, accidents, and noncompliance (Fig. 34.8).[117]

From the perspective of performance grading, the effects of unmeasured risk factors such as symptomatic hypotension,

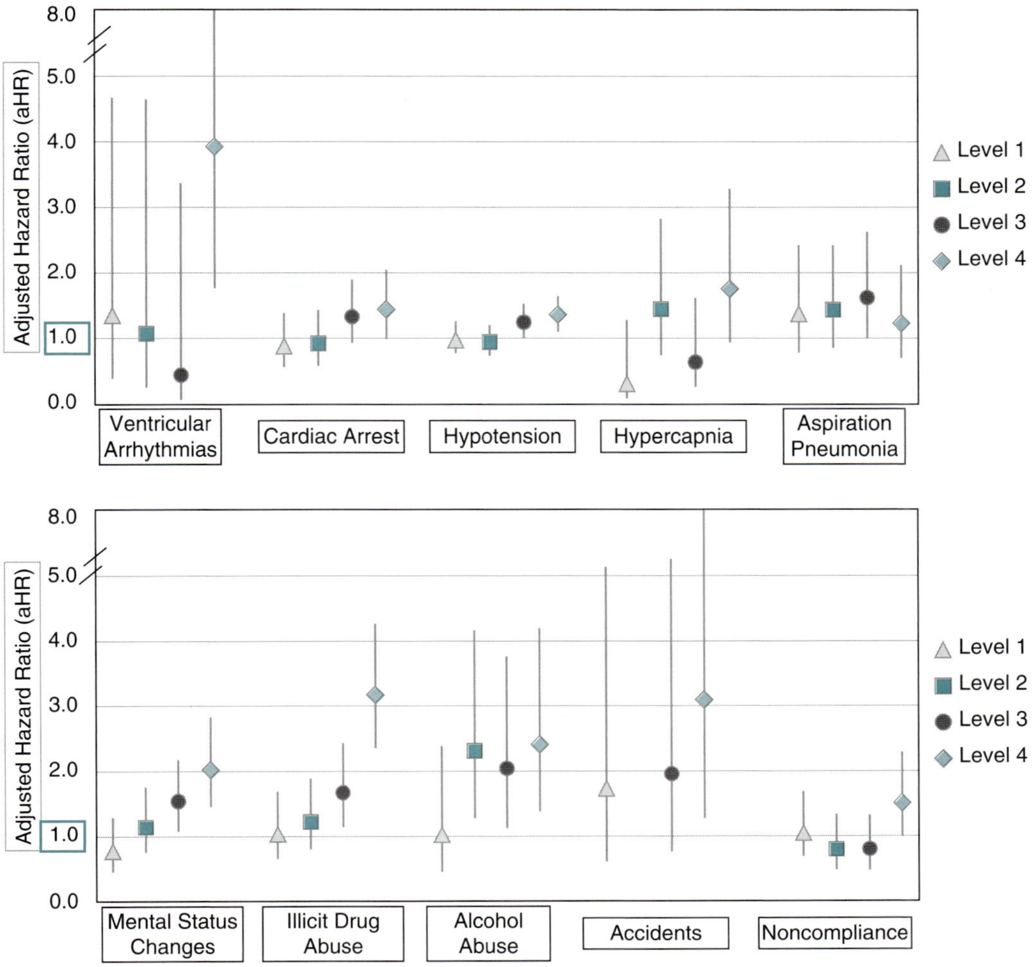

FIG. 34.8 Associations of pretransplant opioid use with posttransplant complications, adjusted for recipient, donor, and transplant factors. (Reproduced with permission from Lentine KL, Lam NN, Xiao H, et al. Associations of pre-transplant prescription narcotic abuse with clinical complications after kidney transplantation. *Am J Nephrol.* 2015;41:165-176.)

CVDS, and opioid use suggest that current risk adjustment methods inadequately characterize risk for transplantation in high-risk patients. Importantly, the SRTR models also do not adjust for risk for innovative practices such as ABO blood type and crossmatch-incompatible transplantation, which increase the odds of posttransplant graft loss, but provide the only meaningful opportunity for transplant for many patients. Although any changes to the OPTN/UNOS data collection is a slow process due to the need to balance considerations of center-reporting burdens and governmental oversight of changes to the registry, supplementation of the registry through data linkages should be considered. Candidates with unmeasured risk factors warrant careful pretransplant evaluation, implementation of strategies to optimize clinical status and mitigate risks (e.g., cessation of opiate use), and focused monitoring of clinical status after transplant to limit the risks for death and graft loss.

ECONOMICS OF KIDNEY TRANSPLANTATION

The many innovations in transplant science have not been matched with parallel developments in the financing of care for patients with ESRD. In this section, we review the history of ESRD care financing, the economic implications of evolving recipient and donor populations, and the economic challenges to practice innovation.

In the early 1960s, neither kidney transplantation nor dialysis was covered by insurance. The costs of both treatments were far in excess of what patients could afford. Therefore access to renal replacement therapy (RRT) was limited to those with private resources and many patients died without treatment.[119] In response, nephrologist Carl Gottschalk was asked to evaluate methods to expand access to dialysis care. The Gottschalk Committee recommended that the federal government subsidize dialysis using the recently created Medicare program as the payment mechanism.[120] When first enacted by Congress in 1972, only 10,000 Americans were on dialysis, with an annual cost of roughly $280 million.[120] By the end of 2014, the number of Americans living with ESRD exceeded 675,000.[121] Nearly 472,000 of the 675,000 Americans currently receiving RRT are on dialysis (hemodialysis or peritoneal dialysis), at an annual cost of nearly $40 billion.[58] Medicare payments for ESRD exceed $30 billion annually, accounting for 7.1% of annual Medicare costs, despite the fact that ESRD affects about 1% of Medicare beneficiaries.[58,122,123] Medicare coverage for chronic kidney disease begins when patients initiate RRT. For patients with existing private health coverage, Medicare remains a secondary payer for the first 30 months of dialysis treatment. After 30 months, Medicare becomes the primary insurer. A small number of patients are covered only by state Medicaid programs despite being on dialysis, if they have not had accrued a sufficient number of working years to quality for Medicare, are not US citizens, or are children.

As early as 1967, Gottschalk's committee concluded that kidney transplantation was preferable to dialysis, based on both its clinical effectiveness and reduced cost.[119] The average payment for a transplant and subsequent care over the first year after transplant was $158,138 for private payers and $99,826 for Medicare.[124] However, in the years following transplant, patients with functioning transplants incur an average annual healthcare spending of only $17,798 and $17,145 for private and Medicare patients, respectively. This compares favorably to annual spending for dialysis and associated care, which exceeds $87,500 per patient per year. In addition, successful transplantation may allow patients to return to work and reduce the rates of rehospitalization and disease progression. Therefore kidney transplant reduces the lifetime cost of ESRD care for payers and society.

ECONOMIC IMPLICATIONS OF RECIPIENT CHARACTERISTICS

Recipient age, comorbidities including obesity, and allosensitization are important factors that affect the clinical and economic benefits of kidney transplant. As noted previously, older patients have been shown to benefit from transplant over dialysis. However, older and frail patients have a greater incidence of complications, prolonged hospital stays, and readmissions with any renal replacement modality, all of which contribute to decreased economic savings in the setting of kidney transplant. Frail patients have 61% higher risk for early hospital readmission posttransplant, as well as a 1.94-fold increased risk for DGF.[125,126] These complications result in higher costs. Patients over the age of 60 years increase the average cost of the transplant episode by $4643 and care during the first year by $18,481.[127]

EPTS scores predict economic as well as clinical outcomes. A recent analysis of cost-accounting data among academic transplant centers captured in the University HealthSystem Consortium found that recipient EPTS was strongly associated with costs incurred during the transplant episode after multivariate adjustment.[128] Compared with patients with EPTS <20, EPTS resulted in significant, graded increases in incremental costs (20 to 50: $1095; 50 to 85 $2292; >85: $5257; $P < 0.005$ for all). Higher cPRA levels also bore strong, graded associations with higher transplant costs, such that cPRA 98 to 100 was associated with $9097 higher incremental expenditure ($P < 0.0001$). Recipient characteristics associated with lower per-transplant costs included polycystic kidney disease, female gender, and working at the time of transplant.

Although obese patients can benefit from transplantation over dialysis, obesity is associated with increased risk for complications and resource utilization during the early and later posttransplant periods. Examination of data for 767 privately insured transplant recipients in 2000 to 2007 found that mean length of stay increased 8.4 days among normal weight to 13.3 days among extremely morbidly obese patients.[129] Another single-center series reported that surgical site infections after kidney transplantation increased from 8.5% of patients with a BMI 20 to 25 kg/m^2 to over 40% in patients with a BMI >40 kg/m^2.[130] Development of a surgical site infection resulted in a $24,454 increase in cost and a $4278 decrease in hospital margin after transplant. Multiple studies have identified association of obesity with increased risk for DGF and the need for dialysis, including a study of registry data for 11,836 recipients reporting graded associations of BMI >25 kg/m^2 with progressively higher DGF risk, such that those with pretransplant BMI >40 kg/m^2 had nearly three times the odds of DGF (adjusted odds ratio [aOR], 2.78; 95% CI, 1.88 to 4.12) after extensive multivariate adjustment, markedly increasing the cost of transplantation.[131]

ECONOMIC IMPLICATIONS OF DONOR CHARACTERISTICS

Although appropriate use of nonstandard kidneys could reduce waiting time and decrease the death rates for patients with high likelihood of waitlist mortality, such as elderly patients, those with diabetes, and those with long expected waiting times for transplantation, many patients who could benefit from listing for nonstandard organs are not listed for consideration of such offers.[132] One barrier to the use of nonstandard kidneys is the significant cost of posttransplant complications, including the need for dialysis, readmission, and decreased allograft survival resulting in an earlier return to dialysis, which do not result in higher payments as the Medicare Diagnosis Related Group (DRG) payment for kidney transplant is not adjusted for complexity.[133] From the transplant center's perspective, these organs result in marked increases in costs without adequate compensation. Analysis of national cost accounting data, demonstrates that older donor age ($62 per year, $P < 0.0001$), death from anoxic injury, higher terminal creatinine ($956 per mg/dL increase, $P < 0.0001$), and DCD ($6182, $P < 0.0001$) were independently associated with higher costs.[127] However, transplants using kidneys placed on a pulsatile perfusion pump are $2039 less expensive in recent practice ($P < 0.0001$).[128]

Living donor kidney transplantation is associated with substantial savings to the healthcare system through provision of the improved long-term recipient survival and reduced early complication rates.[134] Current estimates based on Medicare spending indicate that each living donor transplant performed for a Medicare recipient saves at least $94,579 and adds 3.5 quality-adjusted life years (QALYs) compared with deceased donor transplantation. Considering improved quality of life and functioning, the total economic benefits of living donor transplant have been estimated at $250,000 to $1.3 million per recipient.[134-136] Because living donors themselves incur many types of direct and indirect costs in the donation process, including for travel, medications, lost income, and dependent care,[137] removing financial disincentives to donation for all donors is an important priority.[138] Although some endorse trials of financial incentives as the most potentially impactful approach to increase living donation,[136,139,140] testing of incentives in the United States would require amendment of NOTA, which prohibits organ exchange for "valuable consideration."[141] Importantly, NOTA does not prohibit "reasonable payments associated with the expenses of travel, housing, and lost wages incurred by the donor," and a new trial assessing the impact of reimbursement of lost wages, supported by the National Living Donor Assistance Act, was announced in December 2016.[71]

ECONOMIC IMPLICATIONS OF THE CURRENT KIDNEY ALLOCATION SYSTEM

The use of the KDPI and EPTS to explicitly direct young donor organs into healthier recipients with improved long-term survival incorporated into the new KAS has important clinical and economic implications.[142,143] Under previous allocation policy, average lifetime costs and benefits per transplanted patient, discounted to 2012 US dollars, was estimated at $342,799 and 5.42 QALY, yielding US $63,775 in costs per QALY gained. The KAS system is expected to reduce lifetime costs by $2090 and increase lifetime QALYs by 0.03, further reducing this cost per QALY.[37] Because graft survival is improved in candidates in the top 20% of life expectancy (EPTS <20%) compared with those in the bottom 80%, and rates of return to dialysis are lower, simulations of KAS predict a 7% increase in average median patient life-years per transplant and a 2.8% increase in average median allograft survival.[144] The value of avoiding additional ESRD care of the current policy is expected to be $271 million during the first year and $55 million during each subsequent year.[37] These savings are expected to accrue primarily to Medicare, which would have covered patients with long waiting times, because under the new policy candidates with EPTS <20% are more likely to undergo transplant with a better organ and to have a lower incidence of graft failure requiring retransplantation. There is expected to be a small or modest increase in total private payer ESRD costs. The current KAS was based on historical organ acceptance and decline patterns, and future organ behavior will be an important factor in the ultimate long-term benefits of the revised KAS.

ECONOMIC IMPLICATIONS OF PRACTICE INNOVATION: ABO- AND HLA-INCOMPATIBLE KIDNEY TRANSPLANTATION

Recently large registry analyses in Japan, Europe, and the United States demonstrated that long-term outcomes following ABO incompatible (ABOi) kidney transplant are similar to outcomes of ABO compatible transplantation at 10 years, although the incidence of some early complications is higher.[145] Among the perceived barriers to the expanded use of ABOi transplantation is the cost of the treatment protocols. A 2011 US registry analysis identified 738 patients who had undergone living donor ABOi transplants from 1995 to 2010, representing only 1.5% of all US living donor transplant procedures.[146] The average overall cost of the transplant episode, excluding organ acquisition, was significantly higher for ABOi transplantation ($65,080 vs. $32,039; $P < 0.001$).[147] In addition, ABOi transplantation was independently associated with incrementally higher posttransplant spending (year 1: $25,044; year 2: $10,496; year 3: $7307; $P < 0.01$) (Fig. 34.9). The use of KPD programs is more cost-effective than ABOi; however, for cases for whom a compatible exchange cannot be found, ABOi is less expensive than long-term dialysis.

As already discussed, access to kidney transplantation remains severely limited in highly sensitized patients, such that currently, sensitized recipients (PRA >80%) comprise >14% of the active deceased donor waiting list.[7] Incompatible living donor kidney transplantation (ILDKT) is enabled by desensitization procedures using transplant plasmapheresis and intravenous immunoglobulin, with/without rituximab (anti-CD20) administration.[148,149] After transplant, these patients frequently require additional plasmapheresis treatments and potentially expensive adjunctive therapies. Despite higher rates of graft loss than compatible living donor transplants, multicenter clinical registry studies have confirmed an overall survival advantage of ILDKT recipients compared with matched waitlist controls: 80.6% at 8 years for ILDKT compared with 30.5% at 8 years for those remaining on the waiting list.[148] A recent study of a national cohort of ILDKT recipients with linked hospital cost accounting data from the University HealthSystem Consortium and Medicare claims highlight the increased costs of ILDKT.[150] Overall, ILKDT was associated with an increase in the hospital cost to perform the transplant ($151,024 vs. $106,636) compared with matched compatible transplant controls.[150] The differential in cost between ILDKT and compatible transplantation increased with donor-specific antibody titer levels. The cost was 20% higher in patients with low titer (Luminex assay positive but negative-flow cytometric crossmatch), 26% higher for moderate titer (positive-flow cytometric crossmatch but negative cytotoxic crossmatch), and 39% higher for high titer (positive cytotoxic crossmatch) ILDKT compared with costs for compatible transplants. Although Medicare payment was incrementally higher for these transplants, the additional payment did not compensate for the additional cost of care in most cases.

CONCLUSIONS

Kidney transplantation, especially from a living donor, remains the best treatment for kidney failure and improves the quality and quantity of life over dialysis at the lowest costs to the healthcare system. As disparities in the demand for and the available supply of donated organs continue to grow, there is a need for increased attention to resolving disparities in transplant access based on factors such as socioeconomic status and place of residence. This growth in the waiting list has been associated with greater complexity of the

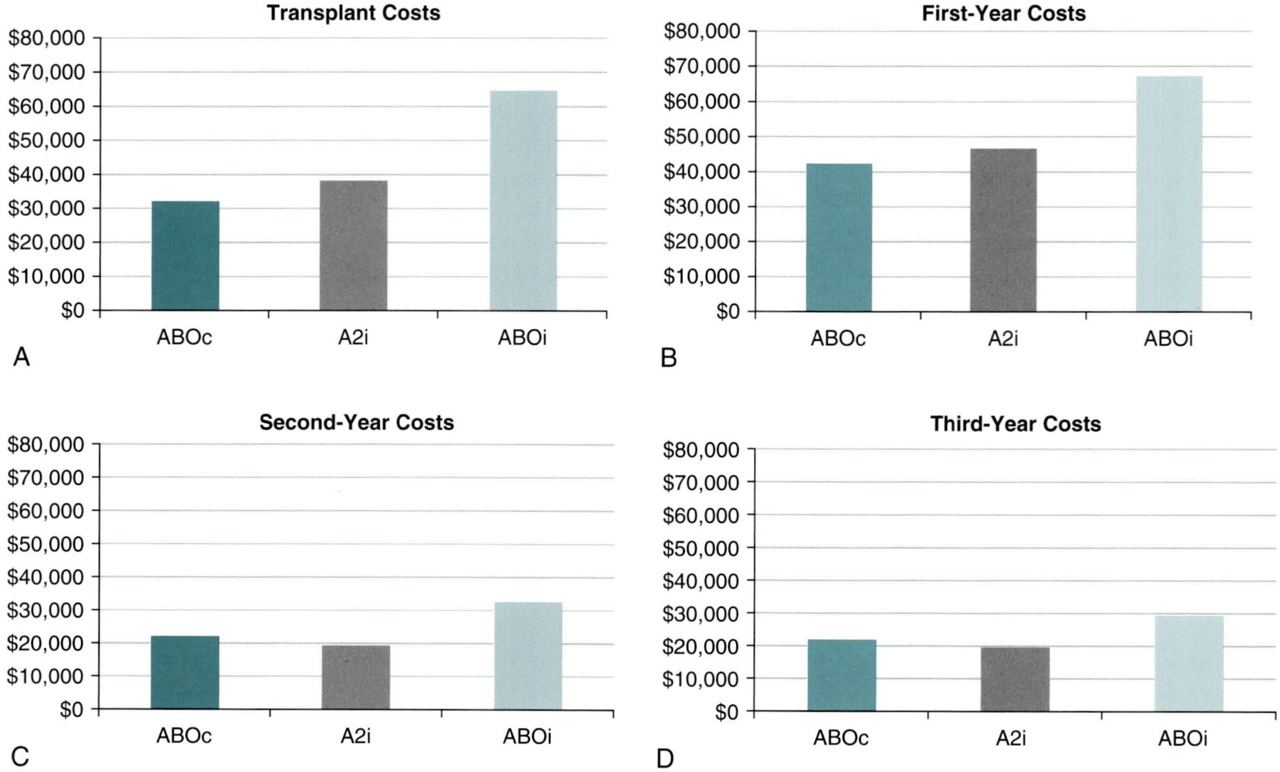

FIG. 34.9 Average adjusted costs according to donor-recipient blood type compatibility during the transplant events and posttransplant periods. (Reproduced with permission from Axelrod D, Segev DL, Xiao H, et al. Economic impacts of ABO-incompatible live donor kidney transplantation: a national study of Medicare-insured recipients. *Am J Transplant.* 2016;16:1465-1473.)

population in need of transplant and pressure to increase use of nonstandard organs, which in turn increase the risks and costs of transplantation. Increased regulatory oversight and performance grading is intended to optimize use of scarce organs, but can lead to unintended consequences of risk aversion, higher discard rates, and decreased access for higher risk patients. Attention to uncaptured risk in performance grading is needed to sustain innovation in transplant practice without penalizing centers that attempt to advance the science of transplantation. Despite the clear long-term benefit of transplantation, transplant centers face significant economic disincentives to develop innovative protocols, use nonstandard organs, and employ novel technologies. Policymakers should consider the creation of risk-adjusted payment for renal transplant, similar to that of liver and heart transplant, to ensure that access is preserved for all candidates. The inclusion of supplemental payments for providers that successfully use organs from higher risk donors (e.g., KPDI >85) would ensure that financial considerations no longer contribute to organ discard but, instead, drive innovation.

ACKNOWLEDGMENTS

DA and KLL received support from NIH/NIDDK R01DK102981 “Choosing Immune Suppression in Renal Transplantation by Efficacy and Morbidity.” The authors acknowledge R01 coinvestigators, including Vikas Dharnidharka, Mark Schnitzler, Daniel Brennan, and Dorry Segev. They acknowledge Bertram Kasiske and the SRTR for their valuable collaboration, and transplant outcomes research collaborators including Abhijit Naik, Ngan Lam, Henry Randall, Rosemary Ouseph, Huiling Xiao, and Zidong Zhang.

A full list of references is available at www.expertconsult.com.

35

Transplantation Immunobiology

Nader Najafian, MD, and Leonardo V. Riella, MD, PhD

OUTLINE

When an organ or tissue from one member of a species is transplanted into a nonidentical member of the same species, an immune response ensues. This response is termed the *alloimmune response*, and it is primarily orchestrated by initial T-cell recognition of alloantigens (allorecognition, signal 1). However, full activation of T cells requires in addition to signal 1 two other sequential signals: signal 2 delivered by ligation of costimulatory receptors on T cells by ligands on antigen-expressing cells (APCs); and signal 3 delivered by multiple cytokines that regulate cell proliferation, differentiation, and survival/death. The first part of this chapter reviews the process of T-cell allorecognition with particular emphasis on recent advances in our understanding of T-cell costimulatory pathways and novel cytokines in regulating different phases of T-cell responses in transplant rejection. Activation of alloreactive T cells subsequently leads to the initiation of the effector mechanisms of the immune system, resulting in allograft destruction. Recently, B cells and alloantibodies against human leukocyte antigen (HLA) and non-HLA targets have been increasingly recognized as critical in the pathogenesis of acute and chronic allograft dysfunction. Furthermore, although T cells alone are necessary and sufficient for the rejection of allografts, evidence is accumulating on the role of humoral and cellular components of the innate immune system in allograft rejection and prevention of tolerance. The second part of this chapter focuses on the various effector mechanisms of allograft rejection. The ultimate goal in clinical transplantation is to induce a state of donor-specific immunological tolerance, where recipients can accept organs without the need of exogenous immunosuppression. The final part of this chapter reviews the most promising approaches to inducing transplantation tolerance. In particular, we highlight the biological basis and putative mechanisms of tolerance and discuss some of the major stumbling blocks to the induction and maintenance of tolerance in clinical transplantation.

THE ALLOIMMUNE RESPONSE

A. Transplantation Antigens

Major Histocompatibility Complex

The major histocompatibility complex (MHC) antigens are the strongest and most polymorphic transplantation antigens, and they can stimulate the primary immune response without priming. The recipient T-cell receptor's recognition of donor MHC/peptide complexes is the central event in the initiation of an alloimmune response, with the allogeneic donor HLA antigens being the main immunological targets of different effector arms on the immune system. In some cases, antibodies against donor HLA antigens may have been previously generated because of pregnancies, blood transfusions, or previous transplantation. These preformed antibodies may cause hyperacute or accelerated acute graft rejection at the time of transplantation, though immunological testing has reduced the frequency of this type of rejection. Later after transplantation, the appearance of de novo donor-specific antibodies has been linked to chronic allograft dysfunction.

T lymphocytes recognize foreign (nonself) antigens in the context of self cell-surface molecules encoded in the MHC.[1] In humans, this genetic region is located in a 3.5 million base-pair region on the short arm of chromosome 6. This locus is further subdivided into three clusters based on the structure and function of the proteins encoded by the genes. Human MHC molecules are called HLAs, and the three regions have been designated HLA class I, class II, and class III (Fig. 35.1).

HLA *class I* molecules (classic HLA-A, -B, and -C, and other nonclassic molecules) are composed of a 44-kD heavy chain and a 12-kD light chain (Fig. 35.2).[1,2] The amino terminus portion of the heavy chain that extends into the extracellular space is composed of three domains: alpha1, alpha2, and alpha3. The alpha1 and alpha2 domains interact to form the sides of a cleft (or groove). The cleft is the site where foreign proteins bind to MHC molecules for presentation to T cells. The highly variable amino acid residues located in the groove

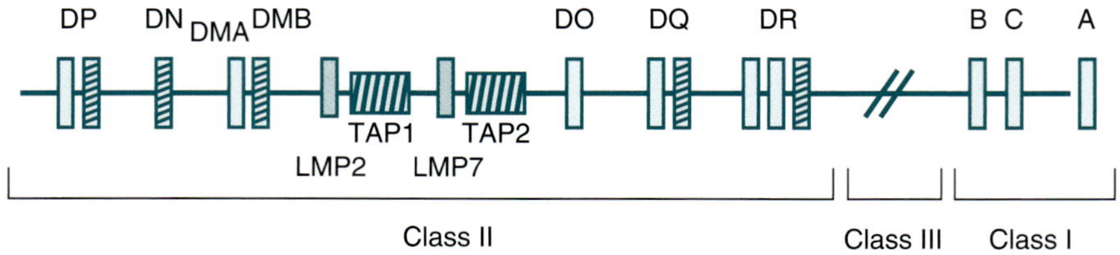

FIG. 35.1 Genomic organization of the human major histocompatibility complex (MHC). See text for explanation. (From Noessner E, Krensky AM. HLA and antigen presentation. In: Tilney NL, Strom TB, Paul LC, eds. *Transplantation Biology: Cellular and Molecular Aspects.* New York: Lippincott-Raven: 31.1.)

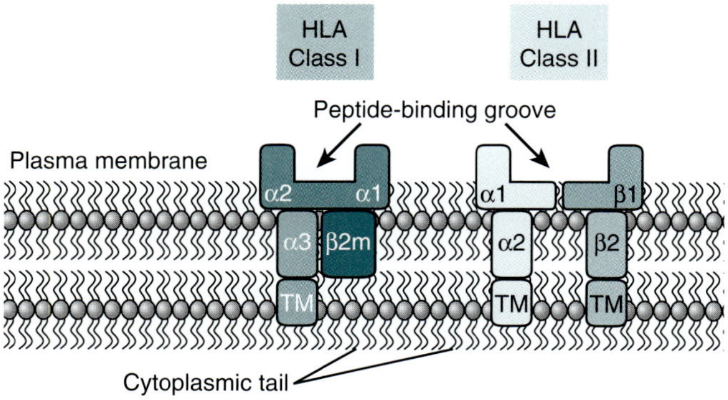

FIG. 35.2 Structure of HLA class I and class II molecules. HLA class I molecules consist of heavy chains made up of three polypeptide domains (α1, α2, α3) and a noncovalently associated light chain, β2-microglobulin. HLA class II molecules are heterodimers of α and β chains with a very similar overall structure and peptide-binding surface. *TM,* Transmembrane region.

determine the specificity of peptide binding and T-cell antigen recognition. The light chain, β_2-microglobulin, stabilizes the heavy chain such that displacement of β_2-microglobulin from the class I molecule causes a loss of heavy chain native structure. Class I molecules are expressed on essentially all nucleated cells. The function of intact class I molecules is to present antigenic peptides as protein fragments (peptides) in the context of self to T lymphocytes. HLA class I molecules are highly polymorphic. This polymorphism aids in maximizing the potential for peptide binding by the species. Peptides bind within the HLA class I groove (see Fig. 35.2) based on the sequence of amino acids in the peptide-binding region.[3] HLA class I molecules tend to bind peptides of 9 to 11 amino acids in length. These peptides fit tightly into the groove and do not extend out of the ends of the molecule. MHC class I molecules generally present endogenous proteins (Fig. 35.3).[4] These proteins, such as viruses and normal self proteins, are degraded in the cytoplasm in proteasomes. Short peptide sequences are then moved to the endoplasmic reticulum through specific transporters associated with antigen presentation (TAP transporters). In the endoplasmic reticulum, these peptides associate with class I heavy chain and β_2-microglobulin, and the mature complex is transported to the cell surface, where it can be recognized by T lymphocytes. Peptides sit in the middle of the groove and run the length of the cleft. The rules for peptide binding are restricted to certain "motifs" based on the polymorphisms described earlier but are lax enough to permit the binding of many different peptides to a single HLA type (allele). Antigens associated with class I molecules are recognized by cytotoxic $CD8^+$ T lymphocytes.

The second major region of the MHC is called the *class II locus* (see Fig. 35.1).[1] HLA class II molecules—HLA-DP, DQ, and DR—are composed of polymorphic α and β chains of about 35 and 31 kD, respectively. These two chains associate to form a peptide-binding region, but unlike class I molecules, determinants of the peptide-binding region are contributed by both chains (Fig. 35.2B).[2] MHC class II molecules bind longer peptides—typically 12 to 28 amino acids. In contrast to class I, MHC class II molecules have binding grooves that are open at the ends, permitting peptides of greater lengths to extend beyond the groove (see Fig. 35.3).[5] Class II molecules tend to bind antigens that are derived from the exogenous pathway (see Fig. 35.3). MHC class II α and β chains associate in the endoplasmic reticulum with an invariant chain, a portion of which binds in the antigen-binding groove. This invariant chain appears to both protect the groove from peptide binding and permit proper folding of the class II complex. A nonomeric form exits the endoplasmic reticulum and moves through the Golgi apparatus and into an endosomal compartment. Within the endosome, the invariant chain is degraded, leaving a shorter class II–associated invariant chain peptide (CLIP) fragment in the groove. Peptides from the extracellular space are taken up into endosomes by endocytosis and targeted to the "compartment for peptide loading." Within this specialized intracellular compartment, exogenous peptides displace CLIP, and the mature heterotrimeric complex (α, β, and peptide) is transported to the cell surface, where it can be recognized by T lymphocytes. Class II molecules are only expressed on specialized cells such as professional APCs and endothelial cells, and antigens bound to class II MHC molecules are usually recognized by $CD4^+$ helper T cells. In addition to the classic class II antigens, the MHC class II region encodes proteins that make up the proteasome (low-molecular-weight proteins LMP-2 and LMP-7) and the TAP transporters (TAP-1 and TAP-2) (see Fig. 35.1). Polymorphisms associated with these structures probably also contribute to the specificity and diversity of peptide binding and antigen presentation. The class III region encodes a variety of proteins of immunological relevance (see Fig. 35.1). These include the tumor necrosis factor (TNF) and the complement proteins factor B and C4.

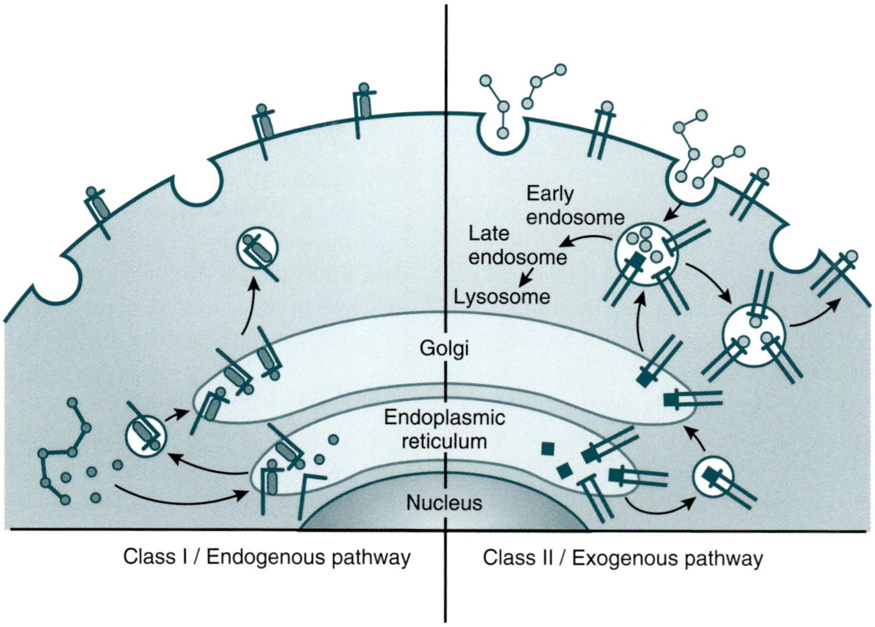

FIG. 35.3 Antigen processing and presentation. In the endogenous pathway *(left)*, HLA class I molecules bind to peptides from endogenous antigens. The proteasome breaks up cytoplasmic proteins into peptides that enter the endoplasmic reticulum via specific transporters. In the endoplasmic reticulum, peptides associate with HLA class I molecules and from the mature complex that is exported through the Golgi apparatus to the plasma membrane. In the exogenous pathway *(right)*, HLA class II molecules bind peptides from exogenous antigens. Exogenous proteins enter the cell by endocytosis and are degraded to peptides in endosomes and lysosomes. Class II molecules bind peptides in the "compartment for peptide loading" and are transported to the plasma membrane.

As just outlined, MHC molecules are highly polymorphic, because each MHC locus can express any one of hundreds of different molecules encoded by various *alleles*. The set of different alleles expressed on one chromosome is called a *haplotype*. Each parental chromosome 6 provides a haplotype to the offspring. Haplotypes are usually inherited intact from each parent, although crossover between the A and B locus occurs in about 2% of offspring, resulting in a recombination and a new haplotype. A genotype is the sum of two haplotypes. A child is by definition a one-haplotype match to each parent unless recombination has occurred. In addition, the MHC molecules are codominantly expressed—that is, an individual expresses alleles from both chromosomes at each locus. Therefore the MHC genotype of an individual consists of 12 different MHC molecules (two alleles from each of six loci). In clinical transplantation, the most polymorphic MHC genes are HLA-A, -B, and -DR and therefore historically identified as the most important transplant targets. The antigenic determinants of their six alleles are the focus of attempts at HLA matching to improve graft survival. Given the remarkable degree of polymorphism exhibited by MHC genes, there are 88 recognized antigens encoded by more than 1000 distinct alleles, and the number of new alleles is still increasing. The HLA antigens were initially identified using antisera obtained from multiparous women and named in the sequence they were discovered (for example, A1, A2, etc.). However, introducing DNA technologies for HLA testing resulted in the identification of growing numbers of alleles that could be identified by their unique nucleotide sequences within the antigen designations. Thus the serological nomenclature was modified to associate alleles with antigens, and four-digit designations were developed in which the antigen designation makes up the first two digits and the sequential allele designation makes up the third and fourth digits. For example, the first allele for HLA-A1 is HLA-A*0101, which includes the locus (A), an asterisk to indicate the typing was performed by DNA methods, the serological antigen (01), and the allele number (01). As an example, HLA-B has more than 3600 different alleles. Although HLA gene polymorphism plays a critical role in protective immunity by enabling the binding and presentation of a wide variety of microbial peptides to T cells, it creates a practical barrier to successful transplantation. In fact, it has recently been found that differences between MHC molecules by as little as one or two amino acids (called *micropolymorphism*) in the antigen-binding cleft can change the size and diversity of the peptide repertoire presented by each HLA molecule.[6] It is not feasible to select a completely HLA-matched donor for every potential recipient because of the enormous polymorphism of the HLA system. Although allele differences between the donor and the recipient of bone marrow transplants (even micropolymorphism) lead to graft-versus-host disease, HLA mismatches affect primarily the long-term graft survival of kidney transplantation with the best outcomes in six HLA-matched kidneys compared with zero matched kidneys.

The alloimmune response is strong and does not require priming.[7] At least part of the basis for the greater magnitude of the allogeneic response is the relatively high frequency of T-cell precursors that are capable of responding to a foreign MHC antigen. For example, the frequency of specific T cells to conventional antigens is approximately 1 in 10^4 to 10^5, whereas the frequency responding during allogeneic stimulation can be as high as 1 in 10^1 to 10^2. The concept of positive and negative selection in the thymus (see mechanisms of self tolerance) also helps explain the strength of the alloimmune response.[8-10] During development, T cells with receptors of too high an affinity are deleted (negative selection), whereas those with too low an affinity are not selected. The result of this selection is that T-cell receptors (TCRs) of intermediate affinity exit the thymus and enter the periphery. Within an individual, clonal deletion occurs early in development. Potentially, autoreactive clones (with too high an affinity for self) are deleted; failure of deletion of some clones may lead to autoimmunity. In the case of transplantation across an allelic difference, however, the recipient's T cells do not contact allo-MHC molecules during development in the thymus and thus escape the deletion (negative selection) imposed by interaction with self-MHC. Thus the result is the large number of donor MHC/peptide complexes on the graft to which a potential recipient has not been tolerized during ontogeny. Moreover, the relatively low affinity of any given TCR for its ligand suggest that each T cell could potentially recognize more than one MHC/peptide complex.[11] The high density of alloantigens on the surface of an allograft additionally contributes to the strong T-cell response. In addition, because recipient T cells recognize intact allogeneic MHC molecules directly (see following), they are stimulated maximally by the high density of MHC on the surfaces of transplanted cells.

Minor Transplantation Antigens

Studies involving MHC identical grafts in mice indicate that minor histocompatibility antigens can also mediate rejection. Recipient T cells can be directly primed to minor histocompatibility antigens. A minor histocompatibility antigen is molecularly defined as a donor-derived peptide presented on a donor cell by an MHC molecule shared by a donor and a recipient. Note that the donor and the recipient express the same MHC molecules. Donor dendritic cells (DCs) directly prime $CD8^+$ T cells to become effector cells without the need for further antigen processing by recipient APCs. As one illustration, $CD8^+$ T cells from female C57BL/6 mice specific for male-derived H-Y Uty peptide + MHC class I mediate rejection of syngeneic C57/BL6 male skin.[12] In humans, it has been recognized for several years that minor histocompatibility antigens can be immunogenic from observations based on organ graft rejections and bone marrow graft-versus-host reactions in cases of genetically matched HLA antigens. A few cases of donor-directed, HLA class I–restricted, cytotoxic T-cell responses have been demonstrated in such cases.[13,14] Two general families of such antigens have been identified[15]:

1. H-Y antigens are proteins encoded on the Y chromosome. Females of the species may mount an immune response against these proteins.
2. T cells recognize peptidic antigens corresponding to polymorphisms among autosomal proteins expressed by individuals of the species. Examples include mitochondrial proteins and enzymes. In the presence of both major and minor incompatibilities, it is clear that the alloimmune response targeted against the MHC molecules predominates.

Several studies reported a detrimental role for minor H antigen-specific T cells in graft survival. However, some data indicate that minor H antigens might also be clinically involved in preventing rejection of solid organ grafts, possibly by induction of regulatory T cells.[16]

ABO Blood Group Antigens

The A and B groups are glycosylated differentially, whereas group O lacks the enzymes necessary for glycosylation. The antigens are readily recognized by natural antibodies, termed *hemagglutinins* because they cause red cell agglutination. They are relevant to transplantation because they are expressed on other cell types, including the endothelium. Thus they cause hyperacute rejection of vascular allografts because of preformed natural antibodies. Allograft rejection as a result of red blood cell type mismatching can be readily prevented by routine blood typing before transplantation. A2 antigen has significantly lower expression on endothelium, so that transplantation of A2 kidneys to B recipients in the absence of high titers against A2 is feasible. The rhesus (Rh) factor and other red cell antigens are of little concern because they are not expressed on endothelial cells.

Monocyte and Endothelial Cell Antigens

Occasionally, allografts undergo hyperacute rejection, despite appropriate ABO matching. Some of these rejection episodes have been attributed to additional non-ABO antigens expressed on endothelial cells (such as MICA) and monocytes,[17,18] but these antigen systems remain poorly understood. Pretransplant tissue typing does not currently evaluate the endothelial/monocyte antigens because of the apparent rarity of such antibodies and the lack of accurate reagents for typing.

B. Cellular Events Leading to Allograft Rejection

In the context of allograft rejection, T cells play a central role in orchestrating the immune response because they recognize alloantigens through three distinct pathways (see later). Once activated, they secrete cytokines and chemokines to activate and attract various effector cells, such as $CD8^+$ T cells and macrophages into the allograft. They are also able to interact with B cells that will secrete highly specific alloreactive antibodies. These cells in turn mediate the effector mechanisms of allograft destruction (see following). Box 35.1 summarizes

BOX 35.1 Steps in Allograft Rejection

1. Recognition of the alloantigen (direct, semi-direct, and indirect pathways)
2. T-cell and B-cell activation, differentiation, and expansion
3. Effector functions
4. Resolution of the response with residual memory

the steps leading to allograft rejection. Furthermore, although T cells alone are necessary and sufficient for the rejection of allografts, evidence is accumulating about the role of the innate immune system in allograft rejection and prevention of tolerance.

Allorecognition Pathways

The first step in an alloimmune response is the recognition of alloantigens by T cells (priming of alloreactive T cells). In the setting of a transplant, there is the potential for three different cellular mechanisms of allorecognition; these have been called the *direct, semi-direct,* and *indirect* pathways of allorecognition (Fig. 35.4).[19-21]

Direct refers to cell recognition of a whole, intact foreign MHC molecule on the surface of donor cells. Although the specific peptide (typically derived from endogenous proteins, including MHC antigens) bound in the groove of the MHC molecule may be important in this recognition process, it does not restrict this response. The graft, which includes donor bone marrow–derived APCs, usually expresses several class I and class II MHC molecules that differ from the recipient's MHC molecules, and which can directly stimulate recipients T cells. In sum, donor APCs prime $CD4^+$ and $CD8^+$ T cells through the direct pathway. However, as these donor APCs are destroyed during the priming process, direct T-cell priming is likely to be time limited. Thus direct allorecognition may account for early acute cellular rejection. Consistent with this idea, direct alloreactivity was not detectable in the peripheral blood of a cohort of renal allograft recipients with chronic allograft dysfunction several years after transplantation.[22,23] In contrast, *indirect* refers to T-cell recognition of nonself MHC-derived peptides (allopeptides) in the context of self MHC molecules expressed on recipient APCs. In this case, similar to the physiological pathway of antigen recognition, the peptide sequence determines the response. Indirect presentation could occur through a number of mechanisms: soluble donor MHC molecules are shed from the graft and drain through the bloodstream/lymphatics to the recipient secondary lymphoid organs, where they would be processed/presented by recipient APCs to recipient T cells. Alternatively, donor graft cells that migrate to recipient secondary lymphoid organs could be endocytosed by recipient APCs. Third, recipient monocyte/macrophages entering the donor graft could endocytose donor antigens and present the peptides to recipient T cells. Other allopeptides may be derived from minor histocompatibility antigens or tissue-specific antigens. Because recipient monocytes migrating through the allograft can constantly endocytose donor antigen, priming through the indirect pathway could occur for as long as the graft is present in the host. Thus, although indirect alloreactive T cells may participate in acute rejection, they may play a predominant role in chronic rejection.[24] Consistent with this concept, several groups have now provided data correlating the indirect alloreactive T cells with the presence of chronic allograft dysfunction.[25-27] Interestingly, recent emerging data demonstrate that not only $CD4^+$ T cells, as traditionally thought, but also $CD8^+$ T cells can be primed through the indirect pathway of allorecognition and contribute to graft destruction.[28]

Endothelial cells of donor origin are located at the interface between the recipient's blood and the allograft and have been implicated in graft rejection (Fig. 35.5).[20,29] Graft endothelial cells express MHC class I and II molecules and have been found recently to promote direct allorecognition by serving as APCs and as targets for T-cell–mediated

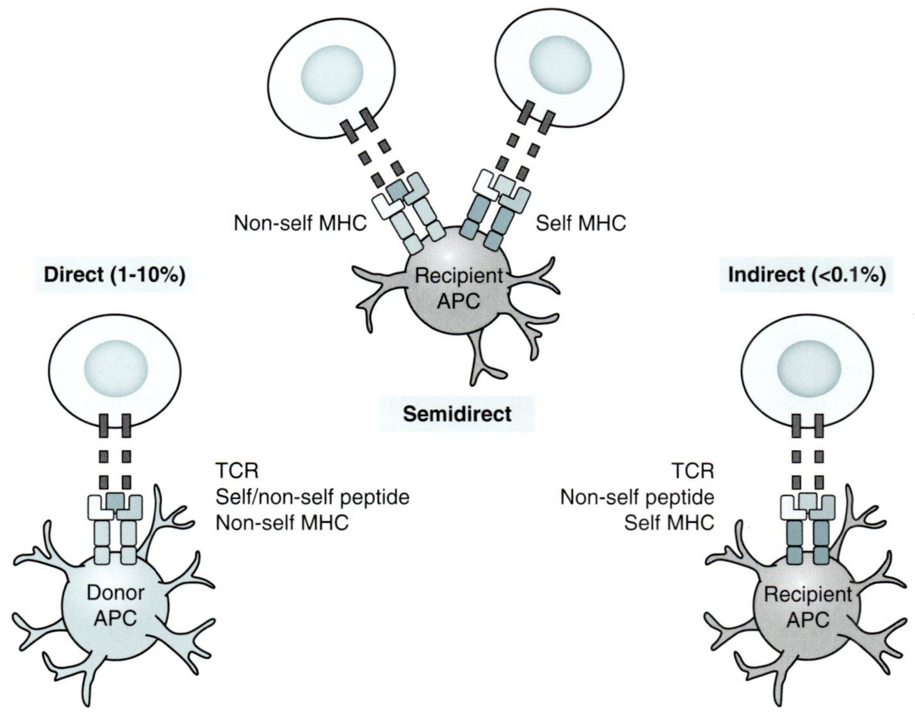

FIG. 35.4 Alloantigen presentation via the direct, semi-direct, and indirect pathways after organ transplantation.

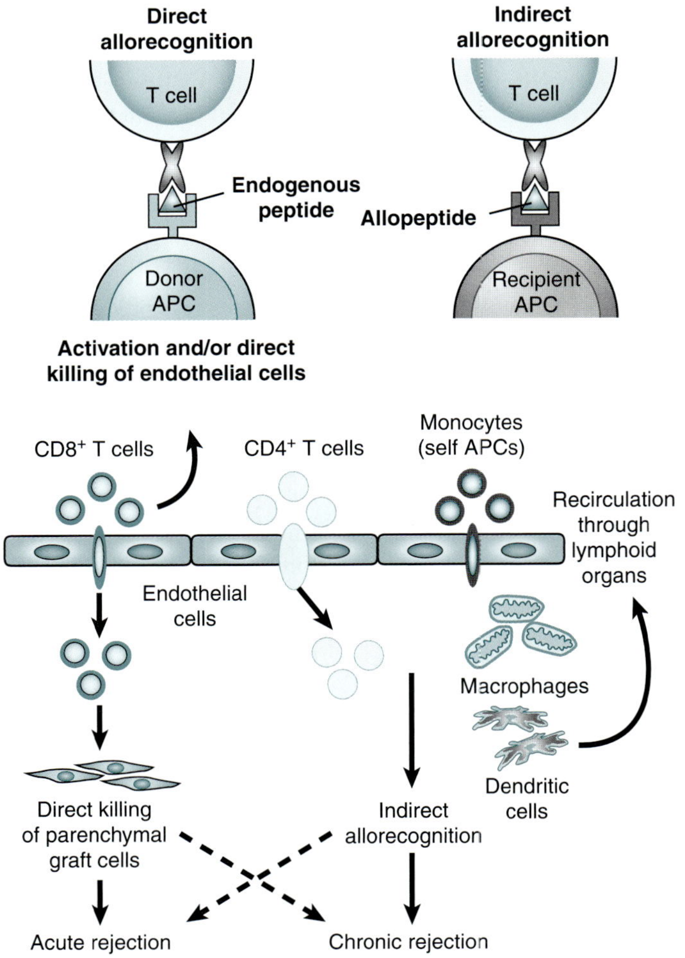

FIG. 35.5 Mechanism of graft rejection. (A) Graft rejection is initiated by CD4+ T cells, which recognize alloantigens. In the direct pathway of allorecognition, the T cell binds to a major histocompatibility complex (MHC) molecule on donor antigen-presenting cells *(left)*. In the indirect pathway, the foreign MHC molecule is processed into allopeptides, which are presented to the T cell by self antigen-presenting cells *(right)*. Activated CD4+ T cells proliferate and secrete a variety of cytokines that act as growth and activation factors for CD8+ cytotoxic T cells, B cells, and macrophages. (B) Interactions among endothelial cells, T cells, and recipient antigen-presenting cells in allograft rejection. Recipient monocytes are recruited by endothelial cells to the graft tissue. They are also transformed to become highly efficient antigen-presenting dendritic cells that may need to recirculate to peripheral lymphoid organs for maturation. The dendritic cells and intragraft macrophages present donor peptides via the indirect pathway to recruited CD4+ T cells. CD8+ T cells, on the other hand, are activated by donor endothelial cells and can either directly kill endothelial cells or traverse the endothelium and kill parenchymal graft.

cytotoxicity. In addition, endothelial cells may promote indirect allorecognition by a crosstalk mechanism, which involves the recruitment and transformation of recipient monocytes by endothelial cells into highly efficient antigen-presenting dendritic cells.[20,29]

More recently, a third pathway of alloantigen presentation has been discovered in which recipient APCs acquire intact allogeneic HLA-peptides complexes from donor cells and present them to directly reactive recipient T cells.[30,31] This presentation is called a *semi-direct* or *cross-dressing* pathway to differentiate it from the true direct presentation performed by donor APCs. Marino et al.[31] described a murine model of recipient APC cross-dressing, in which the HLA molecules derived from donor exosomes and donor immune cells were acquired by recipients APCs (see Fig. 35.4). The relative contribution of this pathway to allograft rejection is still not clear.

Finally, the question of where T cells meet the transplant antigens has been the target of much study. The site of alloantigen recognition had been believed to be in the allograft itself, but data seem to indicate that peripheral lymphoid organs are required for allograft rejection.[32] Whether unprimed T cells encounter antigens first outside the allograft in peripheral lymphoid tissue or they migrate to secondary lymphoid organs after they encounter the alloantigens in the graft for further maturation and differentiation remains controversial. Interestingly, primed/effector/memory cells appear to mediate graft rejection independent of peripheral lymphoid organs, suggesting that they are activated by alloantigens in the graft itself.[32]

T-Cell Activation

Allograft rejection is a T-cell–dependent process; animals that lack T cells do not reject an allograft. In particular, $CD4^+$ helper T cells appear to be essential orchestrators of the alloimmune response leading to allograft rejection.[33] T lymphocytes initiate the immune response, which ultimately results in graft rejection. In addition, they can function as regulators and effectors in the immune response (see following). As just discussed, allorecognition is the essential initial step for initiation of the cascade of events that results in rejection of the graft (see Box 35.1). The essential cell-cell interactions between T cells and APCs (donor or self) may involve five classes of receptors: the antigen-specific TCR, the CD4 or CD8 coreceptor, costimulatory molecules, accessory or adhesion molecules, and lymphokine receptors. Members of each class of receptors may present suitable targets for therapeutic and experimental manipulation and are thus discussed next.

T-cell receptor–CD3 complex. T-cell recognition of alloantigens on APCs is the central event that initiates allograft rejection.[21,34] The interaction between T lymphocytes and APCs involves multiple T-cell surface molecules and their counterreceptors expressed by APCs. Antigen specificity is determined by the TCR, which recognizes processed antigens in the form of short peptides that are bound to an MHC molecule. Clonally restricted TCRs are made up of two chains. The major TCR is an α, β heterodimer, and a less commonly expressed TCR consists of γ and δ chains. The TCR consists of constant and variable portions involved in binding to HLA and recognition of the specific alloantigenic targets. Although the TCR allows T cells to recognize antigen-MHC complexes, the cell-surface expression of TCR molecules and the initiation of intracellular signaling depend on a complex of additional peptides known as the CD3 complex. After a given TCR is engaged by alloantigen, the T cell is activated and a signal (signal 1) is transduced through the TCR-CD3 complex. As will be discussed following, full activation of T cells requires two synergistic signals (see Costimulatory Molecules).

Rabbit antithymocyte globulin (rATG; thymoglobulin or ATG), one of the most common induction therapy agents, targets multiple T-cell surface molecules, including CD3. rATG is typically prepared by immunizing pathogen-free rabbits, with a cell suspension of human thymic tissue (thymocytes). After immunization, the serum is harvested from rabbits, and immunoglobulins against thymocytes are isolated and subjected to a number of purification processes. Samples from more than 26,000 immunized rabbits are pooled to achieve a high level of batch-to-batch consistency. The resulting antibodies are polyclonal and target multiple different surface molecules present on T cells. The mechanism of action of ATGs is lymphocyte depletion, predominantly by complement-dependent cells lysis.

CD4 and CD8 T-cell receptor coreceptors. The two major subsets of T cells, cytotoxic $CD8^+$ T cells and helper $CD4^+$ T cells, recognize processed antigens on MHC class I and II molecules, respectively. CD4 and CD8 molecules enhance the interaction between the TCR and APCs through the MHC. By binding class II MHC molecules, the CD4 molecule facilitates TCR-CD3 complex-mediated signal transduction and assists the actions of class II MHC–restricted T cells. Similarly, the CD8 molecule binds to class I MHC molecules and stabilizes the interaction of the class I MHC–restricted T cell with a target cell–mediating signal transduction. Thus CD4/$CD8^+$TCR–CD3 complex proteins function together in initiating the signals for T-cell activation.

Adhesion molecules. Immune cells gain access to the site of inflammation in the graft from nearby lymph nodes and the bloodstream. Associated with transplantation, alloantigens enter local lymph nodes. APCs, such as dendritic cells and tissue macrophages, take up foreign HLA (indirect allorecognition) or exosomes containing foreign HLA (semi-direct allorecognition), or foreign HLA on donor APCs is recognized directly (direct allorecognition). Antigen-specific T cells are activated, differentiate, divide, and enter the bloodstream.

Immune cells move from the bloodstream into the site of inflammation by a three-step process. First, they roll along the vessel wall through interactions between selectins on the endothelium and receptors on the immune cells. Second, they adhere to vessel endothelium. Third, chemoattractant cytokines (chemokines) are released (Fig. 35.6). Adhesion molecules and chemokines are important regulators of rejection and appear to be targets for immunotherapy. Adhesion molecules (integrins) are well known for their ability to facilitate adhesion between cells and between cells and the extracellular matrix. Integrins on T cells include lymphocyte function-associated antigen 1 (LFA-1), which interacts with intercellular adhesion molecules (ICAM) 1 and 2; CD2, which interacts with CD58 (leukocyte function-associated antigen 3 [LFA-3]); and very-late-appearing antigen (VLA-4) (CDw49d, CD29), which interacts with vascular cell adhesion molecule (VCAM-1, CD106). These receptors are of two large structural families. The integrins, including LFA-1 and VLA-4, are made up of α, β heterodimers, whereas members of the immunoglobulin superfamily, including CD2, LFA-3, VCAM-1, and the ICAMs, are made up of disulfide-linked "receptor" domains. The inhibition of adhesion cell function has been found to be immunosuppressive. Previous studies in murine and primate models reported increased graft survival with anti–ICAM-1 monoclonal antibodies; however, in a randomized multicenter trial, short-term use of the anti–ICAM-1 monoclonal antibody enlimomab for induction therapy after renal transplantation did not reduce the rate of acute rejection or delayed graft function.[35] No agents targeting trafficking of T cells are being used in clinical transplantation.

Costimulatory molecules. T cells require two signals for full activation (Fig. 35.7). One signal is provided by the interaction of the TCR with the MHC-peptide complex; the second "costimulatory" signal depends on one or more additional receptor-ligand interactions between T cells and APCs.[36] The two-signal model has gained enormous support, defining several costimulatory pathways, and is now widely accepted.[37] Traditionally these molecules were broadly grouped into two families based on their molecular structures: the immunoglobulin (Ig) superfamily and the tumor necrosis factor

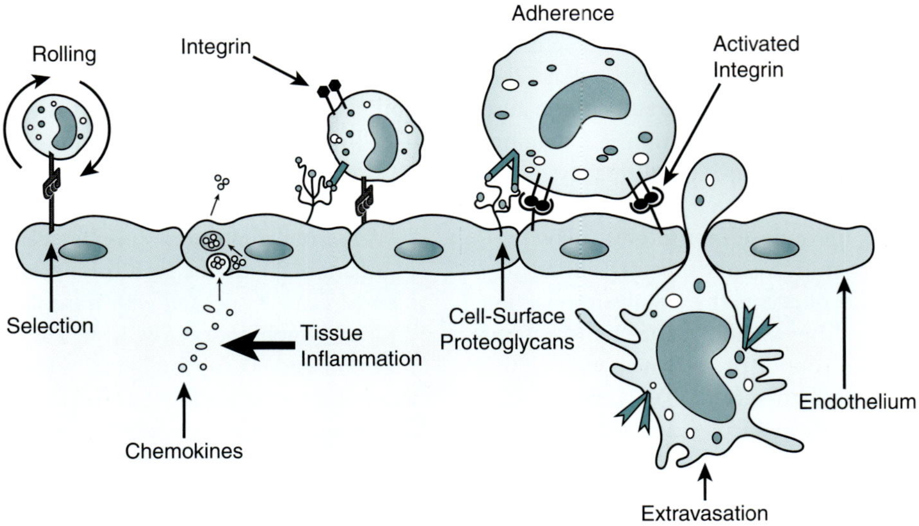

FIG. 35.6 Three-step model of inflammatory cell migration from the bloodstream into the site of rejection. Rolling of monocytes and T lymphocytes along the vascular endothelium is mediated by selectins. Chemokines may be synthesized by the endothelial cell or produced by tissue cells and subsequently transported across the endothelium. Then they bind to glycosaminoglycans on the endothelial cell surface, where they can activate leukocyte chemokine receptors, causing integrin activation, flow arrest, and movement across the endothelial cell barrier into the tissues following the chemoattractant gradient. (From Dong, VM, McDermott DH, Abdi R. Chemokines and diseases. *Eur J Dermatol.* 2003;13(3), 224-230.)

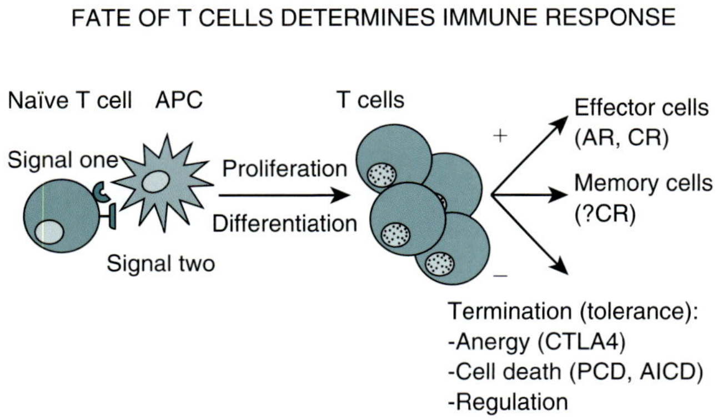

FIG. 35.7 Stimulation of T cells through binding of a peptide–major histocompatibility complex (MHC) to the T-cell receptor (signal 1) in the presence of a costimulatory signal (signal two) leads to proliferation and differentiation of these cells. Apoptosis, cell cycle arrest, and active suppression are known regulators of this immune response. A few antigen-specific cells are spared and become memory cells. (From Najafian N, Khoury SJ, Sayegh MH. T-cell costimulatory blockade as a novel immune intervention in autoimmune diseases, *Clin Dermatol.* 2001;19(5):586-591.)

receptor (TNFR) family. The CD28-B7 (from the Ig superfamily) and CD154-CD40 pathways (from the TNFR family) have been studied the longest and described as the critical costimulatory pathways for T-cell activation. Blockade of these pathways has been reported to regulate both autoimmune and alloimmune responses in experimental models and in human disease. However, studies have indicated that inhibition of these pathways is insufficient to reproducibly induce long-lasting immunological tolerance in some experimental autoimmunity and transplantation models, indicating a role for other costimulatory pathways. In fact, the T-cell immunoglobulin mucin (TIM) family of molecules have been described as having costimulatory properties (see following).

Emerging data suggest that the costimulatory pathways exhibit some redundancy, hierarchy, and unique functions where various costimulatory molecules affect different T-cell populations and act at different times during the course of the immune response.[37] In addition, a growing number of negative T-cell costimulatory or coinhibitory pathways have been found to play an important role in the regulation of T-cell responses.[38] Thus, in the next section, we first review the role of the most widely studied CD28-B7 and CD154-CD40 pathways in transplantation. Thereafter, we review some novel emerging data from studies about the role of costimulatory molecules in transplantation.

The CD28/CTLA4–B7 pathway. Many T-cell molecules may serve as receptors for costimulatory signals; the CD28 molecule is the best characterized of these molecules (Fig. 35.8). According to gene expression studies, CD28 costimulation can lead to significant augmentation of expressions of genes induced by TCR signaling alone. These findings are consistent with a model of costimulation in which CD28 signaling lowers TCR thresholds for activation of cells.[39] CD28 has two known ligands, B7-1 (CD80) and B7-2 (CD86), both of which are expressed primarily on activated professional bone marrow–derived APCs. T cells also express cytotoxic T-lymphocyte-associated protein 4 (CTLA-4), a molecule that is highly homologous to CD28 that also binds CD80 and CD86.[39] However, unlike CD28, CTLA-4 transmits an inhibitory signal that serves to terminate the immune response. Although CD28 is expressed by both resting and activated T cells, CTLA-4 is expressed only on activated T cells. Because CTLA-4 binds B7

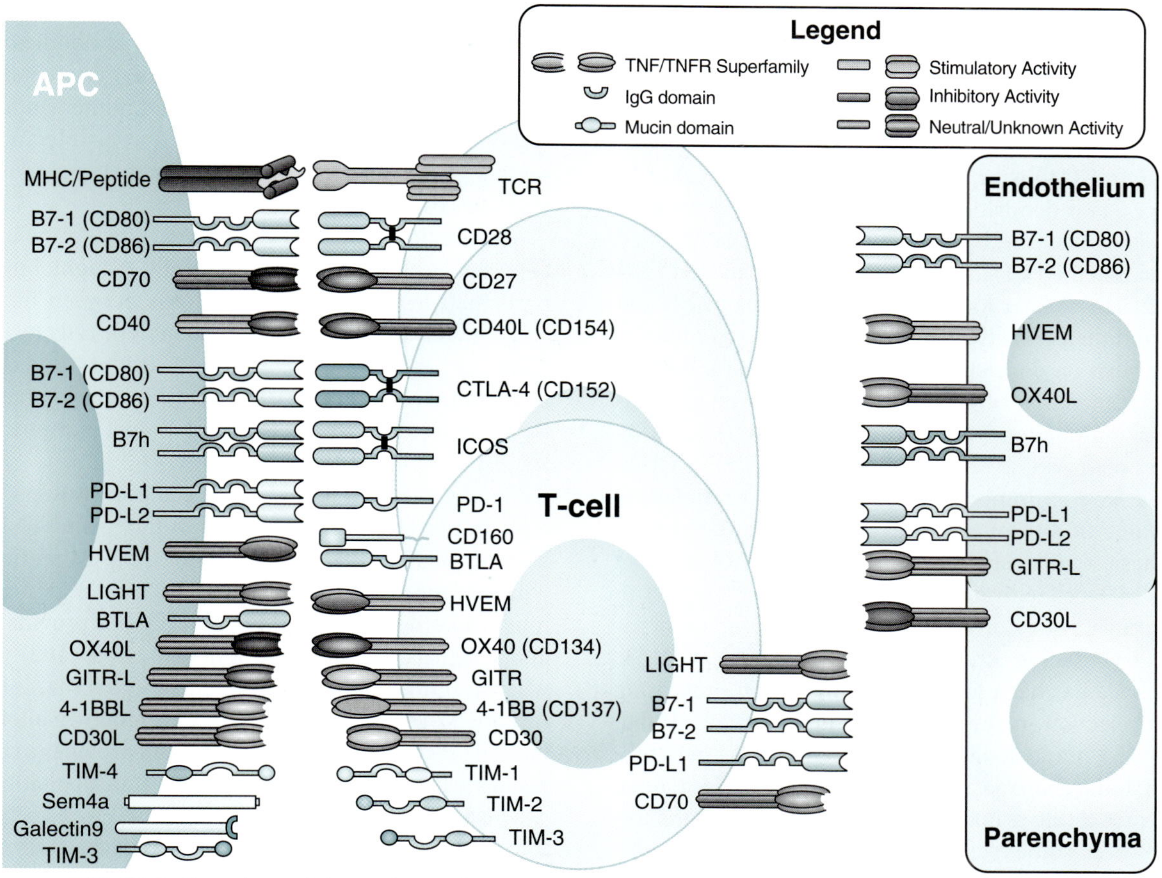

FIG. 35.8 Overview of the main costimulatory molecules. Costimulatory molecules are depicted in general order of their expression by T cells *(center column)*, with constitutive expression by naïve T cells *(top center)*, followed by early activated T cells *(middle center)*, and effector or memory T cells *(bottom center)*. Costimulatory ligands expressed by antigen-presenting cells are depicted to the left. Some of these same molecules are also expressed by activated endothelial cells *(upper right)*, parenchymal cells *(lower right)*, or both *(middle right)*. Finally, activated T cells themselves can express some costimulatory ligands *(center column, right side)*, allowing for additional costimulatory interactions, including those between T cells. The general structure of various family members is depicted by the presence of immunoglobulin G (IgG) domains (Ig superfamily), trimetric structure (tumor necrosis factor superfamily), or mucin domains (T-cell Ig domain and mucin domain family [TIM] family) of each "stalk." Main costimulatory receptors on T cells are: CD28, CD27, CD40L, ICOS, HVEM, OX40, and TIM1. Main inhibitory receptors are: CTLA-4, PD1, GITR, TIM-2, and TIM-3. (From Li XC, Rothstein DM, Sayegh MH. Costimulatory pathways in transplantation: challenges and new developments. *Immunol Rev.* 2009;229(1): 271-293.)

molecules with a higher affinity than does CD28, its inhibitory interaction eventually predominates, leading to the termination of the immune response. The importance of CTLA-4 as a negative regulatory T-cell costimulatory molecule in the physiological termination of T-cell responses is highlighted by the observation that CTLA-4 gene knockout mice develop massive lymphoproliferation and early death. One point that needs to be emphasized is the critical role of costimulation in T-cell responses. In the absence of costimulatory signals, sometimes the T cell simply ignores the peptide–MHC complex presented to it. At other times, the T cell undergoes apoptotic death[40,41] or is rendered anergic for up to several weeks; that is, the T cell is unable to respond to antigens, even when they are presented by APCs that express a costimulatory molecule. Precisely what determines the outcome of the stimulation of T-cell antigen receptors in the absence of costimulation (ignorance, apoptosis, or anergy) is not known. This process is considered one important factor in induction of peripheral tolerance (see following). Thus manipulation of the CD28/B7 pathway has been envisioned as a potential strategy for achieving therapeutically useful immunosuppression or tolerance. T-cell costimulatory blockade in the form of CTLA-4Ig, which blocks CD28 interaction with B7, has been extensively studied as a means of immunosuppression.[42] To improve the biological potency of CTLA4-Ig, CTLA4-Ig was mutated by substituting amino acids at two positions. The resulting protein LEA29Y (belatacept) had a significantly higher affinity for both CD86 and CD80.[43]

The CD154-CD40 pathway. The CD154-CD40 pathway, initially described as having a role in B-cell activation, has been recognized as a key pathway for T-cell activation as well (see Fig. 35.8). CD40 is expressed on APCs, such as B cells, macrophages, and dendritic cells, and other cell types such as endothelial cells. The ligand for CD40 (originally called CD40L and renamed CD154) is expressed on activated CD4 T cells. CD154 was later found on stimulated mast cells and basophils and then on activated platelets in vitro and in vivo and also in vivo on platelets in the process of the thrombus formation. Stimulation of CD40 provides important signals for antibody production by B cells and strongly induces B7 expression on all APCs.[44] In this manner, the CD154-CD40 system may have an important role in T-cell costimulation. Activation of APCs through CD40 also induces the expression of adhesion molecules and inflammatory cytokines that participate in T-cell activation. Therefore CD154 may act in T-cell costimulation by directly providing costimulation, inducing B7, or inducing other costimulatory ligands. CD154-CD40 blockade has been found to be efficient in preventing acute graft rejection in several small animal models. When an anti-CD154 monoclonal antibody was used as part of a strategy to induce mixed allogeneic chimerism in a renal transplant model, the primates developed donor-specific tolerance. However, some recipients developed thromboembolic complications. Such a complication was also found in some human participants entered in the phase I-II transplant trial with the humanized anti-CD154 (Biogen Inc., Cambridge, MA) monoclonal antibody, resulting in premature termination of the trial. Subsequent investigations suggested that these thrombotic events were the result of platelet-derived CD154 either expressed on the surface of platelets or shed in soluble form after platelet activation.[45] Ongoing studies are focused on exploring alternative approaches to disrupting this pathway, such as agents that target CD40.[46]

The role of alternate costimulatory molecules in transplantation. Other molecules belonging to the TNF superfamily and their receptors (TNF-R), including 4-1BB, CD30, CD134 (OX40), and CD27, and their respective ligands, 4-1BBL, CD30L, CD134L, and CD70, also act as efficient costimulatory molecules for various subsets of T cells (see Fig. 35.8).[47,48] CD134/CD134L blockade might be useful for inhibiting activation of $CD4^+$ T cells and blunting the function of effector/memory T cells. In contrast, targeting the 4-1BB pathway may be an attractive approach to manipulating alloreactive $CD8^+$ T cells. Likewise, other members of the B7-CD28 family,[47,48] such as inducible costimulator (ICOS) and its ligand B7h, programmed death 1 (PD-1) and its ligands PD-L1 and PD-L2, and B7-H3 and B7-H4 molecules have all been of major interest. Particularly, the latter three pathways (PD1-PDL, B7-H3, and B7-H4) have been found to transmit negative costimulatory signals to T cells, thus resulting in inhibition of T-cell proliferation and cytokine production either by causing their death or by induction of regulatory T cells that can inhibit the effector T cells. In particular, PD1-PDL seems to be important in peripheral immune regulation after transplant, because the use of anti-PD1 antibodies is capable of precipitating rejection in transplant recipients receiving this agent for cancer therapy.[49] These findings imply that the fate of allografts, like allograft rejection or tolerance, are essentially determined by the interplay between positive and negative costimulatory signals.

Costimulatory signals are not restricted to the interaction between T cells and APC as originally thought, but they also participate in the dialog among T cells, between T and B cells, and between T cells and nonhematopoietic cells such as endothelial or parenchymal cells. In fact, several studies reveal the importance of the graft tissue expression of negative costimulatory molecule PD-L1 in the regulation of immune responses against allografts.[50,51]

Finally, the TIM family of molecules possesses costimulatory properties but is distinct from the Ig and TNFR superfamilies (see Fig. 35.8). Members of the TIM family are type I membrane proteins with an Ig-variable region-like and a mucin-like domain.[52] TIM-1 and TIM-2 provide costimulatory signals that promote T helper cell 2 (Th2) responses, whereas TIM-3 appears to provide a signal that inhibits Th1 responses. The role of TIM family members in alloimmunity has only recently been investigated and provides a compelling rationale for further investigations in transplantation.[53-57]

In summary, studies have contributed to a deeper insight into understanding the functions of costimulatory pathways, but complex interactions between simultaneously activated positive and negative costimulatory pathways among themselves, differential expression of these molecules on different subsets of cells such as effector/memory or regulatory cells, and their expression in parenchymal cells of transplanted tissues clearly affect their functions. Further elucidation of these novel concepts offers new opportunities to apply novel targeting strategies of these pathways to the treatment of human diseases in the near future. A major focus of future research is thus directed at dissecting these functions to provide the rationale for developing novel therapeutic targets and strategies for induction of robust and durable transplantation tolerance.

Cytokines/chemokines. In addition to cell-cell interactions, cell function can be directed through proteins produced by a variety of cell types. These cytokines can function as chemoattractant (chemokines; see following) and growth, activation, and differentiation factors. After antigenic stimulation, $CD4^+$ T cells differentiate into at least four types of distinct populations: Th1, Th2, Th17, T follicular helper cells (Tfh cells), and regulatory T cells (Tregs; see later), each producing its own set of cytokines and mediating separate effector functions.[58,59] *Type 1* helper T (Th1) cells produce interleukin-2 (IL-2) and interferon-γ (IFN-γ) and mediate the activation of macrophages and the induction of delayed-type hypersensitivity (DTH) responses (see following). *Type 2* helper (Th2) cells produce IL-4, IL-5, IL-10, and IL-13, which provide help for B-cell function. However, the functional segregation between the Th1 and Th2 subsets remains incompletely understood. Studies with specific Th1 or Th2 cytokine gene-knockout animals indicate the complexity of the Th1-Th2 paradigm in graft rejection and tolerance.[59-61] Data from animal and human studies indicated that Th2 clones propagated from patients with stable renal transplant function, or animals tolerant to kidney transplants, can regulate a proliferative response from Th1 clones isolated from patients or animals undergoing active rejection.[62,63] Elucidation of a novel lineage of Th17 cells[64,65] has shed light on some of the seemingly inconsistent findings in models of Th1-mediated auto- and alloimmunity where the validity of the Th1/Th2 paradigm has been questioned. Tfh cells are a heterogeneous population of CD4 T cells important for both the survival of memory B cells and the differentiation of B cells into immunoglobulin-producing plasma cells.[66] Tfh cells are mainly present in secondary lymphoid organs, but they can be found also in the tertiary lymphoid organs inside the allograft and in the circulation.[47] In contrast with other T cells, Tfh cells can leave the T-cell area and localize to the B-cell follicle thanks to their concurrent expression of the B-cell zone homing chemokine receptor CXCR5 and downregulation of the T-cell zone homing chemokine receptor CCR7. This close proximity to B cells allows Tfh cells to support their activation, expansion, and differentiation.[48,50,52] This "help" is provided in the form of expression of molecules such as CD40L and cytokines such as IL-21.

IL-17 is a potent proinflammatory cytokine that induces chemokine expression and leukocyte infiltration and mediates tissue inflammation. IL-17 has been implicated in various models of immune-mediated tissue injury, particularly in the absence of a Th1 environment. Our studies have extended this novel paradigm to the transplant setting, enabling us to explain transplant rejection by inflammatory processes mediated by Th17 cells in the absence of Th1-dominant immune responses and found that CD4 Th17 cells mediate cardiac allograft vasculopathy,[67] whereas CD8 T17 cells mediate resistance to cardiac allograft tolerance by costimulation blockade.[57] Indeed, IL-17 has been implicated in both experimental and human renal, vascularized composite allotransplant (VCA), and lung allograft rejection.[68-70] Further, IL-17 neutralization promoted experimental cardiac allograft survival.[71] Except for blockade of the IL-2R, therapeutic strategies in patients that specifically modulated lymphokines have not proved highly effective. Therefore, although manipulation of lymphokine functions may hold promise as a therapeutic modality, we will have to better understand the role of lymphokines in graft rejection and tolerance under physiological conditions if we are to develop effective treatments.

Chemokines are *chemoattractant cytokines*.[72] They are structurally related by amino acid homologies and, in particular, by the placement of cysteines. The nomenclature of chemokines is becoming increasingly complex. Four chemokine families are now recognized, with the majority of members belonging to the C-C chemokine family, represented by RANTES, or the C-X-C chemokine family, typified by IL-8. In general, C-C chemokines attract monocytes and T lymphocytes and C-X-C chemokines attract granulocytes. Detection of altered chemokine messenger RNA (mRNA) in experimental models of rejection suggests that they play an important role in this process, but because of redundancy and differences in the functions of chemokines in rodents and humans, for the most part the exact role that individual chemokines play in an alloimmune response remains unclear. Nevertheless, studies in organ transplantation models in knockout animals and with blocking antibodies indicate key roles for the receptors CXCR3 and CCR5 and selected targeting chemokines.[73,74] Mean cardiac allograft survival of 58 days in CXCR3−/− compared with 7 days in the wild type underline these findings. Similar effects on graft survival were obtained using an anti-CXCR3 antibody in CXCR3+/+ recipients. MHC-disparate cardiac allografts transplanted into CCR5−/− mice show a tripling of graft survival. Although chemokine expression in the heart is primarily by endothelial cells (ECs) or infiltrating mononuclear cells, kidneys have a heterogeneous population of resident cells, which express inflammatory chemokines when stimulated. Further studies of these knockout mice in studies on renal transplantation will help prove the applicability of these data to renal transplantation.

The innate immune system in allograft rejection and tolerance. Historically the focus of transplant immunology has mainly relied on targeting the mechanisms of specific (adaptive) immunity. However, there are emerging data that both rejection and tolerance are influenced by both nonspecific (innate) and adaptive immune responses.[75,76] Factors such as ischemia-reperfusion injury, donor criteria, and brain death serve as danger signals activating the innate immune system. Toll-like receptors (TLRs), natural killer (NK) cells, DCs, monocytes, and soluble components of the innate immune system such as complement are the key players after activation of the innate system.

TLRs are expressed on the surface of various cells, and their engagement is associated with the production of a significant cytokine release, serving to recruit and activate neutrophils and macrophages as part of the innate immune defense system, which in turn has been found to activate the adaptive immune response. NK cells play a multifaceted role in allograft rejection. Although NK cells contribute to graft rejection and play an important role in promoting adaptive immune responses, they do not seem sufficient to reject solid organ transplants. DCs are also members of the innate immune system and are present mainly in tissues. DCs in lymphoid organs remain in an immature or semimature steady state until inflammatory stimuli instigate a complex maturation process, allowing alloantigen presentation. Activated DCs recruit NK and T cells, which then secrete IFN-γ and other inflammatory cytokines that trigger the adaptive immune response. Finally, several other studies have demonstrated that monocytes can precipitate acute rejections after use of T-cell depleting agents in renal transplant recipients.[77,78] Another study demonstrated that the presence of monocytes/macrophages in the follow-up biopsies is one of the factors that may be associated with a bad outcome after antibody-mediated rejection.[79] All in all, these studies suggest a pathogenic role of monocytes in allograft rejection.

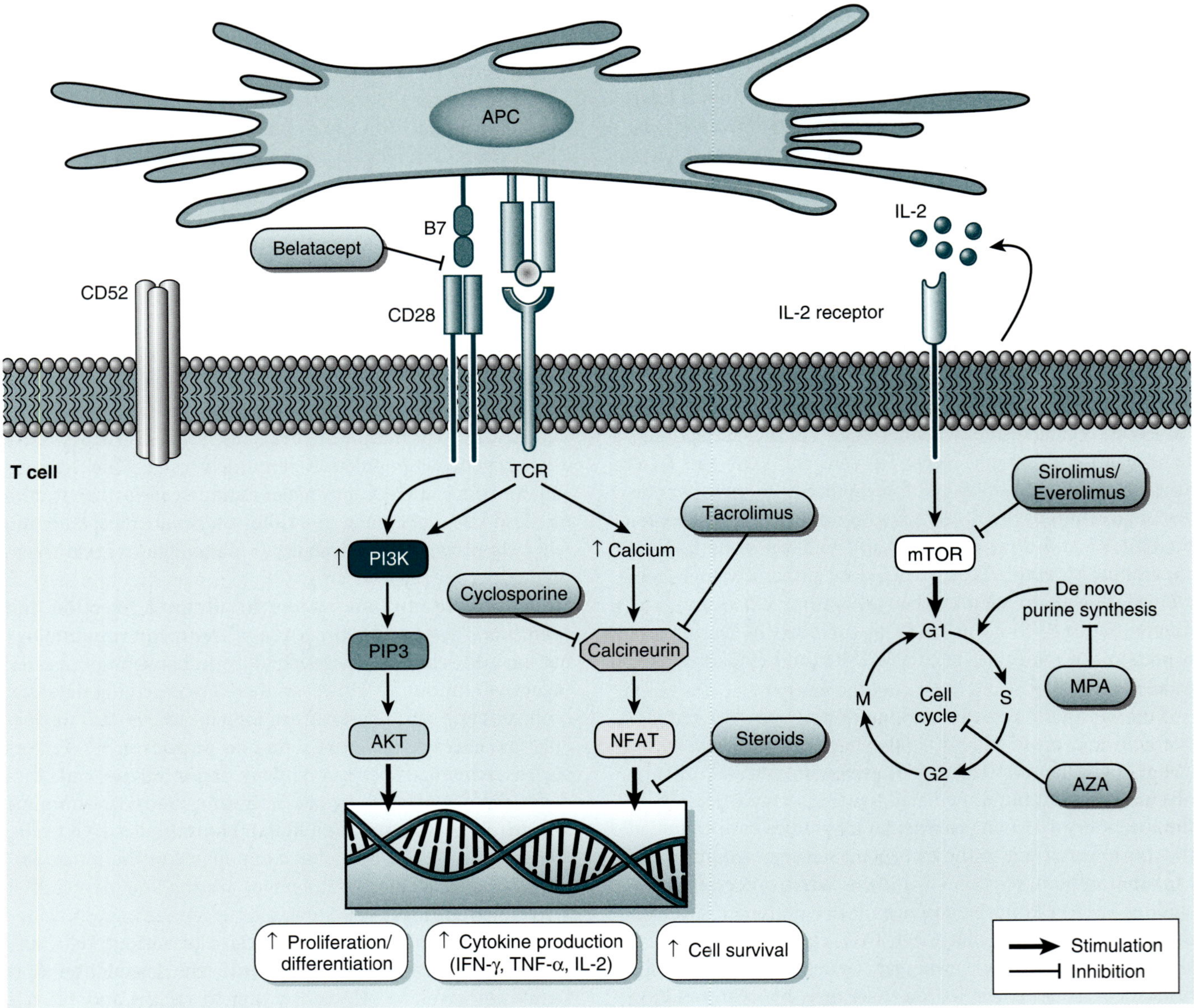

FIG. 35.9 Mechanisms of action of immunosuppressive drugs. (From Riella LV. *Kidney Transplant eBook.* Cupertino, CA: Apple; 2015:274.)

It is clear that innate immune mechanisms are responsible for the initial inflammatory events after engraftment. Although by themselves they are not sufficient to cause graft rejection itself, they are important for optimal adaptive immune responses to the graft and may play a major role in resistance to tolerance induction (see following).

Effector Mechanisms of Allograft Rejection

Transplant rejection has both cellular (DTH responses, cell-mediated cytotoxicity) and humoral components. Once fully activated via the direct, semi-direct, or indirect pathway (see preceding), T cells produce cytokines and chemokines that orchestrate various effector arms of the alloimmune response. The effector mechanisms that are primarily responsible for the rejection process classically involve *Th1 CD4⁺ T cells, cytotoxic CD8⁺ T cells,* and *antibodies.*[80] However, experimental studies revealed alternative mechanisms of rejection that implicate *memory T cells* (see following) and cells belonging to the *innate immune system,* including NK cells, macrophages, and neutrophils. Furthermore, local inflammation associated with rejection is tightly regulated by *Tregs* (see Tolerance). Immunosuppressive drugs currently in use target primarily the T-cell machinery required for activation and proliferation of naïve T cells (Fig. 35.9).

Primed $CD4^+$ T cells can provide help for production of alloantibody and can also provide helper signals required for the induction of $CD8^+$ CTLs,[33,34] both of which can subsequently mediate graft injury. Moreover, $CD4^+$ T cells capable of recognizing donor antigens on donor cells can directly mediate acute graft rejection,[81] but there is some evidence that this outcome is frequency dependent.[82] Below a certain frequency threshold, primed T cells may not reject the transplanted organ but may alternatively be capable of inducing chronic injury that results in fibrosis and vasculopathy, characteristic of chronic allograft dysfunction.[83] Furthermore, directly primed Th1 cells and macrophages can mediate

DTH reactions and contribute to the destruction of the graft. In that setting, it is hypothesized that some of the cytokines produced by T cells and macrophages (TNF-α) may mediate apoptosis of graft cells. The pathology of a transplanted organ may also be dependent on the specific graft cell with which the primed T cells interact. It is tempting to speculate that direct recognition of donor endothelial cells by primed CD8+ T cells may participate in those acute rejections associated with pathological evidence of vasculitis.[84] On the other hand, if intragraft donor parenchymal cells are the predominant targets of the direct alloresponse, acute rejection may appear as the classically described mononuclear cell infiltration with tubulitis. Analogous to T cells functioning through the direct pathway, indirectly primed CD4+ T cells preferentially differentiate into a proinflammatory type 1 cytokine-secreting phenotype[85] and enable helper signals to induce alloantibodies and cytotoxic CD8+ T cells that are capable of injuring the graft.[86-88] In addition, indirectly activated T cells are capable of mediating DTH, and DTH is associated with both acute and chronic graft injury.[89,90] One important question under investigation is whether indirectly primed, proinflammatory T cells can injure a graft even though they cannot interact with any antigen expressed on the graft cells. With skin graft models, it is possible that recipient-derived vascular endothelial cells found on vessels feeding the graft may act as targets of the indirectly primed immune response.[91] The frequency of activated cells may also influence the eventual outcome. Higher frequencies of indirectly primed CD4+ T cells seem to be associated with acute rejection, whereas lower frequencies may mediate fibrosis and vasculopathy.[81]

In summary, the pattern of transplant rejection is not only influenced by the T-cell recognition pathway but also by the frequency, the induced effector functions, and the specific cellular targets of the alloreactive T cells.

B lymphocytes express clonally restricted antigen-specific cell-surface receptors, called *immunoglobulins*.[92] When cell-surface immunoglobulin binds specific antigens in the context of soluble helper factors (such as IL-4, IL-6, and IL-8), B cells are activated. They differentiate, divide, and become plasma cells that secrete soluble forms of antigen-specific antibodies displayed on their cell surface. These antibodies, in turn, can bind allogeneic target antigens and induce graft damage by binding complement or by directing antibody-dependent cellular cytotoxicity. Beside their involvement in the synthesis of alloantibodies, B cells also contribute to rejection by other mechanisms, because the benefits of rituximab treatment do not correlate with reduction of alloantibody levels.[93] B cells infiltrating the graft may actually present graft-derived peptides and contribute to local activation of alloreactive T cells through the indirect pathway of allorecognition.

Both IgM and IgG alloantibodies can be detected in the serum and in the graft of animals and humans undergoing allograft rejection. Preformed anti-HLA class I antibodies and, occasionally, antiendothelial antibodies play an important role in the hyperacute rejection and accelerated vascular rejection seen in previously sensitized transplant recipients. In the case of xenotransplantation, naturally occurring xenoreactive antibodies play a critical role in the hyperacute rejection of xenografts (see Chapter 36). Finally, alloantibodies against both HLA and non-HLA targets are becoming increasingly recognized as critical in the pathogenesis of acute and chronic renal allograft outcomes.[94] Acute and chronic allograft rejection can occur in HLA-identical sibling transplants, implicating the importance of immune response against non-HLA targets.[95]

Other soluble factors induce additional effector mechanisms, including phagocytosis by granulocytes and macrophages, and cell death by NK cells. NK cells express cell-surface receptors called *killer-inhibitory receptors* (KIR) that recognize HLA class I molecules.[96] When self HLA is recognized, NK cells are prevented from killing. If the KIRs do not bind to a self HLA molecule, as in certain tumors or viral infections, the target cell is lysed. In addition, NK cells can lyse certain targets expressing nonself HLA (alloantigens). Although NK cells have been identified in rodent and human allografts undergoing acute rejection, they are neither necessary nor sufficient to drive acute allograft rejection in immunocompetent recipients.[97] It is now thought that NK cells or NK cell subsets do participate in acute rejection of transplanted organs both in mice and humans, particularly when T-cell function is impaired or in the setting of alloantibodies.

Last but not least, as discussed previously, several other studies have demonstrated that monocytes can precipitate acute rejections after use of T-cell depleting agents in renal transplant recipients.[102] Overall, these studies suggest a pathogenic role of monocytes in allograft rejection.

Resolution and Memory

Apoptosis, cell cycle arrest, and active suppression are known regulators leading to a dampening of the induced immune response (see the discussion of peripheral tolerance in the next section).[98] Nevertheless, a few antigen-specific cells are spared, and these become memory cells (see Fig. 35.7). Memory cells have lower activation thresholds than do naïve cells and can respond rapidly to previously encountered antigens. As a result of their survival advantages, rapid reactivation, donor-reactive memory T cells are now recognized as a serious threat for survival of transplanted organs.[99] Human transplant recipients are likely to harbor alloreactive memory T cells resulting from direct allosensitization, cross-reactivity to environmental antigens, or homeostatic proliferation as a result of induced lymphopenia by induction treatment. Memory T cells not only endanger allograft survival by causing both acute and chronic rejection; studies suggest that they impede the induction of transplantation tolerance.[100] Evidence indicates that memory T cells may be the culprit of rejection-resistant costimulatory blockade.[101]

TOLERANCE

Immunological tolerance to an allograft can be defined as normal graft function and histology in the absence of immunosuppression, associated with the absence of a destructive specific alloimmune response to the graft but with an otherwise fully functional immune system.[102,103] Renal transplantation has been made possible by the development of powerful immunosuppressive drugs that can prevent the rejection process but usually require lifelong administration, patient compliance, and the risk for a wide range of unwanted side effects. Although there has been great success in improving short-term allograft survival, chronic allograft nephropathy (CAN) remains the principal cause of late renal allograft failure and may even be accelerated by some immunosuppressive drugs. Immunological tolerance would ideally prevent the side effects of immunosuppression and would hopefully prevent chronic rejection, as demonstrated in several animal models.[104] An individual is usually tolerant to self antigens.

Understanding mechanisms of self tolerance has yielded important information regarding the mechanisms of immune responses and has provided the rationale to develop strategies for induction of acquired tolerance. As discussed previously, the T-cell repertoire is modified through negative and positive selection processes in the thymus to delete potentially self-reactive T-cell clones. Self tolerance is partially mediated by "negative selection" through deletion of autoreactive T-cell clones in the thymus (central tolerance). On the other hand, potentially autoreactive T cells that escaped deletion during intrathymic ontogeny are kept under control by mechanisms of peripheral tolerance. Clonal deletion through apoptosis, anergy, and immunoregulation have all been suggested as non–mutually exclusive and probably complementary mechanisms of peripheral tolerance.[98] Stimulation of lymphocytes through the antigen receptor in the absence of costimulation is not a neutral event and mediates specific inactivation through anergy, a further safeguard against self-reactivity. Thus it has been suggested that the absence of costimulation on resting tissue APCs could serve to induce and maintain T-cell tolerance to self antigens and that aberrant expression of costimulatory molecules on nonprofessional APCs could activate self-reactive T cells, resulting in autoimmunity. Findings suggest that an additional level of regulation may be achieved by the expression of novel inhibitory molecules (CTLA4 and PD1) on T cells that can provide negative signals to terminate immune responses.[47]

Similar to self tolerance, the mechanisms of acquired tolerance are listed in Box 35.2. The two types of acquired tolerance are as follows:

1. *Central tolerance* involves thymic deletional mechanisms analogous to self tolerance.
2. *Peripheral tolerance* is mediated by T-cell anergy and deletion, regulatory/suppressor cells, and/or suppressive cytokines.

BOX 35.2 Mechanisms of Transplantation Tolerance

1. Central tolerance
2. Peripheral tolerance
    a. Anergy
    b. Apoptosis
    c. Regulation (regulatory cells, suppressive cytokines)

The occurrence of natural tolerance was first described by Owen,[102] who found that dizygotic twin cattle that shared a common placenta in utero would continue to have circulating blood cells of their twin specificity after birth. The resultant animals were said to be *chimeric*, and they could not reject skin grafts of the other twin in adult life. This was followed by studies by Billingham, Brent, and Medawar,[106] who demonstrated that it was possible to induce mice to accept skin grafts from a different genetic background if the recipient mice were injected with hematopoietic cells of donor origin while still in utero (or neonatally). This was the first description of acquired tolerance. Neonatal tolerance is thought largely to be due to clonal deletion, whereby T cells reactive with alloantigen are deleted in the thymus, presumably by the same mechanisms that delete self-reactive T cells. Other mechanisms (e.g., immune deviation to Th2 cells), however, have been described as possible mediators of neonatal tolerance.

Anergy is a state of functional inactivation in which antigen-specific T lymphocytes are present but are unable to respond (by proliferating or producing cytokines) to rechallenge with antigens. Anergy is typically induced when T cells do not receive a positive costimulatory signal, when positive costimulatory signals are blocked, or when they receive a negative costimulatory signal. Anergy can sometimes be reversed by IL-2 and thus may not be a desirable clinical approach to induce tolerance, because infections may activate the immune system and reverse anergy.

Another mechanism of peripheral tolerance is through the function of antigen-specific *regulatory or suppressor cells.* Such cells have been demonstrated by in vitro assays and by adoptive transfer experiments in vivo.

Natural regulatory T cells (*natural* Tregs) comprise 5% to 10% of CD4 cells in mice and humans and exhibit potent regulatory activity. They prevent autoimmune diseases, and their depletion can induce de novo autoimmunity in normal mice.[107,108] These cells are selected in the thymus and emerge constitutively, expressing a $CD45RB^{Lo}$ $CD25^{+}$ phenotype. A high proportion also expresses glucocorticoid-induced TNF receptor family–related protein (GITR) and CTLA-4. Although these markers—CD25 in particular—have been extremely useful for identification of natural Tregs, they are also expressed by activated T cells. Moreover a proportion of natural Tregs lack CD25 expression. Foxp3 is a transcription factor with predominance expression by Tregs that can be used to identified this specific CD4 subset[109,110] In humans, this subset of CD4 cells has been identified by expression of CD25 and lack of expression of CD127. In addition to natural Tregs, antigen exposure under various specialized conditions can induce peripheral $CD4^{+}$ T cells to exhibit regulatory activity. Salama and colleagues[111] provided the first evidence of existence of antigen-specific regulatory $CD25^{+}$ T cells that are able to suppress alloresponses to donor HLA peptides in stable renal transplant recipients.

Therefore regulatory $CD4^+CD25^+$ T cells appear to play a role in the regulation of indirect antidonor alloresponse in stable renal transplant patients. An increase was observed in the frequency of $CD4^+CD25high^+$ Tregs in peripheral blood of operationally tolerant patients after living-donor liver transplantation compared with those from age-matched volunteers or patients on immunosuppression.[112] Similarly, the blood cell phenotype of clinically tolerant kidney patients displayed normal levels of $CD25hiCD4^+$ T cells and Foxp3 transcripts compared with healthy individuals.[113] In contrast, recipients with chronic rejection had significantly fewer $CD25hiCD4^+$ T cells and lower levels of Foxp3 transcript compared with clinically tolerant patients.[113] In sum, these studies demonstrate that Tregs exists in human transplant recipients of various organs and may play a crucial role in the maintenance of allograft function in stable and tolerant patients. Indeed, ongoing trials are investigating the infuse of polyclonal Tregs to control inflammation in kidney transplant recipients.[114]

A new, increasingly recognized concept is that Tregs not only have various origins, but like Th cells, they also show plasticity in their development and lineage differentiation. Evidence indicates that depending on the cytokine milieu, $CD4^+CD25^+$ T cells expanded ex vivo in rats displayed functionally distinct phenotypes peculiar to Th1 and Th2 differentiation pathways.[115] Even more striking is the evidence that $CD4^+CD25^+Foxp3^+$ can not only trigger the expansion of IL-17–producing (Th17) T cells but even differentiate themselves into Th17 T cells in vitro in mouse and humans on stimulation with allogeneic antigen-presenting cells.[116,117] It thus seems likely that in vivo the specific conditions at the site of recruitment of Tregs have a significant influence on their eventual role in the inflammatory process.

To achieve tolerance, the interest in tracking and manipulating Tregs seems obvious (see following). In this context, there is increasing evidence about the impact of currently used therapeutic agents on Tregs' frequency and function. For maintenance agents, aggregate data suggest that rapamycin has a more favorable effect than calcineurin inhibitors for both frequency and suppressive activity.[118] In the case of induction agents, looking at the proportion of T cells and especially at the ratio of Teffs to Tregs, it seems that alemtuzumab and ATG do better than anti-IL2R with maintained potency, suggesting that these former agents might reeducate the immune system.[119-121] Manipulation of Tregs by creating alloantigen-specific TCRs may increase the efficiency of the alloimmune response. MacDonald et al.[122] were able to generate Tregs with chimeric antigen receptors (CARs), in which T cells are genetically engineered to express extracellular single-chain Ab (scFv) antigen–binding domains fused to intracellular signaling domains. Specifically, the authors generated CAR Tregs targeting HLA-A2 and tested those Tregs in vitro and in vivo using a xenogeneic GVHD model caused by HLA-A2+ T cells. A2-CAR-Tregs had stable suppressive function and were superior to polyclonal Tregs in inhibiting the alloimmune response.[122]

Novel approaches to induce transplantation tolerance in humans include hematopoietic cell engraftment with the goal of establishment of macrochimerism, lymphocyte depletion strategies, costimulatory blockades, and strategies to expand regulatory T cells ex vivo or in patients.[102] The induction of macrochimerism by marrow transplantation is achievable only in a small number of patients because the morbidity of bone marrow transplantation exceeds that of standard immunosuppression in most patients. Thus investigators have developed strategies to induce mixed chimerism in which the recipient marrow is largely preserved but modified such that both donor and recipient hemopoietic components coexist. Such transferred hematopoietic cells populate the recipient thymus and marrow and facilitate central deletion of donor alloreactive T and B cells. This nonmyeloablative approach has the advantages of being less toxic, preserving immunocompetence, and lessening the risk for graft-versus-host disease. Single-center trials using haplodisparate donor-recipient pairs have indicated that tolerance achievement is possible in a subset of patients.[123,124] Even though promising, mixed chimerism seems to be a practically complex and aggressive approach to tolerance.

Lymphocyte depletion with polyclonal or monoclonal antibodies has been envisioned as a strategy to reduce nonspecifically the precursor frequency of T cells, but effector memory T cells seem to be relatively resistant to depletion. In addition, remaining T cells after depletion undergo homeostatic repopulation, a barrier to the development of tolerance.

As discussed in detail, there is considerable emerging data that costimulation blockade may facilitate tolerance induction, but important limitations and safety issues need to be considered before Treg-based therapy becomes an integral part of clinical armamentarium.

Finally, although the induction of immunological tolerance remains an important clinical goal in transplantation, there are several immunological hurdles that have made it difficult to translate animal studies to humans. These barriers include the large repertoire of alloreactive T cells in the case of transplantation, the limitations of peripheral immune regulatory mechanisms that are commonly exploited to induce tolerance (T-cell deletion, anergy, and suppression), cellular and humoral components of the innate immune system leading to inflammation, and the difficult task of "tolerizing" memory T cells.[102]

SUMMARY

In this chapter we highlighted our understanding of the cellular and molecular mechanisms involved in transplant rejection and acceptance. This information has been important in the design of current therapies and may help usher in a new generation of approaches that will result in immunological tolerance, the ultimate goal of transplantation biologists.

A full list of references are available at www.expertconsult.com.

36

Evaluation of Donors and Recipients

Heidi M. Schaefer, MD, and Beatrice P. Concepcion, MD

OUTLINE

EVALUATION OF THE LIVING DONOR

Living kidney donation has become an increasingly important option because of the ongoing disparity between the number of end-stage renal disease (ESRD) patients listed for kidney transplantation and the availability of deceased donor kidneys. Each year, nearly 6000 transplants are made possible by living donors. As outlined in Box 36.1, living kidney donation has advantages and disadvantages for both the recipient and the donor.[1] Recipients of live donor kidneys have better graft and patient survival compared with deceased donor recipients because donors are healthier, cold ischemia times are shorter, and ischemia-reperfusion injury is minimal. Waiting times for deceased donors organs are typically many years long, so living donation also minimizes or avoids dialysis time for the recipient.

Over the years, the population of living kidney donors has evolved to include biologically unrelated donors and medically complex donors with increasing prevalence. More than 25% of donors are unrelated to the recipient, encompassing spouses, friends, coworkers, and even altruistic donors.[2] With studies showing favorable outcomes related to surgery and long-term health and survival, many centers have relaxed their criteria for living donation and are willing to consider donors with isolated medical abnormalities, including controlled hypertension, obesity, and glucose intolerance, as well as a glomerular filtration rate (GFR) around the lower limits of the normal range. Because living kidney donors are undergoing a surgical procedure without any medical benefit to their own health, it is important that the evaluating physician carefully explain the known risks to the donor during the evaluation process to ensure that informed consent is achieved.

CLINICAL ASSESSMENT OF THE LIVING DONOR

The medical evaluation of the living kidney donor consists of laboratory and radiological studies to confirm excellent health and adequate kidney function. A thorough assessment of the results of these tests, as well as a comprehensive history and physical examination, should be performed by a physician not involved in the care of the recipient to avoid

BOX 36.1 Advantages and Disadvantages of Living Donation

Advantages to Recipient
- Scheduled operation during daytime hours
- No waiting time on the deceased donor waiting list
- Minimal cold ischemia time
- Usual immediate allograft function
- Overall better long-term survival compared with deceased donor kidney transplantation
- Emotional benefits between the donor and recipient

Advantages and Disadvantages to Donor
- Emotional benefits between the donor and recipient
- Sense of altruism and magnanimity for donor
- Potential discovery of unknown health issues
- Invasive operation with potential short- and long-term complications
- Lost wages because of time off from work
- Psychological stress on donor and family

BOX 36.2 Evaluation of the Living Donor

Blood group, HLA typing, and cross-match testing
Complete medical history and physical examination
Chest radiograph
Electrocardiogram
Stress test and echocardiogram as required by the transplant center
Laboratory evaluation with focus on fasting glucose, kidney function, and urinalysis for microscopic hematuria
Hemoglobin A1C and oral glucose tolerance test if high risk for diabetes
Evaluation of GFR
- 24-hour urine for creatinine clearance
- Nuclear medicine renal scan

Estimation of proteinuria
Assessment of renal anatomy usually through computed tomography angiography
Infectious disease screening
Age-appropriate cancer screening
Psychosocial evaluation
Nutritional education

GFR, Glomerular filtration rate; *HLA,* human leukocyte antigen.

potential bias. Most centers require the donor to be at least 18 years of age and able to provide informed consent. The upper limit of age varies among transplant centers and may not be as important as the overall general health of the donor.

Multiple guidelines are available to assist clinicians in the complex process of donor evaluation and selection.[3-5] Recently Kidney Disease: Improving Global Outcomes (KDIGO) has published updated clinical practice guidelines on the evaluation and care of living kidney donors.[6] The history, physical examination, and testing (Box 36.2) should focus on excluding contraindications to donation, ensuring that selected donors are at minimal risk for postdonation complications. It is important that infection and malignancy screening be performed in the potential donor to prevent inadvertent transmission to the intended recipient as a result of the transplant. For the donor candidate, this workup occasionally results in the early detection of diseases that the donor was otherwise unaware of and allows for appropriate treatment and follow-up. Box 36.3 lists the absolute and relative contraindications to living kidney donation.

BOX 36.3 Contraindications to Living Donation

Age <18–25 or >70–75 years
Mentally incapable of making informed decision
Obesity with body mass index >30–35
Hypertension (uncontrolled, end organ damage, non-Caucasian race)
Diabetes (gestational, prediabetes, glucose intolerance)
Significant cardiovascular disease
Low measured GFR or creatinine clearance <80–85 mL/min
Significant proteinuria or microalbuminuria
Malignancy
Nephrolithiasis with high risk for recurrent stones
High risk for infectious disease transmission
Significant psychiatric illness likely to interfere with donation
High suspicion of donor coercion or financial exchange
Withdrawal of donor consent

GFR, Glomerular filtration rate.

Kidney Function

An accurate assessment of predonation kidney function allows physicians to estimate the likely level of residual kidney function that donors would have after donor nephrectomy. Most transplant centers obtain at minimum an estimated GFR (eGFR), although guidelines recommend confirmatory testing either through 24-hour creatinine clearance or radioisotope testing.[3-6] Despite its limitations, measured creatinine clearance is usually the confirmatory test obtained because isotope testing is more costly, more time consuming, and less readily available. If the 24-hour creatinine clearance is marginal, it is recommended that a nuclear study be performed to ensure adequate kidney function before donation. Although previous guidelines recommended a GFR ≥80 mL/min to proceed with kidney donation, KDIGO guidelines have recommend a GFR ≥90 mL/min/1.73 m^2 as the acceptable threshold; most importantly, GFR < 60 mL/min/1.73 m^2 is not acceptable.[7] For GFRs that fall between 60 to 89 mL/min/1.73 m^2, KDIGO recommends that the decision to allow donation should be individualized, taking into account the donor age and other clinical risk factors in relation to the transplant center's risk threshold.

Proteinuria

Proteinuria is usually a sign of renal disease and should be estimated either by 24-hour urine protein excretion or urine protein-to-creatinine ratio. We agree with most guidelines that recommend exclusion of potential live donors with a urine protein excretion of >300 mg/day or >30 mg/mmol on spot protein ratio.[8]

Microscopic Hematuria

Urinalysis and urine microscopy are routinely performed as part of the donor evaluation. Persistent microscopic hematuria, defined as more than 3 to 5 urinary red blood cells per high-power field, can result from many causes, such as infection, glomerular disease, nephrolithiasis, and urothelial carcinoma. To exclude urological disease, investigations can include urine culture, urine cytological testing, imaging of the kidneys and urinary tract through ultrasound or computed tomography (CT) scan, and cystoscopy. If the urological workup is unremarkable, a kidney biopsy should be considered to rule out glomerular disease, which precludes donation with the possible exception of isolated thin basement disease. It is important to distinguish thin basement membrane disease from immunoglobulin A (IgA) nephropathy because progressive renal disease is rarely observed with the former condition but occurs in 15% to 40% of patients with IgA nephropathy.[9] It is important to discuss with prospective donors the additional, albeit small, risk conferred by microhematuria evaluation, in the context of their overall risk and commitment to donate. Although short-term outcomes for donors with persistent microscopic hematuria and no contraindication to donation are reassuring, the long-term outcomes remain to be determined.

Cardiovascular Risk

Cardiovascular risk factors, including assessment for hypertension, diabetes, obesity, hyperlipidemia, tobacco abuse, and family history of early coronary artery disease, should be identified during the initial donor evaluation. Chest x-ray examination and electrocardiogram are also standard. For low-risk donor candidates, further cardiovascular evaluation is not recommended. It is suggested that stress testing should be performed in men aged 50 years or older, women aged 60 years or older, and donor candidates with more than one cardiac risk factor.[10] However, no available evidence exists to support more rigorous cardiac testing than is recommended for nondonors undergoing surgery.

Hypertension

Donors should be screened for hypertension with two or more properly measured seated blood pressure (BP) readings. If there is concern for white-coat hypertension, ambulatory BP monitoring should be performed. Some centers allow for donation in the setting of mild hypertension controlled on one or two agents based on good short-term outcomes in selected donors.[11] Selection criteria of these donors should include absence of end organ damage related to hypertension (left ventricular hypertrophy and retinopathy), absence of proteinuria and microalbuminuria, and normal GFR. The safety of donation under such circumstances has predominantly been studied in Caucasian donors.[11] Available data indicate that hypertensive African American donors should be excluded because of the increased risk for postdonation kidney disease.[12]

Diabetes

Because type 2 diabetes is a major cause of ESRD, most transplant centers do not accept potential donors with glucose impairment or overt diabetes or those with a strong family history of diabetic kidney disease, although it is unclear whether in these settings, donor nephrectomy leads to higher risk for diabetic nephropathy or faster progression of nephropathy. All potential donors should have a fasting plasma glucose, and in those with additional risk factors for diabetes, including first-degree relatives with diabetes, history of gestational diabetes, or body mass index (BMI) >30 kg/m^2, a glucose tolerance test and hemoglobin A1C should be performed. Recently revised American Diabetes Association guidelines should be applied to diagnose diabetes and prediabetes.[13]

Obesity

The majority of transplant centers exclude obese donors with a BMI >35 kg/m^2 because of concern that excess weight is a known risk factor for ESRD.[14] Despite this, the rates of obesity in living donors have increased with >25% considered obese at the time of donation.[15] Obesity may be a risk factor for longer postdonation hospital length of stay and increased rates of postoperative wound complications. Although previous studies have suggested that obesity was not a risk factor for postdonation chronic kidney disease,[16,17] a recent evaluation of Scientific Registry of Transplant Recipients (SRTR) data noted that donor obesity was independently associated with an increased risk for ESRD 20 years after kidney donation.[18] Compared with nonobese living donors, obese donors had a 1.9-fold increased risk for postdonation ESRD.[18] It is prudent to discuss weight loss management strategies and provide informed consent regarding potential short- and long-term risks in obese individuals considering living donation.

Inherited Renal Disease

Potential kidney donors, especially those considering donation to biological relatives, need to be assessed for hereditary kidney disease. It is important to be aware of the cause of the intended recipient's kidney disease and whether other family members are affected. The most common scenario encountered is a family history of autosomal dominant polycystic kidney disease (ADPKD). If the potential donor is older than age 30 years, renal ultrasound or computed tomography of the abdomen and pelvis is highly sensitive in ruling out cystic disease. In younger donors, genetic testing either by linkage analysis or direct deoxyribonucleic acid should be obtained.

Alport syndrome is a genetically heterogeneous disease with X-linked, autosomal recessive, and autosomal dominant variants, with the majority of cases being X-linked. Persons being evaluated for donation with a family history of Alport syndrome need to be screened for hematuria, hypertension, and hearing and eye abnormalities. Male siblings older than age 20 are unlikely to have the disease if hematuria is absent. Sisters of affected male recipients with X-linked disease have a 50% chance of being carriers; a small percentage of such women carrying the abnormal gene do develop renal failure. If hematuria is present, a kidney biopsy should be performed with immunostaining and consideration of genetic consultation.

Nephrolithiasis

A history of urinary tract stones has historically been a relative contraindication to donation because stones tend to recur and obstruction of a solitary kidney could adversely affect function. Despite this risk, there has been increasing acceptance of donors with a history of nephrolithiasis as long as stones are no longer present and no obvious metabolic abnormalities are identified that would increase future stone risk. Although data have shown no difference in the rate of kidney stones requiring surgical intervention or hospitalization in donors compared with nondonors,[19] more studies are needed to evaluate the outcome of stone formers who donate and to identify those in whom donation may contribute to accelerated loss of kidney function or other stone complications.

Psychosocial Evaluation and Informed Consent

Current policy in the United States dictates that an independent live donor advocate (ILDA) must work with potential donors to ensure that they are informed and understand the process, are appropriately motivated, are free from coercion, and can make decisions autonomously, independent of family members or the intended recipient. The donor should not feel overt pressure or undue anxiety about proceeding and must be allowed to stop the evaluation process at any time. In addition, a careful psychosocial evaluation should be conducted by a social worker or psychiatrist. Significant psychiatric illnesses that would either impair the person's ability to give informed consent or that might be negatively affected by the stress of surgery are contraindications to living donation. It is important that the donor have appropriate social support to assist in the postoperative period. If there are signs of secondary gain or financial reimbursement, the donor should be excluded from the process.

SURGICAL TECHNIQUES AND RISKS

The introduction of laparoscopic-assisted kidney donation has been a significant advance in organ donation with most major transplant centers performing this procedure. Before the advent of laparoscopic nephrectomy, donor kidneys were removed through the traditional method of open nephrectomy involving a large flank incision. The advantages of laparoscopic versus open nephrectomy include smaller incision, lower rates of incisional hernia, better wound cosmetics, less postoperative pain, shorter hospitalization, and less time away from work. However, the rates of early allograft dysfunction may be higher with this technique because of higher intraabdominal pressures required during the procedure, longer warm ischemia times, less experience with the technique, a learning curve, and more manipulation of the renal vessels. Despite slower early graft function, a recent Organ Procurement and Transplantation Network (OPTN) database analysis indicated equivalent short- and long-term adult recipient outcomes with either retrieval technique.[20] There are data to suggest that in pediatric recipients, outcomes are inferior with laparoscopically retrieved kidneys.

Despite newer retrieval techniques and changes to the living donor population, including older donors, the surgical mortality has not changed over the past 15 years, with perioperative mortality after donor nephrectomy of approximately 3 per 10,000 cases.[21] Surgical mortality has been noted to be higher in men, African American individuals, and donors with baseline hypertension. These factors are also associated with higher risk for long-term death. Rates of early postoperative complications are low but may include perioperative bleeding requiring blood transfusion, wound complications, and early hospital readmissions.

LONG-TERM RISKS TO THE DONOR

Although many healthy adults are eager and willing to accept the risk for donor nephrectomy to help those in need, the medical community must quantify those risks as best as possible and make this information available during the initial donor evaluation. Fortunately, data have indicated that long-term death rates among living donors are no higher than in a healthy matched cohort,[21] but there are other long-term risks to the donors that must be conveyed.

End-Stage Renal Disease

The overall incidence of ESRD among living kidney donors during the first 10 years after donation is low, with rates of 0.2% to 0.5% reported.[22] Despite this, two studies have suggested that the relative risk for ESRD may be higher in certain populations. A single-center study out of Norway found that 0.47% of donors and 0.07% of nondonors developed ESRD, with all affected donors biologically related to their recipient.[23] In another study performed in the United States comparing living kidney donors to healthy controls, 0.10% of living kidney donors and 0.04% of healthy matched nondonors developed ESRD during follow-up.[24] The incidence of ESRD was noted to be higher among donors aged 60 years and older and African American donors. Although both studies had limitations, it is worthwhile to emphasize that although the absolute risk for postdonation ESRD is low, there may be a slightly higher risk compared with a matched, healthy cohort.

Pregnancy

Multiple studies have found an increased risk for gestational hypertension and preeclampsia after kidney donation in women of childbearing age.[25-27] This raises some concern because preeclampsia may have long-term renal consequences, including increased prevalence of proteinuria and hypertension. Despite these increased risks, maternal and fetal outcomes are comparable to that of the general population, with most having uncomplicated pregnancies. Because women of childbearing age are the largest group of kidney donors, the effects of donation on postdonation pregnancies should be a routine part of the discussion of risks during the initial donor evaluation. Most centers discourage donation in women with a history of pregnancy-induced hypertension or preeclampsia.

Quality of Life

In general, most studies on quality of life after donation report that the majority of donors experience no change or an improvement, with very few experiencing adverse outcomes, including depression and anxiety.[28] On standardized quality-of-life scales such as the Short Form 36 Health Survey, donor and nondonors have scored similarly, even those donors whose recipients had poor outcomes. Most donors would donate again if given the opportunity.

Long-Term Medical Care

In the United States, United Network for Organ Sharing (UNOS) policy requires that the transplant center must maintain contact with the donor for at least 24 months after nephrectomy. Beyond that, recommendations for future medical care and risk modification for a kidney donor are similar to the general population. After donation, kidney donors should undergo routine checkups with a focus on BP and kidney function. Urinary protein excretion should be measured as part of routine follow-up care. Patients should undergo age-appropriate cancer screening and be counseled on the need for weight control, smoking cessation, and abstinence from excessive alcohol. Emphasis should be placed on avoidance of high-protein diets, protein supplements for body building, herbal medications, and excessive use of nonsteroidal antiinflammatory pain medications, all of which may lead to kidney injury.

CONCLUSIONS

Living kidney donation is now commonly practiced worldwide with excellent long-term outcomes and low risk for ESRD. With increasing acceptance of medically complex live donors, including those that are older and those with metabolic abnormalities, obesity, and hypertension, it is important that information regarding the risks of donation is shared with donors during the evaluation process. Ongoing efforts to improve the follow-up of living donors through the development of national registries should continue, with the primary goal to protect their long-term health and survival.

EVALUATION OF THE RECIPIENT

Kidney transplantation is the treatment of choice for patients with advanced kidney disease who have a reasonable medium-term life expectancy and who are medically and surgically fit to undergo the procedure. Transplantation confers a survival advantage over remaining on dialysis even for higher-risk patients such as diabetics and the elderly.[29,30] Evaluation of the patient for transplantation should ideally begin well before the initiation of dialysis.[31] This allows for preemptive transplantation if a living donor is available. Even if living donation is not an option, completion of the evaluation before initiation of dialysis allows the patient to be added to the deceased donor waiting list and begin accruing predialysis waiting time. The initial evaluation must be thorough, and the patient must be educated about the risks and benefits of transplantation.

BOX 36.4 Contraindications to Kidney Transplantation

Absolute Contraindications
Active cancer
Active infection
Active psychiatric illness
Active substance abuse
Ongoing noncompliance with dialysis or medical regimen
Primary hyperoxaluria without liver transplantation

Relative Contraindications*
Major morbidity that would be worsened by transplant or would lead to very short posttransplant survival
High operative risk
Immunological incompatibility†
Severe obesity (e.g., body mass index >40 kg/m^2)
Multiple myeloma without stem cell transplantation
AL amyloidosis without stem cell transplantation
Severe sickle cell disease
Severe scleroderma
Thrombotic thrombocytopenic purpura

* Eligibility varies by transplant center.
† Protocols are available to facilitate transplantation across these barriers.

CLINICAL ASSESSMENT OF THE RECIPIENT

The patient's primary nephrologist usually makes the first assessment as to whether a patient is a potential candidate for transplantation. This most often occurs once renal replacement therapy is expected to be required within the next 12 months[32]; however, in the United States, patients are eligible for listing once the GFR is less than 20 mL/min. Several scoring systems have been proposed to help guide providers in selecting patients who are appropriate for referral to a transplant center,[33,34] and multiple guidelines are available to assist clinicians in the process of evaluating candidates.[5,32,35] Box 36.4 lists absolute and relative contraindications to kidney transplantation. Relative contraindications vary among different transplant centers; therefore it is reasonable for patients who are excluded by one center to seek a second opinion regarding transplant eligibility.[32]

There is no widely accepted age cutoff as far as transplant eligibility is concerned,[5,32,35] though some centers may choose to set an arbitrary age limit, especially for older patients who have no potential living donors and have an expected long waiting time. Ultimately an individualized assessment is ideal because chronological age alone does not necessarily correlate with an individual's overall health status. In general, patients with nonrenal organ failure that is not amenable to intervention are excluded. Other factors that are also considered include a patient's social support and ability to adhere with medical therapy.

History, Physical Examination, and Diagnostic Testing

Once referred to a transplant center, a potential recipient undergoes a thorough medical and psychosocial evaluation to

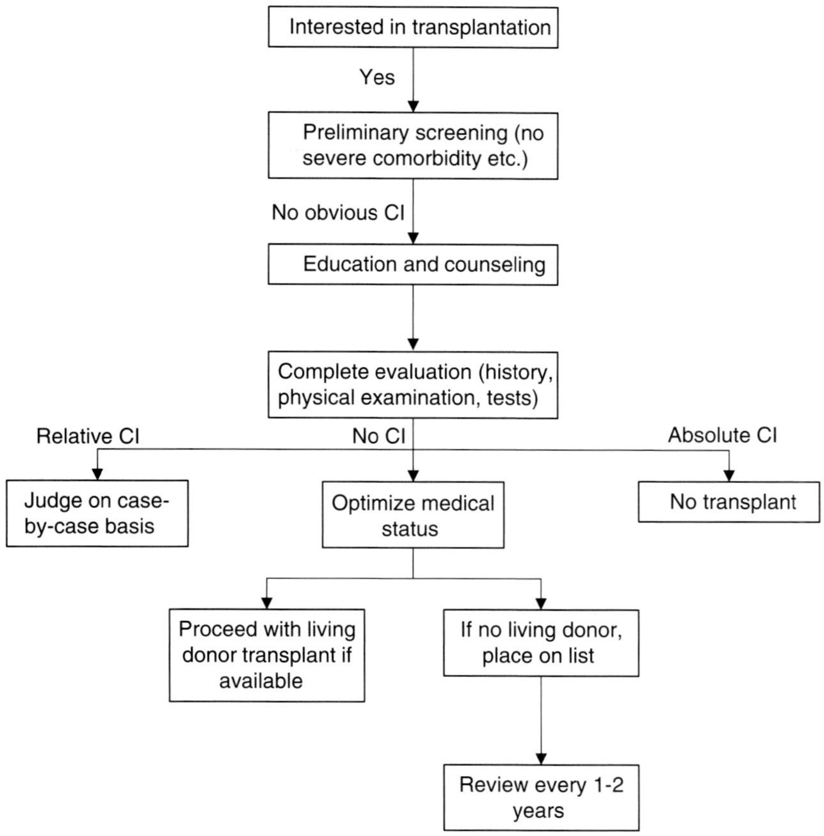

FIG. 36.1 Typical steps in the evaluation of a patient for kidney transplantation. *CI,* Contraindication.

determine suitability for transplantation. The process of evaluating a patient varies among centers but in general includes an education session, a visit with a transplant nephrologist and/or surgeon, a meeting with a social worker and a financial coordinator, and routine diagnostic testing such as bloodwork, a chest radiograph, and an electrocardiogram. The typical steps in the evaluation of a patient for kidney transplantation are shown in Fig. 36.1.

During the physician visit, several important elements in the history should be obtained. This includes establishing the cause of the patient's renal failure if it is known, and if a biopsy was performed, the results should be retrieved and reviewed. Details regarding prior therapy such as immunosuppression should be elicited. For patients who are on dialysis, it is important to ask about current urine output because this will serve as a posttransplant baseline and can also give information regarding a patient's bladder capacity. A thorough investigation of the patient's medical history and comorbidities such as diabetes, cardiovascular disease, chronic lung disease, and chronic liver disease should be elicited, including the duration of each condition and any associated complications. Any history of blood transfusion, pregnancy, venous thrombosis, cancer, infections such as tuberculosis (TB) or fungal infections, hypotension on dialysis, and any prior abdominal or vascular surgeries should be obtained. Review of medications should include a search for drugs that are metabolized by the cytochrome P450 system and thus have a potential drug interaction with calcineurin inhibitors (CNIs) and mammalian target of rapamycin (mTOR) inhibitors. The use of midodrine, usually used for patients with hypotension on dialysis, has recently been identified as a marker for poor outcomes.[36] A thorough review of systems should be performed specifically asking about symptoms of cardiovascular disease and chronic infection. A patient's functional status is also important, and this should include an inquiry on the patient's ability to perform activities of daily living. Finally, the patient's social support system should be evaluated as well as any history of medical nonadherence.

The physical examination should include accurate BP measurements, including a standing BP to screen for orthostatic hypotension. Attention should be given to the cardiovascular examination and should note any signs of fluid overload or murmurs that may suggest congestive heart failure, pulmonary hypertension, or valvular heart disease. To evaluate for peripheral vascular disease, peripheral pulses—particularly the femoral pulses—should be palpated and auscultated and the lower extremities examined for foot ulcerations or ischemic changes. The abdominal examination is important in determining whether obese patients are eligible for transplant, particularly those with a BMI >35 kg/m^2, because distribution of body fat and the size of the pelvis vary among different individuals. For patients with markedly enlarged polycystic kidneys, the abdominal examination can also determine whether there is enough room for a transplant or if a nephrectomy is necessary before transplantation. Finally, a patient's dentition must be examined to ensure there is no active infection that may pose a risk after transplantation.

BOX 36.5 Routine Tests for Potential Kidney Transplant Recipients

ABO blood typing, human leukocyte antigen (HLA) typing, anti-HLA antibodies
Complete blood cell count
Comprehensive metabolic panel
Intact parathyroid hormone
Urinalysis and urine culture if not anuric
Prothrombin time, partial thromboplastin time
Chest radiograph
Electrocardiogram
Tests for human immunodeficiency virus, hepatitis B, hepatitis C, cytomegalovirus, Epstein-Barr virus, syphilis, tuberculosis
If older than 50 years: colonoscopy
Women: Papanicolaou smear; mammogram if older than 40 years
Men: PSA if older than 50 years

PSA, Prostate-specific antigen.

Routine diagnostic testing as listed in Box 36.5 should be obtained in all patients. Based on a patient's history and physical examination, comorbid conditions, and results of the routine testing, supplementary diagnostic tests may be warranted as listed in Table 36.1. Each patient is required to have updated age-appropriate cancer screening such as a colonoscopy, mammogram, Papanicolaou (pap) smear, and prostate-specific antigen, according to conventional guidelines. Based on the results of the evaluation and testing, a determination is then made by a kidney transplant selection committee at each center regarding a patient's suitability for kidney transplantation. The committee is usually composed of transplant nephrologists and surgeons, psychiatrists, pharmacists, nurses, coordinators, social workers, and financial coordinators. Patients who are approved are then activated on the deceased donor waiting list, and for those with available living donors, planning for living donor transplantation can then commence.

TABLE 36.1 Supplementary Tests Sometimes Required for Potential Kidney Transplant Recipients

Indication	Diagnostic Test
Congestive heart failure or valvular heart disease	Echocardiogram
Risk factors for (or known) coronary artery disease	Noninvasive stress testing and/or left-sided heart catheterization
Moderate to severe pulmonary hypertension	Right-sided heart catheterization
Peripheral vascular disease	CT or MR imaging of iliac arteries
Chronic obstructive pulmonary disease	Pulmonary function testing
Cerebrovascular disease	Carotid arterial doppler
Venous or arterial thrombosis or access clotting	Hypercoagulable workup
Systemic lupus erythematosus or history of first trimester spontaneous abortions	Lupus anticoagulant; assessment of disease activity
Polycystic kidney disease	Brain imaging for aneurysms if with family history, native kidney imaging to evaluate kidney size if physical examination is inconclusive
Anti-GBM disease	Anti-GBM antibody titer
History of treatment with cyclophosphamide	Urine cytology or cystoscopy
Failed transplant because of BK nephropathy	Serum BK quantification
End-stage renal disease >5 years	Native kidney imaging for renal cell carcinoma screening
Multiple prior kidney transplants	CT or MR angiogram of abdomen/pelvis

CT, Computed tomography; *GBM,* glomerular basement membrane; *MR,* magnetic resonance.

SELECTED ISSUES IN THE RECIPIENT EVALUATION

Cardiovascular Disease

The high prevalence of cardiovascular disease in patients with chronic kidney disease is well known and among kidney transplant recipients, it remains the leading cause of allograft loss and death after transplantation.[1] An evaluation for cardiovascular disease is imperative before transplantation to determine the risk for perioperative adverse cardiac events and to optimize cardiac function. In addition, detection of a severe burden of cardiovascular disease may render a patient an unacceptable candidate for transplantation because of overall poor life expectancy.

Coronary Artery Disease

A proposed algorithm for the screening of kidney transplant candidates for coronary artery disease is shown in Fig. 36.2. The screening process may vary depending on the transplant center. In general, low-risk patients can proceed without additional testing if they have no risk factors, the electrocardiogram is normal, and they are asymptomatic. For patients who are at moderate risk, noninvasive stress testing is performed whether by nuclear or echocardiographic imaging depending on center expertise. For those with an abnormal stress test or for patients who are at high risk (e.g., known coronary artery disease with prior revascularization or longstanding diabetes), coronary angiography is pursued. Revascularization is determined by current guidelines. Patients with active ischemia and a culprit coronary artery lesion that is not amenable to intervention are often excluded from transplantation. In addition, if there is severe burden of disease found on catheterization (e.g., three-vessel disease), a patient may similarly be excluded especially when revascularization is not feasible and other comorbidities are present. It must be noted, however, that many uncertainties exist regarding pretransplant coronary artery disease screening and management.[34] This is due to the suboptimal sensitivity and specificity of noninvasive cardiac stress testing in patients with chronic kidney

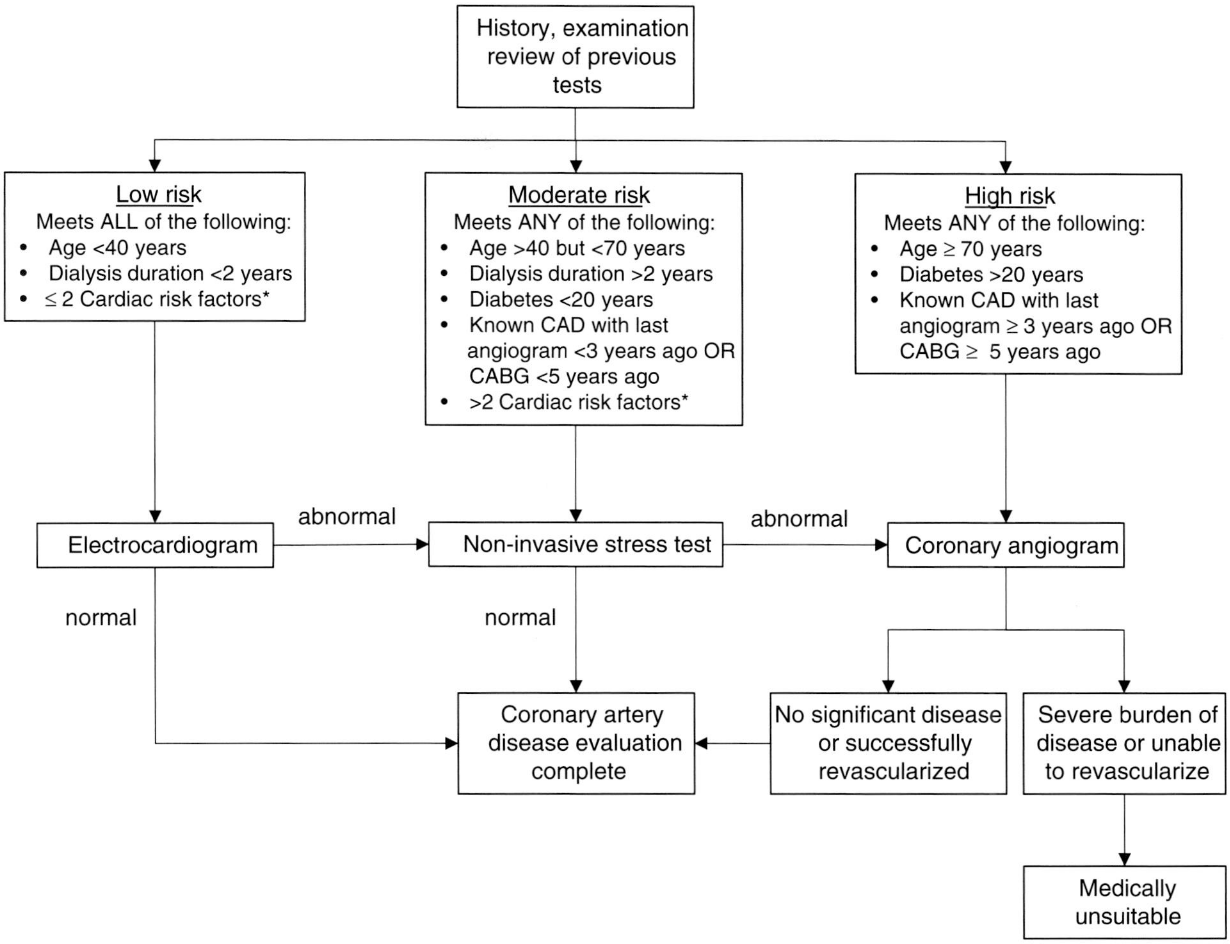

FIG. 36.2 Suggested algorithm for pretransplant cardiovascular screening. *Hypertension, hyperlipidemia, body mass index >35 kg/m^2, smoking. *CABG,* Coronary artery bypass grafting; *CAD,* coronary artery disease.

disease and end-stage renal disease, the conflicting data from observational studies regarding the prognostic value of noninvasive testing and coronary angiography in predicting major adverse cardiac events, and the lack of evidence that revascularization in asymptomatic patients improves outcomes.[37-40]

Congestive Heart Failure and Valvular Heart Disease

In patients who have signs or symptoms of volume overload or an abnormal cardiac examination, an echocardiogram is usually obtained to evaluate for systolic heart failure and valvular heart disease and to screen for the presence of severe pulmonary hypertension. Patients with markedly reduced ejection fractions and no evidence of coronary artery disease can still be considered for transplantation if the cardiomyopathy is thought to be due to the uremic milieu because cardiac function would be expected to improve after transplantation. Patients with severe ischemic cardiomyopathy are excluded unless they are also candidates for heart transplantation. Patients with significant valvular dysfunction may need intervention before transplantation.

Peripheral Vascular Disease

Imaging of the aortoiliac vessels through a CT angiogram or magnetic resonance angiogram (MRA) without contrast to evaluate for peripheral vascular disease is warranted for patients with poor femoral pulses on examination or who have a history of leg claudication or foot ulcerations. For patients who have had long-standing diabetes or are of advanced age (e.g., 70 years or older), a noncontrast CT scan of the abdomen and pelvis may be obtained to screen for severe or circumferential iliac calcifications that would exclude a patient from transplantation.

Diabetes Mellitus

It is important to note that diabetic patients gain a significant survival advantage with transplantation compared with those diabetics remaining on dialysis on the waiting list.[30] All diabetic transplant candidates should undergo careful screening particularly for cardiovascular disease, and this should be aggressively treated. Patients with type 1 diabetes should also be considered for pancreas transplantation—either simultaneous kidney-pancreas or pancreas after kidney transplantation.[41]

Pulmonary Disease

Obstructive and Restrictive Lung Disease

Patients with a history of chronic lung disease should be evaluated with pulmonary function testing and oximetry. Patients who have a forced expiratory volume 1 that is less than 25% of predicted are generally excluded. Similarly, patients on home oxygen or those who have hypoxia (Sao_2 <90% on room air) are not candidates for kidney transplantation.[32] All patients should be counseled to stop smoking.

Pulmonary Hypertension

The presence of severe pulmonary hypertension in a kidney transplant recipient may portend a poor posttransplant outcome.[42,43] Patients with echocardiographic findings of right ventricular pressure overload or a right ventricular systolic pressure more than 45 mmHg may need further evaluation by right-sided heart catheterization to help characterize the type of pulmonary hypertension that is present.[38,44] If volume overload is found to be the driver, aggressive ultrafiltration or diuresis and correction of the pulmonary hypertension before transplantation should be pursued. If a secondary cause for pulmonary hypertension such as obstructive sleep apnea is identified, this should be aggressively treated as well. Transplant centers vary in their cutoffs for acceptable pulmonary artery pressures, and if the severe pulmonary hypertension is not amenable to correction, a patient is usually excluded from transplantation.

Cancer

The presence of an active malignancy is an absolute contraindication to transplantation. Age-appropriate screening tests used in the general population such as a colonoscopy, pap smear, mammogram, and prostate-specific antigen are obtained as part of the pretransplant evaluation. Patients who have had ESRD for several years may benefit from radiographic imaging of the native kidneys to screen for renal cell carcinoma. Those who have a risk factor for bladder cancer such as history of prior treatment with cyclophosphamide can be screened by obtaining urine cytological testing or, if anuric, undergoing cystoscopy.

Several guidelines exist on the appropriate waiting time required before pursuing a kidney transplant for patients with a history of cancer.[32,35,45] Patients with small incidentally diagnosed renal cell carcinomas, basal cell skin cancers, and in-situ cervical cancers that have been adequately treated do not require a waiting period. For most other malignancies, however, a waiting period of 2 to 5 years is required. This is to ensure the absence of cancer recurrence or progression and to establish that the patient is essentially cured of the malignancy and has a reasonable life expectancy. For certain malignancies, particularly lymphoproliferative disease, there is also a concern that immunosuppression can promote cancer recurrence or progression.

Obesity

Obesity is a risk factor for surgical complications such as impaired wound healing, delayed graft function, cardiovascular disease, higher mortality, and inferior posttransplant allograft function.[46,47] Nevertheless, obese patients derive a survival benefit from transplantation as opposed to remaining on dialysis, though this may be less in patients with a BMI ≥40 kg/m^2.[48-50] Severe obesity can also make it physically impossible for a surgeon to implant a kidney into a recipient. Centers vary on the upper limit of BMI that they would consider transplantable, and this usually ranges from 35 to 40 kg/m^2, with some centers considering those between 40 to 45 kg/m^2 on an individual basis. An abdominal examination is important when evaluating obese candidates because fat distribution may vary significantly among individuals. For patients who are deemed ineligible for transplantation because of obesity, they should be counseled on available medical or surgical weight loss therapeutic options that if effective could assist in ultimately getting them to transplantation. Regardless of eligibility, all obese patients should be strongly encouraged to lose weight, with a goal BMI of less than 30 kg/m^2.[32]

Infections

Hepatitis C

Kidney transplantation is associated with superior outcomes compared with dialysis in hepatitis C virus (HCV)–infected ESRD patients. The suggested algorithm for the pretransplant evaluation and management of an HCV-infected kidney transplant candidate is shown in Fig. 36.3.[51] All kidney transplant candidates in high-prevalence regions should be screened for hepatitis C by nucleic acid (HCV RNA) testing. In areas where HCV has a low prevalence, hepatitis C antibody (HCV Ab) testing, followed by HCV RNA testing for seropositive individuals, is recommended. Liver biopsy has traditionally been a requirement for patients with confirmed infection to ensure the absence of cirrhosis; however, the emergence of noninvasive techniques may render this unnecessary for most patients in the future. HCV genotyping has similarly been necessary to guide treatment options. However, it remains to be seen whether this will still be needed going forward given the advent of pangenotypic direct-acting antivirals (DAAs) to treat hepatitis C. Moreover, the option of safely using DAAs posttransplant affords HCV-positive kidney transplant candidates the option to receive a kidney from an HCV-infected donor and be treated for infection after transplantation. By doing so, patients can reduce their waiting time by several years. Emerging data indicate that HCV cure rates greater than 95% after transplantation are being achieved.[52]

Hepatitis B

Kidney transplant candidates are screened for hepatitis B virus (HBV) by checking a hepatitis B surface antigen (HbsAg), hepatitis B surface antibody (HbsAb), and hepatitis B core antibody (HbcAb). Those who have no evidence of exposure to the virus (HBsAb and HbcAb negative) and have not been vaccinated should be vaccinated. For patients with a positive HbsAg or HbcAb, hepatitis B DNA polymerase chain reaction testing should be performed to evaluate for active viremia. Patients with confirmed active infection should undergo a liver biopsy to ensure the absence of cirrhosis and a need for simultaneous liver-kidney transplantation. Liver imaging and an α-fetoprotein level should also be obtained to screen for hepatocellular carcinoma. Patients with active viremia should be treated with antiviral agents such as lamivudine, entecavir, or tenofovir before transplantation because of the risk for developing fulminant

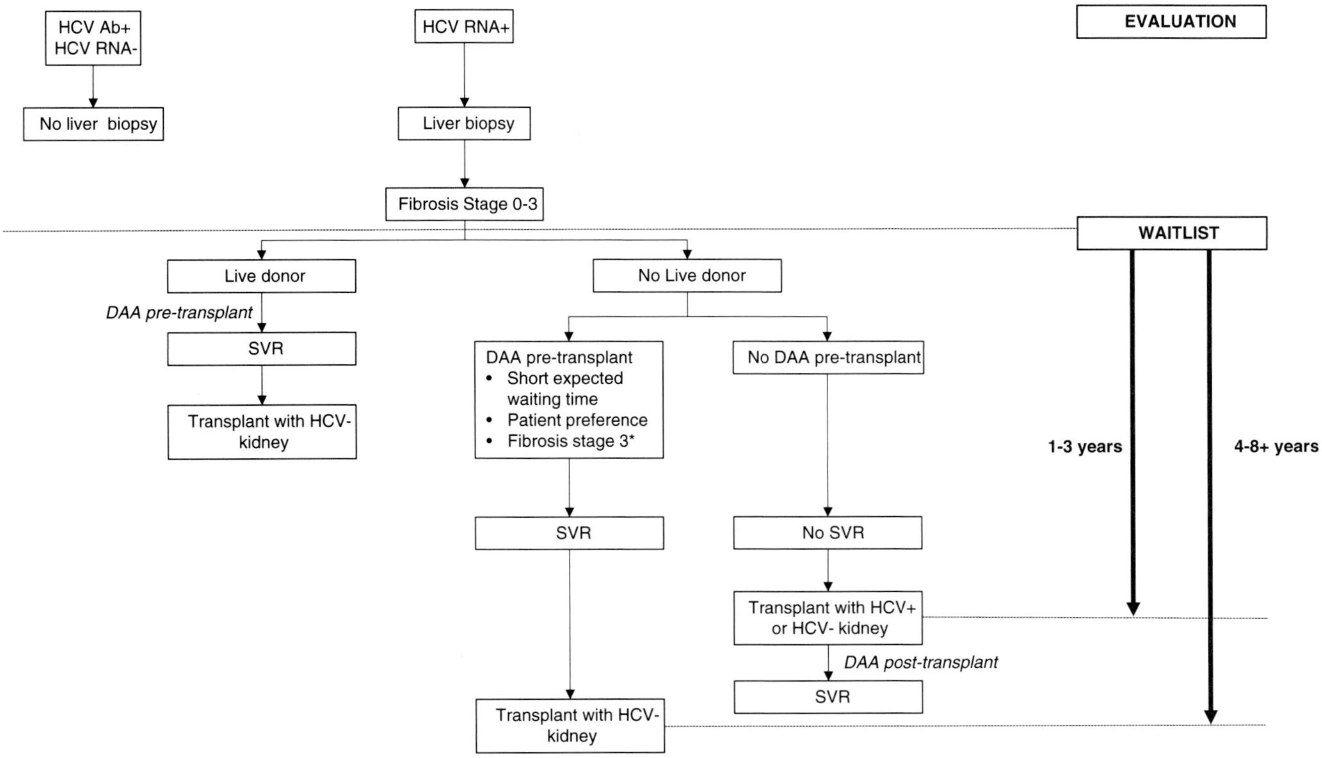

FIG. 36.3 Management of the hepatitis C–positive patient being considered for kidney transplant. *For patients listed in transplant centers with long wait times. *Ab*, Antibody; *DAA*, direct-acting antiviral; *HCV*, hepatitis C; *RNA*, ribonucleic acid; *SVR*, sustained virological response. (Adapted from Sawinski D, Bloom RD. Novel hepatitis C treatment and the impact on kidney transplantation. *Transplantation.* 2015;99:2458-2466.)

hepatitis with immunosuppression. Antivirals should be continued indefinitely after transplantation and an annual HBV DNA PCR should be obtained to ensure appropriate viral suppression.

Human Immunodeficiency Virus

Patients infected with HIV derive benefit from transplantation compared with remaining on the waiting list.[53] Long-term allograft outcomes in these patients are excellent and comparable to noninfected counterparts,[54,55] though patients coinfected with HCV seem to do worse.[56] In addition, an increased rate of acute rejection has been reported,[54] though the reason for this is unknown. Some have posited that avoidance of depleting antibody induction, cautious dosing of maintenance therapies resulting in underimmunosuppression, or drug-drug interactions between antiretrovirals and CNIs may be contributory.[56] To be eligible for transplantation, patients must have an undetectable HIV viral load and a CD4 count of more than 200/mm^3 for at least 3 to 6 months on stable antiretroviral therapy with no intercurrent opportunistic infections. [5,54] Protease inhibitors have a potent inhibitory effect on the cytochrome P450 system; hence a thorough review of the patient's antiretroviral therapy should be performed so that adequate planning regarding posttransplantation CNI or mTOR dosing can be made. Some centers elect to transition patients to protease inhibitor-free regimens to allow for more traditional CNI or mTOR dosing.[56]

Tuberculosis

All kidney transplant candidates should be screened for TB through a careful history of exposures, risk factors, and symptoms.[57] Diagnostic testing using either tuberculin skin testing (TST) (positive if there is ≥5 mm of induration at 48 to 72 hours) or interferon-γ release assays (IGRA) is performed as a screening test, and a chest radiograph is also reviewed for findings that are suggestive of old or active TB infection.[58] Patients who have a positive TST or IGRA should be referred to the local health department and evaluated for active TB because these tests cannot differentiate between active and latent TB infection. If a patient is diagnosed with latent TB, he or she should be treated for latent TB with 9 months of isoniazid or other alternative regimens ideally before transplantation. A patient can generally proceed to transplantation while on latent TB therapy or can also begin treatment posttransplant. However, if a patient is diagnosed with active TB, transplantation should be postponed until the patient completes adequate therapy, which usually consists of at least three drugs and a 9-month course of therapy.

Systemic Diseases

Table 36.2 summarizes the considerations for transplant eligibility for specific systemic diseases not discussed earlier.[32]

TABLE 36.2 Considerations for Transplant Eligibility of Specific Systemic Diseases

Systemic Disease	Considerations
Primary hyperoxaluria	Consider isolated renal transplantation if pyridoxine sensitive and minimal oxalate deposition; Combined liver-kidney transplantation if with severe systemic disease
Fabry disease	Consider if systemic disease not severe
Sickle cell disease	Consider if systemic disease not severe
Systemic lupus erythematosus	Consider if clinically quiescent disease for at least 6 months off cytotoxic agents
Vasculitis	Consider if quiescent disease for at least 12 months off cytotoxic agents; pretransplant antineutrophil cytoplasmic antibodies are not predictive of outcome and may be positive at time of transplantation
Scleroderma	Consider if clinically quiescent disease for at least 6 months off cytotoxic agents and have limited extrarenal disease
Antiglomerular basement membrane (anti-GBM)	Consider if anti-GBM antibody is undetectable and quiescent disease off cytotoxic agents for at least 6 months posttreatment
Thrombotic thrombocytopenic purpura	Consider if quiescent disease
Atypical (complement-mediated) hemolytic uremic syndrome	Consider renal transplantation after evaluation for genetic mutations or culprit antibodies, consider concurrent use of eculizumab*
Cystinosis	Consider for renal transplantation
Congenital nephrotic syndrome	Consider after undergoing bilateral nephrectomy
Autosomal recessive polycystic kidney disease	Consider after screening for evidence of portal hypertension and evaluation for unilateral or bilateral nephrectomy

*Authors' recommendation.
Adapted from Knoll G, Cockfield S, Blydt-Hansen T, et al. Canadian Society of Transplantation consensus guidelines on eligibility for kidney transplantation. *CMAJ*. 2005;173(10):1181-1184.

Emerging Risk Factors That May Affect Kidney Transplant Candidacy

Hypotension on Hemodialysis

Patients with a history of hypotension on dialysis requiring midodrine use are at increased risk for allograft thrombosis, primary nonfunction, delayed graft function, and inferior allograft outcomes.[36] It is prudent to review BPs on dialysis flowsheets for all candidates who are on hemodialysis, especially those on midodrine, or with low or low-normal BP at the time of evaluation. At times, resolution of hypotension can be achieved simply by adjustment of the dry weight. If patients with persistent hypotension are deemed to be suitable transplant candidates, careful selection of a donor kidney may be required, specifically avoiding those at higher risk for developing delayed graft function.

BOX 36.6 Definition of Frailty*

Component
Shrinking
Weakness
Exhaustion
Low physical activity
Slowed walking speed

*The presence of three or more components signifies frailty.
Adapted from Fried LP, Tangen CM, Walston J, et al. Frailty in older adults: evidence for a phenotype. *J Gerontol A Biol Sci Med Sci.* 2001;56:M146-M156.

Frailty and Functional Status

Frailty has emerged as a risk factor for inferior kidney transplantation outcomes, including an increased risk for early hospital readmission, mycophenolate mofetil (MMF) intolerance, delayed graft function, and mortality.[59-61] The definition of frailty[62] is shown in Box 36.6. Similarly, a patient's self-reported functional status has also been correlated with transplant outcomes.[63] These studies support the notion that evaluation of physiological age through these nontraditional measures may have an important role in risk-stratifying potential candidates. For patients who are found to be frail or have suboptimal functional status, there may be a role for rehabilitation before transplantation, termed *prehabilitation*. How this affects posttransplant outcomes remains to be determined.

History of a Failed Allograft

Patients with a history of a failed allograft have improved survival with retransplantation compared with remaining on the waiting list.[64] In evaluating these patients, the reason for graft loss must be determined and risk factors identified, and if a biopsy was performed, the results should be reviewed. A transplant nephrectomy is usually not required before retransplantation unless there is an anatomical indication or a patient has symptoms suggestive of acute allograft rejection such as gross hematuria and allograft pain.

If graft loss was due to acute rejection, factors that may have contributed to this, including medical nonadherence, should be investigated. Rejection treatment that the patient received must be ascertained, particularly lymphocyte-depleting agents such as antithymocyte globulin, because this may have implications for the choice of induction agent for the subsequent transplant.

If the graft was lost due to polyoma virus nephropathy, a patient's serum BK must be undetectable before retransplantation. There is no consensus as to the benefit of a transplant nephrectomy before retransplantation in these patients.

For patients with prior grafts lost because of disease recurrence, counseling is important due to the high risk for a similar outcome, particularly in cases where there is no planned alteration in pre- or posttransplant management from the prior transplant. The decision to proceed with retransplantation may depend on the rapidity by which the prior graft was lost and any available interventions that could be employed to improve outcomes. For patients with rapid failure of an allograft because of recurrent disease, the decision to proceed with retransplantation should be based on shared decision making between the patient and the transplant center. In general, living donor transplantation is avoided in these patients.

High Sensitization to Human Leukocyte Antigens

Human leukocyte antigen (HLA) typing and measurement of class I and class II panel reactive antibodies (PRA) are performed during the transplant evaluation, and PRAs are thereafter periodically measured. Patients who are highly sensitized are less likely to find an immunologically compatible donor and historically have experienced long waiting times. Patients who have an immunologically incompatible living donor can enroll in a paired donor exchange program, undergo desensitization if the levels of HLA antibody are permissible, or wait for a compatible deceased donor.[65] Paired donor exchange can occur within a single transplant center or through kidney exchange programs to increase the chances of finding a compatible pair. Desensitization is another option, and it has been reported that transplantation with an immunologically incompatible live donor offers superior survival compared with waiting on the deceased donor list for a compatible donor.[66] The new Kidney Allocation System, however, has been successful in increasing the number of deceased donor transplants for patients with a PRA of 98% to 100%.[67,68] With this new system, it is difficult to estimate how long patients with PRA 98% to 100% will need to wait on the deceased donor list, because immunological compatibility and not dialysis vintage is the main driver for organ allocation in these patients.

Psychosocial Issues

Psychiatric illness is only a contraindication if it is severe enough to impair understanding of the risks and benefits of transplantation and to prevent normal posttransplant follow-up and adherence. Addiction to alcohol or other drugs should be successfully treated before transplantation. Intellectual disability is not a contraindication if adequate posttransplant support is available. The issue of informed consent for surgery, however, can be difficult.

The recipient evaluation should also examine a patient's ability to adhere to medical therapy and a patient's social and financial support. This may involve probing into a patient's history of dialysis and medication adherence. It is also important to evaluate a patient's ability to travel to the transplant center not only for the transplant procedure but also for posttransplant clinic visits. Patients must understand the costs associated with pursuing a transplant, including potential copays for medications, travel and lodging costs, and costs related to time away from work for both the patient and the support person.

Counseling and Education

All patients who undergo a medical evaluation for transplantation also receive counseling and education. This is often carried out in a formal education class usually conducted in groups. During the physician visit, it is important to address any concerns or questions that may arise from the class. In addition, counseling should be individualized and include a discussion on the specific risks a patient faces in pursuing transplantation, such as rejection, infection, and disease recurrence. These risks must be weighed against the risk for remaining on dialysis. Also, specific transplant options should be discussed. This must include education about the benefits of undergoing preemptive and living donor transplantation as opposed to deceased donor transplantation, including the expected waiting time at the patient's transplant center. In addition, an individualized discussion should take place regarding the risks and benefits of listing for a deceased donor kidney with a kidney donor profile index >85%. Finally, counseling should take place regarding the risks and benefits of listing for Public Health Services increased-risk donor kidneys and A2 to B transplantation (for eligible patients).

Management of the Waiting List

Patients who have no living donor options must wait on a deceased donor kidney, which usually takes several years. In the United States the median waiting time to deceased donor transplant was 5.5 years in 2003 and 7.6 years in 2007.[2] Transplant centers face the challenge of ensuring candidates are medically and surgically suitable for transplantation once an acceptable donor kidney becomes available. While waiting on the list, a patient's medical condition may deteriorate such that he or she may require additional testing or may no longer be eligible for transplantation. The processes for reevaluating candidates and managing the waiting list vary among transplant centers. Some centers ask patients to return for a reevaluation once they are predicted to be close to being called for a transplant, whereas others elect to see patients every 1 to 2 years. Regardless of the process, it is important for the patient, the primary nephrologist, the dialysis unit, and the transplant center to maintain close communication at all times.

CONCLUSIONS

The evaluation of kidney transplant candidates aims to identify patients who would do well with a kidney transplant and ultimately derive a survival benefit and improvement in quality of life. The evaluation also identifies patients who may need medical optimization before transplantation, thus giving them the best chance at a successful outcome. An evaluation must include a thorough medical, surgical, and psychosocial assessment of the patient. Importantly, it should be used as a venue to facilitate shared decision making by educating and counseling patients regarding the risks and benefits of kidney transplantation and discussing the advantages and disadvantages of the different transplant options that are available to them.

37

Surgical Management of the Renal Transplant Recipient

Sophoclis Alexopoulos, MD, FACS, Lea Matsuoka, MD, FACS, and Seth J. Karp, MD

OUTLINE

Before the success of hemodialysis and kidney transplantation, end-stage renal disease (ESRD) was a fatal diagnosis. Interestingly, critical advances in both technologies developed simultaneously in the 1950 to 1960s. Individual hemodialysis treatments for acute renal failure first became available in the 1950s based on the research and ingenuity of Willem Kolff. However, the ability to treat chronic renal failure awaited progress in the field of vascular access. The development of the external Teflon-based arteriovenous (AV) fistula by Belding Scribner at the University of Washington in 1960 and the subcutaneous AV fistula by James Cimino and Michael Brescia in 1966 heralded the successful treatment of ESRD with repeat intermittent hemodialysis.[1] In 1972 Congress authorized Medicare approval of hemodialysis for the treatment of all patients with ESRD.[2] The development of hemodialysis represented the culmination of countless decades of research by hundreds of physicians and scientists. Rapid progress in the field of transplantation was occurring simultaneously. In 1954 the first successful human kidney transplant was performed between identical twins at the Peter Bent Brigham Hospital in Boston. However, over the next 30 years, immunological constraints would prevent widespread adoption of the technique for nonhaploidentical individuals. Institution of calcineurin-based immunosuppressive regimens—first with cyclosporine and subsequently with FK506—revolutionized the field by producing dramatic improvement in both patient and graft survival, and comparisons started being made between ESRD patients treated with chronic dialysis and those treated with kidney transplantation. The conclusive demonstration of the increased life expectancy associated with successful kidney transplantation compared with chronic hemodialysis by Wolfe and colleagues in 1999 resulted in kidney transplantation becoming the standard of care for the treatment of ESRD in selected patients.[3]

In 2016 there were 19,060 kidney transplants performed in the United States, with 13,431 from deceased donors and 3765 from living donors.[4] Surgeons play an important role in the evaluation and care of the kidney transplant recipient and in the evaluation and management of kidney live donors. This chapter focuses on the surgical aspects of live kidney donation and the kidney transplant recipient.

LIVE DONOR KIDNEY TRANSPLANTATION

Since the first live donor kidney transplant performed between identical twins, the technology has provided recipients shorter wait times, less time on dialysis, and superior graft survival. Many studies have been performed in attempts to quantify the risks related with kidney donation. Early studies were retrospective and had limited follow-up, but for the most part demonstrated donors were not at increased risk for mortality or the development of ESRD.[5,6] However, in 2014, Muzaale et al. studied 96,217 live kidney donors who donated a kidney between 1994 and 2011.[7] The study found a small but statistically significant increased risk of <0.5% for the development of ESRD in kidney donors over 15 years. An important part of the live donor process is to thoroughly screen and evaluate potential live donors to minimize their risk related to kidney donation.

Live Donor Evaluation

The donor evaluation is composed of medical and psychosocial components. In the United States, the United Network for Organ Sharing (UNOS) mandates certain aspects of the donor evaluation, whereas other criteria and policies vary among transplant centers. In general, however, donor evaluation includes assessments of overall health, kidney structure and function, and the risk for development of kidney disease, the presence of blood disorders, malignancies and infections, histocompatibility with the intended recipient, and psychosocial evaluation. The team must feel the donor's decision to donate is free of coercion and the donor understands the risks and benefits of donation. In addition, an independent donor advocate meets with potential donors to affirm informed consent. A multidisciplinary team approves live donor candidates.

A critical aspect of the surgical evaluation is the renal anatomy. Most commonly, assessment of live donor anatomy uses multidetector computed tomography (MDCT) imaging with three-dimensional reconstruction. MDCT has an accuracy of 95% to 100% in the delineation of renal anatomy and vasculature.[8,9] The importance of the MDCT cannot be overemphasized. Any nonstandard anatomy introduces technical challenges in both the donor and recipient. Only 70% to 75% of patients have single renal arteries bilaterally.[10] Renal vein anatomy is more uniform, with the right renal veins having more variation than the left. Complete or partial ureteral duplication occurs in 1% of the population.[9] Other considerations include the presence of a mass, stone, atherosclerosis, and the size of the kidneys. MDCT-based volumes have been shown to correlate with nuclear split renal function measurements, and can therefore be used as a reflection of renal function.[8] Depending on the results, 4% to 16% of kidney donors will be excluded secondary to renal findings on imaging studies.[10] Particular concerns are multiple small arteries or the presence of a small lower pole artery that supplies the ureter and therefore places the transplant at risk for ureteral necrosis.

In general, removal of the left kidney is preferred since the longer vascular pedicle makes the operation easier and safer. However, the overriding goal must be to minimize the donor operative risk and preserve long-term donor kidney function. If there is a size discrepancy in the kidneys, a functional study can be performed to ensure that both kidneys will be adequate over the long term.

Live Donor Nephrectomy

The traditional open flank incision for donor nephrectomy has been replaced by minimally invasive techniques. The first laparoscopic donor nephrectomy (LDN) was reported in 1995 by Ratner et al.[11] The LDN provides smaller incisions with improved cosmetic outcome, decreased postoperative pain, decreased hospital length of stay, and earlier return to work.[12,13] In addition, the advent of LDN has led to an increase in rate of live donation and has been adopted as the standard of care.[14] Alternative techniques such as hand-assisted LDN, single-port LDN, mini-incision open nephrectomy, retroperitoneoscopic, and robotic donor nephrectomy have evolved and are supported by individual centers and surgeons.[15-19] These approaches have been reported to result in similar donor and recipient outcomes.[15-19]

LDN is performed with the patient in a lateral decubitus position. In the pure laparoscopic approach to left nephrectomy, trochars are placed in the left upper quadrant and subxiphoid midline. When the hand-assisted approach is used, the hand port is typically placed in the suprapubic midline or via a Pfannenstiel incision. After identification of the vessels and mobilization of the ureter and kidney, the vessels are ligated using a stapling device and the kidney is removed via the hand port site or a Pfannenstiel incision. When the right kidney is removed via a laparoscopic approach, the vein tends to be shorter and the recipient surgeon may need to alter the implantation technique.

LDN has a reported mortality rate of 0.03%, an overall complication rate of 5% to 8%, and a conversion to open rate of <1%.[12,13]

RECIPIENT EVALUATION

Recipient evaluation is driven by whether the patient will benefit from renal transplant measured by both mortality and quality of life. For most patients, renal transplant trades a small upfront increased mortality and surgical discomfort for a potentially dramatic increase in life span and improvement in quality of life versus ongoing dialysis. There is a second ethical consideration in evaluating each patient: organ stewardship. With nearly 100,000 patients on the list, eliminating futile transplants that do not provide significant benefit to the recipient must be a priority.

Patients with a glomerular filtration rate of less than 20 to 30 m/min/m^2 should be considered for referral to a transplant center. Referral before initiation of dialysis is preferred. Complete evaluation of all options, including access placement and live donation, can take 6 months or longer.

In general, patients with ESRD as evidenced by measured creatinine clearance or calculated glomerular filtration rate (GFR) ≤20 mL/min/m^2 or who are on dialysis are candidates for renal transplant. Selected patients with a higher GFR can be considered for transplant depending on symptomatology.

Each patient should undergo a detailed history and physical examination. A comprehensive description of the workup is beyond the scope of this chapter, so we will focus on a few essential and unique elements. The high incidence of graft loss from cardiac disease after transplant mandates careful assessment of cardiac risk. Critical aspects of the history are onset and etiology of renal failure and symptomatology including level of activity, edema, shortness of breath, and fatigue. Evidence of coagulopathy should be sought. Other medical problems including diabetes, hypertension, heart disease, pulmonary disease, lupus, previous cancer, and renal calculi affect the decision to transplant as well as postoperative care. Surgical history including surgery on the kidneys, ureters or bladder, large and small bowel, and abdominal wall hernias affect surgical and postoperative planning.

Family history of renal disease can point out congenital etiologies. In some cases, for example, in patients with polycystic renal disease, this may lead to suggesting other family members undergo testing. Family cardiac history also is critical to assess recipient risk.

Physical examination focuses on cardiac and pulmonary risk and should include assessment of congestive heart failure by pulmonary and cardiac auscultation, palpation, percussion, and assessment of jugular venous pressure and the presence of generalized and peripheral edema. Careful examination of the abdomen for renal size and intraabdominal pathology is essential.

A unique feature of the transplant evaluation involves assessment of the ability of the patient to care for the graft postsurgery and reflects the central imperative regarding organ stewardship. Assessment of medical compliance and social support provide the basis for this decision. A critical component of the recipient evaluation includes evaluation by licensed social work professionals.

Relative contraindications to transplant are advanced age and severe obesity. Cutoffs vary by center but few centers are routinely performing transplants in patients over 80 years of age or with a body mass index higher than 50 kg/m^2. This relates to the well-documented increased complication rates and lower life expectancy in these groups. Each patient should be considered on a case-by-case basis.

It is important to establish a plan for urinary drainage. Inadequate bladder capacity or lack of urinary conduit precludes operation. A general guideline would be a bladder size of at least 75 cc. In patients with a smaller capacity, bladder stretching procedures, augmentations, or urinary conduits can be considered. Urological consultation is highly recommended in these situations.

Previous malignancy requires a variable waiting period before transplant due to risk for recurrence and concerns that immunosuppression may inhibit host immunological control of certain cancers. The Israel Penn registry contains information about cancer recurrence in transplant patients and can be a helpful resource to determine appropriate waiting times.[20]

Description of successful transplantation in patients infected with HIV occurred in the early 2000s, and selected patients with low viral load and adequate CD4 counts (typically >200/mL) may benefit from transplantation.[21,22]

Absolute contraindications for renal transplant include active systemic infection, active substance abuse, significant psychiatric illness likely to interfere with compliance, severe cardiac disease, severe peripheral vascular disease, cirrhotic liver disease (grade 3 or 4 fibrosis), noncompliance with current medical regimen, significant pulmonary disease or oxygen dependence, oxalosis (usually requires liver/kidney transplant), and inadequate family or social support.

As discussed, cardiovascular morbidity and mortality frequently leads to graft loss, and testing to determine risk enhances decision making. A low threshold for nuclear stress testing to determine cardiac ischemia with progression to cardiac catheterization for equivocal results provides invaluable input for risk adjustment. Although data are limited, in general, patients with significant areas of cardiac ischemia should not be offered renal transplantation without some type of coronary revascularization.

Other recommended testing includes pulmonary function tests, cancer screening at appropriate intervals and serological testing for hepatitis, cytomegalovirus, and Epstein-Barr virus. Other preoperative testing is dependent on the underlying cause of renal disease and comorbidities. Abdominal imaging is useful to assess vascular calcifications, size of kidneys in patients with polycystic renal disease, and anatomy in patients with prior surgery or congential anomalies. Carotid Doppler in patients with vascular disease and cerebral imaging in patients with polycystic renal disease to look for intracerebral aneurysms should be considered.

Given the typical comorbidities and risk for disease progression in patients on dialysis combined with extended waiting periods, following patients on the waiting list is essential. Patients should be seen at regular intervals and after significant medical events for reevaluation.

A multidisciplinary team reviews all data and determines suitability for renal transplantation. The selection committee should comprise representatives from transplant surgery, nephrology, social work, human leukocyte antigen (HLA) laboratory, pre- and posttransplant nursing, pharmacy, dietary, psychological services, and finance. Input from all these professional groups ensures the most consistent and evidence-based decision making.

DECEASED DONOR KIDNEY EVALUATION: KIDNEY DONOR PROFILE INDEX

Multiple factors determine the suitability of a particular deceased donor kidney to an individual. The ability of a particular allograft to meet a recipient's demands is a function of the maximal glomerular filtration the kidney can provide with respect to the recipient's body surface area, metabolic demand, and lean muscle mass. The maximal glomerular filtration a kidney can provide depends on both the absolute number of glomeruli and their ability to increase their filtration capacity through hyperperfusion and hypertrophy.[23] Age, height, sex, obesity, and hypertension all significantly affect glomerular mass.[24] Specifically, there is a progressive decline in absolute glomerular mass with increasing age.[25] Several scoring systems have been developed to assess the quality of a deceased donor allograft and assist in clinical decision making. The scoring system currently used in the allocation of deceased donor kidneys in the United States is the Kidney Donor Risk Index (KDRI).[4,26] The KDRI uses donor factors to calculate a score that estimates the relative risk for posttransplant graft failure (Table 37.1). The Kidney Donor Profile Index (KDPI) allows for a continuous assessment of allograft quality compared with the prior designation of standard criteria donor (SCD) or extended criteria donor (ECD) system. For example, a KDPI 1% deceased donor kidney has an 83.3% 5-year predicted graft survival compared with a 46.9% graft survival for a KDPI 99% deceased donor kidney based on data from 2004 to 2011 and scaled to a reference population of all deceased donor kidneys allocated by UNOS in 2013. Unfortunately, no systems account for recipient factors in combination with donor factors.

SURGICAL TECHNIQUE

The technical aspects of kidney transplantation are well described and have not significantly changed in the past several decades.[27,28] Laterality does not significantly affect the approach. A curvilinear incision (hockey stick) is typically made from the level of the anterior superior iliac spine to immediately cephalad to the lateral aspect of the pubic tubercle, while staying lateral to the rectus abdominis and linea semilunaris

TABLE 37.1 KDRI Donor Factors

KDRI Donor Factors	Applies to
Age (integer years)	All donors
Height (cm)	All donors
Weight (kg)	All donors <80 kg
Ethnicity	African American donors
History of hypertension	Hypertensive donors
Cause of death	CVA
Serum creatinine	All donors
HCV status	HCV-positive donors
DCD status	DCD donors

CVA, Cerebrovascular accident; *DCD*, donation after cardiac death; *HCV*, hepatitis C virus; *KDPI*, Kidney Donor Profile Index; *KDRI*, Kidney Donor Risk Index.

muscles. Care is taken to protect the spermatic cord in men. In women, the round ligament is routinely ligated. There are a variety of ways to enter the retroperitoneal space, which is then widely exposed. The inferior epigastric artery and vein are typically encountered caudally and divided to allow better exposure to the bladder. This exposure allows visualization of the external iliac artery and vein. The perivascular lymphoconnective tissue is typically ligated and divided to minimize the risk for lymphocele formation. The external iliac artery and vein are exposed and clamps placed. Typically, the venous anastomosis is performed first, followed by the arterial anastomosis. Both anastomoses are done in an end-to-side fashion. For deceased donors, the donor artery uses a Carrel patch of aorta to minimize the risk for stenosis, and for live donors, an arterial punch may be used to increase the diameter of the arteriotomy in the recipient for the same reason. Immunosuppression is typically administered before reperfusion. A well-perfused kidney should immediately become pink with a palpable arterial pulsation and thrill (Fig. 37.1). Furosemide and mannitol may be administered at this time per surgeon preference. After ensuring adequate hemostasis, the bladder is filled with irrigant to help identification. Typical anastomotic technique is the Lich-Greigor, which is a mucosal-to-mucosal anastomosis. A drain may be placed per surgeon preference.

IMMEDIATE POSTOPERATIVE MANAGEMENT

Postoperative graft function is dependent on numerous factors related to both the donor and the recipient. Recipients can most broadly be categorized into two groups based on the presence or absence of delayed graft function (DGF) defined as the need for dialysis within the first week posttransplant. However, heterogeneity exists within these groups and the rate of decline of a recipient's serum creatinine may be a more accurate reflection of postoperative allograft function (Fig. 37.2).[29] In general, acute kidney injury (AKI) present in the donor will be exacerbated by the procurement and transplant events, and recipients of these organs should be anticipated to have DGF. Additional donor factors influencing graft function include the quality of the organ with the DGF rate increasing from 16.3% in KDPI 0% to 20% kidneys to 39.2% in KDPI 86% to 100%

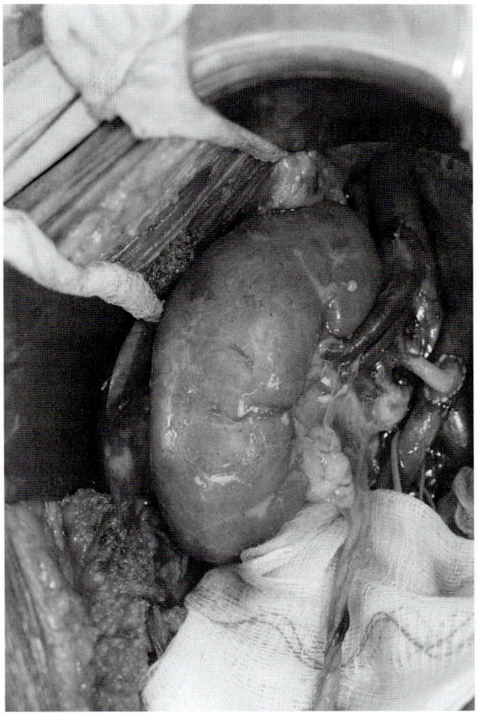

FIG. 37.1 Intraoperative photo of a kidney after transplant reperfusion.

kidneys.[30] A progressive increase is seen in DGF rates when comparing living donor, brain dead donor, and donation after cardiac death (DCD) organs. Recipient factors influencing postoperative graft function include diabetes and duration of time on dialysis as well as the degree of immunological compatibility.[31] Finally, both the cold and warm ischemia times (CIT and WIT, respectively) affect immediate allograft function due to increased ischemia/reperfusion insults (Box 37.1). Specifically, the rate of DGR increases with increasing CIT and appears to compound the effect of increasing donor age or DCD donation.[32-34] Interestingly, however, overall kidney quality as determined by prognostic scores such as KDPI and the overall functional glomerular mass are much more important determinants of long-term outcome than the presence of DGF. It is important to assess risk factors for DGF to anticipate expected kidney allograft function after transplantation.

The most immediate indicator of graft function is the presence or absence of urine production postreperfusion. High-quality allografts such as those obtained from living donors or deceased donors with a low KDPI may begin producing a large volume of urine immediately postreperfusion (see Fig. 37.2).[35] However, kidneys from DCD or high KDPI donors or those with prolonged CIT or WIT, or prerecovery AKI with anuria or oliguria may not produce any urine postreperfusion. It is important for the surgical team to document whether the transplanted kidney produced urine postreperfusion, as this will help guide the patient's postoperative management. The goal of the postoperative management of the kidney transplant recipient is to maintain adequate perfusion to the allograft. This requires a state of euvolemia with an adequate arterial perfusion pressure. Any hypotension

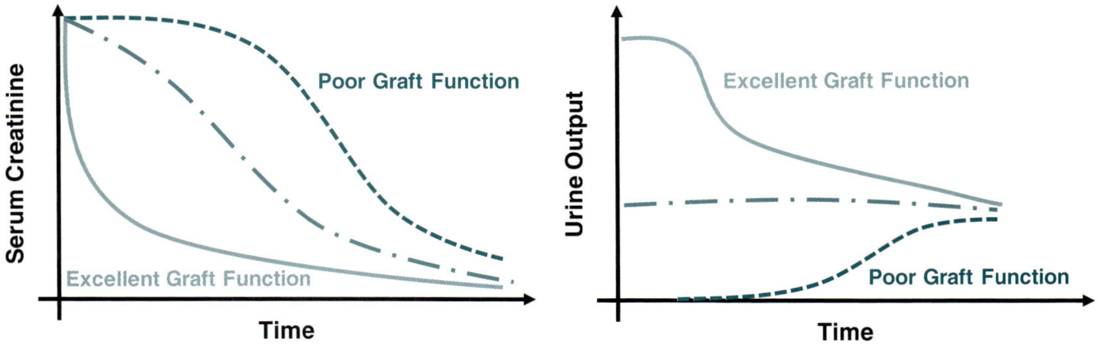

FIG. 37.2 Serum creatinine and urine output over time as a reflection of kidney allograft function after kidney transplantation.

BOX 37.1 Delayed Graft Function (DGF) Risk Factors

Donor age
Cold ischemia time
Warm ischemia time
Donation after cardiac death donor
Donor terminal creatinine
Donor Kidney Donor Profile Index
Immunological compatibility
Recipient diabetes
Recipient dialysis and type
Recipient cardiovascular disease

should trigger an immediate assessment and treatment of volume status and acute blood loss, with cardiac evaluation if volume status is adequate.

The production of urine in combination with a decline in serum creatinine in a recipient who was anuric before transplantation is typically an indicator of adequate allograft perfusion. Recipients of living donor or high-quality donation after brain death (DBD) or DCD allografts can frequently produce up to 1 L per hour of urine during the first 24 hours postreperfusion and should be placed on replacement intravenous fluids to prevent dehydration due to the dysregulation of renal homeostasis occurring immediately posttransplant. Fig. 37.3 shows an algorithm for the management of an euvolemic allograft with low urine output. A sudden decrease in urine output should be immediately evaluated for vascular thrombosis after ensuring patency of the urinary catheter. In addition, all living donor kidney recipients who are anuric/oliguric posttransplant should be promptly evaluated for vascular thrombosis. Doppler interrogation of the transplant allograft is the best first diagnostic test to ensure adequacy of arterial and venous blood flow. A slow progressive decline in urine output can first be managed with a volume challenge followed by administration of a loop diuretic such as furosemide to maintain urine output. However, persistently low urine output in the setting of a normal Doppler examination is often indicative of progressive acute tubular necrosis (ATN) reflective of either ischemia/reperfusion insults or immunological injury. Nearly one-third of deceased donor recipients will have DGF posttransplant and this will frequently be associated with anuria/oliguria. An ultrasound with Doppler interrogation of the vasculature within the first 24 hours is reasonable to ensure adequate perfusion to such allografts. Patients at low immunological risk who are euvolemic with a normal ultrasound examination can be observed while awaiting the resolution of ATN. Patients at high immunological risk should be considered for allograft biopsy if ATN fails to resolve within the first week posttransplantation.

Most kidney transplants can be performed in the retroperitoneal space without peritoneal violation or intestinal manipulation resulting in ileus. Oral intake and oral pain control medication can be introduced within the first 24 hours after recovery from anesthesia and allows for earlier discharge from the hospital. Early ambulation should be encouraged. In addition, there is no data to support prolonged urinary catheter drainage and early catheter removal on postoperative day 2 or 3 should be well tolerated in patients without an obstructive urological process.[36-38]

POSTOPERATIVE COMPLICATIONS

Surgical complications after kidney transplantation can be categorized as vascular, ureteral, and incisional. Vascular complications can involve either the renal arterial or venous anastomosis or the recipient artery itself. Ureteral complications include leaks or strictures of the ureteroneocystostomy or ureteroureterostomy. Wound-related complications include lymphoceles of the retroperitoneal space. These are discussed individually later.

Vascular Complications

Transplant Renal Artery Stenosis

Hypertension in the renal transplant recipient is common, reported in up to 85% of renal transplant patients.[39] There are many risk factors associated with hypertension after renal transplant, with transplant renal artery stenosis (TRAS) being the most common cause of secondary renal hypertension. TRAS is reported to occur in 1% to 23% of renal transplant patients and can lead to allograft dysfunction and decreased allograft survival.[39-41]

TRAS should be suspected in kidney transplant patients with worsening hypertension, hypokalemia, and declining graft function. Patients should undergo duplex ultrasound

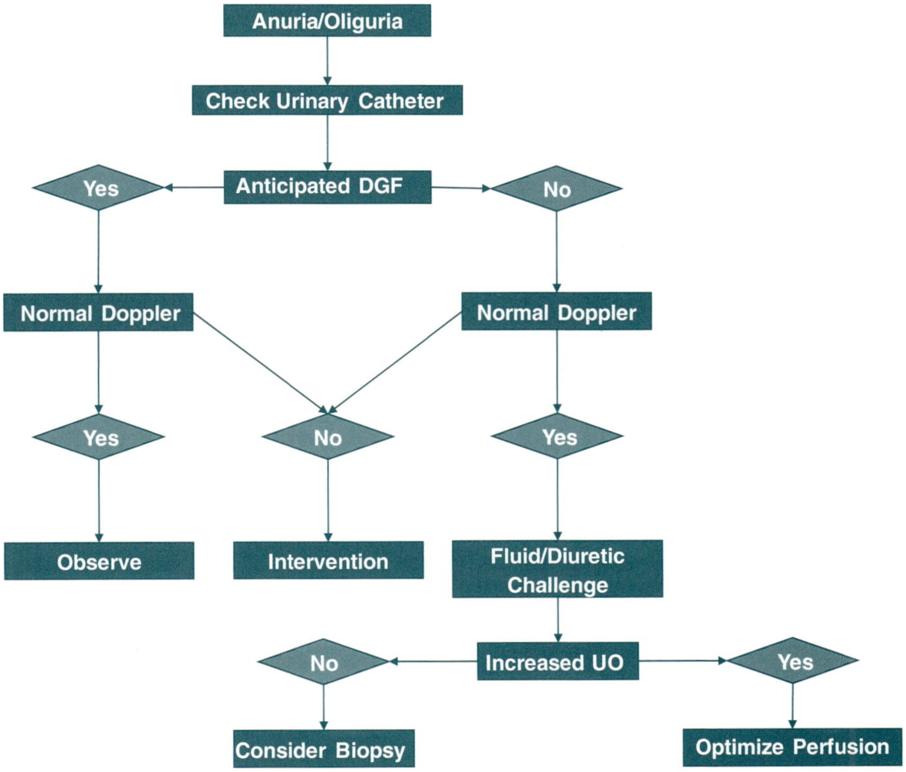

FIG. 37.3 Algorithm for the management of a kidney transplantation patient who develops anuria/oligura.

of the transplanted kidney as the first diagnostic study. Ultrasound is easily accessible, cost-effective, and avoids the risks associated with contrast administration. Criteria for suspicion for TRAS include peak systolic velocity in the renal artery >200 to 300 cm/s, distal spectral broadening, and intraparenchymal arterial acceleration >0.1 s.[42,43] Ultrasound evaluation for TRAS has a sensitivity of 90% to 100% and a specificity of 87% to 100%.[44] TRAS can occur at the site of the anastomosis, at the area of a bend or kink in the artery, or distally along the artery (postanastomotic stricture). Stricture etiologies may vary according to location; anastomotic strictures often are technical complications, whereas postanastomotic strictures are thought to be related to atherosclerotic disease and immunological-mediated factors.[45]

Reported risk factors for TRAS vary but include DGF, cytomegalovirus infection, older recipient age, ECD kidneys, acute rejection, ischemic heart disease, and de novo class II donor-specific antigens.[40,45,46]

TRAS can be treated with percutaneous intervention.[40,41,45,47-50] TRAS lesions were initially treated with percutaneous transluminal angioplasty. However, reported restenosis rate ranges from 20% to 40%.[40,41,49,50] Biederman et al. described 45 patients who underwent 50 interventions for the treatment of TRAS.[41] Eighteen patients received drug-eluting stents, 26 received bare metal stents, and 6 underwent angioplasty alone. Improvement in allograft function was observed in all patients. Patency was significantly higher with stent placement than with angioplasty alone. Complications of stent placement, however, include stent migration and misplaced deployment can lead to dissection or thrombosis. To date, there are no randomized controlled studies comparing angioplasty alone with drug-eluting or bare metal stent placement, so no definitive recommendations can be made. Surgical intervention is warranted if percutaneous intervention fails or there is a complicated stenosis that cannot be approached through percutaneous intervention. Surgical correction has been associated with increased rates of graft loss, reoperation, and mortality.[47]

Renal Vein Thrombosis

Renal vein thrombosis (RVT) is an infrequent complication with an incidence of less than 5% in the perioperative period.[51-53] However, its occurrence frequently results in graft loss and early diagnosis with immediate intervention is paramount for any chance at graft salvage. Many cases of RVT involve a technical problem with the venous anastomosis. A long renal vein can twist or kink, resulting in obstruction and thrombosis. A short renal vein may limit the positioning of the kidney and result in compression during closure. In addition, the renal artery may traverse and compress the renal vein. Uncommonly, the actual anastomosis between the donor renal vein and recipient iliac vein may be narrowed or obstructed. This scenario may be more common when a reconstruction of multiple renal veins has been performed. Data suggests that living donor right renal allografts are at higher risk for RVT than left renal allografts.[54,55] The implication is that a shorter renal vein is associated with a higher RVT rate than a longer renal vein. This may be due to limits

Inverted M Waveform in Renal Vein Thrombosis

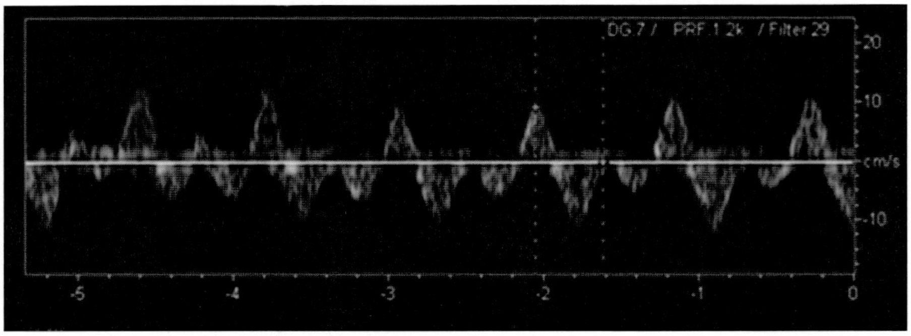

FIG. 37.4 Doppler waveform in a patient with renal vein thrombosis.

positioning an allograft associated with a short renal vein. Other risk factors for RVT include a hypercoagulable state, severe ATN, or severe acute cellular rejection[51,52]; the latter two conditions resulting in severe graft edema, decreased allograft blood flow, and risk for thrombosis. Cases of hyperacute rejection also can present with RVT in the immediate postoperative setting.

Diagnosis of RVT requires a high index of suspicion and should be considered whenever there is sudden onset anuria, oliguria, or hematuria in a previously functioning graft. Patients also may present with acute swelling and tenderness over the graft. Laboratory examination also may reveal development of thrombocytopenia related to platelet consumption in the thrombosed graft. The first and best study for diagnosis of RVT should be Doppler ultrasound of the allograft. Lack of visualization of the renal vein in combination with diastolic flow reversal in the renal artery, although not specific, is highly suspicious for RVT and should prompt contrast venography or operative exploration.[56] The degree of diastolic flow reversal can range from a transient "spike" waveform or continuous or "plateau" waveform to an inverted "M" waveform (Fig. 37.4).[51] Transient diastolic flow reversal also can be seen in severe ATN or rejection when edema results in increased resistance to arterial flow within the graft but this should be a diagnosis of exclusion.[56,57]

Acute complete RVT uniformly results in allograft loss and requires nephrectomy. A kidney cannot tolerate absence of blood flow for more than 45 to 60 minutes. In the operating room, the allograft appears swollen with hemorrhagic infarction. Rare instances of salvage of kidneys with RVT have been described both with surgical and endovascular techniques.[58]

Ureteral Complications

Urine Leak

Urine leaks occur in 1% to 6% of kidney transplant recipients and usually are diagnosed in the early postoperative period.[43,59,60] Urine leaks arise secondary to technical complications or ischemia of the ureter. Reported risk factors include single U-stitch technique, male and African American recipients, donor age, multiple renal arteries, and delayed graft function.[59,60] Patients may present with tenderness at the graft site, fever, decreased urine output, and elevated creatinine levels.

In the evaluation of these patients, perinephric fluid collections usually are detected by ultrasound and appear hypoechoic or anechoic, sometimes with internal debris. These fluid collections are difficult to differentiate on ultrasound from lymphomas, seromas, or hematomas. On noncontrast imaging with CT scan or magnetic resonance imaging (MRI), urinomas also have the same attenuation as simple fluid. Contrast imaging or nuclear medicine studies may be performed to detect a urine leak. Alternatively, fluid collections that are enlarging or symptomatic may be percutaneous drained. The fluid can then be sent for creatinine level to diagnose a urine leak.

Small leaks from the ureteral anastomosis or collecting system may heal with nephrostomy tube and stent placement. Similarly, small leaks from the bladder may heal with Foley catheter placement and decompression. However, large or persistent leaks or leaks occurring in the very early postoperative period often require surgical intervention. Englesbe et al. studied 1698 consecutive kidney transplants and found urine leaks in 27 (1.6%) patients.[59] Patients with urine leaks during the immediate postoperative period underwent surgical repair. Patients presenting at a later time after kidney transplant underwent placement of a nephroureteral stent, which was successful in 66% of patients. The remaining patients subsequently underwent surgical repair. Berli et al. examined 2671 kidney transplants and found that 51 patients underwent intervention for ureteral complications.[60] Of these patients, 43% had surgical intervention within 60 days of the operation, which were all for management of urine leaks. Surgical techniques included anastomotic repair or revision and reimplantation of the ureter.

Urinary Obstruction

Primary urinary obstruction after kidney transplantation occurs in 2% to 6% of patients and is usually secondary to a ureteral stricture.[43,59,60] The majority of these strictures occur in the distal ureter.[61] Patients often are found to have hydronephrosis on ultrasound before any clinical symptoms. Advanced cases may present with decreased urine output, elevated creatinine levels, and abdominal discomfort.

The presumed etiology for ureteral stricture is technical factors or ischemia caused by disruption to the surrounding fatty tissues that contain the ureteral blood supply. Reported risk factors include multiple renal arteries, delayed graft function, donor age, urinary tract infection, acute rejection, and BK virus.[60,62,63] After ultrasound, a percutaneous nephrogram can diagnose the site and severity of the stricture.

The approach to treatment of ureteral stricture after kidney transplant has traditionally been open surgical intervention, but the advent of percutaneous endourological techniques has led to an increase in potential treatment options.[64] A systematic review by Kwong et al. examined 34 articles on ureteral strictures after kidney transplant.[61] The open approach, most commonly ureteric reimplantation, had an 85.4% success rate compared with 64.3% for the endourological approach. The most common endourological approach was dilation alone, although reported techniques included dilation with laser, electrocautery, and endoureterotomy. Englesbe et al. described ureteral strictures in 2.8% of their 1698 patients who underwent kidney transplant.[59] Of patients with ureteral strictures, 68% were treated with percutaneous nephroureteral stents with or without balloon ureteroplasty and the remaining patients underwent surgical repair. Saeb-Parsy et al. reported a 2.3% incidence of ureteral stricture after kidney transplant in 898 patients.[62] All patients were treated with open reimplantation of the ureter, with a 17% restenosis rate.

Other Complications

Lymphocele

The vast majority of kidney transplants are performed using a retroperitoneal approach to avoid intestinal complications that arise from intraabdominal placement. Lymphocele formation is unique to the retroperitoneal placement of renal transplants and does not occur when the allograft is placed intraabdominally. Lymphoceles arise when lymphatic fluid accumulates in the nonepithelialized retroperitoneal space from transected perivascular lymphatics. Small, stable fluid collections are frequently identified on routine postoperative examination of the renal transplant. Many of these collections may represent fluid accumulation from a transient perioperative lymphatic leak that has resolved. Ongoing lymphatic leakage into the retroperitoneal space can result in massive lymphoceles that manifest symptoms due to compression of adjacent structures including venous compression resulting in lower extremity edema, ureteral obstruction associated with allograft dysfunction and abdominal pain.[65] A recent metaanalysis suggests an incidence of symptomatic lymphocele of 5%.[66]

The goal in the treatment of the symptomatic lymphocele is to decompress the collection and prevent its recurrence. This can be achieved either through percutaneous drainage or surgical fenestration of the fluid collection into the peritoneal cavity. Several treatment options accomplish this with varying levels of invasiveness and efficacy. Aspiration of the fluid collection is the least morbid procedure but results in recurrence in 59% of patients. The addition of a sclerosant decreases the recurrence rate to 31%. Laparoscopic transabdominal fenestration results in a recurrence rate of 8% but is

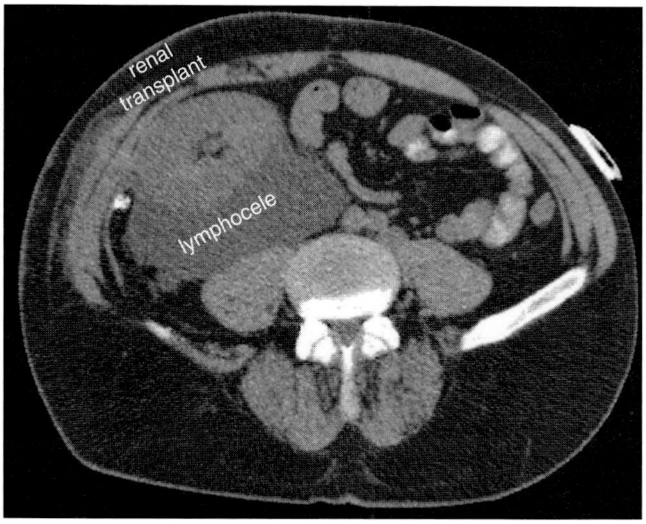

FIG. 37.5 Computed tomography image of a lymphocele after kidney transplant.

more invasive.[66] A reasonable approach to the treatment of the symptomatic lymphocele is to initially aspirate the collection. If the collection recurs, CT or MRI should be obtained to better define the anatomical location of the collection and its relationship to the peritoneum. The majority of symptomatic lymphoceles will abut and displace the peritoneum and provide an approach for fenestration (Fig. 37.5). A percutaneous drainage catheter can be placed to control the accumulation of lymph while laparoscopic fenestration is planned. At the time of laparoscopic fenestration, the catheter can be used to distend the lymphocele with methylene blue and assist in identification of the peritoneum to be fenestrated. In challenging cases, laparoscopic ultrasound can be used to visualize the fluid collection containing the catheter. Care should be taken to avoid injuring the bladder or donor ureter during this procedure and a Foley catheter should be placed preoperatively.

Surgical Site Infection

Patients undergoing kidney transplant are an increased risk for surgical site infections (SSIs) because of their multiple comorbidities and need for immunosuppression after transplant. The incidence of SSIs after kidney transplant ranges from 5% to 27%.[67,68] Reported recipient and postoperative risk factors for wound complications after kidney transplant include older age, higher body mass index, urinary tract infections, prolonged wound drainage, reoperation, diabetes, delayed graft function, and acute rejection.[67-74] Surgical risk factors for SSIs consist of prolonged cold ischemia time and length of surgery, transfusion requirements, use of ureteral stent, and induction agent choice.[75,76] The effect of wound complications on graft and patient survival is controversial, with studies reporting varying results. However, wound complications after kidney transplant can lead to prolonged hospitalization and increased costs, as well as patient discomfort. A study out of the University of Michigan found that SSIs after kidney transplant increased payer outlay by 13%.[68]

CONCLUSIONS

The current approach to kidney transplantation is the culmination of more than 50 years of basic and translational investigation. This treatment provides remarkable improvement in quality of life and decreases mortality for properly selected patients. Evaluation and management requires active collaboration between diverse professionals with specific skills, and each is critical to achieve optimal outcomes. Successful short-term results are now expected; however, urgent issues remain. The shortage of organs for transplantation must be addressed with novel technologies and higher rates of donation. Long-term graft survival remains unacceptably poor due to chronic allograft nephropathy. Solutions await better understanding of the root cause of this difficult to study entity.

A full list of references is available at www.expertconsult.com.

38

Immunosuppressive Therapy

Mary Ann Lim, MD, and Roy D. Bloom, MD

OUTLINE

INTRODUCTION

Significant advances have been made in the field of transplantation since the first successful kidney transplant between identical twins in 1954. A better understanding of immunobiology and immunosuppression not only resulted in transplantation between genetically nonidentical individuals, but has led to declining rates of acute allograft rejection and incrementally improved long-term allograft and recipient outcomes. With close to 18,000 kidney transplants performed in the United States in 2015, this form of therapy is considered the treatment of choice for most patients with end stage renal disease.[1] Optimal care of kidney recipients requires a clear understanding of the nuances of immunosuppressive therapy tailored to each individual patient's needs, as underdosing can lead to rejection and graft loss, whereas excessive immunosuppression can result in serious infections, malignancy, and even death.

In this chapter, we present a brief historical perspective on the evolution of transplantation and immunosuppression. We discuss the importance of individualizing therapy and offer a framework for doing this. We then consider contemporary immunosuppressive therapy, summarizing individual agents, and stressing landmark trials that have led to current treatment standards. We end with a commentary on the use of generic immunosuppression, and explore emerging therapies and future prospects for immunosuppression.

HISTORICAL PERSPECTIVE

When viewed through the lens of medical history, kidney transplantation can be subdivided into four distinct periods, each preceded by a unique technological or medical innovation.

Early Era (1954–1962)

The first human-to-human kidney transplantation was performed by Russian surgeon Yu Yu Voronoy in 1933 across major blood group mismatch, and it resulted in prompt allograft failure.[2] Interest in organ transplantation remained, but it was largely done experimentally among animals until 1954, when the first successful kidney transplantation between identical twins was performed by Joseph Murray.[2] This event heralded intensified interest in the technical and immunobiological aspects of organ transplantation, along with efforts to prevent allograft rejection. Immunosuppressive agents were very limited during this era, primarily comprising corticosteroids and total body irradiation.[3] In the absence of effective immunosuppression, immunological matching between donors and recipients played a central role in transplantation, with most transplants occurring between identical twins and siblings. Consequently, this era was characterized by high rejection rates and dismal 1-year graft survival rates of less than 10%.[3]

The Azathioprine Era (1962–1980)

First synthesized in 1957 as a chemotherapeutic agent, azathioprine (AZA) was found to suppress antibody formation in rabbits exposed to antigens and to extend canine allograft survival.[4,5] The use of AZA in human kidney transplantation was slow to catch on because initial experience with AZA monotherapy was associated with poor outcomes.[2] However, the discovery that combining AZA with prednisone resulted in improved 1-year graft survival (of up to 70%) made this combination the standard immunosuppressive therapy of this era, and ushered in the concept of maintenance chemical immunosuppression.[2,3,6]

The Cyclosporine Era (1980s–1990s)

After the initial isolation of calcineurin inhibitors (CNIs) in 1976, cyclosporine soon became the next therapeutic tool to advance the immunosuppression arsenal.[7] The addition of cyclosporine to combination prednisone and AZA therapy decreased 1-year rejection rates to <50% and improved graft survival rates to >85%.

The Contemporary Era (1990s–Present)

The contemporary era of transplantation began with the discovery that tacrolimus, another CNI, was more efficacious than cyclosporine at clinically relevant dosing, resulting in its approval for organ transplantation in 1994.[8] The approval of mycophenolate mofetil (MMF) shortly thereafter, followed by interleukin (IL)–2 receptor blockers (basiliximab and daclizumab) and then rabbit antithymocyte globulin (rATG) around the millennium, catalyzed the emergence of a variety of new treatment combinations. Now entering the third decade since these contemporary agents were introduced into the clinical arena, they remain the gold standard against which all subsequent comparator immunosuppressive drugs in development have failed to show equivalent, let alone superior, effectiveness. Transplant recipients enjoy significantly lower 1-year rejection rates of 10% to 15% and 1-year graft survival in excess of 95%. As discussed later, challenges in the contemporary era include combating chronic rejection, minimizing side effects of current therapy, and improving long-term graft and patient outcomes.

RISK STRATIFICATION

Before embarking on a comprehensive discussion of current immunosuppressive therapy, the importance of tailoring treatment regimens to an individual recipient's health and personal risk factors needs to be emphasized. Successful management of immunosuppression not only means preventing allograft rejection, but also means keeping the recipient healthy. This entails minimizing or avoiding opportunistic infections and malignancies wherever possible, as well as containing drug-specific side effects. Multiple factors need to be considered when choosing a specific regimen, with the main goal being to balance the benefit of preventing rejections (and thus allograft survival) against the risk for overimmunosuppression. As not every patient has the same risk profile in terms of rejection, infection, and malignancy, it is absolutely vital that an individualized approach is made when it comes to selecting immunosuppressive agents. We believe that the choice of a regimen should be guided by overall efficacy, taking into account the potential toxicities of the drug combinations in the context of immunological and medical risks in individual patients or subpopulations.

Immunological Risk

In the 2009 Kidney Disease Improving Global Outcomes (KDIGO) transplant guidelines, potential recipients are stratified into "high" or "low" immunological risk depending on their risk for rejection.[9] Patients who are younger, have anti-human leukocyte antigen (HLA) antibodies, or, are of African descent are considered high risk for rejection, whereas patients who are older, nonsensitized, of Asian or non-African ancestry, or have received closely HLA-matched kidneys are considered low risk. KDIGO recommends that high-risk patients receive more intensified immunosuppression than would otherwise be administered to low-risk recipients. Although this immunological risk stratification may be broadly applicable, an optimal risk-stratified treatment regimen has not been established because of the lack of standardization with calculated panel reactive antibodies (CPRAs), degree of HLA-mismatch, or demographic factors in immunosuppression studies.

Medical Risk

Patients' medical history, as well as their functional and nutritional status must also be considered in the dosing and choice of immunosuppressants. For example, belatacept use in patients who are Epstein-Barr virus (EBV) seronegative is contraindicated because of the risk for posttransplant lymphoproliferative disease (PTLD). Some transplant professionals consider minimizing or avoiding tacrolimus in elderly recipients because of the potential risk for increased neurotoxicity, or consider a steroid-sparing regimen in patients with bipolar disorder because of risk for exacerbation.

Overall Efficacy

An evidence-based approach of overall efficacy using high-quality studies and randomized trials (whenever possible) should guide immunosuppression management. In transplant recipients, efficacy of therapy should translate into lower rates of rejection and improved graft and patient survival. As we review contemporary therapies and landmark trials that led to current standards, it should be kept in mind that although registries offer the benefit of generalizations from large patient cohorts, they usually are limited by incomplete information related to indication for use/nonuse of certain agents, dose adjustment or drug concentrations/exposures, and inadequate information on specific complications. On the other hand, although prospective randomized trials eliminate these shortcomings, many of these trials are constrained by small cohorts in single centers.

CONTEMPORARY IMMUNOSUPPRESSIVE THERAPY

A clear grasp of the alloimmune response should simplify understanding of how specific immunosuppressive agents work. The reader is referred to Chapter 35 for a detailed review of transplant immunobiology. T-cell activation will be briefly summarized here because most pharmacological targets are aimed against T-cell activation.

After an antigen-presenting cell (APC) interacts with a T cell, three distinct and sequential signals occur to activate the T cell (Fig. 38.1). Signal 1 is delivered when the major histocompatibility complex on the APC binds to the T-cell receptor. Signal 2, or costimulation, is delivered by B7 proteins (CD80 and CD86) on APCs binding to CD28 on T cells. These two signals activate the calcium–calcineurin pathway, the Ras–mitogen–activated protein kinase pathway, and the nuclear factor kappa B pathway, resulting in the expression of IL-2 and other cytokines. Signal 3 is generated by IL-2 binding to its receptor, leading to the activation of the mammalian target of rapamycin (mTOR), and subsequent T-cell proliferation and amplification. By targeting one or more of these signals, immunosuppressive agents disrupt the normal adaptive immune response, preventing allograft rejection and improving transplant outcomes.

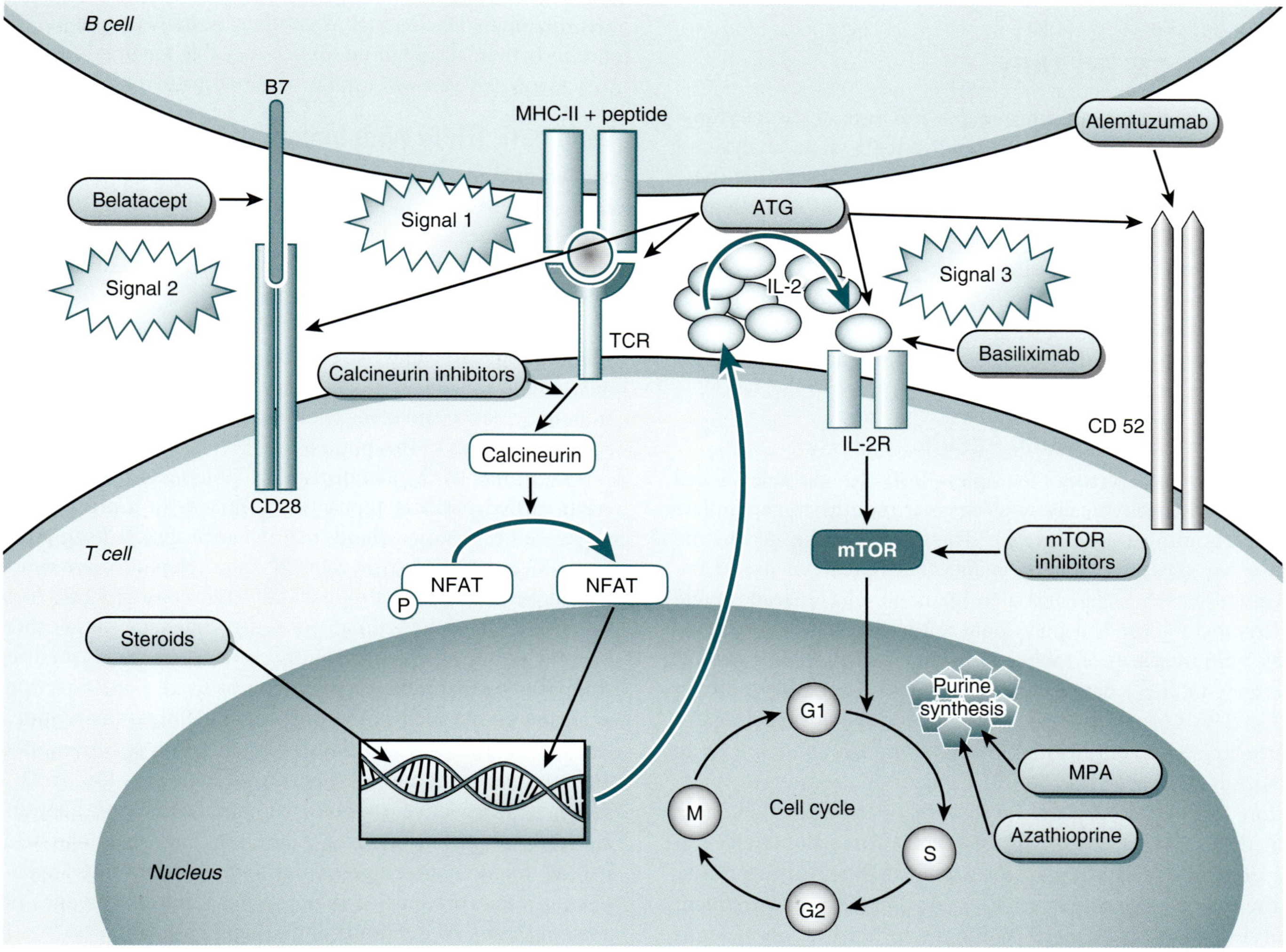

FIG. 38.1 T-cell activation pathways and targets of immunosuppression. The three signals involved in T-cell activation and the specific targets of currently used immunosuppression are depicted in this figure. Alemtuzumab and basiliximab are monoclonal antibodies, whereas ATG, as a polyclonal antibody, has multiple specificities. All three are used as induction agents. Steroids, CNIs, MPA, AZA, mTOR inhibitors, and belatacept comprise maintenance-immunosuppressive agents. Steroids inhibit transcription of inflammatory cytokines, CNIs bind to proteins forming complexes that prevent release of calcineurin, inhibiting NFAT dephosphorylation and ultimately IL-2 transcription, MPA inhibits inosine-5′-monophosphate dehydrogenase and prevents purine synthesis, mTOR inhibitors inhibit signal transduction through mTOR and leads to cell cycle arrest, azathioprine inhibits de novo purine synthesis pathway through suppression of the enzyme glutamine phosphoribosyl pyrophosphate aminotransferase, belatacept binds to CD28, blocking signal 2. *ATG*, Antithymocyte globulin; *AZA*, azathioprine; *CNI*, calcineurin inhibitor; *IL*, interleukin-; *IL-2R*, IL-2 receptor; *MHC*, major histocompatibility complex class; *MPA*, mycophenolic acid; *mTOR*, mammalian target of rapamycin; *NFAT*, nuclear factor of activated T cells; *TCR*, T-cell receptor.

The highest rates of acute rejection and graft loss usually occur within the first several months after engraftment. For this reason, the majority of kidney transplant recipients receive more intensive immunosuppression at the time of transplant (induction therapy) and in the early posttransplant setting, with progressive reduction in the dosing and stringency of maintenance immunosuppressive therapy over time. We discuss the therapies used for induction and maintenance immunosuppression in the following section. A description of each agent, followed by their mechanisms of action and common side effects precede an examination of landmark trials that illustrate efficacy and safety of current therapies.

INDUCTION THERAPY

Induction therapy, administered at the time of kidney transplantation, first gained popularity after a meta-analysis of available trials concluded that regimens incorporating these agents were associated with reduced rejection and allograft loss at 2 years posttransplant.[10] Since then, the use of induction agents has steadily increased, with more than 80% of transplant recipients in the United States receiving some form of induction therapy.[11] In general, induction agents can be divided into lymphocyte-depleting agents and nonlymphocyte-depleting agents.

Lymphocyte-Depleting Agents

Lymphocyte-depleting therapies lead to durable T-cell depletion that typically takes several months to repopulate to preadministration levels.[12] This section is limited to the two lymphocyte-depleting agents that remain in use in the United States: rATG and alemtuzumab. rATG (trade name Thymoglobulin) is a polyclonal antibody preparation made by immunization of rabbits with human lymphoid tissue. It targets multiple pathways in T-cell activation and results in T-cell lysis (see Fig. 38.1). Initially developed decades ago to *treat* rejection, but only approved by the US Food and Drug Administration (FDA) in 2017 specifically to *prevent* rejection, rATG has been the most widely used induction agent in the United States for many years.[11] It usually is given at a dose of 1 to 1.5 mg/kg for a total of three to five doses. The major early side effect is serum sickness, an infrequent occurrence because of concomitant administration of high-dose steroids. Other side effects include constitutional symptoms such as fever, chills or arthralgias, hematological side effects such as leukopenia, thrombocytopenia and clotting of dialysis accesses, and a propensity for certain infections and malignancies. Alemtuzumab (trade name Campath 1H), initially developed to treat chronic lymphocytic leukemia, also has been used for induction therapy, although it is not FDA-approved for this latter indication. It is a recombinant DNA-derived humanized monoclonal antibody (mAb) against cell surface glycoprotein CD52 in T and B cells, and results in profound and prolonged depletion of peripheral and central lymphoid cells (see Fig. 38.1). It usually is given as a single intraoperative dose, allowing ease of administration and shorter hospital stay. Side effects include infusion reactions such as fever, chills, nausea, and rash. Profound lymphocyte depletion also can lead to serious infections.

Interleukin-2 Receptor Blockers

Basiliximab (brand name Simulect) is currently the only non-lymphocyte-depleting agent used in kidney transplantation. It is a chimeric monoclonal anti-CD25 antibody that targets CD25 on the IL-2 receptor, effectively preventing delivery of signal 3 need for T-cell activation (see Fig. 38.1). It is given in two 20-mg doses, usually given 4 days apart. It has few side effects, but because it prevents T-cell proliferation rather than causing depletion, it is considered less potent than rATG or alemtuzumab. Daclizumab is another humanized anti-CD25 antibody that, although no longer available for use, is of historical interest as it was used in some of the pivotal trials.

Landmark Trials With Induction Therapy

Most induction trials have been limited by being underpowered, with wide variation regarding accompanying maintenance therapies used, short follow-up, and primary endpoints largely focused on reduced acute rejection rates. In this section, we review the most pertinent studies.

The superiority of rATG over IL-2 receptor blockade in immunologically high-risk recipients has been demonstrated in two randomized controlled trials (RCTs), showing a reduction in incidence and severity of rejection, as well as improved 5-year outcomes in this population.[12,13]

Compared with alemtuzumab, outcomes for basiliximab-treated patients appear to be mixed. In a prospective single-center study, where maintenance immunosuppression differed in each arm, rates of acute rejection were similar but chronic allograft injury and death-censored graft loss was higher in alemtuzumab-treated recipients.[14] In another prospective, single-center study, where uniform prednisone-sparing maintenance regimen was used, acute rejection occurred earlier after basiliximab than alemtuzumab induction (51 ± 83 vs. 148 ± 82 days), but 12-month rejection rates and survival outcomes were similar.[15] A third study, the 3C study, a prospective randomized trial, compared alemtuzumab with prednisone-free, tacrolimus-mycophenolic acid (MPA) maintenance against basiliximab-tacrolimus-mycophenolic acid-prednisone therapy, and found lower rates of acute rejection by 6 months in the alemtuzumab group.[16]

Alemtuzumab also was compared with basiliximab in low immunological risk patients and to rATG in high-risk recipients in a prospective randomized trial in which all patients received maintenance therapy with tacrolimus-MMF after early prednisone withdrawal.[17] At 3 years posttransplant, alemtuzumab was superior to basiliximab in preventing rejection in low-risk patients (10% vs. 22%; $P = 0.003$), whereas alemtuzumab and rATG fared similarly in high-risk recipients (18% vs. 15%). Adverse reactions were similar in all treatment groups.

Several retrospective analyses have compared alemtuzumab with rATG, with results generally favoring the latter induction agent. In one study of deceased donor kidney recipients, patient survival and adjusted allograft survival were inferior in alemtuzumab-treated patients.[18] A registry analysis examined outcomes in lower immunological-risk live kidney recipients, stratified by use or nonuse of steroids together with tacrolimus-MPA maintenance immunosuppression.[19] Among recipients on steroid-free regimens, acute rejection was lower with rATG (odds ratio [OR], 0.73; 95% confidence interval [CI], 0.59 to 0.90) and alemtuzumab (OR, 0.53; 95% CI, 0.42 to 0.67) than IL-2 receptor blocker; however, there was an increased risk for allograft failure with alemtuzumab (hazard ratio [HR], 1.27; 95% CI, 1.03 to 1.56) but not rATG compared with IL-2 blocker.[19] Among those on a steroid-containing regimen, rATG use was associated with lower rejection rates than IL-2 receptor antibodies (OR, 0.78; $P = 0.001$), although this did not translate into a graft survival advantage.[19]

In a more recent study where Organ Procurement and Transplantation Network data were linked with Medicare claims, outcomes were compared after 1:1 matching of recipient pairs of alemtuzumab versus rATG and rATG versus basiliximab.[20] Compared with recipients treated with rATG, the risk for death or allograft failure was increased by 18% with alemtuzumab and 8% with basiliximab.[20]

In summary, most studies show that compared with lymphocyte-depleting agents, basiliximab may have a better safety profile comparable to placebo, although in high-risk recipients, it is associated with higher rates of rejection and donor-specific antibody formation.[12,13,17,21,22] KDIGO transplant guidelines recommend basiliximab induction in low immunological risk recipients and lymphocyte-depleting therapies in high immunological risk recipients.[9] We generally endorse KDIGO recommendations, although favor rATG over alemtuzumab as the lymphocyte-depleting therapy of choice based on the data just described.

MAINTENANCE IMMUNOSUPPRESSIVE THERAPY

The main goal of maintenance immunosuppression is to prevent rejection and safely preserve allograft function on a chronic basis. Contemporary maintenance immunosuppressive therapy in most US transplant centers is based on a combination of six mechanistically different agents: prednisone, CNIs, AZA, MMF/MPA, mTOR inhibitors, and belatacept. These agents will first be discussed individually, focusing on their mechanisms of action and side effects. This will be followed by a discussion of landmark trials that culminated in the emergence of the current standard of care therapies.

Corticosteroids

Corticosteroids have been used since the early days of organ transplantation and remain a basic component of many immunosuppression protocols. Corticosteroids act by blocking T-cell derived and APC-derived cytokine and cytokine expression via different mechanisms.[23-28] After passive diffusion across the cell membrane, steroids bind to intracellular glucocorticoid receptors forming complexes that then translocate into the nucleus. These complexes interact with glucocorticoid-responsive elements, resulting in altered transcription of various cytokines (see Fig. 38.1).[23-28] By affecting posttranslational events, steroids also inhibit secretion of inflammatory cytokines.[28] High-dose steroids are typically administered intravenously in the perioperative period as part of the induction regimen, followed by oral dose tapering. Although some centers completely eliminate maintenance prednisone using an avoidance or early posttransplant withdrawal approach (steroid-sparing regimens), most continue low-dose maintenance prednisone (e.g., tapered to 5 mg/day by 1 to 2 months posttransplant). High-dose corticosteroid therapy is associated with several adverse effects such as growth retardation in children, glucose intolerance and diabetes, osteoporosis, avascular necrosis, dyslipidemia, hypertension, impaired wound healing, skin fragility, and cataracts.

Calcineurin Inhibitors

CNIs have dramatically affected allograft outcomes. The two CNIs used in transplant are cyclosporine and tacrolimus, with tacrolimus considered more potent at clinically relevant dosing. Calcineurin dephosphorylates transcription factors, including nuclear factor of activated T cells, which can then translocate into the nucleus and induce gene transcription (see Fig. 38.1). Cyclosporine and tacrolimus bind to cyclophilin and FK-binding protein, respectively, forming active complexes that inhibit calcineurin release and thereby block subsequent T-cell activation. Cyclosporine and tacrolimus have similar side-effect profiles with few differences detailed in Table 38.1. Both undergo gut and hepatic metabolism via cytochrome P450 enzymes. Because several drugs commonly used in transplantation (e.g., macrolides, azoles, dihydropyridine calcium channel blockers, amiodarone, and HIV medications) are metabolized by this enzyme system, mindfulness for drug–drug interactions is required in patients receiving CNIs.

Historically, CNIs were manufactured as twice-daily formulations. Two tacrolimus formulations that require only once-daily dosing have recently been approved in several countries. Tacrolimus-ER (brand name Astagraf XL in the United States, Advagraf in Europe) and LCP-tacrolimus (brand name Envarsus XR), demonstrated to be noninferior to twice-daily tacrolimus in conversion and de novo RCTs, offer the

TABLE 38.1 Potential Adverse Effects of Calcineurin-Inhibitors

Adverse Effects	Cyclosporine	Tacrolimus
Nephrotoxicity	+++	+
Hypertension	++	+
Hyperkalemia	++	++
Hypomagnesemia	++	++
Hyperuricemia	+++	+
Neurotoxicity	+	+++
Posttransplant diabetes	+	+++
Hyperlipidemia	++	+
Hair changes	Hirsutism	Alopecia
Thrombotic microangiopathy	Rare	Rare
Gingival hyperplasia	+	-
Hepatotoxicity	Rare	Rare

potential of improved patient adherence.[29-33] Pharmacokinetic differences between the once- and twice-daily formulations often impact the total daily tacrolimus dose requirement for patients. When switching between formulations, we recommend monitoring through tacrolimus levels at 1 and 3 weeks postconversion and dose titration as indicated.

Mycophenolic Acid

MPA is a noncompetitive inhibitor of the rate-limiting enzyme inosine monophosphate dehydrogenase in the de novo purine biosynthesis pathway (see Fig. 38.1). Because lymphocytes cannot efficiently use the salvage pathway and are highly dependent on the de novo pathway of purine synthesis, MPA effectively inhibits the proliferation of T and B lymphocytes. MPA is poorly absorbed after oral administration and is therefore formulated as a prodrug to improve drug bioavailability, as either MMF (brand name CellCept) or mycophenolate sodium (MPS, brand name Myfortic). MMF, a semisynthetic derivative of MPA produced by the fungus *Penicillium,* was first approved by the FDA in 1995 for use in kidney transplantation, whereas MPS was approved about a decade later. After oral administration, MMF is rapidly and completely converted to MPA in the stomach; this process is delayed with MPS, occurring more distally in the gastrointestinal tract. Although not bioequivalent, MMF and MPS have been demonstrated to have very similar efficacy and safety profiles. Common side effects include nausea, vomiting, and diarrhea, occasional severe esophagitis and gastritis, oral ulcers and leukopenia.

Azathioprine

AZA is a purine analog that inhibits the de novo purine synthesis pathway through suppression of the enzyme glutamine phosphoribosyl pyrophosphate aminotransferase (see Fig. 38.1). Purine nucleotides form key elements of DNA and RNA; inhibition of purine synthesis therefore affects DNA synthesis required for cell proliferation, and RNA transcription required for protein synthesis. In addition, purines are needed for the glycosylation of adhesion molecules and the activation of lymphocytes and macrophages. AZA usually is given at a maintenance dose of 1 to 2 mg/kg daily as a single oral dose, with dose adjusted to white blood cell count >3500 cells/mm^3. Side effects of AZA include bone marrow suppression (usually reversed by decreasing the dose), hepatitis, pancreatitis, and hair loss. It is metabolized in the liver to 6-mercaptopurine, which is subsequently converted to inactive 6-thiouric acid by xanthine oxidase. Because of this, simultaneous administration with a xanthine oxidase inhibitor such as allopurinol can lead to significantly high levels of AZA and profound and long-lasting neutropenia; therefore AZA dose should be reduced when combined with allopurinol or the combination avoided if possible.

mTOR Inhibitors

The mTOR inhibitors form complexes with the FK-binding protein that subsequently bind to mTOR, causing dephosphorylation and inactivation of p70S6 kinase. By inhibiting G1 to S phase of the cell cycle, this effectively blocks cytokine-driven T-cell proliferation. The two mTOR inhibitors used in clinical transplantation are sirolimus and everolimus. Side effects in the early posttransplant period include delayed graft function, poor wound healing, and lymphoceles, whereas longer-term side effects include severe edema, proteinuria, hyperlipidemia, thrombocytopenia, leukopenia, and anemia.

Belatacept

Belatacept is a fusion protein that binds to CD80/CD86 on APCs, thereby effectively blocking the costimulatory signal required for T-cell activation (see Fig. 38.1). The most important reported side effects are increased risk for central nervous system PTLD and progressive multifocal leukoencephalopathy (PML), especially in EBV-seronegative recipients. As a result, belatacept is now contraindicated in patients whose EBV serostatus is unknown or negative.

Combination Therapies and Trials That Led to Current Standards

Because the combination of AZA with prednisone was shown to be safer and more efficacious than either agent alone more than 5 decades ago, clinical trials have focused on using combination therapies with each new agent that came along for several reasons. First, since T-cell activation is complex, combination therapies provide the opportunity to simultaneously target multiple steps involved in the process of activation and thereby circumvent potentially redundant pathways. Furthermore, combination therapies can bring about a state of adequate overall immunosuppression at submaximal doses of individual agents, therefore minimizing drug-specific toxicities that might occur with use of individual therapies at higher doses.

Most centers currently use a multidrug maintenance regimen comprising one agent from each column in Table 38.2, although use of prednisone is quite variable. As a result of RCTs demonstrating lower rates of rejection and better allograft and patient survival compared with cyclosporine, tacrolimus has been the predominant CNI since the turn of the century. MPA-based therapies are typically used in conjunction with tacrolimus based on comparative trials demonstrating less acute rejection than AZA.[34-39] According to US Registry data, regimens comprising tacrolimus-MPA (with or without prednisone) were used in 93% of all de novo kidney

TABLE 38.2 Combination Immunosuppression Therapies

Combination Therapies Usually Consist of An Agent From Column I, An Agent From Column II, With or Without Prednisone

I	II	III
Tacrolimus	Mycophenolate mofetil	Prednisone
Cyclosporine	Azathioprine	
Sirolimus	Sirolimus	
Belatacept	Everolimus	

transplants in 2015, thereby constituting the contemporary gold standard against which both existing and investigational therapies are tested.[11]

Because contemporary regimens have resulted in significant declines in acute rejection rates and improved allograft survival, clinical trials have focused on minimizing deleterious adverse effects of long-term maintenance immunosuppression. Outside of cancer and infection, risks that are associated with all immunosuppressive drugs, common drug-specific side effects include nephrotoxicity and neurotoxicity with CNIs, as well as metabolic and cardiovascular effects with steroids, CNIs, and mTOR inhibitors. To mitigate the risk for these adverse effects, clinical investigation has focused on regimens that minimize or avoid exposure to CNIs and steroids.

CNI-SPARING THERAPIES

Four different CNI-sparing strategies have been proposed: (1) minimization, where the CNI dose administered is reduced (either de novo or later posttransplant); (2) conversion, where the CNI is typically weaned and replaced with an alternative; (3) withdrawal/elimination, where CNIs are initially administered at standard or minimized dose, then eliminated or weaned at a defined point posttransplant with no replacement agent added; and (4) avoidance, where CNIs are completely avoided from time of transplant. CNI-sparing strategies by definition rely on the alternative therapies, MPA regimens, mTOR inhibitors, and belatacept to provide adequate immunosuppression coverage.

A summary of landmark, prospective RCTs of CNI-sparing regimens is presented in Table 38.3. Most trials using CNI-avoidance or elimination therapy under coverage of MPA-based therapy have shown higher rejection rates and worse graft outcomes. Consequently, regimens based primarily on MPA are seldom used in clinical transplant practice. ELITE-Symphony (Efficacy Limiting Toxicity Elimination-Symphony) was a very large, four-arm multicontinental RCT that compared CNI minimization in two arms and avoidance with use of sirolimus in one arm against standard cyclosporine-based therapy. Although outcomes were best in the minimized tacrolimus group, it is worth noting that achieved tacrolimus levels were higher than the prespecified targets.[36,40-42]

Among trials using mTOR inhibitors to spare CNI exposure de novo, most have shown inferior outcomes, more postoperative complications, and higher treatment failure rates in patients randomized to the mTOR arms, with either sirolimus- or everolimus-based therapy.[36,43-52] De novo use of mTORs has largely fallen by the wayside because of issues with wound healing and higher rates of delayed graft function and acute rejection. Several trials have evaluated conversion from CNI to mTOR inhibitors, often in the setting of allograft dysfunction. Although some studies have demonstrated small improvements in kidney function after conversion, from cyclosporine in particular, most have been associated with increased rates of treatment failure, and no overall outcomes improvement. Patients with either proteinuria or an estimated glomerular filtration rate <40 mL/min at the time of conversion, appear to be at heightened risk for more rapid progression of chronic allograft injury. For this reason, KDIGO transplant guidelines only recommend using mTOR inhibitor in patients whose kidney function exceeds this kidney function threshold and with a urine protein/creatinine ratio <0.5 g/g.[9]

The pivotal BENEFIT (Belatacept Evaluation of Nephroprotection and Efficacy as First-line Immunosuppresion Trial) and BENEFIT-EXT (Extended Criteria Donors) trials, which evaluated efficacy and safety of belatacept, have compared its use in a CNI-avoidance manner to cyclosporine-based therapy, predominantly in low immunological recipients. Although the belatacept arms had higher rates of early posttransplant rejection, both long-term graft survival and kidney function were significantly better in the patients randomized to costimulation blockade.[53-57] To date, the single published prospective, randomized trial that compared belatacept with tacrolimus-based therapy in low immunological risk, live donor recipients demonstrated that acute rejection was more frequent and more severe in belatacept-treated patients.[58] At 12 months, there was no significant difference in kidney function between the two regimens. The findings of this study do have to be tempered by the small sample size and short follow-up. Conversion from CNI- to belatacept-based therapy in stable kidney recipients has been investigated in a phase II RCT and demonstrated mild improvement in renal function 12 months postconversion despite higher risk for rejection.[59] These findings notwithstanding, belatacept has not been very widely used in organ transplantation. In addition to higher rates of rejection, concerns include that the control arms in the pivotal trials were cyclosporine-based, study populations have been low immunological risk, and the absence of large RCTs undertaken to compare belatacept with tacrolimus-MMF–based therapy. In addition, belatacept incurs greater cost than generic regimens and requires an infusion. Despite some of the attractive attributes of belatacept that emerged from BENEFIT, unless large-scale multicenter safety and efficacy RCTs are performed that compare it with tacrolimus, it will likely struggle to gain traction in the transplant community. Finally, the safety and efficacy of minimized tacrolimus used together with belatacept remains to be determined.

A systematic review and metaanalysis of CNI-sparing regimens in kidney transplantation concluded that there is moderate- to high-strength evidence to suggest that minimization strategies result in better clinical outcomes and that CNI conversion to mTOR inhibitors or belatacept was associated with better renal function but higher rejection risk.[60] However, because most of the studies evaluated cyclosporine-sparing regimens in lower-immunological risk populations, the generalizability of these data to the current era where the gold standard is tacrolimus-MMF–based therapy is limited.

A consistent theme of CNI-sparing regimens pertains to their role in attenuating nephrotoxicity.[61] Most studies have demonstrated that tacrolimus is less nephrotoxic than

TABLE 38.3 **Summary of Randomized Controlled Trials of CNI-Sparing Therapies**

Trial Name/ Author	Study Design	Treatment Arms	Primary Endpoint(s)	Efficacy Outcomes	Comments
USING MYCOPHENOLIC ACID					
CAESAR/ Ekberg[40]	Prospective, multicenter open-label RCT, lower immunological risk, 536 de novo recipients.	(1) Low CyA (levels 50–100 ng/mL), (2) Low CyA for 4 mo, then weaned off at 6 mo, (3) Standard CyA levels.	eGFR at 12 mo posttransplant.	At 12 mo: (1) eGFR similar. (2) AR 38% in withdrawal arm vs. 25.4% (low CyA) and 27.5% (standard), $P <$ 0.05.	All patients received daclizumab, MMF, and prednisone.
ELITE-SYM-PHONY /Ekberg[36]	Prospective, multicenter open-label RCT, 1645 de novo recipients.	(1) Standard CyA, (2) Low Tac (target level 3–7 ng/mL), (3) Low CyA (target level 50–100 ng/mL), (4) SRL (target trough level 4–8 ng/mL).	eGFR at 12 mo posttransplant.	At 12 mo, $P < 0.05$: (1) eGFR highest in Tac arm, lowest in SRL arm. (2) AR lowest in Tac arm, highest in SRL arm. (3) Allograft survival highest in the Tac arm.	(1) MMF-prednisone used in all patients. (2) Daclizumab in arms 2–4. (3) Mean Tac level at 12 mo was 6.4 + 2.4 ng/mL.
ELITE-SYM-PHONY extension Ekberg [41]	Observational follow-up, 958 participants for additional 24 mo.		eGFR at 36 mo posttransplant.	At 36 mo: (1) eGFR highest in Tac arm, lowest in SRL arm, *P* value not significant. (2) AR lowest in Tac arm, highest in SRL arm. (3) Allograft survival highest in the Tac arm.	(1) Differences were less striking than at 12 mo. (2) Mean Tac level at 36 mo was 6.5 + 2.3 ng/mL.
OPTICEPT/ Gaston[42]	Prospective open-label, multicenter trial, 720 recipients.	(1) Concentration-controlled MMF + low CNI, (2) concentration-controlled MMF + standard CNI arm, (3) Fixed dose MMF + standard CNI dosing.	Treatment failure (death, graft loss, rejection) at 12 mo.	At 1 y: (1) No difference in AR, graft loss or death. (2) eGFR similar in all groups.	(1) ~80% treated with Tac. (2) Achieved levels in the low Tac arm were ~7 ng/mL (at 3 mo) and ~6 ng/mL (12 mo), higher than prespecified targets (4–6 ng/mL and 3–5 ng/mL). (3) MPA levels did not impact outcomes in Tac-treated patients.
USING MTOR-INHIBITORS					
ORION/ Flechner[43]	Open-label, multinational, 443 de novo recipients.	(1) Control (Tac-MMF), (2) CNI-avoidance (SRL-MMF) and, (3) CNI-elimination (Tac-SRL, then Tac elimination at week 13).	eGFR at 12 mo posttransplant.	Overall 1- and 2-y AR rates were higher in both Tac-sparing regimens compared with Tac-MMF, with no eGFR benefit.	CNI-avoidance arm was prematurely terminated because of high rejection rates.
Chan[44]	Prospective, multicenter, open-label, 6-mo trial of 92 low-risk, de novo recipients.	(1) Standard Tac (8–11 ng/mL, months 0–3; 7–10 ng/mL, months 4–6), (2) Low Tac (4–7 ng/mL, months 0–3; 3–6 ng/mL, months 4–6).	Serum creatinine and acute rejection at 6 mo.	Mean 6-mo creatinine levels and acute rejection rates at 6 mo were not statistically different between groups.	(1)All received basiliximab, everolimus and steroids. (2) Despite prespecified levels, achieved Tac levels were similar (~7 ng/mL) in both arms.

ASSET/ Langer[45]	Open-label, 12-mo trial of 224 low-risk de novo kidney recipients.	(1) Low Tac (trough 4–7 ng/mL), (2) Very low Tac (trough 1.5–3 ng/mL) levels.	eGFR at 12 mo posttransplant.	At 12 mo: (1) eGFR did not differ between arms. (2) Efficacy failure rates (rejection, graft loss, death or loss to follow-up) were increased in the very low-level group.	(1) All received basiliximab, everolimus and steroids. (2) Mean Tac levels at 12 mo were within range in the low Tac arm, but above target in the very low Tac arm.
Spare-the-Nephron (STN)/ Weir[46]	2-y, open-label, multicenter trial of 299 patients randomized at 115 d posttransplant.	(1) MMF + CNI, (2) MMF + SRL.	eGFR change after 2 y.	At 2 y, similar measures of renal function but with fewer deaths in the MMF-SRL arm.	Of 151 patients on CNI: 120 on tac, 31 on CyA.
Weir[47]	Prospective, observational study of 128 patients from STN Study who had a functioning graft at 2 y.			At 8 y posttransplant, eGFR was similar, but patients in MMF-SRL arm had more cardiovascular events.	
Silva[48]	Multicenter, open-label, 283 de novo kidney recipients randomized at 3 mo posttransplant.	(1) Tacrolimus (n = 107), (2) Sirolimus (n = 91).	eGFR at 24 mo.	(1) No difference in eGFR. (2) No difference in the severity of chronic sclerosing lesions scores in 24-mo protocol biopsies. (3) Higher mean urinary protein-to-creatinine ratio and higher incidence of treated acute rejection between months 3 and 24 (13.4% vs. 4.7%, P = 0.047) in SRL compared with Tac group.	(1) All treated with Tac-MMF-prednisone initially. (2) A third group (n = 79) comprised of patients who were not allowed to undergo conversion for various reasons.
ZEUS/ Budde[49]	3-y follow-up of an open-label, multicenter ZEUS study of 300 kidney transplant recipients randomized at 4.5 mo.	(1) Continue CyA, (2) Convert to everolimus.	eGFR at 24 and 36 mo.	(1) Everolimus arm had better eGFR at 24 and 26 mo (7.5 mL/min/1.73m^2 more, P < 0.001). (2) Everolimus arm had higher incidence of AR at 36 mo (13% vs. 4.8%, P = 0.015). (3) Patient and graft survival, incidences of malignancy, severe infections and hospitalization, were similar between groups.	CNI therapy was reintroduced in 28.4% of everolimus patients by month 36.
CONVERT/ Schena[50]	24-mo efficacy and safety data of phase IIIB prospective, multicenter trial.	(1) Maintenance of CNI therapy (n = 275), (2) Conversion to SRL maintenance therapy (n = 555).	eGFR and cumulative rates of AR, graft loss, or death at 12 mo.	(1) Intent-to-treat analyses at 12 and 24 mo showed no difference in GFR in patients with baseline GFR >40 mL/min. (2) On-therapy analysis showed higher GFR in SRL group. (3) Rejection rate, graft and patient survival were similar between groups. (4) SRL group had worse urinary protein-to-creatinine ratios but lower malignancy rates.	(1) Enrollment of patients with a GFR of 20–40 mL/min was stopped when the primary safety endpoint was reached (16.7% of in SRL, 0/25 of the CNI continuation patients). (2) Significantly greater treatment-emergent adverse events in the overall SRL conversion group.

Continued

TABLE 38.3 Summary of Randomized Controlled Trials of CNI-Sparing Therapies—cont'd

Trial Name/ Author	Study Design	Treatment Arms	Primary Endpoint(s)	Efficacy Outcomes	Comments
SOCRATES/ Chadban[51]	36-mo, prospective, multinational, open-label trial of 126 de novo recipients randomized at 14 days posttransplant.	(1) Initiation of everolimus and withdrawal of MMF and CNI (CNI-WD), (2) Initiation of everolimus and withdrawal of MMF and steroids (steroid-WD), (3) Continuation of initial therapy (control).	eGFR at 12 mo.	At 12 mo: (1) Similar eGFR in CNI-WD and control. (2) AR higher in CNI-WD group (31% vs. control 13%, $P = 0.048$). (3) Trend toward higher composite treatment failure (rejection, graft loss, death, loss to follow-up) in CNI-WD group.	(1) All received 14 d of CyA + MMF + steroids before randomization. (2) Steroid-WD arm was terminated prematurely because of excess discontinuations.
Büchler [52]	Prospective, RCT, 145 renal recipients.	(1) MMF + steroids + SRL, (2) MMF + steroids + CyA.	eGFR at 12 mo.	At 12 mo: (1) Intention-to-treat analyses showed eGFR and AR were similar between the two groups. (2) Proteinuria >0.5 g/24 h was higher (38.8% vs. 5.6%, $P < 0.001$) in SRL-treated patients. (3) Analysis of patients who remained on treatment showed better eGFR in SRL group (69 vs. 60 mL/min, $P = 0.01$).	(1) All received polyclonal antilymphocyte antibodies induction. (2) Higher drug discontinuation rate in the SRL arm.
USING BELATACEPT					
BENEFIT/ Vincenti[53,54]	3-y, prospective study, lower-risk live and deceased donor kidney recipients.	(1) More-intensive (MI) belatacept-based CNI-free regimen, (2) Less-intensive (LI) belatacept-based CNI-free regimen, (3) CyA-based maintenance regimen.	Patient/graft survival, AR and a composite kidney function endpoint at 12 mo posttransplant.	At 12 mo: (1) Patient and graft survival were similar for all three cohorts. (2) Composite kidney function endpoint was superior in both belatacept arms compared with CyA. (3) Iothalamate GFR was superior in both belatacept arms compared with CyA (65, 63, and 50 mL/min for MI, LI, and CyA; $P \leq 0.001$ MI or LI vs. CyA). (4) Both belatacept groups had more rejection (MI: 22%, LI: 17%, and CyA: 7%) and higher rejection grades than CyA group. At 36 months: (1) Patient/graft survival remained similar between groups. (2) eGFR improved by about 1 mL/1.73 m^2 per year in each belatacept groups vs. 2 mL/1.73 m^2 per year decline in CyA group.	(1) All patients received basiliximab, MMF, and prednisone. (2) More cases of PTLD occurred in belatacept-treated patients, mostly in patients with EBV antibody-negative patients.
Vincenti[55]	Extension study of BENEFIT with 84-mo follow-up, 70% of belatacept-treated patients and 60% of the CyA-randomized cohort had evaluable data			Belatacept was associated with a 43% lower risk for death/graft loss, and superior kidney function at 84 mo, compared with CyA (70 mL/min in belatacept arms vs 44 mL/min in CyA, $P < 0.001$).	Both belatacept groups had lower donor-specific antibody formation rates as well (MI: 1.9%, LI: 4.6%, CyA:17.8; $P < 0.001$).

BENEFIT-EXT[56, 57]	3-y study of recipients of extended-criteria donor kidneys, or those with cold ischemia times over 24 h.	(1) MI belatacept-based CNI-free regimen, (2) LI belatacept-based CNI-free regimen, (3) CyA-based maintenance regimen.		(1) At 12 mo, patient and graft survival were similar for all three cohorts. (2) At 36 mo, rates of treatment failure (~40%), death, graft loss, and acute rejection were similar across both belatacept and CyA groups. (3) Kidney function was better in the belatacept arms, although with more PTLD.	
de Graav[58]	Prospective, RCT, 40 kidney-transplant recipients.	Basiliximab, MMF, and prednisolone combined with: (1) belatacept or, (2) Tac.	1-y incidence of biopsy-proven rejection.	At 1 y, AR higher in belatacept group: 55% vs. 10%; $P = 0.006$.	All three graft losses, due to rejection, occurred in the belatacept group.
Rostaing[59]	Randomized, open-label phase II trial, renal transplant patients with stable graft function and on a CNI-based regimen, 85–90 patients in each arm.	At 6–36 mo posttransplant: (1) Continuation of CNI, (2) Conversion from a CNI to belatacept-based regimen.	Change in eGFR from baseline to month 12.	At month 12, the mean change from baseline in cGFR was higher in the belatacept group (7.0 mL/min) than the CNI group (2.1 mL/min).	Six belatacept-conversion patients experienced reversible rejection, all within the first 6 mo.

AR, Acute rejection; *ATG*, antithymocyte globulin; *CNI*, calcineurin inhibitor; *CyA*, cyclosporine A; *EBV*, Epstein-Barr virus; *eGFR*, estimated glomerular filtration rate; *MMF*, mycophenolate mofetil; *MPA*, mycophenolic acid; *mTOR*, mammalian target of rapamycin; *PTLD*, posttransplant lymphoproliferative disease; *RCT*, randomized controlled trial; *SRL*, sirolimus; *Tac*, tacrolimus.

cyclosporine at clinically relevant dosing and also offers the advantage of lower rejection rates and better renal function than non–tacrolimus-based therapies.[62-67] In most CNI minimization studies targeting "low-dose tacrolimus," achieved levels have typically ranged between 6 and 8 ng/mL. Despite these achieved levels exceeding, or being near the upper limit of the target range, tacrolimus has been associated with superior renal outcomes.[41,42] We are not aware of studies showing improved safety and efficacy when achieved 12-month posttransplant tacrolimus levels are less than approximately 6 ng/mL. In fact, in one RCT where target tacrolimus levels less than 5 ng/mL were achieved (3.4 ± 1.4 ng/mL) there was increased efficacy failure without any benefit on kidney function.[45] Finally, large observational biopsy-based cohort studies have demonstrated that CNI nephropathy is an uncommon primary cause of graft failure.[68,69] Although tacrolimus is not devoid of nephrotoxicity, we believe that the concern for this complication at modest target levels (e.g., 5 to 7 ng/mL) is exaggerated and suggest that the focus should be on combating other potential side effects including neurotoxicity and the development of posttransplant diabetes.

STEROID-SPARING REGIMENS

The rationale for minimizing long-term steroid use is related to mitigating its multiple undesirable side effects. Concerns regarding chronic steroid toxicity has fueled trials of steroid-sparing regimens for several decades. The advent of cyclosporine in the 1980s and tacrolimus in the 1990s permitted use of regimens with much lower prednisone dosing than in the preceding era and contributed to reduced steroid-associated toxicity. The emergence of routine use of induction therapy and more efficacious maintenance regimens popularized efforts to withdraw (within the first few weeks) or altogether avoid steroids after transplant, a practice supported by uncontrolled and retrospective studies showing that elimination could be successfully accomplished in low immunological risk patients without compromising outcomes.[70,71]

Although KDIGO guidelines suggest rapid corticosteroid withdrawal in low immunological risk kidney recipients, more than 70% of transplant patients in 2015 remain on steroids at 1 year posttransplant.[9,11] RCTs on steroid-sparing therapies are summarized in Table 38.4. Reluctance to embrace steroid-eliminating regimens comes from results of two RCTs demonstrating increased rejection in steroid-free or steroid-withdrawal groups without any major metabolic or cardiovascular benefit, as well as a single-center, prospective study showing increased fibrosis on 12-month posttransplant protocol allograft biopsies of recipients who underwent early steroid withdrawal.[72-74]

A limitation of these studies is that the investigators relied on reports of adverse events to document incident new-onset posttransplant diabetes. Harmony, a more recent RCT, used American Diabetes Association criteria to diagnose new diabetes in low immunological risk recipients, randomized to either steroid maintenance or one of two steroid withdrawal regimens (under basiliximab and rATG induction, respectively). The incidence of posttransplant diabetes was lower in the steroid-withdrawal arms without increased rejection rates at 12 months.[75] Although the short-term results of this study are promising, we caution against generalizing its results with low immunological risk recipients to all transplant recipients. Another trial comparing steroid withdrawal with steroid avoidance did not show any benefit in posttransplant diabetes at 6 months, but showed higher rates of rejection in the steroid-avoidance arm and higher overall rejection rates.[76] Longer-term follow-up of the Harmony cohort should help to further inform future practice with regard to chronic steroid use.

OUR RECOMMENATIONS

Until studies demonstrate equivalent efficacy and superior safety using alternative regimens, our recommendation is to base long-term maintenance regimens around tacrolimus, targeting levels 5 to 7 ng/mL beyond 6 months titrated to immunological risk. To minimize tacrolimus-specific toxicity, we incorporate depleting antibody induction, reduced-dose MPA, and prednisone (tapered to 5 mg/day by 4 weeks posttransplant). In low immunological risk recipients, a steroid-withdrawal regimen may be considered.

GENERIC IMMUNOSUPPRESSION

Generic immunosuppression formulations have been available for tacrolimus, cyclosporine, MPA, AZA, and sirolimus and offer more affordable alternatives. However, because regulatory requirement for approval of generic medications typically involves a one-time, single-dose pharmacokinetic evaluation of the generic compared with the innovator formulation in healthy individuals, concerns have been voiced on the use of generic formulations and unquantified adverse effects of switching to generic formulations in uncontrolled circumstances.[77,78] Box 38.1 summarizes these concerns. Two studies that showed contradictory findings of generic to brand-name bioequivalence further highlight the concerns of the transplant community.[79,80] Because registration criteria for generic immunosuppressive drugs are unlikely to change and payers will continue to dictate the medication formulations patients receive, we favor a multifaceted approach to safeguard against potential concerns associated with uncontrolled changes in formulations. This involves educating patients about the possibility of different formulations, asking them to visually compare the appearance of immunosuppression capsules from one refill to the next, having them inform the transplant center of changes, and monitoring kidney function and relevant CNI or sirolimus levels at 1 and 3 weeks postconversion.

LOOKING FORWARD

Improvement in immunosuppression strategies have contributed to significantly improved allograft survival. This high bar that needs to be surpassed, coupled with the emergence of

TABLE 38.4 Randomized-Controlled Trial on Steroid-Sparing Regimens

Trial Name/ Author	Study Design	Treatment Arms	Primary Endpoint(s)	Efficacy Outcomes	Comments
ATLAS/ Krämer[72]	6-mo, open-label, prospective multicenter RCT, 457 patients.	(1) Tac/basiliximab, (2) Tac/ MMF, (3) Tac/MMF/steroids.	Incidences of AR, patient and graft survival and eGFR.	(1) First 6 mo: more AR in both steroid-free arms. (2) 6 mo–3 years: AR low and similar in all groups. (3) No difference in renal function or cardiovascular risk factors at 3 y.	Diabetes was diagnosed by adverse-event reporting.
Woodle[73]	Prospective, double-blind, double-dummy study of 386 lower-risk adult recipients.	(1) Tac/MMF + maintenance prednisone (tapered to 5 mg/d by 6 mo posttransplant) or, (2) Tac/MMF + steroid withdrawal at day 7.	Composite of death, graft loss, or moderate/ severe acute rejection.	(1) At 5 y, AR higher in the steroid withdrawal arm, although allograft survival and function were similar. (2) No significant differences in weight change, new diabetes, blood pressure, antihypertensive use, low-density lipoprotein, Framingham cardiovascular risk scores and fracture rates between the groups.	(1) Two-thirds of the patients received rATG for induction. (2) Patients were followed in a double-blinded manner for the 5-y duration of the study. (3) Diabetes was diagnosed by adverse-event reporting.
Laftavi[74]	Prospective, single-center trial of 60 patients on Tac/MMF randomized at 7 d posttransplant.	(1) Maintenance steroids, (2) Steroid withdrawal.	eGFR, AR, and biopsy findings.	(1) Clinical rejections higher in steroid withdrawal arm (13% vs. 11%), but renal function equivalent in both groups. (2) Serial protocol biopsies demonstrated increased allograft fibrosis over time in both groups, but was most significant at 1 y in the steroid withdrawal group.	All patients received rATG induction.
HARMONY/ Thomusch[75]	Open-label, multicenter trial of 615 low-risk renal transplant recipients.	(1) Basiliximab + Tac/MMF + steroid maintenance therapy (arm A), (2) Basiliximab + Tac/MMF + rapid corticosteroid withdrawal on day 8 (arm B), (3) rATG + Tac/MMF + rapid corticosteroid withdrawal on day 8 (arm C).	AR in the first year of transplant.	(1) AR similar in all groups. (2) Posttransplant diabetes rates were lower in both steroid-withdrawal arms (24% and 23% vs. 39% in control arm A, $P = 0.0004$). (3) 12-mo patient and death-censored graft survival were similar in all arms.	(1) Posttransplant diabetes defined by ADA criteria. (2) Study participants were low immunological risk: 96% de novo kidney recipients, 88% with 0% panel-reactive antibodies, average cold ischemic time is 710 min.
ADVANCE/ Mourad[76]	Open-label, multicenter, prospective, 24-wk study of 1081 patients.	(1) Tapered corticosteroids, stopped after day 10, (2) no steroids after the intraoperative bolus.	Diagnosis of posttransplant diabetes per ADA criteria.	(1) At 24 wk, posttransplant diabetes similar in both arms. (2) Incidence of composite efficacy failure, graft and patient survival, and mean eGFR were comparable between arms. (3) AR (13.6% vs. 8.7%, $P = 0.006$) and biopsy-proven AR (25.9% vs. 18.2%, $P = 0.001$) higher in arm 2 vs. 1.	(1) All patients received basiliximab + prolonged-release Tac + MMF and 1 bolus of intraoperative corticosteroids. (2) Posttransplant diabetes defined by ADA criteria. Study participants were low immunological risk: patients with panel reactive antibodies >20% were excluded, retransplant recipients with first transplant lost from rejection were excluded.

ADA, American Diabetes Association; *AR*, acute rejection; *eGFR*, estimated glomerular filtration rate; *MMF*, mycophenolate mofetil; *rATG*, rabbit antithymocyte globulin; *Tac*, tacrolimus.

BOX 38.1 Concerns Regarding Generic Formulations of Immunosuppressive Agents

1. Unproven generalizability of bioequivalence testing in healthy individuals to organ recipients.
2. Absence of assessment of intrapatient variability.
3. Lack of evidence that different generic formulations of the same innovator drug are bioequivalent to each other.
4. Lack of consideration for subpopulation pharmacogenetic variability.
5. Absence of requirements for comparative safety and efficacy trials of generics with the innovator drug.
6. Substitution of generic for innovator, or generic from one manufacturer for generic drug from another manufacturer is seldom at the prescribing clinician's discretion.

generics driving down the cost of maintenance immunosuppression, have hindered therapeutic innovations and led to a slim pipeline of new immunosuppressive medications. Most alloimmune-targeting therapies currently in early clinical investigation are either biological or cell-based.

Costimulation blockade, with the goal of preventing T-cell activation, remains a target of interest. ASKP1240, an anti-CD40 mAb has recently been tested in CNI-free and CNI-minimization regimens and compared with tacrolimus-based therapy in a phase Ib study; however, because the CNI-free regimen had higher rates of acute rejection and both ASKP1240 arms had higher rates of infection than the control arm, the future of this drug is uncertain.[81] CFZ533, a fully human, Fc-silent, anti-CD40 mAb has demonstrated efficacy and safety in nonhuman primate studies, and is currently being investigated in humans (clinicaltrials.gov NCT02217410). Belimumab, a human mAb that inhibits B cell-activating factor and is approved for treatment of lupus, is under investigation for prevention of acute antibody-mediated rejection in de novo kidney transplants and to lower donor-specific antibody titers in sensitized patients (clinicaltrials.gov NCT02500251).

Cell-based immunosuppression hopes to provide long-term engraftment while avoiding immunosuppression-related side effects via the induction of donor-specific unresponsiveness either in the setting of operational tolerance or mixed chimerism. This process involves ex vivo generation of autologous or donor-derived hematopoietic stem cells transplanted concomitantly with a kidney in live-donor recipients. By migrating to sites of antigenic reactivity, mesenchymal stem cells, which are multipotent progenitor cells with the capacity to self-renew and differentiate into cells of different lineages, exhibit their immunoregulatory effects through both cell–cell interaction as well as the release of soluble factors, resulting in effector T-cell suppression and promotion of regulatory T cells.[82] Also currently under investigation are naturally occurring regulatory T cells, purified from live-donor recipients and expanded in culture, that are then infused peritransplant to recipients to prevent rejection. Theoretically, the immunoregulatory properties of regulatory T cells will facilitate donor-specific unresponsiveness and a reduction in conventional immunosuppression in transplant recipients. Although the concept of cell-based therapeutic approaches is revolutionary and early trials are encouraging, these will need to be validated in larger, multicenter RCTs from the standpoints of safety, efficacy, and cost–benefit in comparison to conventional immunosuppression therapies.[83-86]

Finally, research looking at the development of reliable biomarkers (individually or in combination) to monitor patient's alloimmunity may hold the key in individualizing therapy and move the field closer to precision medicine.[87]

CONCLUSION

Advances in immunosuppression have catalyzed the progression of kidney transplantation from an intellectual curiosity in 1954 to a mature clinical discipline in the 21st century. Contemporary standard-of-care therapies are highly effective, have been widely embraced by transplant clinicians for almost 2 decades, and involve T-cell depleting induction therapy with tacrolimus-MPA–based maintenance therapy, with novel regimens focused on minimizing drug-specific side effects. As precision medicine moves into the mainstream, biotechnological advancement has fueled the development of cell-based therapies with potential for achieving donor-specific unresponsiveness and ultimately withdrawal of conventional immunosuppression.

A full list of references is available at www.expertsonsult.com.

39

Diagnosis and Therapy of Graft Dysfunction

Deirdre Sawinski, MD, and Simin Goral, MD

OUTLINE

INTRODUCTION

Despite being a well-established procedure, kidney transplantation is associated with risk for complications. Depending on the period since transplant, the etiology and management of graft dysfunction will vary. Hence, the differential diagnosis is best approached by considering the different posttransplant periods. In this chapter, graft dysfunction will be discussed in three phases:

1. *Delayed graft function* (DGF), occurring in the immediate posttransplant period
2. *Early graft dysfunction,* occurring within the first 3 posttransplant months
3. *Late graft dysfunction,* occurring beyond the first 3 months posttransplant

DELAYED GRAFT FUNCTION

Definition

The term *delayed graft function* (DGF) has been used to describe marginally functioning grafts that take several days to weeks to recover function. DGF must be distinguished from *primary nonfunction,* where the kidney allografts never function and allograft nephrectomy is usually indicated. Various indices, including urine volume, dialysis requirement, and serum creatinine (SCr), have been used to define DGF.

From the standpoint of registry reporting, DGF is defined by the requirement for dialysis in the first posttransplant week. Using the need for dialysis alone to define DGF, however, may lead to underdiagnosis, particularly if there is some

BOX 39.1 Differential Diagnosis of Delayed Graft Function

1. **Prerenal**
   - Volume depletion
   - Nephrotoxic drugs and high CNI levels
2. **Vascular complications**
   - Arterial or venous thrombosis
   - Renal artery stenosis
3. **Intrinsic renal**
   - Acute tubular necrosis
   - Accelerated or acute rejection
   - Thrombotic microangiopathy
   - Recurrence of primary glomerular disease (particularly FSGS)
4. **Postrenal**
   - Catheter obstruction
   - Perinephric fluid collection (lymphocele, urine leak, hematoma)
   - Ureteral obstruction
   - Intrinsic (blood clots, technical issues, ureteral slough)
   - Extrinsic (ureteral kinking)
   - Neurogenic bladder
   - Benign prostatic hypertrophy

CNI, Calcineurin inhibitor; *FSGS*, focal segmental glomerular sclerosis.

residual native kidney function. In studies evaluating the causes and management of DGF, a modified definition of "the need for more than one dialysis session" is sometimes applied to take into account the need for a single postoperative dialysis session for the management of hyperkalemia, or diuretic-resistant volume overload.[1] An elevated SCr concentration of greater than 400 mmol/L (>4.5 mg/dL) 1 week after transplantation has been suggested to be a more sensitive and specific measure of DGF.[2]

A urine output greater than 20 mL/kg/day in the immediate postoperative period is generally a good clinical indicator of adequate kidney function; however, it is limited in cases where large urine volume is still produced by the native kidneys. Alternatively, no increase in urine output postoperatively does not necessarily indicate DGF. The term *slow graft function* (SGF) is sometimes used to describe nonoliguric patients who usually do not require dialysis but who experience a delayed fall in SCr.

Differential Diagnosis

Although most kidneys with DGF when biopsied demonstrate findings consistent with acute tubular necrosis (ATN), it should be noted that these terms are not synonymous. Unless an allograft biopsy is performed, posttransplant ATN should be a diagnosis of exclusion. The differential diagnosis of DGF is shown in Box 39.1. Similar to nontransplant acute kidney injury, a systematic approach to the evaluation of DGF may be divided into prerenal, intrinsic, and postrenal causes. Although uncommon, vascular causes of DGF must be excluded, particularly in the early postoperative period.

Prerenal causes such as intravascular volume depletion or a significant hypotension are usually suggested by a careful review of patients' preoperative history and intraoperative report. Knowing the dialysis dry weight and preoperative weight may aid in assessing recipient volume status in the immediate postoperative period.

Because calcineurin inhibitors (CNIs) cyclosporine and tacrolimus cause a dose-related reversible afferent arteriolar vasoconstriction that may temporarily worsen kidney function, it is possible, though unproven, that these agents could delay recovery of allograft function in the immediate posttransplant period as well. Target of rapamycin (TOR) inhibitors have been found to delay recovery from DGF and are seldom used in the early posttransplant setting.

Intrinsic renal causes of DGF typically include ATN, acute rejection, infection, thrombotic microangiopathy, and recurrence of glomerular diseases affecting the native kidneys. The incidence of ATN varies widely among centers and has been reported to occur in 20% to 25% of patients.[3-10] The difference in reported incidence may in part be related to variation in use of marginal donor organs across centers. Both donor and recipient factors are important determinants of early allograft dysfunction.

ATN found in the posttransplant setting is an ischemic injury that may be synergistically enhanced by both immunological and nephrotoxic insults. All transplanted kidneys are subjected to injury stressors at various stages from donor death to organ procurement, surgical reanastomosis, and in the early postoperative period. The kidney encounters ischemia during organ procurement and storage and then reperfusion when transplanted; this process upregulates endothelial human leukocyte antigen (HLA) expression, causing the release of chemokines, cytokines, and adhesion molecules within the allograft, which leads to the activation and recruitment of T lymphocytes. In a multicenter cohort study[11] of deceased-donor kidney transplants procured from March 2010 through April 2012 by participating organ procurement organizations (OPOs), it was found that preimplant biopsy-reported ATN was modestly associated with the development of DGF only in donation after cardiac death (DCD) kidneys. Their findings suggested that there was substantial variability in pathology reports and that acute structural injury was often underreported.

Although ischemic injury is a major risk factor for the development of posttransplant ATN and DGF, several lines of evidence suggest that immunological factors contribute as well. DGF is more prevalent in retransplant compared with primary transplant recipients, particularly in highly sensitized patients.[3,12]

Some data suggest that ischemic injury may contribute to the upregulation of inflammatory cytokines and increase expression of class I and II major histocompatibility complex antigens, thus increasing the immunogenicity of the transplanted kidney.[13,14] Nitric oxide produced by the inducible nitric oxide synthase enzymes in response to ischemic cell injury has been suggested as a link between ischemic reperfusion injury and graft rejection.[15] Renal epithelial regeneration mediated by growth factors and cytokines, such as epidermal growth factor and transforming growth factor β, after ischemic damage may culminate in low-grade inflammation and fibrosis observed with chronic rejection.[16]

The stress of donor brain death itself likely has a similar effect to ATN on the risk for allograft rejection. In one animal study,[17] brain death was found to be associated with upregulation of macrophage (interleukin-1 [IL-1], IL-6, and tumor necrosis factor α [TNFα]) and T-cell–associated products (IL-2 and interferon-α [IF-α]) in peripheral organs, rendering them more susceptible to host inflammatory and immunological responses.

Immunohistochemical analysis of pretransplant living and deceased donor biopsy specimens demonstrated increased E-selectin expression and interstitial leukocyte accumulation in deceased compared with living donor kidneys, suggesting that brain death initiates an inflammatory reaction in the human kidney.[18] Highly matched kidneys have been suggested to be less susceptible to the harmful effects of DGF, presumably because ATN exposes the mismatched kidney to a more aggressive immune attack.[19]

A number of studies have found that developing posttransplant ATN does not have long-term consequences provided that rejection does not occur, lending support to the theory that it is the immunological consequences of ATN that are responsible for its prognostic significance.[20]

Studies also suggest that there is a sex-based difference in DGF risk, with the female hormonal milieu being protective. Aufhauser et al.[21] demonstrated in a rodent transplant model that female recipient sex was protective against DGF, regardless of donor sex, and supplemental estrogen given to female mice was further protective. Analyses of the United Network of Organ Sharing (UNOS) data set found greater risks of DGF in male transplant recipients, and this difference was not explained by variation in body weight between donor and recipient or nephron dosing. Trials examining supplemental estrogen as a means of reducing DGF rates are underway.

Histologically, allograft and native kidney ATN are similar. Tubular epithelial cells show necrosis, often with sloughed, degenerated, or apoptotic epithelial cells in the tubular lumina.[22] Proximal cell brush border staining of proximal tubular epithelium is focally absent with flattening of tubular cells, and there may be regeneration in the form of mitotic figures (Fig. 39.1).[23] Calcium oxalate deposition in tubular lumina is associated with early graft dysfunction and ATN prolongation.[24] The interstitium is variably edematous, with a minimal or patchy interstitial lymphocytic infiltrate; however, there is no associated tubulitis or glomerular or vascular changes.

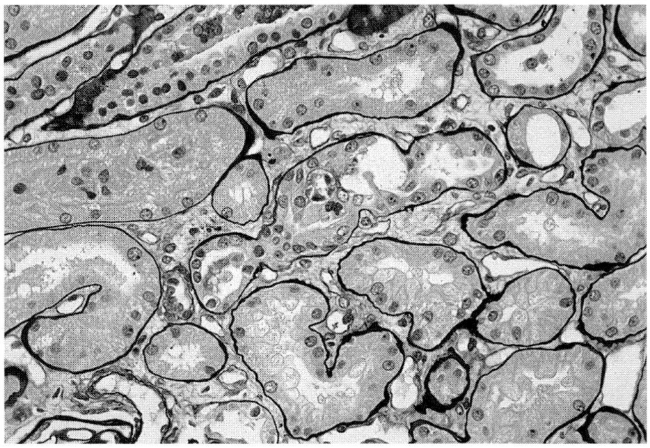

FIG. 39.1 Acute tubular necrosis. Tubular cells show flattening and necrosis and focally are desquamated into the tubular lumina. The central tubule contains calcium oxalate in the lumen, a product of cellular debris (Jones methenamine silver ×250).

Prediction and Prevention of Delayed Graft Function

The uncontrolled circumstances surrounding brain death, as well as the complex deceased donor organ procurement process, inevitably result in varying degrees of ischemic damage that adversely affect allograft function.

Preexisting donor factors are important predictors of early and late graft function. Kidneys from older donors have a higher incidence of ATN,[25] attributed to the diminished capacity of the aging vasculature to vasodilate adequately to protect the kidney from anoxic damage. For this reason, these organs were historically rejected by most centers. However, the critical shortage of organs has resulted in increased use of kidneys from more marginal donors. Until recently, these were labeled "expanded criteria donor" kidneys and were associated with a 70% greater risk for allograft failure compared with kidneys from young, healthy donors. This terminology has since been supplanted by the Kidney Donor Profile Index (KDPI), which incorporates into its assessment of donor "quality" the characteristics of age, height, weight, race/ethnicity, history of hypertension, history of diabetes, hepatitis C status, cause of death, and brain versus cardiac death.[26] KDPI helps understand how long a deceased donor kidney is expected to function relative to all the kidneys recovered in the United States during the last year. Lower KDPI scores are associated with longer estimated graft function, whereas higher KDPI scores are associated with shorter estimated graft function.

To optimize allograft outcomes using these "marginal" kidneys, UNOS has implemented a system to expedite high KDPI kidney placement. Despite the efforts to decrease cold ischemia time, the use of these kidneys inevitably increases the incidence of posttransplantation ATN. Similarly, the use of DCD kidneys, which are exposed to increased warm ischemia in addition to cold ischemia, has resulted in an increased incidence of DGF. In a single-center study of 456 renal transplants,[27] DGF occurred in 17% of heart-beating deceased donor kidneys compared with 95% of DCD kidneys. Nonetheless, graft survival in the DCD recipients with DGF was significantly better compared with recipients of a heart-beating donor kidney transplant that developed DGF at 3 years (84% vs. 73%, respectively; $P < 0.05$) and 6 years (84% vs. 62%, respectively). Although this appears to be paradoxical, it has been proposed that brainstem death causes cytokine release and inflammatory reactions, events that do not occur in donation after cardiac death.[27] In addition, surgeons may be more cautious in accepting organs that have experienced additional "insults" and therefore may select only the "best" DCD organs for transplantation. Analysis of data from the United States Renal Data System revealed that recipients of DCD kidneys experienced nearly twice the incidence of DGF compared with donation after brain death (DBD) kidneys (42.3% vs. 23.3%, respectively). Nonetheless, DCD kidneys had comparable allograft survival to kidneys from DBD donors at 6 years of follow-up (73.2% vs. 72.5%, respectively; P = NS). Significant risk factors for allograft loss for DCD kidney recipients included retransplant, DGF, donor age older than 35 years, and head trauma as a cause of death.[28]

Because the potential for ischemic injury to kidney transplants begins with procurement, the goal of donor management during this period is to maintain adequate organ perfusion before rapid cooling and flushing of the kidneys to minimize warm ischemia. *Warm ischemia time* refers to the period between circulatory arrest and the commencement of cold storage.[29] Ischemia at body temperature can be tolerated for only a few minutes, after which irreversible injury begins to occur and the organ becomes nonviable within 30 minutes. *Cold ischemia time* refers to the period from initiation of cold storage or machine perfusion (MP) until the transplanted kidney is reperfused in vivo. For the purpose of transplantation, anaerobic metabolism can maintain renal cellular energy requirements for up to 48 hours, provided the organ is cooled to about 4°C with an appropriate preservation solution.[30] Increasing warm and cold ischemic time both can result in higher rates of DGF and a progressive decline in graft survival. Ideally, kidneys are transplanted without significant warm ischemia and with cold ischemia time less than 24 hours. In DCD donation, rapid institution of donor cooling to reduce warm ischemia is particularly vital because of the absence of blood circulation. Hypothermia-induced reduction in tissue metabolism (for every 10°C of organ cooling, metabolism is decreased by approximately 50%) alleviates ischemic injury.[31,32]

Pulsatile hypothermic machine perfusion, first developed by Belzer in the late 1960s, was used by many centers to preserve kidneys until EuroCollins preservation solution was introduced in 1969. There has been renewed interest in using MP because of its reported beneficial effects in lowering the DGF incidence and improvement in allograft function.[33,34] A metaanalysis on the effectiveness of MP versus cold storage found that MP led to a 20% reduction in the incidence of DGF in both DBD and DCD kidneys compared with cold storage,[35] with no significant difference in 1-year graft survival between the two preservation methods. Nonetheless, MP may permit identification of kidneys at high risk for primary nonfunction, thus sparing potential recipients the morbidity associated with the transplant operation and the development of allosensitization.[33] The perfusion index (PFI) is used to assess organ function while being perfused.

Because ATN may render allografts more susceptible to immunological injury, the use of lymphodepleting antibody induction may have a beneficial effect on DGF rates. Intraoperative thymoglobulin administration has been reported to be associated with significantly less DGF and better early allograft function compared with administration initiated postoperatively, attributed to modulation and attenuation of ischemia-reperfusion injury.[36] A small molecule mimetic of hepatocyte growth factor/scatter factor (HGF/SF) whose activity is expected to preserve tissue viability and attenuate dysfunction in the setting of organ injury is being tested in kidney transplant recipients to decrease the rates of DGF. HGF/SF is a renotrophic factor that exerts significant cytoprotective, antifibrotic, and antiapoptotic effects in renal epithelial cells. The molecule being tested was found to be efficacious in animal models of ischemia-reperfusion injury as well as toxin-induced injury.

Management of Delayed Graft Function

Most patients with DGF are oliguric or anuric. As discussed earlier, information about both native kidney urine output and donor kidney characteristics is essential. For example, if postoperative oliguria occurs immediately after living donor kidney transplantation, surgical complications such as arterial or venous thrombosis must be immediately considered. In contrast, when a patient receives a deceased donor kidney from a high KDPI donor, DGF may be anticipated. The mate kidney from a deceased donor often behaves in a similar manner, and information on its function can be useful.[1]

Oliguria in the peritransplant period typically refers to a urine output of less than 50 mL/h. Evaluation of oliguria should commence with assessment of volume status, fluid balance, and Foley catheter patency. If clots are present, the catheter should be removed while gentle suction is applied in an attempt to capture the clot. Thereafter, replacement with a larger catheter may be required. For patients with hypervolemia, high-dose furosemide may be given intravenously. If the patient is judged to be hypovolemic, or if a clinical assessment cannot be made, a trial of isotonic saline infusion may be given, with or without subsequent administration of furosemide as dictated by the patient's response to saline infusion alone.

Indications for dialysis in the transplant recipient with DGF are essentially the same as in any patient with postoperative kidney dysfunction. Hyperkalemia must be monitored closely and treated aggressively. It is usually safest to dialyze patient if the potassium level is greater than 5.5 mg/dL. Temporizing measures, such as intravenous calcium and glucose with insulin, can be used but do not obviate the need for dialysis. Sodium polystyrene sulfonate (Kayexalate) should not be administered perioperatively because its use has been associated with gut ischemia.[37]

Patients with DGF often become volume overloaded in the early posttransplant period. Ultrafiltration with or without dialysis may be required. When dialyzing patients who have DGF, care must be taken to avoid hypotension, which may plausibly perpetuate graft dysfunction. In patients with established DGF, dialysis requirements should be assessed daily until graft function improves.

Diagnostic Studies in Persistent Oliguria or Anuria

Failure to respond to volume challenge and furosemide administration warrants further evaluation to determine the cause of the early posttransplant oligo/anuric state.

Imaging studies are used to confirm the presence of blood flow to the graft and the absence of a urine leak or obstruction. Blood flow studies are performed scintigraphically or by Doppler ultrasound.[38] The typical scintigraphic finding in ATN is relatively good flow to the graft but with poor excretion. If the Doppler reveals no demonstrable blood flow, a prompt surgical reexploration is necessary to evaluate the allograft vasculature. Kidneys without arterial circulation are seldom salvageable and are usually removed during reexploration. If imaging studies indicate adequate blood flow to the allograft, the possibility of ureteral obstruction or urinary leak needs to be considered and can be evaluated by the same modalities. In the first 24 hours after transplantation, as long as the Foley catheter has been providing good bladder drainage, the obstruction or leak is almost always at the ureterovesical junction and represents a technical problem that requires surgical correction.[29]

OTHER CAUSES OF GRAFT DYSFUNCTION DURING THE FIRST WEEK AFTER TRANSPLANTATION

Rejection

Hyperacute Rejection

Hyperacute rejection occurs immediately after transplantation and is due to preformed antibodies, usually to blood group antigens or donor HLAs. The rejection occurs after an amnestic response where a critical level of antibodies is produced and results in an irreversible vascular damage. Hyperacute rejection may be evident at reperfusion or may be "hidden," manifesting as primary nonfunction of the kidney allograft.[39] Patients are usually anuric or oliguric and might have associated graft tenderness. The renal scan shows little or no uptake, a finding that differentiates this cause of graft dysfunction from ATN. There may be evidence of intravascular coagulation. Prompt surgical exploration of the allograft is often indicated, and often an intraoperative biopsy is performed to determine viability.

In hyperacute rejection, preformed antibodies activate the complement cascade. Nephrectomy specimens have arterial and glomerular thrombi, which often contain neutrophils. The interstitium is edematous and variable parenchymal necrosis or infarction is observed, depending on the length of time from thrombosis to nephrectomy. There is no significant vascular or tubulointerstitial inflammation. Immunofluorescence microscopy reveals fibrin within the intravascular thrombi, and immunoglobulin M (IgM), IgG, C3, and fibrin may be found in arterial and capillary lumina or lining or within the intimas.[40] Most allografts are nonviable and need to be removed. With advances in crossmatching techniques incorporating flow cytometry and Luminex bead-based assays,[41,42] hyperacute rejection is very rare.

Accelerated Acute Rejection

Accelerated acute rejection or delayed hyperacute rejection typically occurs within 24 hours to a few days after transplantation and may involve both antibody-mediated and cellular immune mechanisms. Accelerated acute rejection probably represents a delayed amnestic response to prior sensitization. It is most commonly observed after ABO- and HLA-incompatible transplants and may also be seen after donor-specific transfusions in recipients of living-donor transplant as a result of a primed T-cell response.[43] HLA sensitization through repeat transplants, multiple pregnancies, or multiple transfusions are well-substantiated risk factors for hyperacute or accelerated acute rejection.

Early T-Cell Acute Rejection

Early T-cell rejection, with a typical interstitial mononuclear cell infiltrate and tubulitis, including CD4 and CD8 T cells, can rarely be detected in the latter part of the first week after transplantation, although it typically occurs somewhat later. It may be difficult to recognize clinically in patients with DGF. If suspected, there should be a low threshold to perform an allograft biopsy. The prognosis for long-term function of these grafts is poor, although adequate function may be achieved, if the ATN reverses and the rejection responds to intensification of immunosuppression.

Nonimmunological Causes

Nonimmunological causes of DGF (other than ATN) may occur in the first posttransplant week or any time thereafter and are discussed under Graft Dysfunction in the Early Posttransplant Period.

Long-Term Impact of Immediate Graft Dysfunction

Studies on the impact of DGF on long-term graft function have yielded conflicting results.[5,7,44,45] Transplant registry data revealed that DGF reduced 1-year graft survival from 91% to 75% ($P < 0.001$) and graft half-life from 12.9 to 8 years, independent of early acute rejection episodes. This deleterious effect of DGF remained significant after adjusting for discharge SCr less than 2.5 mg/dL as well. DGF has also been found to abrogate the survival advantage of well-matched kidneys (0 to 1 mismatch) over those with lesser degrees of matching (5 to 6 mismatches).[44] Some investigators have found that DGF, when combined with rejection, had an additive negative effect on allograft survival, whereas others suggested that DGF is deleterious to graft outcome only when associated with reduced renal mass and hyperfiltration injury.[45,46] A metaanalysis of 33 DGF studies found that DGF was associated with a 41% increased risk for graft loss (risk ratio [RR] 1.41, 95% confidence interval [CI], 1.27 to 1.56) with no clear deleterious effect on patient survival (RR 1.14, 95% CI, 0.94 to 1.39). Patients who experienced DGF had higher posttransplant SCr levels and an increased risk for rejection (RR 1.38, 95% CI, 1.29 to 1.47).[47] The harmful effect of DGF may also be more pronounced when marginal donor kidneys are used.

There are several explanations for the contradictory findings in these studies. First, most studies did not incorporate transplant biopsies and DGF was attributed to ATN; second, there is no universally defined criteria for DGF; third, donor and recipient characteristics were quite variable across studies.

In addition, the duration of DGF has also been suggested to be impactful on outcomes.[48,49] For example, in one study,[49] 5-year graft survival for patients with immediate function and DGF lasting 8 days or less was similar (89%, 85%) and higher than in patients with DGF lasting for more than 8 days (50%). Given the impact of DGF on morbidity and health resource use, trials are underway to prevent or attenuate this detrimental complication.

Graft Dysfunction in the Early Posttransplant Period

The early posttransplant period typically spans the period after discharge from the transplant hospitalization until the end of the third month, by when most patients have achieved stable graft function and immunosuppressive regimen. Although a somewhat arbitrary differentiation, most acute rejection episodes and surgery-related complications occur during this period as well.

By the second week, DGF caused by ATN typically begins to improve, although some patients remain dialysis dependent for several weeks. In dialysis-independent patients, SCr measurement is the main indicator of allograft function and outcome predictor and should be evaluated in the context of the donor type, size mismatch between donor and recipient, and function of the mate kidney if applicable. The SCr level reached by the second week may predict long-term graft function; a baseline level greater than 2 mg/dL warrants further investigation.

Elevations in SCr greater than 25% from baseline almost always indicate a clinically significant and potentially graft-endangering event, and it is advisable to repeat within 48 hours. The clinical algorithm in approaching SCr elevations (or failure to reach a low baseline value) is similar, in principle, to that used in the nontransplant setting: "prerenal," "renal," and "postrenal" causes need to be considered. In the early posttransplantation period, acute rejection is the most important potentially reversible threat to graft function. In addition, anatomical or surgical problems must also be considered before medical diagnoses are sought to explain deteriorating graft function.

ACUTE REJECTION

Clinical Presentation

Acute rejection conventionally describes the cellular and/or humoral immune response to the transplant that produces enough inflammation and destruction to cause detectable allograft dysfunction. The majority of patients with acute rejection are asymptomatic, and clinical suspicion arises on the basis of SCr elevation. In symptomatic patients a concomitant search for alternative causes of graft dysfunction is warranted. For example, a tender, swollen allograft with a rising SCr concentration and fever is a typical presentation of acute transplant pyelonephritis.[50] For this reason, a thorough history, physical examination, standard laboratory tests, and evaluation for infection must be obtained before the diagnosis and treatment of rejection. Because of the interplay between rejection and viral infections, testing for cytomegalovirus (CMV) and BK virus via polymerase chain reaction (PCR) is also a reasonable part of the evaluation of allograft dysfunction.

Although SCr can define the occurrence of allograft dysfunction and is highly convenient, it is insensitive in detecting subclinical rejection. Approximately 15% to 80% of protocol biopsy specimens acquired in the first 3 to 6 months posttransplant in patients with well-functioning grafts have been reported to have histopathological lesions of acute rejection, although this varies markedly depending on the induction and maintenance immunosuppression regimens used.[51,52] Although it may be a risk for chronic rejection and progressive allograft failure,[48,53] treatment of subclinical rejection has not been consistently found to prevent late allograft deterioration or fibrosis in studies with serial biopsies[54-56]; controlled trials in this area are lacking.

Imaging Studies

Although nonspecific for demonstrating rejection, imaging studies are performed to exclude alternative causes of acute allograft dysfunction. In mild acute rejection episodes, imaging studies may be normal.[38,57] The resistive index can be elevated, though this can be observed in other causes of graft dysfunction that result in increased intrarenal vascular resistance.

Given the current radiological limitations, allograft biopsy, although invasive, remains the gold standard for differentiating acute rejection from other causes of acute allograft function.

Core Biopsy

Biopsy evaluation for acute rejection should be performed in unscarred portions of the renal cortex. Rejection can present focally and may be missed on biopsy; therefore at least two cores with two arteries and seven slides of tissue are required for adequate assessment.[58]

Histopathological Diagnosis

The timing and frequency of kidney biopsies vary among centers. We advocate for transplant biopsy to be performed in any patient with elevated SCr for whom an explanation is not apparent, to determine the presence and severity of rejection and its subsequent treatment.

TYPES OF ACUTE REJECTION

On the basis of the underlying immunopathogenic mechanisms (discussed in Chapter 35), acute rejection can be divided into T-cell–mediated and antibody-mediated rejection. The vast majority of acute rejection episodes are T-cell mediated, whereas 12% to 37% of all acute rejection episodes have a humoral component.[59,60] It should be noted that the histopathological findings of acute T-cell rejection and acute antibody-mediated rejection (ABMR) may occur in a renal biopsy simultaneously. The diagnostic criteria for cellular and ABMR are set forth in the Banff classification schema, which are regularly updated.

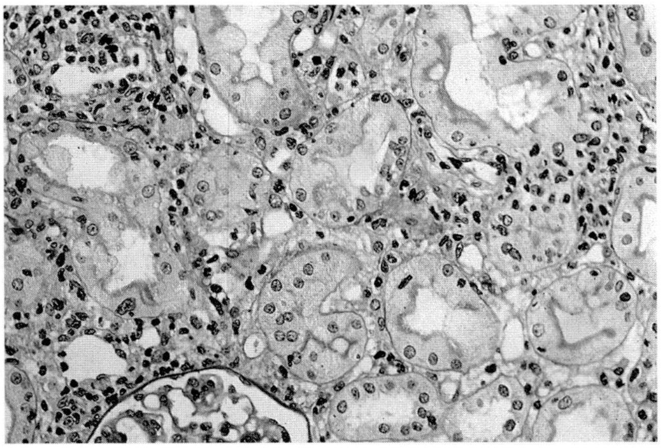

FIG. 39.2 Acute cell-mediated tubulointerstitial rejection. There are interstitial edema and lymphocytes, with lymphocytes in the walls of most tubules (tubulitis) (periodic acid–Schiff ×300).

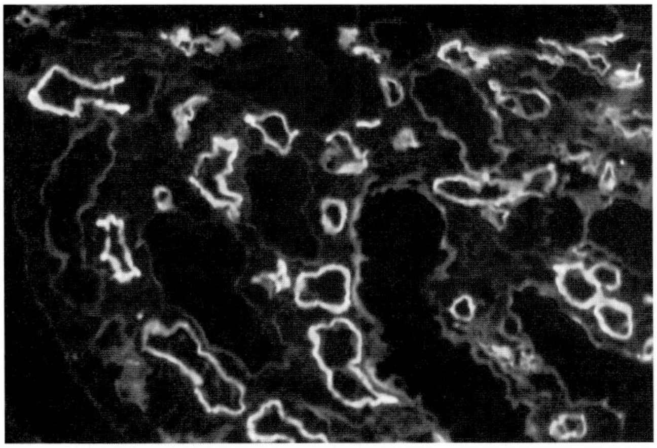

FIG. 39.3 Acute antibody-mediated (humoral) rejection. There is bright staining of peritubular capillaries for C4d in a linear pattern (C4d immunofluorescence ×300).

Acute T-Cell–Mediated Rejection

The 2015 Banff update to the classification of acute T-cell–mediated rejection (TCMR) recognizes category 3, borderline changes suspicious for acute TCMR, and category 4, acute TCMR. "Borderline" changes consist of foci of tubulitis or interstitial inflammation present on biopsy but not meeting category 4 criteria. Depending on the clinical scenario and indication for biopsy, clinicians may choose not to treat borderline rejections, augment maintenance immunosuppression, or give intravenous steroids. In one study[61] in which researchers performed follow-up biopsies for 24 patients with "borderline" TCMR findings on the initial specimen, nearly 80% had mild or moderate cellular rejection on repeat sampling, calling into question the supposedly benign nature of the finding.

Acute TCMR (category 4) can be further subdivided on the basis of the severity of inflammation and the involvement of blood vessels (Fig. 39.2). Grades Ia and Ib acute TCMR both require an interstitial inflammatory infiltrate that involves more than 25% of the cortex with tubulitis (>4 lymphocytes/tubular cross section for Ia and >10 lymphocytes for Ib). Some practitioners treat with steroids alone, though some use lymphocyte-depleting therapy as well. Grade II rejections are characterized by the presence of intimal arteritis (>25% luminal area compromised for IIb) and do not necessarily require interstitial inflammation or tubulitis; these rejections are treated with lymphodepleting antibodies. Grade III rejections are less common and display fibrinoid necrosis changes along with transmural arteritis; these severe rejections require prompt treatment with lymphocyte depleting therapies but often portend irreparable damage to the allograft.

Acute Antibody-Mediated Rejection

The diagnosis of acute ABMR, according to the 2013 update to the Banff criteria,[62] requires evidence of renal parenchymal injury (microvascular inflammation, arteritis, thrombotic microangiopathy, or acute tubular injury), antibody interaction with the vascular endothelium (C4d staining in the peritubular capillaries, microvascular inflammation, or increased expression of endothelial injury gene transcripts), and the presence of donor-specific antibodies (DSAs) (Fig. 39.3).[63] These may occur with or without features of acute TCMR. Furthermore, C4d is not always pathological and can be identified in allograft biopsy specimens lacking morphological evidence of rejection, such as immune accommodation in ABO incompatible transplants.[64]

Noninvasive Diagnostic Biomarkers

Over the last decade, gene analysis using molecular biology techniques such as reverse transcription–PCR has been studied as a noninvasive tool in the diagnosis of acute rejection. Elevated peripheral blood or urine levels of perforin, granzyme B, Fas ligand, and serpin proteinase inhibitor 9 have variably been reported to indicate the presence of ongoing acute TCMR.[65] It has also been suggested that measurement of urine perforin messenger RNA (mRNA) and granzyme B mRNA may offer a noninvasive means of diagnosing acute TCMR, with a sensitivity of 79% to 83% and a specificity of 77% to 83% in one study.[66] In one single-center study,[67] perforin and granzyme B had sensitivities of 50% and specificities of 95% in predicting rejection when a cutoff value of 140 was used.

There have been other attempts at developing noninvasive markers of rejection, including measurement of donor-derived cell-free DNA (dd-cfDNA). Cellular damage leads to the release into the recipient's circulation of donor-derived DNA, termed *cell-free DNA*.[68] This DNA can be amplified by digital droplet PCR or massive parallel shotgun sequencing. A study of 102 kidney transplant recipients correlated plasma dd-cfDNA results with allograft biopsy specimens; a dd-cfDNA greater than 1% was predictive of acute rejection on biopsy (area under the curve [AUC] 0.74, 95% CI, 0.61 to 0.86).[69] Although there was a trend toward increasing dd-cfDNA levels with more severe rejections by Banff classification, the study was underpowered to demonstrate this.

$CD4^+$ $CD25^+$ FoxP3 regulatory T cells (Treg) are involved in the maintenance of immune homeostasis and tolerance to self and nonself antigens.[70] A single-center study[65] in kidney recipients with DGF suggested that measurement of *FOXP3* gene (X-linked forkhead/winged helix transcription factor) in peripheral blood leukocytes and urinary cells provides an accurate marker of acute rejection with a reported sensitivity, specificity, and positive and negative predictive values between 94% and 100%. In a single-center case-control study[71] of stable recipients undergoing tacrolimus dose reduction with ultimate withdrawal of the drug, it was demonstrated that before tacrolimus dose reduction, the $CD8^+$:Treg ratio was higher in rejectors compared with nonrejectors. Rejectors also had a higher memory $CD4^+$: Treg ratio. In rejectors, an increase over time was observed in the percentage of naïve T cells in the peripheral blood, with a reciprocal decrease in the percentage of effector T cells. Whether the combination of the memory T cells:Treg ratio and the changes in T-cell subsets over time might prove useful in the detection of acute rejection remains to be studied. The use of immune monitoring as a noninvasive tool in the prediction and diagnosis of acute rejection is a subject of intense, ongoing research. But despite these encouraging preliminary results, noninvasive methods have failed to supplant biopsy in the diagnosis of rejection.

CALCINEURIN INHIBITOR-MEDIATED NEPHROTOXICITY

CNIs cyclosporine and tacrolimus are two potent immunosuppressive agents with similar mechanisms of action (see Chapter 38 on immunosuppression) and pathological patterns of nephrotoxicity. CNIs produce a dose-related, reversible, renal vasoconstriction that particularly affects the afferent arteriole, manifesting clinically as a blood-level–dependent elevation in SCr concentration that may be difficult to distinguish from other causes of graft dysfunction. High blood levels of CNIs do not preclude a diagnosis of rejection. In the acute phase, tubular function is intact.

CNI nephrotoxicity may develop at low drug levels, especially in malnourished patients with diminished protein binding where the free drug concentration is increased; some degree of toxicity may be intrinsic to their use. In practice, particularly when SCr elevation is modest, it is reasonable to initially presume that a patient with a very high CNI level probably has nephrotoxicity and that a patient with deteriorating graft function and a very low drug level is likely undergoing rejection. CNI toxicity usually resolves within 24 to 48 hours of dose reduction. Progressive elevation of the plasma creatinine level, even in the face of persistently high drug levels, warrants consideration of rejection.

CNI levels are most commonly measured using mass spectrometry and immunoassays. Although mass spectrometry–based measurements are more accurate, these techniques are not standardized across institutions, leading to interlaboratory variability. Immunoassays also have limitations because they are prone to measuring metabolites in addition to the parent drug and may overestimate CNI levels.[72] It is important for clinicians to be aware of which testing methodology their laboratory uses and encourage patients to be consistent in the laboratory they use, especially in the early posttransplant period when CNI levels are highly variable and therapeutic dosing is most critical.

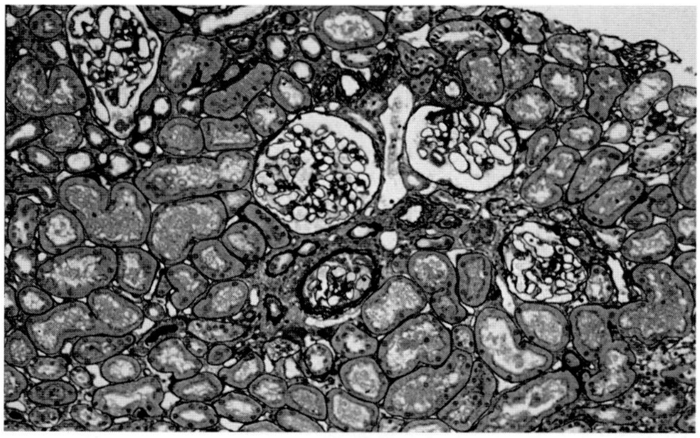

FIG. 39.4 Chronic calcineurin-inhibitor nephrotoxicity. There is "striped" tubular atrophy with interstitial fibrosis, without a significant lymphocytic infiltrate. The intervening tubules are unremarkable, as are the majority of glomeruli. The small glomerulus has mild ischemic features (Jones methenamine silver ×125).

Histological Features of Calcineurin Inhibitor-Mediated Nephrotoxicity

Cyclosporine and tacrolimus nephrotoxicity have similar appearances in renal allografts. The most common form of acute toxicity is a variant of ATN, with scattered individual necrotic tubular cells, considerable dilatation of tubular lumina, and epithelial cell flattening without extensive loss of brush border staining.[73,74] The characteristic feature, often not present, is isometric vacuolization of proximal tubular cell cytoplasm, which tends to involve all tubular cells in few tubular profiles.[74] There is mild interstitial edema without significant inflammation or with focal aggregates of inactive lymphocytes often in perivenous locations; tubulitis is absent. There are no specific glomerular abnormalities. Early in the course of toxicity, arterioles have muscular hypertrophy and individual smooth muscle cells may undergo necrosis; in these locations there is accumulation of rounded plasma protein collections (insudates) in the outer aspect of the muscular walls. The juxtaglomerular apparatus are enlarged.

Chronic CNI toxicity is characterized by focal "striped" interstitial fibrosis, thought to be cortical medullary rays[75] with associated tubular atrophy and little interstitial or tubular inflammation.[76] Arteries are normal, but arterioles may have muscular hypertrophy and rounded insudates in the walls, particularly the outer portion (Fig. 39.4). The glomeruli are unremarkable or have mild ischemic change.[74,76]

THROMBOTIC MICROANGIOPATHY

Thrombotic microangiopathy (TMA) is a rare transplant-related complication that can cause acute graft dysfunction starting as early as 4 days postoperatively. Patients with full-blown manifestations may have previously undiagnosed atypical hemolytic uremic syndrome (aHUS). However, TMA related to CNIs or mammalian target of rapamycin (mTOR)

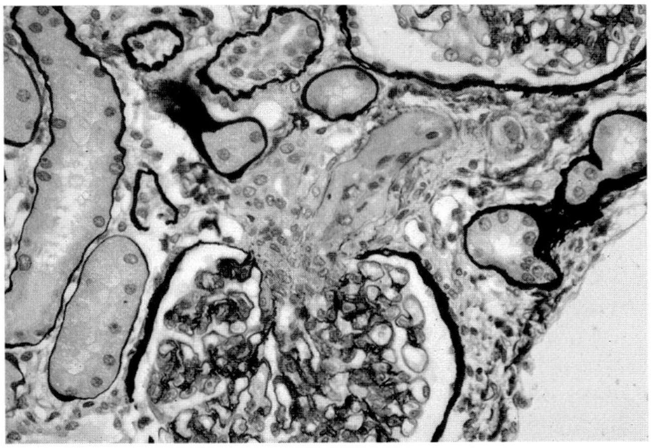

FIG. 39.5 Thrombotic microangiopathic form of acute calcineurin-inhibitor nephrotoxicity. The glomerulus has bland thrombosis of many capillary lumina with few capillary leukocytes (Masson trichrome ×350).

inhibitors has been described in several case series as well, often presenting with renal-limited disease diagnosed by allograft biopsy and none of the classic TMA laboratory findings.[77] Although CNIs can have negative effects on endothelial function, it is possible that many historic cases of posttransplant TMA were not drug related but rather misdiagnosed ABMR or aHUS that coincidentally responded to maneuvers such as changing cyclosporine or sirolimus to tacrolimus,[78-80] or use of plasma exchange or plasmapheresis. The best evidence linking CNIs to TMA comes from case series in nonrenal transplant recipients, which are not confounded by the possibility of renal allograft rejection,[81] although in these cases underlying aHUS has generally not been excluded either. The exact pathogenical mechanism of CNI-mediated TMA is multifactorial and is discussed elsewhere.

Sirolimus has also been associated with posttransplant TMA.[82] Sirolimus administration results in decreased expression of renal vascular endothelial growth factor (VEGF), crucial to the preservation and repair of endothelial cells in the glomerular and peritubular capillaries.[83-85] A "two-hit model" of injury has been suggested where VEGF levels are reduced in all sirolimus-treated patients, but only those with concomitant endothelial injury caused by other insults develop TMA.

Histologically, TMA associated with the CNIs and TOR inhibitors has the usual features of this entity, including glomerular capillary, arteriolar, and occasionally arterial thrombosis (Fig. 39.5).[73,74] Vascular walls display muscular hypertrophy, loose mucoid intimal thickening, and fibrin deposition with luminal narrowing. The thrombotic microangiopathies associated with CNIs have a broad array of kidney involvement, ranging from a patchy and subtle process involving only a few glomerular capillaries to widespread injury with extensive vascular thrombosis and associated cortical infarction.

Although there have been no controlled trials comparing the different treatment modalities of this condition, dose reduction or discontinuation of the offending agent appears to be pivotal in cases where aHUS or AMR have been excluded. Adjunctive plasmapheresis with FFP replacement may offer survival advantages. In transplant recipients with cyclosporine-associated TMA, successful use of tacrolimus immunosuppression has been reported.[77] Indeed, clinicians must remain vigilant for signs and symptoms of recurrence of TMA in patients who are switched from one CNI to another or to an mTOR inhibitor as TMA treatment. For patients who have true drug-related TMA, conversion to belatacept may represent another option.

Other less common transplant-associated causes of post-transplant-associated TMA include viral infections such as CMV, parvovirus B19, influenza A virus,[77] and hepatitis C virus infection occurring concurrently and anticardiolipin antibody positivity.[86]

INFECTION

The most common infections in the early posttransplantation period that are associated with graft dysfunction are urinary tract infection (UTI) and BK and CMV infections. Uncomplicated UTIs do not usually lead to graft dysfunction unless they are complicated by pyelonephritis or urosepsis. Recurrent UTIs can lead to chronic allograft dysfunction. In a large registry study of 28,942 kidney transplant recipients, Abbott et al.[87] reported that the cumulative incidence of UTI during the first 6 months after kidney transplantation was 17% (equivalent for both men and women), but at 3 years it was 60% for women and 47% for men ($P < 0.001$).[87] In addition, late UTI was significantly associated with an increased risk for subsequent death ($P < 0.001$; adjusted hazard ratio [aHR], 2.93; 95% CI, 2.22 to 3.85).

There is no consensus as to the best preventative strategy for recurrent UTIs in transplant recipients. Adequate hydration and frequent voiding can help reduce infections, but for some patients with recurrent infections, consultation with a transplant infectious disease specialist may be required. We generally try to avoid chronic antibiotic use to prevent infections, instead preferring maneuvers to change the urine pH such as methenamine. It is also prudent to consider a formal urological evaluation to investigate mechanical causes of bladder dysfunction.

VASCULAR COMPLICATIONS

Renal Artery Stenosis

Transplant renal artery stenosis (RAS) may occur as early as the first week, but it is usually a late complication, occurring 3 months to 2 years posttransplant, with a reported prevalence of 1% to 23%.[88] Clinically, patients may present with new onset or accelerated hypertension, acute deterioration of graft function or severe hypotension associated with the use of renin-angiotensin-aldosterone system (RAAS) blockade, recurrent pulmonary edema or refractory edema in the absence of heavy proteinuria, and/or erythrocytosis. The presence of a bruit over the allograft is neither sensitive nor specific for the diagnosis of graft renovascular disease. However, a change in the intensity of the bruit or the detection of new bruits warrants an evaluation. The approach to management of transplant RAS is addressed in detail in Chapter 37.

Allograft Thrombosis

Arterial or venous thrombosis almost always occurs within the first 2 to 3 postoperative days but may occur as long as 2 months posttransplant. In most series reported, the incidence of graft thrombosis ranges from 0.5% to as high as 8%, with arterial thrombosis accounting for one-third and venous thrombosis for two-thirds of cases.[29,89] Thrombosis occurring early after transplantation most often is due to technical surgical complications, whereas the later onset generally is due to acute rejection.[29] In patients with initial good allograft function, thrombosis is generally heralded by the acute onset of oliguria or anuria associated with deterioration of allograft function. Abnormal laboratory findings may include thrombocytopenia, hyperkalemia, and a rising lactate dehydrogenase level. Clinically the patient may present with graft swelling or tenderness and/or gross hematuria. In patients with DGF and good residual urine output from the native kidneys, there may be no overt signs or symptoms, and the diagnosis rests on clinical suspicion and prompt imaging studies. The diagnosis is usually made by Doppler ultrasound or isotope flow scan. Confirmed arterial or venous thrombosis typically necessitates allograft nephrectomy. In recipients of kidneys with multiple arteries, thrombosis may occur in a single branch, and depending on the extent of renal parenchymal supplied, adequate residual functioning tissue may remain.

Suggested predisposing factors for vascular thrombosis include arteriosclerotic involvement of the donor or recipient vessels, intimal injury of graft vessels, kidneys with multiple arteries, history of recurrent thrombosis, thrombocytosis, younger recipient and/or donor age, and the presence of a hypercoagulable state such as antiphospholipid antibody (anticardiolipin antibody and/or lupus anticoagulant).[88] There has been no consensus on the optimal management of recipients with abnormal hypercoagulability profile, such as abnormal activated protein C resistance ratio or factor V Leiden mutation, antiphospholipid antibody positivity, protein C or protein S deficiency, or antithrombin III deficiency, but unless contraindicated, perioperative and/or postoperative prophylactic anticoagulation should be considered, particularly in patients with a history of recurrent thrombotic events. Transplant of pediatric en bloc kidneys into adult recipient with a history of thrombosis should probably be avoided. The duration of anticoagulation has not been well defined, but lifelong anticoagulation should be considered in high-risk candidates.[88] The diagnosis and management of transplant renal vein thrombosis is discussed in Chapter 37.

Ureteral Obstruction

Ureteral obstruction occurs in 2% to 6% of kidney transplants.[90] Because this generally occurs as a complication of the transplant surgery, the reader is directed to Chapter 37 for a more detailed overview on this topic. It is important to keep in mind that hydronephrosis may be minimal or absent in early obstruction, whereas low-grade dilatation of the collecting system secondary to edema at the ureterovesical anastomosis may be seen in early posttransplantation and does not necessarily indicate obstruction. Moreover, a full bladder may also cause mild calyceal dilatation because of ureteral reflux, and repeat ultrasound with an empty bladder should be carried out. Persistent or increasing hydronephrosis on repeat ultrasound examinations is highly suggestive of obstruction. Because transplant ureteral strictures have been associated with BK virus infection, BK viral load should be checked in these patients.[91] Calculi are uncommon causes of ureteral obstruction,[29] but when this situation occurs it can be managed by endourological techniques or by extracorporeal shock wave lithotripsy.

Perinephric Fluid Collections

Symptomatic perinephric fluid collections in the early postoperative period can be due to lymphoceles, hematoma, urinoma, or abscesses. Lymphoceles, collections of lymph caused by leakage from severed lymphatics, typically develop within weeks after transplantation. Most lymphoceles are small and asymptomatic and no intervention is required. Generally the larger the lymphocele, the more likely it is to produce mechanical effects and require treatment (reviewed in Chapter 37). Lymphoceles can also cause compression of the iliac vein leading to ipsilateral leg swelling or deep-vein thrombosis or even to urinary incontinence as a result of bladder compression.[29]

An obstructed hematoma is best managed by surgical evacuation. Urinoma or evidence of a urine leak should be treated without delay. A small leak can be managed expectantly with insertion of a Foley catheter to reduce intravesical pressure. This maneuver may occasionally reduce or stop the leak altogether. Persistent allograft dysfunction, particularly in a symptomatic patient, often necessitates early surgical exploration and repair. Infected perinephric fluid collections should be treated by external drainage or open surgery in conjunction with systemic antibiotics.

LATE GRAFT DYSFUNCTION

Late graft loss after kidney transplantation remains a major problem. Both immunological and nonimmunological factors related to donor and recipient characteristics have been suggested to play an interactive role in the development of late allograft dysfunction. In addition, deterioration of kidney function can be insidious, leading to biopsies being done late in the clinical course with the finding of mostly irreversible scar tissue. Patients usually have slow loss of function along with hypertension and variable proteinuria. The term *chronic allograft nephropathy* (CAN) first appeared in the Banff schema in 1991 to replace the often misleading term *chronic rejection*. Although initially succeeding in reversing the misconception that not all late scarring of the graft was due to alloimmune injury, the term *CAN* was increasingly misused to the point where it was generally regarded as "the disease" rather than a generic term to describe nonspecific renal parenchymal scarring.[92] For this reason, the term *CAN* was eschewed in the Banff nomenclature in 2005 in favor of more specific histological descriptions such as BK nephropathy, recurrent or de novo glomerulonephritis, hypertension, or CNI toxicity. In the 2015 Banff update, biopsy results that were once classified as CAN now most commonly fall under category 5, interstitial fibrosis and tubular atrophy (IF/TA), or category 6, other changes not caused by acute or chronic rejection. This latter category includes BK virus nephropathy, posttransplant lymphoproliferative disorders, CNI toxicity, ATN, recurrent glomerular disease, de novo glomerulonephritis, pyelonephritis, and drug-induced interstitial nephritis. Biopsy results indicating changes consistent with IF/TA are very challenging because no specific therapy for graft fibrosis/scar tissue exists and allograft survival is inversely proportional to the percentage of cortical area that is affected.

Differential Diagnosis of Chronic Allograft Injury

Chronic rejection, either T-cell mediated or antibody mediated, needs to be differentiated from other causes of late graft dysfunction. The absence of a history of rejection, DSA, hypertension, and proteinuria should raise diagnostic skepticism. A renal ultrasound with Doppler should be performed at least once to exclude obstructive causes of graft dysfunction and the possibility of RAS particularly in the setting of new or worsened hypertension or erythrocytosis. Kidney biopsy provides a definitive diagnosis and a good estimate of the severity of the lesion.

Causes of late graft failure have been investigated in detail by El-Zoghby et al.[93] in 1317 kidney transplant recipients by reviewing their clinical and histological information. During an average of 50 months of follow-up, 330 grafts were lost (25.0%); 138 (10.4%) because of death with function, 39 (2.9%) because of primary nonfunction, and 153 (11.6%) because of graft failure censored for death. Interestingly, they found that most cases of graft loss had an identifiable cause that was not idiopathic fibrosis/atrophy or CNI toxicity; they found glomerular diseases in 36.6%, fibrosis/atrophy in 30.7%, medical/surgical conditions in 16.3%, acute rejection in 11.8%, and unclassifiable in only 4.6% of their patients. Glomerular pathological conditions leading to failure included recurrent disease (n = 23), transplant glomerulopathy (n = 23), and presumed nonrecurrent disease (n = 10).

In another study[94] of 315 allograft recipients who underwent indication biopsies at 6 days to 32 years posttransplant, 60 kidneys progressed to failure in the follow-up period (median 31.4 months); 56 of the failures were attributed to four main causes: rejection in 36 (64%), glomerulonephritis in 10 (18%), BK nephropathy in 4 (7%), and intercurrent events in 6 (11%). Every case of loss caused by rejection had evidence of ABMR by the time of failure. As seen in most of the centers, in this particular study, nonadherence was more common in patients who progressed to failure (32%) versus those who survived (3%).

Similar to pretransplant CKD, chronic graft dysfunction (CGD) has been associated with graft loss and death. In a prospective study[95] of 2336 transplants, CGD was associated with significant risk for death-censored graft failure and CGD phenotype with concomitant inflammation was associated with increased risk for allograft failure. Among 366 transplant recipients with CGD, 91% had inflammation on biopsy scores; 94 (26%) had inflammatory changes with concomitant acute rejection. Single nucleotide polymorphisms (SNPs) in *FM06* and *FM03*, potential drug metabolism genes, were associated with CGD after accounting for multiple testing, leading the way to larger new studies.

Antigen-Dependent Causes of Late Graft Loss

Acute rejection episodes, poor HLA matching, prior sensitization, inadequate immunosuppression, and noncompliance have all been implicated in the development of de novo DSA, chronic antibody-mediated rejection, and late graft loss. Schinstock et al.[96] retrospectively studied adult kidney transplant recipients who had serial protocol biopsies from 2007 to 2014.[96] Patients with DSA had reduced death-censored allograft survival (87.0% vs. 97.0% no DSA, $P < 0.01$). AMR was present in 25.0% and 52.9% of patients at DSA detection and at 1 year, respectively. Patients with both class I and II DSA had the highest rate of allograft loss. The authors argued that patients with DSA without AMR at time of detection might benefit from a follow-up biopsy within 1 year because AMR can be missed initially and follow-up biopsies could actually identify patients at risk for late graft loss.

Using single antigen bead antibody testing in 83 patients with failed kidney transplants, Süsal et al.[97] also found that the posttransplant presence of persistent or de novo HLA antibodies, especially if C1q binding, is associated with graft loss, even if the antibodies are not specific for mismatched donor HLA.

Hill et al.[98] also reported that among DSA-positive patients, arteriosclerosis significantly progressed between month 3 and month 12 after transplant on protocol biopsies; in contrast, among DSA-negative patients, they did not detect a statistically significant progression during the same time frame. In these protocol biopsies, accelerated arteriosclerosis was significantly associated with peritubular capillary leukocytic infiltration, glomerulitis, subclinical antibody-mediated rejection, and interstitial inflammation.[98]

Many transplant recipients are at risk to develop rejection and late graft loss. Conventional biopsy assessment might not be helpful all the time because of sampling issues and interobserver disagreements. Therefore numerous microarray-based molecular tests are being tested to help with the diagnosis, activity, and prognosis.

Halloran et al.[99] prospectively collected 703 specimens from biopsies of 564 kidneys performed for clinical indications 3 days to 35 years posttransplant and studied them with conventional biopsy assessment as well as microarrays. They noted that kidneys that progressed to failure after the biopsy more commonly presented with decreasing function, had DSA, and were from patients not on tacrolimus-mycophenolate–based immunosuppression. Interestingly, in Cox regression analysis of death-censored 3-year survival, the kidneys of patients with conventional diagnoses of pure TCMR or borderline changes did not have increased risk for failure compared with those with relatively normal biopsy results, whereas kidneys with pure ABMR had worse survival than those with relatively normal biopsy results. Another striking finding was the disappearance of TCMR from indication biopsies after 10 years posttransplant. In this particular study the molecular tests strongly agreed with conventional assessment (accuracy of 91% for pure TCMR and 83% for pure ABMR) and the pattern of rejection over time was similar by conventional and molecular assessments, supporting the idea that combining molecular with conventional assessment could improve our understanding of troubled kidney transplants and help predict which kidneys would fail.

In the prospective, multicenter Genomics of Chronic Allograft Rejection (GoCAR) study,[100] a set of 13 genes that was independently predictive for the development of fibrosis at 1 year was identified by O'Connell et al. They collected protocol biopsy specimens from 204 kidney transplant recipients with stable renal function 3 months after transplantation and used microarray analysis to investigate gene expression in 159 of these tissue samples. Although routine pathological variables were unable to identify which histologically normal allografts would progress to fibrosis (AUC 0.754), the predictive set of 13 genes accurately discriminated between transplants at high and low risk for progression (AUC 0.916). Once validated in large-scale trials and developed for clinic use, this tool could be used to identify transplant recipients at risk for graft loss before the development of irreversible damage. Transplant physicians could then modify their therapies to prevent further progression.

Numerous retrospective studies have found that acute rejection episodes that are severe, recurrent, or happen late have been associated with late graft loss. Several studies have also found that subclinical rejection might be associated with chronic tubulointerstitial damage and subsequent graft dysfunction leading to reduced graft survival. An analysis of the UNOS database involving 105,742 adult transplant recipients performed between 1988 and 1998 revealed that posttransplant SCr greater than 1.5 mg/dL at 1 year significantly decreased graft half-life irrespective of acute rejection episodes.[101]

In a small study,[102] treatment of subclinical rejection with high-dose corticosteroids was found to be associated with an improved outcome; compared with control participants, patients in the biopsy group had a significant decrease in early and late acute rejection episodes, had less chronic damage at month 6, and had a lower SCr at 2 years.

In a recent observational prospective cohort study[103] of 1001 patients who had a kidney biopsy at 1-year posttransplant, three groups of patients were identified at the 1-year screening: 73% patients without rejection, 13% patients with subclinical TCMR, and 14% patients with subclinical ABMR. Patients with subclinical ABMR had the poorest graft survival at 8 years posttransplant (56%) compared with subclinical TCMR (88%) and patients without rejection (90%) ($P < 0.001$). It has also been found that subclinical ABMR at 1 year was independently associated with a 3.5-fold increase in graft loss along with decreased estimated glomerular filtration rate (eGFR) and proteinuria ($P < 0.001$).

An analysis of the Collaborative Transplant Study database consisting of more than 28,000 deceased donor kidney transplants performed between 1995 and 2005 found that the time point of occurrence and the degree of functional recovery after rejection treatment significantly influence the impact of acute rejection episodes on long-term graft survival. Compared with patients who did not receive rejection treatment during the first posttransplant year, the hazard ratios for graft survival for patients with rejection during three different periods after transplantation—namely, 0 to 90 days, 91 to 189 days, and 181 to 365 days—were 1.35, 2.05, and 2.74, respectively ($P < 0.001$ for all three time intervals studied).[104] These findings are consistent with an analysis of UNOS data involving 105,742 adult recipients transplanted between 1988 and 1998 revealed that posttransplant SCr greater than 1.5 mg/dL at 1 year significantly decreased graft half-life.[101]

Histocompatibility

HLA matching is one of the most important predictors for graft survival of both living and deceased donor renal allografts.[105] Among living donor transplants, the half-life for two-haplotype-matched transplants has been estimated to be 22.7 years compared with 13.1 years for one-haplotype-matched transplants, which in turn tend to function longer than zero-haplotype-matched transplants and those from living, unrelated donors.[106] The importance of matching is particularly evident for deceased donor transplants: Six-antigen-matched or zero-mismatched deceased donor transplants have a 5-year survival rate approaching 80% and a half-life approaching 13 years, compared with about 50% and 8 years, respectively, for completely mismatched transplants.[107]

With the advent of more potent immunosuppressive therapy and a decrease in the incidence of acute rejection in recent years, the relevance of matching donor and recipient HLA antigens has been questioned. In an analysis of the Collaborate Transplant Study database, Opelz et al.[108] reported that although graft survival rates have improved overall over time, the relative impact of HLA matching on the graft survival rates has remained strong and highly significant. Both the need for posttransplant rejection treatment and the graft survival rates had statistically highly significant associations with HLA matching regardless of the interval analyzed ($P < 0.001$). Among transplants performed between 1985 and 1994, transplants with no HLA mismatches showed a risk ratio of graft failure of 0.76 (95% CI, 0.71 to 0.8), compared with 0.83 for transplants performed in the 1995–2004 decade. The increased risk for failure associated with six HLA antigen mismatches was 1.23 (CI, 1.14 to 1.32) for those transplanted between 1985 and 1994 and 1.16 (CI, 1.05 to 1.27) for those transplanted in the 1995–2004 decade. Analysis of death-censored graft survival indicated a similar beneficial effect of HLA matches. Although matching is important, the excellent short-term and long-term results of living, unrelated transplants suggest that the condition of the kidney at the time of transplantation is a critical, non–alloantigen-dependent factor.

Prior Sensitization

It has long been recognized that the presence of high levels of preformed, panel-reactive antibodies (PRA) against HLA antigens before transplantation is associated with an increased incidence of rejection episodes and decreased graft survival. In the Collaborative Transplant Study, Opelz et al.[109] reported significantly higher 10-year graft survival among HLA-identical sibling transplants with 0% PRA compared with those receiving HLA-identical sibling transplants with 1% to 50% PRA, or those with greater than 50% PRA. Ten-year graft survival rates were 72.4% vs. 63.3% vs. 55.5%, respectively ($P = 0.0006$ for 0% PRA compared with 1% to 50% PRA, and $P < 0.0001$ for 0% compared with >50% PRA). The strong association between PRA reactivity and long-term graft loss in HLA-identical sibling donors suggests that non-HLA immunity may play a more important role in clinical transplantation than previously suggested.

Alloantigen-Independent Factors

Alloantigen-independent factors can be classified as donor related or recipient related. The former may include donor age, nephron dose relative to recipient's metabolic demand, and donor premorbid conditions such as hypertension, diabetes, or preexisting donor kidney dysfunction. Recipient factors include age, ethnicity, cause of native kidney disease, hypertension, diabetes, dyslipidemia, CNI nephrotoxicity, end-stage kidney disease vintage, proteinuria, and concomitant infections. Over the last decade, BK nephropathy has emerged as an important cause of allograft dysfunction and graft loss. Selected alloantigen-independent factors are discussed next.

Donor Age

The association between donor age and the development of chronic allograft dysfunction has been well described. In a retrospective study consisting of 40,289 primary solitary white adult kidney transplants, older donor and recipient age were found to have an independent yet equally detrimental effect on renal allograft survival.[110]

Chronic CNI Nephrotoxicity

Chronic CNI toxicity generally occurs months to years after transplantation. It may be characterized by an insidious rise in SCr and varying degrees of hypertension and proteinuria. A longitudinal cohort study of 200 patients examined the histological evidence for CNI nephrotoxicity from normal donor kidneys of successful kidney-pancreas transplant recipients transplanted during cyclosporine and tacrolimus eras.[111] The series included 1622 prospective protocol (84.3%) and indication (15.7%) kidney biopsies. Biopsy results from the tacrolimus era indicated less rejection and reduced early immune-mediated tubular damage compared with cyclosporine ($P < 0.001$). In this particular study, a tacrolimus-based regimen appeared superior to the cyclosporine era, with less early CNI nephrotoxicity and fewer rejection episodes but comparable chronic arteriolar toxicity/arteriolar hyalinosis.

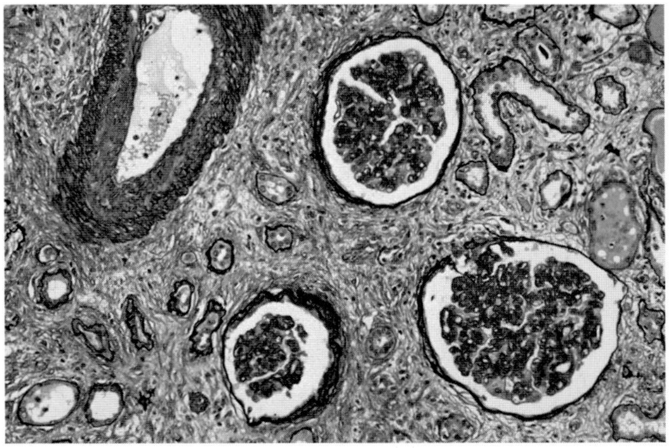

FIG. 39.6 Chronic changes. Arterial intimal fibrosis, tubular atrophy with interstitial fibrosis, interstitial lymphocytes, and chronic transplant glomerulopathy are present (periodic acid–methenamine silver ×125).

Despite a suggested correlation between CNI dose and the severity of chronic CNI toxicity, dosage reduction does not predictably reverse or halt the progression of established chronic kidney dysfunction. Accordingly, studies examining protocol biopsy results have not consistently identified a correlation between CNI blood concentration levels and chronic histological changes.[112]

Histopathological Features of Chronic Graft Dysfunction

As with acute rejection, chronic transplant rejection has cell-mediated and antibody-mediated pathogenetic mechanisms. The typical findings in chronic rejection include intimal fibrosis of arteries with entrapped mononuclear leukocytes in the thickened vascular wall, disruption of the internal elastic lamina, and narrowing of the lumens.[113] There is tubular atrophy with interstitial fibrosis. Glomeruli may be normal, may be ischemic, or may indicate chronic transplant glomerulopathy, a lesion consisting of capillary wall double contours, mesangial widening with mild hypercellularity, mesangiolysis, and leukocytes in capillary lumina; segmental glomerulosclerosis may also be present (Fig. 39.6).[114] These glomeruli have variable deposition of IgM, complement, and fibrin focally in capillary walls identified by immunofluorescence. The features more specifically associated with antibody-mediated chronic rejection include multilayering of glomerular and peritubular capillary basement membranes (Fig. 39.7).[115] Approximately 50% of patients with chronic transplant glomerulopathy will demonstrate concomitant positive C4d staining in peritubular capillaries, indicating a chronic active ABMR process.[116] However, a number of patients with chronic transplant glomerulopathy have no history of DSA or C4d positivity, and complement activation may not be required for the development of this lesion; in these patients it may be a cell-mediated process.[117,118]

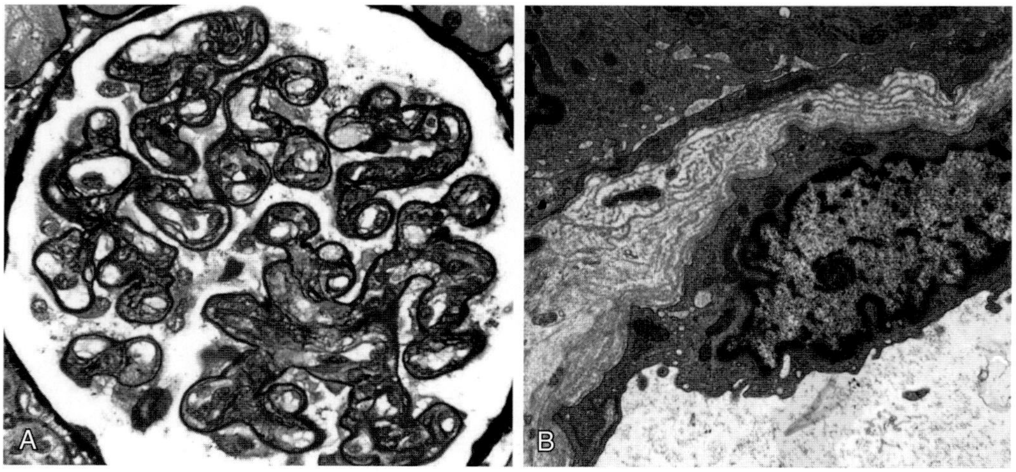

FIG. 39.7 Biopsy features of chronic antibody-mediated rejection. (A) Chronic transplant glomerulopathy with reduplicated capillary walls and segmental mesangial expansion (periodic acid–methenamine silver ×350). (B) Peritubular capillary with multilayered basement membrane and swollen endothelial cell (×14,000).

Strategies to Prevent Late Graft Loss (Also See Chapter 44)

Proceeding to biopsy early in the course of graft dysfunction may help identify rejection and other reversible causes of graft dysfunction. Monitoring for complications of over- or underimmunosuppression, such as the development of BK viremia or de novo DSA, are being increasingly incorporated into standard clinical practice and follow-up of transplant recipients. New tools such as urine biomarkers, signatures from transcriptomics and proteomics profiles, enzyme-linked immunospot (ELISPOT) assay and cell-free donor-derived DNA detection are all promising adjuncts to current practice but require prospective validation and standardization before they can be implemented widely in the clinic. Improvements in HLA matching methodology, the development of new maintenance immunosuppressive drugs such as specific anti–B-cell therapies and inhibitors of complement pathways, and identification of tolerance signatures will all help promote longer-term graft survival in the near future.

To detect and diagnose late allograft dysfunction, clinicians should monitor patients for subtle changes in SCr or eGFR, development of proteinuria (especially an increase in proteinuria of >0.5 g per 24 h) and alterations in blood pressure control over time. Investigations of CGD should include an ultrasound with Doppler studies, serum BK PCR, DSA screening, and a kidney biopsy to investigate for common and treatable causes.

It is well established that uncontrolled hypertension is a significant risk factor not only for late graft loss but also patient mortality. Adequate blood pressure control as well as aggressive management of dyslipidemia and proteinuria are mandatory for a healthy graft, and the reader is referred to Chapter 41 for a detailed review of this topic.

The beneficial effects of angiotensin-converting enzyme inhibitor or angiotensin receptor blocker on posttransplant patient and graft survival have not been consistently demonstrated. Randomized controlled trials have been performed but have been underpowered with inadequate follow-up to draw meaningful conclusions. In a metaanalysis of eight randomized controlled trials (n = 1502 patients), RAAS blockade did not significantly alter all-cause mortality (RR, 0.96; 95% CI, 0.62 to 1.51), transplant failure (RR, 0.76; 95% CI, 0.49 to 1.18), or doubling of SCr (RR, 0.84; 95% CI, 0.51 to 1.39) compared with the control group.[119] There was significantly higher risk for hyperkalemia with RAAS blockade. Definitive data may never be available; the authors calculated that a trial with more than 10,000 patients would be needed to definitively answer whether RAAS blockade reduces graft loss in the transplant population.

In the absence of convincing clinical data, we cannot recommend using RAAS blockade in all kidney transplant recipients. One must balance the putative cardiovascular and "renoprotective" benefits afforded by RAAS blockade with the potential for worsening GFR, anemia, and hyperkalemia. An acutely rising SCr in a patient recently started on RAAS blockade should alert clinicians to a likely causal relationship.

In addition to pharmacological treatment, emphasis should be placed on lifestyle modifications, including decrease in dietary sodium and saturated fat intake, regular aerobic exercise, weight reduction, and tobacco avoidance. Similar to chronic kidney disease in the nontransplant settings, the management of CGD requires a multidisciplinary approach where every potentially complicating factor must be closely monitored and treated. Studies such as the multicenter, observational Long-Term Deterioration of Kidney Allograft Function (DeKAF) Study should help identify and characterize the exact cause of late (defined as >90 days) kidney allograft dysfunction and failure in providing the basis for future therapeutic trials.

For patients whose CGD has no identifiable cause, optimal immunosuppression management remains unclear. If attributed to CNI nephrotoxicity, minimizing exposure

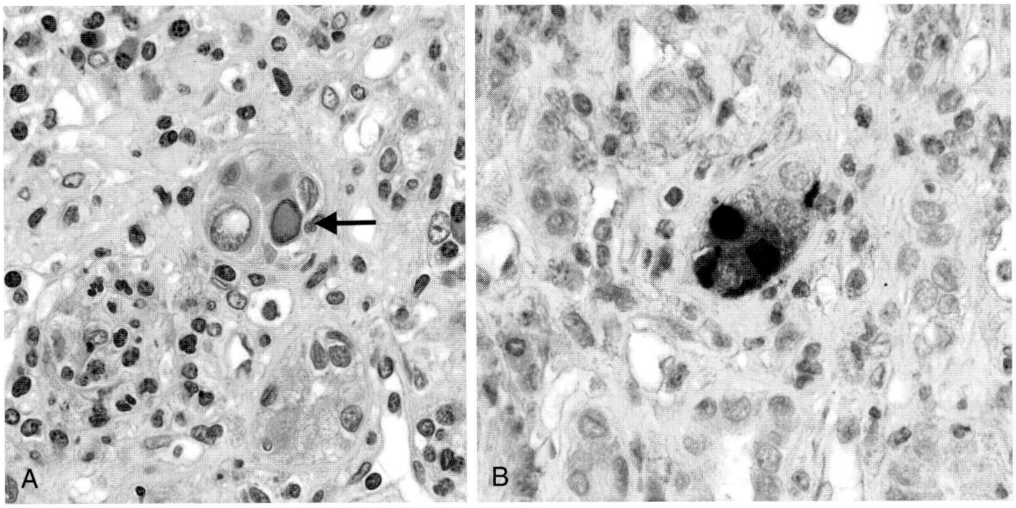

FIG. 39.8 Polyoma virus (BK) nephropathy. (A) Enlarged tubular epithelial cells with an intranuclear viral inclusion *(arrow)* and mononuclear inflammation in the tubules and interstitium (hematoxylin and eosin ×350). (B) Immunohistochemical stain for polyoma virus (SV40) demonstrating an intranuclear viral antigen in a tubule (×350).

and/or conversion to other immunosuppressive agents have been used but not definitely established to be associated with improved outcomes. Some trials have evaluated conversion from CNI to TOR inhibitors in the setting of allograft dysfunction (discussed in detail in Chapter 38 on Immunosuppression). Although kidney function may improve after conversion, from cyclosporine in particular, most trials have reported increased treatment failure rates and no overall outcomes improvement in patients randomly assigned to TOR inhibitors. Because patients with an eGFR less than 40 mL/min at conversion are at risk for faster progression of chronic allograft injury, Kidney Disease: Improving Global Outcomes (KDIGO) transplant guidelines only recommend using mTOR inhibitor in patients whose eGFR exceeds this level of kidney function. In a metaanalysis of 21 randomized trials, sirolimus compared with control was associated with a 40% reduction in the risk for malignancy (aHR 0.60, 95% CI, 0.39 to 0.93) and a 56% reduction in the risk for nonmelanoma skin cancer (0.44, 0.30 to 0.63) but a significantly increased risk for death (1.43, 1.21 to 1.71).[120] Further research is needed to determine whether different populations, such as those at high risk for cancer, might benefit from sirolimus, but not most patients with a kidney transplant.

BK Nephropathy

Over the last two decades, BK virus nephropathy (BKN) has emerged as an important cause of allograft dysfunction after kidney transplantation. BK is a human polyoma virus, and at least six genotypes with varying geographical distribution have been identified; genotype I is the most common worldwide.[121] Primary infection is often acquired in childhood, and patients are asymptomatic as the virus establishes latency in the uroepithelium; it reactivates in the setting of immunosuppression. Established risk factors for BK viremia and nephropathy include the overall state of immunosuppression, including treatment for rejection episodes and degree of HLA mismatch, older age, male gender, and use of ureteral stents. Since the widespread adoption of lymphocyte-depleting antibodies for kidney transplant induction and maintenance immunosuppression regimens based on tacrolimus and mycophenolate mofetil, rates of BK infection have been on the rise[122]; this finding was bolstered by a secondary analysis of the DIRECT trial data, which indicated a higher incidence of BK viremia and higher viral loads in the tacrolimus arm.

BK nephropathy most commonly presents within the first posttransplant year, with peaks of incidence at 3 and 12 months.[123] Because there is no effective antiviral prophylaxis for BK infection, we advocate for a universal screening protocol for kidney transplant recipients. At our center we screen patients using serum PCR; this assay has a sensitivity and specificity >90% for the prediction of BK nephropathy. Although screening urine by PCR for BK DNA or the presence of decoy cells is an alternative approach, confirmatory serum PCR testing is required because only about one-third of patients with BK viruria have BK viremia.[124,125]

The diagnosis of BKN is made by allograft biopsy, which demonstrates BK viral inclusions in renal tubular cell nuclei and occasionally in glomerular parietal epithelium.[126,127] Biopsy specimens often have variable degrees of interstitial mononuclear inflammation with plasma cells, degenerative changes in tubules, and focal tubulitis that can mimic acute rejection (Fig. 39.8); these areas of tubulointerstitial inflammation are often focal and correspond to foci of viral infection. Additional studies including immunohistochemistry or in situ hybridization for viral particles are helpful to confirm the diagnosis. BK infection and acute rejection may occur simultaneously, and distinguishing among BKN, acute rejection, and the concomitant presence of both processes can be a diagnostic challenge. There is a histological classification system for BKN based on the degree of active inflammation, acute tubular injury, and tubulointerstitial scarring, which may have prognostic significance.[128]

The treatment of choice for BK viremia and nephropathy treatment is the careful reduction of maintenance immunosuppression. Studies from Schaub et al.[129] and Hardinger et al.[130] both found that immunosuppression reduction after BK detection resulted in preservation of allograft function and BK viral control, even after 5 years of follow-up. Specific immunosuppression reduction strategies vary across centers and include discontinuation of antimetabolite, CNI dose reduction, and/or conversion to or addition of TOR inhibitor. Two recent studies have highlighted the unintended consequences of reducing immunosuppression to treat BK viremia; whereas longer-term follow-up has indicated that immunosuppression reduction is safe and effective at BK viral clearance, patients with BK viremia are more likely to develop DSAs and immune responses to kidney self-antigens such as fibronectin and collagen IV.[131,132]

There have been several single-center case reports of using cidofovir, leflunomide, or intravenous immunoglobulin in addition to or instead of immunosuppression reduction for the treatment of BK nephropathy; however, no prospective data exist to support this practice.[133-137] Two prospective, placebo-controlled studies of fluoroquinolones for prevention or treatment of BK nephropathy also failed to find a beneficial effect; the course of BK infection was unchanged, but there was an increase in fluoroquinolone-resistant infections and tendonitis in the prophylaxis study.[137,138]

Patients who lose their allografts because of BKN can safely be retransplanted with posttransplant outcomes comparable to those who did not lose a prior allograft to BK, and transplant nephrectomy is not required; however, the BK viral load must be negative before retransplantation.[139]

Recurrent Diseases

Although recurrent diseases are important causes of CGD and allograft failure, this topic is beyond the scope of this chapter and the reader is referred to Chapter 42, where this is extensively discussed.

Nonadherence

Immunosuppression nonadherence is recognized as a cause of both early and late allograft dysfunction, with data suggesting that longer time since transplant is an important risk factor. It is estimated that 22% of kidney transplant recipients experience some degree of nonadherence and it is responsible for 36% of allograft losses.[140] It was suggested in one study by Nevins et al.[141] that missing as little as 5% of immunosuppression doses could significantly increase risk for graft loss.

The definition of nonadherence varies across studies, and it is notoriously difficult to measure. Failure to take medications or taking them at improper intervals can both be considered nonadherence. Electronic pill bottle opening remains the gold standard measurement, acknowledging that opening a pill bottle does not guarantee a patient has consumed the medication.[142,143] Self-report, pill counts, refill records, and drug levels have all been used to assess adherence, and each measure has its own drawbacks. Three phenotypes of nonadherent patients have been described—the accidental, the invulnerable, and the decisive; each type needs to be addressed with a different approach. Increasing the complexity of medication regimens with multiple dosing intervals and increasing total numbers of pills augments the likelihood of noncompliance; this is amplified by unpleasant medication side effects and issues with prescription coverage or insurance.[144] Certain populations have been identified as being at increased risk—adolescents, the elderly, recipients of living donors, and those who are farther out from transplant. This is an area of great interest and study because it is a preventable cause of graft failure.

ACKNOWLEDGMENTS

The authors would like to thank Phuong-Thu T. Pham, MD, Cynthia C. Nast, MD, Phuong-Chi T. Pham, MD, and Gabriel Danovitch, MD, for their contributions to this chapter in the previous edition.

A full list of references is available at www.expertsonsult.com.

40

Infection in Renal Transplant Recipients

Deirdre Sawinski, MD, and Emily A. Blumberg, MD

OUTLINE

INTRODUCTION

Infections are a significant cause of morbidity and mortality after kidney transplantation and have been implicated in allograft dysfunction, rejection, and loss. Both opportunistic and traditional organisms are important causes of infection. The risk for specific infections varies with timing posttransplant, exposures, and the degree of immunosuppression. Because the array of pathogens is diverse, the risk factors not necessarily modifiable, and the causative exposures not consistently anticipated, prevention of infection is a complicated and imperfect process. Moreover, the clinical presentation of infection may be atypical in the setting of immunosuppression, making diagnosis more difficult. Concurrent coinfections with multiple organisms can occur, and in some cases, it is difficult to differentiate infectious from noninfectious causes of patient presentations. Because transplant recipients are chronically maintained on immunosuppression, they are at especial risk for more severe presentations of infection, even with organisms traditionally associated with more benign courses. Prompt and accurate diagnosis is imperative to ensure optimal outcomes.

Infections in kidney transplant recipients can be viewed as the balance of the host interaction with the environment as mediated by prophylactic strategies.[1] Transplant recipients may have underlying conditions associated with depressed host immunity before the administration of the exogenous immunosuppression required to maintain allograft function. The choice of immunosuppression plays an important role in specific infection risks. For example, T-cell depleting therapies, including antithymocyte globulin, increase the risk for opportunistic infection, and mammalian target of rapamycin (mTOR) inhibitors have been associated with skin and soft tissue infections (Table 40.1).[2] The risk for infection also reflects a recipient's exposures. This includes pretransplant infections that have the potential for latency (e.g., herpesvirus infections, tuberculosis [TB]) as well as infections associated with the transplant including donor-derived and hospital-acquired infections. In the posttransplant setting, new exposures related to environmental and community interactions need to be considered. In some cases, these exposures can be anticipated based on predictive risk periods posttransplant and appropriate prophylaxis can be administered during the highest risk period to reduce the risk for infection; antivirals directed against cytomegalovirus (CMV) are an example of risk mitigation. A thorough evaluation of all potential recipients and donors is critical to manage infection risks.

PRETRANSPLANT RECIPIENT EVALUATION

All potential transplant candidates should undergo screening to identify both active infections that may have an effect on transplant eligibility and latent infections that may reactivate after transplant and affect patient outcomes (Table 40.2).[3] The screening process should include a thorough history of prior infections, environmental exposures associated with infection risks (including current and prior locations of residence, occupations, hobbies, and pets), and close contacts with communicable diseases such as TB. A careful physical

TABLE 40.1 **Common Immunosuppressive Agents and Select Infection Risks***

Immunosuppressive	Mechanism of Action	Associated Infections
Alemtuzumab	Bind to CD52 on lymphocytes, monocytes, macrophages, natural killer cells, and potentially granulocytes to disrupt their function	Opportunistic infections, including bacterial and fungal infections (including PJP), CMV, EBV/PTLD
Antithymocyte globulin	Cause lysis of lymphocytes with prolonged lymphocyte depletion	Opportunistic infections, including bacterial, CMV, EBV/PTLD, BK, fungal infection (including PJP, *Cryptococcus*)
Basiliximab/Daclizumab	Block IL-2 receptor	Risk for opportunistic infections does not appear to be increased and may be decreased with these agents
Belatacept	Disrupt T-cell costimulation and consequently activation	Associated with EBV/PTLD in EBV-seronegative recipients of seropositive organs
Tacrolimus	Inhibit cytokine production, primarily IL-2, by CD4-positive T-cells	Possible increase in BK, intracellular pathogens
Cyclosporine	Inhibit cytokine production, primarily IL-2, by CD4-positive T-cells	Intracellular pathogens
Mycophenolate	Impair T- and B-cell proliferation and function	Early bacterial infections, late CMV, BK
Azathioprine	Impair T- and B-cell proliferation and function	Possibly papillomavirus
Corticosteroids	Inhibit inflammatory responses and impair T-cell activation	Bacterial pathogens, PJP, Hepatitis B and C
Sirolimus/Everolimus	Inhibit cell cycle proliferation	Wound infections, may reduce risk for viral infections
Rituximab	Bind to CD20 to disrupt B-cell function	Reactivation of hepatitis B, possible increased risk for PJP
Eculizumab	Binds complement protein C5	Increased risk for meningococcal infection

CMV, Cytomegalovirus; *EBV*, Epstein-Barr virus; *IL*, interleukin; *PJP*, *Pneumocystis jirovecii* infection; *PTLD*, posttransplant lymphoproliferative disease.
*This includes risk when agents are used for induction or treatment of rejection; the risk may vary based on timing of administration.

TABLE 40.2 **Standard Candidate and Donor Laboratory Screening**

Organism	Candidate	Donor
Cytomegalovirus	Serology	Serology
Herpes simplex	Serology	ND
Epstein-Barr Virus	Serology	Serology
Varicella zoster	Serology	ND
HIV	Serology, NAT if positive serology or risk for window period infection	Serology, NAT if positive serology or risk for window period infection
Hepatitis B	Hepatitis B surface antigen, core antibody, surface antibody; NAT if surface antigen positive, isolated core antibody positive or at risk for window period infection	Hepatitis B surface antigen, core antibody; NAT if surface antigen positive, isolated core antibody positive or at risk for window period infection
Hepatitis C	Serology, NAT if increased risk for infection or unexplained liver enzyme abnormalities	Serology, NAT if increased risk for window period infection
West Nile Virus	Optional for at-risk individuals (seasonal)	Optional for at-risk individuals (seasonal)
Treponema pallidum (Syphilis)	Serology	Serology
Mycobacterium tuberculosis	Intradermal PPD or interferon gamma release assay	Live donors only
Toxoplasmosis	Serology	Serology
Strongyloides stercoralis	Serology for at at-risk individuals	Serology for at-risk individuals
Trypoanosoma cruzi	Serology for at-risk individuals	Serology for at-risk individuals
Coccidioides immitis	Serology for at-risk individuals	Serology for at-risk individuals
Histoplasmosis	Serology for at-risk individuals	Optional serology for at-risk individuals

NAT, Nucleic acid testing; *ND*, not done; *PPD*, purified protein derivative.

examination should be performed. Laboratory testing should include serological testing for herpesviruses (CMV, herpes simplex virus, varicella zoster virus, and Epstein-Barr virus [EBV]), human immunodeficiency virus (HIV), hepatitis B virus (HBV), hepatitis C virus (HCV), syphilis, and *Toxoplasma gondii*. In situations where window period infections for HIV, HBV, or HCV may be suspected or if there is concern regarding underlying immunodeficiency that may reduce the sensitivity of serological testing, nucleic acid antibody testing should be obtained. Tuberculin testing is especially important; either interferon gamma release assays (IGRAs) or intradermal tuberculin purified protein

TABLE 40.3 Recommended Immunizations for Adult Transplant Candidates and Recipients

Vaccine	Pretransplant	Posttransplant	Comments
Influenza	Annual	Annual	Posttransplant, may delay immunization to late fall if transplanted in the summer and no local influenza activity. Household contacts should be immunized
Streptococcus pneumonia	Conjugate vaccine followed by polysaccharide capsule vaccine	If not given pretransplant, should give posttransplant	Schedule as per ACIP recommendations*
TDAP	Give if not previously given	Give if not previously given	Tetanus toxoid should be given every 10 y thereafter
Hepatitis B	Give high dose on regular schedule to patients without prior history of hepatitis B	Safe to give posttransplant	All patients with ESRD should have response to hepatitis B vaccine assessed after completing series and if not immune, should administer full series again at increased dose
Hepatitis A	Give to individuals at increased risk	Safe to give posttransplant	
HPV	Give to eligible individuals	Safe to give posttransplant	
Meningococcal conjugate vaccine	For at-risk individuals	Safe for att-risk individuals	Indicated for patients receiving eculizumab
Zoster	Consider live attenuated or subunit vaccine	Subunit vaccine if not immunized before transplant	
Polio vaccine	Inactivated vaccine recommended for travelers to at-risk countries	Inactivated vaccine recommended for travelers to at-risk countries	Assess before immunization status to determine whether indicated
Yellow fever vaccine	For at-risk travelers	Contraindicated	
Salmonella typhi	For at-risk travelers	For at-risk travelers	Posttransplant and candidates receiving immunosuppression should receive injectable vaccine; oral vaccine acceptable pretransplant. Reimmunization may be indicated for subsequent travel

ACIP, Advisory Committee on Immunization Practices; *DTAP*, Tetanus, diphtheria, and acellular pertussis; *ESRD*, end-stage renal disease; *HPV*, human papillomavirus.

*From Kim DK, Riley LE, Harriman KH, et al. Advisory Committee on Immunization Practices Recommended Immunization Schedule for Adults Aged 19 Years or Older - United States, 2017. *MMWR Morb Mortal Wkly Rep.* 2017;66(5):136-138.

derivative (PPD) placement can be performed. Since both tests have reduced sensitivity in patients with end-stage renal disease, a detailed history focusing on common risk factors and radiography are important components of this evaluation.[4] For patients with a history of birth or prolonged residency in places where there are increased risks for geographically associated infections (e.g., strongyloidiasis, Chagas disease, coccidioidomycosis, and histoplasmosis), additional serological testing for the specific organism should be considered.[3] During the pretransplant evaluation, immunization histories should be reviewed and vaccines updated as appropriate (see immunization section; Table 40.3).

DONOR EVALUATION

Donor-derived infections occur rarely.[5-7] Nevertheless, both living and deceased organ donors have been implicated in donor-derived infections; transmissible pathogens are diverse and include bacteria (e.g., pyogenic organisms and *Mycobacterium tuberculosis*), fungi (especially endemic mycoses and Candida), viruses (most commonly herpesviruses), and parasitical organisms (including strongyloides).[5,7] Standard evaluations of both should include a thorough history of past infections and exposures associated with transmissible infections.[3,6] Because deceased donor histories are provided by surrogates, they are generally less detailed; however, the increased use of paired kidney exchange has led to increased numbers of evaluations being obtained outside the recipient's center. Whether this impacts on the quality of donor information is unknown. In both cases, laboratory testing should mirror that of the transplant candidate with specific attention to active infections at the time of deceased donation and infections that may reactivate in an immunosuppressed transplant recipient (including herpesviruses, endemic mycoses, and parasitical infections) in both living and deceased donors (see Table 40.2). Live donors may be evaluated for latent TB using either intradermal tuberculin PPD testing or IGRA.[8] Given the limitations of TB testing in the setting of deceased donor evaluation, it is especially important to obtain historical information and radiography to assess the potential for deceased donor latent infection.[8] The presence of potentially transmissible donor infections may not exclude a donor from transplantation. Donors with bacteremia, meningitis, or other bacterial infections that do

TABLE 40.4 **The 2013 Criteria for Defining Public Health Service Increased Risk Donors**

Infection at Risk	Risk Behaviors	Time Frame of Risk Behavior
HIV, HCV, HBV	Persons exchanging sex for money or drugs	Past 12 mo
HIV, HCV, HBV	Persons who inject drugs	Past 12 mo
HIV, HCV, HBV	Persons who have been incarcerated for >72 h	Past 12 mo
HIV, HCV, HBV	Persons with syphilis, gonorrhea, chlamydia, or genital ulcers	Past 12 mo
HIV, HCV, HBV	Men who have sex with men	Past 12 mo
HIV, HCV, HBV	Persons having sex with a person with known or suspected HIV, HCV, or HBV	Past 12 mo
HIV, HCV, HBV	Persons having sex with a person who injects drugs	Past 12 mo
HIV, HCV, HBV	Women who have sex with men who have a history of sex with men	Past 12 mo
HIV, HCV, HBV	Child <18 mo old born to a mother known or suspected to have HIV, HCV, or HBV	Past 12 mo
HIV, HCV, HBV	Child breastfeeding from a mother known or suspected to have HIV, HCV, or HBV infection	Past 12 mo
HCV	Persons on hemodialysis	Past 12 mo

HBV, Hepatitis B virus; *HCV*, hepatitis C virus.

not involve the kidney have been successfully used and may be considered, assuming that the donor has been appropriately treated for 24 to 48 hours and there are acceptable antimicrobial treatment options. [6,9-11] Latent infections in the donor including TB and endemic mycoses may be treated with appropriate antimicrobials after transplantation. Donors who are actively infected with organisms that do not have effective treatment options should be excluded. Special attention should be paid to deceased donors with undiagnosed central nervous system (CNS) processes as these donors have been implicated in severe and fatal donor-derived infections, including West Nile Virus, rabies, and *Cryptococcus*; consequently the risks associated with using these donors must be balanced with the need for transplantation.[12]

Recent publications have focused on donors who pose an increased risk for blood-borne viral disease transmission because of behaviors associated with recent acquisition of HIV and HCV[13] (Table 40.4). Depending on the screening methodology used (serological vs. nucleic acid testing), there is a window of variable duration during which infection may be present but cannot yet be detected. The Public Health Service (PHS) increased risk donor (IRD) criteria attempt to identify donors at risk for window period infections and disease transmission. The absolute risk for disease transmission overall is quite small, but varies based on the risk behavior, the infection in question, and the testing methodology; for example the risk for HIV transmission from a donor who was incarcerated with negative nucleic acid testing (NAT) and antibody testing is 0.9 per 10,000 but the risk for HCV infection from a donor with active intravenous (IV) drug abuse and antibody testing alone is 300 per 10,000.[14-16] The prevalence of PHS IRDs is increasing and IV drug users represent the largest proportion of this group of donors.[17-19] Compared with deceased donors overall, PHS IRDs are more likely to be young and male and less likely to meet expanded donor criteria[20]; despite the better organ quality afforded by these donors, these organs are more likely to be discarded (odds ratio [OR], 0.67; 95% confidence interval [CI], 0.61 to 0.74).[20] However, for recipients who accept these organs, outcomes are equivalent to those observed with non-PHS IRDs.[18,20]

The updated guidelines and Organ Procurement and Transplantation Network policies require NAT testing for all IRDs as well as specify testing for living donors to be performed within the 28 days before the transplant surgery.[13] There was also greater emphasis placed on the informed consent process for recipients and clarification regarding the assays and intervals for posttransplant testing; recipients of PHS IRDs should have serological and NAT testing for HIV, HBV, and HCV performed between 1 and 3 months after transplant and testing for HBV at 1 year.

As the opioid epidemic continues to affect large parts of the United States, and PHS IRDs continue to contribute a substantial number of organs to the donor pool, it is important that patients are counseled about the acceptable posttransplant outcomes as well infectious risks associated with these organ offers, compared with the risk for death and disease transmission on dialysis; in recognition of the high prevalence of HCV infection among the population with end-stage renal disease (ESRD), hemodialysis patients themselves are considered PHS IRDs. It has been shown that patients will consider these organ offers. In one study, younger donor age, exposure to dialysis, and longer wait times for an organ were associated with increased acceptance of PHS IRD.[21]

TIMELINE OF INFECTION

Infection risks may be anticipated based on the net state of immunosuppression, patient exposures (defined as active and latent infections in donor and recipient, and health-care and community environmental and personal contacts), and prophylactic measures (Fig. 40.1). Standard immunosuppression protocols have allowed for the development of a timeline of anticipated infection that provides a starting point for infection assessment[1] (Table 40.5). Infections in transplant patients may be more severe, especially during periods of more intense immunosuppression. They also may be more difficult to recognize due to the absence of typical features of infection (e.g., fever) in patients on immunosuppressive agents, and noninfectious syndromes occasionally mimic infections. Consequently, this timeline should be

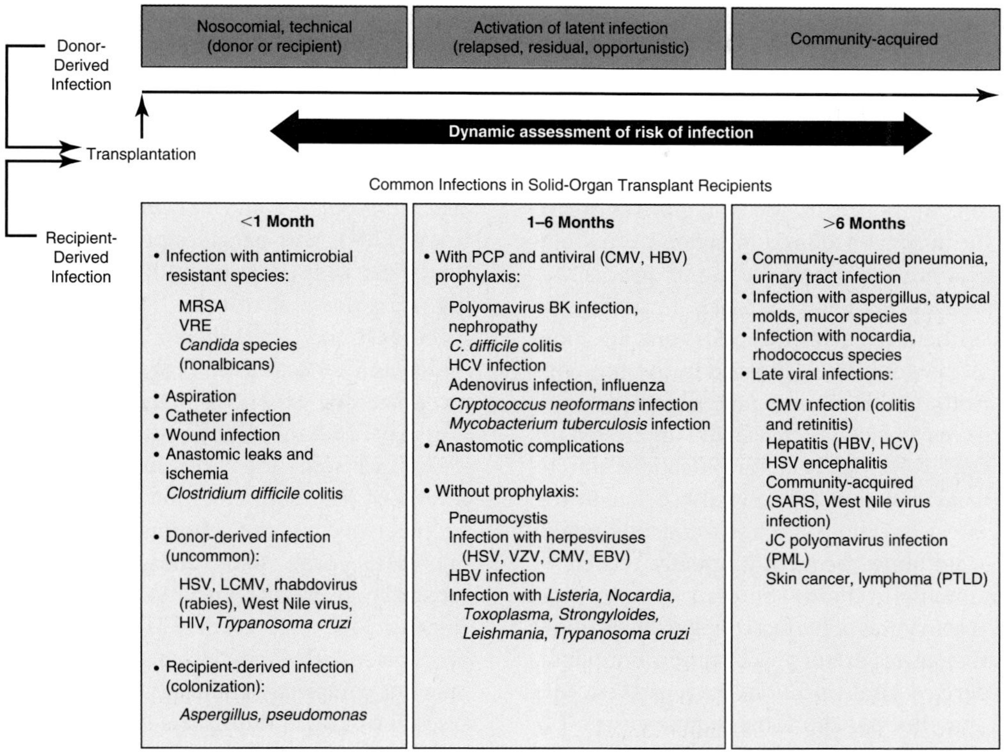

FIG. 40.1 The timeline of posttransplantation infections. (Adapted from Fishman JA. Infection in solid-organ transplant recipients. *N Engl J Med.* 2007;357(25):2601–2614.) *HBV,* Hepatitis B virus; *HIV,* human immunodeficiency virus; *HSV,* herpes simplex virus; *LCMV,* lymphocytic choriomeningitis virus; *MRSA,* methicillin-resistant staphylococcus aureus; *PCP,* pneumocystis jiroveci pneumonia; *PML,* progressive multifocal leukoencephalopathy; *PTLD,* posttransplantation lymphoproliferative disorder; *SARS,* severe acute respiratory syndrome; *VRE,* vancomycin-resistant Enterococcus faecalis; and *VZV,* varicella-zoster virus.

TABLE 40.5 Infection Risk Based on Timing Posttransplant*

	Days 1–30	Months 1–6	>6 Mo
Bacteria	Hospital acquired, includes surgical site and device related; may involve resistant donor-derived pyogenic organisms	Opportunistic bacteria including listeria, nocardia, tuberculosis, and non-tuberculous mycobacteria Donor-derived bacteria	Encapsulated organisms, especially sinopulmonary; Urinary tract infections; Pancreaticobiliary and diverticular-associated infections
Viral	Herpes simplex Healthcare-associated respiratory viruses Donor-derived (LCMV, WNV, etc)	CMV EBV/PTLD Varicella zoster/herpes zoster Polyomaviruses (especially BK) Donor-derived	Community-acquired respiratory viruses CMV (delayed onset due to prophylaxis) EBV/PTLD (less common after year 1)
Fungal	Candida Donor derived	Molds, especially aspergillus *Cryptococcus* PJP if no prophylaxis	Endemic/environmental mycoses *Cryptococcus*
Parasitical/ Protozoal	Donor derived (e.g., balamuthia)	Strongyloides Toxoplasmosis *Trypanosoma cruzi*	Variable risk based on exposures

CMV, Cytomegalovirus; *EBV,* Epsterin-Barr virus; *LCMV,* latent cytomegalovirus; *PTLD,* posttransplant lymphoproliferative disease; *WNV,* West Nile Virus.

*Timing presumes no rejection and limited prophylaxis. For patients who are treated for rejection, risk for opportunistic pathogens increases. Prophylactic interventions may delay the onset of opportunistic infections. New exposures (e.g., environmental) may affect timing of infection.

regarded as a starting point and individual patient circumstances should be carefully considered to determine the optimal patient evaluation.

The Early Posttransplant Period (Month 0 to 1)

Although immunosuppressive therapies are initiated at maximal doses at the time of transplant, the early posttransplant period is notable for hospital-acquired infections, especially related to the surgical procedure and the use of devices that disrupt the host's mucocutaneous barriers, including IV and urinary tract catheters.[22] Bacterial infections are most common and given the antibiotic exposure in the pre- and peritransplant period, multidrug-resistant organisms and *Clostridium difficile* have been increasingly implicated in recent years.[23-25] Donor-derived bacterial infections due to pyogenic organisms are rare but typically also occur in the first month.[5,6,11] Fungal infections are less frequently noted; *Candida* species occur most frequently, usually related to devices or less commonly to donor sources.[1,7,26] Early viral infections include reactivation of herpes simplex, nosocomial transmission of seasonal respiratory viruses and norovirus, and rarely donor-derived viral infections such as West Nile Virus, rabies, and lymphocytic choriomeningitis virus.[1,27-30] It is especially unusual to see parasitical infections in the first month; rare cases of donor-derived infections including balamuthia and microsporida have been reported.[31-33]

Months 1 to 6

This intermediate period posttransplant is typically considered to be the highest risk period for the occurrence of opportunistic infections.[1] During this time, the effects of exogenous immunosuppression required to prevent rejection are maximal, enhancing the net state of immunosuppression. Further immune modulation may occur in the setting of coinfection with immunomodulating viruses, such as CMV, or related to metabolic derangements (especially diabetes) that are common during this period. Reactivation of latent infections and acquisition of new infections from the environment, other individuals, and the donor may occur; the resulting infections may be more severe in the immunosuppressed host.

The pathogens seen during this intermediate period are diverse and in the absence of prophylaxis, include bacteria (e.g., *Nocardia* species, *Listeria monocytogenes*, and mycobacteria, especially TB), fungi (e.g., *Aspergillus* species, *Cryptococcus*, and *Pneumocystis jirovecii*), viruses (e.g., CMV, EBV), and parasites/protozoa (e.g., toxoplasmosis).[1] Infections with geographically restricted pathogens including *Strongyloides stercoralis*, *Trypanosoma cruzi*, and endemic mycoses (*Coccidioides immitis*, *Blastomyces dermatitidis*, and *Histoplasmosis capsulatum*) also may occur. It is important to recognize that exposures both before and after transplantation may result in infections during this period.

Because some infections may be predictably anticipated, several of the more common opportunistic infections may be prevented by the administration of prophylactic antimicrobials (Table 40.6). The use of trimethoprim sulfamethoxazole to prevent *Pneumocystis jirovecii* pneumonia and valganciclovir to prevent CMV are examples of successful prophylactic strategies. However, prophylactic antimicrobials may not completely eradicate the risk for infection; in some cases, the onset of the disease is merely delayed until after the prophylaxis is discontinued. The changing nature of immunosuppressive strategies and treatment of rejection also may affect the timing and presentation of common opportunistic infections. Consequently, the risk period for opportunistic infections may extend beyond this intermediate risk period.

Beyond 6 Months

In stable recipients, the time frame beyond the first 6 months is typically a period of stable allograft function when infections are less frequently noted. Those that occur are typically community acquired infections caused by typical community acquired bacterial and viral infections.[1] Urinary tract infections (UTIs) are especially common and typically caused by *Enterobacteriaceae*, especially *Escherichia coli*.[34] Respiratory tract infections also occur, often due to community-acquired

TABLE 40.6 Prophylactic Antimicrobials Commonly Used Following Kidney Transplantation

Pathogen	Antimicrobial	Duration	Comments
Cytomegalovirus	Valganciclovir	Varies based on risk CMV D+/R– 6 mo CMV R + 3 mo	Alternative strategies include valacyclovir for lower risk, monitoring (preemptive therapy) for lower risk (includes CMV D–/R– who do not need valganciclovir)
Herpes simplex	Valacyclovir or Acyclovir	3 mo or prolonged if history of HSV recurrences	Not indicated if patient on valganciclovir
Pneumocystis jirovecii	Trimethoprim sulfamethoxazole or Atovaquone or Dapsone	6–12 mo	Consider longer if patient with increased immunosuppression
Candida	Nystatin or Clotrimazole	30 d	Clotrimazole has been associated with increased calcineurin inhibitor levels

CMV, Cytomegalovirus; *D–*, donor negative; *D+*, donor positive; *HSV*, herpes simplex virus; *R-*, recipient-negative.

viruses (influenza, parainfluenza, respiratory syncytial virus, adenovirus, and human metapneumoviruses); these may be more severe with prolonged viral shedding, increased risk for lower tract disease, morbidity, and allograft rejection.[35-37] Bacterial pathogens including legionella and *Pneumococcus* also occur and transplant patients are at a 12.8-fold greater risk for invasive pneumococcal disease than the general population.[38,39]

Although this late period is not considered to be a high-risk period for opportunistic infections, some may occur after augmentation of immunosuppression.[1] It is important to recognize that the net state of immunosuppression cannot be estimated solely by considering the specific medications, doses, and levels; patient responses may vary considerably. Moreover, there are episodes of later rejection that require additional augmentation of immunosuppression and diabetes mellitus, infections, and malignancies may further increase the risk for later opportunistic infections. One of the more common late-onset opportunists is CMV, which usually occurs following suspension of prophylaxis, especially in CMV-seronegative recipients of CMV-seropositive donor organs.[40] Reactivation of latent infections whose control was dependent on normal T-cell function may occur during this period. For example, histoplasmosis and TB have both been reported; the risk for TB is 20% to 74% higher in transplant recipients than in the general population.[4,41-43]

The late period is also notable for the occurrence of healthcare-associated infections. Transplant patients are at increased risk for comorbidities, such as malignancy, diabetes mellitus, and vascular disease, conditions that often require additional interventions in healthcare facilities. These have led to infection with hospital-acquired pathogens, including multidrug-resistant bacteria and *Clostridium difficile*. Diabetic foot infections also may be seen.

SELECTED INFECTIONS OF IMPORTANCE

Recognition of infections in the posttransplant period requires consideration of specific recipient and donor exposures, the net state of immunosuppression, comorbidities, and the timing of the infection. Because the list of potential pathogens can be diverse and diagnoses may be obscured in the setting of immunosuppression, broad-spectrum empiric antimicrobial therapy with concurrent detailed evaluation involving laboratory and radiographic evaluations may be necessary to prevent bad outcomes. We provide more in-depth information regarding some of the more common infections encountered after kidney transplantation.

Cytomegalovirus

CMV is the most common opportunistic pathogen after kidney transplantation. Notable for both direct and indirect effects, it typically occurs in months 1 to 4 posttransplant if no prophylactic antivirals are administered.[40] If prophylactic antivirals are used, the onset of infection is delayed until the antiviral is suspended; post-prophylaxis CMV may occur in posttransplant months 6 to 12.[44] Rarely the onset of CMV is further delayed (late onset), occurring beyond at least 6 months after cessation of prophylaxis.[44-46] These later infections are differentiated from those occurring shortly after suspension of prophylaxis by their later acquisition, worse allograft function, higher mortality, and absence of association with CMV donor-positive, recipient-negative (D+/R–) serostatus.[44-46]

The manifestations of CMV are diverse.[1,40] The most common direct effects are asymptomatic viremia; CMV syndrome, which can include fever, malaise, and cytopenias (usually leukopenia and/or thrombocytopenia); and gastrointestinal (GI) symptoms (including anorexia, diarrhea, abdominal pain, bleeding, ulcerations, and perforation). Disseminated infection, hepatitis, pneumonitis, pancreatitis, and nephritis occur less frequently and chorioretinitis is a rare late manifestation. Of special concern are the indirect manifestations of CMV related to its impact on the host's immune system; decreased allograft and patient survival, increased risk for rejection, and increased risk for opportunistic infections (including fungal infections), posttransplant lymphoproliferative disease (PTLD), and bacteremia have all been noted.[47,48] Although the association between CMV and rejection and allograft damage has been recognized for years, the exact mechanism is not known.[49] Some possible mechanisms include upregulation of the inflammatory response with alterations in the expression of cytokines, proinflammatory growth factors, and chemokines and an increase in proinflammatory adhesion molecules. Increased antigen processing and presentation associated with the major histocompatibility complex (MHC), alterations in the T-cell subset composition, smooth muscle proliferation with induction of intracellular reactive oxygen species, and increased procoagulant activity have been noted.[47,50,51] Notably administration of antiviral prophylaxis to CMV-seronegative recipients of CMV-seropositive organs has been associated with a 50% reduction in organ rejection and improved patient and allograft survival at 3 years, observations that provide further support for the critical role played by CMV with respect to allograft function.[52,53]

Patterns of transmission

CMV may occur as a result of primary infection, reactivation of latent infection, or superinfection. Primary infection occurs frequently when a CMV-seronegative recipient receives a CMV-seropositive donor kidney with clinically apparent infection in approximately 45% of recipients in the absence of prophylaxis.[52] Infrequently, primary infection is the result of blood transfusion or close/intimate contact with an individual shedding CMV in their secretions (community acquired). Recipients with primary infection due to organ transplantation are more likely to experience CMV shortly after cessation of prophylaxis. When recognized early, these infections may have limited symptoms with viremia as the most common manifestation. Community-acquired CMV may occur at any time after transplant and because it often is unanticipated, may be more severe. Since the majority of adults are CMV seropositive at the time of transplant, this mode of acquisition is more common in pediatric settings.

Reactivation of latent- recipient CMV is less common with rates varying based on the choice of immunosuppression; induction with antilymphocyte therapies is associated with a higher incidence of CMV. There are multiple genotypes of CMV; *gB 1* is most common.[54] Superinfection typically occurs when both donor and recipient are CMV positive. Because CMV genotyping is not typically performed, the true incidence of CMV superinfection is not known. However, as CMV occurs more commonly in D+/R+ recipients than in D−/R+ recipients, it is likely that the donor strain is the causative agent of the majority of these infections.[55]

Pathogenesis/Risk Factors

MHC-restricted, virus-specific, cytotoxic T lymphocytes play a major role in the control of CMV; consequently immunosuppressive agents that interfere with this host response increase the risk for CMV.[56] Specifically, the use of antilymphocyte antibodies (a frequent component of induction therapy) that ablate lymphocyte function for prolonged periods and prompt the elaboration of proinflammatory cytokines is associated with CMV, as they both allow for reactivation of latent virus and enhance viral replication. Viral reactivation may be promoted by azathioprine, mycophenolate, and cyclophosphamide. Although calcineurin inhibitors (CNIs) are not drivers of reactivation, they do allow for amplification of reactivated virus; tacrolimus is more potent than cyclosporine.[57] The use of mTOR inhibitors may reduce the risk for reactivation.[58] In addition to the net state of immunosuppression as defined by the choice of immunosuppression, risk factors for the development of CMV include CMV-seropositive donor, especially if the recipient is CMV seronegative, allograft rejection, coinfections with other viruses (HHV 6), host factors (including genetic factors), and severe hypogammaglobulinemia.[44,59] Recently, assays designed to assess the cell-mediated immune (CMI) response have been used to assess the risk for CMV. One example of this is the QuantiFERON-CMV assay, which assesses cell-mediated immunity by measuring interferon (IFN)-gamma levels produced by CD8-positive T cells following in vitro stimulation with CMV antigens.[60] Individuals with reduced responses to CMV stimulation were at greater risk for CMV; those who failed to respond to any stimulation were at the highest risk. Allograft rejection and CMV have a uniquely bidirectional interaction, whereby the proinflammatory environment created by rejection and the additional treatment with immunosuppressive agents prompt the reactivation and amplification of CMV and CMV upregulates antigens that promote alloreactivity leading to acute and chronic rejection syndromes.[40,48,61]

Diagnosis

Prompt recognition of CMV is imperative to prevent complications and to improve outcomes. This requires initial consideration based on the clinical presentation and risk assessment. Recipients presenting with unexplained cytopenias, GI complaints, or both should be assessed for CMV, especially if they have risk factors and have recently suspended prophylaxis. Currently, assays targeted at detection of viremia are most commonly used for diagnosis.[62] In particular, NAT uses polymerase chain reaction (PCR) technology to measure CMV DNA in plasma to rapidly and accurately determine the presence of CMV in the blood. This assay is quantifiable and higher values typically correlate with more severe disease. It also can be used to follow the course of treatment as effective treatment is accompanied by resolution of viremia. NAT has been notable for interlaboratory variability but the development of an international standard has reduced this variability; regardless comparison of values between different laboratories can still be confusing.[63,64] Antigenemia testing (a semiquantitative fluorescent assay that stains circulating neutrophils for CMV early antigen [pp65]) can be used to assess viremia. Similar to NAT, this assay can be used to follow the response to treatment. Both assays may be negative in the presence of active infection, especially GI, neurological, and retinal CMV.[62] Consequently, histopathological diagnosis remains the gold standard for CMV diagnosis and patients with consistent clinical syndromes and negative tests for viremia should undergo tissue biopsy.[40,62] Because of the delay in diagnosis and lower sensitivity, neither culture nor serological testing is routinely used for CMV diagnosis.

Prevention

Because CMV has been associated with worse outcomes in kidney transplant recipients, risk-based prevention is essential. Universal prophylaxis and preemptive therapy have been used routinely. Universal prophylaxis involves administration of an antiviral during a risk period typically defined by the recipient and donor's CMV serostatus. The preemptive approach uses quantitative assays to monitor for CMV reactivation/infection at specified time points posttransplant. Patients with evidence of CMV are then treated with antivirals. There are advantages and disadvantages to both strategies.[62] Prophylaxis may reduce the indirect effects of allograft rejection and opportunistic infection and decrease the risk for infection with other herpesviruses; the cost and toxicity of prolonged antivirals may be impediments to this approach. The preemptive strategy may reduce the cost of medications and the medication-related adverse events and it also may allow for more effective recovery of the host immune response. But coordination of care and the cost of monitoring may affect the feasibility of this strategy. Notably, neither approach has prevented infection with resistant CMV strains.

Current guidelines recommend that patients at highest risk for CMV receive antiviral prophylaxis for 3 to 6 months after transplant, with many centers opting for 6 months prophylaxis based on a study comparing 3 to 6 months in a group of CMV D+/R− kidney recipients.[40,62,65] Although there are studies supporting the use of acyclovir, valacyclovir, and ganciclovir, the majority of centers currently use valganciclovir for prophylaxis, given the ease of administration and improved outcomes.[52,66-68] The optimal dose of valganciclovir for prophylaxis is not known. For CMV-seropositive recipients, some centers use 450 mg daily rather than the recommended dose of 900 mg, but at least one center has suggested that the lower dose may not be appropriate for

CMV D+/R– recipients.[69,70] Regardless, valganciclovir dosing should be determined solely on the basis of kidney function and dose reductions should not be made because of medication-related toxicities, including cytopenias.[62]

Treatment

Treatment of CMV requires administration of an effective antiviral until all signs and symptoms have resolved; a minimum of 2 to 3 weeks is considered standard.[62] The vast majority of CMV isolates are susceptible to ganciclovir and IV ganciclovir (dose 5 mg/kg every 12 hours, dose adjusted for kidney dysfunction) is the standard regimen.[40,62] For mild to moderate disease, valganciclovir (dose 900 mg/kg twice daily, dose adjusted for kidney dysfunction) can be considered.[71] Because CMV infection often is a consequence of "overimmunosuppression," it is important to reassess the immunosuppressive regimen and consider if this can be reduced. Reduction in dose or suspension of mycophenolate or azathioprine is most commonly considered. During treatment, weekly monitoring of CMV viral loads is recommended to determine response to treatment. At 2 weeks, a log decrease in viral load should be demonstrated. If the viral load does not decline by 2 weeks, the patient should undergo testing for CMV resistance using a genotypic assay.[40,62] Risk factors for resistance include CMV D+/R– status and prolonged subtherapeutic exposure to ganciclovir or valganciclovir.[62,72] Ganciclovir-resistant patients may be treated with foscarnet or cidofovir; investigational agents also may be available.[40,62] Both foscarnet and cidofovir are nephrotoxic and close monitoring of kidney function and electrolytes during therapy is critical.

There are several concerns regarding treatment of CMV. In some cases (especially involving the GI tract), viral loads do not accurately reflect the extent of CMV disease.[62] Endoscopic evaluation should be performed before suspension of treatment to ensure eradication of infection. In addition, recurrent disease can occur following completion of treatment. Although guidelines have suggested that there may be a role for either secondary prophylaxis or monitoring for relapse with viral load monitoring, there are no trials demonstrating that either approach is beneficial.[62] If CMV occurs during usual risk periods, prophylaxis may be resumed after completion of therapy. Regardless of which approach is chosen, the risks and benefits of additional prophylaxis and monitoring should be balanced against observation and standard care.

Epstein-Barr Virus and Posttransplant Lymphoproliferative Disease

Similar to CMV, EBV is a member of the herpesvirus family. Acquired in childhood by person-to-person spread primarily via saliva, the vast majority of adult kidney recipients are seropositive before transplant. In the normal host, EBV first infects oropharyngeal epithelial cells then B lymphocytes, where it establishes latency. After kidney transplant, EBV can manifest in diverse ways.[73] Most commonly, it reactivates asymptomatically, but infectious mononucleosis-like syndromes and PTLD also can occur. EBV viremia is common after kidney transplant, with one study showing that 40% of 383 kidney recipients monitored regularly experienced EBV viremia with median time to viremia of 31 days.[74] Viremia is most common in EBV-seronegative recipients of seropositive donor kidneys and has been associated with allograft loss and an increased risk for opportunistic and bacterial infections.[75]

Posttransplant Lymphoproliferative Disease

The most significant complication of EBV infection is EBV-associated PTLD. Adult kidney transplant recipients are at lower risk for this compared with other organ transplants, with an estimated incidence of 1% to 2%.[76] The major risk factors for PTLD include primary infection (EBV D+/R–) and the net state of immunosuppression.[73,76] The choice of immunosuppressive agent used in induction has been an important factor in the subsequent development of PTLD; antithymocyte globulin and belatacept have both been implicated and EBV-seronegative status is a contraindication to the use of belatacept.[77,78] PTLD is generally divided into early PTLD (occurring in the first year posttransplant)—which is more likely to be associated with primary EBV infection, polymorphic, and involve the allograft—and late PTLD (occurring after the first year), which is usually a disease of older recipients, EBV negative, and monoclonal.[73]

Diagnosis of Epstein-Barr Virus and Posttransplant Lymphoproliferative Disease

The clinical presentation of EBV and PTLD can be quite variable.[73] A cause of fever of undetermined origin, it can also present with a mononucleosis-like syndrome. Cytopenias may occur and involvement of the allograft, GI tract, lungs, liver, and CNS have all been described; extranodal disease is especially common with late PTLD. Constitutional B symptoms are sometimes present. Quantitative NAT of whole blood, peripheral blood mononuclear cells (PBMCs), plasma, or serum is often used as the first step for the diagnosis of acute EBV and PTLD, but there are a number of issues that limit the utility of this assay for diagnostic purposes.[73,76] It is important to recognize that specimen selection has a major effect on viral load measurements, since higher viral loads will be seen with whole blood cells or PBMCs. Furthermore, there is still some interlaboratory variability related to the absence of an international reference standard, making it difficult to compare results obtained from different laboratories. Finally, it is important to recognize that PTLD can occur in the absence of viremia and in the presence of viremia may occur in the absence of PTLD. Histopathological diagnosis is ultimately required to make the diagnosis. The World Health Organization has devised criteria for staging PTLD based on the clinical presentation, with early (stage I) disease defined as benign polyclonal proliferation, stage II polymorphic disease, stage III monomorphic B- or T-cell lymphoma/neoplasms, and stage IV disease defined as classical Hodgkin lymphoma.[79]

Treatment and Prognosis of Posttransplant Lymphoproliferative Disease

Because PTLD often is a reflection of a more immunosuppressed state, a key component of treatment is the reduction of immunosuppression, which may result in a significant reduction in disease burden for some individuals.[80] However, this does increase the risk for rejection and many patients will require additional interventions, including rituximab, chemotherapy, surgery, and/or radiation oncology.[76,80] Although PTLD is often EBV associated, there is no role for antivirals.[76] A multidisciplinary approach, involving transplant physicians, oncologists, and infectious disease specialists is recommended to optimally manage these patients.[76]

Prevention

Prevention of PTLD should include a multitiered approach.[73,76] For seronegative recipients, belatacept should be avoided. Serial viral load monitoring can be used to titrate immunosuppression, especially during the first year posttransplant. Prevention of CMV may help decrease the risk as CMV has been identified as a potential cofactor for the development of PTLD. Rituximab has been used for some patients with persistently elevated EBV viral loads, but is associated with an increased risk for other infections and, in the absence of controlled trials, is not currently recommended.[81,82] More recently, there has been interest in using T cell–based therapies directed specifically against EBV.[83,84] Not universally available yet, this approach offers promise for future therapeutic intervention.

BK Virus

BK virus is a common posttransplant viral infection, affecting predominantly kidney transplant recipients, although case reports have implicated it as a cause of acute kidney injury in solid organ recipients. It was first identified in the urine of a kidney transplant recipient with ureteral stenosis in 1971. The virus is a member of the polyoma family, which includes JC virus, Saint Louis polyomavirus, and New Jersey polyomavirus.[85] There are at least six different genotypes identified, and each has a different geographical predominance. Genotype I is the most common worldwide, and the primers utilized in PCR detection assays are based off this strain.[86,87] Most adults are seropositive for BK, which after primary infection in childhood establishes latency in the uroepithelium. It reactivates in the setting of immunosuppression, leading to viruria, which if unchecked progresses to viremia and BK nephropathy. Approximately one-third of kidney transplant recipients develop BK viruria, about 20% develop viremia, and <10% develop BK nephropathy.[88,89]

Risk Factors

Several common risk factors for BK viremia and nephropathy have been identified. The overall degree of immunosuppression is probably the most important factor, as the prevalence of BK infection has increased as more potent immunosuppression has been introduced and factors augmenting the cumulative immunosuppressive burden, such as rejection episodes or greater HLA mismatching also increase the risk.[90,91] Older age, male sex, diabetes, and use of ureteral stents also have been implicated as BK risk factors. There is growing evidence to suggest that the infection is donor derived and the absence of prior recipient infection may increase the risk for nephropathy.[92] In one study, donor, but not recipient BK antibody titers were predictive of BK viremia and nephropathy; recipients of high antibody titer donor kidneys had a 10-fold increased risk for BK viremia (10.1; 95% CI, 3.5 to 29; $P < 0.001$), corroborating earlier work by Bohl et al.[93]

Viral Load Monitoring, Diagnosis, and Prevention of BK Nephropathy

BK antibodies are not protective and no effective antiviral prophylaxis has yet been identified. Most centers screen prospectively for BK infection by measuring BK viral loads in plasma or urine. Since the majority of BK infections are detected in the first year after transplant, screening is concentrated in the early posttransplant period, although late BK infections have been reported and BK infection should be included in any investigation of allograft dysfunction.[94,95] The American Society of Transplantation (AST) consensus guidelines recommend screening patients for BK viremia every 1 to 3 months for the first 2 years posttransplant.[91] The majority of transplant centers screen using serum BK PCR but this approach is not mandated and urine BK PCR remains a popular alternative.[96] Due to the lack of a universal standard assay for real-time BK PCR, there is significant interlaboratory variability in the assay's quantification; therefore consistency in the laboratory used for viral load monitoring is important and results that are inconsistent with a patient's clinical course should be questioned.[97] Although a BK viral load >4 log copies/mL is "presumed" BK nephropathy, this diagnosis can only be made by kidney biopsy. Although biopsy may not change management, it does provide useful information regarding the degree of inflammation and fibrosis, and by extension, the risk for allograft loss.[98,99] BK nephropathy on biopsy can be mistaken for acute cellular rejection with a lymphocytic infiltrate and tubulitis, and definitive diagnosis is made by demonstrating the presence of immunohistochemical stains directed at the SV-40 large T antigen or VP-1 capsid protein (PAB-597 stain).[100,101]

Treatment

The cornerstone of BK viremia and nephropathy treatment is the careful reduction of immunosuppression.[102-104] A variety of approaches have been employed to achieve this, including discontinuation of the antimetabolite, dose reduction of the CNI, switching CNIs or replacing them with another agent altogether. In vitro data suggest that sirolimus and cyclosporine may have inhibitory effects on BK viral replication, whereas tacrolimus is permissive, suggesting that reduction of tacrolimus may be most beneficial in eradicating BK infection.[105] Both short- and longer-term data suggest that immunosuppression reduction results in BK viral clearance in the majority of patients and does not have a negative effect on allograft or patient survival.[104,106,107] At our center, we discontinue the antimetabolite and monitor BK viral loads every

2 to 4 weeks thereafter; if the viral load does not respond, we then decrease the CNI, aiming for a 25% reduction in the trough level. Anecdotally, we have had success in clearing BK infection in patients with persistent viremia despite tacrolimus trough levels in the 4 to 5 ng/mL range by switching them to cyclosporine and aiming for a trough level of 50 to 75 mg/dL. Serum creatinine must be monitored closely during this period of reduced immunosuppression.

Although retrospective data had suggested a role for fluoroquinolone antibiotics in the prevention of BK infection, a prospective, double-blind, randomized trial of levofloxacin prophylaxis to prevent BK infection in kidney transplant recipients failed to find any such benefit.[108,109] After 3 months of treatment in the 154 patients enrolled in the study, there was no difference in the incidence of BK viruria (29% vs. 33.3%; $P = 0.58$) but there were significantly more quinolone-resistant bacterial infections and tendonitis in the levofloxacin group.

There have been case series reporting success in treating BK with leflunomide, cidofovir, levofloxacin, and IV immunoglobulin, often in conjunction with immunosuppression reduction, but no large-scale, prospective trials to advocate for the use of any of these agents.[91,110-112] There are also several reports of lower rates of BK viremia in patients maintained on sirolimus and increased viral clearance with conversion to mTOR inhibitors; however, given the increased risk for death demonstrated with sirolimus use in the kidney transplant population, we do not advocate for this as a first-line treatment approach.[113-116]

Hepatitis C

Recent data from the National Health and Nutrition Examination Survey (NHANES) indicates that the prevalence of HCV infection in the general US population is low (~1%), but the ESRD population is enriched for HCV with a prevalence that ranges from 2.6% to 22.9% depending on the series.[117,118] The DOPPS (Dialysis Outcomes Practice Patterns Study) identified length of time on maintenance dialysis as one of the most important predictors of HCV infection, with HCV seroprevalence of greater than 50% in those with more than 20 years of ESRD; blood transfusions, prior transplantation, and IV drug use were other risks for HCV acquisition.[119] HCV transmission in dialysis units has been well described, emphasizing the importance of universal precautions without a need for patient isolation; in recognition of these risks, maintenance hemodialysis patients are categorized as PHS IRDs.[13]

It is recommended by the Kidney Disease Initiative to Improve Global Outcomes (KDIGO) guidelines to screen all kidney transplant candidates for HCV infection.[120] NAT for HCV RNA in the blood is preferred over antibody screening in high-prevalence areas, patients with unexplained elevations in hepatic transaminases, or in immunosuppressed populations who may be viral load-positive but never mount an antibody response (antibody-negative but NAT-positive); additionally NAT enables identification of patients who have spontaneously cleared the infection (antibody-positive but NAT-negative) and those with early infection. All patients who are HCV NAT-positive should be referred to a hepatologist for an assessment of liver disease severity before transplantation.

Kidney Transplantation in Hepatitis C Virus-positive Patients

Kidney transplantation offers a survival benefit for HCV-positive patients over remaining on maintenance dialysis; in contemporary case series, cardiovascular disease, rather than cirrhosis, was the predominant cause of death on the waitlist.[121] Although early case series suggested that posttransplant patient and allograft outcomes for HCV-positive patients were similar to HCV-negative recipients, more contemporary data and metaanalyses have indicated that outcomes are in fact worse.[122] Older studies had identified cirrhosis as the main cause of death for HCV-positive transplant recipients, but newer data suggests that cardiovascular disease and diabetes are significant contributors to mortality.[123] Allograft survival is also negatively affected by recipient HCV-positive status with a metaanalysis reporting a hazard ratio (HR) of 1.7 (95% CI, 1.46 to 2.11) for graft loss, but not all studies have consistently shown a negative effect of HCV infection on kidney allograft survival.[122]

There has been concern that the immunosuppression required for kidney transplantation could accelerate liver disease in HCV-positive recipients; HCV viral loads have been shown to increase after transplantation and historically cirrhosis was a main cause of patient mortality. However, in the limited case series that have had both pre- and posttransplant liver biopsies available, this was not the case. In a series report of 31 patients by Roth et al., 77% (24) had stable or improved histology on follow-up biopsy and only 23% had interval worsening of their liver fibrosis.[124] Another series from France, with sequential posttransplant biopsies in 36 patients, showed a similarly benign posttransplant course; despite increased viral loads, >60% of patients in the study had stable liver fibrosis on repeat biopsy and only 3 patients developed cirrhosis by 20 years of follow-up.[125]

Infections may be one source of the increased mortality observed in HCV-positive transplant recipients. Although some reports identified sepsis as an important cause of death in their HCV-positive patients, a recent prospective study from Spain did not observe a difference in the overall incidence of infection among HCV-positive and HCV-negative patients.[126,127] However, they did observe a significant increase in bacteremia in HCV-positive recipients (HR, 3.14; 95% CI, 1.19 to 8.24; $P = 0.02$).[127]

Use of Hepatitis C Virus-positive Donors

Long waits for transplantation in the United States and the overall shortage of suitable donor kidneys have led many centers to explore means of expanding the donor pool by using "nonstandard" donors, such as those with HCV infection. The growing opioid abuse epidemic has increased HCV infection rates in certain regions of the United States, leading to an increase in both overdose deaths and donors with HCV infection. Historically, the use of HCV-positive organs has been restricted to recipients with genotype 1 infection. Because donor HCV genotyping is not available before transplantation, clinicians assume HCV-positive deceased donors have genotype 1 infection, since this the most prevalent genotype in the United States. However, superinfection with other HCV genotypes is possible. Since pan-genotypic, IFN-free, direct-acting antiviral (DAA) agents to cure HCV exist, this limitation to genotype 1 recipients may be outdated.

One of largest published single series describing the use of HCV-positive donors comes from Spain. Morales and colleagues reported the outcomes for 162 HCV-positive recipients of HCV-positive kidneys compared with 306 HCV-positive recipients of HCV-negative donors.[128] Patient survival at 5 years was similar (84.8% in D+/R+ vs. 86.6% in D−/R+; P = 0.25) but allograft survival was diminished (5-year allograft survival 58.9% in D+/R+ compared with D−/R+ 65.5%; P = 0.006). A recent propensity score matched analysis performed using United Network for Organ Sharing (UNOS) data to address this question found that transplantation with a HCV-positive donor was associated with an increased risk for death (HR, 1.43; 95% CI, 1.18 to 1.76; P < 0.001) and graft loss (HR, 1.39; 95% CI, 1.16 to 1.67; P < 0.001) among HCV-positive recipients, an effect that was not explained by differences in acute rejection (OR, 1.16; 95% CI, 0.84 to 1.61; P = 0.35).[129] Given the time frame of the study, it is unknown if DAA eradication of HCV would have changed the outcome. The use of HCV-positive donors for HCV-positive individuals is associated with shorter wait times to transplantation (~1 year less on average) but recipients should be counseled about the risks and benefits associated with the use of these donors.[130] Whether HCV-positive donors may be safely used for HCV-negative recipients is currently an area of study now that the potential treatment options for HCV have expanded.[131] Presumably, donors who are not viremic are much less likely to transmit HCV via transplantation; consequently there has been increasing interest in using these donors. More data are needed to determine the safety of HCV-positive donors.

Treatment of Hepatitis C Virus With Direct-Acting Antiviral

The initial KDIGO guidelines, during the era before DAA therapy, recommended treatment of HCV in all kidney transplant candidates.[120] Until recently, this meant pretransplant treatment with IFN-based regimens, which have modest response rates to therapy and poor tolerability; treatment with IFN after kidney transplant has been associated with unacceptably high rates of acute rejection and graft loss. Since 2013 there has been a rapid expansion in the number of IFN-free DAA regimens approved to treat HCV infection. These regimens have been associated with HCV cure rates in excess of 95% in the general population and have demonstrated efficacy in kidney transplant recipients as well.[132]

DAA regimen selection for kidney transplant recipients is complex. Currently, the greatest number of therapeutic options exist for patients with genotype 1 infection, but this area is rapidly changing (the American Association for the Study of Liver Diseases [AASLD]/Infectious Diseases Society of America [IDSA] guidelines provide the most current treatment recommendations and are continuously updated as new information becomes available).[133] Kidney function and DAA-immunosuppression drug–drug interactions must be taken into account when a DAA regimen is being selected. Sofosbuvir-containing regimens are not approved for use in patients with a glomerular filtration rate less than 30 mL/min. Regimens that contain simeprevir can increase cyclosporine levels and elbasvir/grazeprovir, when coadministered with cyclosporine increases grazeprovir levels. In addition, regimens that require ritonavir boosting (such as dasabuvir/ombitasvir/paritaprevir) will result in major increases in CNI blood levels and require significant CNI dose adjustment; these regimens are generally avoided in the posttransplant setting. CNI levels have been shown to fluctuate even after DAA treatment is completed, highlighting the need for careful monitoring of kidney function and drug levels both during and after therapy. Prescribers also need to be aware of issues of viral resistance, with appropriate testing for *NS5a* resistance mutations of genotype 1a patients depending on the regimen selected, as well as reports of hepatitis B reactivation while on HCV therapy. Treatment of HCV in kidney transplant recipients should be managed carefully with combined efforts by hepatologists, infectious disease specialists, and transplant nephrologists.

Hepatitis B

Unlike HCV, the prevalence of HBV in the US ESRD population is low (estimated to be around 1%), and likely due to efforts to vaccinate all chronic kidney disease (CKD) patients before their start of dialysis, improved infection control in dialysis units, and more widespread use of erythropoietin-stimulating agents rather than transfusions to manage anemia.[134] All kidney transplant candidates should be screened for HBV infection at the time of transplant evaluation with measurement of hepatitis B surface antigen (HBsAg), hepatitis B surface antibody (HBsAb), and core antibody (HBcAb), in addition to the regular screening conducted in dialysis units. Patients who are HBsAg-positive or have detectable HBV DNA should be referred to hepatology for evaluation and treatment. Patients who are HBsAb-positive have immunity, whether from vaccination or cleared infection (the latter if the presence of HBcAb is detected). Patients who are not immune should be vaccinated, preferably before the initiation of renal replacement therapy.

The initial outcomes for kidney transplantation in hepatitis B-infected recipients were poor. Ten-year patient survival was 55% and 10-year allograft survival was 36%.[135] Cirrhosis was a frequent complication, developing in 28% by 5 years of posttransplant follow-up and hepatocellular carcinoma was common.[136] However, the introduction of effective HBV therapies into routine clinical practice improved outcomes significantly. In a study of 1346 HBsAg-positive recipients transplanted from 2001 to 2007, 5-year patient survival was 85.3% and allograft survival was 74.9%, which was not significantly different from contemporary HBV-negative controls.[137] A fivefold increased risk for hepatic decompensation among the HBV-positive recipients was observed; however, this complication only occurred in 1.3% of patients overall.

Before transplant, candidates with chronic HBV infection should be screened for cirrhosis as well as coinfection with HCV and hepatitis A and counseled to avoid other hepatotoxins (including alcohol). Because there is currently no cure for HBV infection, patients who are HBsAg-positive and/or DNA-positive should receive lifelong antiviral therapy and routinely screened for complications of chronic infection, including cirrhosis and hepatocellular carcinoma. Individuals who are HBcAb-positive may be at risk for reactivation of HBV after intense periods of immunosuppression, especially when B-cell depleting agents, such as rituximab, are used. In anticipation of rituximab treatment, all patients should be checked for hepatitis B and prophylactic antivirals considered for HBcAb- and/or HBsAg-positive individuals.[138]

Treatment of Hepatitis B Virus

The improved outcomes for patients are due to a multitude of antiviral agents now available to treat HBV.[139] Lamivudine is among the most widely used, but is not recommended for long-term prophylaxis due to its low barrier to resistance. Tenofovir difumarate is both highly potent and has a high barrier to resistance, but nephrotoxicity and its association with bone loss makes it an unattractive choice for chronic use in kidney transplant patients. Tenofovir alafenamide is a newer formulation that is effective against HBV and has a lower risk for associated kidney impairment and osteopenia. Entecavir is also highly effective and has a high barrier to resistance without nephrotoxicity, and is therefore often used for kidney transplant recipients who will require chronic HBV therapy.

Use of Hepatitis B Virus-positive Donors

HBV-positive kidneys have been explored as a means to increase the available donor pool and guidelines for their use have been developed by a work group from the American Society of Transplantation.[140] The risk for transmission of HBV depends on several factors including the particular organ being transplanted, recipient HBV immunity, and the HBV prophylaxis strategy employed.[140] HBsAg-positive donors are used least frequently and represent <1% of all deceased donors. They can be used in HBsAg-positive recipients, who will require lifelong treatment with entecavir or tenofovir regardless due to recipient HBV status; additionally, hepatitis B immunoglobulin (HBIG) administration could be considered if HBsAb titers are low. HBsAg-positive kidneys have been used in HBsAb-positive recipients with and without antiviral prophylaxis with minimal transmission risks. The use of HBsAg-positive donors in HBV-naive or unvaccinated patients is not advised. HBcAb-positive donors can be used in HBcAb-positive and/or HBsAb-positive recipients and no prophylaxis is required. Hepatitis B-naive or unvaccinated recipients can also receive HBcAb-positive kidneys since the risk for transmission is low but guidelines suggest lamivudine may be considered for 1 year posttransplant as prophylaxis. All recipients receiving kidneys from HBV-positive donors should have posttransplant monitoring with HBV DNA viral loads, surface antigen, and core antibody (for individuals without prior infection), regardless of their immune status.

Human Immunodeficiency Virus

HIV infection is a known risk factor for the development of CKD and ESRD. Widespread adoption of potent antiretroviral therapy (ARV) has contributed to a decline in ESRD among whites with HIV infection, but rates of ESRD are still disproportionately higher among affected blacks.[141] Kidney transplantation is accepted as the ideal therapy for ESRD, even among HIV-positive individuals, but HIV-positive patients have diminished access to the waiting list and are less likely to achieve kidney transplantation. Of the 309 HIV-positive patients evaluated at a single transplant center from 2000 to 2007, only 20% achieved wait-listing compared with 73% of HIV-negative patients during the same time period.[142] A study of waitlist outcomes for HIV-positive patients demonstrated that although waitlist mortality was similar to HIV-negative patients (adjusted hazard ratio [aHR], 1.03; 95% CI, 0.89 to 1.20; $P = 0.67$), HIV-positive candidates were less like to receive a deceased donor transplant (aHR, 0.87; 95% CI, 0.74 to 1.01; $P = 0.07$) and significantly less likely to achieve living donor transplantation (aHR, 0.53; 95% CI, 0.44 to 0.64; $P < 0.001$).[143] However, kidney transplantation is associated with a survival benefit, compared with remaining on the waitlist (adjusted risk ratio [aRR], 0.21; 95% CI, 0.10 to 0.42; $P < 0.001$), for HIV-positive patients, as has been observed for other high-risk patient groups.[144]

Due to high patient mortality and high rates of allograft failure in HIV-positive patients transplanted in the pre-ARV era, HIV was once considered a relative contraindication to transplantation. However, with improved HIV patient survival after the widespread implementation of potent ARV therapy, this relative contraindication was reconsidered. After numerous case series reporting promising results, the National Institutes of Health (NIH) funded a multicenter prospective trial to assess feasibility of kidney transplantation in HIV-positive patients; this study enrolled 150 patients at 19 centers across the United States and followed them for 3 years.[145] Patient survival was 88% and allograft survival was 73.7% at 3 years, similar to outcomes for older kidney recipients as reported in the Scientific Registry of Transplant Recipients (SRTR), but outcomes were worse for HCV-coinfected recipients. Since the publication of the results of the NIH trial, several groups have examined the national experience with HIV-positive transplantation, using registry data. One study compared outcomes for 492 recipients with HIV and 147 recipients with HIV/HCV coinfection to an uninfected reference group. HIV monoinfected patient mortality (HR, 0.90; 95% CI, 0.66 to 1.24) and allograft loss (HR, 0.60; 95% CI, 0.40 to 0.88) were not statistically different, but there was an increased risk for death (HR, 2.26; 95%, 1.45 to 3.52) and graft loss (HR, 2.59; 95% CI, 1.60 to 4.19) in the HIV/HCV coinfected patients.[146] A "mate kidney" analysis, to control for donor quality, found similar results, as did a study matching HIV-positive recipients with HIV-negative controls.[147,148] Interestingly, Locke et al. demonstrated that experience in HIV-positive transplantation, as reflected in a center's participation in the NIH multicenter trial, did not affect outcomes (patient survival aHR, 1.13; $P = 0.63$ and allograft survival aHR, 1.08; $P = 0.71$), but there was an era effect, with patients transplanted between 2008 and 2011 having better outcomes than those transplanted earlier.[149]

Acute Rejection

Despite the fact that HIV infection is a state of overall immunosuppression, higher than expected rates of acute rejection have been consistently observed. In the NIH multicenter trial, the incidence of rejection was 31% in the first year, compared with the expected Scientific Registry of Transplant Recipients (SRTR) 1-year rejection rate of 12.3% in HIV-negative kidney transplant recipients.[145] A similarly high incidence of rejection has been reported in multiple subsequent case series from the United States and Europe.[150,151]

Excess acute rejection risk may not be entirely due to immune dysregulation from HIV infection; drug–drug interactions, selection of induction and maintenance immunosuppression as well as viral suppression likely also play a role. A recent study demonstrated that patients who had undetectable viral loads for less than 2 years before transplant were 2.48-fold more likely to experience acute rejection after kidney transplantation.[152] An analysis of the SRTR database revealed that HIV-positive patients are less likely to receive lymphocyte-depleting induction therapy than HIV-negative controls (31.4% vs. 55.5%), but use of antithymocyte globulin was associated with a lower risk for rejection (RR, 0.39; 95% CI, 0.18 to 0.87; $P = 0.02$). Maintenance immunosuppression is also important. In that same study, patients on maintenance sirolimus had a higher risk for rejection (aRR 2.15; 95% CI, 1.20 to 3.87) than those on a CNI.[153] Data from a single-center case series suggested that tacrolimus use in HIV-positive recipients is associated with a lower acute rejection risk (21%) than cyclosporine (58%; $P = 0.003$).[154]

Drug–Drug Interactions

Drug–drug interactions between ARVs and CNIs are complex. Protease inhibitors (PIs), historically a main component of ARV regimens, are potent inhibitors of the cytochrome P450 (CYP)3A enzyme system, which is the main metabolic pathway for CNIs. When PIs and CNIs are coadministered, the result is higher CNI levels, necessitating CNI dose reductions. For patients on a PI and cyclosporine this means a four- to fivefold lower cyclosporine dose with a 50% increase in the dosing interval, whereas patients on tacrolimus and a PI require an 80% dose decrease and a sevenfold increase in the dosing interval.[155] Non-nucleoside reverse transcriptase inhibitors (NNRTI) generally induce CYP3A enzyme activity and cause subtherapeutic levels, but individual effects can vary by NNRTI; this can be more easily overcome by increasing the CNI dose to achieve the desired trough level. In light of these complex interactions, many transplant professionals prefer the use of PI-free regimens whenever possible, favoring regimens based on integrase inhibitors, which permit more "traditional" CNI dosing and have been shown to be both safe and effective in the transplant setting.[156] Alternatively, one could consider using belatacept in EBV seropositive recipients to avoid CNI–PI interactions, which has been described in several case reports.[157]

Infection

Infection is a common complication of HIV-negative transplantation and of special concern in the HIV-positive recipient. In the NIH trial, 38% of patients had an infectious complication requiring hospitalization, with the majority of these infections being bacterial in nature. The most common sites involved were the genitourinary tract (26%), the respiratory tract (20%), and the bloodstream (19%).[145] The authors noted that infections of any type were twice as common among recipients who received antithymocyte globulin induction. Of 150 recipients, 5 developed BK nephropathy, similar to the prevalence observed in the HIV-negative transplant population. A more contemporary study using SRTR data linked to Medicare claims failed to find an increased risk for infection associated with induction immunosuppression in HIV-positive kidney transplant recipients; rates of infections overall in the first year were similar among HIV-positive patients who received no induction, antithymocyte globulin or anti-interleukin-2 receptor antibodies.[158] The most common infection in this national cohort was of the urinary tract. Importantly, patients who received induction of either type spent fewer days in the hospital, had fewer readmissions overall, and had superior death-censored graft survival than those who did not receive induction immunosuppression.

Opportunistic infection prophylaxis for HIV-positive recipients is similar to the approaches used in HIV-negative patients; no HIV-specific data exists to suggest the need for more aggressive prophylaxis. The American Society of Transplantation Infectious Diseases guidelines outline one approach.[159] The authors suggest lifelong prophylaxis against *Pneumocystis* pneumonia, ideally with trimethoprim-sulfamethoxazole but atovaquone or dapsone can be substituted for patients with sulfa allergies. CMV prophylaxis is also recommended for at-risk recipients and either valganciclovir or ganciclovir can be used; at many centers the dosing (450 vs. 900 mg/d) and duration of therapy (3 vs. 6 months) mirrors that which is used in the HIV-negative population. Although fluconazole was used selectively by some centers in the NIH trial as antifungal prophylaxis, many centers prefer nystatin to avoid drug–drug interactions with CNIs. Prophylaxis for infections such as toxoplasmosis (when CD4 ≤200 cells/mm^3) with trimethoprim-sulfamethoxazole and *Mycobacterium avium* complex (when CD4 ≤75 cells/mm^3) with azithromycin is also recommended, but since most HIV-positive transplant recipients have robust CD4 counts pretransplantation and rarely have prolonged periods of severe lymphocytopenia posttransplant, this is rarely required. Nine months of isoniazid therapy for any patient with previously untreated latent *Mycobacterium* TB is strongly advised.

Use of Human Immunodeficiency Virus-positive Donors

Whether HIV-positive individuals will be a safe and significant contributor to the donor pool is unknown. The most extensive experience using HIV-positive donors comes from South Africa. Muller et al. reported the results of 27 patients transplanted with kidneys from HIV-positive deceased donors, all with lymphocyte-depleting induction and tacrolimus-based immunosuppression.[160] Acceptable outcomes were reported, with patient and allograft survival both 84% at 3 years. Although these results provide evidence of feasibility for HIV-positive to HIV-positive transplantation, the HIV-positive population in the United States is quite different.

In the United States the National Organ Transplantation Act, passed in 1984 specifically prohibited organ donation by HIV-positive individuals and the signage of the HIV Organ Policy Equity (HOPE) Act in November 2013 was a significant departure from this policy. The HOPE Act authorizes research in the area of HIV-positive to HIV-positive organ donation and specific research criteria for studies employing these organs have been established, with provisions for both living and deceased donors.[161] To date, no living HIV-positive individual has served as a kidney donor but several deceased HIV-positive donor kidney transplants have been performed both in the United States and in Europe.

Using data from the Nationwide Inpatient Sample, the HIV Research Network, and UNOS, it was estimated that there were 500 potential HIV-positive donors in the United States per year; but these sources lacked necessary information to assess donor organ quality.[162] A study of HIV-positive patients who died "in HIV care" in Philadelphia with more granular clinical information was only able to identify 13 potentially suitable HIV-positive donors over 5 years.[163] The median kidney donor profile index (KDPI), a measure of organ quality, was 95%, indicating that these organs would be considered marginal kidneys. Use of HIV-positive donors in the United States has the potential to increase access to transplantation for HIV-positive individuals, but the extent to which these organs will contribute to the donor pool remains unknown and organ quality may be of concern. A multicenter trial using HIV-positive donors is underway and should provide useful information to guide future use of HIV-positive donors.

FUNGAL PATHOGENS

Kidney transplant patients are at increased risk for opportunistic infections due to diverse fungal pathogens, including *Candida* species, *Aspergillus*, *Cryptococcus*, and *Pneumocystis*. A US national survey of fungal infections revealed *Candida* infections to be most common (accounting for 49% of all infections); *Cryptococcus* occurred in 15% and *Aspergillus* in 14% of surveyed patients.[26] Endemic mycoses were seen in 10% and *Pneumocystis* was relatively uncommon, accounting for 1% of infections in kidney recipients. Risk factors and clinical presentation vary based on the pathogen and the prophylactic strategy.

Candida

In the Transnet multicenter survey, *Candida albicans* was the most common *Candida* species found after transplantation and bloodstream infections were the most common site of infection.[164] Because of the methodology used to collect cases in Transnet, mucocutaneous infections, the most common manifestation of *Candida*, were not captured. *Candida* also has been associated with intraabdominal infections (more commonly in kidney pancreas recipients), UTIs, and device-related infections.[165] Candiduria poses a unique situation in the kidney transplant recipient. Because this may simply represent colonization, especially in women, it is important to differentiate infection from colonization. Guidelines recommend against treatment of asymptomatic candiduria.[166] It is important to recognize symptomatic infection and fungus balls that can result in obstructive uropathy especially in recipients with poor bladder function or will be undergoing urinary tract manipulation; treatment is indicated in these circumstances.[165]

Risk factors for *Candida* infections are similar to those found in the general population and include diabetes mellitus, renal replacement therapy, broad-spectrum antibiotic use, parenteral nutrition, central venous catheters, and neutropenia.[162] Kidney pancreas transplant recipients who undergo enteric drainage are at increased risk for *Candida* infections due to the surgical procedure. Overall mortality in transplant recipients with *Candida* infections in the Transnet survey was 25% with mortality highest in patients infected with non-albicans *Candida* species.[164] Additional risk factors for mortality in kidney recipients included the presence or hepatic and/or renal insufficiency, congestive heart failure, and the use of amphotericin B.

Optimal treatment of *Candida* infections depends on the site and species.[165,166] It is important to remove any implicated devices (e.g., IV catheters) whenever possible. Fungus balls may require surgical removal. The choice of antifungal should be determined based on the species. Empiric treatment with echinocandins can be considered until the species is identified; however, these agents do not penetrate well into the urinary tract and consequently should be avoided for UTIs. Azoles are preferred for the treatment of UTIs. The vast majority of *C. albicans* species are susceptible to fluconazole; treatment of the less-susceptible non-albicans species may require treatment with echinocandins, voriconazole, or amphotericin B (lipid formulation). If azoles are used, it is important to consider the potential for drug interactions with CNIs and with mTOR inhibitors and dose adjustments of the immunosuppressive agents are often required at the time of initiation of azole therapy.

Cryptococcus

The multicenter epidemiological study of fungal infections in transplant patients (Transnet) identified *Cryptococcus* as the second most common invasive fungal infection in kidney transplant recipients.[26] This opportunistic infection typically occurs late after transplant with a median time of onset of 575 days posttransplant.[26] The most common manifestations are CNS disease (basilar meningitis) and pneumonia.[167] Risk factors for the disease include end-stage liver disease and lymphocyte depletion secondary to alemtuzumab or antithymocyte globulin.[167] Given the late onset of infection, environmental exposure may also play a role. Mortality associated with this infection is high; Transnet revealed a 12-month mortality of 27% although other studies estimated mortality of approximately 14% with baseline kidney failure a risk factor for mortality.[26,168]

Prompt recognition and treatment of cryptococcal infection is critical to patient survival. Many patients present with typical signs and symptoms of basilar meningitis, including headache and visual symptoms, including diplopia. Pulmonary nodules, skin nodules, liver, renal, and rarely bone and joint disease have also been described.[167] Because of the predilection of *Cryptococcus* for CNS involvement, patients with extraneural disease should undergo lumbar puncture to exclude meningeal involvement. Lumbar punctures should include measurement of opening pressure (an important prognostic indicator) as well as glucose, protein, cell count, fungal culture, and cryptococcal antigen. A serum cryptococcal antigen can be performed but a negative serum antigen does not exclude the possibility of *Cryptococcal* disease and lumbar puncture and/or tissue biopsy may still be warranted in patients suspected of infection.[167]

Optimal treatment of infection depends on the site of disease but ideally includes a 2-week induction phase with a lipid-based amphotericin and 5-flucytosine, followed by fluconazole, for patients with CNS or more severe disease.[167] The optimal duration of therapy is unknown and it is important to follow patients with repeat lumbar punctures and imaging as appropriate to ensure disease resolution. An important complication of cryptococcal infection has been the development of immune reconstitution inflammatory syndrome (IRIS), especially associated with rapid tapering of immune suppression.[169] This has been manifested by worsening of cryptococcal symptoms and findings; serial lumbar punctures have been required in the presence of IRIS and meningitis to decrease the intracranial pressure. There is no specific treatment for this complication but corticosteroids have been beneficial in anecdotal reports.[167]

Aspergillus

Aspergillus was noted to cause 14% of invasive fungal infections in kidney recipients in the Transnet study.[26] Typically seen in the first 6 to 9 months posttransplant, mortality is high; Transnet reported a 12-month mortality of 41% for invasive aspergillosis, a rate similar to that seen in a large multicenter multinational study.[26,170] Notably, graft loss was also high, affecting 20% of patients with invasive aspergillus.[170] The majority of infections involve the lungs, although extrapulmonary and disseminated infection can occur. Risk factors for the development of invasive pulmonary aspergillus in the multinational study include pretransplant chronic obstructive pulmonary disease, serious posttransplant infections, and impaired allograft function.[171] Additional risk factors include hemodialysis and intensified immunosuppression, including prolonged high doses of corticosteroids.[172] Diagnosis requires differentiation of colonization from infection; consequently pulmonary infection requires a combination of imaging (typically computed tomography) and respiratory tract microbiological sampling. Extrapulmonary sites often require tissue biopsy for pathology and culture. Galactomannan obtained from serum or bronchoalveolar lavage can be a useful adjunct to diagnosis but a negative serum galactomannan does not exclude the diagnosis.[172] The treatment of choice has been voriconazole, although there are significant drug interactions that must be managed, especially with CNIs and mTOR inhibitors.[172] In addition, the IV formulation of voriconazole includes a cyclodextran base that can cause hyperviscosity when administered to individuals with CKD. Other azoles, including posaconazole and isavuconazole, echinocandins, and lipid formulation of amphotericin also are effective. It is unknown whether combination therapy will improve outcomes, but the multinational study did not show any benefit in their cohort of renal transplant recipients.[170]

Pneumocystis jirovecii

Pneumocystis jirovecii (formerly known as *Pneumocystis carinii*) is an uncommon cause of pneumonia in kidney transplant recipients, accounting for 1% of fungal infections in the Transnet study.[26] This low incidence likely reflects the common use of trimethoprim sulfamethoxazole in the early posttransplant period. Although relatively uncommon, mortality can be quite high. Increased immunosuppression, especially with agents that reduce the absolute CD4 count, high doses of corticosteroids, CMV, rejection, and proximity to other patients with *P. jirovecii pneumonia* (PJP) are all recognized risk factors for PJP.[173] Radiographic findings are variable and diagnosis of PJP requires sampling of respiratory secretions, typically via bronchoscopy; cytology and PCR often will provide the diagnosis. Because the burden of organisms is lower than seen with patients with HIV infection, biopsy may be required to exclude the diagnosis.[173] Serum beta D-glucan is often very elevated and this may be a clue to the diagnosis. The treatment of choice is high-dose trimethoprim sulfamethoxazole coupled with a tapering course of higher-dose corticosteroids.[173] Given the potentially poor outcomes in patients with PJP, it is important to provide prophylaxis to at-risk individuals. Commonly 6 to 12 months of trimethoprim sulfamethoxazole is recommended after transplant but longer courses should be considered for patients requiring higher doses of immunosuppression, including for the treatment of rejection. Individuals with CMV are also at increased risk for PJP, so some centers reinstitute PJP prophylaxis for patients who develop CMV infection. Alternative regimens, including atovaquone and dapsone (for patients with normal G6PD levels), can be considered for patients who are allergic to trimethoprim sulfamethoxazole.[173]

BACTERIAL INFECTIONS

Bacterial infections are a major cause of morbidity and mortality after transplant. Surgical site infections, pneumonias, and diabetic foot infections are all seen, but the most common infections are those related to the urinary tract. The involved site may be anticipated based on the timing after transplant with surgical site infections occurring in the first month and pneumonias occurring related to hospital acquisition early and to more typical bacterial pathogens (e.g., *Streptococcus pneumonia* and *Legionella* species) in the later period. Kidney transplant recipients are at increased risk for reactivation of TB and opportunistic bacterial infections, including with *Nocardia* species. It is important to consider the diversity of pathogens when evaluating patients presenting with signs and symptoms of infection. The net state of immunosuppression, latent infections, and new environmental exposures all should be considered when developing a diagnostic plan. In many cases, more invasive testing may be required to confirm a diagnosis.

Urinary Tract Infections

UTIs are the most common bacterial infection seen in kidney transplant recipients with a prevalence of 23% to 75%.[34] Although most commonly seen in the early posttransplant period, it is important to realize that UTIs can occur at any time following transplant, especially in women.[174] Pyelonephritis and bloodstream infections are commonly seen; in one survey of bloodstream infections after kidney transplant, 75% were attributed to UTIs.[175] Whether UTIs have a significant effect on long-term allograft function is controversial. The varying definitions for UTI, variable findings based on timing of infection posttransplant, and lack of uniform measures to assess kidney function used in clinical studies make it difficult to assess the overall effect. Regardless, these infections have been associated with increased mortality and at least acute impairment of kidney function and possibly long-term allograft damage.[34,175] Risk factors for UTI vary with timing after transplant and include female sex, diabetes mellitus, ureteral stents, urinary tract catheterization, urinary tract abnormalities (including reflux), immunosuppression (antithymocyte globulin, mycophenolate), reduced allograft function, *en bloc* double kidney transplants, deceased donors, and acute rejection.[34,176]

It may be difficult to recognize UTI in kidney transplant recipients because the usual symptoms may not be present given the disruption of the usual neural pathways. Allograft tenderness is often seen. Standard definitions of UTI reflect those used in nontransplant recipients and include the demonstration of both pyuria and bacteriuria.[34] *E. coli* remains the most common organism causing UTIs.[34] It is important to perform susceptibility testing for urinary tract isolates since there have been increasingly frequent reports of multidrug-resistant pathogens.[34,177,178] Ultrasound and computed tomography imaging may confirm the diagnosis of pyelonephritis and reveal structural abnormalities that increase the risk for UTIs.

Treatment of infection should be based on the suspected site of infection, something that can be difficult given the atypical presentation of infection. Shorter durations (i.e., 5 to 7 days) are recommended for lower tract infection; pyelonephritis should be treated with 14 days of antibacterials, and relapsed/recurrent infection with the same organism warrants prolonged treatment (>4 weeks).[34] The choice of antimicrobial should consider the potential for resistance, the severity of illness, and drug interactions, especially with immunosuppressive agents; IV therapy should be initiated for more severe infections. Patients with frequent or persistent UTIs should be assessed for structural abnormalities and surgical interventions considered as appropriate. A significant area of controversy has been the management of asymptomatic bacteriuria. A recent prospective trial of treatment of asymptomatic bacteriuria commencing 2 months posttransplant failed to show a benefit from treating asymptomatic bacteriuria and current guidelines do not recommend treating these patients, especially given the potential risk for adverse events including increased antibacterial resistance and *C. difficile*.[34,179] The optimal management of patients with recurrent infections is unknown. Correction of structural and functional abnormalities should be performed. Postmenopausal women may benefit from vaginal estrogen and urinary acidification also has been employed. Chronic or prolonged antimicrobials should be reserved for recipients who have had more complicated courses since there is a significant potential for adverse effects from antibiotics.[34]

PREVENTION

Successful transplantation is more likely when candidates are carefully evaluated for infection risk before transplant. That includes assessing their home and work environments, including prior living arrangements, their personal contacts, pets, and their hobbies.[180] Because of the potential for TB and endemic diseases such as coccidioides and strongyloides to reactivate after the transplant, it is important to evaluate patients for diseases that may have been acquired earlier due to residence in areas where these infections were endemic. Especially important is the need to evaluate candidates for TB, because this infection may reactivate after transplant and diagnosis and treatment is complicated by immunosuppressive therapy. This should include taking a thorough history, obtaining chest radiography, and performing either an intradermal skin test using PPD or an IGRA.[4] Given the reduced sensitivity of these tests in patients with CKD, it is important to assess the individual's risk for infection by taking a careful history and reviewing chest radiography for signs of prior infection. Patients who have evidence of latent TB who have not completed prior prophylactic therapy should be treated with 9 months of isoniazid either before or after transplant. Shorter-course rifampicin containing regimens can be considered in the pretransplant setting if there are no significant drug interactions that will prevent its use.

Immunization

One especially important intervention in the pretransplant setting is the review and updating of vaccine status.[181] Given the potentially reduced immunogenicity and efficacy of vaccines administered after transplant and the increased risk for transplant recipients for vaccine-preventable infections, this is especially important. Recommended vaccines are included in Table 40.3. Hepatitis B vaccine is especially important for patients who are listed for transplantation since there is an increased risk for transmission in dialysis centers and patients who are immune may be more safely transplanted with kidneys from donors with a history of hepatitis B or those at increased risk for new hepatitis B infections. Patients with

CKD should receive a double dose of the recombinant vaccine and hepatitis B surface antibody levels should be measured following completion of the vaccine series.[182] Historically, there have been some concerns regarding an increased risk for rejection after influenza vaccine due to the development of low level *de novo* anti-HLA antibodies after immunization.[183] However, the linkage of vaccination to rejection has not been demonstrated and a study examining Medicare claims data in the first year after kidney transplant demonstrated that influenza vaccination was associated with reduced allograft loss and death.[184] Ideally, all vaccines should be updated before transplantation; however, nonlive virus vaccines may be safely administered after transplant.[181] If possible, it may be advisable to delay posttransplant immunization for 6 months to improve vaccine response; if a patient is transplanted immediately before influenza season, vaccines may be given sooner after transplant. Because transplant recipients may have suboptimal vaccine responses, it is important to vaccinate household contacts as well. CKD and transplantation have both been associated with reduced vaccine responsiveness; these individuals should receive conjugate pneumococcal vaccine followed by the pneumococcal polysaccharide capsule vaccine to maximize vaccine response.[185] Vaccine schedules are updated annually; it is important to review to ensure appropriate immunizations are administered.[186]

Although kidney transplant recipients are at increased risk for infection, careful consideration of specific infection risks, implementation of preventive measures, and early recognition of infections may mitigate this risk. Given the ever-changing nature of transplantation, ongoing consideration of preventive strategies, including antimicrobials, immunization, and environmental assessments and utilization of directed diagnostic strategies for prompt recognition of infection is essential to optimize posttransplant outcomes.

A full list of references is available at www.expertconsult.com.

41

Noninfectious Complications After Kidney Transplantation

Monica Grafals, MD, MPH, John P. Vella, MD, FACP, FRCP, FASN, FAST, and Anil Chandraker, MD, FRCP

OUTLINE

INTRODUCTION

Kidney transplantation is the treatment of choice for selected patients with end-stage renal disease (ESRD) because of improvements in patient survival, quality of life, and reduced long-term health costs.[1,2] Clearly, the success of transplantation is founded upon the use of potent immunotherapies that prevent allograft rejection and permit long-term engraftment. The complex pathophysiological changes that occurred during kidney failure before transplantation are often compounded by complications that are directly induced by suppression of the immune system. As patient and graft survival rates have improved, attention has been directed to strategies that mitigate the relatively high burden of morbidity and mortality. Cardiovascular disease, infection, and malignancy are the dominant causes of mortality after kidney transplantation.[3,4] This chapter will focus on the noninfectious complications that develop after transplantation and their management strategies. Complications range in severity from to those that are relatively minor events to those that are allograft- or life-threatening.

CARDIOVASCULAR DISEASE

Atherosclerotic cardiovascular disease (ASCVD) is the leading cause of mortality in dialysis and transplant patients,[5] accounting for at least one-third of all deaths in transplant recipients,[6-9] and remains the most common cause of graft loss.[10] ASCVD before kidney transplantation is three to four times more prevalent in the ESRD compared with the general population and has been shown to be the single most important predictor of cardiovascular mortality after transplantation.[11] Vanrenterghem and colleagues reexplored this topic to define current trends.[12] In a cohort of more than 2000 primary allograft recipients, the incidence of cardiovascular events increased over time. Within 15 years of transplantation, only 47% of surviving patients had not experienced any cardiovascular events. Risk factors associated with cardiovascular complications were male gender, age, hypertension (HTN) before transplantation, longer duration of pretransplantation dialysis, cardiovascular event before transplantation, older era of transplantation, center-specific effect, posttransplant diabetes mellitus, increased pulse pressure after transplantation, use of corticosteroids and azathioprine, lower serum albumin after transplantation, and higher serum triglyceride levels after transplantation. The risk for death was also increased in patients with low or elevated hematocrit, whereas it was minimal with values of about 38%. Numerous other reports have underscored the prevalence and importance of "traditional" risk factors for ASCVD in transplant recipients.[11,13-19]

In spite of those issues, kidney transplantation has repeatedly been shown to reduce cardiovascular and all-cause mortality compared with dialysis. For example, Meier-Kriesche and associates[20] compared the cardiovascular death (CVD) rates of more than 60,000 adult first kidney transplant recipients with those of 67,000 waitlisted patients over the same time period. A progressive decline in CVD rates was seen in the transplant recipients compared with the opposite trend for patients who remained on the waiting list. Even though CVD rates were higher in the early postoperative period, by 3 months posttransplantation, rates were lower than for dialysis patients.

Nontraditional Risk Factors

So what is it about transplantation that lowers cardiovascular risk? Recently, attention has focused on nontraditional cardiovascular risk factors that are prevalent in patients with chronic kidney disease (CKD) and that are not effectively controlled by dialysis. An overview of the effect of traditional and nontraditional risk factors is provided in Fig. 41.1. *Oxidative stress* is now known to be an important factor in the pathogenesis of ASCVD in patients with ESRD.[21,22] Uremic oxidative stress is characterized biologically by an increase in lipid peroxidation products and reactive aldehyde groups as well as by retention of oxidized thiols.[23,24] The pathophysiology of oxidative stress in uremia is multifactorial, but the retention of oxidized solute by the loss of kidney function is probably a major contributor. Simmons et al. evaluated time-dependent changes in biomarkers of oxidative stress before and after living donor transplantation.[25] Pretransplantation levels of the proinflammatory proteins interleukin-6 (IL-6), tumor necrosis factor-alpha (TNF-α), and C-reactive protein (CRP), and the oxidative stress markers plasma protein carbonyls and F_2-isoprostanes, were significantly elevated in CKD patients compared with healthy control subjects. There was a rapid and sustained decline in all of these biomarkers after transplantation, and by 2 months posttransplantation, levels had reached those of the controls. Cueto-Manzano and colleagues also reported increased levels of inflammatory markers pretransplantation that initially fell posttransplantation and, in the case of CRP, remained low, whereas levels of TNF-α and IL-6 fell, only to rise by the first posttransplantation year.[26] Ducloux and associates recorded coronary events in 8% of 344 consecutive kidney transplant patients who were free of vascular disease at the time of transplantation.[19] In addition to "traditional" Framingham risk factors, CRP and homocystinemia were found to be independent risk factors for ischemic heart disease events. Sezer and colleagues retrospectively analyzed the predictive role of CRP on the development of chronic allograft dysfunction.[27] No difference was found between the pretransplantation levels of CRP between those transplant recipients who were destined to develop allograft dysfunction and those who were not. However, CRP levels were significantly higher in patients with allograft dysfunction by 1 month posttransplantation and at the time of diagnosis of allograft dysfunction.

Hypertension

About 70% of transplant recipients are hypertensive.[28] HTN after transplantation is associated with numerous factors that include pretransplantation HTN, cause of primary disease, as well as posttransplantation factors such as delayed graft function, immunosuppression therapy, rejection, transplant renal artery stenosis, acquired glomerular filtration rate (GFR), chronic immune and nonimmune injury, recurrent or *de novo* allograft glomerulonephritis, and weight gain.[28,29] HTN is a risk factor for premature allograft failure, ASCVD, and death with a functioning graft.

It is known that calcineurin inhibitors (CIs) and steroids induce or exacerbate HTN after transplantation. The CIs disrupt the normal balance between endogenous vasodilators and vasoconstrictors, leading to afferent arteriolar

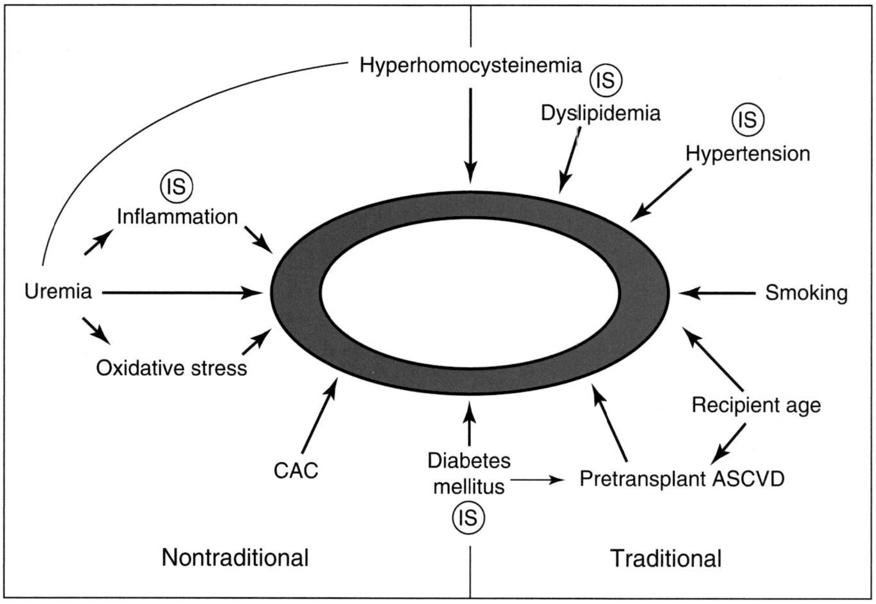

FIG. 41.1 Pathogenesis of atherosclerosis after kidney transplantation. Numerous processes interplay to induce atherosclerosis after transplantation, including traditional (or Framingham) and nontraditional factors. *ASCVD,* Atherosclerotic cardiovascular disease; *CAC,* coronary artery calcification; *IS,* immunosuppression.

vasoconstriction and thus HTN. In part, this effect is mediated via activation of the sympathetic nervous system[30,31] and also increased expression of endothelin.[32] Watschinger and Sayegh described the pathogenic role of endothelin in this setting by[33] administering an endothelin receptor antagonist that blunted the rise in blood pressure induced by cyclosporin A (CsA) in vivo. Vasoconstriction is compounded by depressed nitric oxide–induced vasodilatory activity.[34] A recent report described a novel mechanism by which CsA causes sodium retention in the thick ascending limb of the loop of Henle, leading to HTN.[35]

It should be recognized that not all CIs induce HTN to the same extent. For example, numerous clinical trials have shown that tacrolimus is associated with a significantly reduced requirement for medications to control HTN compared with CsA.[36-38] Similarly, ISA 247, a novel CI currently undergoing clinical trials, may also be associated with less HTN compared with CsA.[39] HTN has also been shown to resolve on converting patients from CsA to tacrolimus and to increase again when switched back to CsA treatment.[40] In addition, individuals without kidney disease are more likely to develop HTN when given CsA compared with tacrolimus.[41]

Steroids also elevate blood pressure via mineralocorticoid-induced sodium retention. The effects are dose related, and the relatively low doses of steroids currently used after the first 6 to 12 months are thought to have a small effect on blood pressure. Patients with preexisting HTN appear to be more susceptible to this adverse effect of chronic steroid use.[42] Steroids are associated with multiple complications including HTN, obesity, glucose intolerance, osteoporosis, avascular necrosis, glaucoma, cataracts, myopathy, and neuropsychiatric complications after transplantation.[43] In various older studies, steroid withdrawal was shown to improve blood pressure, glycemic control, and lipid profiles.[44-46] In truth, although steroid avoidance or early steroid withdrawal is now routinely practiced by many centers in the United States, there are no data to indicate that such a practice has any beneficial effect on patient or graft survival.[47,48] Furthermore, such practices have been shown to increase the early rejection rate and may adversely affect long-term graft function in at least some patient groups.[49,50]

Smoking

Smoking remains an important remediable cardiovascular risk factor that is associated in kidney transplant recipients with an increased burden of cardiovascular disease and an increased risk for premature graft failure.[51] In a recent cross-sectional single-center study analyzing smoking habits, it was found that kidney transplantation is a strong incentive for patients to quit.[52] Morphologically, the main allograft lesion associated with smoking is fibrous intimal thickening of small arteries.[53] A recent cross-sectional analysis demonstrated that 76% of the waitlisted patients and 87% of allograft recipients were nonsmokers at the time of investigation.[52] Among the nonsmoking waitlisted patients, only 31% had never smoked, whereas 41% of the allograft recipients had never smoked. Of former smoking patients, only 28% had stopped smoking after transplantation. Patients younger than 55 years of age and females were more likely to quit than older or male patients. Smokers were significantly less likely to be transplanted compared with nonsmokers. Detection of smoking habits is typically dependent on patient self-reporting, seemingly a rather unreliable practice. In a cohort of 233 kidney transplant recipients, 45% were reported never to have smoked. In this group, serum cotinine serum levels were unrecordable.[54] Among the 55% with a lifetime history of smoking, cotinine level was diagnostic of current smoking in 32 (25%). However, only 66% of the current smokers admitted to the nephrologist that they had continued smoking, and 34% claimed to be nonsmokers. The authors concluded that identification of current smokers among kidney transplant recipients should start with questioning about lifetime history of smoking; if positive, cotinine serum level should be measured.

Dyslipidemia

After transplantation, the prevalence of hypercholesterolemia is 60% and hypertriglyceridemia is 35%.[55] Most immunosuppressive drugs, with the exception of the antimetabolites and belatacept, adversely affect dyslipidemia. Various reviews have described the differential effects of sirolimus, cyclosporine, and tacrolimus on dyslipidemia, which range in severity from most to least, respectively.[3,4] Approximately 70% of CsA-treated kidney transplant patients have serum cholesterol levels higher than 200 mg/dL, and 30% have levels higher than 250 mg/dL.[56] In addition, low-density lipoprotein (LDL) oxidation is increased in patients treated with cyclosporine.[57,58] Oxidized LDL is thought to play a crucial role in the development of arteriosclerotic lesions because it is toxic for endothelial cells and triggers endothelial dysfunction.[59] Kidney transplant recipients, and particularly those treated by CsA, have an increased incidence of endothelial dysfunction, which is revealed by impaired endothelium-dependent vasodilatation.[60,61]

Because cardiovascular disease is so prevalent in kidney transplant recipients, it is reasonable to consider the kidney transplantation state to be a "coronary heart disease risk equivalent" when applying guidelines.[62,63] This implies targeting plasma LDL cholesterol to less than 100 mg/dL via a combination of therapeutic lifestyle changes and drug therapy. Changing immunotherapy may also affect dyslipidemia in a beneficial manner. For example, switching to tacrolimus from sirolimus or cyclosporine and withdrawing steroids may permit normalization of lipid levels without any other pharmacological intervention.

Statins are the lipid-lowering drugs of choice in transplant recipients. A recently published trial that investigated the use of fluvastatin in kidney transplant recipients (Assessment of Lescol in Renal Transplantation [ALERT]) demonstrated efficacy in lowering cholesterol levels.[64] More importantly, cardiac deaths and nonfatal myocardial infarcts, although not overall mortality, were also significantly reduced after a mean of 6.7 years of follow-up. Of note, earlier reports of this study that failed to demonstrate use in reducing cardiovascular events should remind the reader that most statin trials reveal divergent outcomes only after 5 or more years of follow-up.

The reader is reminded that statin metabolism is at least partly inhibited by CI therapy that can lead to elevated blood and tissue concentrations and risk for adverse effects such as rhabdomyolysis. It is currently recommended that statins be used at reduced doses in CI-treated transplant recipients. This interaction is further enhanced if additional inhibitors of cytochrome P-450, such as diltiazem, are administered. Other measures that are often considered to minimize the risk for toxicity include the use of pravastatin or fluvastatin (which appear to have the least interaction with CIs), avoidance of other inhibitors of the cytochrome P-450 system, and avoidance of fibrates; periodic checking of plasma creatine kinase and liver function tests is also advisable.[65] Early reports indicating that pravastatin may reduce the risk for rejection in kidney and heart transplant recipients are probably of less relevance in the current era of "modern" immunosuppression.[66,67] Rarely, nonstatin drugs are used to lower plasma lipids in transplant patients. Bile acid sequestrants, if used, should be taken separately from CI because they impair absorption of these drugs. Fibrates should be prescribed with extreme caution to patients on statins and CI.

New-Onset Diabetes After Transplantation

The development of new-onset diabetes after transplantation (NODAT) is a serious complication of transplantation that is associated with dyslipidemia, chronic allograft dysfunction, cardiovascular morbidity, and death.[68,69] The incidence of NODAT is definition dependent and ranges from 2% to 53%.[70,71] Risk factors include obesity, weight gain, hepatitis C, steroids, tacrolimus, and restoration of insulin metabolism by the kidney allograft.[72] For reasons that are unclear, autosomal dominant polycystic kidney disease (ADPKD) is also a risk factor for NODAT.[73] The causative pathophysiological mechanisms include a decrease in the number and binding affinity of insulin receptors, malabsorption of glucose in peripheral organs, and activation of the glucose/fatty acid pathway. Such mechanisms appear particularly important in those with significant posttransplantation weight gain.[74]

The introduction of CI therapy, particularly tacrolimus, increases the risk for NODAT.[75] Early studies indicated that up to 20% of tacrolimus-treated patients developed diabetes and required insulin, although the generally accepted number currently is about 7%.[3,4] Both in vitro and biopsy studies indicate that CI impair pancreatic β-cell function, causing islet cell injury[76]; this leads to diminished insulin synthesis or secretion, or both.[77-81] Tacrolimus previously has been shown to impair first-phase (or early) insulin secretion,[82] whereas CsA has been shown to impair second-phase (or later, sustained) insulin secretion.[83] The clinical significance of the latter observation is unclear.

Steroids induce hyperglycemia primarily by causing insulin resistance by increasing hepatic gluconeogenesis, inhibiting peripheral glucose uptake, and also by impairing insulin secretion.[84,85] Reducing or withdrawing steroids has been shown to ameliorate hyperglycemia.[86,87]

The prognosis of NODAT is variable, although some studies indicate that up to one-third of patients ultimately regain euglycemia off treatment.[88] This figure may be higher if such patients undergo steroid minimization or withdrawal along with a reduction or change in CI therapy.[89] However, most patients require a long-term approach to management that includes therapeutic lifestyle change, oral hypoglycemics or insulin, or both. Tight control of blood sugars has been shown to slow the progression of end organ damage in diabetes; similar benefits are likely in kidney transplantation patients. It should be remembered that in spite of beneficial effects of tacrolimus on parameters such as HTN, GFR, and lipids, registry data indicate that there is no difference in patient or graft survival between those patients who receive cyclosporine and tacrolimus.[90] This observation is probably explained by the deleterious effect of tacrolimus-induced NODAT on long-term patient survival.

Metabolic Syndrome

The metabolic syndrome (MS) is known to be a risk for cardiovascular disease in the general population. In a study of more than 300 transplant recipients, 32% met criteria for MS at 1 year.[91] Predictive factors for MS included older age, male gender, pretransplantation high body mass index (BMI), and an increase in BMI after transplantation. In addition, the cumulative incidence of adverse events was more than three times greater in patients with MS compared with others without MS. In another study, MS was present in 54% of transplant recipients.[92] In this cohort, there was a significant correlation between the various components of the MS and the severity of coronary artery calcification (CAC). Median CAC scores were 0, 33, 98, and 262 for patients with one, two, three, and four or more positive components of the MS, respectively. It has also been suggested that MS is related to inflammation as measured by CRP levels in transplant recipients.[93] The effect of a 12-month dietary regimen on the nutritional status and metabolic outcome of kidney transplant recipients in the first posttransplantation year was reported by Rike and colleagues.[94] Forty-six deceased-donor kidney transplant recipients were enrolled during the first posttransplant year and followed prospectively for a further 12 months. Compliance with dietary recommendations was related to gender (male better than female) and was associated with weight loss primarily due to a decrease in fat mass, with decrease in total cholesterol and glucose plasma levels and with a concomitant rise in serum albumin concentrations.

Obesity

The epidemic of obesity in the United States has not spared kidney transplant candidates. Obesity trends in transplant recipients tend to mimic those in the general population, 65% of which is now defined as overweight (BMI greater than 25 kg/m^2). Several factors contribute to weight gain, including steroid use, removal of dietary restrictions after transplantation, and physical inactivity. Obesity is an established risk factor for atherosclerotic heart disease and increases the risk for diabetes, dyslipidemia, and HTN.[95] Obesity is also known to be associated with depression after transplantation.[96] Bosma and colleagues described an association between obesity and iothalamate-determined glomerular hyperfiltration in

838 kidney transplants.[97] With higher BMI, estimated GFR (eGFR) and filtration fraction (FF) increased significantly. Multivariate analysis supported the effect of BMI on eGFR and determined that this association was not explained by diabetes mellitus. On Cox regression analysis, lower eGFR and higher FF were independent determinants of graft loss and patient mortality. It is now known that the likelihood of receiving a transplant decreases with increasing degree of obesity compared with nonobese patients.[98] Similarly, the likelihood of being bypassed when an organ becomes available increases in a graded manner with category of obesity. The defining questions about obesity and transplantation are whether the former affects outcomes and whether weight loss before transplantation is a mitigating factor. In a study of 5700 patients, obesity was associated with poor graft survival. Patient survival was inferior only in univariate and not in multivariate analyses.[99] Perhaps surprisingly, underweight patients had greater late death-censored graft loss, mainly due to chronic allograft nephropathy. However, obesity was associated with greater odds risk (OR) for delayed graft function and 6-month risk for acute rejection. Management of obesity includes lifestyle changes, dietary modifications, and in some cases gastric bypass or banding, for which the published experiences in transplant recipients are limited.[100,101]

Peripheral and Cerebrovascular Disease

Dialyzed and kidney-transplanted patients have a higher rate of peripheral vascular complications than the general population.[1,109,110] Although transplantation is associated with significantly better survival than maintenance dialysis,[111] kidney transplant recipients still remain at high risk for vascular complications.[112-114] This risk can be enhanced by immunosuppressive drugs.[115] Kasiske and associates[55] reported a 15% prevalence of peripheral vascular disease at 15 years posttransplantation. Sung and associates[116] retrospectively studied 664 adult recipients and found a cumulative 5- and 10-year incidence of 4% and 6%, respectively; the presence of peripheral vascular disease was independently associated with poorer recipient survival. There is also some evidence from registry data that peripheral vascular disease is a risk factor for poor graft outcomes.[117] It therefore seems reasonable to aggressively treat patients with this condition with measures, such as aspirin, statins, smoking cessation, and revascularization where appropriate.

Posttransplantation Anemia

Posttransplantation anemia is present in more than 50% of kidney recipients at some stage after surgery.[102,103] Immediately posttransplantation, anemia is a consequence of postoperative blood loss, the use of myelosuppressive immunosuppressive medications such as antimetabolites, sirolimus and antithymocyte globulins (ATG), inflammation, and defective erythropoietin production by the transplanted kidney.[104,105] Furthermore, anemia can persist months after transplantation due to several factors including antiviral therapy, allograft dysfunction, or infection.[106] Table 41.1 summarizes the major causes of anemia in kidney transplant recipients and their mechanisms.

Angiotensin-converting enzyme (ACE) inhibitors and angiotensin receptor blockers (ARBs) exacerbate or induce anemia in the transplant patient, although for reasons that are incompletely understood.[107] In the Transplant European Survey on Anemia Management (TRESAM) study, data from 4263 patients from 72 transplant centers in Europe was collected 6 months to 5 years posttransplantation.[108] The mean hemoglobin levels before transplantation were significantly higher in the more recently transplanted recipients. At enrollment, 39% of patients were found to be anemic. Of the 8.5% of patients who were considered severely anemic, only 18% were treated with recombinant human erythropoietin (rHuEpo). Anemia was associated with impaired kidney function and use of azathioprine, ACE inhibitors, and ARB therapy.

Recombinant human erythropoietin is often administered to patients with CKD and more frequently to patients on maintenance dialysis. The use of rHuEpo after kidney transplantation remains to be defined. Van Biesen and associates reported

TABLE 41.1 Causes of Anemia in Kidney Transplant Recipients

Cause	Mediated by	Ultimate Effect
Allograft dysfunction Hyperparathyroidism-Inflammation	Erythropoietin deficiency	Decreased bone marrow production of RBCs
Azathioprine MMF/MPA SRL TMP-SMX-(val) ganciclovir Antithymocyte globulins	Myelosuppression	Decreased bone marrow production of RBCs
ACE inhibitors ARB	Impaired production of, or resistance to, erythropoietin	Decreased bone marrow production of RBCs
Iron deficiency	Impaired synthesis of hemoglobin	Decreased bone marrow production of RBCs
Minor ABO incompatibility	Donor antibodies	RBC hemolysis
Posttransplantation hemolytic uremic syndrome	Multiple factors, including genetic defects, viral infection, calcineurin inhibitors, antiphospholipid antibodies	RBC hemolysis
Gastrointestinal or other bleeding	RBC	RBC losses exceed production

This table shows only the more common causes of anemia posttransplantation. Frequently, more than one is present in the individual recipient. *ACE,* Angiotensin-converting enzyme; *ARB,* angiotensin receptor blockers; *MMF/MPA,* mycophenolic mofetil/mycophenolic acid; *RBC,* red blood cell; *SRL,* sirolimus; *TMP-SMX,* trimethoprim-sulfamethoxazole.

the results of a trial in which patients were randomized to either receive rHuEpo three times a week immediately after transplantation or not. The time to reach a hemoglobin level greater than 12.5 g/dL was 66 days in the rHuEpo group compared with 57 days in the control group. The authors concluded that although the administration of rHuEpo reduced the duration of anemia, this effect was marginal, and the doses needed were high.[104] There was no difference in harder endpoints such as length of stay or patient or graft survival between the groups.

Evaluation of Atherosclerotic Cardiovascular Disease Before Transplantation

Given the high incidence of preexisting ASCVD in the ESRD population, screening for such disease remains an important part of the transplant evaluation before surgery. Such investigations generally include electrocardiography, echocardiography, provocative stress testing, and cardiac catheterization when needed as the standard of care. Nevertheless, the efficacy of such an approach has been debated because patients awaiting transplantation have high mortality rates despite careful preselection. Hage and coworkers examined mortality outcomes in 3700 patients with ESRD referred to a single center for transplantation.[118] The mean age of the cohort was 48 years, and 42% were female. Stress myocardial perfusion imaging (MPI) was performed in 60% and coronary angiography in 7%. Over a period of 30 months, 17% of the cohort died. Interestingly, neither the presence nor severity of coronary disease as defined by angiography predicted survival. Coronary revascularization did not affect survival, either, except in patients with three-vessel disease. The best predictor of death was left ventricular ejection fraction (LVEF), as measured by gated myocardial perfusion imaging, with 2.7% mortality increase for each 1% ejection fraction decrease. Conversely, Bergeron and colleagues studied the outcome of 485 patients with CKD who had undergone dobutamine stress echocardiography (DSE) as part of an evaluation for transplantation and who were followed for more than 2 years.[119] Almost 40% of the patients died during the follow-up period. Patients with more extensive ischemia had inferior outcomes compared with those with lesser degrees of ischemia and also those with a normal stress testing. By multivariate analyses, the percentage of ischemic segments on DSE was an independent predictor of all-cause mortality. Vanrenterghem et al. reported the prognostic power of stress MPI in 150 patients with ESRD being evaluated for kidney transplantation with known coronary anatomy based on angiography.[12] An abnormal MPI result was present in 85% of patients, 30% had LVEF of less than 40%, and 40% had multivessel coronary artery disease using angiography. After 3 years, 35% of patients had died. Low ejection fraction, left ventricular dilatation, and diabetes mellitus were all associated with higher mortality. In a multivariate model, abnormal MPI results (low LVEF or abnormal perfusion) and diabetes alone were independent predictors of death, whereas number of narrowed arteries using coronary angiography was not. Thus MPI was a strong predictor of all-cause mortality in patients with ESRD. In truth, as a consequence of the observation that cardiovascular disease is the major cause of mortality in the peritransplant period, most transplant programs insist on echocardiography and provocative stress testing as a prerequisite for listing.

Hickson et al. reported a different approach to cardiac risk stratification using cardiac troponin T (cTnT) from a cohort of 644 patients, of whom 61% had elevated levels.[120] Higher levels related to diabetes, longer time on dialysis, history of ASCVD, and low serum albumin. High cTnT levels related to specific cardiac anomalies including left ventricular hypertrophy, wall motion abnormalities, and stress-inducible ischemia. Importantly, increasing cTnT levels were associated with reduced patient survival independent of serum albumin. In this study, the results of the stress testing or coronary angiography, or both, did not affect survival. However, high cTnT identified patients with abnormal echocardiogram findings and poor survival. Wait-listed patients with normal cTnT had excellent survival irrespective of other factors.

It has been suggested that normalization of GFR may alter CAC after transplantation. Schankel et al. studied this issue by performing electron beam computed tomography (CT) in 82 subjects at the time of transplantation and at least 1 year later.[121] Curiously, calcification scores actually increased over time. In multivariate analysis, diastolic blood pressure, Caucasian race, GFR, months posttransplant, BMI, and baseline CAC score were independent predictors of annualized rate of CAC change. Consequently, it seems that reasons other than arterial calcification are responsible for the favorable outcome–associated transplantation from a cardiovascular perspective.

Table 41.2 summarizes the adverse effects associated with the various immunosuppressant medications currently in clinical use.

MALIGNANCY AFTER KIDNEY TRANSPLANTATION

Improvements in patient and graft survival rates in renal transplantation remain overshadowed by the long-term risk for malignancy. With the exception of skin cancer, recipients of kidney transplants are about three to four times more likely to develop neoplastic disorders than the general population.[122] In general, three types of malignancy have features specific to the transplanted population:

- Posttransplant lymphoproliferative disease (PTLD)
- Nonmelanoma skin cancer
- Kidney cell carcinoma arising from (atrophic) native kidneys

The relationship between the nature and intensity of immunotherapy and subsequent malignancy is well defined and has been described in prior reviews.[4,123] It remains clear that the incidence of all types of cancer is higher for allograft recipients than for the general population. In a recent study of more than 2000 kidney transplant recipients with 20 or more years of graft function, more than 40% had developed skin cancer and more than 10% had developed cancer at other sites.[124] Importantly, cancer was the second most common cause of death after cardiovascular disease.

TABLE 41.2 **Adverse Effects of Immunotherapy**

Biological Effect	CsA	Tac	SRL	Pred	MMF/MPA
Hypertension	++	+	–	++	–
Nephrotoxicity	+++	++	+	++	–
Dyslipidemia	++	+	++++	++	–
Hyperglycemia	+	++	–	++	–
Hyperkalemia	++	+++	–	–	–
GI side effects	–	+	++	–	++
Tremor	+	++	–	–	–
Malignancy	+	+	Less	–	?
Osteoporosis	+	+	+	++	–
Hirsutism	+	–	–	–	–
Gingival hypertrophy	–	+	–	–	–
Alopecia	–	+	–	–	–

CsA, Cyclosporine; *GI,* gastrointestinal; *MMF/MPA,* mycophenolic mofetil/mycophenolic acid; *Pred,* prednisone; *SRL,* sirolimus; *Tac,* tacrolimus.

In another study, the cumulative incidence of cancer after 25 years was 49% for all tumors.[125] The most frequent tumors observed were nonmelanoma skin cancer (21%), kidney cancer (12%), and cancers of the pharynx, larynx, or oral cavity (8%). The increase in cancer risk was 4.3-fold. Webster and associates reported standardized ratios of cancer in transplant recipients compared with the general population using the Australia and New Zealand Dialysis and Transplant Registry data.[126] Over a 20-year period, 11% of 15,000 recipients developed cancer. The risk for cancer was found to be inversely related to age, and women aged 25 to 29 years had rates equivalent to those in women aged 55 to 59 years from the general population. Within the transplanted population, the cancer risk was affected by age differently for each sex and was elevated by prior malignancy but reduced by diabetes. The authors concluded that cancer rates in kidney recipients are similar to those in people in the general population that are 20 to 30 years older, but the absolute risk differs across patient groups.

The increase in cancer risk after transplantation is thought to result from the complex interplay of numerous factors that include cumulative exposure to immunosuppression that leads to disruption of both antitumor and antiviral immune surveillance.[126,127] In addition, some drugs may promote carcinogenesis by mechanisms independent of their immunosuppressive effects. Viral infections (particularly herpes, hepatitis, and papilloma viruses) are clearly linked to some malignancies, and chronic antigen stimulation from the transplanted organ, repeated infections, and transfusions of blood products have also been implicated.

Effect of Immunosuppression

It has been suggested that the use of antilymphocyte antibody therapy and tacrolimus increases the risk for PTLD.[128,129] Hardinger and associates recently reported the 10-year follow-up of a randomized trial of Thymoglobulin (Genzyme, Cambridge, MA) or ATGAM (Pharmacia-Upjohn, NY) induction.[130] Event-free survival was significantly higher with Thymoglobulin compared with ATGAM (48% vs. 29%). At 10 years, patient and graft survival rates were similar, whereas acute rejection remained lower (11% vs. 42%) in the Thymoglobulin group. The incidence of all types of cancer was numerically although not significantly lower with Thymoglobulin compared with ATGAM (8% vs. 21%). There were no posttransplant lymphoproliferative disorder cases in the Thymoglobulin group, and there were two cases in the ATGAM group. Kidney function and measures of quality of life were found to be higher in the Thymoglobulin compared with ATGAM group. Wimmer and colleagues reported that the use of IL-2 receptor antagonists as induction therapy significantly reduced the cancer risk for transplant recipients.[125] With the exception of mammalian target of rapamycin (mTOR) inhibitors (sirolimus and everolimus), tumor risk between immunosuppressive drugs typically used for maintenance immunosuppression was not significantly different. However, mTOR inhibitor–based immunosuppressive protocols showed a clear tendency for lower malignancy rates.[131,132] Acknowledging the potential anticancer actions of the mTOR inhibitors demonstrated in clinical studies, de Fijter analyzed the effect of conversion from CIs in 53 renal transplant recipients developing nonmelanoma skin cancer after transplantation.[133] Remission was observed in 37 patients, and therapy was generally well tolerated with minimal adverse events reported. Fifteen patients developed new lesions after conversion. Drug levels did not seem to affect the outcomes of conversion. Interestingly, the use of sirolimus has recently been shown to reduce levels of prostate-specific antigen by 50% in patients without prostate cancer.[134] Why this occurs is unknown.

Reports continue to accumulate indicating that Kaposi sarcoma (KS) after transplantation is exquisitely sensitive to conversion from CI to mTOR inhibitor therapy. As an example, Campistol and Schena reported that conversion to either everolimus or sirolimus led to regression of KS lesions in 11 out of 12 patients.[135] Conversion was generally well tolerated, stable kidney function was maintained in most patients, and there was no rejection. Similarly, Di Paolo and colleagues studied mTOR-signaling pathways in 10 renal transplant patients with KS who successfully responded to mTOR inhibitor conversion therapy.[136] Patients with KS showed markedly increased basal P70 (S6K) activation and depressed phosphorylation of AKT. Long-term treatment with sirolimus was associated with marked inhibition of phosphorylation of both AKT and P70 (S6K), in parallel with regression of the dermal neoplasm.

In spite of the benefits described earlier, mTOR inhibitors have failed to gain traction because of the high incidence of symptomatic adverse effects, including increased risk for infection, wound problems, edema, mouth ulcers, and proteinuria, which are seen in up to 25% of patients and lead to conversion to alternate immunotherapy. Nevertheless, for those recipients suffering from cancer after transplantation, such agents may be useful. The reader's attention is directed to a report prepared by an international group pertaining to the use of "proliferation signal inhibitors" (referred to earlier as mTOR inhibitors), everolimus and sirolimus, and their antioncogenic effects.[128]

Posttransplantation Lymphoproliferative Disease

Transplant recipients are at the greatest risk for developing PTLD within the first year after transplantation. Most cases of PTLD are induced by Epstein-Barr virus (EBV) infection causing uncontrolled proliferation of B cells. The incidence is higher in EBV-seronegative children who receive seropositive grafts from adult donors. Heart-lung transplants showed the highest relative risk among various types of organ transplants.[3] The use of tacrolimus and induction or rescue therapy with OKT3 or ATG is known to increase the risk for PTLD.

Although EBV infection is known to be associated with the development of PTLD, the prognosis of such transplant recipients has been less clear. Smith and colleagues described the outcomes of pediatric kidney transplant recipients with PCR-defined EBV infection after ganciclovir prophylaxis.[137] Primary infection developed in 46 patients, of whom 50% were asymptomatic, 26% were symptomatic, and 24% developed PTLD. Adolescents were more likely to develop PTLD than younger transplant recipients. Among the 11 cases of PTLD, there were 2 deaths and 2 graft failures, all in adolescent recipients. Suzuki and colleagues performed a prospective study of 32 tacrolimus-treated kidney transplant recipients that included EBV serology and PCR testing.[138] Seroconversion occurred in five of six patients approximately 22 weeks after transplantation. The viral load was significantly higher in seronegative compared with seropositive patients.

The diagnosis of PTLD is generally suggested by clinical symptoms (organ involvement or fever, or both) and imaging study results. The clinical symptoms that patients complain of are extremely variable and depend on the site and stage of PTLD. Traditionally, CT scanning with oral and intravenous contrast has been the test of choice for defining the presence and extent of PTLD. It has been suggested that fluorodeoxyglucose-positron emission tomography (FDG-PET) in-line with CT scanning may be a superior methodology.[139] In a report of four transplant recipients with histologically confirmed PTLD, scans at diagnosis showed increased FDG uptake in all examined PTLD lesions, and the disease was upstaged on the basis of FDG-PET/CT scan results over conventional CT scanning in one patient. Furthermore, PET/CT scans no longer demonstrated FDG uptake in the original PTLD lesions in all patients at the end of treatment.

Treatment of Posttransplant Lymphoproliferative Disease

The current approach to the treatment of PTLD involves a number of therapeutic options that include:

- Reduction of basal immunosuppression
- Antiviral treatment in the case of EBV-positive B-cell lymphoma
- Rituximab in the case of CD20-positive lymphomas
- Cyclophosphamide, hydroxydaunomycin/doxorubicin, Oncovin, prednisone (CHOP) chemotherapy alone or in combination with rituximab for diffuse lymphoma or incomplete response to previous treatment

Swinnen and associates reported the results of a prospective, multicenter study that examined the efficacy of a PTLD treatment algorithm that started with a defined course of reduced immunotherapy and escalated to interferon-α2b, and finally to chemotherapy.[140] Intravenous acyclovir was given to all patients. The CI was reduced by 50% for 2 weeks and then by another 50% unless the patient was in complete remission. Sixteen patients with biopsy-proven PTLD were eligible to participate in the study; 13 had received heart transplants, and 3 had received kidney transplants. Reduced immunotherapy resulted in only 1 of 16 partial responses and no complete remissions. Progressive disease developed in half, and 40% experienced rejection. Only 1 of 13 patients achieved durable remission with interferon. Five of seven patients who received chemotherapy achieved remission. The applicability of such a study to kidney transplantation remains uncertain, because most patients in that study were heart transplant recipients. The authors concluded, "A strong case can be made for adding rituximab to RI [reduction in immunosuppressives] as initial therapy." Trappe and colleagues performed a retrospective analysis to determine the efficacy and safety of salvage therapy in recipients of solid organ transplants with progression of PTLD after rituximab first-line therapy.[141] Eleven patients who had received reduced immunotherapy and single-agent rituximab were analyzed. Of these, 10 had received CHOP. This cohort seems to have been quite different from the usual PTLD cohort in that most of these patients had late disease (median onset of disease 145 months posttransplant) and had monomorphic histology, and only 36% were associated with EBV. CHOP therapy achieved complete remission in 50% of patients at 44 months posttreatment and partial remission of 20% of patients. The median overall survival was 46.5 months.

ELECTROLYTE DISORDERS

Electrolyte disorders are common after kidney transplant. Hyperkalemia can be induced by poor graft function, CIs, particularly tacrolimus, and by other drugs such as ACE inhibitors, ARBs, or beta blockers. Treatment is similar to that of hyperkalemia in CKD: reduction in potassium intake, adjustment in medications, and administration of loop diuretics. Kayexalate should be avoided immediately posttransplantation because of a rare but potentially catastrophic complication of colonic perforation.[142,143] Therefore refractory hyperkalemia complicating delayed graft function is best treated with dialysis.

Hypophosphatemia is almost universal after kidney transplantation once good graft function is achieved. It generally lasts for a few months and is often of sufficient severity to warrant oral and occasionally parenteral phosphorus supplementation. It was generally thought to be to persistent hyperparathyroidism. However, hypophosphatemia can occur despite low parathyroid hormone (PTH) levels and can persist after high PTH levels normalize. A novel growth factor, fibroblast growth factor-23 (FGF-23), which induces phosphaturia, inhibits calcitriol synthesis, and accumulates in CKD, has recently been implicated as a dominant cause of hypophosphatemia after transplantation.[144-146] Bhan and associates studied 27 living donor transplant recipients, of whom 85% developed hypophosphatemia.[145] FGF-23 levels dropped by more than 50% within the first week after transplantation, although they still remained higher than normal. Furthermore, FGF-23 was independently associated with serum phosphate, urinary excretion of phosphate, and calcitriol levels; PTH was not independently associated with any of these parameters. Similarly, Evenepoel and associates studied 41 patients before and 3 months after transplantation.[144] In this cohort, FGF-23, but none of the other mineral metabolism indices, was an independent predictor of the phosphate nadir in the early posttransplant period.

MUSCULOSKELETAL COMPLICATIONS OF TRANSPLANTATION

Immunotherapy and secondary hyperparathyroidism are considered among the more important pathogenetic factors leading to post kidney transplantation bone disease. Other implicated causes include preexisting uremic osteodystrophy (hyperparathyroidism and diabetic osteopathy), poor kidney function, and ongoing secondary hyperparathyroidism, hyperphosphaturia, and pathogenic vitamin D alleles. The main syndromes are bone loss with a consequent fracture rate of 3% per year, osteonecrosis of the hip, and bone pain.[147] The bone of a typical kidney transplant patient will pass through four phases:

1. The development of uremic osteodystrophy before kidney transplantation
2. Exacerbation immediately after kidney transplantation caused by high-dose immunosuppressive therapy and continuing homeostatic disturbances
3. A phase of stabilization secondary to immunosuppressive dose reduction and reestablishment of normal homeostasis
4. The return of uremic osteodystrophy caused by failing graft function[147]

Osteopenia and Osteoporosis Posttransplantation

Bone loss is particularly pronounced during the first year after transplantation, leads to about a 9% reduction in bone mineral density, and may persist for several years, even in patients with adequate kidney function. Recent studies indicate that osteoblast apoptosis and impaired osteoblastogenesis play important roles in the pathogenesis of glucocorticoid-induced osteoporosis. In a study of 20 patients with a mean age of 36 years who were subjected to bone biopsy after kidney transplantation, the main alterations in posttransplant biopsies were a decrease in osteoid and osteoblast surfaces, adjusted bone formation rate, and prolonged mineralization lag time.[148] In contrast with pretransplant biopsies, terminal deoxynucleotidyl transferase dUTP nick end labeling (TUNEL)-positive cells in the proximity of osteoid seams or in the medullary space were observed, indicating that impaired osteoblastogenesis and early osteoblast apoptosis may play important roles in the pathogenesis of posttransplant osteoporosis.

Although steroids have typically been implicated as the dominant cause of osteoporosis posttransplantation, animal studies have previously indicated that cyclosporine therapy may be an inducer of bone disease even in the absence of corticosteroids.[149] A recent study compared bone densitometry and histomorphometry in patients receiving cyclosporine monotherapy versus those receiving azathioprine and steroid therapy.[150] Bone mineral density was low in both immunosuppressive regimens, and there were no significant differences between the groups. Histopathological analysis indicated that mixed uremic bone disease was present in 42%, adynamic bone in 29%, and hyperparathyroid disease in 17%. Normal bone was seen in only 12%. Patients showed a slight increase in osteoclast number and function, decreased osteoblast number and function, and retardation of dynamic parameters. No differences in histopathological diagnosis or histomorphometrical findings were observed between the immunosuppressive therapy groups. The authors concluded that both cyclosporine and steroid therapies were associated with slight osteoclast stimulation and osteoblast suppression and with marked retardation of mineral apposition and bone formation rates. Both drugs also were associated with reduced bone density.

Treatment of Posttransplant Osteopenia and Osteoporosis

One of the problems with the clinical trials in preventing bone disease posttransplantation is the focus on secondary endpoints such as biochemical changes, alterations in bone density, or occasionally histology as against a primary endpoint such as fracture risk. One such study examined intravenous pamidronate compared with vitamin D and calcium.[151] Patients on pamidronate demonstrated preservation of bone mass at 6 and 12 months as measured by bone densitometry, whereas control patients lost bone mass. Of some concern, all of the pamidronate- treated patients had histological evidence of adynamic bone disease at 6 months, whereas 50% of control patients continued to have or developed decreased bone turnover. There was no reported difference in fracture risk.

A metaanalysis was recently reported of 23 clinical trials of posttransplant bone disease with a total of 1209 patients.[152] Significant improvements in spinal and femoral bone mineral density (BMD) were reported with the use of bisphosphonates and vitamin D analogs. Calcitonin improved spinal, though not femoral neck bone mineral density. The incidence of reported toxicity was low. No trial found a reduction in fracture risk.

Another recent trial examined the use of two doses of zoledronate at 2 and 12 weeks posttransplantation in a cohort of 20 patients.[153] Although zoledronate was associated with an early improvement in bone density, this benefit was not sustained at 3 years. Increasingly, investigators are examining the effect of bone intervention strategies in children who have been transplanted. For example, one study examined 30 children or adolescents with low BMD at 48 months posttransplantation.[154] The patients were randomized to take either daily alfacalcidol 0.25 mcg or placebo. After 12 months of treatment, bone density was significantly worse in the placebo group compared with a significant improvement in the treatment group. Enthusiasm for the widespread use of bisphosphonates in transplant patients most recently has been tempered by reports of significant adverse effects. For example, reports of collapsing glomerulopathy and other glomerular epithelial cell disorders are accumulating with the use of high-dose pamidronate.[155] Most recently, hundreds of cases of jaw osteonecrosis related to bisphosphonate therapy have been reported from around the world.[156] Admittedly, most such cases have occurred to patients receiving high-dose parenteral therapy in the setting of hematological malignancy frequently precipitated or realized at the time of dental extraction.

Another reported approach to the management of osteoporosis after transplantation is the avoidance or minimization of steroids. In a study of 364 transplant recipients, ter Meulen and coworkers randomized patients to steroid-free therapy or prednisone (0.3 mg/kg per day tapered to 0 mg at week 16) after transplantation.[157] All patients received tacrolimus, mycophenolate mofetil, daclizumab, and, during the first 3 days, 100 mg prednisolone intravenously. Lumbar spine bone density decreased somewhat in both groups during the first 3 months following transplantation. No difference between the groups was found at either 3 months or 12 months after transplantation. The authors concluded that moderate-dose steroid has little effect on bone density within the first posttransplant year.

Osteonecrosis post kidney transplantation has been largely attributed to the use of steroids. However, other risk factors such as microvascular thrombosis, hyperlipidemia, and alternate immunotherapies have been described. The incidence of hospitalized osteonecrosis reported to the United States Renal Data System (USRDS) is 7.1 episodes/1000 person-years.[158] A single-center radiological survey of 49 patients revealed an osteonecrosis incidence of 4% by plain radiograph and magnetic resonance imaging (MRI).[159] In a recent report based on analysis of the USRDS, 3.5% of patients who received the combination of sirolimus and cyclosporine developed osteonecrosis, compared with 1.4% of patients who received the combination of sirolimus and tacrolimus.[159] In a multivariate analysis, the use of cyclosporine compared with tacrolimus was independently associated with an increased risk for osteonecrosis.

Matas and associates recently reported data from a 5-year trial of prednisone-free maintenance immunosuppression.[160] In this study, almost 600 kidney transplant recipients were treated with a protocol that involved discontinuation of their prednisone on postoperative day 6. At 5 years, the actuarial patient survival was 91%; graft survival, 84%; death-censored graft survival, 92%; acute rejection–free graft survival, 84%; and chronic rejection–free graft survival, 87%. In all, 86% of kidney recipients with functioning grafts remain prednisone-free. Compared with historical controls, recipients on prednisone-free maintenance immunosuppression had a significantly lower rate of avascular necrosis and fractures.

Osteoarticular Pain Posttransplantation

Osteoarticular pain posttransplantation occurs in up to 10% of patients soon after transplantation and typically affects the lower extremities.[161-163] This complication has been described in patients taking both cyclosporine and tacrolimus. The clinical evaluation is unremarkable, and the described radiological features include:

- Epiphyseal patchy osteoporosis at radiograph
- Increased focal or diffuse uptake of the tracer at bone scintigraphy
- Areas of low signal intensity at T1-weighted images on MRI

The MRI abnormalities are generally believed to be consistent with areas of medullary edema, although some authors suggest that the syndrome may be related to "microfractures" or impaction and may be related to subclinical trauma.[162] Clinical recovery is the rule and usually occurs within several weeks. It has been suggested that patients should refrain from excessive physical activity shortly after transplantation to minimize risk for locomotor injury.

Tendonitis

Achilles tendonitis with ruptures was initially described in patients taking high-dose quinolone antibiotics more than a decade ago. More recently, a case-control study reported a fourfold overall increased risk for tendonitis and ruptures in patients taking steroids.[164] This study identified a sixfold increase in OR in patients aged 60 to 79 years and a 20-fold increase in OR in patients aged 80 years or older. In persons aged 60 years and older, the OR was 28 for current exposure to ofloxacin. Approximately 2% to 6% of all Achilles tendon ruptures in people older than 60 years can be attributed to quinolones. An ultrastructural study of tenocytes from rats exposed to quinolones exhibited degenerative changes such as multiple vacuoles and large vesicles in the cytoplasm that resulted from swelling and dilatation of cell organelles (mitochondria, endoplasmic reticulum).[165] The nucleus became dense, and the chromatin had clumped to form rough plaques. The cells detached from the extracellular matrix. Other important findings were a general decrease of the fibril diameter and an increase in the distance between the collagenous fibrils. Consequently, high-dose quinolones should be used with caution in older patients on steroids.

NEUROPSYCHIATRIC COMPLICATIONS OF TRANSPLANTATION

The development of ESRD combined with the realization that life may no longer be possible without medical intervention may lead to anxiety, depression, nonadherence with diet or medications, sexual dysfunction, and suicide in the transplantation patient.[166] Immunotherapy has also been implicated in causing psychiatric disturbances that may include euphoria, delirium, generalized anxiety disorder, and occasionally hallucinations.[167] Such disorders often require intervention with psychopharmacological agents. However, psychotropic drug administration may be hazardous because of pharmacokinetic interactions with immunosuppressive drugs.[168]

Depression

ESRD and transplantation are associated with depression, which affects adversely upon compliance and may be associated with decreased longevity.[169,170] In the kidney transplant population, depression occurs early after transplantation and is associated with both acute and chronic rejection.[169] Depression is also common in recipients of other organ transplants. Among heart transplant patients, for example, the incidence of depression was as high as 34% beyond the first posttransplant year.[171] Similarly, 43% of patients with end-stage liver disease presented at least one psychiatric diagnosis. Child-Pugh score and previous psychiatric diagnoses were independent significant predictors of depressive disorders.[172] The specific factors that increase a heart transplant recipient's risk for depression and anxiety-related disorders include the following:

- Pretransplant psychiatric history
- Poor social support
- The use of avoidance coping strategies for managing health problems
- Low self-esteem

Other factors that may lead to depression include the disfiguring effects of immunosuppressive medication, such as high-dose corticosteroid therapy, and antihypertensive treatment with beta blockers.

Suicide

In one study, the crude suicide rate in kidney transplant recipients from 1995 to 2001 was 24 per 100,000 patient-years, a finding that was 84% higher than in the general population.[166] In multivariate models, age greater than 75 years, male gender, white or Asian race, geographical region, alcohol or drug dependence, and recent hospitalization with mental illness were significant independent predictors of death as a result of suicide.

Nonadherence

Nonadherence (or noncompliance) with diet and medication is a major risk factor for rejection and is responsible for up to 25% of deaths after the initial recovery period.[169] In one study, the risk for acute graft rejection was 4.2 times greater among recipients who were noncompliant with medications.[173] The numerous factors implicated include psychiatric disturbances, adverse effects of medications, lack of knowledge concerning the need for medications, and financial concerns. This problem is particularly prevalent in adolescents and young adults. An overview of the literature reported that certain patient characteristics were closely linked to noncompliance among solid organ transplant recipients[169]:

- Younger and older age, and nonmarried
- Anxious individuals and those prone to denial, and those who have severe personality disorders or who are mentally retarded
- History of substance abuse

Additional factors underlying compliance include the particular transplant center and dosing frequencies of immunosuppressive medications, with higher dosing frequencies resulting in decreased adherence.

Psychopharmacology

Previous therapeutic options for depression were hampered by the adverse effects associated with traditional agents. By comparison, newer antidepressant medications are more effective and safer in both the general population and medically ill patients. This diverse group of compounds possesses distinct pharmacokinetic properties that are unrelated to either the tricyclic/tetracyclic antidepressants or the monoamine oxidase inhibitors. These newer agents include selective serotonin reuptake inhibitors (SSRIs) such as fluoxetine, paroxetine, sertraline, trazodone, and fluvoxamine. Agents with serotonin reuptake activity that also prevent the uptake of other neurotransmitters (such as norepinephrine and dopamine) include nefazodone, bupropion, and venlafaxine.

A problem associated with the use of these agents may be drug interactions resulting in elevated CI levels due to alterations in the cytochrome CYP3A4 isoenzyme system. Among the newer antidepressant medications, fluvoxamine and nefazodone have the strongest inhibitory action on the CYP3A4 isoenzyme. In fact, we have previously reported interactions between cyclosporine and nefazodone or fluvoxamine that led to severe CI nephrotoxicity, allograft dysfunction, and uncontrolled HTN.[168] The corollary of such observations is that agents with minimal inhibitory effects on the CYP3A4 isoenzyme, such as paroxetine and sertraline, would not be expected to cause a pharmacokinetic interaction. Although fluoxetine has moderate inhibitory potency, it has not been implicated in causing such interactions. Information is lacking for trazodone, venlafaxine, and bupropion. Caution dictates that levels of affected drugs should be carefully monitored in any transplant patient who requires treatment for major affective disorders. Appropriate dosage adjustments should be performed as necessary to circumvent toxicity. For patients who require antidepressant medications, fluoxetine or bupropion are often used as first-line therapy because these agents have not been shown to have significant interactions with CIs.

Psychotherapy has also been studied in a cohort of approximately 80 recipients of primary deceased-donor kidney transplants.[170] In this report, patients were randomized to receive either group therapy or individual psychotherapy without psychopharmacological intervention. Standardized depression scores improved in both groups, although patients who received individualized therapy had the greatest improvement in the depression score.

Neurological Complications

Tremors after transplantation are extremely common and are generally related to CI therapy. Cyclosporine has long been known to activate the sympathetic nervous system and to increase circulating catechol levels. It is now understood that tacrolimus is an even greater offender in this regard.[38] Most often, such tremors are related to the higher levels that are required early posttransplantation to prevent allograft rejection. In general terms, tremors abate over time as the levels are allowed to run at a lower range.[174] A new-onset tremor in a transplant recipient may be a clue to CI toxicity and should prompt a measurement of the drug level. Sirolimus and the antimetabolite immunosuppressive agents are not generally associated with this adverse event.

VISUAL DISTURBANCES AFTER TRANSPLANTATION

Ocular complications after transplantation are frequently encountered and range in severity from blurred vision from poorly controlled hyperglycemia to sight-threatening steroid-induced retinopathy. Cataracts develop in approximately 40% of transplant patients and lead to surgery in many of those afflicted.[175] Risk factors include diabetes mellitus, older age, and the use of corticosteroids. Diabetic retinopathy is often "burned out" by the time a diabetic comes to transplantation. However, for type 1 diabetics undergoing pancreas transplantation, active retinopathy may regress. Ocular infections consequent on immunotherapy such as cytomegalovirus or toxoplasmosis are, fortunately, rare in the organ transplant population. Because visual disturbances after solid organ transplantation may be sight threatening, any new symptoms are most appropriately evaluated by ophthalmology. Routine ophthalmological examinations are currently recommended for high-risk patients on an annual basis.

SUMMARY AND CONCLUSION

Although the introduction of more potent immunosuppressive agents has reduced the rates of acute rejection and early graft loss, late graft loss and premature death continue to limit the long-term success of transplantation. Morbidity from posttransplant diabetes, malignancy, and bone disease is substantial. More attention is therefore being paid to preventing and treating these medical complications of transplantation. In many ways, kidney transplant recipients need to be managed similarly to those with CKD. More effective intervention at the predialysis or dialysis stage also is needed to reduce the burden of morbidity in transplant patients. It is also of vital importance that nephrologists refer patients for transplant evaluation before beginning dialysis because patients can be listed for a kidney transplant once their GFR is less than 20 mL/min, and it is well known that mortality decreases the earlier a patient is transplanted. Finally, reduction in long-term immunosuppression should be strongly considered in all patients.

A full list of references is available at www.expertconsult.com.

Recurrent and De Novo Renal Diseases After Kidney Transplantation

Neil Sheerin, MBBS, PhD, FRCP, and Greg Knoll, MD, MSc, FRCPC

OUTLINE

Despite the introduction of new immunosuppression, reduced acute rejection rates, and the improvement in short-term outcomes, long-term kidney allograft survival has not improved significantly in the past 30 years.[1] Recurrent or de novo disease is increasingly recognized as important causes of graft loss and are only behind chronic rejection and death with a functioning graft as a cause of overall graft loss.[2] Recurrent disease is reported in 10% to 20% of cases and accounts for up to 5% to 10% of graft failures (Fig. 42.1 and Table 42.1). Glomerular diseases are the cause of renal failure in 30% to 50% of patients undergoing transplantation[2,3] and are the most likely to recur. Patients with end-stage kidney disease (ESKD) due to glomerular disease are twice as likely to develop glomerulonephritis (GN) in their transplant.[4] These patients often are younger than patients with other diagnoses and therefore the effect of recurrent or de novo disease is likely to be greater and perhaps contributes to the higher rate of graft loss reported in younger patients.[5] When recurrent or de novo disease is diagnosed, treatment options are very limited, with little evidence that strategies to either prevent or treat recurrent disease are effective (Table 42.2).

There is a wide variation in the reported rates of recurrent and de novo diseases for a number of reasons. The primary cause of renal failure is often unknown, with only 20% of transplant recipients having had a biopsy of their native kidneys. Therefore in many cases it is not possible to accurately categorize disease as recurrent or de novo. Studies that report the rate of recurrent or de novo disease in patients undergoing biopsy because of graft dysfunction will miss patients with asymptomatic, subclinical disease. As such, the incidence of GN is generally higher in series using protocol biopsies compared with "for-cause" biopsies. The timing of biopsy is also important. The incidence of glomerular disease increases with time after transplantation, with a reported rate of 4% in early (median 0.8 months) compared with 13% of late (median 7.5 years) transplant biopsies.[6] In addition, multiple pathologies can coexist in a transplanted kidney, failing grafts often are not biopsied because of the lack of effective interventions and transplant biopsies may not routinely undergo immunofluorescence and electron microscopical analysis.

THE EFFECT OF RECURRENT OR DE NOVO DISEASE ON TRANSPLANT OUTCOME

Although it is recognized that recurrent or de novo disease is common, perhaps more important is understanding the effect that this has on patient and allograft outcomes. This is not without its challenges, not the least of which is the lack of a diagnosis for the cause of ESKD. There are several ways of addressing this question.[4] First, what is the rate of

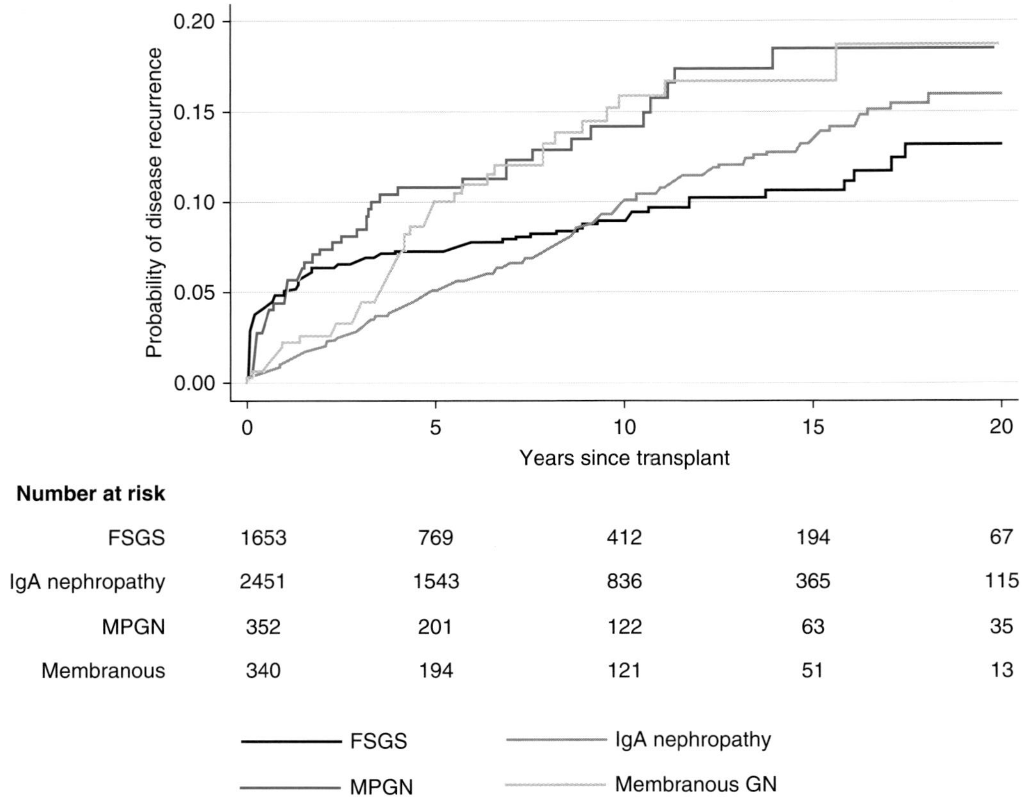

FIG. 42.1 Kaplan–Meier estimates of disease recurrence by glomerulonephritis type. (Adapted from Allen PJ, Chadban SJ, Craig JC, et al: Recurrent glomerulonephritis after kidney transplantation: risk factors and allograft outcomes. *Kidney Int.* 2017;92(2):461-469.)

TABLE 42.1 Risk for Recurrent Disease and Graft Loss Due to Recurrence

Disease	Risk for recurrence, %	Risk for graft loss in patients with recurrent disease, %
FSGS	30	30–50
Membranous nephropathy	30–60	10
IgA nephropathy	30	10
Immune complex MPGN	40	10–20
C3 glomerulopathy	50–100	30
Anti-GBM disease	<10	Rare
SLE	5	Rare
ANCA-associated vasculitis	10–20	Rare
Systemic sclerosis	5–20	Rare
Atypical HUS	10–80	50
Fibrillary immunotactoid glomerulopathy	50	30–50

ANCA, Antineutrophil cytoplasmic antibody; *FSGS*, focal segmental glomerulosclerosis; *GBM*, glomerular basement membrane; *HUS*, hemolytic uremic syndrome; *IgA*, immunoglobulin A; *MPGN*, mesangioproliferative glomerulonephritis; *SLE*, systemic lupus erythematosus.

Adapted from Fairhead, T, Knoll, G: Recurrent glomerular disease after kidney transplantation. *Curr Opin Nephrol Hypertens.* 2010;19:578-585.

death-censored graft loss attributable to recurrent disease. This is estimated at 5% to 10%.[6-8] Second, are there causes of ESKD that are associated with a higher rate of graft failure after transplantation compared with the general recipient population? If so, this would imply that the primary disease is influencing graft survival. This analysis has been performed using data from the Australia and New Zealand Dialysis and Transplant Registry[2] and the United Network for Organ Sharing (UNOS).[9] Of the primary glomerular diseases, graft survival is worse in patients with focal segmental glomerulosclerosis (FSGS) and membranoproliferative glomerulonephritis (MPGN).[2,9] Graft survival is also worse in some systemic diseases including sickle cell nephropathy (SCN), amyloidosis, and scleroderma.[9]

The effect on graft survival in recipients who develop recurrent disease also can be assessed. If all patients with glomerular disease as a cause of ESKD are considered, those with recurrent disease have a two- to threefold higher risk for death-censored graft loss,[4,7] with a death-censored 5-year graft survival of 55% (Fig. 42.2).[10] Performing the same analysis by disease type, recurrence of MPGN had the greatest effect, but recurrence of FSGS and immunoglobulin (Ig)A nephropathy also had an adverse effect on graft outcome.[4] It is also relevant to consider the cause of graft failure loss in patients who develop recurrent disease. In a study of transplant recipients with a primary diagnosis of membranous nephropathy (MN), overall transplant survival was

TABLE 42.2 Options for the Prevention or Treatment of Recurrent Disease

Type of Glomerulonephritis	Prevention and Treatment Options
IgA nephropathy	ACEI and/or ARB use posttransplantation
FSGS	Acute and/or chronic plasmapheresis for early recurrence Consider rituximab or cyclophosphamide in severe cases
Membranous nephropathy	Consider rituximab
Immune complex MPGN	Identification and treatment of any underlying cause
C3 glomerulopathy	Eculizumab may be useful for treatment of recurrent disease
ANCA glomerulonephritis	Defer transplant until quiescent disease Cyclophosphamide ± plasmapheresis for recurrence
SLE	Defer transplant until disease quiescent Continue full-dose immunosuppression if recurrence
Anti-GBM	Defer transplant until disease quiescent Cyclophosphamide ± plasmapheresis for recurrence
Fibrillary immunotactoid glomerulopathy	No effective preventative or treatment measures

ACEI, Angiotensin-converting enzyme inhibitor; *ANCA*, antineutrophil cytoplasmic antibody; *ARB*, angiotensin receptor blocker; *FSGS*, focal segmental glomerulosclerosis; *GBM*, glomerular basement membrane; *IgA*, immunoglobulin A; *MPGN*, mesangioproliferative glomerulonephritis; *SLE*, systemic lupus erythematosus.

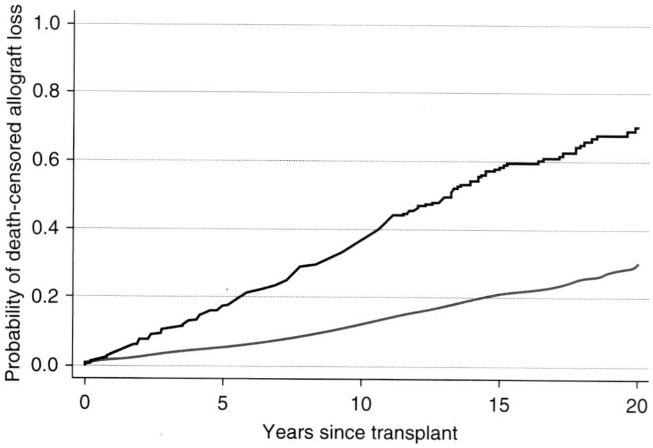

FIG. 42.2 Death-censored graft loss in patients with recurrent glomerulonephritis. (Adapted from Allen PJ, Chadban SJ, Craig JC, et al: Recurrent glomerulonephritis after kidney transplantation: risk factors and allograft outcomes. *Kidney Int.* 2017;92(2):461-469.)

similar to recipients with a primary diagnosis of polycystic kidney disease. However, 5 of the 11 graft losses in patients with recurrent MN lost their graft due to recurrent disease,[11] suggesting recurrent disease must contribute to graft loss. Similarly, in a registry study, 61% of patients with recurrent GN lost their allografts due to disease recurrence, whereas death with a functioning graft accounted for only 8% of graft losses.[7]

PRIMARY GLOMERULOPATHIES

Focal Segmental Glomerulosclerosis

FSGS is a histological diagnosis that includes primary (idiopathic) variants and secondary cases, in which an underlying cause can be identified. There are also an increasing number of genetic causes of FSGS, identified in patients with both familial and sporadic FSGS and usually affecting proteins found in the podocyte split diaphragm. Recurrence of primary FSGS is reported in 10% to 56 % of first transplants,[12-14] with a true recurrence rate of approximately 30%.[4] Some reports suggest a lower rate. For example, a recent report from the Australian and New Zealand Dialysis and Transplant Registry suggested a recurrence rate of biopsy-proven primary FSGS of 10% to 11%.[7,15] When disease recurs, graft loss attributed to recurrence is reported in 30% to 50% of cases. Therefore, in transplant recipients with primary FSGS, approximately 10% to 20% of grafts are lost due to recurrent disease, with a reported relative risk for graft loss of 2.03 compared with other glomerular diseases.[2] In the Australian and New Zealand registry data, 5-year graft survival in recipients with FSGS was 52% in patients with recurrent FSGS compared with 83% in patients without recurrent disease.[2,15]

Factors that have been reported as associated with an increased risk for recurrent FSGS included young age,[14,15] non-white ethnicity,[15] live donor transplantation,[15] mesangial hypercellularity,[12] rapid progression to ESKD,[16] high levels of pretransplant proteinuria, and recurrence of FSGS in a previous graft. However, clinical assessment of recurrence risk lacks specificity. A circulating factor(s) that mediates recurrence is likely, but has not been identified. The concentration of soluble urokinase plasminogen activator receptor has been proposed as a predictor of recurrence,[17] but this has not been replicated.[18] Despite living donation being an independent risk factor for disease recurrence, allograft survival is generally equivalent or superior to deceased donor grafts.[15] Living donation, therefore, is not contraindicated for recipients with FSGS. Most reports suggest that genetic forms of the disease have a lower rate of recurrence,[19,20] although this is not invariably so and recurrence does occur.[21] The lower rate reported by most authors would suggest that genetic screening is indicated before transplantation in younger patients with steroid-resistant nephrotic syndrome to stratify for recurrence risk. In patients who have previously lost a transplant due to recurrent disease, the risk for subsequent recurrence is high, on the order of 80%.[4] The benefits of retransplantation with likely recurrence compared with long-term, maintenance dialysis should be considered on a case-by-case basis.

Plasmapheresis often is used to treat recurrent disease and there are case series that report a beneficial effect. In approximately half of patients, proteinuria can be reduced, particularly if treatment is started early.[12,22,23] There are reports of a beneficial effect of plasmapheresis before transplantation, reducing the rate of recurrence from 66% to 37%[24] and potentially modifying risk in patients who have previously lost grafts due to recurrent disease.[25] Good data to support a beneficial effect of plasma exchange on long-term allograft outcome are not available and not all studies report a benefit of plasmapheresis without other interventions.[14] There are reports of the effectiveness of rituximab in treating recurrent FSGS,[14,26] but again this is at the level of case reports and series and there also are reports of no benefit.[27,28] Therefore there is insufficient evidence to recommend the routine use of rituximab to prevent recurrence.

FSGS has been reported as the leading form of de novo glomerular disease.[29] Although it is possible for primary FSGS to occur de novo in a transplant kidney, many of these cases probably represent secondary cases. Clinically, de novo FSGS is associated with proteinuria typically occurring late (>12 months) after transplantation. The presence of de novo FSGS is a negative predictor of graft survival,[30] although it follows a less aggressive clinical course than recurrent primary disease. A 5-year survival of 40% has been reported in patients with de novo FSGS,[30] but the contribution of glomerular disease to graft failure is unclear.

Drugs have been implicated in the development of de novo FSGS. FSGS-like lesions can be seen in the glomeruli of patients with calcineurin inhibitor (CNI) nephropathy, due to the vasoconstrictor effects of CNIs on the microvasculature or increased growth factor expression.[31] Sirolimus treatment can lead to heavy proteinuria, particularly if started in patients with preexisting proteinuria, with FSGS-like changes on biopsy. Sirolimus appears to have an effect on podocyte function, altering the expression of proteins associated with podocyte differentiation.

The collapsing variant of FSGS also has been described in transplanted kidneys, occurring in 0.6% of transplants.[32] In most cases, the etiology is not known but has been reported in association with cytomegalovirus,[33] parvovirus B19 infection,[34] and antibodies to angiotensin II receptor type 1.[35] De novo collapsing carries a worse prognosis than noncollapsing variants with all 10 grafts lost within 3 years in one series.[36] There is no specific treatment for de novo FSGS, but treatment of any ongoing cause of renal injury, management of blood pressure, and renin–angiotensin system inhibition may be beneficial.

Membranous Nephropathy

MN is the most common cause of nephrotic syndrome in adults and progresses to ESKD in 20% to 30% of cases. MN occurs in both primary (previously idiopathic) and secondary forms. Recently, autoantibodies to the M-type phospholipase A2 receptor (PLA2R) have been identified. PLA2R appears to be the main immune target in primary disease,[37] although other targets have been reported. Anti-PLA2R antibodies are present in about 70% of patients with primary MN[37] and in a similar proportion of transplant candidates with a primary diagnosis of MN.[11,38]

There is substantial variation in the reported recurrence of MN ranging from 10% to 50%,[8,11,39,40] with rates varying due to duration of follow-up and the use of for-cause or protocol biopsy strategies. Dabade and colleagues identified recurrence in 8 of 19 patients (42%) in protocol biopsies 2 to 61 months after transplantation.[39] Clinical features of disease were mild or absent. Grupper et al. identified a similar rate (48%) in protocol biopsies at 1 year.[11] In contrast, when patients were biopsied due to proteinuria, a recurrence rate of 7% was reported.[41] Patients who are anti-PLA2R antibody positive have a higher risk for recurrence (60% to 83%) compared with those who are antibody negative (28% to 53%).[11,38,42] There is insufficient data to know whether the same is true when antibodies are directed against other antigenic targets. Heavy proteinuria at the time of transplantation is also a risk factor for recurrent disease.

Recurrent disease usually occurs within the first 2 years after a transplant and unlike disease in native kidneys, it rarely remits spontaneously. The effect of recurrent primary MN on allograft outcome is unclear with reports of both worse[40] or equivalent[11] outcomes in patients with recurrent primary MN. This difference may reflect whether recurrence is diagnosed on protocol biopsies and newer treatment strategies. It is clear that recurrent primary MN can lead to graft failure and when it does recur, up to 50% of death-censored graft losses can be attributed to recurrent disease.[11]

There is accumulating evidence for the use anti-CD20 therapy (rituximab) for the treatment of recurrent primary MN. Complete or partial clinical remission has been reported in 80% of cases treated with rituximab.[8,11,43,44] There is currently insufficient data to determine whether the presence of anti-PLA2R antibodies is predictive of the response to anti-CD20 treatment and treatment should be considered regardless of antibody status. Alkylating agents have been used to treat recurrent primary MN similar to the treatment of native kidney disease. There is no evidence at present for the preemptive treatment of transplant candidates with either rituximab or alkylating agents to prevent recurrent primary MN.

De novo MN has been reported in about 2% of allografts.[45] It can occur months or years after transplantation and can vary in presentation from asymptomatic disease to severe nephrotic syndrome. The etiology of de novo MN may be different from primary or recurrent disease with anti-PLA2R antibodies being less common in patients with de novo MN. Debiec and colleagues reported the presence of anti-PLA2R antibodies in 50% of patients with recurrent MN but not in any of the patients with de novo MN (n = 9).[46] In addition, staining for PLA2R, which is frequently seen in primary and recurrent MN, is much less frequently observed in de novo disease.[47] This suggests that antibodies in de novo MN are targeted against different antigens than those responsible for primary or recurrent disease, but these antigens remain to be identified. The effect of de novo MN on transplant survival, with some reports of high rates of allograft failure[48] and others reporting that the allograft survival is not affected[49] by the presence of de novo MN. The development of de novo MN is not a contraindication to retransplantation.

IgA Nephropathy

There is significant variability in the reported rate of recurrence of IgA nephropathy after transplantation. As with other conditions, this relates to the criteria for biopsy (protocol or clinical) and the duration of follow-up. Clinical recurrence occurs in approximately 30% of cases.[50] Histological recurrence is more common and probably occurs in >50% or cases, with this percentage increasing the longer the period between transplantation and biopsy.[4,51]

Generally, the outcome of transplantation in patients with IgA nephropathy is equivalent to or better than other primary diagnoses.[51,52] However, despite good outcome overall in patients with IgA nephropathy, recurrence is associated with a higher risk for allograft failure,[53] suggesting that recurrent IgA nephropathy does damage the allograft. Early recurrence of IgA nephropathy has been reported and this may be more common in younger transplant recipients with rapidly progressive, crescentic disease in their native kidneys.[54]

De novo IgA nephropathy has been reported, but this has to be distinguished from undiagnosed recurrence or donor disease if the biopsy is performed early after transplantation.[31] Crescentic de novo disease has been described, which is associated with a poor prognosis.[24]

Antiglomerular Basement Membrane Disease

Antiglomerular basement membrane (anti-GBM) disease is a rare cause of ESKD. If transplant is performed when circulating anti-GBM antibodies are still detectable histological recurrence (linear IgG deposition in the capillary wall) is detectable in up to 55% of transplant biopsies. However, even in these patients with histological recurrence, clinical recurrence is uncommon,[55] probably affecting less than 10% of recipients and transplant loss is rare.[56] When clinical recurrence does occur, it is in patients who have circulating anti-GBM antibodies. Therefore it is recommended that transplantation be delayed until immunological remission and 6 to 12 months since disease was active.[57] If relapse does occur some cases can be salvaged by treatment with cyclophosphamide and plasmapheresis, but the outcome is poor.[58]

Although primary anti-GBM disease could occur in a transplant, it is a very rare disease and although reported,[59] this is unlikely. The context in which anti-GBM disease can occur is in transplant recipients with a primary diagnosis of Alport syndrome.[60] This condition results from a mutation in the gene encoding the α5 chain of type IV collagen, a major component within the GBM. Because of the abnormality in α5, collagen IV is not assembled correctly into a network of α3, α4, and α5. Therefore α3, the antigenic target in anti-GBM disease, is also not present in the GBM of patients with Alport syndrome.[61] Thus, after transplantation, the recipient encounters α3 for the first time and generates antibodies against this target. Linear deposition of IgG along the GBM occurs commonly but the development of full-blown anti-GBM disease is rare. In a series of 30 patients, 15 had a renal biopsy and linear IgG deposition was seen in 5.[62] No patient had other evidence of disease. The risk for de novo anti-GBM disease does not have an adverse effect on graft survival. In a series of 62 patients with Alport syndrome, Kelly and colleagues reported a 47% 20-year graft survival (better than the control cohort),[63] although no patient developed anti-GBM disease in this series.

Membranoproliferative Glomerulonephritis and C3 Glomerulopathy

Recent progress in the understanding of the pathogenesis of MPGN has led to a revision of the classification depending on the presence of Ig-containing immune complexes (IC-MPGN) or dominant C3 (C3 glomerulopathy). The risk for recurrent disease and the potential impact on graft survival is dependent on the type of MPGN and therefore studies that do not differentiate between the different types of MPGN have to be interpreted with caution. Overall, the rate of recurrence is high for these diseases and recurrence is associated with an inferior graft outcome.[64,65]

Using protocol biopsies, Lorenz and colleagues reported a risk for recurrent IC-MPGN of 41%, with a higher risk in those patients with monoclonal IgG deposition.[65,66] Recurrence of MPGN with monoclonal deposition is associated with a poor prognosis. Only a minority of patients will have a detectable paraprotein (30%) and have a low risk for progression to multiple myeloma. The risk for recurrent disease in cases with polyclonal IgG deposition, including type I cryoglobulinemia, is lower provided the underlying cause is adequately treated.

C3 glomerulopathy, where there is dominant deposition of C3 in the glomerulus, is further divided into two diseases depending primarily on the electron microscopy appearance; dense deposit disease and C3 GN. The rate of recurrence of both subtypes of C3 glomerulopathy is high—70% in C3 GN[67-69] and 50% to 100% in dense deposit disease.[67,68] Recurrence of C3 glomerulopathy has an effect on transplant survival. A study using data from the North American Pediatric Renal Transplant Cooperative Study reported a 5-year graft survival of 50% in patients with a primary diagnosis of dense deposit disease compared with the database as a whole (74%).[70] This 5-year survival is consistent with other reports in the literature.[71] A similar 5-year allograft survival is reported for patients with C3 GN.[69] In patients with either C3 GN or dense deposit disease, 5-year allograft survival of >50% is expected; therefore, transplantation is a realistic option for this patient cohort despite the risk for recurrence.

The cause of primary disease should be assessed in potential transplant recipients with a primary diagnosis of C3 glomerulopathy.[72] However, insufficient data are available to comment on whether the cause of complement dysregulation (genetic or acquired) predicts risk for recurrence. Several factors have been reported to predict a higher risk for recurrence and poor outcome including low complement (C3 and C4) levels at the time of transplant in some,[65,73] but not all reports.[70,74] Young age, heavy proteinuria, and crescentic primary disease are also risk factors.[70] There are reports of a response to treatment with the complement (C5) inhibitor eculizumab in patients with recurrent C3 glomerulopathy, particularly when there is biopsy evidence of glomerular inflammation.[75]

De novo IC-MPGN is uncommon after transplantation and was found in only 13 of 399 (3.3%) renal transplant recipients in a French series.[76] De novo disease is commonly associated with hepatitis C infection[77] or in other systemic illnesses. The clinical presentation can vary from persistent subnephrotic proteinuria to nephrotic syndrome, declining renal function and graft loss.[78] Any underlying condition should be sought and treated if found. When no cause is identified, augmented immunosuppression, usually including corticosteroids, has been used with inconsistent benefit.

SECONDARY GLOMERULOPATHIES

Systemic Lupus Erythematosus

Systemic lupus erythematosus (SLE) is a rare cause of ESKD accounting for 1% of cases with a suggestion that disease activity is reduced once patients develop ESKD.[79] The reported incidence of SLE recurrence after transplantation varies widely, from 2.5% to 54%. The variation will depend on whether clinical recurrence or biopsy recurrence is reported.[80-83] A retrospective analysis of the UNOS database suggests that the disease recurrence rate is low, affecting 2.4% of patients (167 of 6850).[84] In contrast, a recurrence rate of 54% was reported when surveillance biopsies were performed.[85] Clinically relevant recurrence is likely to be in the range reported from registry data (<5%).

From the UNOS data, the risk for graft failure is increased fourfold higher in patients who develop recurrence than in those without recurrence.[84] However, the estimated attributable risk for graft failure due to recurrent disease is low at 7%. Although some studies have suggested that the outcome is worse in patients with SLE,[86] most studies report a low rate graft loss as a result of recurrent lupus and equivalent transplant survival compared with patients with other primary diseases.[80-82,87,88]

The UNOS data suggest that black race, female sex, and young age increase the risk for recurrence.[89] There are cases of successful transplantation in patients with serologically active lupus[90]; however, there are reports that the risk for recurrence is higher in patients with clinical or serological disease activity at the time of transplantation than in those without.[91] Therefore it is generally accepted that disease should be quiescent, or at least stable, and patients should be on minimal or no immunosuppression before transplantation. There is no relationship between time on dialysis before transplantation[80] and risk for recurrence, so there is no indication that transplantation should be delayed if disease is quiescent. Although a period on dialysis before transplantation has been suggested,[91,92] there is limited evidence to support this. One report suggested an increased risk for recurrent SLE in living related donor kidneys[81]; however, this has not been confirmed in other case series.[86] The use of mycophenolate mofetil, which is known to be effective in native lupus nephritis, appears to reduce the rate of recurrent SLE.[87]

Antiphospholipid Syndrome

Primary or secondary (most commonly in association with SLE) antiphospholipid syndrome (APS) can cause acute intrarenal vasoocclusive disease (thrombotic microangiopathy) or more chronic vascular changes, ultimately leading to ESKD. In patients undergoing renal transplantation, APS is associated with arterial and venous thrombosis, bleeding at the time of transplant, recurrence of nephropathy, and catastrophic APS. Consequently, laboratory evidence of active disease with antiphospholipid antibodies, lupus anticoagulant, or abnormal coagulation, is associated with worse allograft and patient survival.[93] Given the association of SLE with APS, patients with a primary diagnosis of SLE should be screened for the presence of antiphospholipid antibodies. Plasma exchange and peri- and postoperative anticoagulation have been successfully used but anticoagulation is associated with an increased risk for bleeding.[94] The relevance of isolated positive antibody tests, particularly anticardiolipin antibodies, in the absence of clinical features of APS, is less clear as anticardiolipin antibodies can be found in up to one-third of dialysis patients and do not increase the risk for adverse outcomes after transplantation.[95]

Antineutrophil Cytoplasmic Antibody-Associated Vasculitis

ESKD develops in approximately 20% of patients with antineutrophil cytoplasmic antibody (ANCA)-associated vasculitis.[96] Disease can relapse after transplantation with the reported rate of relapse ranging between 9% and 37%,[97-99] with a pooled analysis suggesting a recurrence rate of 17%.[98] The difference in reported rates is due to different regimens used to treat primary disease and the criteria used for diagnosis of recurrence. A more recent series of 35 patients, with patients on modern posttransplant immunosuppression (including tacrolimus and mycophenolate mofetil) reported a lower rate of recurrence (9%) during a 5-year follow-up period and only extrarenal manifestations were observed.[100] Therefore the outcome after transplantation is favorable for patients with ANCA-associated vasculitis with 10-year patient and death-censored allograft survival of 87% and 70% to 84%, respectively.[97,101,102] Graft loss due to recurrent disease is rare.

The risk for relapse is not influenced by the pattern of original disease (granulomatosis with polyangiitis or microscopical polyarteritis or whether the disease is renal localized) or ANCA type (proteinase-3 or myeloperoxidase specific).[98] There are reports of relapse if transplantation is performed in patients with active disease[103] or with high ANCA titers.[104] Despite this, it is generally accepted that ANCA positivity at the time of transplant does not increase risk for recurrent disease or graft loss and is not a contraindication to transplantation.[98,100,102] Of 35 cases (15 of whom were ANCA positive at the time of transplant) reported by Gera et al., none developed disease recurrence.[100] Similarly, changes in ANCA titer posttransplant are not an accurate predictor of disease activity.[105] Routine monitoring of ANCA titers either before or after transplant is therefore not justified. There is some evidence that the risk for relapse is increased if transplantation is performed within 1 year of clinical remission.[102] A period of pretransplant disease quiescence is recommended in published guidelines, although the evidence supporting this is not strong.[106] If recurrent disease does occur, there are reports of successful treatment with cyclophosphamide, plasmapheresis, and rituximab.[98,107]

Henoch-Schonlein Purpura

Generally, the outlook after renal transplantation for patients with a primary diagnosis of Henoch-Schonlein purpura (HSP) is good, with similar death-censored graft survival compared with patients with other diagnoses. The risk for recurrence is lower than for IgA nephropathy with a rate of only 12% at 10 years reported in a multicenter European study.[108] The proportion of graft losses attributed to recurrent HSP was 7.5% to 13.6% in the European series and UNOS database studies.[108,109]

Systemic Sclerosis

Systemic sclerosis (SS) is a multisystem disease that that can cause acute kidney injury (scleroderma renal crisis) or a more indolent decline in function and is a rare cause of ESKD. A UNOS report suggested that although transplantation improved the outcome of patients with SS (68% 1-year graft survival) compared with remaining on dialysis, survival was less favorable than for other transplant recipients.[9,110] More recently, a French Registry study reported the outcome of 36 transplants in 34 patients with a primary diagnosis of SS. Patient survival was 82.5% at 5 years, with death-censored graft survival of 92.8% at 5 years.[111] There were three cases of renal crisis in this cohort and cardiac and gastrointestinal disease worsened in 45% and 26% of patients, respectively. A similar low rate of recurrent disease was reported from the UNOS registry with graft loss attributed to recurrent disease in only 3 of 142 transplants.[110] Rapid loss of native renal function with progression to ESKD within 1 year of scleroderma renal crisis increased the likelihood of recurrence that may manifest early with an increase in nonrenal disease manifestations.[112] The risk for recurrence does not appear to be related to posttransplant immunosuppression.

Hemolytic Uremic Syndrome and Other Thrombotic Microangiopathies

Thrombotic microangiopathy (TMA) is characterized by microangiopathic hemolysis and thrombocytopenia. End-organ damage occurs due to thrombi occluding small vessels and vascular injury to small and medium-sized arteries. TMAs were originally classified according to their clinical presentation, with hemolytic uremic syndrome (HUS) typically affecting the kidney and thrombotic thrombocytopenic purpura (TTP), typically causing neurological disease. It is clear that this does not reliably distinguish between these two diseases and diagnostic tests are now available that can help distinguish HUS and TTP. An inherited or acquired deficiency in ADAMTS13 is responsible for TTP, which can cause acute kidney injury, but rarely causes ESKD. Recurrence of previously undiagnosed TTP after renal transplantation has been reported.[113]

HUS is most commonly due to infection with a Shigatoxin producing *Escherichia coli* (STEC HUS, 90% of cases). STEC HUS is a self-limiting illness that only rarely results in ESKD, although lesser degrees of CKD are common. The remaining 10% of cases, referred to as *atypical HUS*, are most commonly (60% of cases) due to an abnormality of complement activation, although other genetic or acquired abnormalities can cause atypical HUS. STEC HUS recurs very rarely after transplantation (0% to 1%)[114] and is therefore not a contraindication to transplantation. The low rate of ESKD in patients with STEC HUS raises the possibility of an alternative diagnosis when ESKD occurs after an episode of STEC HUS, particularly an atypical, complement-mediated form of disease. In this situation, a genetic or acquired defect in complement regulation should be excluded.[115] Similarly, if presumed STEC HUS recurs after a transplantation, alternative diagnoses should be considered. Alberti et al. described genetic defects in complement regulation in two patients with recurrent HUS, despite evidence of STEC infection during the initial presentation.[115]

Unlike with STEC HUS, the renal prognosis of atypical HUS has historically been reported as poor, with 50% of patients developing ESKD.[116] Patients with a pathological variant of complement factor H (CFH), complement factor I (CFI), C3, complement factor B (CFB), or high titer anti-CFH autoantibodies have an 80% to 90 % risk for recurrence and, without treatment with a complement inhibitor, most grafts are lost after recurrence.[117,118] Patients with a variant membrane cofactor protein (which is expressed normally on the donor endothelium), low titer, or historical anti-CFH antibodies can be considered for transplantation as the recurrence risk is low.[117,118] Patients in whom no cause of atypical HUS has been identified are at intermediate risk for recurrent disease.[119] Recurrence typically occurs early after transplantation (60% in the first month), perhaps due to ischemia or drugs (calcineurin or mammalian target of rapamycin [mTOR] inhibitors) causing endothelial activation and precipitating disease.[118] Recurrence of disease has been reported in patients treated with both calcineurin inhibitors and mTOR inhibitors, with higher rates of disease reported in patients receiving sirolimus.[120]

The therapeutic use of complement inhibition to either treat or prevent recurrent disease, is effective and improves the prognosis of patients with atypical HUS undergoing transplantation.[121-123] Prophylactic treatment has been recommended if disease is likely to recur.[122] Recently, however, favorable outcomes have been reported for atypical HUS patients undergoing living donor kidney transplantation without prophylactic eculizumab.[124] For patients with a genetic defect in proteins primarily synthesized in the liver (CFH, CFI, C3, and CFB) an additional option is combined liver and kidney transplantation. This restores normal complement inhibitor function and avoids the need for complement inhibitor therapy; however, it is associated with significant perioperative morbidity and mortality.[125]

De novo posttransplant TMA can develop in the absence of previous atypical HUS or any known susceptibility factor. However, the relationship between atypical HUS and de novo TMA in transplanted kidneys is complex. Approximately 30% of patients who develop de novo post-transplant TMA carry mutations in complement regulatory proteins.[126] In these cases, it may be difficult to distinguish between de novo and recurrent disease. The reported rate of de novo disease varies, with registry data usually reporting lower rates (<1%)[120] than single-center studies (4% to 14%)[127,128] De novo TMA is associated with both CNI[129] and mTOR inhibitor[130] treatment and can occur as a manifestation of acute antibody-mediated rejection. Typically, de novo TMA occurs early after transplantation and hematological features are less marked than when the TMA affects native kidneys. The diagnosis may only be apparent on kidney biopsy. Treatment will depend on the likely precipitant; reduction or withdrawal of CNI or sirolimus may be effective. A response to plasma exchange has been reported[127,131] but is inconsistent. There have been reports of a response to eculizumab,[132] but this should only be considered when ESKD could have been due to a TMA.

Diabetic Nephropathy

Diabetic nephropathy (DN) is the most common cause of ESKD in developed countries and therefore is the main reason why patients require renal transplantation. After transplantation, DN can develop in the graft as either recurrent or de novo disease.[133,134] Histological recurrence can be seen within 2 to 4 years in patients with diabetes.[134] DN in a transplant kidney presents with proteinuria and a slow decline in renal function over many years. Because of the slow decline in function, DN rarely causes allograft failure; patients are more likely to die with a functioning graft or have graft failure due to other causes.[135]

In a prospective study of 48 patients with type 1 diabetes mellitus, tight glycemic control reduced the histological changes of DN after transplantation.[136] Similarly, glycemic control achieved by simultaneous pancreas transplant protects against the development of DN in the transplanted kidney.[137] Interventions that slow progression of disease DN in native kidneys, including blood pressure control and angiotensin-converting enzyme inhibition, may benefit but are not proven to slow disease progression in transplant recipients with DN.[138,139]

De novo DN can develop in patients with new-onset diabetes after transplant and histological evidence has been reported 5 to 6 years after transplantation.[9] Poorer graft and patient survival has been reported in patients who develop diabetes after transplant,[140] although not in all series[141,142] and not in children.[143] The contribution of de novo DN to the reported increased risk for graft loss is not clear. Treatment should include optimizing glycemic control both to reduce the risk for nephropathy and other complications associated with diabetes.

GLOMERULAR DEPOSITION DISEASES

Diseases Associated With Plasma Cell Dyscrasia

Renal manifestations of plasma cell dyscrasias are common, are evident in approximately 25% of patients with a plasma cell dyscrasia at the time of presentation, and occur in 50% of patients at some point in their disease.[144,145] The most common renal manifestations of a plasma cell dyscrasia are cast nephropathy, monoclonal Ig deposition disease, and amyloid light-chain (AL) amyloidosis. These are found in 40% to 63%, 19% to 26%, and 7% to 30%, respectively, in patients with plasma cell dyscrasia. Patient survival depends on the type of renal disease present and the level of kidney function at presentation. Cast nephropathy, AL amyloid, and monoclonal Ig deposition disease have a median survival of 6, 22, and 48 months, respectively.

AL Amyloidosis

AL amyloidosis is a multisystem disorder with a significant rate of cardiac involvement. Patients with AL amyloidosis can be considered for transplantation unless it is precluded by severe extrarenal disease. Two published case series of patients with AL amyloidosis reported renal allograft survival in 41 patients from 18 to 72 months.[146,147] Recurrent disease could be detected by scintillography or biopsy in a minority of cases (7 of 41) but no grafts were lost due to recurrent AL amyloidosis. The majority of these patients had received treatment for their plasma cell dyscrasia consisting of chemotherapy with or without autologous stem cell transplantation (auto-SCT) and had maintained good functional status. A study from the UK National Amyloidosis Center reported the outcome of 25 patients with AL amyloidosis who received a kidney transplant. Median patient survival was 7.3 years and median graft survival was 5.8 years. No graft was lost due to recurrent AL amyloidosis. Survival was improved if there was at least a partial response to treatment aimed at suppression of the precursor fibril load (median survival 8.9 vs. 5.2 years in those patients with no response).[148] An alternative approach is to perform an auto-SCT after renal function has been improved by kidney transplantation. Leung et al. described five cases treated with this strategy. After a median follow-up period of 18 months, renal function was stable with no evidence of recurrent disease.[149]

Multiple Myeloma/Cast Nephropathy

Multiple myeloma with cast nephropathy is generally regarded as a contraindication to transplantation because of the high risk for recurrence and poor survival due to the underlying myeloma.[106] However, there are a number of case series and reports describing survival in patients with myeloma.[150] In a series of nine myeloma patients who received a kidney transplant, patients survived between 14 and 114 months, and this was before the introduction of new treatment strategies.[151] Three patients died of recurrent disease and three from sepsis. No graft was lost due to recurrent cast nephropathy. The European Renal Association–European Dialysis and Transplant Association (EDTA) registry identified 35 myeloma patients undergoing transplantation with a median survival of 9.6 years.[152] There is no information about disease or patient characteristics, but this is likely to represent a highly selected group of patients. There is no evidence to inform the wait time between induction of myeloma remission and transplantation. Successful outcomes have been reported after HLA-matched, combined kidney and stem cell transplantation. In a series of seven cases reported in 2011, four remained disease free after 4 years.[153]

Light-Chain Deposition Disease

Light-chain deposition disease (LCDD) is the most common form of Ig deposition disease and has been considered as a contraindication to transplant. Myeloma is common in patients with LCDD and may be present in 60% of cases, and, as with cast nephropathy, poor outcomes have been reported after kidney transplantation. In a series reported by Leung et al., seven patients received a kidney transplant, with a median allograft survival of 37 months. Disease recurred in five patients, four of whom died.[154] Aggressive treatment of the underlying plasma cell dyscrasia, including auto-SCT, can induce remission, and successful renal transplantation has been reported in patients who achieve hematological remission.[155-157]

Amyloid A and Other Amyloidoses

Most patients with amyloidosis who undergo transplantation have amyloid A (AA) amyloidosis.[158] Histological evidence of recurrent disease is relatively common, and amyloid deposition in the graft can be seen in up to 25% of cases by 12 months.[159] There is conflicting data on the outcome of kidney transplantation with a primary diagnosis of AA amyloidosis, with both equivalent[160] and inferior[161] graft and patient survival reported. A multicenter study reported inferior 10-year patient survival in patients with AA amyloidosis (62% vs. 83%) but equivalent death-censored graft survival.[162] This suggests an effect of nonrenal manifestations of AA amyloidosis on patient survival, and in support of this, the major cause of graft loss was death with a functioning graft in one series.[163]

Fibrillary-Immunotactoid Glomerulopathy

Fibrillary-immunotactoid glomerulopathy is characterized by the glomerular deposition of microfibrillary or microtubular deposits in the glomerulus. Clinically it has a poor prognosis, with 50% of patients progressing to ESKD by 5 years. It is clear that a significant proportion of patients with fibrillary deposits will also have a monoclonal gammopathy.[89] There is limited experience of transplantation in this patient group, but initial reports suggested a high risk for recurrence and graft failure.[164] However, recent series suggest that posttransplant recurrence may be lower, with slower progression than seen in native kidneys. Samaniego et al. reported the transplant outcome of 14 patients with fibrillary glomerulopathy.[165] Recurrent disease occurred in 6 patients and led to graft loss in 2 patients. The remaining grafts functioned for 4 to 13 years. In a second series, Pronovost et al. reported recurrence in three of five allografts that were followed for 4 to 11 years, with slow progression of recurrent disease.[166] The risk for recurrence appears to depend on whether there is a coexisting monoclonal gammopathy. In 12 patients with ESKD due to fibrillary glomerulopathy, 7 had evidence of a monoclonal gammopathy. After transplantation, recurrence was diagnosed in 5 patients, all of whom had a monoclonal gammopathy, indicating the potential need to treat the underlying disorder before proceeding to renal transplantation.[89]

NONGLOMERULAR DISEASES

Oxalosis

Primary hyperoxalurias are a group of three autosomal recessive diseases that lead to the accumulation of oxalate. Type 1 primary hyperoxaluria is the most common (80% of cases) and results from mutations in the gene encoding the pyridoxine-dependent liver enzyme alanine-glyoxolate aminotransferase (AGT). Excess oxalate is produced and excreted through the kidneys causing renal injury due to tubular crystal deposition and renal stone disease. The consequence is progressive renal damage and finally ESKD, which develops in 50% of cases by 40 years of age.[167] As renal disease progresses (glomerular filtration rate [GFR] <40 mL/min/1.73 m^2), oxalate production exceeds excretion and tissue accumulation occurs. Dialysis, unfortunately, does not remove sufficient oxalate to prevent accumulation in other organs including the heart and bones. Oxalate accumulation can be prevented by liver transplantation or pyridoxine supplementation in patients who are sensitive.

If kidney transplant alone is performed in patients with primary hyperoxaluria, the graft is exposed to both newly synthesised oxalate and tissue stores that are mobilized on restoration of renal function.[168] Early reports of kidney transplantation in primary hyperoxaluria suggested poor outcomes. Data from the EDTA registry published in 1990 reported a 3-year graft survival of 23% from living donors and 17% from deceased donors.[169] A more recent publication from the International Primary Hyperoxaluria Registry reported better but still poor graft survival of 45% at 5 years.[170] To improve graft survival, oxalate load should be minimized before transplantation. This can be achieved by pyridoxine treatment in those patients who respond. Oxalate accumulation also can be reduced by early preemptive renal transplantation or intensive dialysis started early in the course of disease, even with a GFR >20 mL/min/1.73 m^2.[171]

Liver transplantation will reverse the metabolic abnormality responsible for primary hyperoxaluria type 1. Combined liver and kidney transplantation offers superior death-censored graft survival compared with kidney transplant alone.[170,172] Although the metabolic defect is corrected, high oxalate levels may persist after transplantation due to mobilization of tissues stores.[168] To prevent this, sequential liver and kidney transplantation can be performed.[173] The liver transplant restores AGT tissue, which results in a reduction in body oxalate stores reducing injury to the renal allograft.

Fabry Disease

Fabry disease is an X-linked lysosomal disease resulting from a deficiency in α-galactosidase, which leads to an accumulation of glycosphingolipids in lysosomes. This results in progressive renal failure and extrarenal manifestations, particularly cardiac disease that leads to premature death in the fourth to fifth decade of life.

The outcome after transplantation is good, with a 5-year graft survival of 75% reported in a series of 197 transplant recipients[174] and 66% in a smaller study of 10 patients.[175] Allograft survival was similar to a matched cohort but patient survival was inferior, probably relating to extrarenal manifestations.[174] Accumulation of glycosphingolipids can be seen in endothelial and tubular cells in transplanted kidneys but clinical disease recurrence does not occur.[176] Data on the use of enzyme replacement therapy after renal transplantation is limited. Patients on replacement therapy maintain GFR and do not develop significant proteinuria, but this would be expected as clinically significant recurrence is not seen.[177,178] Consistent with this, the European Best Practice Guideline recommends enzyme replacement therapy after transplantation only for nonrenal manifestations of disease.[179]

Cystinosis

Cystinosis is an autosomal recessively inherited disorder of lysosomal cystine metabolism that often leads to renal failure. Cystinosis does not recur in the kidney after transplantation and therefore transplantation is an effective treatment for the renal manifestations of cystiniosis.[180] However, the systemic effects of cystinosis will persist after renal transplantation and are responsible for posttransplant morbidity and mortality.

Sarcoidosis

Sarcoidosis is a rare cause of ESKD. Renal transplantation is a good option for these patients although recurrence has been reported.[181] A multicenter French study identified 10 patients with a primary diagnosis of renal sarcoidosis who had received a renal transplant. Renal sarcoidosis recurred in three patients and although renal function was inferior, graft loss was not reported.[182]

Sickle Cell Disease

SCN can recur after transplantation[183] and early experience of renal transplantation suggested a poor outcome in this patient group.[184] Graft loss can occur during an acute vasoocclusive crisis or from recurrent vasoocclusive events in the microvasculature leading to progressive loss of function. More recent reports suggest that graft and patient survival, certainly in the early stages, are similar for patients with sickle cell compared with other causes of ESKD. One-year graft survival of 78% to 89% and patient survival of 89% to 91% have been reported.[9,185,186] Longer-term outcome in patients with sickle cell are less favorable with a higher rate of graft loss observed at 3 years (48% vs. 60% in matched controls) and higher mortality rates.[9,186]

There is a risk for vasoocclusive crisis during the transplant procedure itself. Brennan et al. published a suggested protocol for the preoperative management of sickle cell patients in 1995. This includes preoperative transfusion (or exchange transfusion) to reduce the proportion of hemoglobin S, recipient preoxygenation, and warming of the graft before reperfusion.[187] There is also evidence that acute vasoocclusive crises are more common after transplantation, presumably because of improved erythropoiesis and increased blood viscosity.

A full list of references is available at www.expertconsult.com.

43

Pediatric Renal Transplantation

Vikas R. Dharnidharka, MD, MPH

OUTLINE

ROLE OF TRANSPLANTATION

Chronic dialysis and renal transplantation are both effective treatments for end-stage renal disease (ESRD). The majority of adults with ESRD are receiving dialysis rather than undergoing renal transplantation, although the number seeking renal transplantation continues to rise.[1] Renal transplantation was recognized as the better form of treatment for children with ESRD many decades ago,[2] and it is known to provide a survival benefit for this population.[3] Both peritoneal dialysis and hemodialysis are not optimal for catch-up growth after the deceleration that occurs in ESRD.[4] Data from the dialysis component of the North American Pediatric Renal Trials and Collaborative Studies (NAPRTCS) registry,[5] now over 30 years, and from 6842 patients showed that children were significantly behind their peers in somatic linear height at dialysis initiation and did not show much catch-up growth on dialysis without growth hormone therapy. Fluid and dietary restrictions are many; appetite is also generally worse on dialysis than with a transplant. In addition, children do not tolerate being dependent on any modality, and maintenance dialysis induces loss of self-esteem and emotional maladjustment.[6] Also, ESRD of childhood is associated with an impaired cognitive and educational attainment in adulthood.[7] Long duration of dialysis may enhance intellectual impairment, which may not be reversible after renal transplantation.[8] In contrast, the mobility and freedom from dietary restrictions afforded by a functioning renal transplant enable children to live nearly normal lives. Although renal transplantation has not lived up to the promise of normal growth for all children, dramatic short-term improvements in height can be seen in many, and final adult height is improving after transplantation.[9] Most importantly, successful transplantation permits the child to attend school and to develop normally. School function testing improves dramatically after transplantation.[10] Importantly, young children now have the best long-term outcomes of all ages of transplant recipients, verifying the utility of transplantation in this age group.[11] For all of these reasons, successful renal transplantation remains the primary goal of programs that care for children with ESRD. Pediatric recipients of kidney transplants have the highest percentages of living donors (LDs), and they receive preference on the deceased donor (DD) transplant waiting list,[12] leading to relatively short waiting times. Thus pediatric patients with ESRD should not have substantial delays in undergoing renal transplantation after developing ESRD.

TABLE 43.1 Distribution of Children Getting a Renal Transplant by Age Group, Gender, Race, and Primary Diagnosis

	AGE AT TRANSPLANTATION					
	0–1 yr (percent)	2–5 yr (percent)	6–12 yr (percent)	13–17 yr (percent)	≥18 yr (percent)	Total
Gender						
Male	69.2	65.5	58.7	56.4	55.9	59.2
Female	30.8	34.5	41.3	43.6	44.1	40.8
Race						
White	73.6	63.0	60.3	56.1	51.7	59.2
Black	8.2	14.4	14.7	19.8	25.0	17.0
Hispanic	11.9	16.2	18.2	17.6	15.7	17.1
Other	6.3	6.4	6.9	6.5	7.6	6.7
Primary Diagnosis						
Renal	29.0	23.5	16.6	11.3	9.6	15.8
Plasias						
Obstructive	18.6	20.6	16.0	13.2	10.1	15.3
Uropathy						
FSGS	0.7	8.4	12.3	13.2	16.6	11.7
Other	51.7	47.4	55.1	62.2	63.7	57.1

FSGS, Focal segmental glomerulosclerosis.

Incidence and Frequency of Pediatric Renal Transplantation

In 2016 about 19,000 kidney transplants were performed in the United States,[13] and about 700 of these were in children younger than 18 years. In most years, pediatric patients comprise <5% of all transplant recipients. Although the number of pediatric transplants performed each year has generally varied by no more than 10%, the donor origin has undergone substantial changes. Living kidney donation is generally more prominent in children due to parental motivation to donate. With policies that increased availability to deceased donors for children, living donations fell.[14] In 2016 living donation accounted for 39% of all kidney transplants in the United States, but for 65% of kidney transplants to children.[13] Most of these are living-related, but similar to the adult population, increasing percentages of living-unrelated or paired-exchange donors are being reported.[15,16]

In the 1980s there was a tendency to preferentially place kidneys recovered from infants into infant recipients (size matching), with high thrombosis rates and disastrous consequences for patient and graft survival.[17] As a result of widespread dissemination of these data, there has been a marked change in practice. The majority of DD kidneys for children are now recovered from adult donors. This change in allocation of kidneys from young donors led to improvement in graft survival. Many programs reserve grafts from very young donors for en bloc transplantation into older recipients.[18,19]

Etiology of End-Stage Renal Disease in Children

ESRD in children is generally due to congenital or inherited diseases. In reviewing 11,603 transplants in the NAPRTCS database,[9] the most common congenital diagnoses found are aplastic/hypoplastic/dysplastic kidneys and obstructive uropathy, with each representing about 15% of the patients (Table 43.1). Among glomerular disorders, focal segmental glomerulosclerosis (FSGS) is the most common at 11%. The primary diagnosis also varies with the race of the recipient. Caucasian children account for 59% of all recipients; however, Caucasian children account for less than 50% of the children transplanted for FSGS. Table 43.1 shows the primary diagnoses by gender and race of 10,632 children who received a transplant as recorded by NAPRTCS since 1987 and the percentage of biopsy-proven diagnoses. It is important to observe that the biopsy confirmation of the primary diagnosis was made in 94% of FSGS, in 87% of systemic immunological diseases, and in 90% of congenital nephrotic syndrome patients. The information regarding primary diagnosis is critical in predicting graft survival and recurrence of the original disease, as discussed later.

Indications for Renal Transplantation in Children

There has been a substantial change in long-term renal allograft outcome for children across the world during the past three decades.[9,11,20-22] Previously, young children were thought to have poor short- and long-term graft survival related to several factors, most prominently a proposed heightened immune response, especially in infants.[23] The most recent comprehensive registry reviews have clearly demonstrated a dramatic reversal in outcomes with marked improvements in patient and kidney graft survival for infants and young children.[9,11,20,21,24] Indeed, several analyses have identified these very young recipients as now having the best long-term survivals of all age groups.[11,25] Thus children of all ages are excellent transplant candidates. Therefore by the time that the child has reached chronic kidney disease (CKD) stage 4 to 5, planning for kidney transplantation and pretransplant preparation should have begun. There are very few contraindications to kidney transplantation in children. Perhaps the only two are the presence of another otherwise-fatal condition with a short projected survival, such as metastatic Wilms' tumor and severe neurological compromise. About 75% of children are treated with a course of chronic dialysis before renal transplantation, but unless there is a need for specific pretransplant preparation, there is no advantage to pretransplant dialysis. For adults, preemptive renal transplantation has a survival advantage, whereas in children, although advantage is harder to show, there is no detriment.[22,26]

PRETRANSPLANT PREPARATION

Recipient Age at Transplantation

Kidney transplantation before 6 months of age or in a recipient who weighs less than 6 kg is very unusual. Since 1987, NAPRTCS has recorded approximately 560 transplants performed in children younger than 12 months, around 5.3% of the total.[9] The yearly number has dropped in more recent years. Because infants and adolescents have different risk factors for both patient and graft survival, children frequently have been grouped into five age categories: 0 to 1 year, 2 to 5 years, 6 to 12 years, 13 to 17 years, and 18 to 21 years of age. In 1987 25% of all pediatric transplants were performed in children 0 to 5 years of age,[20] whereas by 2010 the same age group accounted for 20%.[9] The decreased number of transplants in this group is likely due to greater surgical challenges in these small recipients, combined with the development of better dialysis for infants. However, excellent results have been obtained in very young patients in some individual centers.[25,27,28] The concept of a heightened immune response in young recipients is controversial.[23,29] Thus the unique problems associated with transplantation in young recipients may be related to infections,[30] technical issues,[24] and differences in pharmacokinetics[31] rather than to their immune response.

There has been a substantial change in long-term renal allograft outcome for children during the past three decades.[11,20,32] Infants have flipped from poor long-term allograft survival to the best long-term survival.[11] Conversely, however, adolescents were subsequently noted to have a higher rate of late acute rejections[33]; infants may have a lower rate of acute rejection than older children.[9] An important analysis of the United Network for Organ Sharing (UNOS) data demonstrated that in the mid-1990s, short-term pediatric renal transplant survival rates became comparable to those in adults.[33] The most recent comprehensive registry reviews have clearly demonstrated a dramatic reversal in outcomes. Improvements in surgical technique,[28,34,35] donor selection,[36] immunosuppression practices,[37-40] the enhanced experience of specialized pediatric transplant teams,[41] and the development of multicenter research consortia have all led to marked improvements in patient and kidney graft survival for infants and young children.

Currently, pediatric recipients have 5-year allograft survival rates of 86.5% if from an LD and 83.2% if from a DD,[9] which is comparable to rates seen in adults.[11] Unfortunately, this excellent outcome is not seen in adolescents, whose 5-year graft survivals are less than 80% and whose 10-year graft survival is only 50%, worse than all other age groups except the most elderly.[5] The graft failure risk dramatically increases between the ages of 11 and 24.[42]

Recipient Preparation

Before a child can undergo renal transplantation, the problems caused by CKD must be addressed and optimized if possible. In those cases where ESRD is due to urological abnormalities, corrective reconstructive surgery should be undertaken, especially to the lower urinary tract, before transplantation. Two of the major consequences of CKD are anemia[43-51] and growth retardation,[52-55] both of which should be addressed before transplantation. A recent report of final adult height in pediatric renal transplant recipients suggests that the current improvement in final adult height posttransplantation is more related to improving height deficits before transplantation than to any net gains achieved after transplantation.[55,56] Uremia also leads to wasting and malnutrition in the child, and this can compromise the success of the procedure. For example, prophylactic native nephrectomy and reversal of protein wasting and malnutrition improve the outcome of transplantation in children with congenital nephrotic syndrome.[57] Careful preparation is particularly important in children undergoing preemptive transplants. Because live viral vaccines are generally not indicated in chronically immunosuppressed patients, children should receive all appropriate vaccines pretransplantation. Whereas guidelines exist for the evaluation of the adult transplant recipient,[58] there are no similar published reports for pediatric patients.

Urological Preparation

Children with the developmental diagnoses described in Table 43.1 require a thorough urological evaluation before transplantation, and they frequently require pretransplant reconstructive urological surgery. Lower urinary tract abnormalities are present in as many as 25% of pediatric kidney transplant recipients. For all such patients, a history of voiding pattern before development of renal failure is most helpful. In pretransplant testing, urinary flow rate should be at least 15 mL per second, the postvoid residual volume should be less than 30 mL, and urinary bladder pressures should not exceed 40 cm H_2O.[59] Further investigations would consist of urethrocystoscopy in patients suspected of a urethral stricture, and a voiding cystometrogram is essential for complete assessment of bladder function.[59] This provides information about bladder capacity, pressure rise, and the efficiency of voiding. Still more information can be obtained by combining the urodynamic studies with radioisotope imaging. Routine voiding cystourethrogram is not indicated in older children with no symptoms related to the urinary tract.

A bladder with a very small capacity may not be adequate for a functioning transplant. Occasionally a small-capacity bladder may be seen in patients with prolonged oligoanuria. However, if the bladder is distensible and the bladder wall compliant, such a bladder may be used safely for kidney transplantation. When a bladder fails to empty completely, infection and obstruction are potential complications that may shorten graft survival. Clean intermittent self-catheterization, which is widely used in urological practice, can be safely used posttransplantation in patients where the primary abnormality is an inefficient and uncoordinated detrusor function.[59]

Most pediatric patients have a urinary bladder that will adapt to the new kidney. Although the bladder may not appear to have the capacity, especially in patients on long-term dialysis before transplantation, it will most often distend with usage. However, in patients with a truly low-capacity or high-pressure bladder, augmentation may be necessary before transplantation. The goal of modern reconstructive pediatric urology is to have a competent low-pressure urinary reservoir that can be emptied by voiding or at least by intermittent catheterization. Augmentation cystoplasty consists of adding bowel or gastric wall to the bladder, whereas substitution cystoplasty is performed when most of the bladder is excised and replaced with bowel. Gastric remnants have been popular for augmentation; however, they do tend to cause excessive loss of acid in the urine, leading to discomfort and metabolic alkalosis.[60] These augments typically are performed pre–kidney transplant. In patients in whom augmentation has been performed, long-term antibiotic therapy and intermittent catheterization may have to be carried out to prevent urine stasis and infection. In general, the incidence of urinary tract infection (UTI) and other complications is higher in these recipients; their graft survival may also be slightly worse than in pediatric recipients without urological abnormalities.[61]

If native kidneys in children with ESRD are causing hypertension, chronic infections, or excess losses of protein, urine, or other substances, there should be serious consideration for nephrectomy before or at the time of transplantation.[59] About 25% of children have native nephrectomies before transplantation.

Donor Preparation

Donor Selection

The selection of the appropriate donor is an integral part of the transplantation procedure and may be a limiting factor in the long-term outcome of kidney transplantation for any individual child. The use of LDs has generally been much more common in pediatric kidney transplantation than in adults.[11] In general, the choice of an LD is a good one because, on average, graft survival can be twice as long when an LD is used compared with a DD.[62] There are limitations to the use of LDs, however, such as donor suitability, blood group incompatibility, and age; thus not every child may have a suitable LD. When DDs are used for children, careful attention should be paid to using low-risk donors because the mortality risk for children after kidney transplantation is low[11] and children are expected to require the grafts for long periods of time.

THE TRANSPLANTATION PROCEDURE

Technical Issues in Transplantation

The operative technique differs based on the weight of the child. For children less than 15 kg, the transplant is performed through a midline incision, and the large abdominal vessels are used.[24] After reflection of the right colon, the aorta and the inferior vena cava are exposed. The aorta is mobilized from above the inferior mesenteric artery to the external iliac artery on the right side. After the lumbar branches are ligated and divided, the iliac arteries and the inferior mesenteric are encircled. Next the inferior vena cava is mobilized from the left renal vein to the iliac veins. After the lumbar veins are ligated, the iliac veins are encircled. The donor renal vein is anastomosed to the recipient vena cava in an end-to-side technique. The donor renal artery is then anastomosed to the recipient aorta in an end-to-side fashion. Careful attention must be paid to the recipient's hemodynamic response upon clamping and unclamping of the major vessels, and it is desirable to maintain a central venous pressure of 15 to 18 cm H_2O before unclamping.[35] The perfusion of the transplanted kidney may be slow because a large adult kidney will take up a significant portion of the normal pediatric blood volume.[32] Hemodynamic studies suggest that the cardiac output of infants must double to perfuse the adult donor kidney adequately. Thus volume replacement is critical when the kidney is large relative to the infant's body (Fig. 43.1). The ureteral anastomosis is performed by implanting the donor's ureter into the recipient's bladder, most commonly these days via a nonrefluxing extravesical

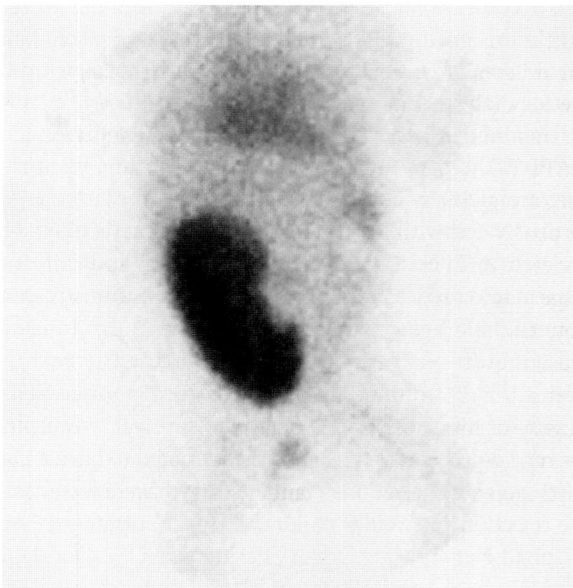

FIG. 43.1 ^{99m}Tc-MAG3 radionuclide renal scan in a 9-month-old infant who received a living donor renal transplant from his father. The graft is intraperitoneal and occupies most of the right side of the peritoneal space. Note the relative sizes of the graft and the heart. (From Smith JM, Martz K, Blydt-Hansen TD: Pediatric kidney transplant practice patterns and outcome benchmarks, 1987-2010: a report of the North American Pediatric Renal Trials and Collaborative Studies. *Pediatr Transplant.* 2013;17(2):149-157.)

(Lich-Grégoire) approach rather than an intravesical approach (Politano-Leadbetter procedure) because it is faster, a separate cystotomy is not required, and less ureteral length is necessary, thus assuring a distal ureteral blood supply.[63]

The transplantation technique used in children with a body weight greater than 15 kg is similar to that employed in adults. Unlike the transperitoneal approach necessary in younger children, this transplant is extraperitoneal, with the renal vein anastomosed to the common iliac or the external iliac vein. The arterial anastomosis can be to either the common iliac or internal iliac artery. The ureterovesicular anastomosis is performed using the techniques described earlier.

Evaluation of Graft Dysfunction

At the completion of the vascular anastomosis and release of the vascular clamps, immediate function of the transplanted kidney is demonstrated by the production of urine. Various causes, however, may prevent initial function, and evaluation of immediate nonfunction and the differential diagnosis of this condition are critical components of the transplant physician's role (see Chapter 36).

Delayed Graft Function

A well-functioning kidney graft should lead to normal renal function within 2 to 3 days. The lack of attainment of normal renal function, as would be demonstrated by a fall of the serum creatinine to normal levels, is termed delayed graft function (DGF). There is no consensus concerning the definition of DGF.[64] In some settings, DGF is used only to distinguish recipients who require dialysis after transplantation, but that is a very stringent definition. Acute tubular necrosis (ATN) represents the most frequent cause of immediate graft nonfunction in children. Current data from the NAPRTCS show that ATN was observed in 4.8% of LD and in 14.7% of DD index transplants (Karen Martz, personal communication). Because the NAPRTCS definition for ATN is the stringent "requiring the use of dialysis in the first posttransplant week," these figures probably underrepresent the actual incidence of ATN. The risk for early ATN is related to factors such as prior transplants, prolonged cold ischemia, absence of prophylactic antibody therapy, and the use of more than five pretransplant blood transfusions. The diagnosis is confirmed in most cases by Doppler sonography or the use of radionuclide scan (Fig. 43.2). If recovery of graft function is delayed, however, a transplant biopsy may be necessary, because other diagnostic tests cannot distinguish between ATN and rejection or recurrence of primary disease. Importantly, early acute rejection can mimic ATN or coexist with it.[65] The presence of ATN does not auger well for the transplant, because the acute rejection rate jumps from ~20% to 30% in LD and 40% in DD transplants to children.[65] Long term, there is a 15% to 20% drop in graft survival in children if ATN occurs immediately posttransplant.[65]

Importantly, although the incidence of DGF is increased when a donation after cardiac death (DCD) donor is used, the detrimental effect of DGF on long-term outcomes in this setting does not appear to be as severe as when it occurs after living donation or after transplantation from brain-dead DDs.[64]

Graft Thrombosis

Graft thrombosis is an almost unique complication of Pediatric Transplantation. Although usually a major cause of immediate graft nonfunction, it can be seen later on in the course and has been recorded to occur as late as 15 days posttransplantation after initial engraftment and function. Graft thrombosis has been the third most common cause of graft failure in pediatric renal transplantation[36] and may rise to second as acute rejection rates continue to fall. The critical nature of this complication can be appreciated from the fact that it accounts for ~10% of graft failure in index transplantation and 12% in repeat transplants in the NAPRTCS registry.[9] A dreaded event, this condition is irreversible in most cases and necessitates removal of the graft. Graft thrombosis should be suspected in cases where there has been immediate function followed by the development of oligoanuria. The diagnosis is established by sonography or radionuclide scan using diethylenetriamine pentaacetic acid (DTPA) or MAG3, which reveals a photopenic defect with no uptake by the transplant kidney (Fig. 43.3).

Because the outcome of graft thrombosis is uniformly dismal, numerous studies have been conducted in an attempt to understand and anticipate this complication. The etiology of graft thrombosis is multifactorial, but it is more commonly seen in young recipients.[66] In a special study of 2060 LD and 2334 DD kidneys, the NAPRTCS has shown that a history of prior transplantation increases the risk, whereas increasing recipient age has a protective effect for LD kidneys.[17] The prophylactic use of antilymphocyte antibody also decreases the risk, and this may be particularly true for the monoclonal interleukin-2 receptor (IL-2r) antibodies.[67] For DD kidneys, a cold ischemia time longer than 24 hours increases the risk for thrombosis. The use of antibody induction therapy, the use of donors older than 5 years of age, and increasing recipient age were factors that decreased the risk for thrombosis.

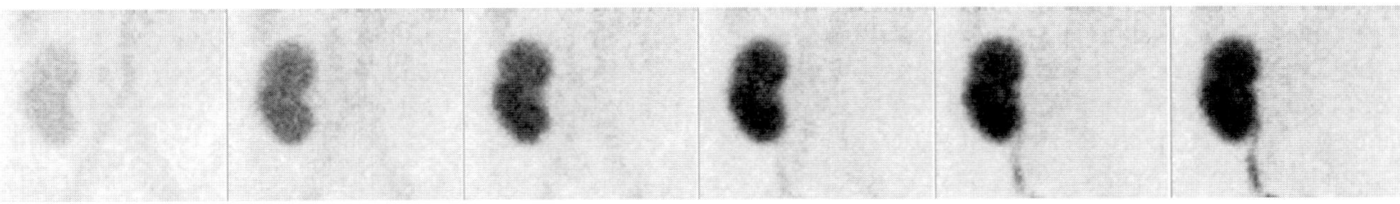

FIG. 43.2 ^{99m}Tc-MAG3 radionuclide renal scan of a deceased donor renal transplant in a 15-year-old boy performed on the first postoperative day. The cold ischemia time exceeded 24 hours, and the recipient experienced oliguric acute tubular necrosis. Note the good perfusion, followed by little excretion and "washout" of the tracer from the graft.

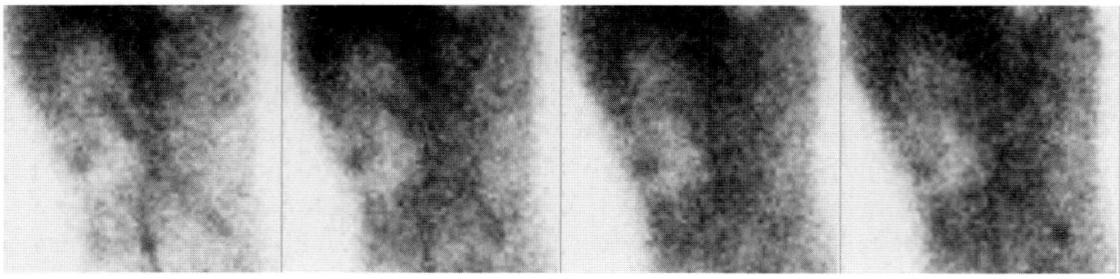

FIG. 43.3 ^{99m}Tc-MAG3 radionuclide renal scan in a 6-year-old girl with focal segmental glomerulosclerosis who received a living donor renal transplant, performed 16 hours postoperation. Note the photopenic area in the right abdomen, indicating thrombosis of the graft with no perfusion.

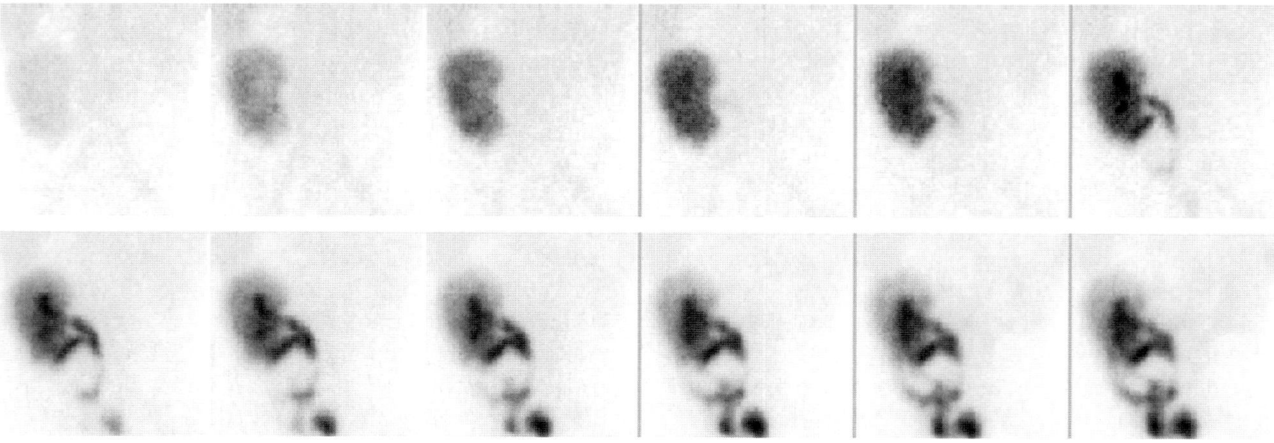

FIG. 43.4 ^{99m}Tc-MAG3 radionuclide renal scan in an 8-year-old girl who received a deceased donor renal transplant, performed 12 hours postoperation. Note the good perfusion of the graft and the rapid concentration and excretion from the kidney. Tracer, however, rapidly accumulates in the right lower quadrant, outside of the bladder. Investigation demonstrated a traumatic bladder rupture.

One study showed that centers that performed fewer infant transplants had higher rates of graft thrombosis,[41] and other studies suggested that pretransplant use of peritoneal dialysis increased the risk for thrombosis.[68,69] Some centers routinely administer anticoagulants to pediatric recipients at high risk for graft thrombosis, but no clinical studies of their effectiveness have been performed, and their use is not without complications.[70]

Obstruction, Urinary Leak, and Urological Complications

An uncommon but correctable cause of immediate graft dysfunction is obstruction of the urinary flow, which presents as decreasing urine output and the development of hydronephrosis. An ultrasound or radionuclide scan with a furosemide washout enables the clinician to establish this diagnosis. Obstruction can be due to kinking of the ureter, to edema or blockage of the implantation site of the ureter, or to development of a lymphocele. A more ominous cause of immediate nonfunction is the rare case of urinary leak due to disintegration of the distal ureter or rupture of the bladder. This condition is extremely painful due to the extravasation of urine into the pelvis or peritoneal cavity and is established by radionuclide scan (Fig. 43.4). The appearance of the tracer in the peritoneal cavity or in the scrotal, vulvar, or inguinal area clinches the diagnosis, and immediate surgical correction is necessary.

Immunosuppression Strategies

Between 80% and 90% of pediatric kidney transplant recipients currently receive antibody-based induction therapy after kidney transplantation, with the majority of those receiving T-cell depleting agents.[71] In addition, most children receive triple maintenance immunosuppression with tacrolimus, mycophenolate mofetil (MMF), and steroids.[71] As shown in the NAPRTCS annual report, the "typical" immunosuppression protocols have changed frequently over the past two decades (Fig. 43.5). However, it also appears as though children who begin treatment under one combination stay on that regimen. Several recent multicenter research efforts have been directed toward an attempt to decrease the number of types of chronic immunosuppression, with corticosteroids and calcineurin inhibitors (CNIs) being the most common medications targeted for removal.[11] Several multicenter trials[38,39,72] have reported success in avoiding or withdrawing corticosteroids, although some of these have had substantial adverse effects.[73,74] There have also been reports of avoidance of CNI in children, a move designed to prevent nephrotoxicity. At least one of these trials resulted in excellent long-term graft function but had a high rate of early acute rejections.[75] In general, children metabolize immunosuppressive drugs faster than adults. Thus data show that young children often need cyclosporine dosing three times a day[76] or sirolimus twice a

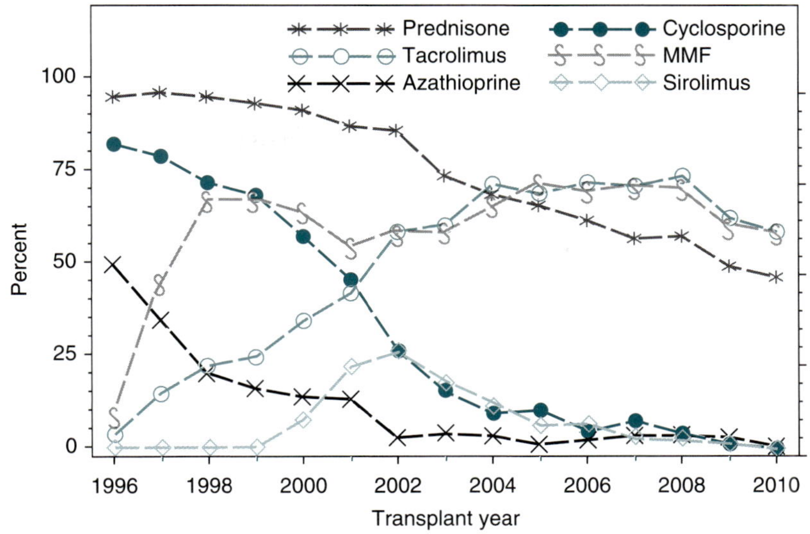

FIG. 43.5 Maintenance immunosuppression in pediatric living donor renal transplant recipients by transplant year. (From Smith JM, Martz K, Blydt-Hansen TD. Pediatric kidney transplant practice patterns and outcome benchmarks, 1987-2010: a report of the North American Pediatric Renal Trials and Collaborative Studies. *Pediatr Transplant.* 2013;17(2):149-157.)

day,[31] versus the standard dosing used in adults. Body surface area dosing of drugs may be more accurate than per-kilogram dosing in young children.[77]

ALLOGRAFT DYSFUNCTION

In the absence of tolerance, the renal allograft is destined for loss by some form of rejection. Rejections are classified as hyperacute (occurring immediately upon grafting), accelerated acute (occurring within the first week after transplantation), acute (generally occurring within the first year of transplantation), late acute (occurring after the first year), and chronic, for which the time sequence is difficult to establish, because it may occur as early as 3 months but generally occurs years later in the course of the transplant. The original disease that caused the native kidneys to fail may also affect the transplanted kidney.

Hyperacute Rejection

Hyperacute rejection is the result of specific recurrent antidonor antibodies against human leukocyte antigen (HLA), ABO, or other antigens. Irreversible rapid destruction of the graft occurs. Histologically there is glomerular thrombosis, fibrinoid necrosis, and polymorphonuclear leukocyte infiltration. In the early years of transplantation, when the HLA-matching techniques were not well developed, hyperacute rejection was more common. As in adults, hyperacute rejection has become exceedingly rare in children. The only treatment is surgical removal of the allograft. Graft failure from hyperacute rejection is reported in only 0.7% of all index or subsequent transplants in the last NAPRTCS report.[9]

Acute Rejection

Information regarding the incidence and outcome of acute rejection in pediatric renal transplantation is available from the NAPRTCS data. Because NAPRTCS receives data from multiple centers that use different diagnostic and treatment protocols, the definition of a rejection episode is based upon the circumstance of a patient having been treated with antirejection therapy, although biopsy confirmation is becoming more common. A remarkable decrease in the incidence of acute rejection has occurred over the past 30 years (Table 43.2). In a study of two cohorts of pediatric renal transplant recipients (1469 in 1987–89; 1189 in 1997–99), the rejection ratios dropped from 1.6 to 0.7 per patient.[78] Sixty percent of the latter group were rejection-free compared with 29% of the former, and 1-year graft survival was 94% compared with 80%. Historically, more than half of the patients experienced a rejection in the first post-transplant weeks; now the great majority of patients experience

TABLE 43.2 **Percent of Recipients Experiencing an Acute Rejection Episode in the First Transplant Year, Stratified by Living Donor or Deceased Donor and by Transplant Year Cohorts, Demonstrating a Dramatic Drop in Percent in More Recent Cohorts**

	LIVING DONOR		DECEASED DONOR	
Transplant Year	**%**	**SE**	**%**	**SE**
1987–1990	54.2	1.7	68.9	1.5
1991–1994	44.9	1.5	60.3	1.6
1995–1998	33.0	1.4	40.5	1.7
1999–2002	21.9	1.3	26.6	1.8
2003–2006	12.8	1.3	17.1	1.5
2007–2010	8.6	1.8	16.6	2.1

SE, standard error.
From Smith JM, Martz K, Blydt-Hansen TD: Pediatric kidney transplant practice patterns and outcome benchmarks, 1987-2010: a report of the North American Pediatric Renal Trials and Collaborative Studies. *Pediatr Transplant.* 2013;17(2):149-157.

a rejection-free first year. In the most recent cohorts, the 1-year acute rejection rates are 8.6% for LD transplants and 16.6% for DD transplants.[9]

Risk factors for rejection after DD transplantation include the absence of prophylactic depleting antibody induction therapy, donor age younger than 5 years, African American race, and no antigen D–related (DR) matches. Risk factors for rejection after LD transplantation are the absence of lymphocyte-depleting antibody induction and one or two DR mismatches, African American race, and ATN. In an earlier study, the NAPRTCS noted that when reviewed by age groupings, rejection ratios, time to first rejection, and the mean number of rejection episodes were not different; however, for the initial rejection episode, recipients younger than 6 years of age had significantly increased irreversible rejections leading to graft loss.[79] On the other hand, data from surveillance transplant biopsies suggest equivalent rejection responses in all groups.[29,80] Most recent Scientific Registry of Transplant Recipients (SRTR) data demonstrated that infants and young children now have the best outcomes of all age groups.[11] Thus either the proposed heightened immune response has been overcome by improved immunosuppression or the cause of previously poor outcome was related to other factors.

Diagnosis of Acute Rejection

Rejection is suspected when there is decreasing urinary outflow and a rising serum creatinine. In the past, classical signs of acute rejection included fever and graft tenderness. Under CNI and prophylactic antibody therapy, however, these signs are rarely seen; thus early evidence of graft dysfunction should initiate concern. The differential diagnosis consists of ureteral obstruction, renal vascular compromise from stenosis, urinary leak, and an infectious process. When rejection is suspected, a urinalysis and urine culture should be performed to assess the possibility of infection. The urinalysis is also helpful if it suggests intragraft inflammation or immune response as evidenced by proteinuria and the presence of leukocytes and other cells in the sediment. Blood or urinary cytokine/gene expression analyses may also be useful for diagnosing rejection, although they are not used on a routine clinical basis.[81] Examination of the urine sediment may be useful in detecting reasons for graft dysfunction, such as infection or recurrence of the primary kidney disease. An ultrasound is performed to rule out anatomical obstruction. Obstruction can be the result of a lymphocele, hematoma or, rarely, an abscess. The ultrasound can also provide information about intragraft blood flow and pressure. A radionuclide renal scan, using a tracer such as ^{99m}Tc-MAG3, is a very helpful tool in establishing some diagnoses (see Figs. 43.3 through 43.5). Rejection is suggested by rapid uptake of the tracer by the kidney, but with a delayed excretion. Unfortunately, radionuclide scans cannot distinguish among various causes of intragraft dysfunction, such as rejection, cyclosporine toxicity, and ATN. Thus a definitive diagnosis of rejection requires a transplant biopsy.

Pediatric Renal Transplant Biopsy

The renal transplant biopsy procedure is very easy and safe when conscious sedation and ultrasound guidance are used. Data evaluating renal transplant biopsies, including some in intraperitoneal kidneys and many performed during the first week posttransplantation, have demonstrated a very low risk for major complications.[82-84] A major factor in reducing post-biopsy bleeding is the use of an automated biopsy device using a small (18 gauge) rather than a standard (15 gauge) needle. Biopsies should be performed in pediatric renal transplant recipients whenever the diagnosis of rejection is in doubt.

Treatment of Acute Rejection

The standard initial treatment of an episode of acute rejection is still intravenous methylprednisolone in a single daily dose of 10 to 20 mg/kg (maximum dose: 0.5 g) for three consecutive days. Most Banff grade I and II rejections will respond to steroid therapy. Steroid-resistant rejection episodes are treated with lymphocyte-depleting antibody therapy, such as the polyclonal rabbit antithymocyte globulin Thymoglobulin. Thymoglobulin is now given in a dose of 1.0 to 1.5 mg/kg/dose for a total of 5 to 14 days, generally not exceeding 7.5 mg/kg in more recent cohorts. It may be advisable to monitor $CD3^+$ cells during treatment and to restrict the frequency of dosing to days when the count is greater than 20 cells/mm^3.[85] All antibodies have several side effects. Precaution against the potential anaphylactic reaction related to polyclonal antibodies consists of using 500 mg of methylprednisone with the infusion of the antibody and administering an antihistamine such as diphenhydramine (Benadryl) 30 minutes to an hour before drug administration.

Reversibility of Acute Rejection

From the recent NAPRTCS data it was observed that among LD kidneys, 52% of rejection episodes were completely reversed, 44% were partially reversed, and 5% ended in graft failure. Similar figures for DD kidneys are 45%, 48%, and 7%, respectively.[9] When stratified by age, young transplant recipients have irreversible rejection episodes more frequently. Ten percent of acute rejections among infants receiving an LD kidney ended in graft failure, compared with 4% for older children. For DD kidneys the rate of graft failure in infants was 15%, compared with 7% for older children. Molecular or genomic characterization of rejection biopsies, many derived from pediatric cohorts, may become more helpful in describing different types of acute rejection.[81,86-92]

In those patients for whom neither steroids nor antibody therapy has successfully reversed a rejection episode, conversion to an alternative CNI or to other immunosuppressants may be warranted. There have been no controlled studies in children to document reversal of rejection with conversion to tacrolimus; however, anecdotal reports do suggest that in some cases conversion helps stabilize graft function.[93]

Chronic Allograft Dysfunction

The gradation from acute to chronic rejection is gradual; however, many biopsies may show features of both, and some characteristic vascular changes of chronic rejection may be seen early.[80] The clinical picture is that of gradually declining renal function together with varying degrees of proteinuria and hypertension.[94] The clinical condition may be referred to as transplant glomerulopathy, chronic rejection, chronic allograft dysfunction (CAD), chronic allograft nephropathy (CAN), or interstitial fibrosis and tubular atrophy (IFTA).[95] The succession of names reflects lack of clarity of the etiology, clinical course, or treatment of this disorder. Nonetheless, this process, which will be referred to as CAD in this chapter, is the leading cause of graft loss after kidney transplantation in children.

An ongoing controversy exists as to whether the changes seen in chronic rejection are immune mediated, secondary responses to infection, ischemic in nature, or nonimmunological injury due to hyperfiltration.[96] Data in children have shown clearly that acute rejection is a predictor of chronic rejection.[97] In a study of 1699 LD and 1795 DD recipients, NAPRTCS noted that acute rejection was a relative risk (RR) factor for chronic rejection (RR = 3.1) and that multiple acute rejections increased the RR to 4.3.[97] Late acute rejections are also clinical correlates of chronic rejection.[98] Even if acute rejection is the most critical element in the genesis of chronic rejection, other immune mechanisms may mediate its progression, such as antibodies directed against the donor, major histocompatibility complex class I–related chain A (MICA), endothelial cells, and B lymphoblasts. Gene expression profiles in graft biopsies of patients with established CAD demonstrate upregulation of profibrotic and growth factors, and now such profiles may be able to predict later CAD.[99]

Symptomatic therapy is currently the only available method of dealing with CAD. Hypertension should be controlled, and the proteinuria may occasionally respond to angiotensin-converting enzyme (ACE) inhibitors; however, renal function will generally continue to decline. In children, CAD produces an additional burden because decreased renal function will result in deceleration of growth. It is in this context that prevention of chronic rejection by early aggressive therapy in patients who have had an episode of acute rejection may be rewarding. Because currently available immunosuppressive medications have been unsuccessful in preventing or slowing the progression of chronic rejection, the use of regimens without steroids[38,40] or immunosuppressives other than those currently approved may be reasonable, such as the use of costimulation blockade rather than nephrotoxic CNIs.[100,101] Although some programs have concluded that these techniques might be beneficial after CAN is established,[102] there may be a point at which substitution of non-nephrotoxic agents is not helpful.[103] The presence of heavy proteinuria in recipients with CAD may also predict lack of benefit of changing chronic immunosuppression.[104]

Recurrent Kidney Disease

Some diseases will recur in a transplanted kidney, and the recurrent disease may lead to loss of the graft, as it had done to the native kidneys previously. Recurrence of the original disease is the cause of 7% of all graft losses, and it is the cause of up to 9.5% of graft losses in subsequent transplants.[9] Thus recurrence is one of the top four causes of all graft losses to children, which is unlike graft losses to adults. The 5-year LD graft survival for children with FSGS is 71%, and for children with glomerulonephritis it is 77%, in contrast to all other causes of ESRD, in which 5-year graft survival is greater than 83%.[105] Several other pediatric diseases also recur posttransplant. In particular, atypical hemolytic uremic syndrome (HUS) from genetic deficiencies of complement inhibitors can recur in 20% to 80% and is the attributable cause of graft loss in 10% to 80%, especially for factor H mutations. Membranoproliferative glomerulonephritis (MPGN) type II, also related to complement cascade, has very high recurrence rates of 66% to 100% and attributable graft loss rates of 25% to 60%. Hyperoxaluria or oxalosis, a genetic disease, recurs in 80% to 100% and is the attributable cause for graft loss in 90% to 100%.[106] More details are described later.

Focal Segmental Glomerulosclerosis

FSGS is the most common cause of steroid-resistant nephrotic syndrome leading to ESRD and is the most common acquired cause of ESRD in children. Reports of recurrence of FSGS vary from 15% to 50%, and about 50% of the recurrences lead to graft loss.[105-107] FSGS is a pathological diagnosis and represents the appearance of a large number of diseases that might be due to immunological, genetic, or other causes. The genetic diseases do not seem to recur in a graft. Risk factors for recurrence include early onset of nephrotic syndrome, rapid progression to ESRD (<3 years), resistance to treatment, Caucasian or Asian race, recurrence in a previous transplant, and possible presence of a circulating glomerular permeability factor.[108,109] Recurrence can occur immediately after transplantation and result in massive proteinuria, ATN, and even graft failure related to small vessel thrombosis. Typical FSGS lesions on pathological examination, other than foot process fusion, may not appear early in the course of recurrence but may follow early thereafter. In general, children with active nephrotic syndrome are not candidates for preemptive transplant because of the heavy proteinuria and consequent risk for graft thrombosis and delayed diagnosis of recurrence. Many programs will perform native nephrectomy and will maintain the children on chronic dialysis for some period of time, certainly to improve nutritional status and to normalize the serum albumin. There is no benefit to LD transplantation in children with recurrent FSGS; although graft loss due to rejection is lower in recipients of LD transplants, graft loss due to recurrence is higher, leading to equivalent graft survivals in LD and DD transplants.[110] Whether this is the result of a higher frequency of recurrence in LD recipients, a more aggressive course in those recipients, or simply a higher rate of rejection in the DD recipients is not known. Plasmapheresis is often used prophylactically before transplantation or immediately after it to attempt to prevent or treat recurrence of FSGS,[111] and some programs report complete remission in up to 60% treated in that manner. Rituximab has also been used to treat recurrent FSGS in children, with mixed results.[112]

Hemolytic Uremic Syndrome

HUS in children is most commonly caused by enteropathic bacteria and Shiga toxin, and this version of the disease typically does not cause ESRD or recurrence in a kidney transplant. On the other hand, children with atypical or non-Shiga toxin-associated HUS have a much higher incidence of progression to ESRD and recurrence of the disease after transplantation.[106] In patients with factors H or I or with B mutations, the recurrence rate appears to be high, and transplantation may be deferred.[106] Eculizumab therapy at transplant can reduce or treat recurrence.[113-115]

Membranoproliferative Glomerulonephritis, Types I and II

Both forms of MPGN can recur in transplants, with variable frequency from 30% to 60%.[106] Type II seems to be more severe, and neither form seems to be treatable after recurrence.[116,117]

Oxalosis, Methylmalonic Acidemia, and Metabolic Diseases

Primary oxalosis recurs almost immediately and universally after kidney transplantation and was once considered a contraindication to kidney transplantation. However, treatment with intensive pretransplant and posttransplant plasmapheresis to lower the body burden of oxalate, along with the use of combined kidney-liver transplantation, has led to substantially better outcomes.[118] If liver transplantation is being considered, however, careful consideration must be paid to determining whether the child has a variant that might be responsive to lifelong treatment with pyridoxine rather than liver transplantation.[106] Methylmalonic acidemia may be partially ameliorated by kidney transplantation, but full treatment may require liver transplantation in select recipients.[106] Certain inherited diseases, including insulin-dependent diabetes mellitus and sickle cell disease, may recur in a kidney transplant, but this almost universally happens during adulthood, many years after the primary transplant in a child.

Other Autoimmune Diseases

Immunoglobulin A (IgA) nephropathy, Henoch-Schönlein purpura, lupus nephritis, and antineutrophil cytoplasmic antibody (ANCA)-associated vasculitis may recur after kidney transplantation in children, but these recurrences may be minimally apparent and less frequently lead to graft loss.[106] Surprisingly, lupus nephritis does not recur to any great extent after renal transplantation. Patients with lupus have similar outcomes compared with other patients,[119,120] except for a slight increase in mortality,[119] an increase in incidence of recurrent rejections, and a slight tendency to graft failure in those patients receiving DD grafts after peritoneal dialysis.[120]

Cystinosis

ESRD is typically the earliest organ failure in children with cystinosis and often accounted for the bulk of deaths from this disorder. However, the use of kidney transplantation and cystine-depleting therapy with cysteamine has extended their life expectancy to the fifth decade.[121,122] Although cystine may accumulate in the interstitium of renal grafts, it does not cause graft failure. However, the unremitting accumulation of cystine results in substantial nonrenal morbidity and mortality.[121,122]

GRAFT SURVIVAL

Pediatric renal centers reporting graft survival show varying results. Because the number of patients at any one center is small, such data cannot represent the pediatric transplant population at large. Furthermore, multiple factors affect graft survival, such as donor and recipient age, histocompatibility matching, recipient race, and so forth. Thus there cannot be accurate descriptions of graft survival rates without classification of the important variables. To obtain a proper population mix representing gender, age, and racial diversity, multicenter registry results such as SRTR and NAPRTCS annual reports have been used.

NAPRTCS has recorded that a total of 2920 graft failures occurred between 1987 and 2010, representing about 25% of all transplants in that time frame.[9] Of the failures, about 9% were deaths with a functioning graft, 84% were returned to dialysis, and 7% were retransplanted at the time of failure. With increased length of follow-up, chronic rejection continues to increase in importance; it is now the most common cause of graft failure. Overall, 48% of graft failures are caused by rejection with chronic rejection accounting for 35% and acute rejection accounting for 13%. Recurrence of original disease as a cause of graft failure was observed 202 times, accounting for 7% of graft failures. The specific diseases include: FSGS accounted for 44% of these graft losses, MPGN type II 9%, HUS 9%, oxalosis 5%, chronic glomerulonephritis 4%, others 28%. Vascular thrombosis remains a major cause of failure, and 378 graft failures (13.5%) were attributed to primary nonfunction, vascular thrombosis, or miscellaneous technical causes. Considering just transplants that have been performed since January 1, 2000, chronic rejection is the leading cause of graft loss (41.3%), followed by vascular thrombosis (8%), recurrent disease (7.9%), acute rejection (6.3%), and medication discontinuation (6.3%).

Expected graft survival for index transplants performed in the most recent 2003 to 2010 cohort at 1, 3, and 5 years for LD kidneys is 96%, 91%, and 84%, respectively, and for DD kidneys it is 95%, 84%, and 78%.[9] Similar numbers for the corresponding cohorts are reported by ANZDATA and the Collaborative Transplant Study.[23] There has been a continuous improvement in short- and midterm graft survival rates, mostly due to marked improvements in early graft survival rates. This may be related to the decreased frequency of acute rejection rates and to the decreased incidence of acute rejection as a cause of graft loss. It is notable, however, that the slopes of the graft survival curves have not changed significantly over the past two decades. These important trends in improved graft survival in pediatric LD and DD renal transplantation outcomes have been reported frequently over the past decade by sources such as SRTR, ANZDATA, and the Collaborative Transplant Study.[11]

Table 43.3 shows relative hazards (RH) for graft failure for selected transplant characteristics for both living and deceased kidneys. Relative risks of graft failure are derived using Cox proportional hazards regression models. For recipients of LD grafts between 1996 and 2010, the most influential

TABLE 43.3 **Relative Hazard Analysis for Graft Failure in Multivariate Proportional Hazards Model**

			LIVING DONOR			DECEASED DONOR		
Characteristic	**Comparison Group**	**Reference Group**	**RH**	**95% CI**	**p-value**	**RH**	**95% CI**	***P-value***
Recipient race	Black	Nonblack	1.05	0.85–1.30	0.628	1.43	1.21–1.70	<0.001
Recipient age	<24 months	≥24 months	0.51	0.36–0.71	<0.001	0.89	0.50–1.59	0.700
HLA-DR mismatch	1 mismatch	None	1.31	1.04–1.63	0.020	1.27	0.93–1.73	0.137
	2 mismatches		1.01	0.79–1.30	0.929	1.20	0.88–1.62	0.253
Induction therapy	No	Yes	1.15	1.00–1.32	0.060	0.89	0.75–1.06	0.191
Prior random transfusions	1–5	None	1.02	0.87–1.19	0.811	1.00	0.84–1.20	0.995
	>5		1.00	0.77–1.31	0.985	0.92	0.69–1.22	0.543
Donor-specific transfusions	Yes	No	0.52	0.26–1.06	0.070	—	—	—
Preoperative immunotherapy	Yes	No	1.05	0.91–1.20	0.538	—	—	—
Cold storage time	>24 h	≤24 h	—	—	—	1.11	0.88–1.41	0.366
Transplant year	1996–2010		0.91	0.89–0.93	<0.001	0.93	0.90–0.95	<0.001

CI, Confidence interval; *HLA-DR,* human leukocyte antigen D related; *RH,* relative hazards.
From Smith JM, Martz K, Blydt-Hansen TD: Pediatric kidney transplant practice patterns and outcome benchmarks, 1987-2010: a report of the North American Pediatric Renal Trials and Collaborative Studies. *Pediatr Transplant.* 2013;17(2):149-157.

poor prognostic variables of index graft survival are recipient age >24 months, receipt race black, prior transplant, prior transfusions, prior dialysis, prior native nephrectomy, no induction therapy, older transplant year, and higher HLA-B but not DR mismatches. Conversely, for DD recipients, the important worse prognostic factors include the same factors, but recipient age *less* than 24 months and *both* HLA-B and DR mismatches; however, induction antibody use is not significant.[9] Some of these associations may reflect other confounding factors.

Although assessment of graft survival is a reasonable measure of transplant outcome, it does not include an accurate portrayal of the course of CAD. The usual course of a kidney transplant includes an inexorable and continuous decline in renal function over many years. Thus many kidney transplant recipients suffer from the consequences of CKD for many years as graft function deteriorates. Projected graft half-lives have continued to improve for children in recent eras,[123] largely driven by improvements in early graft failure. However, there have been much fewer to minimal improvements in late allograft survival, similar to that in adults.[124] The DD allograft half-life in children was only 5 years in 1989 and is now approximately 10 years in 2005. Percent attrition rates remain constant between 5% and 10% in the 1- to 3-, 3- to 5-, and 5- to 10-year periods posttransplant over time.[123] As noted previously, the various causes for decrease in kidney function include immunological, such as immune response or rejection and recurrent disease; and nonimmunological, such as nephrotoxic medications, infection, perfusion injury, and so forth. Studies designed to identify the causes and ameliorate any etiological causes are clearly indicated.

The primary disease causing ESRD can have an effect on graft survival. In many of the rare diseases that are more preponderant in children, improvements in transplant success rate have been dramatic. Children with oxalosis used to have very bad outcomes, to the extent that the diagnosis was considered a contraindication to transplantation. However, improvements in outcome related to combined liver-kidney transplantation have been encouraging after using intensive hemodialysis before and immediately after transplantation and performing the procedure before complications of the disease have caused multiple organ damage in the recipient.[118] Similarly, infants with congenital nephrotic syndrome often had very poor outcomes, but strategies designed to reduce the risk for thrombosis and to improve nutrition pretransplantation have led to marked improvements.[61] Children or adults with sickle cell disease and ESRD can receive kidney transplants successfully,[125,126] as can those with Down syndrome.[127,128]

GROWTH AFTER TRANSPLANTATION

A major distinguishing feature of pediatric from adult recipients is the need for children to grow. Growth in children with CKD/transplant has to be measured relative to growth in normal children, and must be adjusted for the changing age between serial measurements and the changing height velocities in different phases of childhood. Thus Z-scores are used to compare children with CKD to normal children, and the change or delta between Z-scores is used to judge catch-up growth.

The growth failure commonly observed in children at the time of transplantation is multifactorial; however, the most important cause is the reduced response to endogenous growth hormone[129] through perturbations in the growth hormone/insulin-like growth factor 1 axis.[4,130] Other important mechanisms include poor appetite and nutrition, elevated metabolic rate, the combination of the two leading to cachexia, low-level inflammation, persistent metabolic acidosis, and renal osteodystrophy.[130]

Growth failure often begins insidiously early in the course of CKD. From NAPRTCS data, of children with CKD (glomerular filtration rate <75 mL/min/m^2), more than one-third had a height deficit of more than two Z-scores.[131] Chronic renal insufficiency beginning in infancy leads to permanent reduction in growth potential.[4] Growth retardation continues in children on a dialysis regimen, whether the mode of dialysis is peritoneal or hemodialysis.[5] Though a functioning transplant achieves some catch-up growth, the final height of the group remains below the population average.[132]

The most recent NAPRTCS data show that the mean height deficit at the time of transplantation is −1.75.[9,11] Males (−1.78) and younger recipients have greater height deficits at the time of transplantation. Younger children can show catch-up growth with complete inversion of Z-score up to 0.6 at 2 years for those younger than 5 years of age at transplant.[9,11] Older children may grow at a normal rate but rarely show catch-up growth. Final adult height for children with ESRD is improving, but all of the improvements seem to be related to the gains achieved during treatment for CKD rather than after transplantation. On a positive note, however, there has been an improvement in the height deficit at the time of transplantation: In 1987 children receiving their initial kidney transplant were an average of 2.43 standard deviations (SD) below average, whereas in the 2010 cohort the deficit was only 1.23 SD below average.[9,11] As a result, the final adult height of children transplanted more recently is much better than that of those transplanted years ago, in the range of −1.0 to −1.8 Z-score.

Individual center and multicenter randomized studies have adopted a variety of techniques to improve growth posttransplant. Steroids affect growth hormone secretion and inhibit growth.[133] Measurements of pulsatile and pharmacologically stimulated hormone release reveal that steroids play an inhibitory role.[134] Therefore many pediatric programs have focused on steroid dose reduction, such as early discontinuation[39,135] or late withdrawal of prednisone,[72] alternate-day steroid therapy,[136] or steroid avoidance.[38] Although each approach appears to help in catch-up growth, longer-term 3-year results from one randomized multicenter trial suggest that eventual catch-up growth is similar with or without steroids, except perhaps in the younger children.[38]

An alternative method of attaining catch-up growth posttransplantation would be the use of growth hormone. Based on a landmark randomized placebo-controlled trial,[137] recombinant human growth hormone (rhGH) has been approved for children with chronic kidney failure, but it has not actually been approved for use in children posttransplantation. Despite the lack of formal regulatory approval, studies have shown its ability to accelerate growth in this setting.[138] Several complications of the use of rhGH posttransplantation have been suggested, including acute rejection diabetes, worsening of preexisting scoliosis, and pseudotumor cerebri,[139] but the controlled trials demonstrated that it could be used safely and effectively.[137,138] Although one report suggested that the pretransplant use of rhGH may be associated with subsequent posttransplant lymphoproliferative disorder (PTLD), its use posttransplantation had no such association.[140]

COMPLICATIONS OF PEDIATRIC RENAL TRANSPLANTATION

There are multiple complications of the transplant surgery and of chronic immunosuppression. These complications tend to diminish the success of kidney transplantation. The complications include multiple types of infections; cardiovascular complications, including hypertension and vascular problems; metabolic abnormalities such as hyperglycemia and dyslipidemias; obesity; growth deficiency; and complications of orthopedic, gastrointestinal, neurological, pulmonary, and hematological systems.

Adherence to Chronic Immunosuppression Treatment

Nonadherence dramatically increases the risk for earlier graft loss in pediatric renal transplant recipients, especially adolescents.[42,141,142] A major reason for nonadherence was thought to be the alteration in appearance that accompanies immunosuppressive medications, including the cushingoid facies and growth retardation related to long-term daily corticosteroid administration and the hirsutism and gingival hypertrophy associated with cyclosporine. However, even with steroid-sparing strategies and change from cyclosporine to tacrolimus, nonadherence remains prevalent. The true incidence of nonadherence is unknown. Nonadherence rates of 22%,[143] 44%,[144] and as high as 64%[145] in adolescents have been reported. Some factors, such as young age, adolescence, poor socioeconomic status, psychiatric illness, and family stress, have been associated with increased levels of nonadherence.[142,146] Importantly, however, healthcare workers are not able to identify a significant proportion of nonadherent patients.[147] Change to lower-frequency medications has not been helpful in improving adherence.[148] Many other strategies to improve adherence are being tried, including the use of age-appropriate communication and technology.[149,150]

Hospitalization

The median duration of hospitalization at the time of LD transplantation during the first posttransplant month in the most recent NAPRTCS report was 8.7 days, with longer stays required for young patients and for recipients of DD transplants.[65] The mean length of hospital stay has shortened over time. The rehospitalization rates after the initial discharge after renal transplantation have also fallen over time; 45% of LD recipients and 52% of DD recipients are hospitalized in months 1 to 5 posttransplant.[9] The most common reason for hospitalization in months 1 to 5 is still for treatment of rejection, but now treatment of viral and bacterial infections is the most common reason in the 6- to 24-month period.[151]

Posttransplant Lymphoproliferative Disorder and Malignancy

PTLD has been a major complication of pediatric organ transplantation for many decades.[152] Though the cumulative incidence in adult kidney transplants (<1% in 5 years) tends to be lower than for other organs,[153] children with a kidney transplant have a proportionately higher risk, in part due to higher incidence of recipient seronegativity for Epstein-Barr virus (EBV) and early EBV-positive PTLD. The cumulative 5-year incidence of PTLD rose into the 4% to 5% range as children received more potent immunosuppression protocols,[73] but it now has dropped again to 2% to 3% with a shift to minimization protocols.[11]

PTLD often appears within lymph nodes, but it can be extranodal, frequently occurring within the gastrointestinal tract or within the graft.[154] Presentation of PTLD within the central nervous system is often devastating and rapidly fatal.[155] Approximately 50% to 80% of PTLD cases associate with and likely emanate from an EBV infection. In several reports, the incidence rate of PTLD for EBV-seronegative recipients was many times higher than for EBV-seropositive recipients,[156-158] representing an absence of prior immunity to EBV in these recipients. A higher overall intensity of immunosuppression, rather than specific drugs, are considered to increase the risk for PTLD. However, the use of one agent OKT3, as either induction or antirejection therapy, increased the risk for developing PTLD.[159] The diagnosis of PTLD has generally been made on the basis of characteristic pathological findings on biopsy, and the diagnosis cannot be made without biopsy material. Advances in detection of EBV DNA have permitted early detection of patients at high risk to develop PTLD.[160] Surveillance of blood and prospective adjustment of immunosuppression has been proposed, but there are no universally accepted standards in this area.[160]

The initial treatment of PTLD is the reduction or discontinuation of immunosuppression.[161,162] Of interest, in a number of these cases, the graft is not rejected, despite the marked lowering or discontinuation of immunosuppressive medications. Based on recent results from the PTLD-1 trial[163] and a trial in children,[164] combinations of rituximab with either reduced or full-dose sequential chemotherapy are the current standard of care next step, with remission rates in the 66% to 75% range. Therapies such as interferon-alfa are no longer used, whereas the use of antiviral agents such as ganciclovir remains controversial.[165,166] The morbidity and mortality are lower in children than in adults and have improved in recent years.[167]

Other Infections

Immunosuppression renders the recipient susceptible to numerous viral and bacterial infections, especially opportunistic organisms. Infections account for the majority of complications posttransplantation in children and are the principal cause of morbidity. Prophylactic therapy against the more common infections seen in the context of a renal transplantation is employed by most centers.

Cytomegalovirus

Cytomegalovirus (CMV) is an extremely important cause of infectious complications affecting transplant recipients.[168] Unlike the situation seen in nonimmunocompromised individuals, CMV infection in renal allograft recipients more often causes serious symptoms. CMV presents as a primary infection in seronegative patients; in seropositive patients the infection is secondary due to reactivation of the patient's own latent virus. As with other herpesviruses such as EBV, clinically the two types cannot be distinguished, although the former is generally more severe. CMV can also lead to acute rejection[169] and chronic allograft vasculopathy.[170] Because of the high risk to the patient and renal allograft, prophylactic therapy is indicated for all seronegative patients who receive a seropositive kidney and for all patients who receive induction with a T-cell antibody. Although some studies[171] suggest a benefit to preemptive therapy (starting therapy as soon as first sign of viral replication on serial monitoring) over prophylaxis, most studies and therefore guidelines recommend universal prophylaxis. Such prophylaxis can be carried out with either specific antiviral therapy or with high-titer CMV immunoglobulin,[172] or both. Oral valganciclovir chemoprophylaxis has been proven effective and is considered the standard of care today. Extending the duration of prophylaxis from 100 to 200 days posttransplant reduces the overall 1-year infection and disease rate,[173] though some of the infections are merely shifted to the second half of the first year. The dose of oral valganciclovir in children is given by the formula (7 × body surface area × creatinine clearance) with a maximum of 900 mg once per day.[174] There have been no controlled trials of CMV immunoglobulin versus antiviral agents, so the relative merits and indications of the two strategies are unknown. CMV can also develop resistance to first-line antiviral agents through *UL97* gene mutations; in such cases more toxic therapies such as foscarnet are needed.[168] Interlaboratory variation between CMV polymerase chain reaction (PCR) assays was found to be high,[175] but serial monitoring of CMV has become more consistent with the introduction of an international CMV standard.

Pneumocystis Carinii

Because of their defective cellular immunity, transplant patients are susceptible to respiratory infections by opportunistic organisms that are not of concern to normal children. Pneumonia is a common cause of morbidity in children with a renal allograft, and *Pneumocystis carinii* used to be the most important cause, occurring in about 3% of all renal transplant recipients in the early days.[176] Though prophylaxis with trimethoprim-sulfamethoxazole (Bactrim) has dramatically reduced the incidence, breakthrough outbreaks are still known.[177] Pneumocystis produces a diffuse pneumonia in which shortness of breath and hypoxemia, with a paucity of examination findings, are salient features. If diagnosed quickly, it can be treated effectively; however, delay can be fatal, and hence prophylaxis is standard therapy in most centers. More recent kidney transplant guidelines use the same drug for dual-purpose UTI prophylaxis.[178]

Varicella

Chickenpox is one of the constant worries of both the transplant physician and the patient's family, because exposure in the pediatric age range is extremely high.[179] The rash in an immunocompromised patient may become confluent, bullous, and hemorrhagic. If the disease becomes systemic, the fatality rate can be high.[180] Treatment of varicella in immunocompromised children generally consists of intravenous acyclovir at least until all lesions are crusted.[181] Prophylaxis, consisting of the administration of varicella zoster immunoglobulin (VZIG), is carried out routinely in all transplanted seronegative children upon exposure.[181] The administration of varicella vaccine (Varivax) before transplantation substantially reduces the frequency and severity of the disease posttransplantation.[182] The use of varicella vaccine posttransplantation has been reported in only a small series,[183] but it is likely safe, although not uniformly successful.

Urinary Tract Infection

UTIs are extremely common during the first 3 months posttransplantation and may be seen in as many as 50% of patients in the first 3 years after transplant.[184-186] In randomized trials in pediatric kidney transplant, UTI rates were 13% to 35% in the first 1 to 3 years.[39,40,187,188] Children who practice clean intermittent catheterization are at higher risk. During the first 3 months, UTI may be a common source of bacteremia. Whether early or late, UTIs can lead to higher risks for patient death and allograft damage.[189,190] The Kidney Disease: Improving Global Outcomes (KDIGO) guidelines recommend that all kidney transplant recipients receive UTI prophylaxis with daily trimethoprim-sulfamethoxazole for at least 6 months after transplantation.[178] They further suggest that for allograft pyelonephritis, treatment should involve initial hospitalization and treatment with intravenous antibiotics.[178] For patients with urological primary disease or bladder dysfunction, prophylaxis is often continued longer.

Polyomavirus

Polyoma BK virus infection has emerged in the past two decades to become an increasingly important cause of graft dysfunction and graft loss after renal transplantation.[191] In the landmark prospective study, viruria occurred in the first year in 40%, viremia in ~15%, and frank nephropathy in 3% to 5%.[192] Children are affected by BK virus nephropathy at least as much as adults, and the rate may even be higher given that the same D+/R− mismatch applies to this infection as well.[193-195] In a special NAPRTCS analysis, BK virus nephropathy was reported in 25 (4.6%) of 542 patients at a median onset of 10.1 months after transplantation.[196] More intense immunosuppression, as with other opportunistic viruses, is a major risk factor for this infection.[191,197,198] In addition, because this virus lives in the uroepithelium (including the donor ureter), ureteral stenting is another risk factor.[198-201] The clinical symptoms in kidney transplant recipients may be negligible, with elevation in serum creatinine often the only laboratory abnormality. Hemorrhagic cystitis is more often seen in bone marrow transplant patients. The diagnosis of nephropathy is made by demonstration of BK viral inclusions in the renal transplant medulla on either standard stains or more specific immunohistochemistry, preferably with associated surrounding inflammation. With the development of PCR assays for urine and blood,[202] routine screening in the first year posttransplant is proposed by several guidelines.[191,203,204] Routine monitoring may allow for reduction of immunosuppression before viremia exceeds 10,000 copies/mL, a level at which the risk for nephropathy is deemed very high.[191] Although no effective treatment for BK virus nephropathy is proven, agents that have been tried include intravenous immunoglobulin (IVIG), cidofovir, leflunomide, and ciprofloxacin.[205-207] Established nephropathy is a major risk for earlier graft loss.[194] Retransplants after the first graft failed from BK virus nephropathy have shown good results.[208] No effective chemoprophylaxis or immunization exists, with levofloxacin failing to reduce viral replication or nephropathy in randomized trials.[209,210]

Hypertension

Hypertension is extremely common in children with chronic renal failure and remains common after a kidney transplant. The incidence of needing antihypertensive medications posttransplant in an older NAPRTCS study was 70% at 1 month and 59% at 24 months.[211] Hypertension posttransplantation is related primarily to the side effects of drug therapy. The two most widely used immunosuppressives, CNI and prednisone, exacerbate preexisting hypertension. In more recent randomized trials, the hypertension incidence is from 25% to 69%, but in the lower ranges of 25% to 35% in the more recent trials of steroid withdrawal or avoidance that also used lower CNI target levels.[38-40,72,187,188] Hypertension has been correlated with multiple complications of transplantation, including reduced graft survival and cardiovascular complications.[212,213]

With dose reduction of prednisone and CNI, almost all hypertensive patients can be managed, though multiple-drug regimens may be necessary in some patients. An effective and safe drug to use is a calcium channel blocker, such as nifedipine, which also reduces cyclosporine toxicity.[214] Another drug particularly favored in adolescent patients because of concerns of noncompliance is clonidine, which is available in a transdermal patch. Clonidine may induce drowsiness, and sudden withdrawal tends to produce rebound hypertension. In patients who complain of palpitations due to drug-induced reflex tachycardia, prazosin is more effective because it induces the least amount of tachycardia. Minoxidil, an acute vasodilator, should be used only with severe hypertension and for only a limited duration because it causes hirsutism.

Hyperlipidemia/Dyslipidemia

Steroids, CNIs, and mammalian target of rapamycin inhibitors (mTORi) such as sirolimus and everolimus induce hyperlipidemia or dyslipidemia, especially the latter class of drugs.[215] The rise in obesity in developed countries has exacerbated this problem.[216] As in adults, posttransplantation hyperlipidemia in children has an adverse effect on cardiovascular morbidity.[216] In the randomized steroid avoidance SNS01 study, hypertriglyceridemia was common at baseline in both groups, with mean levels 160 to 177 mg/dL.[38] Serum cholesterol levels were significantly lower in the group randomized to steroid avoidance, but triglyceride levels were not different.[38] In cases with higher serum lipid levels, 3-hydroxy 3-methylglutaryl (HMG) coenzyme (CoA) reductase inhibitors are particularly effective in reducing total cholesterol levels and may help reduce cardiovascular morbidity.[217]

Posttransplantation Diabetes Mellitus

Hyperglycemia and posttransplant diabetes mellitus (PTDM) after kidney transplant are much less frequent in children than in adults. In randomized trials, the incidence of sustained PTDM was 2% to 5%.[38-40,72,187,188] A NAPRTCS study described an overall incidence of less than 3% of pediatric renal transplant recipients, with African Americans at higher risk.[218] Corticosteroid use leads to peripheral insulin insensitivity and hyperglycemia that is relatively insensitive to exogenous insulin. Tacrolimus may diminish insulin secretion.[219] Steroid withdrawal or avoidance may lead to improvements in this condition, though results in trials are not statistically different.[38,72] Treatments for PTDM are the same as in adults, including insulin, and may be aided by reducing or eliminating corticosteroid or CNI doses.

LONG-TERM OUTCOMES OF PEDIATRIC RENAL TRANSPLANTATION

Rehabilitation

Organ transplantation typically results in dramatic improvement of all aspects of physical, emotional, and social functioning.[220] Very early, transplant professionals recognized that cognitive skills improve after successful renal transplantation,[221] suggesting stabilization of neurophysiological functioning. Health-related quality-of-life measures are generally good,[222] especially in older children and adolescents,[223] although all ages report some problems with usual activities. Important measures for these children include: becoming full-time students again, being gainfully employed, and eventually getting married and having children,[224] all of which remain below the rates in a general population.[225] A majority still end up below normal height,[132] and up to one-third were dissatisfied with their body appearance.

TABLE 43.4 Patient Survival After Kidney Transplant, Stratified by Living Donor or Deceased Donor and by Transplant Year Cohorts, Demonstrating a Dramatic Increase in Survival in More Recent Cohorts

	LIVING DONOR			DECEASED DONOR		
Cohort Group	**1 yr**	**3 yr**	**5 yr**	**1 yr**	**3 yr**	**5 yr**
1987–1990	89.4	81.1	74.6	75.1	63.4	54.8
1991–1994	91.7	85.3	80.3	85.2	76.4	69.5
1995–1998	94.0	90.7	85.2	90.7	81.9	74.2
1999–2002	96.0	91.6	86.8	92.8	83.9	79.2
2003–2010	96.5	91.5	84.3	95.1	84.1	78.0

From Smith JM, Martz K, Blydt-Hansen TD: Pediatric kidney transplant practice patterns and outcome benchmarks, 1987-2010: a report of the North American Pediatric Renal Trials and Collaborative Studies. *Pediatr Transplant.* 2013;17(2):149-157.

Mortality

The overall mortality after kidney transplant is much lower in children than in adults,[11] likely due to lower cardiovascular comorbidities. Current 1-, 5-, and 7-year patient survival rates for pediatric LD kidney transplants are 98%, 96%, and 94% (Table 43.4), and for pediatric DD transplants they are 97%, 93%, and 91%, respectively.[9] Infection is generally the major cause of death (28%), particularly in the first posttransplant years.[9] Other major causes include cancer or malignancy (11%), cardiopulmonary causes (15%), and dialysis-related complications (3%). Over time, the patient survival has improved for LD and DD transplants,[226] and the gap in survival between the two has diminished.[9] Young infants tend to have slightly worse survival than older children, but they have also shown marked improvement over the years.

A full list of references is available at www.expertconsult.com.

44

Chronic Kidney Disease in the Kidney Transplant Recipient

John S. Gill, MD, FRCPC, MS, FAST, Habib Mawad, MD, FRCPC, and Olwyn Johnston, MB, MRCPI, MD, MHSc

OUTLINE

INTRODUCTION

There now are more than 200,000 prevalent kidney transplant recipients (KTRs) in the United States, more than double the number of patients in 2000.[1] A significant proportion of prevalent KTRs will have decreased kidney function and be at risk for complications related to chronic kidney disease (CKD), including cardiovascular disease, mineral and bone disorders, metabolic acidosis, hypoalbuminemia, and anemia. Even among patients with "normal" kidney function, the burden of previous exposure to uremia and dialysis often carries through to the posttransplant period. In this chapter, we will review the current classification of CKD, potential advantages for including patients in the CKD classification, and the applicability of the CKD classification in KTRs, as well as the relevant clinical management considerations before transplantation, during the period of allograft function, and after allograft failure.

The Chronic Kidney Disease Classification

The National Kidney Foundation's Kidney Disease Outcomes Quality Initiative (NKF K/DOQI) clinical practice guidelines published in 2002 defined CKD as either kidney damage or glomerular filtration rate (GFR) <60 mL/min/1.73 m^2 for ≥3 months, irrespective of cause.[2] Kidney damage was defined by structural or functional abnormalities of the kidney, with or without decreased GFR, as manifested by either pathological abnormalities or markers of kidney damage (i.e., abnormalities on blood or urine tests or abnormal imaging tests). These guidelines also proposed a classification of CKD based solely on the level of GFR. Five stages of CKD were defined, and each stage had an associated action plan. The initial NKF K/DOQI CKD guidelines recommend referral to a specialist if the clinical action plan cannot be prepared, or if the prescribed evaluation or recommended treatment cannot be carried out.[2] The guidelines further recommend that, in general, patients with GFR <30 mL/min/1.73 m^2 be referred to a nephrologist.

In the initial NKF K/DOQI CKD classification, KTRs were not specifically addressed.[2] The inclusion of KTRs was subsequently emphasized in a position statement from a Kidney Disease: Improving Global Outcomes (KDIGO) initiative.[3] This KDIGO position statement recommended that all KTRs be considered to have CKD, irrespective of GFR or the presence or absence of markers of kidney damage, and highlighted the inclusion of KTRs with the designation "T" to indicate transplantation. In a consensus conference on the care of KTRs, organized by the NKF and KDIGO, it was recommended that the clinical action plan in the initial NKF K/DOQI CKD classification be amended for KTRs.[4] Table 44.1 summarizes both the initial NKF K/DOQI classification and the revised KDIGO classification, which included a transplant-specific clinical action plan.[4] First, estimation of progression of CKD (originally recommended in patients with CKD stage ≥2) and evaluation and treatment of CKD-related complications (originally recommended in those with CKD stage ≥3) should be applied in all KTRs (CKD stage 1 to 5). The rationale for this modification is that KTRs carry the burden of preexisting CKD (i.e., hyperparathyroidism, anemia, cardiovascular disease), and consequently these complications should be addressed even if the GFR is relatively normal. Second, preparation for kidney

TABLE 44.1 Stages of Chronic Kidney Disease (CKD) and Action Plan for Nontransplant CKD (−T) and Transplant CKD (+T)

		CLINICAL ACTION PLAN[a]	
CKD Stage	**Definition**	**Non-Tx CKD (−T)**	**Tx CKD (+T)**
1	Kidney damage or post-Tx with normal or ↑ GFR(≥90 mL/min/1.73 m^2)	Diagnosis and treatment Treatment of comorbid conditions Slowing progression CVD risk reduction	Diagnosis and treatment Treatment of comorbid conditions Slowing progression CVD risk reduction
2	Kidney damage or post-Tx with mild ↓ GFR (60–89 mL/min/1.73 m^2)	Estimating progression	Estimating progression Evaluating and treating complications due to CKD before and after Tx
3	Moderate ↓ GFR(30–59 mL/min/1.73 m^2)	Evaluating and treating complications	Managing Tx-specific issues
4	Severe ↓ GFR(15–29 mL/min/1.73 m^2)	Preparation for kidney replacement therapy	If evidence of CKD progression, preparation for kidney replacement therapy (patient and family education, dialysis access, preemptive Tx)
5	Kidney failure(<15 mL/min/1.73 m^2)	Replacement (if uremia present)	Replacement (if uremia present)

[a]Includes actions from preceding stages.
CVD, Cardiovascular disease; *GFR,* glomerular filtration rate; *Tx,* transplant.

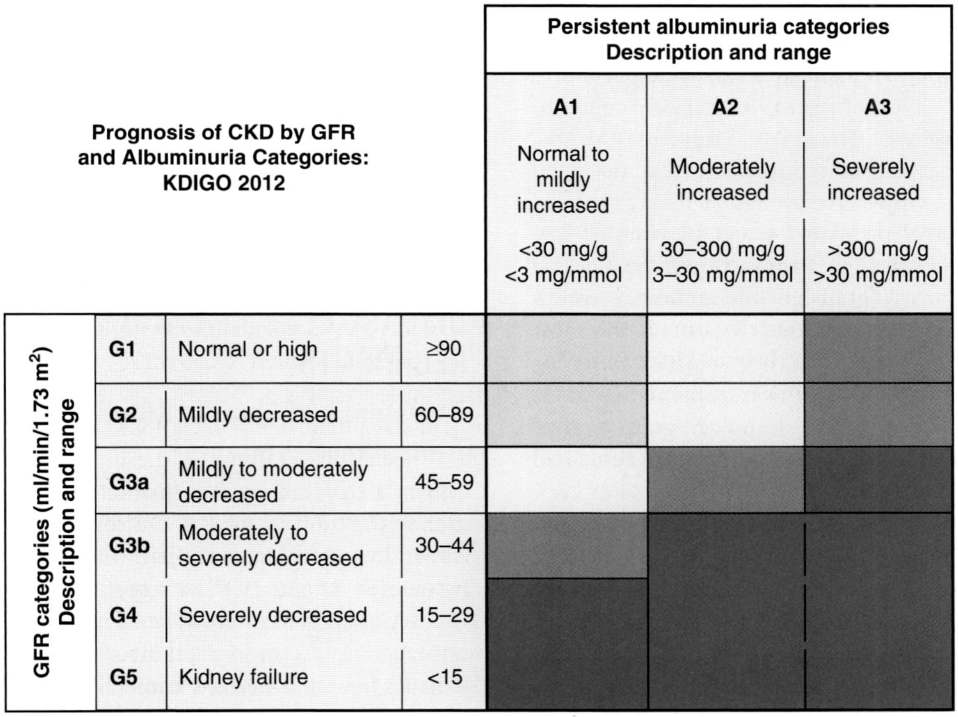

Dark gray: low risk (if no other markers of kidney disease, no CKD); light gray: moderatety increased risk; light green: high risk; dark green: very high risk.

FIG. 44.1 Kidney Disease: Improving Global Outcomes Classification of Chronic Kidney Disease. The revised Chronic Kidney Disease classification includes consideration of the etiology of disease as well as the severity of proteinuria. (From Kidney Disease: Improving Global Outcomes (KDIGO) CKD Work Group: KDIGO 2012 Clinical Practice Guideline for the Evaluation and Management of Chronic Kidney Disease. *Kidney Int.* 2013;3(1):1–150.)

replacement therapy (originally recommended in those with CKD stage ≥4) should apply only to KTRs with stage ≥4 CKD *with* evidence of progressive GFR decline. The rationale for this modification is the recognition that the rate of CKD progression in KTRs may differ from that in other forms of nontransplant CKD, and that KTRs can maintain a stable but low GFR for many years.[5,6]

In subsequent KDIGO guidelines published in 2012, stage 3 CKD was divided into stage 3a (GFR 45 to 59 mL/min/1.73 m^2) and stage 3b (GFR 30 to 44 mL/min/1.73 m^2) based on data supporting different outcomes in these subgroups.[7] In addition the 2012 KDIGO guidelines recommended staging based on cause, GFR category, and albuminuria category (Fig. 44.1)[7] based on evidence that proteinuria is an independent predictor of mortality and progression to end-stage kidney disease in transplant-naïve patients with CKD.[8] Importantly, the 2012 KDIGO guidelines continued to include KTRs irrespective of the level of GFR or the presence of markers of kidney damage. The rationale for this designation is that biopsies in KTRs frequently show pathological abnormalities even in patients without decreased GFR or albuminuria, and that KTRs have an increased risk for mortality and kidney failure compared with the general population and require specialized medical care.[7] It is important to note that KTRs were not included in the study cohorts that informed the recommendations to include the cause of CKD and the severity of proteinuria in the 2012 KDIGO CKD guidelines.

Rationale for Including Kidney Transplant Recipients in the Chronic Kidney Disease Classification

Over the past decades, there has been remarkable improvement in the 1-year graft survival rate, which is now well in excess of 90%.[1] This improvement is attributed to advances in immunosuppression and reduction in acute rejection. Unfortunately, transplant survival beyond the first year has showed only modest improvement over the same period.[9,10] Among 252,910 adult KTRs between 1989 and 2005 reported by the Scientific Registry of Transplant Recipients (SRTR), allograft half-life increased from 6.6 to 8.8 years in deceased donor (DD) recipients, whereas these figures barely changed for living donor (LD) recipients (11.4 to 11.9 years).[11] The most significant improvement was among lower-quality DD transplant recipients, where graft half-life increased from 3 to 6.4 years during the study period.[11] Based on the most recent data provided by the SRTR, 10-year graft failure for transplants in 2005 was 53% for DD transplants and 37% for LD transplants.[1] Although death-censored graft survival improved over time, death with a functioning graft remained relatively constant.[1]

These observations suggest the need for novel strategies beyond optimization of immunosuppression to improve the long-term survival of KTRs. The potential importance of treating CKD-related complications in improving long-term allograft survival is suggested by studies demonstrating that the high levels of serum phosphate, calcium-phosphate product, fibroblast growth factor 23, and metabolic acidosis are independently associated with a greater risk for allograft loss.[12,13] Similarly, the importance of optimal treatment of cardiovascular risk factors such as hypertension is emphasized by the fact that cardiovascular disease is the leading cause of death among adult KTRs. Nonetheless, controlled studies demonstrating that aggressive treatment of CKD-related complications improves allograft or patient survival are lacking.

There are a number of additional potential advantages to including KTRs in the CKD classification.[14] Increased recognition of CKD may facilitate implementation of therapeutic strategies to delay progression of kidney function decline or to prevent CKD-related metabolic complications. Inclusion of KTRs in a simple severity-based kidney disease classification schema may improve communication between clinicians, enhance public education, and facilitate research. Finally, a uniform disease classification and action plan including all patients, irrespective of the need or type of renal replacement therapy (i.e., dialysis or transplantation), may enhance the continuity of patient care.

Transplant recipients have multiple care providers before, during, and after transplantation. Recent publications have shown that transplant recipients are at increased risk for death during transitions between different forms of renal replacement therapy[15] (i.e., during the transition from dialysis to transplantation and the transition back to dialysis after transplant failure), suggesting that maintenance of continuity of care in these patients is a significant concern. Because aggressive CKD care should begin before transplantation and continue after allograft failure, it may be appropriate for a nontransplant physician to direct the CKD care of transplant recipients. The advantages of an integrated multidisciplinary care model in the management of CKD-related complications are well established in patients with native kidney disease. In addition to improving the proportion of patients who meet treatment targets for CKD-related complications, multidisciplinary care models have also been associated with a slower rate of decline of GFR.[16-18] The effect of similar models in KTRs has yet to be evaluated. Irrespective of who assumes the responsibility for CKD care, communication between the multiple responsible care providers is essential to ensure continuity of care, and this may be enabled by the use of the CKD classification.

APPLICABILITY OF THE CHRONIC KIDNEY DISEASE CLASSIFICATION IN TRANSPLANT RECIPIENTS

Prevalence of Chronic Kidney Disease in Kidney Transplant Recipients

The fact that kidney transplantation incompletely restores kidney function in most KTRs is well recognized. Fig. 44.2 shows the prevalence of CKD in 69,394 adult first KTRs between 1987 and 1997 with graft survival of at least 1 year in the United States Renal Data System (USRDS).[19] GFR was estimated at 1, 3, and 5 years after the time of transplantation with an equation derived from the Modification of Diet in Renal Disease (MDRD) study,[20] and patients were classified by K/DOQI CKD stage.[2] At each time point, the mean GFR was approximately 50 mL/min/1.73 m^2 and the prevalence of K/DOQI CKD stage 3, 4, or 5 was greater than 70%. More recent information demonstrates that although GFR at 1 year after transplantation has modestly improved in the current era, these data remain valid: Among a cohort of 189,944 adult first KTRs between 2001 and 2013 in the SRTR, the mean estimated GFR at 1 year after transplantation was 56 mL/min/1.73 m^2, and most patients would still be classified as having CKD stage 3 or greater disease.[21] Given the reality of the organ shortage and the necessity to utilize DD kidneys of lower quality as well as the increasing use of kidneys from older-age living donors, we can expect that CKD will be an increasingly important issue for KTRs in the future.

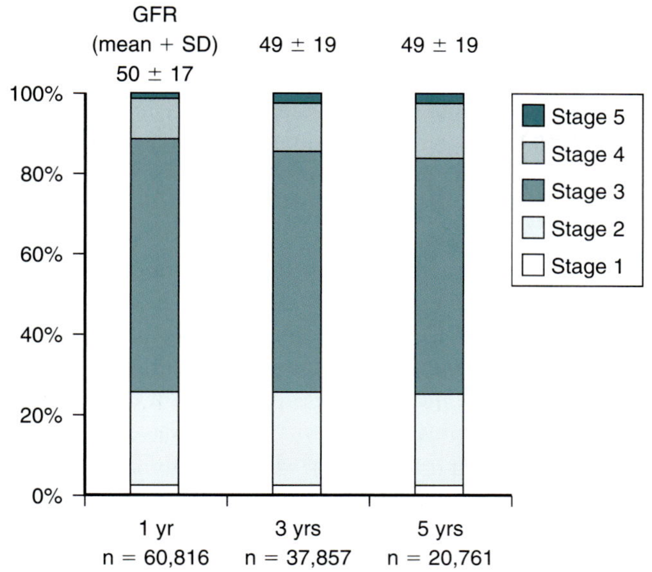

FIG. 44.2 Glomerular filtration rate and prevalence of chronic kidney disease in patients with functioning transplants. Mean ± standard deviation (SD) of estimated glomerular filtration rate (GFR) (mL/min/1.73 m^2) and prevalence of Kidney Disease Outcomes Quality Initiative (K/DOQI) chronic kidney disease stages among adult first transplant recipients in the United States between 1987 and 1997 at 1, 3, and 5 years after transplantation. (Adapted from Gill J, Mix C, Pereira BJG: Glomerular filtration rate and the prevalence of chronic kidney disease in transplant recipients. *Am J Transplant.* 2002;2(Supplement 3):417.)

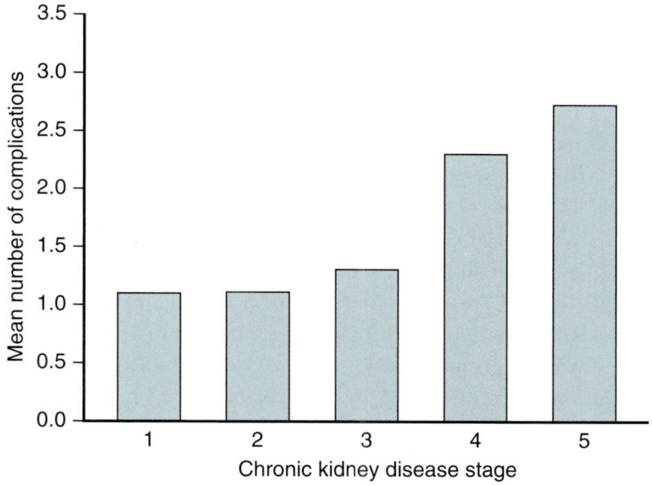

FIG. 44.3 The mean number of chronic kidney disease (CKD) complications per patient by CKD stage. The complications included hypertension (blood pressure ≥140/90 mmHg), serum calcium <8.5 mg/dL, serum phosphorus >4.5 mg/dL, hemoglobin <11 g/dL, serum albumin <3.5 g/dL, low-density lipoproteins >100 mg/dL, and total CO_2 <22 mEq/L. (Adapted from Karthikeyan V, Karpinski J, Nair RC, Knoll G: The burden of chronic kidney disease in renal transplant recipients. *Am J Transplant.* 2004;4(2):262-269.)

Prevalence of Chronic Kidney Disease–Related Complications in Kidney Transplant Recipients

As in patients with native kidney disease, the prevalence of CKD-related complications including anemia, hypertension, hyperphosphatemia, hypoalbuminemia, and acidosis increases with declining GFR in transplant recipients. Fig. 44.3 shows the mean number of CKD complications per patient in a stable kidney transplant population at a single Canadian center.[22] Similar findings have recently been reported in patient cohorts from the United Kingdom[23] and Spain.[24]

The Predictive Value of Chronic Kidney Disease Staging for Outcomes Among Kidney Transplant Recipients

The association of CKD stage based on GFR estimation at 1 year after transplantation with long-term allograft survival was evaluated in over 13,000 KTRs.[25] Compared with stage 2 disease, increasing CKD stage was associated with a progressively higher risk for all-cause graft failure. However, patients with CKD stage 1 disease were also at higher risk for all-cause graft failure (hazard ratio [HR], 1.41 [1.13 to 1.75], $P = 0.002$), which may be due to serum creatinine–based associations independent of kidney function. The association of CKD stage with death-censored graft failure was stronger and showed a more consistent dose-response pattern than did the association with death with a functioning allograft.[25] Although proteinuria has been associated with decreased kidney allograft survival and with increased risk for cardiovascular events and death in KTRs,[26] the predictive value of the 2012 KDIGO CKD classification that recommends consideration of the cause of CKD and the level of kidney function and proteinuria has not been rigorously evaluated in KTRs. Furthermore, the cause of decreased kidney allograft function is frequently uncertain, multifactorial, and/or due to complex pathogenic processes that are incompletely understood from a mechanistic perspective, and therefore the prognostic value of the current CKD classification in KTRs remains unclear.

Previous work has shown that although kidney allograft function at 1 year after transplantation is independently associated with outcomes including allograft failure and patient death,[25,27-29] GFR at 1 year has limited predictive value for long-term outcomes in individual patients. Previous work has also shown a disconnect between the level of kidney function achieved at 1 year after transplantation and the subsequent decline in kidney function.[5] This has precluded the use of early measures of kidney allograft function as a surrogate for outcomes in clinical trials.[30] In contrast, the stability of kidney function may hold more promise for use as surrogate outcome in clinical trials in KTRs. A recent study using data from the Australia and New Zealand Dialysis and Transplant Registry[31] evaluated different surrogate endpoints in 7949 adult first KTRs from 1995 to 2009 with graft survival of at least 3 years. A decline in GFR ≥30% between years 1 and 3 after transplant was found to be superior to all other surrogates, including 1-year GFR.[31] The advantages of using a ≥30% decline in GFR over 2 years compared with doubling of serum creatinine as a surrogate were recently demonstrated in transplant-naïve CKD cohorts as part of a workshop sponsored by the NKF and the US Food and Drug Administration (FDA).[32,33] Further work is needed to advance stability of kidney allograft function and/or measures of proteinuria as surrogate endpoints for clinical trials.

CHRONIC KIDNEY DISEASE MANAGEMENT

Chronic Kidney Disease Care Before Transplantation

The clinical manifestations of CKD in a given transplant recipient will depend on the duration and burden of CKD before transplantation and the level of kidney function achieved after transplantation. Exposure to immunosuppressive medications after transplantation may exacerbate CKD-related complications such as hypertension, diabetes, dyslipidemia, and anemia. Early recognition and treatment of CKD-related complications, maximization of allograft function, and minimization of immunosuppressive-related side effects should decrease the effect of CKD in transplant recipients.

Aggressive CKD care should begin before transplantation, because the preexisting burden of CKD present at the time of transplantation will not necessarily be undone by the provision of a functional allograft. In contrast, many of the complications of CKD, such as hypertension, dyslipidemia, anemia, and malnutrition, can be minimized by early detection and treatment before transplantation.[34] Prolonged exposure to dialysis before transplantation has been associated with reduced allograft survival,[35,36] and preemptive transplant recipients have an allograft survival advantage.[37,38] The reasons underlying these associations are somewhat uncertain; however, a lower burden of CKD complications in patients with no or limited dialysis exposure is a plausible explanation.[39] Reducing dialysis exposure through LD transplantation and preemptive transplantation should be encouraged.

Chronic Kidney Disease Care in the Peritransplant Period

Transplant recipients are at increased risk for mortality in the peritransplant period compared with wait-listed patients who remain on dialysis. Data from the USRDS and Medicare claims were used to describe the incidence of cardiovascular morbidity and mortality after transplantation.[40] There was a marked increase in the rate of all cardiovascular events (death, myocardial infarction, congestive heart failure, coronary revascularization, and stroke) during the early posttransplant period. The estimated probability of myocardial infarction, cardiac arrest, and congestive heart failure in DD transplant recipients in the first posttransplant month was 1.2%, 1.1%, and 5.2%, respectively. Approximately 5% of first KTRs will die within the first posttransplant year.[40] The majority of deaths are due to cardiac causes and comorbid disease (diabetes, peripheral vascular disease, angina), and patients with a longer duration of CKD are at increased risk. These deaths could be regarded as failures of CKD management rather than as failures of transplantation because they result from the accumulated burden of CKD before transplantation that might have been prevented by aggressive pretransplant CKD care. Posttransplant factors including the incidence of acute rejection and delayed graft function may contribute to the excess morbidity and mortality in the peritransplant period.[41,42] Whether more rigorous attention to volume status, standardization of the use of dialysis, and immunosuppression in the setting of delayed graft function would reduce peritransplant morbidity and mortality merits further study. Ideally, patients who consent to accept lower-quality DD kidneys should undergo transplantation rapidly, allowing for close wait-list surveillance and optimal management of comorbid conditions, which may also help reduce the risk for perioperative morbidity and mortality.[43]

Chronic Kidney Disease Care in Patients With a Functioning Allograft

Cardiovascular disease is one of the most important threats to long-term patient survival after transplantation. The management of cardiovascular disease in transplant recipients will continue to be an important component of posttransplant CKD care because of the increasing age and burden of CKD in these patients. Comprehensive reviews of posttransplant cardiovascular disease as well as treatment guidelines for cardiovascular risk reduction are available (see Chapter 39), and therefore a detailed discussion of these issues is not provided here.[44-46] There is significant interest in the effect of immunosuppressive agents on the development and progression of cardiovascular disease. For example, new-onset diabetes mellitus after transplantation (NODAT) is now recognized as a common immunosuppression-related complication[47] that is associated with an increased risk for graft loss, with the risk being comparable to that of acute rejection.[48] Randomized studies of early steroid withdrawal showed surprisingly little effect on NODAT.[49,50] However, a modest decrease in NODAT was observed in patients randomized to receive cyclosporine rather than tacrolimus.[51] In the BENEFIT trial, KTRs randomized to treatment with belatacept had better metabolic and cardiovascular risk profiles compared with those randomized to cyclosporine (i.e., less NODAT, lower blood pressure, and lower serum lipids).[52,53] The mean 5-year GFR was also significantly higher.[53] At 7 years posttransplantation, there was a 43% reduction in the risk for death and graft loss compared with cyclosporine, despite a greater incidence of acute rejection.[54] A comparison of the specific causes of death in the trial revealed a trend in favor of fewer cardiovascular events in the belatacept-treated group.[54,55] In summary, the choice of immunosuppression continues to be determined by center-specific protocols that are dominated by considerations of immune risk rather than cardiovascular risk. Although there are important differences between immunosuppressive drugs that may mitigate the risk for posttransplant cardiovascular disease, early and aggressive treatment of cardiovascular risk factors is likely the most important strategy to minimize the risk for cardiovascular disease after transplantation.

The level of kidney function achieved after transplantation has been associated with both patient and allograft survival and with the development of hospitalized heart disease.[28,56] Because of these associations, it is important that an accurate assessment of allograft function be made. A key component of CKD care in transplant recipients is recognition of the fact that patients who are typically thought of as having "good graft function" actually have significantly impaired kidney transplant function and are at risk for the complications of CKD. Serum creatinine alone is not an accurate index of kidney function, and an estimate of the GFR is the preferred measure of kidney function. There are a number of prediction equations available to estimate kidney function in transplant recipients, and a review of the accuracy and limitations of these equations is beyond the scope of this discussion. The latest KDIGO guidelines recommend the use of the Chronic Kidney Disease–Epidemiologic Prognosis Initiative (CKD-EPI) equation in adult patients.[7] The CKD-EPI equation uses the same four variables as the MDRD equation (i.e., gender, race, age, and serum creatinine) but has been shown to perform better, especially at higher GFR.[57] In the transplant setting, the superiority of CKD-EPI over MDRD is less clear.[58-62] In a recent study performed in 3622 solid organ transplant recipients, including 53% adult KTRs, the CKD-EPI and MDRD equations performed similarly.[63] Although both the CKD-EPI and the MDRD equations performed better than all other creatinine-based equations, both the CKD-EPI and the MDRD equations misestimated true GFR by more than 30% in 1 of 5 patients in the study.[63,64] The use of cystatin C as an alternative or a complement to creatinine may improve the accuracy and precision of the estimation of GFR in KTRs. Cystatin C–based equations have been shown to perform better than creatinine-based equations in some[59] but not all studies.[65]

The level of kidney function achieved after transplantation is determined largely by donor and immunological factors. Because the mean level of kidney function established after 1 year of transplantation is only about 56 mL/min/1.73 m^2,[21] preservation of kidney function is an important aspect of CKD management in transplant recipients. Recent studies of administrative data sets as well as experience in single centers have described the change in kidney function after transplantation.[66-68] Of importance is the observation that transplant recipients have a mean rate of kidney function decline that is slower than that in patients with native kidney disease with similar levels of kidney function.[69] This is surprising given the fact that KTRs are at increased risk for kidney failure. There have been secular improvements in the rate of kidney function decline after transplantation over the last decade,[6,68] but the reasons for this improvement have remained somewhat uncertain in these reports.

It would appear that there are only relatively small differences in the rate of kidney function decline between patients treated with cyclosporine and tacrolimus-based maintenance immunosuppressive regimens.[70] In contrast, calcineurin-free maintenance immunosuppressive regimens using belatacept have shown stability in kidney allograft function compared with cyclosporine-based regimens. In the latest analysis of the BENEFIT trial, the mean GFR for KTRs treated with belatacept increased at an approximate rate of +1.35 mL/min/1.73 m^2 per year over the first 7 years after transplantation.[54] In comparison, among KTRs treated with cyclosporine, there was a decline in GFR at a rate of −1.04 mL/min/1.73 m^2 per year.[54] Because tacrolimus is used in the vast majority of new transplant recipients, robust studies comparing belatacept- and tacrolimus-based maintenance regimens are needed.

Proteinuria and hypertension are associated with a loss of kidney function in KTRs. Although renin-angiotensin system (RAS) blockade has been proven effective at lowering blood pressure and proteinuria in KTRs, its role in preservation of kidney transplant function remains unclear.[71,72] A recent metaanalysis of existing trials failed to show that RAS blockade improves clinical outcomes in KTRs.[73] Evidence regarding the role of anemia in the progression of kidney function decline is relatively sparse.[74] Although associations between anemia and adverse graft outcomes have been reported in observational studies, correction of anemia to preserve allograft function and survival is not recommended. Further studies are needed to determine the optimal blood pressure and the role of proteinuria and other modifiable CKD factors in the rate of kidney function decline after transplantation. In the absence of direct evidence in KTRs, treatment of these factors based on their established role in the progression of native kidney disease is justified, especially because many of these factors also increase the risk for cardiovascular disease.

Chronic Kidney Disease Care in Patients With Transplant Failure

Patients with transplant failure now make up about 15% of the waiting list in the United States.[1] A number of studies have demonstrated that patients with transplant failure who return to dialysis are at increased risk for death compared with patients who maintain transplant function,[15,75] and that their mortality is higher than that of transplant-naïve patients initiating dialysis for the first time.[76] The survival of transplant failure patients who initiate hemodialysis and peritoneal dialysis is similar.[77] Older patients and those with comorbid conditions such as peripheral vascular disease and diabetes have a higher risk for mortality after transplant failure.[15,78] Surprisingly, however, survival after transplant failure is not significantly affected by transplant-related factors such as acute rejection, antibody induction, donor source, duration of graft survival, and the maximum attained GFR during transplantation.[78]

Repeat transplantation is associated with a survival benefit in transplant failure patients compared with treatment with dialysis.[79] Preemptive repeat transplantation is associated with a lower risk for allograft failure from any cause including death, and death with a functioning graft but a similar risk for death-censored graft loss compared with nonpreemptive repeat transplantation.[80] The benefits of preemptive transplantation were evident in patients with first transplant survival ≥1 year; however, there was a 34% increased risk for death-censored graft loss in preemptive recipients when first transplant survival was <1 year.[80] When preemptive repeat transplantation is not possible, planning for dialysis should be undertaken in a timely fashion and include optimization of CKD parameters and vascular access creation if hemodialysis is chosen. The optimal timing of dialysis initiation after transplant failure remains uncertain.

Despite being known to physicians with knowledge of CKD, recipients of failed transplant in the United States initiate dialysis with levels of hematocrit, albumin, erythropoietin use, and residual renal function that are suboptimal and similar to those in the general incident dialysis population.[81] In addition, based on recent data from the USRDS, the rate of central venous catheter use in patients with allograft failure initiating dialysis was about 65%.[82] Recent studies have demonstrated a higher rate of sepsis after dialysis initiation in transplant failure patients compared with nontransplant failure patients.[83] The role of continued immunosuppression and temporary vascular

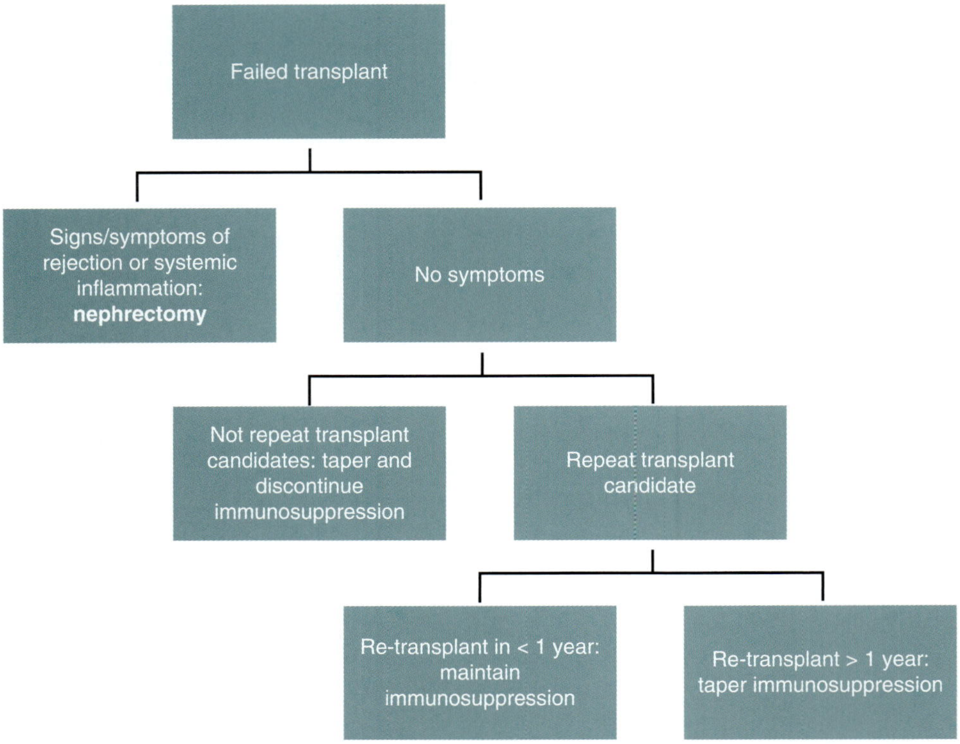

FIG. 44.4 Suggested management of transplant failure patients. The speed of immunosuppressant drug tapering will vary depending on risk of rejection and patient tolerance of immunosuppressant medications (see text for details). (Adapted from Gill JS: Managing patients with a failed kidney transplant: how can we do better? *Curr Opin Nephrol Hypertens*. 2011;20(6):616-621.)

access was not specifically assessed but may have contributed to the higher rate of sepsis in the transplant failure group. These findings demonstrate that there are significant opportunities to improve the CKD management of transplant recipients and that there is a need for increased awareness of CKD among the medical professionals involved in the care of these patients.

Management of immunosuppression after transplant failure is dependent on the patient's suitability for repeat transplantation.[84] There is no consensus on the optimal management of immunosuppression after transplant failure.[84-87] In patients who are not repeat transplant candidates, immunosuppression should generally be tapered with the long-term objective of complete withdrawal or long-term treatment with minimal doses of corticosteroids to avoid adrenal insufficiency.[84] Some nephrologists may continue immunosuppression with the goal of preserving residual renal function.[86] To date, no study has formally evaluated the effect of maintenance of residual allograft function on outcomes in patients with kidney transplant failure. The rate at which immunosuppression is tapered in transplant failure patients is also an area of uncertainty. The key considerations are avoiding acute rejection that would require therapeutic nephrectomy and/or manifest more subtly as fatigue, weight loss, and resistance to erythropoietic-stimulating agents.[84,88,89] In addition to factors noted with close patient monitoring, clinical and laboratory factors that may indicate the need for a slower pace of tapering include early transplant failure and rejection as the mechanism of transplant failure, as well as the patient's pretransplant and current level of sensitization against anti–human leukocyte antigen antibodies. Nephrectomy traditionally has been reserved for patients with acute symptoms related to rejection of the failed allograft. Although observational data have suggested that nephrectomy is associated with improved survival in transplant failure patients who return to dialysis, these findings may be confounded by other factors, and the role of elective nephrectomy in the management of transplant failure patients warrants further study.[90,91]

In patients who are repeat transplant candidates, the timing of repeat transplantation is a key consideration. In general, some degree of immunosuppression should be continued to avoid allosensitization. In transplant candidates who are not expected to undergo repeat transplantation rapidly (i.e., within 1 year of transplant failure), an individualized approach is recommended. In general, patients who are at relatively low risk for sensitization or the development of symptoms in the failed allograft and who have prolonged waiting times for repeat transplantation may be suitable for tapering of immunosuppressive medications over a period of 6 months to a year.[84] Whether such patients should completely discontinue all drugs or be maintained on low-dose prednisone is unknown. Patients thought to be at higher risk for sensitization and/or rejection in the retained allograft may require ongoing immunosuppressive medications for longer time periods. The amount of immunosuppressant medication required would be determined empirically with ongoing monitoring for signs or symptoms suggestive of inadequate immunosuppression and for drug-related complications. Fig. 44.4 summarizes a suggested management approach.[84]

A full list of references is available at www.expertsonsult.com.

SECTION V

Acute Kidney Injury

45

The Epidemiology of Acute Kidney Injury

Anand Srivastava, MD, MPH, and Sushrut S. Waikar, MD, MPH

OUTLINE

> *"The disease seems in general to come suddenly. The peculiar symptom is a sudden diminution of secretion of urine, which soon amounts to a complete suspension of it. The affliction is probably first considered as retention; but the catheter being employed, the bladder is found to be empty.... [A]fter several days, the patient begins to talk incoherently, and shows a tendency to stupor. This increases gradually to perfect coma, which in a few days is fatal...."*
>
> **John Abercrombie (1780–1828),**
> **"Observations on Ischuria Renalis."[1]**

Acute kidney injury (AKI) is characterized by sudden (i.e., hours to days) impairment of kidney function. Descriptions of syndromes consistent with AKI date back to the ancient Greek period,[2] when the diagnosis was possible only by observing a reduction in urine volume. Initial descriptions of AKI from the early 20th century centered around specific conditions such as crush injuries,[3] war nephritis,[4] and falciparum malaria.[5] Sir William Osler in 1912 described several recognizable causes of AKI under the heading of "acute Bright's disease," including sepsis, pregnancy, burns, and toxins.[6]

The modern-day conception of AKI has evolved alongside developments in pathology and clinical biochemistry that have permitted clinicopathological correlations and earlier diagnosis.[7] AKI is not a single disease but rather a designation for a heterogeneous group of conditions that share common diagnostic features: specifically, an increase in the blood urea nitrogen (BUN) concentration, an increase in the serum or plasma creatinine concentration, a reduction in urine volume, or some combination of these. The causes of AKI have traditionally been divided into three broad categories: prerenal azotemia, intrinsic renal parenchymal disease, and postrenal obstruction. In prerenal azotemia, glomerular filtration falls as a result of inadequate kidney perfusion from hypovolemia, decreased cardiac output, or renal vasoconstriction. Prerenal azotemia is considered to be functional in nature and reversible with restoration of renal perfusion. Intrinsic renal diseases can be subdivided into those affecting the glomeruli (e.g., glomerulonephritis), tubules (e.g., acute tubular necrosis [ATN]), interstitium (e.g., acute interstitial nephritis), or blood vessels (e.g., thrombotic microangiopathy). Postrenal obstruction results from mechanical disturbance to the normal flow of urine from the kidneys to the ureter to the bladder and finally to the urethra for elimination.

DEFINITION OF ACUTE KIDNEY INJURY

The specific quantitative criteria for diagnosing AKI—as defined by a rise in serum creatinine (SCr) concentration—ranges widely in the published literature, with more than two dozen definitions in use. An international panel of experts in nephrology and critical care medicine proposed a consensus definition of AKI in the Kidney Disease Improving Global Outcomes (KDIGO) Clinical Practice Guidelines for Acute Kidney Injury.

AKI is stratified into three stages, and each of the three stages can be reached either by a rise in SCr or a reduction in urine output. Stage 1 AKI can be reached by an increase in SCr of 0.3 mg/dL, 1.5 to 1.9 times the baseline SCr, or a reduction in urine output to <0.5 mL/kg/h for 6 to 12 hours. SCr-based definitions for stages 2 and 3 AKI can be reached by a doubling or tripling of baseline SCr, respectively. The urine output–based definitions for stage 2 are reached by sustaining <0.5 mL/kg/h for at least 12 hours, and for stage 3 they are reached with <0.3 mL/kg/h for at least 24 hours or anuria for at least 12 hours. The KDIGO criteria for the diagnosis of AKI are compared with other definitions of AKI in Table 45.1.

There are several limitations of any SCr-based definition of AKI. First, the baseline SCr is often not known, making it impossible to gauge the absolute or percentage rise from

TABLE 45.1 Serum Creatinine–Based Definitions of Acute Kidney Injury

Acute Kidney Injury Network[88]	Stage 1: increase of ≥0.3 mg/dL *or* 50% increase over baseline within 48 h Stage 2: ≥100% increase over baseline (doubling) Stage 3: ≥200% increase over baseline *or* 0.5 mg/dL increase to at least 4 mg/dL
Acute Dialysis Quality Initiative[89]	RIFLE "R": ≥50% increase over baseline RIFLE "I": ≥100% increase over baseline (doubling) RIFLE "F": ≥200% increase over baseline *or* ≥0.5 mg/dL increase to at least 4 mg/dL
Kidney Disease Improving Global Outcomes (KDIGO)[90]	Stage 1: increase in SCr ≥0.3 mg/dL *or* ≥1.5 times; urine output <0.5 mL/kg/h for ≥6 h Stage 2: increase in SCr ≥2 times; urine output <0.5 mL/kg/h for ≥12 h Stage 3: increase in SCr ≥3 times, *or* SCr >4 mg/dL, or initiation of renal replacement therapy; urine output <0.3 mL/kg/h for ≥24 h *or* anuria for ≥12 h
International Ascites Club for AKI in Cirrhosis[91]	Baseline SCr: stable SCr ≤3 mo ; if not available, a stable SCr closest to current one; if no previous SCr at all, use admission SCr Definition of AKI: increase in SCr ≥0.3 mg/dL ≤48 h, *or* increase of 50% from baseline Stage 1: increase in SCr ≥0.3 mg/dL *or* increase in SCr ≥1.5–2 times baseline Stage 2: increase in SCr >2.0–3 times baseline Stage 3: increase in SCr >3 times baseline, SCr ≥4.0 mg/dL with increase ≥0.3 mg/dL, *or* initiation of renal replacement therapy
Contrast nephropathy[50]	≥0.5 mg/dL increase *or* 25% increase over baseline within 48 hours of receiving contrast

RIFLE, Risk, injury, failure, loss of kidney function, and end-stage kidney disease; *SCr,* serum creatinine.

baseline.[8] Second, creatinine itself is an inadequate biomarker of kidney injury because of tubular secretion, the need for steady state determinations for accurate estimates of glomerular filtration rate (GFR), and the confounding influences of muscle mass and changes in volume of distribution, the latter particularly in the setting of acute illness.[9] Assessment of GFR by gold standards such as iothalamate or inulin clearance is cumbersome and impractical in the acute setting but may be facilitated by technological developments.[10] In patients with prerenal azotemia, creatinine may rise in the absence of any structural injury to the kidneys. In patients with severe parenchymal kidney injury, such as lupus nephritis, SCr may not rise at all.

Recent investigation into tubular injury biomarkers may herald a paradigm shift in the definition of AKI, similar to that seen over the past several decades in the definition of acute myocardial infarction (MI) (see Chapter 47). Acute MI is defined on the basis of myocardial injury markers, including troponin, without the requirement for a functional decrease in myocardial function such as cardiac output. It is possible that AKI may eventually be defined on the basis of sensitive injury biomarkers that rise well before the complex sequence of events and before an ultimate reduction in GFR, followed thereafter by a rise in SCr.

Early Cohort Studies of Acute Kidney Injury

Hou and colleagues[11] in 1983 published one of the first chart review–based cohort studies of AKI. These investigators focused on hospital-acquired disease and therefore excluded patients with established AKI on admission. Over a 5-month period beginning in 1978, a total of 2216 consecutive medical and surgical admissions to Tufts Medical Center in Boston were followed for the development of AKI. The definition of AKI in this study was based on an absolute increase in SCr depending on the admission SCr: increase in SCr of greater than 0.5 mg/dL if admission SCr was less than 1.9 mg/dL; increase of greater than 1 mg/dL for admission SCr of 2 to 4.9; or an increase of greater than 1.5 mg/dL for admission SCr of greater than 5 mg/dL. Overall, 4.9% of patients met criteria for AKI. The major causes of hospital-acquired AKI were decreased renal perfusion (42%), major surgery (18%), contrast nephropathy (12%), and aminoglycoside antibiotics (7%). The crude in-hospital mortality rate was 32%, and the degree of kidney injury as assessed by change in SCr was noted to be important. In-hospital mortality was 3.8% in patients with an increase in SCr of 0.5 to 0.9 mg/dL and increased progressively to 75% in patients with a greater than 4 mg/dL increase who were not treated with renal replacement therapy. This study was also one of the first to establish the association between oliguria and mortality in patients with AKI (52% vs. 17% with and without oliguria, $P < 0.01$).

Shusterman and associates[12] performed a case-control study of hospital-acquired AKI in patients admitted during 1 month to the Hospital of the University of Pennsylvania in Philadelphia in 1981. The definition of AKI was different from that employed by Hou et al. 4 years earlier. AKI was defined as a greater than 0.9 mg/dL increase in SCr with baseline SCr of less than 2 mg/dL, or a greater than 1.5 mg/dL increase in SCr with baseline SCr of greater than 2 mg/dL; the incidence was 1.9% among patients on medical, surgical, and gynecological services. The 34 AKI cases were matched to 57 controls without AKI. From this small group of cases and controls, the authors found volume depletion, aminoglycoside use, septic shock, congestive heart failure, and intravenous contrast administration as risk factors for AKI. They also found a 10-fold increased odds of death and a doubling of the length of stay among patients with AKI.

Nash and colleagues[13] published a follow-up report of hospital-acquired AKI almost two decades later, using similar methodology and definitions to the earlier publication. Over a 4-month period in 1996, they prospectively followed 4622 medical and surgical admissions at Rush Presbyterian–St. Luke's

Medical Center in Chicago for the development of AKI, defined as in their earlier study. They identified 332 patients (7.2% of admissions) who developed AKI, higher than the 4.9% in the original study performed at a different institution. The in-hospital mortality rate of 19.4% was somewhat lower than the 25% reported previously. The most common causes of AKI remained decreased renal perfusion (39%; defined broadly to include congestive heart failure, cardiac arrest, and volume contraction), nephrotoxin administration (16%), contrast administration (11%), and major surgery (9%).

In 2016, Leaf and colleagues[14] evaluated diagnostic testing for all adult inpatients who were admitted with or developed AKI during a single calendar year at Brigham and Women's Hospital in Boston, defined using KDIGO criteria. A total of 70.8% of the patients experienced stage 1 AKI, 17.1% had stage 2 AKI, and 12.1% had stage 3 AKI. In a random subset of 100 AKI episodes, the most common underlying causes were ischemic ATN (24%), prerenal azotemia (21%), nephrotoxic ATN (10%), cardiorenal syndrome (8%), glomerulonephritis (5%), obstruction (3%), and hepatorenal syndrome (2%). Notably, the cause of AKI was unknown in 22% of episodes, and the remaining 5% included acute interstitial nephritis, rhabdomyolysis, and tumor lysis syndrome.[14]

Multicenter Cohort Studies of Acute Kidney Injury

Initial cohort studies of AKI shed important light on the frequency, causes, and mortality associated with hospital-acquired AKI. No matter how carefully conducted, single-center studies are inherently limited in terms of sample size and external validity (i.e., generalizability to AKI at other medical centers). Recognizing this limitation, and the heterogeneity of causes of AKI at individual institutions, investigators have conducted multicenter epidemiological investigations of AKI.

Liano and Pascual[15] conducted a prospective, 9-month study of all AKI episodes in 13 tertiary-care hospitals in Madrid, Spain, beginning in 1991. They defined AKI as a sudden rise in SCr of more than 2 mg/dL, excluding patients with preexisting chronic kidney disease (CKD; defined as SCr >3 mg/dL). Unlike the Hou et al.[11] and Nash et al.[13] studies, hospital- and community-acquired cases of AKI were included. Of the 748 episodes of AKI (representing 0.4% of admissions and 21 per 100,000 population), ATN was the most common cause (45%, defined to include diverse causes including surgery, nephrotoxin administration, sepsis, and renal hypoperfusion), followed by prerenal azotemia (21%, defined as the rapid recovery of kidney function after volume administration or restoration of cardiac output), acute-onset chronic renal failure (12.7%, not defined), and urinary tract obstruction (10%). The crude in-hospital mortality rate was 45% overall and as high as 65.9% in patients requiring dialysis (which constituted 36% of all cases of AKI). In a follow-up study, Liano and colleagues[16] provided more details on the specific differences between AKI in and out of the intensive care unit (ICU). Compared with non-ICU patients, those admitted to the ICU were younger, more likely to die in hospital (71.5% vs. 31.5%), and more likely to have ATN from sepsis or renal hypoperfusion than from nephrotoxin administration.

Brivet and colleagues[17] focused on AKI occurring in the ICU in a 20-center, prospective, 6-month study performed in France in 1991. They included all patients with a rise in SCr to at least 3.5 mg/dL or BUN to at least 100 mg/dL, or both, or a 100% increase if there was preexisting CKD. Patients with severe CKD (baseline SCr >3.5 mg/dL) were excluded. Overall, 7% of patients admitted to the ICU developed AKI or had AKI on admission. The major causes of AKI were attributed to sepsis (48%), hemodynamic alterations (32%), nephrotoxin administration (20%), and prerenal factors (17%). Overall in-hospital mortality was 58% and was higher in those with sepsis (73%) and delayed occurrence of AKI after admission (71%). Another group of French investigators performed a similar prospective observational study beginning in 1996.[18] These authors found a 7.7% incidence of AKI in the ICU, defined as SCr of greater than 3.4 mg/dL or the need for dialysis. Overall in-hospital mortality was 66%, and 81% in patients with AKI that developed 1 week after admission to the ICU.

The Program to Improve Care in Acute Renal Disease (PICARD) performed a 31-month-long prospective observational cohort study of patients at five academic medical centers in the United States from 1999 to 2001.[19] Eligible patients were those in the ICU for whom nephrology consultation was obtained; AKI was defined as an increase in SCr of greater than 0.5 mg/dL if baseline was less than 1.5 mg/dL or an increase of greater than 1 if baseline SCr was between 1.6 and 4.9. Unique to PICARD among AKI epidemiological studies to date was the extensive clinical detail captured (more than 800 data elements per patient, including details on dialysis procedures) and limited biological sample collection. A total of 618 patients were enrolled in PICARD. One of the most illustrative findings in PICARD was the degree of heterogeneity of patients with AKI across the five medical centers in terms of baseline characteristics, processes of care, and in-hospital mortality. Even across five academic medical centers, in-hospital mortality associated with AKI from ATN and nephrotoxins ranged from a low of 24% to a high of 62%. Substantial differences in process of care were also evident across the five sites in terms of dialysis modality. Despite the many differences, however, the presumed causes of AKI were relatively similar among institutions. Fifty percent of patients were labeled as having ATN with no specified precipitant. The next most common causes included nephrotoxin administration (26%), cardiac disease (20%, including MI, cardiogenic shock, and congestive heart failure), ATN from hypotension (20%), ATN from sepsis (19%), unresolved prerenal factors (16%), and liver disease (11%). The PICARD cohort has been the subject of subsequent epidemiological studies to derive prediction rules for mortality[20] and to explore the associations between dialysis modality[21] and timing of initiation and survival.[22] The biological samples from subsets of PICARD participants have been used to study urea volume of distribution,[23] insulin resistance,[24] cytokine levels,[25,24] and oxidative stress[26] in patients with AKI.

The Beginning and Ending Supportive Therapy for the Kidney (BEST Kidney) investigators prospectively studied patients admitted to 54 ICUs across 23 countries over 15 months beginning in September 2000.[27] The target population was patients with severe AKI: inclusion criteria were treatment with renal replacement therapy or AKI defined as oliguria (<200 mL in 12 hours) or BUN of greater than 84 mg/dL. Of 29,269 patients admitted to the ICUs, 1738 (5.7%) had AKI. The most common causes of AKI were septic shock (47.5%), major surgery (34%), cardiogenic shock (27%), hypovolemia (26%), and nephrotoxin administration (19%) (multiple causes were allowed on the data collection form, accounting for a total of more than 100%).

The overall in-hospital mortality rate in the BEST Kidney cohort study was 60.2%. As with PICARD, mortality varied widely across centers. Among countries contributing more than 100 patients to the cohort, in-hospital mortality ranged from 50.5% to 76.8%. A multivariable logistic regression model to identify independent correlates of in-hospital mortality yielded several previously identified risk factors also found in PICARD[19] or the French Study Group,[16] or both, including delayed AKI, age, sepsis, and a generic disease severity score that included BUN and urine output. Follow-up studies from the BEST Kidney multinational database have compared severity scoring systems for AKI-related mortality[27] and investigated the relationship between diuretic administration and mortality.[28]

Bagshaw and colleagues[29] performed a retrospective interrogation of prospective data from the Australian New Zealand Intensive Care Society Adult Patient Database (ANZICS APD) to evaluate the incidence, risk factors, and outcomes associated with early AKI in septic ICU patients from January 2000 to December 2005. The patients were from 57 ICUs across Australia. Of the 33,375 patients with a sepsis-related diagnosis (27.8% of all patients admitted to the ICU), 42.1% had concomitant AKI. AKI was defined using a modified RIFLE (risk, injury, failure, loss of kidney function, and end-stage kidney disease) criteria for risk (1.5 times SCr or <35 mL/h urine output), injury (2 times SCr or <21 mL/h urine output), and failure (3 times SCr or ≥0.5 mg/dL if baseline SCr >4.0 mg/dL or <4 mL/h urine output). They found that septic AKI had greater acuity of illness, lower blood pressures, worse pulmonary oxygenation, greater acidemia, and higher white blood cell counts than patients with nonseptic AKI. In addition, septic AKI was associated with greater severity of AKI and 60% increased odds of mortality in the ICU.[29]

In 2013, the FINNAKI study group performed a prospective, observational, multicenter cohort study of adult admissions exceeding 24 hours during a 5-month period in 17 Finnish ICUs.[30] They first defined AKI by the Acute Kidney Injury Network (AKIN) criteria and second with the KDIGO criteria. They arrived at identical classification, and found that in 2901 eligible patients the incidence of AKI was 39.3% (17.2% for stage 1, 8.0% for stage 2, and 14.1% for stage 3). In logistic regression analyses, they found pre-ICU hypovolemia, diuretics, colloids, and CKD were independent risk factors for AKI. The hospital mortality for AKI patients was 25.6%, and the 90-day mortality for AKI patients was 33.7%.[30]

Large Database Studies of Acute Kidney Injury

Medical administrative and claims databases afford investigators the opportunity to study AKI in large numbers of patients admitted to a wide spectrum of hospitals over multiple years, including patients not ordinarily represented in prospective cohort studies. The major limitation of most administrative databases is the lack of detailed clinical and laboratory information. The *International Classification of Diseases, 9th Revision, Clinical Modification* (ICD-9-CM) codes for acute renal failure (ARF) (584.x) and renal replacement therapies (39.95) have been found to be accurate for the identification of patients with severe AKI (defined as AKI requiring dialysis, or AKI-D) but less accurate for AKI not requiring dialysis.[31]

Multiple studies to date have used large administrative or claims databases, or both, to study secular trends in the epidemiology of AKI in the United States. Waikar and colleagues[32] used the Nationwide Inpatient Sample (NIS), a nationally representative database of hospital discharges, to study AKI from 1988 and 2002. Using ICD-9-CM codes to identify AKI, the study found a marked rise in the incidence and fall in the mortality associated with AKI and AKI-D. In the NIS, which includes patients younger than age 65, the incidence of AKI rose from 4 to 21 per 1000 discharges between 1988 and 2002. The study found a statistically significant decline in mortality, in contrast to the prevailing wisdom and a 2005 systematic review,[33] which suggests that mortality rates have remained unchanged over decades.

Hsu and colleagues[34] published studies on the regional and temporal variation in the incidence of AKI in the United States between 2007 and 2009. They found that the incidence of AKI-D was highest in the Midwest (523 cases/million person-years) and lowest in the Northeast (457 cases/million person-years). This incidence pattern differed from the regional variation in the incidence of end-stage renal disease (ESRD) patients requiring renal replacement therapy. Despite this incidence pattern, they found the in-hospital mortality associated with AKI-D was highest in the Northeast (25.9%) and lowest in the Midwest (19.4%).[34] In their analysis of the NIS, Hsu et al. reported that the incidence of AKI-D increased from 222 to 553 cases/million person-years between 2000 and 2009.[35] This increase was evident among all age, sex, and race subgroups evaluated. In addition, the total number of deaths associated with AKI-D more than doubled over this 10-year period.[35] These findings are similar to their previous work reporting a rising incidence of AKI-D in a large integrated administrative and laboratory database from Kaiser Permanente of Northern California between 1996 and 2003.[36] In another analysis of the NIS, Hsu and colleagues[37] investigated the reasons for the increase in AKI-D incidence. They found that six diagnoses accounted for the temporal trend in AKI-D: septicemia, hypertension, respiratory failure, coagulation/hemorrhagic disorders, shock, and liver disease. Temporal changes in procedures commonly associated with AKI-D did not account for the increase in AKI-D rates.

A 2017 study evaluating the incidence of AKI and AKI-D was performed in patients admitted to the Mayo Clinic Hospital in Rochester, Minnesota, between 2006 and 2014 and found differing results.[38] During the 9-year study period, the authors found no significant change in the annual AKI incidence rate, with a relative risk of 0.99 (95% confidence interval [CI], 0.97 to 1.01) for ICU patients and 0.993 per year (0.98 to 1.01) for general floor patients. They found similar results when using ICD-9 codes for the incidence of AKI-D and concluded that the incidence of AKI has been relatively stable over the last decade.[38]

EPIDEMIOLOGY IN DISEASE-SPECIFIC STATES

Estimates of the incidence of AKI and associated mortality have been performed in numerous conditions, including sepsis, contrast nephropathy, major surgery, and nephrotoxic antibiotic administration. Several of the largest studies are summarized in Table 45.2. A striking and consistent finding across all causes studied to date is the marked increase in mortality associated with the development of AKI.

Risk Factors for the Development of Acute Kidney Injury

AKI that occurs in the hospital or outpatient setting can be predicted with limited accuracy. For AKI caused by ischemic or toxic ATN, the severity of injury—for example, duration of hypotension, dose, or duration of nephrotoxin exposure—is an obvious risk factor for AKI. Specific predisposing demographic and clinical variables associated with a heightened risk for AKI have been investigated in a number of studies to help clinicians stratify patients according to the probability of AKI (Table 45.3).

Cardiac surgery has been the most extensively studied clinical setting for risk prediction of AKI. Cardiac surgery may cause AKI through a number of pathophysiological processes, including ischemia-reperfusion injury from hypotension, toxic injury from cardiopulmonary bypass–induced hemolysis with release of hemoglobin, inflammation, and oxidative stress.[39] The existence of large clinical databases from tens of thousands of patients undergoing cardiac surgery has enabled a number of detailed epidemiological studies of risk factors for AKI. The overall risk for AKI depends on the definition used; defined as a 25% increase in SCr, the risk is approximately 15%, whereas the risk for severe AKI requiring dialysis is significantly lower, approximately 1% to 2%. Consistently observed risk factors for severe AKI include higher preoperative SCr (or lower preoperative GFR), valve surgery, and diabetes mellitus. Scoring systems have been developed to assist clinicians to assign expected probabilities for AKI-D; the scoring systems have a moderate predictive ability, with C statistics in the order of 0.8.[40] The dominant risk factor in predicting AKI after cardiac surgery is preoperative kidney function. In scoring systems that assign points for various risk factors for AKI-D, preoperative SCr or estimated glomerular filtration rate (eGFR) are the highest weighted variables.[41,42] The association between preoperative eGFR and the risk for AKI-D is shown graphically in Fig. 45.1. Beginning at eGFR <60 mL/min/1.73 m², the risk for AKI-D increases sharply.

AKI after noncardiac surgery has been less well studied than cardiac surgery. Recent analyses of the National Surgical Quality Improvement Program included 152,244 operations, 762 of which (1%) were complicated by AKI, defined as an increase in SCr of at least 2 mg/dL or the need for dialysis.[43] Independent risk factors for AKI were age older than 56 years, male sex, emergency surgery, intraperitoneal surgery, diabetes mellitus, ascites, hypertension, and preoperative CKD. Similar to cardiac surgery scoring systems for AKI, the C statistic in this study was 0.8. In the same year, Abelha and colleagues[44] evaluated determinants of postoperative AKI in 1166 patients admitted to the postanesthesia care unit without baseline CKD. They defined AKI as an increase of 0.3 mg/dL or >50% change in SCr from baseline or a reduction in urine output of less than 0.5 mL/kg/h over a 6-hour interval within a 48-hour period after adequate volume resuscitation. In multivariate analysis, they found that risk scores such as the American Society of Anesthesiologists (ASA) Physical Status Classification System and Revised Cardiac Risk Index scores were independent preoperative determinants for AKI. In this study, they also found that patients with AKI were at threefold increased odds for hospital mortality.[44] Bell and coworkers[45] developed a prediction model for the risk for AKI after orthopedic surgery in the National Health Service Tayside region of Scotland from 2005 to 2011. AKI was graded using KDIGO criteria. They identified older age, male sex, diabetes, number of prescribed drugs, lower eGFR, use of angiotensin-converting enzyme inhibitors or angiotensin receptor blockers, and ASA grade as independent predictors of AKI. The model's C statistic was 0.74 in the development cohort, and they validated the predictive model in an external cohort of 4395 patients from a third hospital (C statistic, 0.70).[45] In a single-center cohort study of 3646 patients who underwent vascular surgery from 2000 to 2010, Huber and colleagues[46] studied the association between kidney disease and long-term cardiovascular mortality. AKI was defined using KDIGO criteria. They identified that perioperative AKI occurred in 49.4% of the cohort. Patients who experienced AKI had increasing risk for cardiovascular mortality with increasing severity of baseline CKD status.[46]

AKI after the administration of iodinated contrast material for radiological imaging or angiographic procedures (contrast-induced AKI [CI-AKI], or contrast nephropathy) is one of the most common forms of AKI in hospitalized individuals. The risk for CI-AKI depends greatly on the clinical context, with radiographic imaging constituting a significantly lower risk than angiographic imaging, in part because of the volume of administered contrast material. The incidence of CI-AKI after computed tomography (CT) is negligible for those with normal baseline renal function (eGFR >60 mL/min/1.73 m²). In a study of 421 patients with eGFR of less than 60 mL/min/1.73 m², Weisbord and coworkers[47] found an incidence of CI-AKI of 6.5% when defined as a greater than 25% increase in SCr and only 0.5% when defined as a greater than 50% increase in SCr; no patient required postprocedure renal replacement therapy, and fewer than 1% of patients with baseline eGFR >45 mL/min/1.73 m² developed

TABLE 45.2 **Incidence and Mortality of Acute Kidney Injury in Selected Conditions**

Author, Year (Reference)	Setting	Definition of AKI	Incidence	In-Hospital Mortality
Sepsis				
Rangel-Frausto et al., 1995[92]	ICU admissions with sepsis/SIRS (*n* = 2527)	Acute SCr increase to >2 mg/dL, need for dialysis, or doubling of SCr	AKI: 9% for SIRS, 51% for culture + septic shock	3%–46%, depending on severity AKI mortality not reported
Neveu et al., 1996[93]	ICU admissions with AKI and sepsis (*n* = 345)	100% increase in SCr to ≥3.5 mg/dL or BUN ≥100 mg/dL, or 100% increase in BUN or SCr	Not reported; 46% of all AKI was in the setting of sepsis	AKI from sepsis: 74% Nonseptic AKI: 45%
Hoste et al., 2003[94]	Surgical ICU admissions with sepsis (*n* = 185)	SCr rise from ≤1 to ≥2 mg/dL	AKI: 30% AKI-D: 11%	No AKI: 28% AKI: 57%
Yegenaga et al., 2004[95]	ICU admissions with sepsis/SIRS (*n* = 217)	SCr increase to >2 mg/dL	AKI: 13% AKI-D: 6%	No AKI: 24% AKI: 72% AKI-D: 69%
Bagshaw et al., 2008[29]	ICU admissions with sepsis (*n* = 33,375)	Modification of RIFLE criteria, restricted to initial 24 h of admission	AKI: 42.1% RIFLE "F": 9.6%	No AKI: 12.6% AKI: 29.7% RIFLE "F": 35.8%
Lopes et al., 2010[96]	Septic ICU admissions (*n* = 426)	RIFLE criteria	Not reported	No AKI: 15.6%, AKI: 55.8%
Pereira et al., 2017[97]	ICU admission with sepsis/septic shock (*n* = 457)	RIFLE, AKIN, and KDIGO criteria	RIFLE "R": 18.2%, "I": 23.0%, "F": 48.3% AKIN stage 1: 18.2%, stage 2: 30.0%, stage 3: 56.6% KDIGO stage 1: 21.3%, stage 2: 23.3%, stage 3: 48.3%	Not reported
Percutaneous Coronary Intervention (PCI)				
McCullough et al., 1997[98]	PCI (*n* = 1826)	Increase in SCr >25%	AKI: 14% AKI-D: 0.8%	No AKI: 1% AKI: 7% AKI-D: 36%
Rihal et al., 2002[49]	PCI (*n* = 7586)	Increase in SCr ≥0.5 mg/dL	AKI: 3.3% AKI-D: 0.3%	AKI: 22% No AKI: 1%
Marenzi et al., 2004[99]	ST-elevation acute MI treated with primary PCI (*n* = 208)	Increase in SCr >0.5 mg/dL	AKI: 19% AKI-D: 3%	AKI: 31% No AKI: 0.6%
Mehran et al., 2004[50]	PCI (*n* = 8357)	Increase in SCr ≥25% or ≥0.5 mg/dL	AKI: 13%	Not reported
Harjai et al., 2008[100]	PCI (*n* = 985)	Increase in SCr >0.5 mg/dL	AKI: 5.2% AKI-D: 0%	AKI: 40.9% No AKI: 10.2%
Brown et al., 2016[101]	PCI (*n* = 3,633,762)	ICD-9 reported AKI and AKI-D	AKI: 19.6% (2001) to 9.2% (2011) AKI-D: 28.3% (2001) to 19.9% (2011)	Not reported
Marenzi et al., 2016[102]	PCI ST-elevation MI (*n* = 3772)	Increase in SCr by 25% (AKI-25), ≥0.3 mg/dL (AKI-0.3), ≥0.5 mg/dL (AKI-0.5)	AKI-25: 15% AKI-0.3: 17% AKI-0.5: 29%	Not reported
IV Contrast for Radiological Examination				
Mitchell & Kline, 2007[103]	CT angiography to rule out pulmonary embolism in the emergency department (*n* = 1224)	Increase in SCr >25% or 0.5 mg/dL within 7 days	AKI: 4% of entire cohort, 12% of those with two SCr measurements AKI-D: 0%	Not reported
Weisbord et al., 2008[47]	Baseline eGFR <60, nonemergent CT with IV contrast	Increase in SCr ≥25%	AKI: 6.5% AKI-D: 0%	No difference in 30-day mortality for AKI vs. no AKI

Continued

TABLE 45.2 Incidence and Mortality of Acute Kidney Injury in Selected Conditions—cont'd

Author, Year (Reference)	Setting	Definition of AKI	Incidence	In-Hospital Mortality
Cardiac Surgery				
Chertow et al., 1997[104]	CABG or valvular surgery (*n* = 43,642)	Need for dialysis	AKI: not reported AKI-D: 1.1%	(30-day mortality) No AKI: 4.3% AKI: not reported AKI-D: 63.8%
Mangano et al., 1998[105]	CABG or valvular surgery (*n* = 2222)	Increase in SCr ≥0.7 mg/dL to at least 2 mg/dL	AKI: 7.7% AKI-D: 1.4%	No AKI: 0.9% AKI: 19% AKI-D: 63.8%
Ryckwaert et al., 2002[106]	CABG or valvular surgery (*n* = 591)	Increase in SCr ≥20% within 3 days of surgery	AKI: 15.6% AKI-D: 1.4%	No AKI: 1% AKI: 12% AKI-D: 37.5%
Bove et al., 2004[107]	Cardiopulmonary bypass/ CABG (including valve replacement) (*n* = 5068)	Increase in SCr ≥100%	AKI: 3.4% AKI-D: 1.9%	No AKI: 2.7% AKI: 46.2% AKI-D: 63.8%
Loef et al., 2005[108]	CABG or valvular surgery (*n* = 843)	Increase in SCr ≥25% within 7 days of surgery	AKI: 17.2% AKI-D: 0.7%	No AKI: 1.1% AKI: 14.5% AKI-D: 83.3%
Thakar et al., 2005[109]	Open-heart surgery (*n* = 18,838)	Need for dialysis	AKI: not reported AKI-D: 1.7%	Not reported
Mehta et al., 2006[41]	Cardiac surgery (*n* = 449,524)	Need for dialysis	AKI: not reported AKI-D: 1.4%	No AKI-D: 2.3% AKI-D: 43.6%
Brown et al., 2006[110]	Patients undergoing CABG (without valve replacement) (*n* = 1391)	Increase in SCr <25%, 25%–49%, 50%–99%, ≥100%	25%–49%: 16% 50%–99%: 7% ≥100%: 5%	(90-day mortality) Increase in SCr: 25%–49%: 0.5% 50%-99%: 0.8% ≥100%: 4.1%
Robert et al., 2010[111]	Cardiac surgery (*n* = 25,086)	AKIN and RIFLE criteria	AKIN: No AKI: 1.3%, stage 1: 4.1%, stage 2: 14.2%, stage 3: 36.8%; RIFLE: No AKI: 1.4%, "R": 3.3%, "I": 11.1%, "F": 36.4%	Not reported
Nephrotoxic Antibiotics				
Leehey et al., 1993[112]	Aminoglycosides (*n* = 243)	Increase in SCr = 0.5 mg/dL and 100% over baseline	AKI: 20.6% AKI-D: 1.2%	Not reported
Wingard et al., 1999[113]	Amphotericin B for aspergillosis (*n* = 239)	Increase in SCr ≥100%	AKI: 53% AKI-D: 14.5%	No AKI-D: 57% AKI-D: 76%
Bates et al., 2001[114,115]	Amphotericin B (*n* = 707) (64 received liposomal preparation)	Increase in SCr ≥50% to at least 2 mg/dL (severe: peak SCr ≥3 mg/dL)	AKI: 30% Severe AKI: 13%	No AKI: 14% AKI: 54%
Fowler et al., 2006[116]	Daptomycin (*n* = 124) or gentamicin + penicillin or vancomycin (*n* = 126)	Decrease in CrCl to <50 mL/min, or decrease in CrCl of 10 mL/min if <50 at baseline	AKI, daptomycin: 11% AKI, gentamicin: 26.3%	Not reported
Rocha et al., 2015[117]	Amphotericin B (*n* = 160)	AKI-binary criteria (≥2 times baseline, ≥0.3 mg/dL or 1.5 times baseline) KDIGO	No AKI: 21.4% AKI (≥0.3mg/dL or 1.5 times baseline): 44.4% KDIGO: No AKI: 23.9%, stage 1: 18.0%, stage 2: 30.0%, stage 3: 73.3%	No AKI: 23.9% AKI: 30.5%

TABLE 45.2 Incidence and Mortality of Acute Kidney Injury in Selected Conditions—cont'd

Author, Year (Reference)	Setting	Definition of AKI	Incidence	In-Hospital Mortality
Aortic Aneurysm Repair				
Godet et al., 1997[118]	Thoracic or thoracoabdominal aortic surgery (n = 475)	Increase in SCr to >1.7 mg/dL or 30% over baseline	AKI: 25% AKI-D: 8%	AKI (no dialysis): 38% AKI-D: 56%
Ryckwaert et al., 2003[119]	Infrarenal aortic abdominal surgery (n = 215)	Increase in SCr ≥20%	AKI: 20% AKI-D: 2.8%	No AKI: 1.2% AKI: 9.3% AKI-D: 50%
Prinssen et al., 2004[120]	Open (n = 174) or endovascular (n = 171) AAA repair	Increase in SCr ≥20%	AKI: 13% (both groups) AKI-D: not reported	Not reported
Piffaretti et al., 2012[121]	Endovascular TAA (n = 171)	RIFLE	No AKI: 4% AKI: 29%	Not reported

AAA, Abdominal aortic aneurysm; *AKI*, acute kidney injury; *AKIN*, Acute Kidney Injury Network; *BUN*, blood urea nitrogen; *CABG*, coronary artery bypass grafting; *CrCl*, creatinine clearance; *CT*, computed tomography; *DM*, diabetes mellitus; *eGFR*, estimated glomerular filtration; *HR*, hazard ratio; *ICU*, intensive care unit; *IV*, intravenous; *MI*, myocardial infarction; *PCI*, percutaneous coronary intervention; *RIFLE*, risk, injury, failure, loss of kidney function, and end-stage kidney disease; *SCr*, serum creatinine; *SIRS*, systemic inflammatory response syndrome; *TAA*, thoracic aortic aneurysm.

TABLE 45.3 Predictors of the Development of Acute Kidney Injury

Author, Year (Reference)	Clinical Setting	N (% With AKI Outcome)	AKI Definition	Identified Risk Factors in Multivariable Models
Davidson et al., 1989[122]	Diagnostic cardiac catheterization	1162 (6%)	Increase in SCr ≥0.5 mg/dL	Older age and baseline SCr ≥1.2
Rich & Crecelius, 1990[123]	Cardiac catheterization, age ≥70, including percutaneous coronary intervention	183 (11%)	Increase in SCr ≥0.5 mg/dL	Contrast volume ≥200 mL, serum albumin <3.5 mg/dL, DM, serum sodium <135 mmol/L, SCr >1.5, NYHA class III or IV
Lautin et al., 1991[124]	Femoral arteriography	394 (22%)	Increase in SCr >0.3 mg/dL and 20% over baseline	Diabetes, baseline SCr >1.5 mg/dL
McCullough et al., 1997[98]	Percutaneous coronary intervention	1826 (0.77%)	Need for dialysis	Lower baseline CrCl, diabetes, contrast volume
Godet et al., 1997[118]	Thoracoabdominal aortic surgery	475 (25%)	Increase in SCr to at least 1.7 mg/dL or ≥30% increase if preexisting CKD	Age >50, preoperative SCr >1.3, ischemia duration >30 min, use of cell saver, >5 units pRBC transfusion
Chertow et al., 1998[125]	Established AKI (placebo arm of RCT)	256 (57%)	Need for dialysis or death	Oliguria, low serum albumin, acute MI, mechanical ventilation, arrhythmias
Chertow et al., 1998[126]	Cardiac surgery	42,773 (1.1%)	Need for dialysis	Valve surgery, lower preoperative CrCl, IABP, prior heart surgery, NYHA class IV, PVD, LVEF <35%, pulmonary rales, COPD, SBP ≥160 (CABG only)
Gruberg et al., 2001[127]	Percutaneous coronary intervention	7690 (0.66%)	Need for dialysis	Non–Q-wave MI, saphenous vein graft intervention, peak postprocedural SCr, IABP, contrast volume, lower baseline CrCl
Rihal et al., 2002[49]	Percutaneous coronary intervention	7586 (3.3%)	Increase in SCr ≥0.5 mg/dL	Older age, higher baseline SCr, CHF, DM, shock, MI, PVD, contrast volume
Hoste et al., 2003[94]	Sepsis	185 (16%)	Increase in SCr to at least 2 mg/dL	pH <7.3 and SCr >1 mg/dL on day of sepsis diagnosis

Continued

TABLE 45.3 Predictors of the Development of Acute Kidney Injury—cont'd

Author, Year (Reference)	Clinical Setting	N (% With AKI Outcome)	AKI Definition	Identified Risk Factors in Multivariable Models
Mehran et al., 2004[50]	Percutaneous coronary intervention	8357 (13.1%)	Increase in SCr ≥25% or ≥0.5 mg/dL	Hypotension, IABP, CHF, CKD, DM, age >75, anemia, contrast volume
Yegenaga et al., 2004[95]	Sepsis	257 (11%)	Increase in SCr to at least 2 mg/dL or urine output <400 mL/24 h	Older age, higher SCr, higher CVP, serum bilirubin >1.5 mg/dL
Marenzi et al., 2004[99]	Percutaneous coronary intervention for acute MI	208 (19%)	Increase in SCr >0.5 mg/dL	Age ≥75, or older anterior acute MI, time to reperfusion ≥6 h, contrast volume, IABP
Thakar et al., 2005[109]	Cardiac surgery	33,217 (1.7%)	Need for dialysis	Female, CHF, IABP, COPD, insulin-requiring diabetes, previous cardiac surgery, emergency/valve surgery, higher preoperative SCr
Chawla et al., 2005[128]	Sepsis	194 (18%)	>75% increase in SCr (baseline ≤2 mg/dL) or >50% increase (baseline >2 mg/dL)	Low serum albumin, high A-a gradient, active cancer
Chertow et al., 2006[20]	Established AKI	618 (64%)	Need for dialysis	Younger age, oliguria, higher BUN, liver failure
Mehta et al., 2006[41]	Cardiac surgery	449,524 (1.4%)	Need for dialysis	Higher preoperative SCr, older age, type of surgery (±valve), diabetes, recent MI, nonwhite race, chronic lung disease, prior CABG, NYHA class IV, cardiogenic shock
Wijeysundera et al., 2007[42]	Cardiac surgery	20,131 (1.3%–2.2%)	Need for dialysis	Lower preoperative eGFR, diabetes, lower LVEF; previous cardiac surgery, procedure (±valve), urgency, and preoperative IABP
Kheterpal et al., 2009[43]	General surgery	75,952 (1%)	Need for dialysis	Age ≥56 or older man, emergency surgery, intraperitoneal surgery, DM, congestive heart failure, ascites, hypertension, CKD
Plataki et al., 2011[129]	Septic shock	390 (61%)	>50% increase in SCr, 2 times SCr, or urine output <0.5 mg/kg/h × 12 h	Delay to initiate antibiotics, intraabdominal sepsis, blood product transfusion, use of ACEI/ARB, BMI
Soto et al., 2012[129]	ICU—ARDS	751 (62%)	>25% decrease in eGFR or SCr × 1.5	BMI
Darmon et al., 2015[130]	ICU—hematological malignancies	1009 (67%)	≥0.3 mg/dL or 50% increase over baseline within 48 h	Older age, nonrenal SOFA, hypertension, tumor lysis syndrome, nephrotoxic agents, myeloma

A-a, Alveolar-arterial; *ACEI,* angiotensin-converting enzyme inhibitor; *AKI,* acute kidney injury; *ARB,* angiotensin receptor blocker; *ARDS,* acute respiratory distress syndrome; *BMI,* body mass index; *BUN,* blood urea nitrogen; *CABG,* coronary artery bypass grafting; *CHF,* congestive heart failure; *CKD,* chronic kidney disease; *COPD,* chronic obstructive pulmonary disease; *CrCl,* creatinine clearance; *DM,* diabetes mellitus; *eGFR,* estimated glomerular filtration rate; *IABP,* intraaortic balloon pump; *ICU,* intensive care unit; *LVEF,* left ventricular ejection fraction; *NYHA,* New York Heart Association; *pRBC,* packed red blood cells; *PVD,* peripheral vascular disease; *RCT,* randomized controlled trial; *SBP,* systolic blood pressure; *SOFA,* sequential organ failure assessment.

AKI. Risk factors for CI-AKI in this study included congestive heart failure, baseline SCr >1.5 mg/dL, and inpatient versus outpatient status. A 2017 single-center study[48] evaluated 17,934 emergency department visits where patients underwent contrast-enhanced, unenhanced, or no CT scan during 2009–2014 to identify the incidence of AKI. They concluded that the incidence of AKI was similar between the groups, and intravenous contrast was not associated with an increased frequency of AKI.[48] Percutaneous coronary intervention (PCI) carries a significantly higher risk for CI-AKI than CT with iodinated contrast. In 7586 patients undergoing PCI, Rihal and colleagues[49] found a 3.3% overall incidence of CI-AKI,

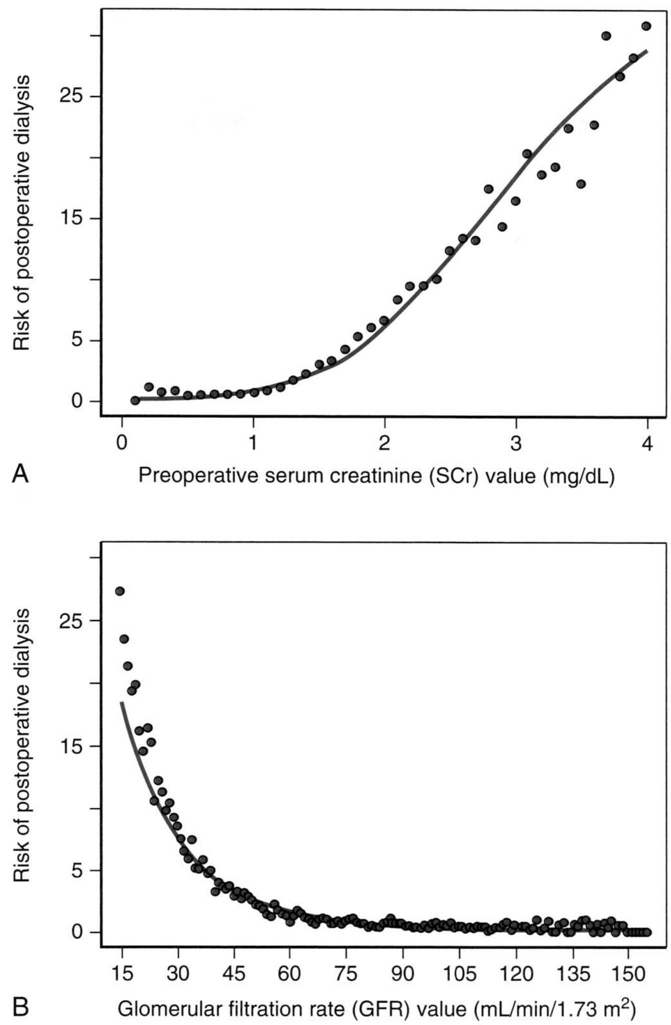

FIG. 45.1 The risk for requiring postoperative dialysis according to (A) preoperative serum creatinine concentration and (B) preoperative estimated glomerular filtration rate.

defined as a greater than 0.5 mg/dL increase in SCr; the incidence was approximately 2.5% in those with baseline SCr of less than 2 mg/dL, 22.4% in those with baseline SCr between 2.1 and 2.9 mg/dL, and 30.6% in those with baseline SCr of greater than 3 mg/dL. Mehran and associates[50] derived a risk score to predict CI-AKI in a study of 8357 patients undergoing PCI: The eight variables that independently predicted the risk were hypotension, intraaortic balloon pump, congestive heart failure, CKD, diabetes, age older than 75 years, anemia, and volume of contrast. In 2014 Tsai and colleagues[51] developed an updated risk score to predict CI-AKI using data from 947,012 patients undergoing PCI at 1253 sites in the National Cardiovascular Data Registry. They found a risk score including 11 variables provided a C statistic of 0.71 for CI-AKI and 0.89 for AKI-D after PCI.[51]

Risk Factors for Mortality Associated With Acute Kidney Injury

An accurate scoring system for risk assessment in individuals with AKI would be of considerable use, given the high mortality rates associated with AKI and extremely high costs of care. Severity scores could assist in shared clinical decision making, monitoring of resource use, and comparison of the quality of care across institutions. A number of general illness severity scores have been developed for use in the critically ill hospitalized population. Validated scoring systems for critically ill patients, such as the Acute Physiologic and Chronic Health Evaluation (APACHE) system, the Simplified Acute Physiologic Score (SAPS), and the Mortality Prediction Model, have excellent calibration and discrimination but perform less well in disease subpopulations such as patients with AKI. Several disease-specific scoring systems have been developed for patients with AKI (Table 45.4). In the PICARD study, Chertow and colleagues[20] developed predictive models in the PICARD cohort and compared them with 11 previously published scoring systems for mortality prediction in AKI. They examined three clinically relevant time points: day of AKI diagnosis, day of nephrology consultation, and, for those with AKI requiring dialysis, the first procedure day. Age, sepsis, central nervous system failure, cardiovascular failure, liver failure, hematological failure, and the need for dialysis were the significant predictors of mortality in time-varying exposure models. Mortality prediction in patients with AKI remains imperfect: The models' areas under the receiver operating characteristics curve (AUC-ROC)—a test of diagnostic performance that ranges from

TABLE 45.4 **Predictors of Mortality After Acute Kidney Injury**

Author, Year (Reference)	Clinical Setting	N (% Mortality)	AKI Definition	Identified Risk Factors for Mortality in Multivariable Models
Liano et al., 1993[132]	Hospital	328 (53%)	Increase in SCr to at least 2.0 mg/dL (baseline <1.5 mg/dL)	Coma, mechanical ventilation, hypotension, oliguria, jaundice, nephrotoxic etiology (protective), normal consciousness (protective)
Mehta & Chertow, 1995[58]	Intensive care unit	132 (70%)	Need for dialysis	Mechanical ventilation, malignancy, nonrespiratory organ system failure
Neveu et al., 1996[93]	Intensive care unit	345 (59%)	Increase in SCr to at least 3.5 mg/dL or BUN to at least 100 mg/dL, or >100% increase in SCr	Sepsis as cause of AKI, occurrence of AKI during ICU stay, oliguria, mechanical ventilation, generic severity of illness score, preadmission health status
Paganini et al., 1996[133]	Intensive care unit	512 (67%)	Need for dialysis	Male gender, mechanical ventilation, hematological dysfunction, bilirubin >2.0 mg/dL, absence of surgery, higher SCr on first dialysis treatment, increasing number of failed organ systems, increased BUN from time of admission
Chertow et al., 1998[125]	Placebo arm of randomized controlled trial	256 (36%)	Increase in SCr of ≥1 mg/dL	Male gender, mechanical ventilation, oliguria, acute myocardial infarction, stroke/seizure, hypertension (protective), low serum bicarbonate
Metnitz et al., 2002[134]	Intensive care unit	839 (63%)	Need for dialysis	Mechanical ventilation, cardiopulmonary resuscitation, treatment of complicated metabolic acidosis/alkalosis, enteral nutrition (protective)
Mehta et al., 2002[135]	Intensive care unit	605 (52%)	BUN >40 mg/dL or SCr ≥2 mg/dL; increase in SCr ≥1 mg/dL if preexisting CKD	Older age, male gender, nonrenal organ failure (respiratory, liver, and hematological), lower SCr, higher BUN, oliguria, higher heart rate
Lins et al., 2004[136]	Intensive care unit	293 (51%)	Increase in SCr to at least 2 mg/dL, or ≥50% increase in SCr if preexisting CKD	Older age, lower serum albumin, higher INR value, mechanical ventilation, CHF, higher serum bilirubin, sepsis, hypotension
Uchino et al., 2005[27]	Intensive care unit	1738 (60%)	BUN >84 mg/dL or oliguria <200 mL in 12 h	Older age, delay between admission and inclusion into study, mechanical ventilation, generic severity of illness score, vasopressor use, metabolic diagnosis (protective), hematological diagnosis, septic shock, cardiogenic shock, hepatorenal syndrome
Chertow et al., 2006[20]	Intensive care unit	618 (37%)	Increase in SCr ≥0.5 or 1 mg/dL if baseline CKD	At diagnosis: older age, CKD stage 4 (protective), high BUN, liver failure, sepsis
Waikar et al., 2007[137]	Hospitalized patients	399,928 (22% white, 19% black)	Acute renal failure ICD-9-CM code	White race (compared with black race)
Macedo et al., 2011[138]	Intensive care unit	317 (6%)	≥0.3 mg/dL or 50% increase over baseline within 48 h	Oliguria
Demirjian et al., 2011[53]	Intensive care unit	1122 (53%)	Need for dialysis	Age, chronic hypoxemia, cardiovascular disease, malignancy, immunosuppressive therapy, ischemic AKI, postoperative AKI, heart rate, mean arterial pressure, urine volume, mechanical ventilation, FiO_2 ≥0.6, interaction of mechanical ventilation and FiO_2 ≥0.6, arterial pH, arterial oxygen partial pressure, SCr, serum bicarbonate, serum phosphate, serum albumin, total bilirubin, INR, platelet count

TABLE 45.4 **Predictors of Mortality After Acute Kidney Injury—cont'd**

Author, Year (Reference)	Clinical Setting	N (% Mortality)	AKI Definition	Identified Risk Factors for Mortality in Multivariable Models
Joyce et al., 2012[139]	Intensive care unit AKI survivors	439 (23%)	Need for dialysis	Health-related qualify of life
Silver et al., 2017[140]	Posthospitalization AKI survivors	156,690 (28%)	Acute kidney injury ICD-10	Older age, female sex, rural locale, nursing home residence, cancer, liver disease, dementia, CKD, gastrointestinal bleed chemotherapy administration, number of hospitalizations, hospital length of stay, healthcare outpatient visits in the year before hospitalization with AKI

AKI, Acute kidney injury; *BUN,* blood urea nitrogen; *CHF,* congestive heart failure; *CKD,* chronic kidney disease; *FiO_2;* fraction of inspired oxygen; *ICD, International Classification of Diseases; ICU,* intensive care unit; *INR,* international normalized ratio; *NYHA,* New York Heart Association.

0.5 (no better than chance alone) to 1 (perfect prediction) and that represents the probability that a randomly selected individual who died will have a higher score than a randomly selected individual who survived—ranged from 0.5 to 0.73 in the PICARD cohort. A single-center study from Brazil[52] using a less strict definition for AKI (50% increase in SCr) examined the performance of five general and three AKI-specific scoring systems in 366 patients and found generally higher AUC-ROCs than in the multicenter PICARD cohort: On the day of nephrology consultation, the best performing general score was the SAPS II and the best performing AKI-specific score was the Stuivenberg Hospital Acute Renal Failure score, with AUC-ROCs of 0.83 and 0.81, respectively. Demirjian and colleagues[53] developed a predictive model for 60-day mortality in patients with AKI requiring renal replacement therapy in the ICU. The model used 21 independent predictors of 60-day mortality and the derived integer risk score had an AUC-ROC of 0.80, which was a better performance than other existing scoring systems.[53] In 2013 Wilson and colleagues[54] evaluated the risk for dialysis, mortality, and a combined endpoint of dialysis or death within 14 days of severe AKI onset (defined as doubling of SCr) in 6119 patients admitted to three centers at the University of Pennsylvania Health System. Their models had an AUC-ROC of 0.89 for dialysis, 0.83 for death, and 0.85 for the combined endpoint.[54]

Acute Kidney Injury in the Setting of Chronic Kidney Disease

It is intuitive that an already damaged organ is at heightened risk for acute injury. Indeed, elevated baseline SCr has been consistently reported to be a risk factor for the development of AKI in a number of settings, including radiocontrast administration, cardiac surgery, and sepsis (see Table 45.3). Patients with CKD constitute a large fraction of patients with AKI in cohort studies. One-third of patients in the PICARD cohort had CKD stage 4 or greater.[20] Similarly, in the BEST Kidney cohort, 30% of patients had impaired kidney function (defined as "any abnormal serum level of creatinine or creatinine clearance prior to hospitalization"), whereas 15% had unknown baseline kidney function.[27] In the cohort study by Nash, 151 of 332 patients with AKI had SCr concentrations of greater than 1.2 at baseline.[13] Interestingly, patients with CKD have been reported in some studies to have lower in-hospital mortality than patients without CKD who develop AKI. This finding has been noted in large database studies and studies to identify predictors of mortality after AKI. For example, among patients included in the NIS, 22% of patients with CKD and AKI-D died in hospital, compared with 30% of patients without CKD.[32] In the PICARD cohort, baseline CKD conferred a 43% (95% CI 16%–61%) lower adjusted odds of in-hospital mortality[20]; CKD was not associated with lower mortality in the BEST Kidney cohort.[27] Used as a continuous variable, higher baseline SCr has also been associated with lower mortality in studies examining outcomes after AKI.[20,55] Reasons that may underlie this seemingly paradoxical finding include confounding by malnutrition (and lower SCr values from low muscle mass) and unrecorded differences in disease severity between those with and without CKD who develop AKI. The latter may reflect relatively less severe kidney injury required in patients with CKD to manifest AKI, as currently diagnosed.

The presence or absence of CKD probably influences long-term outcome in survivors of AKI-D. In a population-based surveillance study of AKI from Calgary, among all patients with AKI who required maintenance dialysis 1 year after hospital admission, 63% had preexisting CKD (median baseline SCr 2.6 mg/dL).[56] Because the presence of CKD influences the risk for AKI, its consequences, and the propensity for the development of ESRD, future studies of AKI epidemiology should use definitions that incorporate baseline CKD stage, as has been suggested by others.[57,58] Likewise, prevention and intervention studies of AKI should be stratified on baseline kidney function.

Long-Term Implications of an Episode of Acute Kidney Injury

Parikh and associates[59] studied the long-term risk for death conferred by an episode of AKI in more than 140,000 elderly patients admitted for acute MI and found a graded association

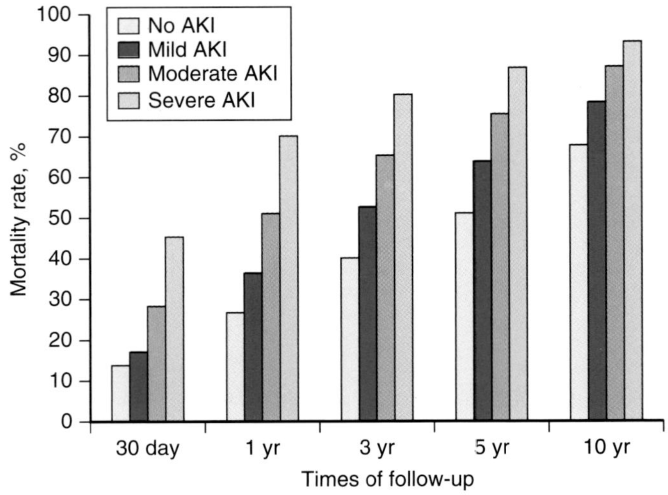

FIG. 45.2 The risk for in-hospital and long-term mortality after an episode of acute kidney injury, by severity of injury. (Modified from Parikh CR, Coca SG, Wang Y, et al., Long-term prognosis of acute kidney injury after acute myocardial infarction. *Arch Intern Med.* 2008;168(9):987-995.)

between the severity of AKI and death up to 10 years after discharge. Compared with those who did not suffer an episode of AKI, the multivariable-adjusted risk for death at 10 years was increased by 15% after mild AKI, 23% after moderate AKI, and 33% after severe AKI (Fig. 45.2). A systematic review and metaanalysis by Coca and colleagues[60] of 48 studies that reported long-term outcomes after AKI confirmed the association between AKI and long-term mortality. A 2017 systematic review by Odutayo and coworkers[61] evaluating 25 studies reported an association between AKI and long-term risks of cardiovascular events and mortality.

The kidney possesses a remarkable capacity for repair after even severe insults sufficient to cause temporary dialysis dependence.[62] The classic teaching has been that the kidneys recover completely after an episode of AKI as a result of ATN. However, even complete recovery to baseline as inferred by the SCr concentration may mask permanent structural damage to kidney parenchyma. Animal studies of AKI have found permanent damage to the microvasculature and the development of tubulointerstitial fibrosis in kidneys that apparently recovered completely from ischemia-reperfusion injury.[63,64] Episodes of AKI may therefore predispose to worsening hypertension, proteinuria, and steeper decline in GFR in survivors of the initial episode.[65]

The large study by Hsu and associates[66] using the Kaiser Permanente of Northern California database sheds light on the long-term risks of renal function decline after an episode of AKI. The investigators tracked more than 39,000 hospitalized individuals with preexisting CKD and examined long-term outcomes in those who did and did not suffer an episode of superimposed AKI. They found that superimposed AKI led to a 30% higher risk for death or ESRD during long-term follow-up of up to 7 years. Another study from the Kaiser Permanente Database examined long-term outcomes of severe AKI requiring dialysis in patients with previously normal or near-normal baseline renal function: Lo and coworkers[67] found that an episode of AKI requiring dialysis conferred a striking 28-fold increased risk for progressive CKD and a more than twofold increase in the risk for death. In a large administrative database study of Medicare beneficiaries, Ishani and associates[68] found that both AKI and CKD (individually and together) were strong predictors for the subsequent development of ESRD. In a study of 3679 patients with diabetes followed from 1999 to 2008, Thakar and co-workers[69] evaluated the effects of AKI episodes during hospitalizations on the risk for CKD. The primary outcome of the study was the development of CKD stage 4 (eGFR <30 mL/min/1.73 m^2), and AKI was defined as >0.3 mg/dL or a 1.5-fold increase in SCr relative to admission. They found that 530 people experienced an AKI episode and 157 experienced more than 1 episode. Experiencing an episode of AKI conferred slightly greater than a 3.5-fold increased hazard for CKD stage 4, and they found that each AKI episode doubled that risk.[69] Wald and colleagues[70] conducted a population-based cohort study between 1996 to 2006 in Ontario of 41,327 patients with AKI not requiring in-hospital dialysis and who survived longer than 30 days after discharge. They matched AKI patients to patients without AKI during their index hospitalization on age, sex, history of CKD, receipt of mechanical ventilation, and a propensity score for developing AKI. They found that patients with AKI had a 2.7-fold increased risk for chronic dialysis, and the absolute risk for death was eight times the rate of chronic dialysis.[70] In the AKI Risk in Derby study, Horne and associates[71] performed a prospective case-control study in a general hospital population. They matched 300 patients in a 1:1 fashion for age and baseline renal function between September 2011 and October 2012. They followed patients and measured eGFR and proteinuria at 3 months, 1 year, and 3 years. A total of 70% of the AKI patients had stage 1 AKI by a modified AKIN criteria. The clinical endpoints were CKD development or progression (defined as ≥25% decline in eGFR associated with a decline in eGFR stage). They found that 24.6% of the patients in the

AKI group versus 7.5% of the patients in the non-AKI group had CKD development or progression at 3 years.[71]

James and colleagues[72] formed a predictive model for the progression of AKI to advanced CKD. They used data to derive the model from 9973 patients hospitalized in Alberta, Canada, from 2004 to 2014 with follow-up to 2015. They externally validated the risk models in a cohort of 2761 patients hospitalized in Ontario, Canada, from 2004 to 2012 with follow-up to 2013. The two populations were based on patients with prehospitalization eGFR >45 mL/min/1.73 m^2 and survived hospitalization with AKI. They defined AKI as a SCr increase during hospitalization of >0.3 mg/dL or >50% of their prehospitalization baseline and defined advanced CKD as a sustained reduction in eGFR <30 mL/min/1.73 m^2 for at least 3 months during the year after discharge. In the derivation cohort, older age, female sex, higher baseline SCr value, albuminuria, greater severity of AKI, and higher SCr at discharge were independently associated with the outcome. The model had a C statistic of 0.81 in the external validation cohort and improved discrimination and reclassification compared with models including fewer variables.[72]

ACUTE KIDNEY INJURY IN THE DEVELOPING WORLD

The epidemiology of AKI differs tremendously between developed and developing countries because of differences in demographics, economics, geography, and comorbid disease burden.[73] Although certain features of AKI are common to both—particularly because urban centers of some developing countries increasingly resemble those in the developed world—many causes of AKI are region specific, such as envenomations from snakes,[74-76] spiders,[77] caterpillars,[78] and bees[79,80]; infectious causes such as malaria[81] and leptospirosis[82]; and crush injuries and resultant rhabdomyolysis from earthquakes.[83-86] A study published in 2015 and conducted between 2008 and 2012 studied AKI among patients in ICUs from nine centers in developed countries and five centers in emerging countries to explore differences in the epidemiology of AKI around the world. The authors found that patients in developed countries were more likely to have sepsis and higher APACHE scores but less likely to have CKD, glomerulonephritis, and interstitial nephritis. Rates of dialysis use were also quite variable, ranging from 15.2% in developed countries to 30.2% in developing countries; there are multiple reasons for these differences, including differences in ICU admission criteria, insurance, and costs of dialysis care.[87]

SUMMARY

AKI is an increasingly common and potentially catastrophic complication in hospitalized patients. Our understanding of the incidence and consequences of AKI has grown considerably, yet mortality rates remain unacceptably high despite significant advances in the care of the critically ill. CKD is a dominant risk factor for AKI, and AKI may contribute to progressive CKD. The rising incidence of AKI and CKD, and their strong associations with poor clinical outcomes, highlight the need for kidney disease prevention and treatment as major public health priorities.

A full list of references is available at www.expertconsult.com.

46

Metabolic and Nutritional Complications of Acute Kidney Injury

Edward D. Siew, MD, MSCI, and Kathleen Liu, MD, PhD, MAS

OUTLINE

The incidence of acute kidney injury (AKI) is growing and remains associated with increased mortality, cardiovascular disease, and long-term loss of kidney function.[1-4] When severe, AKI presents a complicated array of metabolic challenges affected by the underlying precipitant, the systemic response to injury, and derangements resulting from the kidney injury itself and its subsequent therapies. The extent of these abnormalities and the processes that drive them adversely affect the nutritional and metabolic status of patients with AKI and contribute to the high mortality rates observed.[3,5]

Although comorbidity burden and illness severity often are the main focus in determining prognosis, the nutritional status of patients with AKI is an overlooked but likely important determinant of morbidity and mortality. In addition to imbalances in electrolyte, acid-base, and volume status, AKI is associated with alterations in protein, carbohydrate, and lipid metabolism.[6] This chapter details these complications and includes discussion of perturbations of substrate and energy metabolism, their underlying pathophysiological mechanisms, and the challenges of providing nutritional and metabolic support to this population.

TERMINOLOGY

Different definitions have been applied to describe impaired nutritional status in acute and chronic kidney diseases, including uremic wasting, renal cachexia, malnutrition-inflammation complex, and protein-energy malnutrition. This variability has led to the potential for misinterpretation of terms and the available literature. For example, the term *malnutrition* refers specifically to a collection of findings resulting from inadequate nutrient and caloric intake that reverses upon adequate replenishment. It is well recognized, however, that although malnutrition shares some features with those seen in a variety of disease processes, differences in their timing of onset and tendency to persist despite nutritional supplementation makes them distinct from isolated malnutrition[7] (Table 46.1). For example, serum albumin, a classic biochemical marker of nutritional status, often remains relatively preserved during starvation until later stages, whereas decreases in levels during acute disease processes tend to occur earlier despite nutritional resuscitation.[8,9] Among the factors that may explain these apparent defects in nutrient utilization and enhanced catabolic responses in patients with AKI include inflammation, oxidative stress, acidemia, uremic toxin accumulation, dialytic losses, and a variety of hormonal abnormalities including insulin resistance (IR)[10] (Fig. 46.1).

In 2008 the International Society of Renal Nutrition and Metabolism proposed the consensus term *protein-energy wasting* (PEW) to characterize loss of lean body mass and energy reserves observed in kidney disease.[10] Minimum requirements to meet this diagnosis include deficiencies in biochemical (albumin, prealbumin, or cholesterol) and anthropomorphic (body mass index [BMI] <23 kg/m^2 or unintentional weight loss) measures, quantified muscle mass (bioimpedence analysis [BIA]), or midarm muscle circumference), and low dietary protein/energy intake (e.g., <0.6 g/kg/day in patients with chronic kidney disease (CDK) stages 2 to 5)[10] (Box 46.1). These criteria remain to be validated in AKI.

PREVALENCE OF PROTEIN-ENGERY WASTING IN ACUTE KIDNEY INJURY

Components of PEW are prevalent in patients with hospitalized AKI. Fiaccadori et al. observed severe preexisting malnutrition, as assessed by the Subjective Global Assessment (SGA), in 42% of 309 patients with AKI admitted to a renal intermediate care unit.[11] Affected patients experienced a higher likelihood of in-hospital death and more intensive healthcare resource utilization. Another study of 100 retrospectively identified AKI patients demonstrated that hypoalbuminemia (<3.5 g/dL) and hypocholesterolemia (<150 mg/dL) on hospital admission were independently predictive of mortality.[12] Another longitudinal study of prealbumin levels in 161 patients with AKI requiring renal consultation found that low serum prealbumin (<11 mg/dL) independently predicted in-hospital mortality after adjustment for illness severity and AKI stage.[13] Further, every 5 mg/dL increase in prealbumin level was associated with an additional 29% decrease in hospital mortality (hazard ratio [HR], 0.71; 95% confidence interval [CI], 0.52 to 0.96), suggesting its potential as a prognostic marker. It is not clear whether prealbumin and other plasma nutritional markers reflect recent nutritional status or are influenced by the extent of underlying inflammation and illness severity. More importantly, whether treatment and/or prevention of PEW affects outcomes in AKI also remains poorly addressed.

TABLE 46. 1 Common Nutritional Features in Patients With Malnutrition versus a Catabolic Disease Process

Features	Malnutrition	Catabolic Disease State
Appetite	Starving	Anorectic
Metabolic rate	Decreases adaptively	Remains the same or increases
Principal substrate	Lipids/Fatty acids	Lean body mass/ Muscle
Serum albumin	Preserved early	Depressed early
Response to nutrition	Effective	????

DYSMETABOLISM OF ACUTE KIDNEY INJURY

Acute illness can affect a patient's metabolic milieu, the effects of which can be further compounded by loss of kidney homeostatic function in patients who develop AKI. These derangements include dysregulation of the host inflammatory response as well as enhanced oxidative stress, which are implicated in the pathogenesis and outcomes in AKI and associated with abnormalities in carbohydrate, lipid, and protein metabolism (Fig. 46.2).

Inflammation

As AKI rarely occurs in isolation, the inflammation associated with it often is described in the context of the acute

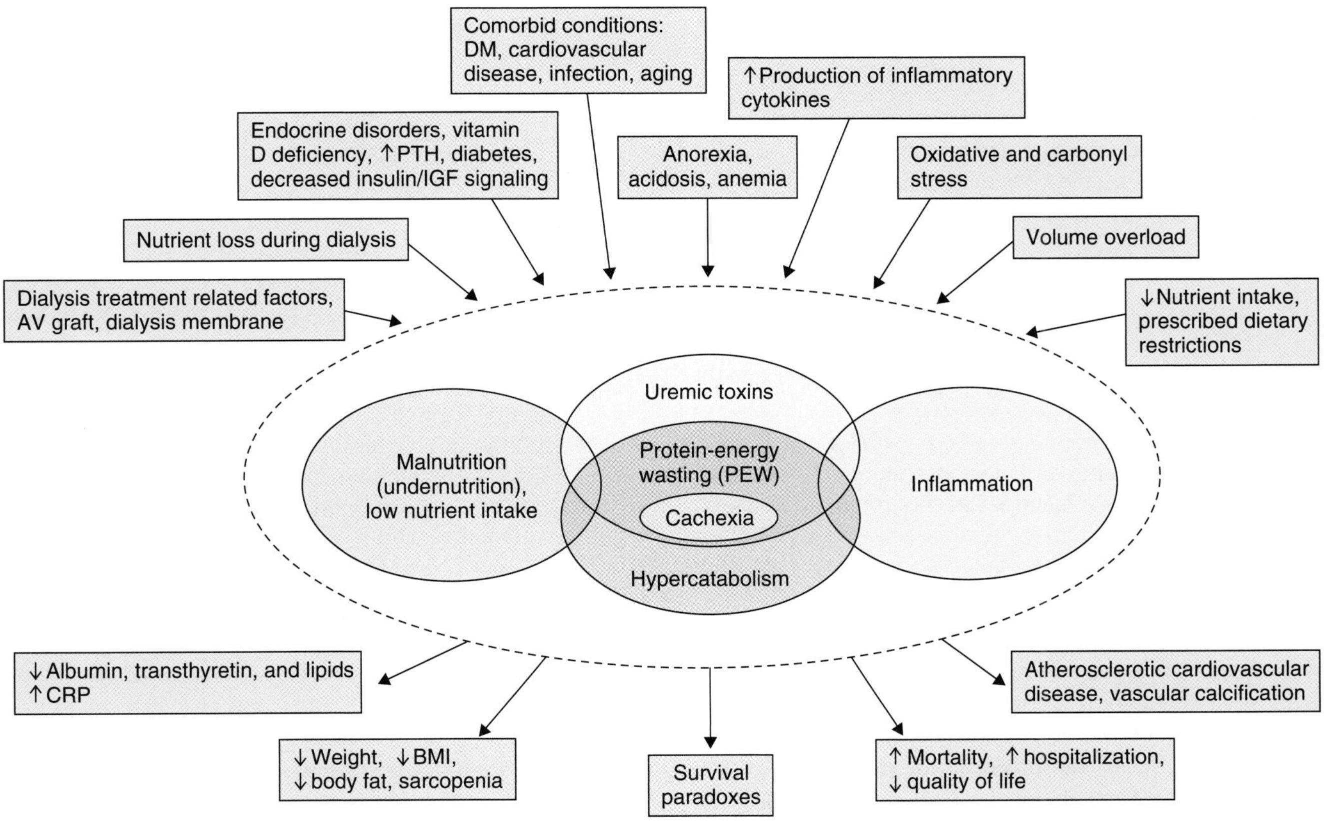

FIG. 46.1 Schematic representation of the causes and manifestations of the protein-energy wasting syndrome in kidney disease. (Reprinted by permission from Macmillan Publishers Ltd. Fouque D, Kalantar-Zadeh, K, Kopple J., et al. A proposed nomenclature and diagnostic criteria for protein-energy wasting in acute and chronic kidney disease. *Kidney Int.* 2008;73:391-398.)

BOX 46.1 Proposed Criteria for the Diagnosis of Protein-Energy Wasting Syndrome in Acute Kidney Injury or Chronic Kidney Disease

Criteria

Serum Chemistry

Serum albumin <3.8 g/100 mL (Bromcresol Green)

Serum prealbumin (transthyretin) <30 mg/100 mL (for maintenance dialysis patients only; levels may vary according to GFR level for patients with CKD stages 2–5)[a]

Serum cholesterol <100 mg/100 mL[a]

Body mass

BMI <23 kg/m^2[b]

Unintentional weight loss over time: 5% over 3 mo or 10% over 6 mo

Total body fat percentage <10%

Muscle mass

Muscle wasting: reduced muscle mass 5% over 3 mo or 10% over 6 mo

Reduced midarm muscle circumference area[c] (reduction >10% in relation to 50th percentile of reference population)

Creatinine appearance[d]

Dietary intake

Unintentional low DPI <0.80 g/kg/d for at least 2 mo[e] for dialysis patients or <0.6 g/kg/d for patients with CKD stages 2–5

Unintentional low DEI <25 kcal kg/d for at least 2 mo[e]

AKI, Acute kidney injury; *BMI*, body mass index; *CKD*, chronic kidney disease; *DEI*, dietary energy intake; *DPI*, dietary protein intake; *GFR*, glomerular filtration rate; *nPCR*, normalized protein catabolic rate; *nPNA*, normalized protein nitrogen appearance; *PEW*, protein-energy wasting.
At least three of the four listed categories (and at least one test in each of the selected category) must be satisfied for the diagnosis of kidney disease–related PEW. Optimally, each criterion should be documented on at least three occasions, preferably 2–4 wk apart.

[a]Not valid if low concentrations are due to abnormally great urinary or gastrointestinal protein losses, liver disease, or cholesterol-lowering medicines.

[b]A lower BMI might be desirable for certain Asian populations; weight must be edema-free mass, for example, postdialysis dry weight. See text for the discussion about the BMI of the healthy population.

[c]Measurement must be performed by a trained anthropometrist.

[d]Creatinine appearance is influenced by both muscle mass and meat intake.

[e]Can be assessed by dietary diaries and interviews, or for protein intake by calculation of normalized protein equivalent of total nitrogen appearance (nPNA or nPCR) as determined by urea kinetic measurements.

(Reprinted by permission from Macmillan Publishers Ltd. Fouque D, Kalantar-Zadeh, K, Kopple J., et al. A proposed nomenclature and diagnostic criteria for protein-energy wasting in acute and chronic kidney disease. *Kidney Int.* 2008;23;391-398.)

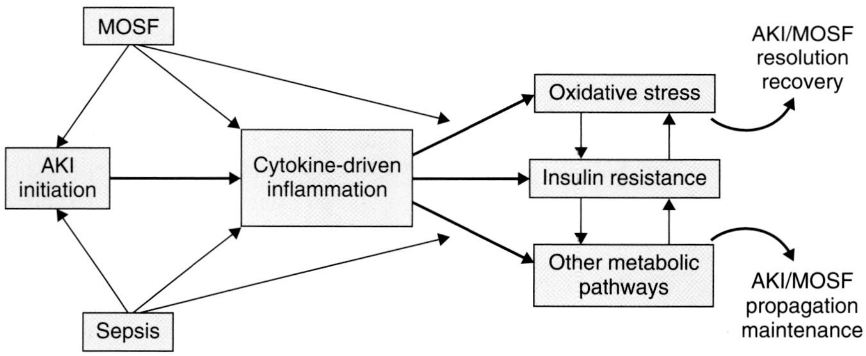

FIG. 46.2 A proposed mechanistic approach to dysmetabolism of AKI. The dysmetabolism of acute illness is exacerbated in AKI owing to loss of kidney homeostatic function. Once established, these metabolic derangements, along with other potential pathways including, but not limited to, endothelial dysfunction, interact with each other to the extent that they may be the decisive factor leading to recovery or death. On the other hand, they also represent intriguing targets for future intervention in patients with AKI. *AKI*, Acute kidney injury. (Reprinted by permission from Macmillan Publishers Ltd. Himmelfarb J, Ikizler TA. Acute kidney injury: changing lexicography, definitions, and epidemiology. *Kidney Int.* 2007;71:971-976.)

physiological disturbance from which it stems. Severe illness of almost any etiology is accompanied by a generalized host inflammatory response, referred to as the *systemic inflammatory response syndrome* (SIRS).[14] Key responses to tissue injury or infection include the elaboration of potent inflammatory mediators such as tumor necrosis factor (TNF)-α, interleukin (IL)-1, and IL-6, as well as compensatory antiinflammatory response (CARS) mediators such as IL-10 into the systemic circulation.[15] Although critical to the modulation of immunity and cellular repair, imbalances of these responses have been postulated to disrupt capillary permeability, endothelial and vasomotor function, and coagulant and complement cascades.[15] When sustained, these imbalances also adversely affect the prognosis of this patient population and possibly contribute to dysfunction in multiple organs.[16,17]

Sepsis remains one of the most potent determinants of the onset and prognosis of AKI and a classic example of the kidney's susceptibility to deranged inflammation.[18,19]

Infusion of TNF-α and IL-1 in animal models produce renal injury by promoting local neutrophil adhesion and activation as well as decrements in renal blood flow via effects on nitric oxide (NO) and prostaglandin synthesis.[20,21] An abundance of evidence implicates a critical role for local inflammation and leukocyte infiltration in the pathogenesis of AKI during sepsis,[18,22] ischemia-reperfusion,[23,24] and nephrotoxic injury.[25]

Several animal models have demonstrated systemic release of inflammatory markers including, but not limited to, TNF-α, IL-1β, C-reactive protein (CRP), and IL-12 after experimentally induced ischemia-reperfusion injury.[26-29] Ischemia-induced AKI recently was shown to result in a rapid increase in serum CRP and granulocyte colony-stimulating factor levels as well as inflammatory and functional changes in the brain not seen with ischemic liver injury. Experimental studies also have found that AKI can induce inflammation in remote organs including the lungs and brain.[29-31] Bilateral nephrectomy also has been used in animals as a model of acute renal loss not confounded by the systemic effects of ischemic injury.[28] Hoke et al. demonstrated an increase in circulating levels of IL-6 and IL-1β after bilateral nephrectomy, which was independently associated with an pulmonary inflammation.[28] Finally, a recent analysis of genomic changes in the kidney and lung after ischemic AKI detected similar upregulation in the transcription of several genes responsible for inflammation and innate immunity in both organs.[24] Functional genomic analysis suggested that increased signaling at the level of IL-6 and IL-10 might be responsible for these remote effects.

The extension of these findings to humans have been described by repeated observations detailing how a proinflammatory phenotype confers high risk for the development of AKI. Chawla et al., for example, demonstrated an independent association between elevations in plasma IL-6 levels and the development of AKI in a cohort of critically ill patients with severe sepsis.[32] Similarly, in examining the ability of inflammatory cytokines to predict AKI in 876 patients with acute respiratory distress syndrome, Liu et al. found elevations of IL-6, soluble TNF receptors, and plasminogen activator inhibitor-1 to be predictive of AKI even after adjusting for age, demographics, intervention, and severity of illness.[33]

In addition to contributing toward the pathogenesis of AKI, the extent of dysregulated inflammation and immune responses also may affect the outcome of patients with established AKI. In a subset of patients from the multicenter PICARD (Program to Improve Care in Acute Renal Disease) study, the association between serum cytokine levels and outcome was compared in critically ill patients with established AKI at the time of nephrology consultation.[34] Relative to healthy controls and patients on chronic hemodialysis, AKI patients experienced a 10- to 20-fold elevation in several proinflammatory cytokines including IL-6, IL-18, TNF-α, CRP, as well as the antiinflammatory cytokine IL-10 (Fig. 46.3). Interestingly, these elevations were observed in AKI patients both with and without evidence of sepsis. Elevations of IL-6 and IL-8 also appeared to independently predict in-hospital mortality. The same group of investigators examined the effect

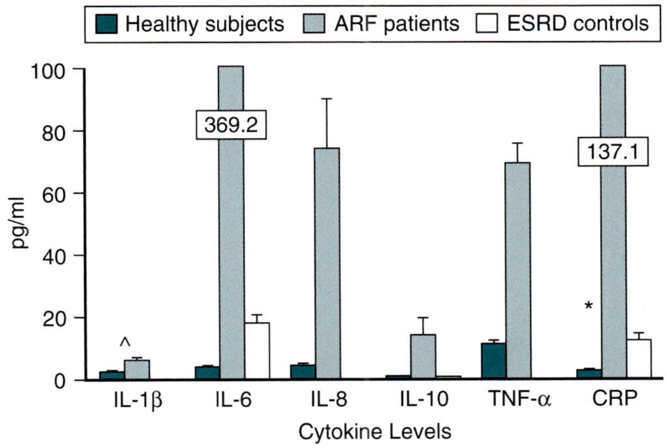

FIG. 46.3 Cytokine levels of critically ill patients with acute kidney injury at the time of nephrology consultation compared with healthy subjects or those with ESRD on chronic hemodialysis. *ESRD*, End-stage renal disease. Bars and error bars represent mean ± SEM for each time point. $P = 0.031$ for interleukin (IL)-1b (AKI study patients vs. healthy subjects); $P < 0.001$ for all other comparisons (AKI study patients vs. healthy subjects and AKI study patients vs. ESRD control patients). *CRP in mg/L. (Reprinted with permission from Macmillan Publishers Ltd. Simmons EM, Himmelfarb J, Sezer MT, et al. Plasma cytokine levels predict mortality in patients with acute renal failure. *Kidney Int.* 2004;65:1357-1365.)

of the systemic cytokine profile on immune function at the cellular level. Lipopolysaccharide stimulation of monocytes from AKI patients resulted in decreased production of inflammatory cytokines including IL-1β, TNF-α, and IL-6 compared with chronic kidney disease and end-stage renal disease patients.[35] This suggests that imbalances in inflammation and immune responses in AKI represent a complex interplay at both a local and systemic level.

In summary, dysregulated expression of pro- and antiinflammatory mediators is central to both the development of AKI as well as its consequences at a local and systemic level. The biological effects of these mediators can be extensive, affecting both distant organ function as well as the capacity to effectively utilize nutritional substrates (see substrate metabolism).

Oxidative Stress

Under normal physiological conditions, cellular injury produces reactive oxygen species (ROS), primarily through mitochondrial oxidative phosphorylation. Detoxification and decomposition of ROS occurs via endogenous antioxidant compounds. Antioxidants are a varied group of molecules with diverse functions. These include enzymes with specific catalytic properties, water- and lipid-soluble chemical moieties with relatively nonspecific scavenging capacity, and metal chelating agents, which can inhibit oxidant production. As a rule, antioxidants control the prevailing relationship between reducing and oxidizing (redox) conditions and biological systems. Once regarded as virtually a medical curiosity, a large body of evidence now implicates ROS as important mediators of ischemic and toxic tissue injury.

In a number of pathological states, increased oxidative stress can occur when an imbalance develops between oxidant production and antioxidant defense. Considerable experimental data point to increased oxidative stress as a contributor to renal tubular epithelial cell injury and AKI.[36] The dysregulated inflammatory response and uremia further potentiate oxidative stress in patients with AKI.[37] Finally, increased systemic oxidative stress may contribute to the development and maintenance of the multiple organ dysfunction syndrome, potentially mediating adverse outcomes in critically ill patients with AKI.

What Is Oxidative Stress?

Oxidative stress often is defined as a disturbance in the balance between oxidant production and antioxidant defense. An imbalance in favor of prooxidants can lead to the oxidation of macromolecules and resultant tissue injury. Oxidative processes predominantly occur within the mitochondria, and the mitochondrial cytochrome oxidase enzyme complex accounts for the majority of metabolized oxygen. The mitochondrial cytochrome enzyme complex contains four redox centers, each of which stores a single electron. Mechanisms for the simultaneous reduction of the four redox centers resulting in the transfer of electrons results are evolutionarily conserved, and limit the production of ROS. Nonetheless, mitochondrial oxygen can leak through the electron transport chain, resulting in the formation of reactive oxygen intermediates and free radicals, which can diffuse out of mitochondria and be a source of oxidative stress.

An additional important in vivo source of excess oxidants occurs through the action of another enzyme complex, nicotinamide adenine dinucleotide phosphate (NADPH) oxidase.[38] The NADPH oxidase system also is highly conserved, and is particularly important within the endothelium and in phagocytic cells for the generation of reactive oxygen intermediates. During an inflammatory response, phagocytes consume high levels of oxygen for the generation of reactive oxygen intermediates as part of the host defense against pathogens via the respiratory burst. Phagocytes contain other enzymes (including superoxide dismutase, nitric oxide synthase [NOS], and myeloperoxidase), which also contribute to the production of hydrogen peroxide, NO, peroxynitrite, and hypochlorous acid, respectively. Other enzyme systems, including xanthine oxidoreductase and uncoupled NOS, also may contribute to increased oxidative stress in the setting of AKI.

Animal Models of Oxidative Stress in Acute Kidney Injury

Sepsis and Endotoxemia: Sepsis is the most common etiology of AKI. Increased ROS production has been demonstrated to contribute to ischemic kidney injury in animal models, likely mediated through intense renal vasoconstriction. In the early phase of endotoxin-induced AKI, vasoconstriction may be mediated via activation of the sympathetic nerves and the renin-angiotensin system. The vasoconstriction can be counterbalanced through the vasodilatory effects of NO. However, increased oxidative stress results in an increase in superoxide anion production, causing NO to be scavenged, thus leading to an imbalance favoring vasoconstriction and ischemic AKI. Wang and colleagues demonstrated that during endotoxemia-related AKI in mice, several antioxidants exert a protective effect by potentiating NO function.[39] Increased tissue levels of peroxynitrite, the end product of the reaction between superoxide anion and NO, have been detected in animal models of AKI.[40]

Ischemic Acute Kidney Injury: The development of increased oxidative stress during acute renal ischemia-reperfusion has been reported in studies ranging over two decades. Furthermore the concept that damaged endothelium contributes to the pathogenesis of AKI in models of renal ischemia goes back several decades to the pioneering work of Alexander Leaf and colleagues.[41] The injured endothelium may directly lead to oxidative and nitrosative stress through activation of endothelial NADPH oxidase, and conversion of xanthine reductase to an oxidase. Increased oxidative stress also may result when injured or activated endothelium promotes infiltration of phagocytic cells into the injured kidney. Overexpression of the cell adhesion molecule ICAM-1 by vascular endothelium is observed in ischemic models of AKI, and blockade of ICAM-1 receptors attenuates injury.[42] A role for iron in mediating AKI through increased generation of oxygen-free radicals has been demonstrated in a number of studies. In a rat model of ischemia-reperfusion injury induced by clamping the renal artery, pretreatment with the iron chelator deferoxamine prevented AKI development. In this study, urinary-free iron concentration increased up to 20-fold during reperfusion.[43] It has been found that labile or catalytic iron are elevated after cardiopulmonary bypass surgery and in critical illness in humans, and are associated with increased risk for AKI and death.[44,45] Acute nitrosative stress also has been demonstrated to accompany increased oxidative stress in a rat model of acute kidney ischemia.[46] In this model system, administration of Ebselen (a scavenger of peroxynitrite), before reperfusion, was able to ameliorate ischemic kidney injury and to reduce lipid peroxidation and DNA damage in ischemic kidneys.

Nephrotoxic AKI: Increased oxidative stress also is contributory to the pathogenesis of nephrotoxic AKI.[47,48] Walker et al. demonstrated that increased oxidative stress also contributes to gentamicin-induced nephrotoxicity. Although the precise mechanisms of gentamicin nephrotoxicity remain unclear, gentamicin alters mitochondrial respiration and increases hydrogen peroxide generation. Gentamicin also has been demonstrated to induce superoxide anion and hydroxyl radical formation in renal cortical tissue.[49] Gentamicin also may mobilize iron from mitochondria, and rats treated with deferoxamine had significantly lower blood urea nitrogen levels and improved histology than untreated rats. Human studies have demonstrated excess iron accumulation in proximal tubule lysosomes in biopsies of patients with AKI.[50]

Injury from increased ROS production also has been demonstrated in models of cisplatin- and cyclosporine A-induced nephrotoxicity. In the glycerol model of myohemoglobinuric kidney injury, the resulting rhabdomyolysis and hemolysis led to the release and tubular cell absorption of heme proteins. Heme-loaded cells produce excess hydrogen peroxide, which can subsequently increase the release of iron from porphyrin compounds, thereby amplifying iron-dependent free radical generation. The resulting injury causes massive lipid peroxidation leading to cell death, a process that can be attenuated both in vitro and in vivo with the use of iron chelators such as deferoxamine.

Biomarkers of Oxidative Stress in Clinical Acute Kidney Injury

In vivo, oxygen intermediates are produced in minute quantities and have very short biological half-lives. The combination of low concentration and extreme reactivity make the in vivo detection of ROS extremely technically difficult. In response to these difficulties, the most effective strategy for understanding the underlying in vivo mechanisms of oxidative injury is to detect stable end products of redox chemistry reaction pathways. These biomarkers of increased oxidative stress measure the oxidation of important macromolecules, including lipids, carbohydrates, proteins, amino acids, and DNA. Elevations in these biomarkers (e.g., plasma protein thiol oxidation and carbonyl content, F2-isoprostanes and isofurans, and erythrocyte superoxide dismutase) provide supporting evidence for clinical AKI as a state of increased oxidative stress.[51-53]

Pro- and Antioxidant Enzyme Gene Polymorphisms in Acute Kidney Injury

In clinical AKI, several gene polymorphisms have been described in key pro- and antioxidant enzymes that could potentially account for interindividual variability in the response to AKI. Perianayagam et al. examined gene polymorphisms associated with the NADPH oxidase enzyme and the antioxidant enzyme catalase (which metabolizes hydrogen peroxide) in a cohort of 200 patients with established AKI.[54] A genotype-phenotype association was demonstrated between the NADPH oxidase genotype and plasma nitrotyrosine levels as a measure of increased oxidative and nitrosative stress. Furthermore, a genotype–phenotype association also was demonstrated between catalase genotypes and whole blood catalase activity. Of possible importance, the inheritance of an NADPH oxidase allele was associated with a 2.1-fold higher odds for dialysis requirement or hospital death.[55] Polymorphisms in the gene encoding heme oxygenase-1, the rate-limiting enzyme in the degradation of heme, which has important antioxidant functions, have been shown to be associated with increased risk for AKI.[56] These data suggest that propensity to increased oxidative stress may contribute to adverse outcomes in patients with established AKI. However, these results need to be confirmed in larger multicenter studies.

NUTRITIONAL DERANGEMENTS IN ACUTE KIDNEY INJURY

A deeper understanding of how nutritional impairment in AKI may contribute toward poor outcomes requires a discussion of its effects on the metabolism of three principle substrates: carbohydrates, protein, and lipids.

Carbohydrate Metabolism

The Kidney and Glucose Metabolism

Glucose metabolism can be impaired by defects in insulin secretion or from defects in cellular sensitivity to insulin. The kidney plays an important role in glucose metabolism. Isotopic dilution studies have demonstrated that the renal cortex is responsible for between >25% of total body glucose appearance, whereas the more metabolically active medulla accounts for up to 20% of systemic glucose utilization.[57-59] As renal function declines, diminished clearance of insulin coupled with decreased glucose utilization likely contribute to the IR observed in uremia.[60] Animal studies have demonstrated that uremia is associated with both decreased hepatic and peripheral glucose uptake and IR.[61-63]

In human studies, DeFronzo et al. used insulin clamp techniques in chronic hemodialysis patients to further characterize a diminished tissue sensitivity to insulin in advanced kidney disease.[64] The site of this altered insulin sensitivity appears to be primarily a postreceptor defect of the phosphatidylinositol 3-kinase (PI3K)-Akt signaling, which is subject to influence from inflammation, oxidative stress, and the accumulation of "uremic toxins."[65,66]

Loss of Kidney Function Alters Insulin Dispersion

The kidney is a major site for the catabolism of plasma proteins with a molecular mass less than 50 kDa. Because most polypeptide hormones have molecular masses greater than 30 kDa, metabolism by the kidney is variable. Renal metabolism of polypeptide hormones after glomerular filtration often involves the binding of the hormone to specific receptors in the luminal membrane of tubular epithelia, which is followed by uptake and either reabsorption or catabolism. The rate of glomerular filtration of peptide hormones is variable and dependent on molecular mass, shape, charge, and the degree of protein binding.

The kidney and liver are the major sites of insulin degradation. In humans, less than 1% of the filtered insulin is freely excreted in the urine. Instead, catabolism of insulin in the kidney occurs after filtration-reabsorption and peritubular uptake. The kidney also catabolizes the insulin precursor proinsulin and C-peptide, with the kidney accounting for most of the catabolism of proinsulin. Renal extraction of each of these peptides is reported to be proportional to arterial concentration. In experimental studies, ligation of the renal pedicle results in a 75% increase in the levels of plasma insulin and a 300% increase in the levels of proinsulin and C-peptide. Conversely, the kidney accounts for only one-third of the metabolic clearance rate of insulin; with liver and muscle accounting for the majority of the dispersion of this peptide. The kidney also accounts for about one-third of the metabolic clearance of glucagon as a counterregulatory hormone.

Growth Hormone and Insulin-like Growth Factor I Axis

Growth hormone (GH; molecular mass, 21.5 kDa) has a somewhat restricted filtration rate of approximately 70% compared with the rate for insulin. However, the kidney accounts for approximately 40% to 70% of the metabolic clearance rate of GH in experimental animal studies; as a result, metabolic clearance is markedly decreased kidney failure. Similar to insulin, less than 1% of filtered hormone is excreted unchanged in the urine. Many of the GH biological effects are mediated by insulin-like growth factors (IGF)-I and IGF-II. GH stimulates the synthesis and release of IGFs, and circulating IGFs exert a negative effect on GH secretion, thereby forming a hormonal axis with negative feedback. Interestingly, the biological effects of IGF-I and IGF-II are blunted when assayed in the presence of uremic serum, suggesting that uremic factors interfere with biological activity.

Insulin Resistance in Critical Illness

Hyperglycemia, along with other aspects of IR, predicts death and morbidity in the critically ill and hallmarks the so-called "diabetes of injury."[67-69] Up to 75% of patients in the intensive care unit (ICU) may have detectable IR on admission as assessed by homeostasis model assessment (HOMA), with approximately two-thirds exhibiting overt hyperglycemia (serum glucose >7 mmol/L or 126 mg/dL).[70] Traditionally, IR and hyperglycemia were considered to be a part of an overall adaptive response to increase substrate and energy availability during physiological stress.[68] However, it has become clear that these responses are unregulated, maladaptive, and may contribute to organ dysfunction, infection, polyneuropathy of critical illness, and mortality.[71-73]

Increased hepatic gluconeogenesis and glycogenolysis and decreased insulin-driven peripheral utilization are the main effectors of this phenomenon.[67,74] Cellular uptake of glucose via the glucose transporter (GLUT) systems, a family of transport proteins distributed broadly among different cell types, are downregulated normally in response to hyperglycemia, presumably to avoid intracellular glucose overload.[75] The GLUT-4 transporter is responsible for insulin-mediated glucose uptake in skeletal muscle, the main site of total body glucose disposal. The function of this transporter is often impaired in the setting of critical illness and hyperglycemia.[75,76] In contrast, the GLUT-1, GLUT-2, and GLUT-3 transporters operate independently of insulin and appear on multiple cell types including neurons, hepatocytes, endothelial cells, gastrointestinal (GI) mucosa, and renal glomerular and tubular cells.[75,77,78] Their upregulation during acute stress may partially account for the observed increase in total body glucose uptake despite frank hyperglycemia and IR in critical illness.[79] Additional evidence suggests that intracellular accumulation of glucose has direct toxic effects on cellular function via enhanced generation of free radicals (oxidative stress) from increased uncoupling of oxidative phosphorylation.[80,81] Furthermore, this process also appears to have deleterious effects on mitochondrial ultrastructure and function within hepatocytes of critically ill patients not receiving intensive insulin therapy.[82]

The mechanisms by which IR ultimately leads to poor outcomes in critical illness are not fully established. As mitochondrial dysfunction and cellular energy depletion in critical illness have been implicated in the genesis of multiple organ failure, it may be that the benefit of avoiding excessive hyperglycemia is due to a reduction in the amount of circulating glucose available for noninsulin-mediated GLUT transport and subsequent cellular glucose toxicity.[68] Indeed, one compelling finding from a post hoc analysis of intensive insulin therapy in the critically ill was a significant reduction in the occurrence of AKI.[83] It also is known that hyperglycemia hampers the immune system, largely through the impairment of neutrophil and macrophage function.[84] Insulin also is known to have an antiapoptotic role as well as antiinflammatory actions. Finally, as anabolic effects are known to extend beyond simple glucose metabolism, IR renders the body unable to effectively incorporate other nutrients.

Counterregulatory Hormones and Inflammation in the "Diabetes of Injury"

Although the mechanisms remain to be completely elucidated, it is clear that excessive counterregulatory hormone and cytokine elaboration often couple to alter glucose metabolism. Elevation of several classic "stress hormones" including glucagon, epi- and norepinephrine, cortisol, and GH oppose some of the normal actions of insulin.[85] Early infusion studies using these hormones result in marked elevation in hepatic glucose production in humans.[86,87] Epinephrine has been demonstrated to have multiple effects on glucose metabolism including impairment of insulin-mediated glucose uptake, increased glycogenolysis, and enhanced gluconeogenesis.[88,89] Glucocorticoids are known to impair insulin-mediated uptake into skeletal muscle, likely via inhibition of GLUT-4 translocation to the plasma membrane.[90] Finally, GH exerts its effect through IGF-1, which has insulin-like effects on cells. In excess, GH down-regulates expression of the insulin receptor and appears to increase gluconeogenesis.[91]

As noted previously, severe illness often induces release of potent inflammatory mediators into the systemic circulation. Many of these mediators are involved in both the pathogenesis of AKI and IR.[18,34,92,93] TNF-α, for example, has been associated with the development of IR in patients with renal impairment and those undergoing acute stress.[94,95] In addition to secretion by macrophages, TNF-α also is found in skeletal muscle, where levels are known to inversely correlate with glucose disposal.[96] Although the mechanism remains to be fully elucidated, one study demonstrated that infusion in humans induces directly suppresses phosphorylation of Akt substrate 160 leading to dysfunction of GLUT-4 translocation and glucose uptake.[97] IL-6 has been shown to inhibit insulin receptor tyrosine phosphorylation and downstream signaling in hepatocytes as well in skeletal muscle in animal models.[98-100] Elevated levels of IL-6 are also associated with IR in patients during cardiac surgery.[95]

Insulin Resistance in Acute Kidney Injury

The high prevalence of AKI in the acutely ill[2,101] and the known impairments of glucose metabolism resulting from loss of kidney function places AKI patients at high risk for IR. A large multicenter observational study of critically ill patients with established AKI recently demonstrated that hyperglycemia and IR are common and independently associated with poor outcomes.[102] In this study, IR, defined by hyperglycemia in the setting of hyperinsulinemia, was associated with increased mortality rates. Moreover, glucose levels over a period of 5 weeks were significantly higher in nonsurvivors than in survivors, and insulin levels were higher in those who died, independent of demographics and severity of illness.

Whether or not hyperglycemia and/or hyperinsulinemia contribute directly to adverse events in patients with AKI or simply reflect the severity of metabolic injury has not been established. In addition to the potential glucotoxic mechanisms, IR may itself influence outcomes through alterations in the IGF-1 and IGF binding protein (bp) axis, a critical component for insulin action. For example, increased levels of IGFbp1, a major binding protein for IGF-1, suggest hepatic IR and appear to be higher in critically ill patients who die than in those who survive.[103] IGFbp3, another binding protein for IGF-1, carries the majority (90% to 95%) of circulating IGF-1 in a ternary complex consisting of IGF-1, IGFbp3, and an acid-labile subunit. Timmins detected that a protease directed against IGFbp3 is induced in critically ill patients diminishing availability of IGF-1 and IGFbp3.[104] In survivors, recovery is associated with decreased protease activity and subsequent levels of IGF-1 and IGFbp3. These findings also are consistent with the aforementioned observational study of AKI where IGFbp3 levels were lower and IGFbp1 levels were higher in those who died.

In summary, IR is a metabolic consequence of AKI with important implications on glucose and energy homeostasis as well as for the utilization of other substrates including protein and lipids. Furthermore, IR often occurs in concert with inflammation and oxidative stress to generate the deranged metabolic milieu in AKI and contribute to the poor outcomes observed.

PROTEIN METABOLISM

A key metabolic challenge facing recovery from illness is the restoration of cellular scaffolding and machinery, functions that are critically dependent on the proper synthesis and assembly of proteins. The substrate for these tasks is amino acids from both the intake of exogenous sources and the catabolism of endogenous ones. The normal adaptive response to dietary protein restriction is to limit oxidative degradation of proteins and essential amino acids.[105] However, in AKI and other acute illness, enhanced protein catabolism often is observed and is marked by excess amino acid release from the skeletal muscle and negative nitrogen balance with protein catabolic rates of 1.4 to 1.8 g/kg/day reported in severe cases.[106-111]Amino acid transport into skeletal muscle for protein synthesis also might be impaired, partly due to hepatic extraction to support gluconeogenesis and the synthesis of acute-phase proteins.[112] The resulting imbalances in the utilization and clearance of both plasma and intracellular amino acid pools support are associated with poor prognosis in patients with AKI.[113,114] Furthermore, deranged protein catabolism also might directly impair endothelial function,[115] increase oxidative stress,[116] and weaken the immune response.[117]

Cellular protein homeostasis depends on the coordinated breakdown of proteins by a highly regulated system known as the *ubiquitin-proteasome system* (Fig. 46.4).[118] In muscle, for example, the enzyme caspase-3 first degrades myofibrillar proteins into component actin and myosin. These proteins are subsequently marked for degradation by covalent linkage to the protein factor ubiquitin by a series of conjugating enzymes. These reactions are repeated, forming a chain of several ubiquitin molecules sufficiently large enough to target the protein for degradation via a large proteolytic complex (the proteasome) into peptides and amino acids. The bulk of these amino acids are then recycled for use as an energy source or by the liver for gluconeogenesis. Several catabolic conditions including renal impairment (acute and chronic), sepsis, cancer, diabetes, AIDS, and Cushing syndrome have been associated with increased activation of the ubiquitin-proteasome proteolytic (UPP) system. In AKI, contributions from hormone imbalances, metabolic acidosis, the dialysis procedure itself, as well as underlying inflammation have been shown to enhance UPP activity and underlie the observed imbalance between protein accretion and breakdown in this disease.[113,119]

Causes of Enhanced Protein Catabolism in Acute Kidney Injury

The mechanisms driving enhanced protein catabolism in AKI have not been well characterized, although several potential contributing factors have been identified.

Inflammation

Experimental infusion studies with TNF-α have demonstrated an enhanced proteolytic effect on muscle protein as well as a reduction in protein synthesis.[120,121] Elevated IL-1 levels also appear to enhance muscle protein breakdown in animal models, which may improve with pharmacological blockade.[122] It has been shown that IL-6 is associated with accelerated muscle atrophy, which may be through direct upregulation of the UPP system and attenuated by administration of IL-6 receptor antibody.[123,124] Furthermore, in maintenance dialysis patients, IL-6 is elaborated from skeletal muscle during hemodialysis, which correlates with protein catabolism independent of amino acid availability.[125] Similarly, IL-6 and CRP levels have been shown to predict decline in serum albumin in stable hemodialysis patients despite protein intake.[126]

Although the exact mechanism by which inflammation affects protein degradation in AKI is not entirely clear, one possibility involves its effects on insulin signaling. We have previously discussed how TNF-α infusion in healthy humans induced IR by suppression of glucose uptake and metabolism in muscle.[97] Inflammation also might contribute to the production of counterregulatory hormones, thereby affecting insulin signaling, which is a key modulator of the UPP system.[127]

Insulin Resistance

Often overshadowed by its role in carbohydrate metabolism, insulin is the body's principle protein anabolic hormone with

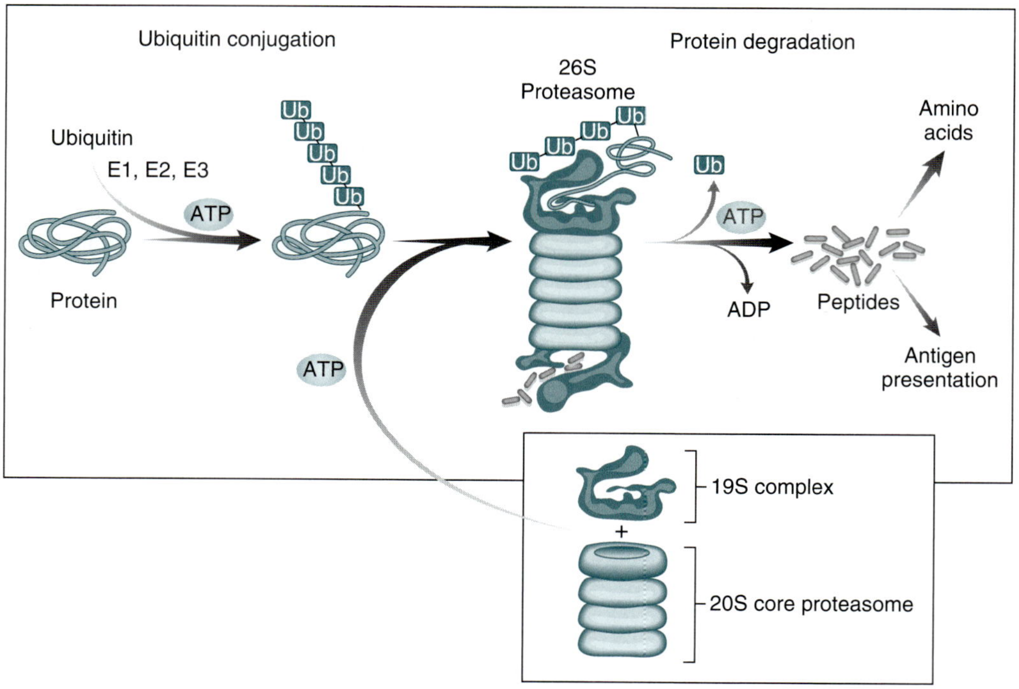

FIG. 46.4 The ubiquitin–proteasome pathway (UPP) of proteolysis. Proteins degraded by the UPP are first conjugated to ubiquitin via activation of ubiquitin via the E1 enzyme in an ATP-dependent reaction. Activated ubiquitin is transferred to an E2 carrier protein and then to the substrate protein, a reaction catalyzed by an E3 enzyme. This process is repeated as multiple ubiquitin molecules are added to form an ubiquitin chain. In ATP-dependent reactions, ubiquitin-conjugated proteins are recognized and bound by the 19S complex, which releases the ubiquitin chain and catalyzes the entry of the protein into the 20S core proteasome. Degradation occurs in the 26S core proteasome, which contains multiple proteolytic sites within its two central rings. Peptides produced by the proteasome are released and rapidly degraded to amino acids by peptidases in the cytoplasm or transported to the endoplasmic reticulum and used in the presentation of class I antigens. (From Mitch WE, Goldberg AL. Mechanisms of muscle wasting. The role of the ubiquitin-proteasome pathway. *N Engl J Med.*1996;335:1897-1905. Copyright © [1996] Massachusetts Medical Society. All rights reserved.)

effects including the suppression of protein breakdown and, to a lesser extent, promotion of amino acid uptake. Classic observations of insulinopenia in humans (i.e., uncontrolled type 1 diabetes mellitus [DM]) illustrated a condition highlighted by negative nitrogen balance, hyperaminoacidemia, and profound lean tissue atrophy, findings now known to be reversible upon the provision of insulin. The underlying mechanism appears to be suppression of insulin receptor substrate-1-associated PI3K activity resulting in stimulation of the UPP system via caspase-3.[66] Investigations using tracer kinetic models and insulin clamp techniques have suggested that the blunting of proteolysis rather than enhanced protein synthesis promote the net protein anabolic effect of insulin in the postabsorptive state.[128,129] The lack of effect on protein synthesis is probably due to the insulin-mediated decrease in amino acid release into the bloodstream. Biolo et al. examined protein metabolism in patients with insulin-dependent DM and healthy individuals and found no differences in protein turnover in the fasting or fed state between the two groups.[130] However, other studies indicate that muscle protein synthesis is sensitive to both insulin and increases in amino acid concentrations administered by IV infusion.[131]

Experimental studies suggest that enhanced protein catabolism not only applies to insulin-deficient states, but to insulin-resistant ones as well. Animal models of IR have demonstrated increased protein degradation in skeletal muscle via enhanced activation of caspase-3 and the UPP system, which are attenuated with the insulin-sensitizer rosiglitazone.[132] In humans, Chevalier et al. demonstrated a greater degree of whole-body protein breakdown and a suppressed protein anabolic response to insulin in relatively healthy obese women compared with their lean counterparts using a hyperinsulinemic, euglycemic, isoaminoacidemic clamp technique.[133] Dialysis patients with type 2 DM have been observed to have a marked increase in skeletal muscle protein breakdown compared with nondiabetic counterparts. As no significant difference in muscle protein synthesis was observed between the groups (at least in the fasting state), the net result was a significantly negative protein balance in the muscle compartment in the DM group.[134] This finding was later supported by prospective data identifying diabetes as a potent independent predictor of loss of lean body mass in chronic hemodialysis patients.[135] The role of IR in this process was examined further in a group of chronic hemodialysis patients without diabetes or severe obesity.[136] Using stable tracer isotope methodology, a positive correlation was noted between the degree of IR as quantified by HOMA score, and the amount of skeletal muscle protein breakdown. An interesting finding from this study was that, although net balance trended toward being more negative in IR, HOMA score also correlated to a lesser degree with protein synthesis. This may reflect an imperfect adaptive mechanism to preserve protein stores in the face of increased substrate availability seen in diseases marked by enhanced catabolism such as AKI. In summary, multiple lines of evidence suggest that IR is evident in AKI, is associated with enhanced protein breakdown, and represents a potential target for metabolic intervention.

Metabolic Acidosis

Metabolic acidosis is a common complication of AKI/uremia and may represent another factor associated with increased protein degradation. Elegant studies in models of acute uremia have demonstrated that acidosis is associated with accelerated skeletal muscle proteolysis and is reversible with bicarbonate supplementation.[137,138] Subsequent mechanistic studies in chronic dialysis patients using tracer isotopes have revealed enhanced whole-body protein degradation, which also was ameliorated upon correction of the acidosis.[139,140] How exactly acidosis contributes to protein catabolism is not entirely clear; however, concomitant glucocorticoid presence may play a permissive role evidenced by their requirement to stimulate degradation in other models of sepsis and acidosis.[137,141] Correction of acidosis with bicarbonate supplementation also has been demonstrated to improve IR. Mak demonstrated that 2 weeks of oral bicarbonate replacement significantly improved IR in eight chronic hemodialysis patients as measured by hyperinsulinemic euglycemic clamp. The mechanism remains unclear but may be mediated through upregulation of vitamin D 1,25(OH)2D3 levels via enhanced renal 1-α hydroxylase activity.[142]

Renal Replacement Therapy

Renal replacement therapy (RRT) engenders negative nitrogen balance through the loss of amino acids and, to a lesser degree, plasma proteins incurred during treatments. A standard intermittent hemodialysis (IHD) run with current high-flux dialysis membranes can result in losses as high as 8 to 10 g of amino acids into the dialysate.[143,144] Amino acid losses from continuous renal replacement therapy (CRRT) have generally been reported to be between 1.2 and 15 g/day, although as high as 20 to 30 g/day have been observed.[145-147] Although heavily influenced by flow and filtration rates, convective clearance of amino acids may exceed that of dialysis by up to 30%.[148] This also has direct implications for nutritional support as up to 17% of amino acids being received during the provision of total parenteral nutrition (PN) may be lost during treatment.[149] Furthermore, studies in chronic hemodialysis patients have demonstrated markedly enhanced whole-body and skeletal muscle protein catabolism during the treatment itself, likely through the induction of inflammation and oxidative stress.[125,150]

In summary, protein metabolism is a dynamic process involving a delicate balance between ongoing synthesis and catabolism. Dysregulation of this process in AKI is described by an imbalance toward the latter, often overriding attempts at increasing synthesis. The net result is ongoing negative nitrogen balance and loss of lean body mass with potential consequences for immune or organ function, liberation from mechanical ventilation, wound healing, and endothelial function. These effects combined with diminished clearance of solutes and nitrogenous wastes in AKI also have implications for the provision of nutritional support.

LIPID METABOLISM

Several studies suggest that lipid metabolism is profoundly altered in the setting of AKI.[151] In particular, the triglyceride (TG) content of lipoproteins is increased, while cholesterol content is decreased. This is true for low-density lipoprotein (LDL) and high-density lipoprotein (HDL). The major cause of impairment in lipid metabolism appears to be due to inhibition of lipolytic enzyme function, including peripheral lipoprotein lipase and hepatic TG lipase.[152] These abnormalities can be exacerbated if heparin is administered, including as an anticoagulant for dialysis therapy.[153] As a result of diminished lipolytic function, fat elimination is impaired. For example, if lipid is administered intravenously as part of PN, clearance of fat emulsion is reduced by as much as 50%. This includes clearance of both long- and medium-chain TGs.[154] Although not well studied, it also appears that plasma concentration in many fat-soluble vitamins (including vitamins A, D, and E) may be decreased in the setting of AKI. In contrast, vitamin K stores appear to be replete in this clinical setting.[155]

Provision of Nutritional Support

Although AKI patients have proven to be susceptible to PEW and its complications, several challenges arise in providing nutritional support to this population. It is well known, for example, that AKI patients are especially prone to fluid and solute overload from aggressive resuscitation, diminished clearance, and third spacing from underlying illness. Not only does this hinder accurate assessment of nutritional status, but it also heightens concerns over the potential consequences of overfeeding including worsening azotemia, hyperglycemia, volume status, hypercapnia, electrolyte abnormalities, lipid toxicity, and increased infections.[156] These concerns, however, must be reconciled with observations that targeted goals of supplementation are often unmet in the ICU and are associated with adverse clinical outcomes.[157-160] Unfortunately, the provision of nutritional support in AKI remains hindered by a paucity of adequate randomized controlled trials targeting hard clinical outcomes. In addition, the heterogeneity in type, timing, and severity of AKI as well as the varying comorbidity burden of these patients makes a uniform set of recommendations for all AKI patients unfeasible. Based on the available evidence, however, several recent reviews have been published,[161-164] and consensus guidelines, based largely on expert opinion, are available for patients with

TABLE 46.2 **Macronutrient Guidelines for Adult Patients With Acute Kidney Injury**

Guidelines	Energy	Protein	Comments
ESPEN Guidelines 2006	20–30 kcal/kg/d Carbohydrate: 3–5 (max 7) g/kg/d Fat: 0.8–1.2 (max 1.5) g/kg/d	Conservative: 0.6–0.8 g/kg/d Extracorporeal therapy: 1.0–1.5 g/kg/d CRRT: ≤1.7 g/kg/d	Adapt to individual needs in cases of underweight/obesity
SCCM/ASPEN 2016	25–30 kcal/kg/d	1.2–2.0 g/kg/d ≤2.5 g/kg/d on RRT	Protein should not be restricted as a means to avoid/delay initiating dialysis therapy

ASPEN, American Society for Parenteral and Enteral Nutrition; *ESPEN*, European Society of Parenteral and Enteral Nutrition; *SCCM*, Society of Critical Care Medicine.

AKI from various nutritional societies including the 2009 European Society for Clinical Nutrition and Metabolism (ESPEN) and the 2016 American Society for Parenteral and Enteral Nutrition (ASPEN)/Society of Critical Care Medicine (SCCM) (Table 46.2).

Energy Requirements

Indirect calorimetry (IC), which measures oxygen consumption and carbon dioxide production, provides an assessment of energy expenditure. It is considered the gold standard in critically ill patients and is preferred over estimating equations, although widespread use may be limited by availability of a metabolic cart, expertise, and cost.[161,163,165,166] Measurements made by IC also can be affected by variations in ventilator and oxygen settings, patient agitation/thermogenesis, hypothermia (especially during CRRT), volume status, and loss of carbon dioxide via dialysis or ventilator/cuff leak. Observational studies using IC suggest that resting energy expenditure (REE) in AKI appears to be principally determined by the acute illness associated with AKI rather than by the renal impairment itself. One study found an approximate 30% relative increase in REE in patients with sepsis-related AKI compared with healthy controls.[74] However, when patients with "isolated" AKI, including such causes as drug-induced interstitial nephritis or glomerulonephritis, were examined, there was no similar increase in REE relative to these same controls. Another study comparing IC with estimating equations in stable mechanically ventilated patients could not demonstrate a marked increase in REE between those with and without kidney injury.[73] Based on these observations, ESPEN has recommended energy intake of 20 to 30 kcal/kg/day (nonprotein calories) depending on estimated requirement. If estimating equations are to be used, it has been recommended that no more than 1.3 times the REE be used to estimate caloric requirement.[162,167] More recently, the 2016 ASPEN/SCCM guidelines recommend a 25 to 30 kcal/kg/day target using standard enteral formulations. However, specialty formulations lower in certain electrolytes can be used if electrolyte abnormalities develop.

Protein Requirement

Standard enteral formulae used broadly in critically ill patients are generally whole-protein solutions. Although many are sufficient in protein content, they often are accompanied by a larger electrolyte burden. Other formulae containing peptides or amino acids in powder form are also available, although they may be limited in terms of nutrient variability, osmolality, and ease of administration. Several enteral formulas with mixed essential and nonessential amino acids have been adapted for use in chronic uremia (i.e., patients with end-stage renal disease) and have been recommended as a "reasonable" option for AKI patients, largely based on lower electrolyte content (potassium/phosphorous).[164,167] Patients with AKI, especially those RRT, can experience enhanced protein catabolism with normalized protein catabolic rates of between 1.4 and 1.8 g/kg/day).[109-111] Optimal dosing of protein in AKI as well as the appropriate target for nitrogen balance remain to be determined. An early observation of 40 patients on continuous veno-venous hemofiltration estimated that between 1.5 and 1.8 g/kg/day of protein would be needed to achieve nitrogen balance.[168] Increases in the dose of protein supplementation also were accompanied by an increase in protein catabolism, although perhaps somewhat less so with lower energy intakes of 25 to 35 kcal/kg/day (Fig. 46.5). A subsequent nonrandomized study of patients on CRRT compared a higher dose of dietary protein supplementation 2.5 g/kg/day to a group of patients receiving standard-of-care 1.2 g/kg/day with both receiving equal amounts of calories.[169] Patients receiving the higher dose of protein were more likely to achieve a positive nitrogen balance at any time during follow-up (53.6% vs. 36.7%; $P < 0.05$) and trended toward having less overall negative nitrogen balance but required more CRRT due to azotemia. Scheinkestel et al. performed a study randomizing patients to either 2 g/kg/day or an escalating regimen of 1.5, 2, and 2.5 g/kg/day of protein supplementation with energy requirements estimated by Schonfield equation or IC.[114] Nitrogen balance was more likely to be positive with doses of greater than 2 g/kg/day and was associated with improved outcome after adjustment for age, sex, and severity of illness. A subsequent study examined the effect of varying energy intakes on achieving positive nitrogen balance using a cross-over design in a small group of patients with AKI.[170] Comparing 30 versus 40 kcal/kg/day using a fixed protein dose of approximating 1.5 g/kg/day, the higher energy regimen did not improve nitrogen balance and was associated with increased fluid administration,

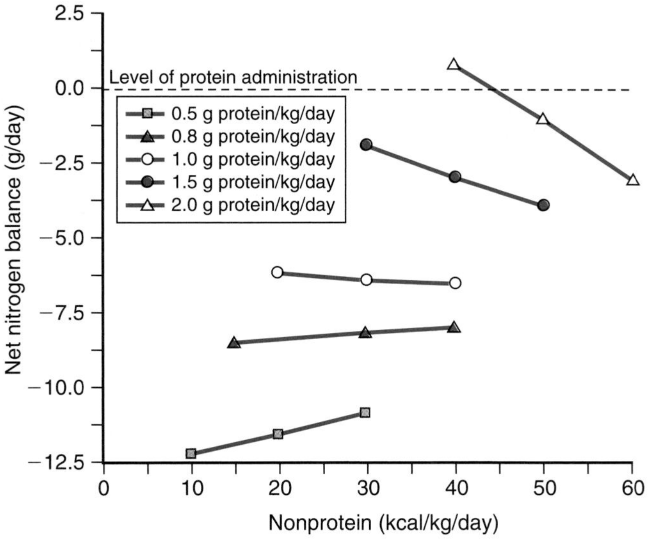

FIG. 46.5 Interaction between net nitrogen balance and non-protein calories at various protein intakes in patients with severe AKI receiving CVVH. Model assumes a patient weight of 68 kg and previous day's nPCR value of 1.59 g protein/kg/day. Net nitrogen balance was calculated using a predicted nPCR for a given level of energy and protein support. This figure illustrates that higher levels of protein may be necessary to achieve positive nitrogen balance in critically ill patients with AKI. *AKI*, Acute kidney injury; *CVVH*, continuous veno-venous hemofiltration; *nPCR*, normalized protein catabolic rate.

serum TG and glucose levels, and insulin requirement. Based on the above data, ESPEN previously recommended protein dosing based on the expected degree of catabolism with 0.6 to 0.8 g/kg/day for conservative therapy, 1 to 1.5 g/kg/day for extracorporeal treatment, and a maximum of 1.7 g/kg/day in hypercatabolism.[167] More recent ASPEN/SCCM guidelines recommend a standard enteral formulation targeting protein intake of 1.2 to 2 g/kg actual body weight per day and up to a maximum of 2.5 g/kg/day among those receiving RRT. Further adequately powered, well-designed trials with clinical endpoints and safety monitoring are required to make more specific recommendations.

Lipids

Impaired lipolysis characterizes the main lipid abnormality of AKI resulting in hypertriglyceridemia, elevated very low-density lipoprotein and LDL levels, and diminished HDL levels. Consequently, it has been recommended that supplementation remain between 0.8 and 1.2 g/kg/day[170] with a general recommendation that total caloric intake from fat calories not exceed 25% to 35%.[162,171] This goal can usually be met with 10% to 30% lipid formulations. The contribution of lipid-based medications such as propofol also should be considered.

Parenteral lipid emulsions usually contain long-chain TGs that are mostly derived from soybean oil, but fat emulsions containing a various mixture of long- and medium-chain TGs (coconut oil) and/or olive oil and/or fish oil are available. Whether a lower content of polyunsaturated fatty acids yields the proposed advantages and a reduction in proinflammatory side effects is unknown. The benefits of medium-chain TGs in PN formulations compared with long-chain TGs also remain unclear and are not widely available.[103] Advantages of IV lipids include their high specific energy content, a low osmolality, provision of essential fatty acids to prevent deficiency syndromes, a lower rate of hepatic lipid accumulation, a lower risk for inducing hyperglycemia, and reduced carbon dioxide production (especially relevant in patients with respiratory failure). Periodic monitoring of TG levels and liver function also are recommended, especially when PN is employed with adjustments made as necessary to avoid problems associated with hypertriglyceridemia.

"Immunonutrition," Micronutrients, and Other Additives

Using additives that modulate inflammatory or immune responses has garnered interest in recent years.[172] Glutamine is a nonessential amino acid that is abundantly synthesized in skeletal muscle under normal conditions that is often regarded as conditionally essential during catabolic illness. The observations that increased utilization by immune cells occurs during critical illness and that low levels associate with poor outcomes have suggested that supplementation may be helpful and led to the concept of "immunonutrition" or "pharmaconutrition." Even less is known about their role in AKI; however, significant losses of glutamine (3.5 to 3.6 g/day) have been demonstrated in patients on CRRT, suggesting the need for supplementation although dose and safety remain undetermined.[173]

A number of small underpowered and relatively heterogeneous trials largely failed to demonstrate significant mortality benefit.[123,128-130,172] A recent large randomized clinical trial examined the effects of treatment with glutamine and antioxidants (selenium, zinc, β-carotene, and vitamins E and C) in 1223 mechanically ventilated patients with two or more organ failures in a 2 × 2 factorial design.[174] Supplements were started within 24 hours of ICU admission and provided enterally and intravenously. Median time to starting nutrition was within 24 hours of the first organ failure. Eighty percent of patients received enteral nutrition (EN) only, and <10% received any PN. There were no differences in the type or amount of calories or protein received in any study arm. A trend toward higher 28-day mortality was observed among those receiving glutamine than those who did not (32.4% vs. 28.2%; $P = 0.05$), with no significant differences observed between those receiving antioxidant supplements and those who did not. No interaction was observed in patients receiving both. Among secondary outcomes, in-hospital and 6-month mortality were higher among patients receiving glutamine than those who did not, as well as longer ICU length of stay. Supplementation with glutamine (enterally or parenterally) is currently not recommended for routine use in critically ill patients; however, some interest remains in the use of these formulations in specific subpopulations with specific pathologies including traumatic brain injury and trauma; additional study remains needed in AKI.

Other antioxidants have been evaluated in the general ICU setting. *N*-acetyl-cysteine, a thiol-containing antioxidant, has minimal toxicity and is routinely used for the treatment of acute liver failure, in particular in the context of acetaminophen overdose. Small trials evaluating its use for treatment of acute lung injury in critically ill patients have yielded mixed results. Although PN enriched with antiinflammatory fish oils and antioxidants was shown in a small trial in patients with acute respiratory distress syndrome to improve clinical outcomes, there was no observed benefit in the larger OMEGA clinical trial, which was stopped for futility.[175] In a single-center randomized clinical trial, patients receiving methylene blue (an inhibitor of the NO pathway) improved oxygen delivery, reduced body temperature, and reduced requirements for pressor support. In animal models of ischemic AKI, edaravone (a free radical scavenger) and mesna (a thiol-containing antioxidant) have demonstrated renoprotective effects and thus may be suitable for clinical trials in patients with AKI. However, the lack of compelling evidence for immunomodulatory nutrition regimens has made them difficult to recommend for routine use in the critically ill or in AKI.[167,176,177]

Alterations in the metabolism of vitamins and trace elements in AKI patients have not been well studied. In patients receiving CRRT, losses of water-soluble vitamins in effluent have been reported, although limited data exist to support specific recommendations for replacement. For example, vitamin C loss can occur during CRRT but concerns over the potential for secondary oxalosis led the ESPEN in 2009 to recommend not exceeding 30 to 50 mg/day in patients on CRRT.[178-180] Similarly, vitamin A may accumulate in renal impairment as a result of diminished clearance of retinol-binding protein and retinol, which also are poorly dialyzed.[181] If supplementation is deemed necessary after careful weighing of the risk and potential benefits, a conservative approach coupled with careful monitoring for signs and symptoms of vitamin A toxicity also has been recommended.[181,182] Folate losses also have been reported in one study to be about 265 ug/day.[179] Thiamine (vitamin B_1), vitamin B_6, selenium, zinc, and copper losses also have been reported in patients undergoing CRRT with suggestions for replacement at doses greater than the recommended dietary allowance.[147,183] Many of these vitamins can be found in commercially available multivitamins tailored to patients with kidney disease.

Lastly, as electrolyte requirements will vary among a heterogeneous AKI population and can change quickly (with and without RRT), there also are currently no "standard" recommendations for electrolyte replacement. Although special formulations lower in potassium and phosphorous may benefit some patients, strategies for replacement should be evaluated on an individual and day-to-day basis with frequent monitoring and in concert with treating providers, including nephrologists and intensivists.

Insulin

Given the discussed adverse effects that hyperglycemia and IR have on clinical outcomes, attempts to control this derangement has been well studied. One early study of intensive insulin therapy designed to maintain blood glucose ≤110 mg/dL was shown to reduce morbidity and mortality in a surgical ICU.[184] Although mortality data in a subsequent study from a medical ICU were equivocal, subgroup analysis suggested that benefit might be derived in those staying in the ICU for greater than 3 days.[185] The effect of intensive insulin therapy in patients with established AKI remain to be determined; however, intensive insulin therapy has been postulated to have a role in the prevention of AKI because a secondary analysis of both Leuven trials, intensive insulin therapy was associated with reductions in the development of subsequent AKI.[83] This effect was seen more prominently in surgical patients than medical, possibly due to lesser severity of illness in the former. Two subsequent trials in mixed ICU populations challenged this potential benefit of intensive insulin therapy, with both terminating early because of increased hypoglycemia in patients receiving intensive insulin therapy with neither showing improvement in short-term mortality.[186,187] Recently, results from a larger multinational prospective randomized trial (NICE-SUGAR Study) were published,[188] confirming the potential harm of overly tight glucose control. This well-powered study randomized 6104 critically ill patients anticipated to remain in the ICU for more than 3 days to tight (81 to 108 mg/dL) or moderate (144 to 180 mg/dL) glycemic control. Using the primary endpoint of death at 90 days, intensive glucose control resulted in a higher rate of death (27.5% vs. 24.9%; $P = 0.02$) with severe hypoglycemia (blood glucose level ≤40) also observed more commonly among patients undergoing intensive therapy (6.8% vs. 0.5%; $P = 0.001$). Of note, no differences in the need for or days of RRT were observed between both groups despite similar renal function at study entry.

Based on these results, the target blood glucose of 140 or 150 to 180 mg/dL for general ICU populations has been recommended. As the attendant risk for hypoglycemia may be even more severe in patients with AKI, especially those requiring RRT,[185] attention to potential contributions from nephrological care to both hypoglycemia and hyperglycemia is warranted. For example, awareness of how changes in delivery/dose of RRT may affect glucose levels in patients receiving insulin therapy as well as the glucose content of dialysate/replacement fluids, PN, and medications are paramount to reducing risk.[189]

Route

Enteral versus parenteral. Traditional teaching promotes EN as the preferred route of supplementation in the acutely ill, with purported benefits including maintenance of intestinal mucosa to minimize bacterial translocation, less infectious risk, and lower cost.[190] In support of this teaching, one observational multicenter study of patients with severe sepsis or septic shock found the use of PN to be independently predictive of mortality (odds ratio, 2.09; 95% CI, 1.29 to 3.37) despite similarities in mean glucose concentrations between those receiving PN and those receiving EN.[191] However, systematic reviews of studies comparing PN with EN have not demonstrated a clear mortality benefit with the latter, although they have suggested less infectious complications, possibly due to a higher incidence of hyperglycemia and the need for central access with PN.[177,192,193] Currently, ESPEN, ASPEN, and the critical care group of Canada remain supportive of the primary use of EN and do not recommend the routine exclusive use of PN in patients with functioning GI tracts.[167,177,194]

However, two recent trials, CALORIES and NUTRIREA-2, have provided further insight into this question. CALORIES was a pragmatic trial that randomized 2388 patients to EN versus PN among patients who were anticipated to be in the ICU for more than 3 days.[195] Target energy replacement was 25 kcal/kg actual body weight within 48 to 72 hours of ICU admission. The amount of protein and caloric intake and adherence rates were similar between groups; however, targets were not met for the majority of patients. No difference in the primary outcome of 30-day mortality (33.1% PN vs. 34.2% EN; P = 0.57) was observed. The mean number of infectious complications also were similar in both groups (0.22 vs. 0.21; P = 0.72). Adverse events differed between groups with patients receiving EN experiencing more vomiting and hypoglycemia, whereas patients receiving PN tended to have more frequent elevation of liver enzymes. Notably, most patients did not have malnutrition defined on the basis of BMI and weight loss over the 5-day duration of the protocol. Another recent multicenter study performed in French ICUs (NUTRIREA-2) randomized 2410 patients to PN or EN targeting 20 to 25 kcal/kg/day within 24 hours of intubation.[196] In contrast to the CALORIES study, this study focused on patients receiving invasive mechanical ventilation and vasopressor support. The trial was stopped early because there was no difference in 28-day mortality (37% EN vs. 35% PN; P = 0.33). Furthermore, no differences in ICU-acquired infections were noted and the EN group experienced higher rates of GI complications including vomiting (34% vs. 20%; P < 0.001, diarrhea (36% vs. 33%; P = 0.009), and bowel ischemia (2% vs. <1; P = 0.007). These studies suggest that the negative effects of PN on clinical outcomes in modern-day practice may be overstated and that in patients who are severely ill, insisting on early initiation of full or near-full doses of EN may even increase the risk for GI complications.

Timing

The optimal timing to initiate nutritional therapy in patients with AKI is not established but has been addressed by recent trials in the critically ill (Table 46.3).[69] The EPaNIC (Early versus Late Parenteral Nutrition in Critically Ill Adults) study randomized 4640 critically ill patients already receiving EN to early initiation of PN within 48 hours of ICU admission versus initiation after day 7.[69,198] The amount of PN was titrated to meet caloric requirements in combination with EN to reach caloric goals. The primary endpoint of the number of ICU days differed between the two groups, with patients in the late-initiation group experiencing a 6.3% reduction in length of stay. Modest reductions in infectious complications (26.2 vs. 22.8 %; P = 0.008), mean cost ($1600), and a median reduction of 3 days in the duration of RRT (P = 0.008) were also observed; however, no difference in mortality at 90 days were noted. In the EDEN randomized trial,[70,199] 1000 adults with acute lung injury requiring mechanical ventilation were randomized to trophic or full enteral feeding for 1 week. Patients were excluded if there was a contraindication to enteral feeding, including high-dose vasopressors. Eligible patients were randomized to initial trophic-feeding (EN at 10 mL/h, or 10 to 20 kcal/h) compared with the full-feeding group, which was initiated at 25 mL/hour and rapidly titrated to a target of 25 to 30 kcal/kg/day of nonprotein calories and 1.2 to 1.6 g/kg/day of protein. No difference in the primary outcome of ventilator-free days nor other important secondary outcomes including 60-day mortality and infectious complications were observed, although the early full-feeding group experienced more vomiting, high gastric residuals, and insulin requirements. A similar study (PermiT) was recently performed in 895 general ICU patients randomized within 48 hours of ICU admission to permissive underfeeding (40% to 60% of caloric requirements until day 14 or initiation of oral feeding) or standard feeding targeting 70% to 100% of caloric requirements with enteral feeds.[71,200] During the intervention period, the average caloric intake was 46% of daily requirements in the underfeeding group versus 71% in the full feeding group. Protein intake did not significantly differ between groups. No difference in 90-day mortality was observed between the groups (27.2% in the underfeeding vs. 28.9% in the full feeding group, P = 0.58) or in days of mechanical ventilation or hypoglycemia. Post hoc analysis suggested that incident RRT was required less frequently in the permissive underfeeding group (7.1% vs. 11.4, P = 0.04), generating an interesting hypothesis about whether caloric restriction might be renoprotective, as has been demonstrated in animal studies, although further research is needed.

In summary, these recent studies suggest that the benefits of early initiation of enteric feeds over PN are likely overemphasized. Early full enteric feeds appear to be associated with more complications than PN, with a small but significant increase in serious complications including bowel ischemia. That said, early enteral support is generally well tolerated in those without contraindication (e.g., anatomical, high-dose vasopressors). There may be little difference in clinical outcomes such as death or time on the ventilator between patients receiving early full versus early trophic feeds in critically ill patients. Furthermore, PN, in the short term, has a comparable safety profile to EN in the overall ICU population, although the risk for infectious

TABLE 46.3 Summary of Recent Clinical Trials of Nutrition in the Critically Ill

Study Name/ Journal/ Date/ Author	Topic	Size	Setting	Intervention	Outcomes
CALORIES, *N Engl J Med* 2014, Harvey[195]	Route	2400	Critically ill adults in the United Kingdom with unplanned admission to the ICU	EN vs. PN within 36 h of admission and used exclusively for 5 d. Energy target = 25 kcal/kg/d within 48–72 h	1. No difference in 30-d mortality (33% PN vs. 34% EN, $P = 0.57$). 2. No differences in infectious complications or mortality at 90 d. Less hypoglycemia and vomiting in PN group. Trend toward more elevation of liver enzymes in the PN group. Caloric intake similar in both groups but target not commonly achieved.
NUTRIREA-2 *Lancet* 2017, Reignier	Early route	2410	Severely critically ill (ventilated and on pressors) in French ICUs	EN vs. PN within 24 h of intubation targeting (20–25 kcal/kg/d)	1. No difference in 28-d mortality (37% EN vs. 35% PN; $P = 0.33$). 2. No difference in incidence of ICU-related infections but EN group had higher rates of vomiting, diarrhea, bowel ischemia, and acute colonic pseudo-obstruction.
EPaNIC, *N Eng J Med* 2011, Casaer	Timing (of PN)	4640	Critically ill adults receiving EN	Early: day 1 400 kcal (20% glucose), day 2, 800 kcal, day 3 PN + EN to meet caloric needs: Late: day 5 initiation of 5% glucose at same volume as early group for hydration, PN on day 8 if insufficient enteral calories	1. ICU length of stay. Late initiation group had a relative 6.3% increase in the likelihood of being discharged alive earlier from the ICU, $P = 0.04$. 2. Late initiation group with relatively lower risk for mechanical ventilation >2 d and a median reduction of 3 d of RRT, and lower cost.
J Am Med Assoc 2011, Rice (OMEGA)	Supplements	272	Critically ill adults with acute lung injury in the United States	ω-3 fatty acids, γ-linolenic acid, and antioxidants until the earliest of 21 d, 48 h of unassisted breathing, or extubation	No difference in ventilator-free days to study day 28. Stopped early for futility.
N Eng J Med 2013, Heyland	Supplements	1223	Critically ill adults in Canada	2 × 2 factorial: glutamine (0.35 g/kg/d IV per IBW) Antioxidants (500 ug selenium, 20 mg zinc + 10 mg β-carotene, 500 mg vitamin E, 1500 mg vitamin C)	1. Trend toward increasing mortality at 28 d among glutamine (32.4% vs. 27.2%; $P = 0.05$). No difference in mortality at 28 d in antioxidant arms (30.8% vs. 28.8%; $P = 0.48$).

complications increases over time. PN can be considered an adjunct if enteral goals are not being met, although it does remain more costly and may lack nonnutritional benefits to the gut.

Conclusion

AKI is a common and complex and disease associated with a wide array of metabolic derangements resulting from the primary injury, the host response, loss of renal homeostatic function, and its associated therapies (i.e., RRT). The effects of these derangements can have profound implications for the utilization and catabolism of key substrates, ultimately hindering the ability of afflicted patients to promote cellular recovery. Although adequately designed and powered studies examining the optimal approach to metabolic and nutritional support specifically targeting patients are lacking, it is clear that nutritional risk is high in this patient population and an important determinant of morbidity and mortality. Consequently, frequent ascertainment of the nutritional and metabolic demands of patients is warranted with an individualized therapeutic approach coupling the best-available evidence and guidelines for patients with comparable illness severity.

A full list of references is available at www.expertconsult.com.

47

Acute Kidney Injury Diagnostics and Biomarkers

Justin M. Belcher, MD, PhD, and Chirag R. Parikh, MD, PhD

OUTLINE

BIOMARKERS IN ACUTE KIDNEY INJURY

Acute kidney injury (AKI), previously referred to as acute renal failure (ARF), represents a common clinical problem with high mortality. It is estimated that the overall incidence of AKI among intensive care unit (ICU) patients is as high as 58%.[1] A multinational study of 29,269 critically ill patients admitted to the ICU revealed an overall occurrence of AKI requiring renal replacement therapy (RRT) of 5.7% with an associated mortality of 60.3%.[2] It is estimated that AKI in high-income countries costs US $1 billion, claims 300,000 lives, results in 170,000 end-stage renal disease (ESRD) diagnoses, and contributes to the development of 300,000 advanced chronic kidney disease (CKD) cases on an annual basis.[3] The poor outcome associated with AKI has not improved in the past few decades despite progress in the understanding of the pathophysiology of AKI and advances in therapeutics and supportive care. AKI has been increasing in frequency[4] and continues to be associated with an unacceptably high in-hospital mortality of 40% to 80% in the intensive care setting.[1,5]

Historically, the definition of AKI was not standardized, with some authors defining it by a change in urine output, others by myriad combinations of an absolute increase in creatinine from baseline, a relative change from baseline, an absolute threshold creatinine had to rise above or even the need for RRT. The barriers to research that such heterogeneity represents are obvious. In an attempt at standardization, several guidelines have been put forth defining AKI using either absolute or relative changes in serum creatinine (sCR) levels or acute changes in urine output. The Acute Dialysis Quality Initiative (ADQI) developed a set of criteria for defining AKI, based on sCR levels and urine output. These are called the RIFLE (*R*isk, *I*njury, *F*ailure, *L*oss, and *E*nd-stage) criteria. RIFLE uses relative changes in sCR and glomerular filtration rate (GFR) as criteria for its first three categories of risk, injury, and failure. In a further effort to standardize the definition of AKI, the ADQI and the Acute Kidney Injury Network (AKIN) modified the RIFLE criteria.[6-8] The AKIN group defined AKI as an abrupt (within 48 hours) reduction in kidney function currently defined as an absolute increase in sCR of ≥0.3 mg/dL (≥25 μmol/L), a percentage increase in sCR of ≥50% (1.5-fold from baseline), or a reduction in urine output (documented oliguria of <0.5 mL/kg/h for >6 hours). Finally, in 2011, the Kidney Disease: Improving Global Outcomes (KDIGO) Clinical Practice Guideline proposed something of a synthesis of these two systems and defined AKI as an increase in creatinine of ≥0.3 mg/dL within 48 hours or an increase to ≥1.5 times baseline within 7 days or urine output ≤0.5 mL/kg for 6 hours.[9] The three classification systems are summarized in Table 47.1.

A biomarker is defined as a characteristic that can be objectively measured and evaluated as an indicator of normal biological or pathogenic processes (a diagnostic biomarker), or pharmacological responses to a therapeutic intervention (a therapeutic biomarker).[10] Any parameter that can be measured—for example, proteins, lipids, genomic or proteomic patterns, imaging methods, blood pressure, electrical signals, and cells present in urine—may serve as a biomarker. Biomarkers are of different types: disease, toxicity, mechanistic, efficacy, predictive, and drug-target interaction biomarkers. Some of these markers can serve as translational markers that can be used in both preclinical and clinical settings. A surrogate endpoint marker is a biomarker that can substitute for a clinical endpoint. A surrogate endpoint marker is expected to predict clinical benefit (or harm or lack of benefit) based on epidemiological, therapeutic, pathophysiological, or other scientific evidence.[10,11] An ideal biomarker is easily measurable, noninvasive, reproducible, sensitive, cost-effective, easily interpretable, and would use readily available specimens (blood and urine). The widely accepted measure of biomarker sensitivity and specificity is the receiver operating characteristic (ROC) curve. An ROC curve is a graphical

TABLE 47.1 Classification Systems and Criteria for the Diagnosis of Acute Kidney Injury

Classification System	Criteria by Changes in Creatinine	Criteria by Changes in Urine Output
RIFLE		
R	150%–200% of baseline creatinine *or* GFR decreased by 25% (within 7 d)	<0.5 mL/kg/h for <6 h
I	200%–300% of baseline sCR *or* GFR decreased by >50%	<0.5 mL/kg/h for >12 h
F	>300% of baseline sCR *or* GFR decreased by >75% *or* sCR of >4 mg/dL in the setting of an increase of ≥0.5 mg/dL	<0.3 mL/kg/h × 24 h *or* anuria × 12 h
L	Complete loss of kidney function requiring dialysis for >4 wk	
E	Complete loss of kidney function requiring dialysis for >3 mo	
AKIN		
Stage 1	150%–200% of baseline sCR *or* increase of ≥0.3 mg/dL (within 48 h)	<0.5 mL/kg/h for >6 h
Stage 2	200%–300% of baseline sCR	< 0.5 mL/kg/h for >12 h
Stage 3	>300% of baseline sCR *or* sCR of >4 mg/dL in the setting of an increase of ≥0.5 mg/dL	<0.3 mL/kg/h × 24 h *or* anuria × 12 h
KDIGO		
Stage 1	150%–200% of baseline creatinine (within 7 d) *or* increase of ≥0.3 mg/dL (within 48 h)	<0.5 mL/kg/h for 6 h
Stage 2	200%–300% of baseline sCR	<0.5 mL/kg/h for 12 h
Stage 3	>300% of baseline sCR *or* increase in sCR to ≥4 mg/dL *or* initiation of renal replacement therapy	<0.3 mL/kg/h for 24 h *or* anuria for ≥12 h

AKIN, Acute Kidney Injury Network; *GFR*, glomerular filtration rate; *KDIGO*, Kidney Disease Improving Global Outcomes; *RIFLE*, Risk, Injury, Failure, Loss of Function, End Stage Renal Disease; *sCR*, serum creatinine.

display of tradeoffs between the true-positive rate (sensitivity) and the false-positive rate (1-specificity), when the biomarker is a continuous variable. A curve is generated; the closer the curve to the left-hand and top borders of the graph, the better the accuracy of the biomarker. The area underneath the ROC curve can range from 0.5 (*useless test performing at the level of chance*) to 1 (*perfect test*).[12] A perfect biomarker will have true-positive rate of 1 and false-positive rate of 0. As will be seen in the evaluation of biomarkers for the diagnosis of AKI, the validity of all such tests is contingent on the validity of the gold standard against which they are compared.

Creatinine as a Biomarker

Creatinine levels in the serum were first reported to be a marker of chronic nephritis more than 100 years ago[13,14] and proposed as a means of distinguishing between what has become known as AKI from CKD soon after.[15] Despite such an impressive run of clinical utility, creatinine as a biomarker of AKI has several widely recognized shortcomings. First, creatinine production and its release into the circulation is highly variable with age, sex, meat intake, muscle mass, and diseases. For example, in certain disease states such as rhabdomyolysis, sCR levels may rise more rapidly, due to the release of preformed creatinine from the damaged muscle. Second, a static measure of creatinine does not depict the real-time changes in GFR resulting from acute changes in kidney function. Given the large amounts of functional renal reserve in a healthy individual and the variable amounts of renal reserve in patients with mild renal diseases, creatinine is not a sensitive marker and does not change until significant renal damage has occurred. When creatinine levels do increase, it often takes 24 to 48 hours after the AKI (as the degree to which serum levels can rise is limited by the daily production), and at this point in most cases the acute event is remote in time and the likelihood that an intervention will alter the patient's course of kidney injury will be markedly diminished. Third, the delay in detection of AKI is exacerbated and the underestimation of its severity potentiated by a decrease in creatinine production in critically ill patients.[16] Fourth, a drug-induced alteration in tubular secretion of creatinine might result in underestimation of renal function. Fifth, the creatinine assay is subject to interference because of intake of certain drugs or because of certain pathophysiological states including hyperbilirubinemia and diabetic ketoacidosis. Finally, and perhaps most importantly, sCR is a marker of renal filtration, not structural injury. An acute rise in creatinine signals only an acute change in GFR. It is a functional rather than structural marker and thus cannot distinguish functional causes of changes in GFR such as prerenal azotemia from those involving frank structural injury such as acute tubular necrosis (ATN). Given the vast differences in mechanistic pathways, appropriate therapies, and ultimate outcomes between such disparate entities, it is likely that the inability of creatinine to distinguish between functional and structural AKI is one of the most fundamental causes of the vexing lack of therapies for acute tubular kidney injury. Urine microscopy is a time-honored test for evaluation of AKI, and seasoned physicians will attest to its value in detecting evidence of structural injury. Nevertheless, the sensitivity of this test as an early indicator of tubular injury in the kidney remains controversial.[17,18] Because of these multiple significant limitations of creatinine as a marker, there has been a great deal of interest in the identification of improved biomarkers for kidney injury.

U.S. Food and Drug Administration Critical Path Initiative

As a major initiative of the U.S. Food and Drug Administration (FDA) focusing on biomarkers, The Critical Path Initiative is an effort to stimulate and facilitate a national effort to modernize the scientific process through which a potential human drug, biological product, or medical device is transformed from a discovery or "proof of concept" into a medical product.[19,20] The FDA has provided guidelines that a biomarker can be considered "valid" only if the following conditions are met: (1) It is measured in an analytical test system with well-established performance characteristics; and (2) there is an established scientific framework or body of evidence that elucidates the physiological, pharmacological, toxicological, or clinical significance of the test result.

Need for New Biomarkers

Clinicians and researchers are in need of new biomarkers of AKI for the following reasons: (1) Rather than being injury markers, the current blood and urine markers are functional consequences of the injury itself[21]; (2) creatinine, a central component of many of the definitions of AKI,[22] is a poor biomarker because of its aforementioned characteristics; and (3) we have an urgent need for novel biomarkers to diagnose AKI at early stages, to predict outcomes in patients with AKI, to identify who will respond to a given intervention, and to ascertain whether the intervention is actually working. Critically, better biomarkers will permit better stratification of patients for clinical trials and potentially lead to identification of new therapeutics for AKI. The absence of sensitive and specific early biomarkers of AKI not only delays the diagnosis of AKI but also greatly impairs early intervention strategies and clinical trial design, thus delaying the initiation of potential therapies. As a marker in changing function, a rise in creatinine after an AKI is analogous to a change in ejection fraction (EF) after a myocardial infarction (MI). Any attempts to develop therapies for MI based solely on changes in EF would be bedeviled by poor sensitivity, poor specificity, and delayed diagnosis. By more accurately phenotyping patients with AKI due to frank structural injury, biomarkers can enhance statistical power at a given sample size by reducing misclassification, reduce trial costs by identifying those patients most likely to have progression of early AKI and prioritizing them for trial enrollment, and serve as potential outcomes measures to identify therapies that deserve further investigation in costly, large, multicenter trials.[23] In summary, the need for new biomarkers can be seen through the following list of potential applications: (1) early diagnosis; (2) to differentiate AKI subtypes (prerenal, intrinsic, postrenal); (3) to identify AKI associated with various etiologies; (4) to determine the primary location of the injury in the kidney; (5) to predict outcomes; and (6) to predict response to various therapies.[24] The same biomarker may not perform in all of these settings.

Blood and urine are two candidate fluids used to measure biomarkers of kidney injury. Urine has the advantage of being readily available noninvasively and amenable to straightforward testing by both healthcare professionals and patients themselves. In addition, the low protein content of the urine in most clinical states makes urine more favorable for proteomic approaches. On the other hand, changes in urine flow rate and concentration will have effects on the concentration of an analyte, and variations in physical and chemical properties of urine may affect the stability of the analyte and reliability of the test. Serum samples are also readily available and may be more stable than urine. The presence of abundant proteins such as albumin and immunoglobulins in the blood leads to high interference and makes proteomic approaches more challenging.

Biomarkers have been proposed to reflect injury to various parts of the nephron or to reflect interstitial disease,[24] although in many cases the specificity of particular biomarkers for specific nephron sites has not been sufficiently studied. The proximal tubule is the primary site of damage for ischemic injury or reperfusion injury as well as with most tubular toxins. Even in those cases where the primary site of injury is more distal in the nephron, the proximal tubule is often secondarily involved as well. Although there are some important exceptions to this generalization, such as lithium toxicity that predominantly occurs at distal nephron, in general a biomarker that is sensitive for proximal injury will be useful in many clinical scenarios.

An ideal AKI biomarker should be (1) easily and reliably measured in a noninvasive or minimally invasive manner; (2) stable; (3) rapidly and reliably measurable at the bedside; (4) inexpensive to measure; (5) able to detect AKI early in the course; and (6) predictive in its ability to forecast the course of AKI and potentially the future implications of AKI.

Specific Biomarkers of Acute Kidney Injury

There are many cellular proteins that are released into the urine and have been used in the past to monitor kidney injury in animals and humans.[25,26] As the concept of kidney injury biomarkers has evolved, new biomarkers have continued to be proposed and some older ones have come to receive less attention.[27] One of the earlier reviews on AKI biomarkers focused on β2-microglobulin (β2M), retinol-binding protein, *N*-acetyl-glucosaminidase (NAG), adenosine deaminase binding protein, and L-alanine aminopeptidase.[28] Since then, a plethora of proteins have been proposed, including but certainly not limited to α1-microglobulin (α1M), α-glutathione *S*-transferase (αGST), kidney injury molecule-1 (KIM-1), neutrophil gelatinase-associated lipocalin (NGAL), interleukin (IL)-18, fatty acid binding protein (FABP), cystatin C (Cys-C), netrin-1, clusterin, trefoil factor-3, osteopontin (OPN), monocyte chemotactic protein-1 (MCP-1), uromodulin, YKL-40, IL-6, IL-10, tissue inhibitor of metalloproteinase 2 (TIMP2) and insulin-like growth factor binding protein 7 (IGFBP7). The location of production and physiological significance of multiple biomarkers are shown in Fig. 47.1. Because of the limitations of the length of this review, we will focus on an overview of important features of some of these markers (particularly urinary rather than serum) without being able to do justice to the data available on the full scope of current research.

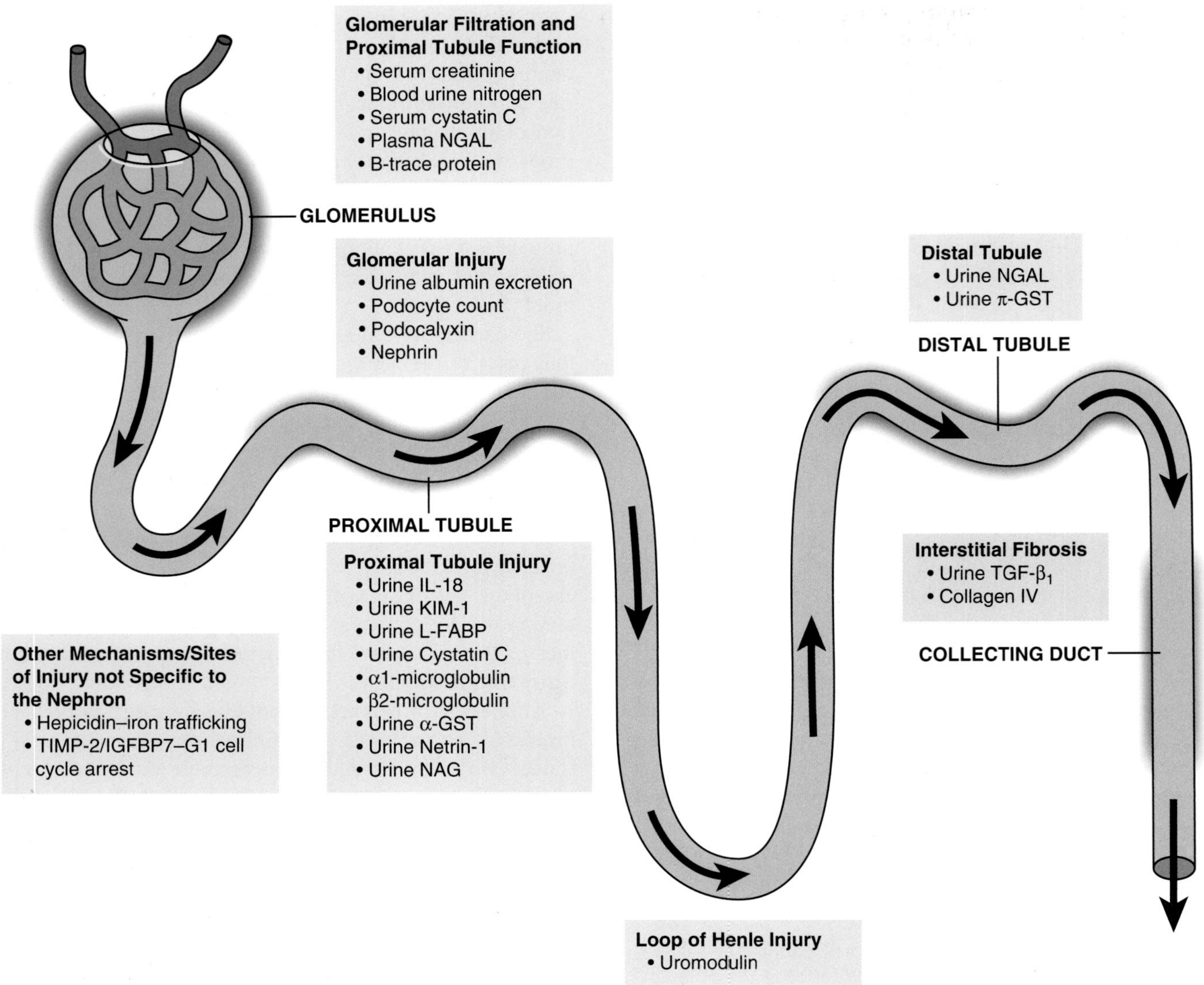

FIG. 47.1 Nephron location and physiological significance of renal biomarkers. The location of production, filtration, or secretion of multiple renal biomarkers is shown. Through consideration of biomarker localization, such markers may not only identify kidney injury but also pinpoint the injury to specific sections of the nephron, thereby enhancing the possibility of targeted therapeutics. (Modified from Koyner JL, Parikh CR. Clinical utility of biomarkers of AKI in cardiac surgery and critical illness. *Clin J Am Soc Nephrol.* 2013; 8(6):1034-1042.)

α1-Microglobulin

α1M is a glycoprotein of approximately 27 to 30 kDa primarily synthesized by liver, available both in free form and as a complex with immunoglobulin A. α1M is freely filtered at the glomerulus and completely reabsorbed and catabolized by the proximal tubule. Megalin mediates the uptake of this protein in the proximal tubule. α1M is more stable than β2M over a range of pH levels in the urine.[29] α1M quantitation in the urine has been reported as a sensitive biomarker for proximal tubule dysfunction in both adults and children.[29–32] In a small cohort of 73 patients, out of which 26 required RRT, comparing α1M, β2M, cys-C, retinol-binding protein, αGST, lactate dehydrogenase, and NAG early in the course of AKI, Herget-Rosenthal et al. found that urinary cys-C and α1M have the highest ability to predict the need for RRT.[33] In addition, α1M also has been reported as a useful marker for proximal tubular damage and recovery in early infancy.[34] In a study of 78 patients undergoing elective cardiac surgery, urinary levels of α1M were moderately predictive of the subsequent development of AKI when corrected for urinary creatinine, area under the curve (AUC) of 0.71.[35] Limitations associated with α1M include the variation in serum levels with age; sex[36]; clinical conditions, including liver diseases,[31] ulcerative colitis,[37] HIV, and mood disorders[31]; and the lack of international standardization.

Interleukin-18

IL-18 is a proinflammatory cytokine that plays an important role in many human diseases and is produced in a number of tissues. Renally, IL-18 is produced in the proximal tubule and is converted from its proform to the active form by caspase-1. Unlike the majority of other novel proteins that serve solely as biomarkers for AKI, IL-18 has been shown to be a potent mediator of ischemic AKI in animal models and has been shown to contribute to tubular damage during ischemia-reperfusion injury.[38] Interestingly, IL-18–deficient mice have been shown to be protected from ischemia/reperfusion-induced AKI.[39] It has been reported that IL-18 levels are elevated in the urine of patients with AKI and delayed graft function (DGF) compared with healthy individuals and patients with prerenal azotemia, urinary tract infection (UTI), CKD, and nephritic syndrome.[40] In the same study, the urinary concentration cutoff for IL-18 at 500 pg/mg creatinine gave an optimal sensitivity (0.85) and selectivity (0.88) for the diagnosis of ATN. Parikh et al. reported that IL-18 is an early predictive biomarker of AKI after cardiopulmonary bypass (CPB), and that NGAL and IL-18 are increased in tandem after CPB.[41] Coca et al., in an analysis of published literature, reported that the urine levels of IL-18 are significantly greater in patients with established ATN (AUC = 0.95) compared with all other types of patients including CKD, UTI, and prerenal azotemia.[42] Furthermore, IL-18 has been shown to be a selective marker for predicting severity of AKI[40] and mortality in adult,[43] and critically ill children.[44] In four studies of urinary IL-18 as an early predictive biomarker of AKI in adults and children,[41–44] authors carried out ROC analysis of biomarker performance. In the four studies, AUCs for IL-18 varied from 0.54 to 0.9, suggesting IL-18 as a biomarker with variable sensitivity but with higher specificity for the early diagnosis of AKI.

A metaanalysis of 11 studies investigating IL-18 was composed of 2796 patients ranging from newborns to elderly.[45] The majority of studies were either set in the ICU or involved cardiac surgery. The overall AUC was 0.77, whereas the diagnostic odds ratio for urinary IL-18 to predict AKI was found to be 5.1 (95% confidence interval [CI], 3.3 to 8.1) with a sensitivity and specificity of 0.51 and 0.79, respectively. IL-18 performed similarly in cardiac surgery patients and those in the ICU. However, it was noted that performance was better in pediatric populations than in adults and, in subgroup analysis, the early (<12 hours) predictive time group had significantly greater odds ratio than the 24- or 48-hour groups.

In an exhaustive study, Arthur et al. investigated 32 potential biomarkers in 95 patients with stage 1 AKI after cardiac surgery to assess for the association with worsening of AKI or death (primary outcome) or stage 3 AKI or death (secondary outcome).[46] IL-18 was the best predictor with AUC of 0.74 and 0.89, respectively. A combination of IL-18 and KIM-1 demonstrated an excellent AUC of 0.93 to predict stage 3 AKIN or death.

Neutrophil Gelatinase-Associated Lipocalin

NGAL, also known as lipocalin-2 or Siderocalin, was first discovered as a 25-kDa protein in granules of human neutrophils. NGAL is currently the most widely studied AKI biomarker and has been investigated in numerous settings including the emergency room, generalized hospital patients, adult cardiac surgery, pediatric cardiac surgery, the ICU, transplant, and in cirrhosis. NGAL is normally expressed at low levels in a number of organs including kidney, breast, liver, small intestine, prostate, stomach, lymphoid cells, thymus, and lungs.[47] NGAL expression is upregulated in several cancers, including pancreas,[47] lung,[47] colon,[47] ovary, breast,[48] and brain.[49] NGAL is markedly elevated in many organs during inflammation[49,50] and ischemia.[41] Systemic NGAL is filtered and reabsorbed in the proximal tubules via a megalin-dependent pathway.[51] Renal NGAL production occurs primarily in the thick ascending loop of Henle and the intercalated cells of the collecting ducts.[52,53] Elevated urine levels with AKI therefore could be secondary to decreased reabsorption by damaged proximal tubule cells or increased production distally. NGAL exists in three distinct isoforms: 25-kDa monomer, 45-kDa homodimer, and 135-kDa heterodimer. Because NGAL can be produced by neutrophils and other organs in addition to the kidney, in clinical conditions such as sepsis or UTIs, the appearance of NGAL in the urine might not directly reflect the severity of kidney injury.[54] However, the heterodimer, which is conjugated to gelatinase, is specific to neutrophils and thus fractionating urinary isoforms should allow for improved isolation of renally produced NGAL.[55]

NGAL binds to iron-siderophore complexes, thereby exerting a bacteriostatic effect by limiting bacterial iron uptake (Fig. 47.2).[56,57] In addition, NGAL provides antiapoptotic effects and enhances proliferation of renal tubular cells, potentially making it protective in AKI.[58] Intriguingly, recent data suggests that recombinant NGAL might be useful prophylactically for the prevention of cisplatin-

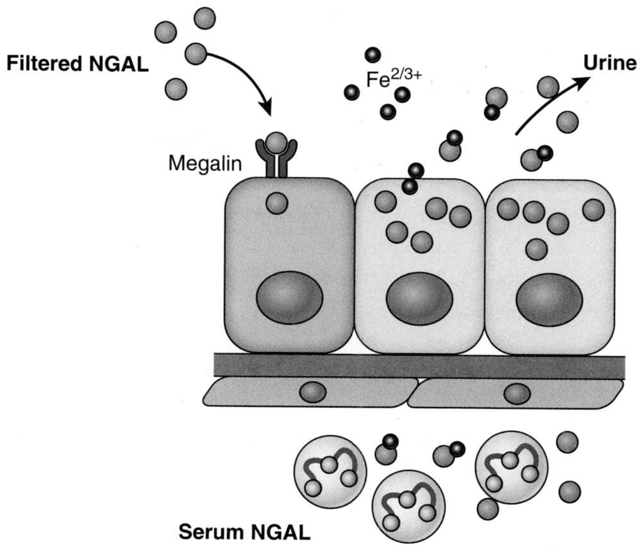

FIG. 47.2 Tubular handling of NGAL. Systemically NGAL is produced by neutrophils as well as being expressed in the liver spleen and kidney. A small amount of NGAL is routinely filtered and taken up proximally by megalin. Upon injury, NGAL production is upregulated and levels rise both in the urine and plasma. NGAL may be renally protective after acute kidney injury through scavenging of iron and thus reducing the production of toxic reactive oxygen species. (From Charlton JR, Portilla D, Okusa MD. A basic science view of acute kidney injury biomarkers. *Nephrol Dial Transplant.* 2014; 29(7):1301-1311, with permission.)

induced AKI.[59] An elevation in urinary NGAL is detectable as early as 3 hours after tubular injury, peaks between 6 to 12 hours, and can persist up to 5 days depending on the severity and resolution (or lack thereof) of the renal insult.[60–62]

The early clinical studies with NGAL were done in children. Mishra and colleagues prospectively obtained serial urine and serum samples from 71 children undergoing CPB for surgical correction of congenital heart disease.[63] Twenty children (28%) developed AKI, defined as a 50% increase in sCR. Both serum and urinary NGAL within 2 to 6 hours after CPB almost perfectly predicted which patients would subsequently develop AKI with an AUC of 0.91 and 0.99 for serum and urine, respectively. A larger follow-up study of 120 children by Dent et al. showed that 2-hour postoperative serum NGAL was predictive of AKI (AUC ROC = 0.96) and correlated with postoperative change in sCR, duration of AKI, and hospital length of stay.[64] At 12 hours, NGAL levels strongly correlated with mortality. In a subsequent prospective study in children by Zappitelli et al.,[65] in which the AKI population was more heterogeneous with unknown timing of AKI, the AUCs of urinary NGAL for prediction of AKI were lower than the AUC reported by Mishra et al.[63] In a study of adults, NGAL levels were measured in a series of patients who entered the hospital via the emergency department.[60] At a cutoff value of 130 mcg/g creatinine, sensitivity and specificity of NGAL for detecting acute injury were 0.9 and 0.995, respectively. These values were better than those for NAG, α1M, α1-acid glycoprotein, fractional excretion of sodium, and sCR, although the AUC was equivalent for NGAL and creatinine.

The most frequently studied setting for NGAL is in cardiac surgery. A recent metaanalysis identified 28 studies investigating AKI biomarkers measured either intraoperatively or immediately postoperatively; 16 of the studies containing 2906 patients measured NGAL.[66] AKI was defined via the AKIN criteria in the majority of studies with the remainder using RIFLE or KDIGO. The composite AUC for NGAL across studies was 0.72. In a large multicenter study of 1191 adults undergoing cardiac surgery, plasma NGAL (drawn both pre- and postoperatively) was assessed with long-term survival at 3 years.[67] In univariate analysis both pre- and postoperative levels were associated with survival but after adjustment only the presurgery level was independently associated.

In addition to being studied for the early detection of AKI, NGAL also has been investigated for differential diagnosis and to predict progression of clinical disease. Singer and colleagues investigated 161 hospitalized patients with established AKI via RIFLE criteria.[68] After 16 patients were excluded due to post-renal obstruction or insufficient information, the remainder were clinically adjudicated as having intrinsic AKI (75), prerenal AKI (32), or indeterminant (38). Urinary NGAL discriminated between intrinsic and prerenal with an AUC of 0.87 (NGAL values in the indeterminate group were very similar to prerenal). An NGAL level >104 μg/L resulted in a likelihood ratio (LR) for intrinsic of 5.97, whereas a level <47 μg/L rendered intrinsic unlikely, LR 0.2. NGAL values were higher in patients who would meet a composite endpoint of progression to a higher RIFLE stage, dialysis, or death than in those who did not. A sampling of the ability of NGAL and other urinary biomarkers to predict prognosis is presented in Table 47.2.

Multiple studies have evaluated urinary biomarkers, including NGAL, as a means of distinguishing between ATN and hepatorenal syndrome (HRS) in patients with cirrhosis. In one of the largest, Belcher and colleagues investigated 110 patients with cirrhosis and AKI, 55 adjudicated as having prerenal azotemia (PRA), 16 with HRS, and 39 with ATN.[81] Median NGAL values for PRA (54 ng/mL) and HRS (115 ng/mL) were significantly less than for ATN (565 ng/mL). At a cutoff of 365 ng/mL, NGAL had an AUC of 0.78 (95% CI, 0.69 to 0.88) to identify ATN. A metaanalysis identified eight studies comprising 1129 patients with cirrhosis and AKI which assessed NGAL for differential diagnosis and prognosis. NGAL performed extremely well in identifying patients with ATN, AUC of 0.89 (95% CI, 0.84 to 0.94) as well as predicting 90-day mortality, AUC of 0.76 (95% CI, 0.71 to 0.82).[82]

Several studies have evaluated urinary NGAL levels in the immediate postoperative period to predict DGF in kidney transplant recipients. Parikh and colleagues found NGAL obtained on day 0 in recipients of kidneys from living or deceased donors performed well in predicting DGF (AUC = 0.9).[54] In a follow-up study, NGAL was able to distinguish between patients who would go on to have immediate graft function, slow graft function, and DGF and could predict at 6 hours postoperatively which patients would require dialysis, AUC of 0.81 (95% CI, 0.70 to 0.92).[84] Overall, NGAL represents a promising candidate as a biomarker for the early diagnosis, differential diagnosis, and prognosis of AKI.

Liver Type Fatty Acid-Binding Protein

L-FABP, also known as fatty acid-binding protein 1 (FABP1) is a 14-kDa protein encoded by the *FABP1* gene in humans. It is expressed not only in the liver but also in the lung, intestine, stomach, and kidney.[85] L-FABP binds and transports fatty acids to mitochondria and peroxisomes and also functions to mitigate H_2O_2-associated oxidative stress.[86,87] In the kidney, L-FABP is expressed in the proximal tubule. Urinary levels of L-FABP are shown to be significantly upregulated in transgenic rodent models of kidney injury, including ischemia-reperfusion, cisplatin, folic acid, adenine, and cephaloridine.[87–92] The levels of L-FABP were markedly elevated as early as 2 hours after cisplatin administration, whereas a rise in creatinine was not detectable until after 72 hours of cisplatin treatment.[92]

Portilla and colleagues[93] reported that in humans, urinary L-FABP levels at 4 hours after surgery were an independent risk indicator for AKI (defined as a 50% increase in creatinine over baseline) with an AUC of 0.81, sensitivity of 0.71, and specificity of 0.68 for a 24-fold increase in urinary L-FABP. Increases in the urinary levels of L-FABP also have been found to predict renal outcomes in idiopathic membranous nephropathy patients with a calculated sensitivity and specificity of 81% and 83%.[94] In a recent study of 12 living kidney transplant related patients, immediately after reperfusion of their transplanted organs, a significant direct correlation was found between urinary L-FABP levels and both

TABLE 47.2 **Prognostic Performance of Acute Kidney Injury Biomarkers**

Biomarkers	Setting	Outcomes
Urine IL-18 (77)	Pediatric cardiac surgery	AUC 0.72 for AKI progression
Urine IL-18 (78)	Cardiac surgery	AUC 0.91 for AKI progression
Urine IL-18 (79)	All hospitalized patients	AUC 0.68 for AKI progression, dialysis, or death
Urine IL-18 (50)	ICU	>100 ρg/mL, HR, 1.6 (95% CI, 0.8–2.9) for death >200 ρg/mL, HR, 2.3 (95% CI, 1.2–4.4) for death >500 ρg/mL, HR, 5.1 (95% CI, 2–13.1) for death
Urine IL-18 (80)	Cardiac surgery	>185 ρg/mL, OR, 3 (95% CI, 1.3–7.3) for AKI progression
Urine IL-18 (81)	ICU	AUC 0.64 for AKI progression, dialysis, or death
Urine IL-18 (82)	Cardiorenal syndrome	OR, 3.6 (95% CI, 1.4–9.5) for AKI progression
Urine IL-18 (83)	AKI in cirrhosis	AUC = 0.71 for AKI progression or death
Urine NGAL (82)	Cardiorenal syndrome	OR, 4.7 (95% CI, 1.7–13.4) for AKI progression
Urine NGAL (81)	ICU	AUC = 0.65 for AKI progression, dialysis, or death
Urine NGAL (79)	All hospitalized patients	AUC = 0.75 for AKI progression, dialysis, or death
Urine NGAL (83)	AKI in cirrhosis	AUC = 0.77 for AKI progression or death
Urine NGAL (77)	Pediatric cardiac surgery	AUC = 0.71 for AKI progression
Urine NGAL (84)	ICU	AUC = 0.70 for AKI progression or dialysis
Urine KIM-1 (79)	All hospitalized patients	AUC = 0.69 for AKI progression, dialysis, or death
Urine KIM-1 (83)	AKI in cirrhosis	AUC = 0.66 for AKI progression or death
Urine KIM-1 (78)	Cardiac surgery	AUC = 0.70 for AKI progression
Urine KIM-1 (79)	All hospitalized patients	AUC = 0.70 for AKI progression
Urine KIM-1 (81)	ICU	AUC = 0.62 for AKI progression, dialysis, or death
Urine L-FABP (83)	AKI in cirrhosis	AUC = 0.76 for AKI progression or death
Urine L-FABP (81)	ICU	AUC = 0.79 (95% CI, 0.70–0.86) for progression, dialysis, or death
Urine L-FABP (86)	Cardiac surgery	AUC = 0.78 for nonrecovery of kidney function
Urinary YKL-40 (87)	All hospitalized patients	OR, 3.4 (95% CI, 1.5–7.7) for AKI progression or death
Urine [TIMP-2]×[IGFBP7] (88)	ICU	>2, HR, 2.16 (95% CI, 1.3–3.5) for death or dialysis

AKI, Acute kidney injury; *AUC,* area under the curve; *CI,* confidence interval; *HR,* hazard ratio; *ICU,* intensive care unit; *IGFBP7,* insulin-like growth factor binding protein 7; *IL,* interleukin; *KIM-1,* kidney injury molecule-1; *L-FABP,* liver-type fatty acid binding protein; *NGAL,* neutrophil gelatinase-associated lipocalin; *OR,* odds ratio; *TIMP-2,* tissue inhibitor of metalloproteinases 2.

peritubular capillary blood flow and the ischemic time of the transplanted kidney.[95] A systematic review and metaanalysis by Susantitahphong and colleagues identified 23 studies evaluating L-FABP and AKI spanning cardiac surgery, cardiac catheterization, ICUs, emergency departments, general hospital wards, liver transplantation, and hematopoietic cell transplantation.[78] Unfortunately, only 7 could be included in a metaanalysis. L-FABP was found to have sensitivity and specificity for AKI diagnosis of 75% and 78%, 69% and 43% for predicting the need for dialysis, and 93% and 79% for in-hospital mortality. More recently, Parr and associates investigated several biomarkers in 152 ICU patients to predict a composite outcome of progression of AKI, dialysis, or death.[73] L-FABP was the only biomarker with a strong ability to predict the composite outcome (AUC = 0.79 compared with NGAL, IL-18, and KIM-1 which were 0.65, 0.64, and 0.62, respectively) and the only one to improve the discrimination when added to a clinical model. The levels of urinary L-FABP should be interpreted with caution, however, as they may be influenced by a number of preexisting renal diseases, such as early diabetic nephropathy, nondiabetic CKD, polycystic kidney disease, and idiopathic focal glomerulosclerosis.[23] Because L-FABP is expressed in other organs such as the liver, urinary L-FABP may lose specificity for kidney disease when there is coexisting liver disease. Nevertheless, L-FABP remains an intriguing candidate biomarker.

Kidney Injury Molecule-1

KIM-1 is a type I cell membrane glycoprotein, which contains in its extracellular portion a novel six-cysteine immunoglobulin-like domain, two *N*-glycosylation sites, and a Thr/Ser/Pro-rich domain characteristic of mucin-like *O*-glycosylated proteins. KIM-1 was initially discovered in rodents when, after an acute ischemic kidney injury, Kim-1 (the rodent counterpart to human KIM-1) mRNA was found to be significantly upregulated in proximal tubules cells 24 to 48 hours postinjury.[96,97] The ectodomain of KIM-1 sheds from cells both in vitro[98] and in vivo into the urine in rodents[99,101] and humans[101] after proximal tubular kidney injury. Elevated levels of soluble KIM-1 ectodomain in the urine also were demonstrated in patients with renal cell carcinoma.[102] KIM-1 appears to act as a scavenger receptor on renal epithelial cells, which converts the normal proximal tubule cell into a phagocyte, facilitates the clearance of dead cells in the lumen, and likely plays an important role in the innate immune response after injury.[103]

KIM-1 is constitutively expressed at very low levels in the kidney as well as other organs, but its expression is significantly upregulated in the kidney after both ischemia-reperfusion and drug-induced AKI. Characteristics of KIM-1 commending it as a biomarker include much higher expression in proximal tubular cells of the kidney than in any other cell of the kidney or any other organ, stability of the soluble ectodomain in the urine over a broad range of pH, sustained expression in proximal tubular epithelial cells until complete recovery, and extremely low levels in the healthy kidney, providing a high signal-to-noise ratio. In one of the first studies linking urinary levels of KIM-1 and AKI, an increased expression of KIM-1 in kidney biopsy specimens was demonstrated from patients with a pathological diagnosis of ATN along with corresponding levels of KIM-1 ectodomain in the urine.[104] Notably, KIM-1 appeared in the urine before the appearance of casts. A subsequent study revealed that KIM-1 expression in transplant was significantly correlated with levels of creatinine and inversely correlated with estimated GFR on the biopsy day.[105] KIM-1 was expressed focally in affected tubules in 92% of kidney biopsies from patients with acute cellular rejection. Focal positive KIM-1 expression was found in 28% of protocol biopsies in the presence of no detectable tubular injury on histological examination. This observation demonstrates the superior sensitivity of KIM-1 expression in detecting proximal tubule injury compared with morphology alone. The clinical significance, however, of increased KIM-1 in this setting remains to be determined. Van Timmeren and coworkers[106] also found that occurrence of renal allograft loss over time increased with rising levels of KIM-1 excretion measured at baseline. High KIM-1 levels were associated with low creatinine clearance, proteinuria, and high donor age. KIM-1 levels predicted graft loss independent of creatinine clearance, proteinuria, and donor age. The pathological basis for this association may have been demonstrated in another study by the same authors where it was found that, in 102 transplant biopsies, the amount of KIM-1 protein expression in proximal tubule cells correlated with tubulointerstitial fibrosis and inflammation.[104]

A number of studies have demonstrated the potential of KIM-1 as a biomarker of AKI. In a cohort of 201 patients with clinically established AKI, Liangos and coworkers evaluated urinary KIM-1 and NAG in predicting adverse clinical outcomes and reported that elevated levels of urinary KIM-1 and NAG were significantly associated with the composite endpoint of death or dialysis, even after adjustment for disease severity or comorbidity.[107] KIM-1 is also a sensitive marker of kidney injury in children undergoing cardiac surgery.[108]

In a study of 1199 adults undergoing cardiac surgery, 407 (34%) developed AKI with 251 (62%) having an AKI duration of 1 to 2 days, 118 (29%) with duration 3 to 6 days, and 38 (9%) ≥7 days.[109] Multiple urinary biomarkers collected 0 to 6 hours postoperatively were independently associated with duration of AKI including IL-18, KIM-1, NGAL, L-FABP, and albumin. Of these, KIM-1 had the highest odds ratio at 1.36 (95% CI, 2.21 to 2.52). Additional prognostic data was found in a study by Jungbauer and associates of 149 patients with chronic heart failure and CKD.[110] Over a 5-year follow-up, 26 (19%) patients developed progression of their CKD. Urinary KIM-1, along with NAG, was associated with CKD progression, and KIM-1 was independently associated with a combined endpoint of CKD progression or death.

In a novel study of 22 marathon runners, Mansour and colleagues investigated multiple urinary injury biomarkers including KIM-1, tumor necrosis factor-α, IL-18, IL-6, IL-8, and NGAL along with putative repair biomarkers YKL-40 and MCP-1 in the periods before and after the race.[111] SCR rose significantly from a median of 0.81 mg/dL (interquartile range [IQR] = 0.76 to 0.95) premarathon to 1.28 mg/dL (IQR = 1.09 to 1.54) immediately after the marathon. By the following day, however, this had returned to baseline, 0.90 mg/dL (IQR = 0.80 to 0.90). All urinary injury and repair biomarkers demonstrated a statistically significant rise after the race from before it but only KIM-1 remained significantly elevated the following day; premarathon 132.6 pg/mL (IQR = 67.6 to 220), after the marathon 723.3 pg/mL (IQR = 459.4 to 970.6), following day 702.4 pg/mL (IQR = 123.3 to 1009; $P < 0.001$).

KIM-1 has primarily been measured by enzyme-linked immunosorbent assay.[100] Importantly, although not yet in widespread clinical practice, a point-of-care dipstick has been developed that can provide semiquantitative results in 15 minutes.[112] This is critical for studies going forward as biomarker research has been consistently hamstrung by the requirement of specialized laboratories for measuring levels.

In recognition of its strong performance relative to traditional biomarkers of kidney injury in preclinical biomarker FDA and European Medicines Agency qualification studies,[113] KIM-1 has been approved by the FDA as an AKI biomarker for preclinical drug development.

Tissue Inhibitor of Metalloproteinase 2 and Insulin-Like Growth Factor-Binding Protein 7

TIMP2 and IGFBP7 are two proteins involved in G1 cell cycle arrest during the very early phases of cellular injury. The cyclin-dependent kinase inhibitor p21 halts cell cycle succession from G1 to S phase. P21-deficient mice have been demonstrated to be more sensitive to cisplatin-induced AKI, develop a more severe injury and have increased mortality, implying that cell cycle arrest is critical both to preventing AKI and abrogating its sequelae.[114] A discovery study identified TIMP2 and IGFBP7 out of 340 potential candidate markers.[115] The authors then validated these biomarkers using the Sapphire cohort. In this study, TIMP2 and IGFBP7, along with [TIMP2]x[IGFBP7], outperformed numerous other biomarkers including NGAL, KIM-1, IL-18, L-FABP, and π-GST in predicting moderate to severe AKI within 12 hours of sample collection. Subsequent studies have confirmed the utility of [TIMP2]x[IGFBP7] to predict stage 2 and 3 AKI with AUC of 0.82[116] and 0.79,[117] respectively. Gocze and colleagues measured [TIMP2]x[IGFBP7] in 107 surgical patients at high risk for AKI, of whom 45 (42%) developed AKI.[118] The AUC for AKI was 0.85; for early use of RRT, it was 0.83; and for 28-day mortality, it was 0.77. In a multivariable model incorporating established perioperative risk factors, [TIMP2]x[IGFBP7] was the strongest predictor of AKI.

Koyner and colleagues again used the Sapphire cohort of ICU adults to evaluate the association between TIMP2 and IGFBP7 with long-term outcomes, assessing them with a composite outcome of death or need for RRT.[80] Data was available for 692 patients, of whom 382 (55%) developed AKI and 217 (31%) met the composite endpoint. On univariate analysis,

[TIMP2]x[IGFBP7] >2 was associated with an increased risk (hazard ratio [HR], 2.11; 95% CI, 1.37 to 2.23). In a significant landmark for biomarker clinical translation, the FDA has allowed marketing of the NephroCheck test, which measures [TIMP2]x[IGFBP7] to determine whether certain critically ill patients are at risk for developing moderate to severe AKI within 12 hours after testing.[119]

Osteopontin

OPN is a multifunctional 44 kDa phosphoprotein, widely distributed in a variety of tissue types ranging from bone to epithelial cells of the gastrointestinal (GI) tract, lungs, breast, salivary glands, inner ear, placenta, and kidneys.[120,121] OPN has been associated with a variety of physiological and pathological functions, including bone modeling, immunity, cell adhesion, and migration. OPN is expressed in ureteric buds and few interstitial cells of fetal kidney, whereas in the normal adult kidney OPN is localized primarily to the distal tubule and thick ascending segments of the loop of Henle.[122] During renal disease, however, OPN has been shown to be upregulated in all tubular segments, including proximal tubules.[129] OPN is secreted in the urine and inhibits the formation of calcium oxalate kidney stones. OPN has been evaluated in various experimental models of kidney injury, and multiple studies have reported the detection of OPN mRNA in regenerating proximal tubules in renal ischemia models.[123,124] The elevated levels of OPN are sustained for 7 days after the injury. In gentamicin-induced ATN in rodents, OPN is detected only in the cortical distal tubules during first few days of the injury, but is markedly elevated in regenerative proximal tubules after day 15.[125]

Recent work has evaluated serum levels of OPN as predictive of survival and renal recovery in patients acutely requiring RRT. Lorsenzen and coworkers measured serum OPN (sOPN) in 109 ICU patients with AKI.[126] Lower sOPN at RRT initiation was independently associated with 28-day survival (AUC = 0.82). Twenty-four of 69 surviving patients (35%) were still dependent on RRT 4 weeks after initiation. sOPN was significantly lower at initiation in those survivors who recovered renal function than in those who did not. In those with recovery, sOPN levels at 4 weeks were significantly lower than at initiation, whereas they were unchanged in those without recovery. In a subsequent study of 102 ICU patients with AKI requiring RRT, sOPN levels on RRT day 1 were evaluated for association with 60-day mortality.[127] After adjusting for a robust panel of variables, including creatinine and urine output when coming off RRT, sOPN levels in the second and third tertiles had adjusted odds ratio for 60-day mortality of 2.3 and 5.3, respectively (AUC = 0.81). In this study, however, sOPN was not associated with renal recovery in survivors.

YKL-40

YKL-40, also known as chitinase-3-like-1 protein, is a 40kDA glycoprotein secreted by a variety of cells and is involved in the activation of the innate immune system, extracellular matrix remodeling, and angiogenesis.[128] YKL-40 is intimately involved in endothelial dysfunction and atherosclerosis[129] and it is independently associated with albuminuria among patients with type 1 and type 2 diabetes mellitus. YKL-40 modulates renal repair mechanisms after ischemic kidney injury and can act as an effective marker of renal injury in the setting of kidney transplantation.[130] Puthumana and associates measured YKL-40 in 1301 deceased kidney donors and ascertained outcomes in the corresponding 2435 recipients, 756 of whom experienced DGF.[131] Donors with existing AKI at the time of kidney recovery had higher urinary YKL-40 and more frequent ATN on procurement biopsy. Elevated donor urinary YKL-40 concentration was independently associated with reduced risk for DGF in both recipients of AKI donor kidneys (adjusted relative risk [aRR], 0.51; 95% CI, 0.32 to 0.80 for the highest versus lowest YKL-40 tertile) and recipients of non-AKI donor kidneys (aRR, 0.79; 95% CI, 0.65 to 0.97). In those patients who suffered GFR, elevated donor urinary YKL-40 concentration associated with higher 6-month estimated GFR (6.75 mL/min/1.73 m^2; 95% CI, 1.49 to 12.02) and lower risk for graft failure (aRR, 0.50; 95% CI, 0.27 to 0.94). These findings suggest that YKL-40 is produced in response to tubular injury and is independently associated with recovery from AKI and DGF.

Hall and associates measured YKL-40 249 hospitalized patients with AKI as defined by AKIN criteria.[132] Seventy-two patients (29%) had progression of their AKI to a higher stage or death. Urinary YKL-40 collected on the first day of AKI was ≥5 ng/mL and had an adjusted odds ratio of 3.4 (95% CI, 1.5 to 7.7) for this combined outcome. In patients deemed at high risk for the combined outcome due to elevated NGAL levels, YKL-40 was able to partition these patients into moderate or very high-risk groups. When added to a clinical model, YKL-40 resulted in a continuous net reclassification improvement of 29% (P = 0.04). In addition, it has been found that YKL-40 is associated with increased mortality among patients with coronary artery disease, type 2 diabetes mellitus, cardiac failure, and peripheral artery disease. Tatar and colleagues evaluated 100 patients with a median of 72 months posttransplant.[133] Patients were divided into tertiles based on serum YKL-40 levels (<42, 42 to 69, >69 ng/mL). SCR increased across tertiles, 1.39, 2.03, 2.45 mg/dL, as did proteinuria, 0.34, 0.74, 1.22 g/g. YKL-40 levels were positively associated with C-reactive protein and negatively with serum albumin. In multivariate analysis, GFR, systolic blood pressure, and YKL-40 were independently associated with levels of proteinuria.

Uromodulin

Uromodulin, also known as Tamm-Horsfall protein, is a glycoprotein expressed exclusively by renal tubular cells lining the thick ascending limb (TAL) of the loop of Henle. It is the only biomarker discussed in this chapter that is primarily produced in this location. Uromodulin has been implicated in the pathophysiology of multiple kidney diseases including polycystic kidney disease, UTIs, and nephrolithiasis.[134,135] Uromodulin has been shown to confer protection to proximal tubules against AKI via a possible crosstalk between the two functionally distinct tubular segments. In a murine model of ischemia-reperfusion AKI, El-Achkar et al. demonstrated that although uromodulin expression in TAL is downregulated at the peak of injury, it is significantly upregulated 48 hours after.[136] Uromodulin expression is redirected from the apical domain to the basolateral and interstitium. This corresponds with increased uromodulin in the serum but not in the urine. Compared with the wild-type, uromodulin (-/-) mice show significantly delayed renal recovery after ischemia-reperfusion, possibly due to reduced suppression by uromodulin of proinflammatory cytokines and chemokines such as MCP-1 during recovery. The redistribution of uromodulin in the TAL after AKI and its increased interstitial presence therefore may downregulate inflammatory signaling in neighboring proximal tubules, thereby augmenting kidney recovery. In a post hoc analysis of 218 patients undergoing on-pump cardiac surgery, Garimella and associates investigated the association between preoperative urinary uromodulin levels and postoperative AKI.[137] Lower urinary uromodulin-to-creatinine ratio was associated with higher odds for AKI (adjusted odds ratio [aOR], 1.43; 95% CI, 0.99 to 2.07). The lowest uromodulin-to-creatinine ratio quartile also was associated with higher odds for AKI relative to the highest quartile (aOR, 2.43; 95% CI, 0.91 to 6.48). Each lower SD in uromodulin-to-creatinine ratio was associated with a higher adjusted mean peak sCR (0.07 mg/dL per SD; 95% CI, 0.02 to 0.13).

Interleukin-6/Interleukin-10

IL-6 and IL-10 are cytokines believed to play critical roles in the inflammatory process mediating the pathophysiology of AKI. IL-6 is one of the main proinflammatory cytokines, whereas IL-10 has anti-inflammatory and immunomodulatory functions related to the regulation of lymphocyte activity. Multiple studies both in children and adults have demonstrated that these cytokines may be potential biomarkers of AKI.[138,139] In animal models, AKI itself, not just the proinflammatory state of sepsis or surgery, induces higher IL-6 and IL-10 levels.[140] IL-6 and IL-10 also are known to play a key role in the systemic inflammatory response to cardiac surgery and CPB. Greenberg and colleagues evaluated 106 children 1 month to 18 years of age undergoing CPB as part of the TRIBE-AKI (Translational Research Investigating Biomarker Endpoints in AKI) cohort, assessing for an association between IL-6 and IL-10 and postoperative AKI.[141] Stage 2/3 AKI, defined by at least a doubling of the baseline sCR concentration or dialysis, was diagnosed in 24 patients (23%). Preoperative serum IL-6 concentrations were significantly higher in patients with stage 2/3 AKI (median 2.6 pg/mL; IQR = 0.6 to 4.9 pg/mL) than in those without stage 2/3 AKI (median 0.6 pg/mL; IQR = 0.6 to 2.2 pg/mL; $P=0.03$). Adjusted for clinical and demographic variables, the highest preoperative IL-6 tertile was associated with a sixfold increased risk for stage 2/3 AKI compared with the lowest tertile (OR, 6.41; 95% CI, 1.16 to 35.35). IL-6 and IL-10 levels increased significantly after surgery, peaking postoperatively on day 1 but did not significantly differ between patients with and without stage 2/3 AKI. In a study of 960 adults undergoing cardiac surgery, preoperative concentrations of IL-6 and IL-10 were not significantly associated with AKI or mortality.[142] However, elevated first postoperative IL-6 concentrations were significantly associated with higher risk for AKI, and the risk increased in a dose-dependent manner (second tertile aOR, 1.61; 95% CI, 1.10 to 2.36; third tertile aOR, 2.13; 95% CI, 1.45 to 3.13). Elevated first postoperative IL-10 concentration was significantly associated with higher risk for AKI (aOR, 1.57; 95% CI, 1.04 to 2.38) and lower risk for mortality (aHR, 0.72; 95% CI, 0.56 to 0.93).

With cytokines such as IL-6 and IL-10 perhaps not only serving as markers of AKI but also as mediators of outcomes, several studies have therefore looked at the effect on outcomes of lowering their levels with dialysis. Park et al. studied 212 patients with sepsis and AKI randomized to receive continuous venovenous hemodiafiltration (CVVHDF) at conventional (40 mL/kg/h) or high (80 mL/kg/h) doses.[143] High-dose, but not conventional, CVVHDF reduced serum IL-6 and IL-10 levels. However, there was no difference in either overall survival or dialysis-free survival at 28 days. A smaller study by Kade and colleagues examined 28 patients receiving continuous venovenous hemodialysis using a high cutoff hemofilter.[144] Cytokine levels were measured before the start of dialysis and after 24 hours of treatment. After 24 hours, IL-10 levels in the serum were significantly lower. Clearance of IL-6 was approximately four times higher than IL-10 yet IL-6 levels rose, significantly correlating with mortality. It remains to be seen whether using this method to remove IL-6 will alter patient outcomes.

Repurposed Biomarkers

Fractional Excretion of Sodium

The fractional excretion of sodium (FENa), defined as [(urine sodium × plasma creatinine)/plasma sodium ×x urine creatinine) × 100], has historically been used to distinguish between prerenal azotemia (functional AKI) and ATN (structural AKI). A FENa <1% indicates both increased sodium avidity and tubular integrity sufficient to meet sodium reabsorptive demands, whereas a value >2% to 3% suggests frank tubular injury. However, in some settings of extreme sodium avidity, such as advanced cirrhosis, virtually all patients, whether they have AKI or not, have a FENa <1% and so the test has historically not been employed. Several recent studies have investigated whether it still might have utility if a different cutoff is used. In a study by Fagundes and associates of 74 patients with cirrhosis and prerenal azotemia (16), CKD (14) HRS (33), and ATN (11), FENa varied significantly across groups and was lowest in HRS (0.2%) and highest with ATN (2.2%).[145] Verna and colleagues studied 118 patients with cirrhosis, 17 of whom had prerenal azotemia, 20 HRS syndrome, and 15 with ATN. FENa was once again significantly lower in the HRS patients (0.17%) than in ATN (0.7%).[146] Similarly, Belcher and associates investigated 110 patients with cirrhosis and AKI who were diagnosed with prerenal azotemia (55), HRS (16), or ATN (39).[81] Once again FENa was significantly

TABLE 47.3 Fractional Excretion of Sodium in Patients With Cirrhosis and Kidney Disease

	CKD	PRA	HRS	ATN
Ariza		0.5% ± 0.4 (*n* = 12)	0.3% ± 0.7 (*n* = 15)	2.1% ± 3.3 (*n* = 12)
Belcher		0.27% (0.13–0.58) (*n* = 55)	0.10% (0.02–0.23) (*n* = 16)	0.31% (0.12–0.65) (*n* = 39)
Fagundes	0.2% (0.1–0.7) (*n* = 14)	0.5% (0.2–1.1) (*n* = 16)	0.08% (0.04–0.3) (*n* = 33)	3.2% (2.1–6.1) (*n* = 11)
Qasem	0.32% ± 0.17 (*n* = 15)	0.54% ± 0.24 (*n* = 17)	0.15% ± 0.07 (*n* = 14)	4.05% ± 1.05 (*n* = 22)
Verna	0.66% (0.27–2) (*n* = 14)	0.22% (0.10–0.77) (*n* = 17)	0.17% (0.09–0.33) (*n* = 20)	0.7% (0.27–2.7) (*n* = 15)

ATN, Acute tubular necrosis; *CKD,* chronic kidney disease; *HRS,* hepatorenal syndrome; *PRA,* prerenal azotemia.

lower for patients with HRS (0.1%) than for those with ATN (0.31%). Table 47.3 presents FENa values for different diagnoses across studies for patients with cirrhosis.

Urine Microscopy

Evaluation of urine sediment is a time-honored and critical component of any evaluation of AKI. Recently, several studies have evaluated microscopy not for differential diagnosis (its historic utility) but rather for prognosis in patients with established AKI. Bagshaw and associates enrolled 83 critically ill patients with septic and nonseptic AKI.[147] A urine microscopy score (UMS) was derived based on the observed quantification of renal tubular cells and casts in the sediment. The UMS was compared between septic and nonseptic AKI and correlated with urinary NGAL, worsening AKI, RRT, and hospital mortality. Septic AKI was present in 43 patients (52%). Septic AKI was associated with higher UMS compared with nonseptic AKI ($P = 0.001$). There was no correlation between UMS and FENa or fractional excretion of urea (FeU). Elevated urine NGAL (uNGAL) correlated with higher UMS ($P < 0.001$). Worsening AKI occurred in 23%; a UMS score ≥3 was associated with increased adjusted odds of worsening AKI (OR, 8; 95% CI, 1.03 to 62.5). For a UMS ≥3, sensitivity and specificity were 0.67 (95% CI, 0.39 to 0.86) and 0.95 (0.84 to 0.99), and positive and negative predictive values were 0.80 (0.49 to 0.94) and 0.91 (0.78 to 0.96) for detecting worsening AKI, respectively. A higher UMS correlated with both need for RRT and in-hospital mortality on univariate analysis but the associated was attenuated on multivariate regression. Hall and colleagues enrolled 284 hospitalized patients on the first day of developing AKI and evaluated urine microscopy as related to a combined outcome of AKI progression, dialysis, or death.[71] A microscopy score was calculated based on the number of granular casts and renal tubular epithelial cells per field. Seventy-two patients (29%) developed the composite outcome. The incidence of the composite outcome increased stepwise with the microscopy score, and patients with a microscopy score ≥3 had an adjusted 3.5-fold higher risk compared with those with a score of 0.

Biomarkers Panels

With urinary biomarkers arising from different tubular locations and exhibiting different time courses, it stands to reason that ultimately they might find clinical use as a panel. Several studies have investigated the performance of biomarker combinations. A cross-sectional study evaluated the diagnostic performance of nine urinary biomarkers of AKI: KIM-1, NGAL, IL-18, hepatocyte growth factor (HGF), Cys-C, NAG, vascular endothelial growth factor (VEGF), chemokine interferon-inducible protein 10 (IP-10; CXCL10), and total protein in 102 patients with AKI of various etiologies and 102 individuals without clinically documented AKI.[148] For each of the urinary proteins, median concentrations were significantly higher in patients with AKI than in those without AKI. A nonbiased logistic regression model approach was used to optimize the combination of biomarkers and derive an algorithm. The resulting algorithm (risk score of 2.93 × [NGAL >5.72 and HGF >0.17] + 2.93 × [PROTEIN >0.22] − 2 × [KIM <0.58]) yielded an AUC of 0.94, which was significantly greater than any individual biomarker. In a study of patients undergoing cardiac surgery, Han and associates reported that prediction of AKI at 3 hours after surgery using KIM-1, NAG, and NGAL significantly improved with use of a combination of biomarkers, compared with the performance of individual biomarkers.[149] In a study of 110 patients with cirrhosis and AKI, Belcher and colleagues adjudicated 39 as having ATN. AUCs and optimal cutoffs were calculated for each biomarker.[89] The relative risk for ATN increased significantly in patients with multiple biomarkers above their cutoff (RR, 4.63, 6.98, 9.78, and 13.33 for 1, 2, 3, or 4 markers, respectively).

The Future of Biomarkers in Acute Kidney Injury

A significant amount of progress has been made over the past few years in the discovery, characterization, and validation of new biomarkers. Additional work, however, still remains to bring these biomarkers successfully to clinical practice for AKI. Studying these biomarkers in animals, one has the luxury of a true gold standard of toxicity-histological analysis of the kidney. In humans, we are often left to evaluate biomarkers using very poor metrics. For example, we rely on sCR for the definition of AKI, knowing that this marker is insensitive and nonspecific for kidney injury. With many patients having significant renal functional reserve, not only is there a delay in the rise of creatinine after an injury, in many cases there is likely subclinical injury without a rise in creatinine at all. In these cases, if biomarkers rose, they would be said to have failed in "predicting" "AKI." What they would have done, however, is detect frank AKI. Therefore relying on AUCs in assessing the performance of biomarkers can be flawed. We should not really want a biomarker with an AUC of 1 for prediction φ Delta-creatinine–defined AKI; such a marker, although allowing for earlier detection, would be no more sensitive or specific for true kidney injury than is creatinine. Therefore prospective studies in humans using modest changes in sCR to determine AKI are going to be subject to ambiguity in interpretation. In addition, researchers must be clear about the context in which they intend to use the biomarker. Are we interested in a biomarker that tells us that there is injury? What if a study shows that this biomarker does not predict outcome? That does not mean it is a bad biomarker. The link between injury and outcome is quite convoluted and often poorly understood.

As AKI is a complex disease with multiple etiologies and often occurs in the setting of systemic diseases, one biomarker may not suffice for early diagnosis and prediction of clinical course. We may benefit from multiple biomarkers (plasma and urine) that can provide early evidence of both risk and injury, and have the ability to distinguish between different types of AKI in both adults and pediatric patients.

SUMMARY

Tremendous progress has been made over the past 15 years in the discovery and validation of novel biomarkers for AKI. It is clear as well that much work remains to find the appropriate clinical role for the biomarkers reviewed in this chapter. However, despite this, it is critical that we do not allow the perfect to become the enemy of the good. The breadth of settings in which biomarkers have shown their worth is compelling. Although still in their adolescence, biomarkers have demonstrated their ability to augment conventional tests in the diagnosis, prognosis, and differential diagnosis of AKI and will hopefully soon be more fully integrated into clinical practice.

DISCLOSURES

Dr. Parikh is supported by NIH grants for development and validation of biomarkers in kidney disease. He is also on the Drug Safety Monitoring Board of clinical trials sponsored by Abbvie and Triceda.

ACKNOWLEDGMENTS

The authors would like to thank Drs. Joseph Bonventre and Venkata Sabbisetti for their contributions from a previous version of this chapter.

A full list of references is available at www.expertconsult.com.

Pharmacological Interventions in Acute Kidney Injury

Tushar Chopra, MD, MBBS, FASN, Rasheed Abiodun Balogun, MBBS, FACP, and Mark Douglas Okusa, MD, FASN

OUTLINE

Pharmacological therapy of acute kidney injury (AKI) continues to be largely unsuccessful despite proven benefits found in preclinical studies. Prevention and treatment of AKI is an important clinical issue because mortality in patients with AKI, especially in critically ill patients, remains high despite substantial advances in techniques of resuscitation and renal replacement therapy. Furthermore, there are a number of studies that suggest that those patients who survive AKI in the hospital develop chronic kidney disease (CKD) or end-stage renal disease (ESRD) (for a review, see Coca et al.[314]). Based on databases of US hospitalizations over the past 10 to 15 years, the incidence of AKI is increasing markedly[1,2,351] as a result of the expansion of invasive medical and surgical procedures and the increasing expectation for aggressive medical management of critically ill patients. In critically ill patients, mortality is 40% to 60%[3-6] and traditionally has been attributed to comorbid conditions. Data suggest, however, that AKI has an independent negative impact on mortality.[7,8] Chertow et al.[9] reported that even a rise of serum creatinine of 0.3 to 0.4 mg/dL was associated with an increase in mortality (multivariable odds ratio [OR], 1.7; 95% confidence interval [CI], 1.2 to 2.6). Standardization of the definition of AKI has led to advancements in the study of clinical AKI. The Acute Dialysis Quality Initiative (ADQI) classification, called RIFLE (*R*isk, *I*njury, *F*ailure, *L*oss, *E*nd-stage kidney disease), and Acute Kidney Injury Network (AKIN) staging (1, 2, and 3) are based on graded levels of rise in serum creatinine or decrease in urine output.[4,10] Even the least severe category, R or AKIN stage 1, was associated with a mortality rate of 30.9% or 30.7%, respectively.[11] In 2012 the Kidney Disease Outcomes Global Initiative (KDIGO) combined the AKIN and RIFLE guidelines into a single definition of AKI. The diagnosis of AKI may be missed when using one or the other classification schemes. However, combining the two criteria into one KDIGO criteria ensured that the diagnosis is captured. KDIGO defined AKI by an absolute serum creatinine increase of ≥0.3 mg/dL occurring within 48 hours (this is similar to AKIN) and a 50% increment of serum creatinine within 7 days (similar to RIFLE).[397] These studies highlight the important effects of a small decline in glomerular filtration rate (GFR) on the overall outcome of critically ill patients.

Although many animal studies have demonstrated that different classes of pharmacological agents are effective in preclinical studies, few have been found to be beneficial in human studies of AKI. For these reasons, and because of the high morbidity and mortality associated with AKI, a better understanding of the barriers to the prevention and treatment of AKI is necessary. Significant efforts are currently being directed in an international and multidisciplinary manner to improve outcomes in such patients by finding ways to prevent AKI, establishing early diagnoses and treatments with both nonpharmacological and pharmacological interventions.[12–14,334,347,352,355,288] With a refined and consistent definition of AKI and point-of-care use of novel biomarkers for the early identification of AKI and predictors of AKI,[12,15,16,384,401,362,432,393,402] new and old pharmacological therapies will require testing (or retesting) in well-designed randomized clinical trials.

This chapter focuses on pharmacological agents that have been used to prevent or treat AKI clinically, with variable levels of proven success (or failures), and also those with promising data from recent experimental studies of AKI in animals and humans.

BARRIERS TO SUCCESSFUL CLINICAL TRIALS IN ACUTE KIDNEY INJURY

Patient and Comorbid Factors

The changing spectrum of human illnesses is an important variable to consider in the outcomes of interventional studies. Recent studies of AKI have noted a trend of increasing severity of comorbid and extrarenal complications.[1,2,17] Those patients with higher comorbidity were associated with a higher incidence of AKI, especially if they were on mechanical ventilation.[2,321] In a multicenter study of 618 patients with AKI in the intensive care unit (ICU) (the Program to Improve Care in Acute Renal Disease Network [PICARD]), the incidence of comorbid conditions was high, including 30% with CKD, 37% with coronary artery disease, 29% with diabetes mellitus (DM), and 21% with chronic liver disease. AKI was accompanied by extrarenal organ system failure in most patients. These comorbid conditions are likely contributors to failed treatment regimens.

Preexisting renal disease is the most important factor in predicting AKI after exposure to radiocontrast agents, major surgery, and other medical conditions.[18] In a recent study, 1764 patients who developed hospital-acquired AKI and were treated with dialysis were compared with more than 600,000 patients who were hospitalized but did not develop AKI requiring dialysis.[19] In the group of patients with AKI requiring dialysis, 74% occurred among patients with an estimated GFR <60 mL/min/1.73 m^2. The more severe the baseline CKD, the greater the risk for AKI: a twofold increase among patients with estimated GFR (eGFR) 45 to 59 mL/min/1.73 m^2 and a fortyfold increase among patients with eGFR <15 mL/min/1.73 m^2. These results, and results from other studies, strongly suggest that underlying CKD may be the single most important risk factor for AKI.

Pathogenesis of Acute Kidney Injury Is Complex

The pathogenesis of AKI is complex; whereas initiating events may be dissimilar (ischemia or toxins are major factors that precipitate injury), subsequent injury responses may involve similar pathways. The complexity of AKI is illustrated in the following example. AKI associated with ischemia caused by a reduction of renal blood flow (RBF) less than the limits of blood flow autoregulation leads to maladaptive molecular responses. These responses lead to endothelial and epithelial cell injury after the onset of reperfusion.[20] Pathogenic factors such as vasoconstriction, leukostasis, vascular congestion, apoptosis, and abnormalities in immune modulators and growth factors have formed the basis of rational therapeutic interventions.[21-25,353,382,398,413] However, many of these targeted therapies have failed, are inconclusive, or have yet to be performed despite the advances made in understanding the pathogenesis of AKI.[26,27,359,318] Given the complexity of the pathogenesis of AKI, it may be naïve to expect that one therapeutic intervention would have success unless that intervention focuses on prevention of AKI and targets a specific initiating cause. Given the multiple overlapping pathways involved in AKI, therapies may need to simultaneously target multiple pathways to achieve success.[28] In addition, despite the advances made in our understanding of the pathogenesis of AKI, translating this information to treat human AKI requires addressing issues such as identification of relevant targets through the analysis of human tissue biopsy and necropsy specimens, development of relevant disease models of AKI, inclusion of proper pharmacokinetic/pharmacodynamics studies and dose-response studies, and, lastly, improvement in preclinical and human clinical trial design.[407,318,398,374]

Acute Kidney Injury Is a Multisystem Disease

If small changes in serum creatinine are independent predictors of increased mortality, why then do these patients with AKI die? In ICUs it is not uncommon to observe complicated medical conditions that arise from the dysfunction of one organ leading to the dysfunction of another. In a cohort of patients with AKI after radiocontrast, many developed complications after the onset of AKI, including sepsis, hemorrhage, central nervous system (CNS) manifestation, and respiratory failure.[8] AKI in some cases is thought to contribute to distant organ dysfunction syndrome, leading to hospital mortality and long-term consequences.[426] Experimental studies provide some insight as to the mechanism by which isolated events leading to the loss of GFR can lead to distant organ dysfunction. Many potential factors may lead to distant organ effects, including circulating factors such as cytokines and chemokines, activated leukocytes, and adhesion molecules leading to immune cell infiltration. Oxidative injury, apoptosis, and cellular necrosis contribute to the final pathway of organ dysfunction. In critically ill patients, coexistent AKI and acute lung injury is associated with high mortality of 58% to 80%.[29,30] Experimental studies demonstrated increased pulmonary vascular permeability, lung edema, alveolar hemorrhage, and leukocyte circulation after ischemic AKI.[31-33,325,290,293,327] These data are scientifically and clinically relevant in defining the complex cross talk between the lung and kidney and will provide insight into human AKI. Recent studies have identified α-Klotho as a circulating factor that has cytoprotective effects in distant organs after AKI.[416,350] The extracellular domain of α-Klotho is cleaved and released into the circulation and has cytoprotective effects in distant organs such as the lung in part through the activation of the nuclear factor erythroid 2–related factor 2 (Nrf2) pathway. Circulating α-Klotho derived mainly from the kidney and ischemia-reperfusion injury (IRI) leads to systemic α-Klotho deficiency and acute lung injury. Purified recombinant α-Klotho has a direct cytoprotective effect on epithelial cells by activating an antioxidant response element reporter and increasing the Nrf2 pathway.[416,350]

Klein and colleagues[34] found that interleukin-6 (IL-6) is a direct mediator of AKI-induced increase in vascular permeability, leukocyte circulation, and increased edema after bilateral IRI or nephrectomies.[34]

Liu and associates[35] reported that mice with AKI exhibited increased brain vascular permeability and an increase in the level of glial fibrillary acidic protein, a marker for activated glial cells during brain inflammation, and activated microglial cells (brain macrophages) that were associated with increased numbers of pyknotic neurons. Thus CNS manifestations of AKI may be the result of distant effects of AKI-induced inflammation.

AKI promotes cardiac injury that is characterized by hypertrophy and fibrosis.[36] AKI has been found to increase cardiac apoptosis and production of IL-1 and tumor necrosis factor (TNF),[31] cardiac hypertrophy and fibrosis,[36] and gene expression for the macrophage chemokine osteopontin. These effects lead to an increase in inflammation[37] and abnormal cardiac function.[31]

There is considerable interest in the role of volume overload after AKI, which predisposes to multiorgan dysfunction and high mortality in the critically ill patient. Salt and water overload is associated with impaired wound healing, bowel edema, pulmonary edema/acute respiratory distress syndrome, lung infection, congestive heart failure, and cerebral edema. Conservative fluid management strategies are associated with improved outcomes.[412,339]

The cholinergic antiinflammatory reflex pathway, an immunomodulatory neuroimmune circuit interfacing the brain with the immune system, has been described as an endogenous homeostatic response to inflammation caused by infection, injury, and trauma.[405] The vagus nerve and the spleen are important components of the efferent limb of the neuroimmune circuit. In experimental models of AKI, splenectomy or denervation of the spleen, which would interrupt this pathway, exacerbate kidney IRI.[333] Importantly, distant organ effects were observed in splenectomized animals. In animals with splenectomy subjected to AKI, there was an increase in lung injury as measured by capillary leak, higher myeloperoxidase activity, and higher chemokine (C-X-C motif) ligand 1 (CXCL1) compared with animals with AKI alone.[292] Activation of the cholinergic antiinflammatory pathway through nonpharmacological approaches attenuates IRI-induced AKI and sepsis-induced AKI[334,335,355,288] and blocks systemic inflammation.[333,355]

In conclusion, although AKI is an independent risk factor for mortality,[7] in most studies of AKI renal failure per se is usually not the cause of death.[28] The potential systemic effects of AKI involve multiple organs and lead to high mortality. Thus the complexity created by the systemic effects of isolated AKI may have contributed to ineffective treatments in past clinical trials. These observations also suggest that potential therapeutic strategies should not be limited to treatment of kidney injury alone but should be broadly based to treat systemic effects of AKI.

PHARMACOLOGICAL INTERVENTIONS

Pharmacological interventions can be expected to be useful when used at various points in the natural history of AKI. Theoretically these would include agents that are used to lower the risk (i.e., prevent) in patients identified with high risk for AKI, agents that are used to limit injury in established AKI, and those that improve outcomes by improving rates of recovery from AKI. More clinical information is available for the prevention of AKI and very scant information for the other categories (Table 48.1).

Diuretics

Both loop diuretics and osmotic diuretics decrease tubular oxygen demand and relieve intratubular obstruction in animals.[38] Intratubular obstruction with debris released from injured or dead tubular epithelial cells from more proximal parts of the nephron increase proximal tubule pressure, further limiting glomerular filtration.[39] This observation, and the belief that nonoliguric AKI predicts better outcomes, made the clinical use of diuretics (especially loop diuretics) in oliguric AKI popular until recent times.[40] Both loop diuretics and osmotic diuretics are of limited use in attenuating the extent of the kidney injury or altering the outcomes in a positive manner.[3,41-44] Furthermore, a prospective observational study in 17 Finnish ICUs reported diuretics as a risk factor for the development of acute kidney injury.[392]

In a retrospective analysis of data from a cohort of 552 patients with AKI in the ICUs of a university hospital, Mehta et al. examined the effect of diuretic use on all-cause hospital mortality, nonrecovery of renal function, and the combined outcome of death or nonrecovery of renal function.[44] In this cohort about 59% of the patients had used diuretics; after adjustments for covariates and propensity scores, this group had a significantly higher risk for death or nonrecovery of renal function (OR, 1.77; 95% CI, 1.14 to 2.76). There have been additional systematic reviews or metaanalyses concerning the role of diuretics in this setting.[45-47] None of these found that diuretics were of any benefit in reducing the incidence of AKI, mortality, or need for renal replacement therapy (RRT).

Other studies have found that diuretics are not associated with higher mortality.[442,339] These results may be related to the importance of volume overload and mortality, and diuretics may provide a pharmacological approach to control fluid overload. In the PICARD study, a >10% fluid accumulation was associated with mortality at the start of renal replacement therapy[304]; there was a 19.6% fluid overload in nonsurvivors versus 10.1% in survivors.[337] In the Fluid and Catheter Treatment Trial (FACTT), which compared liberal versus conservative fluid management strategy using fluid

TABLE 48.1 Agents With Significant Existing Clinical Information

Agent	Clinical Evidence	Comments	References
Loop diuretics	Negative	Not used for prevention or treatment of AKI, but is used in pharmacological management of fluid overload	3,44,46,56 339 442 Uchino 2004 304
Osmotic diuretics	Negative	Not useful in improving mortality	24,41, 42
Antioxidants NAC	Conflicting	Some recommend use in radiocontrast-induced AKI along with isotonic crystalloid administration Not recommended to prevent AKI after cardiac surgery	51–57,60,62, 63 346 356 427
Ascorbic acid	Conflicting	Not enough evidence to support its use in the prevention of radiocontrast-induced AKI	65,66 358
Low-dose dopamine	Negative	No proven role in prevention and treatment	82–88,115
Fenoldopam	Conflicting	No role in prevention and treatment	93,103–115 370 305 335
Vasopressin	Possible	Not enough evidence for a beneficial effect in sepsis (but maybe beneficial in subgroup with less septic shock)	130–134
Terlipressin	Positive	May be useful in bridging for transplantation in hepatorenal syndrome	131,133,134
Angiotensin II	Conflicting	Beneficial in animal studies Also, improved BP in patients with vasodilatory shock	445 365
Calcium channel antagonist	Conflicting	No proven role in prevention and treatment	159–163
Theophylline	Minimal	Possibly useful in decompensated cardiac failure Evidence of reduction of AKI in postterm neonates with severe perinatal asphyxia	139–150 291
Atrial natriuretic peptide	Conflicting	No proven role in prevention and treatment Lower doses may be beneficial by reducing hypotensive episodes	152–156 391 394, 425
Insulin	Conflicting	Intensive insulin therapy not recommended for management of AKI and is associated with severe hypoglycemia	67,68,77,78 330 309
Statins	Negative	Not recommended for prevention of AKI	301
Corticosteroids	Negative	Not recommended for prevention of AKI	449
Recombinant EPO	Negative	Not recommended for prevention of AKI	318 324

AKI, Acute kidney injury; *BP,* blood pressure; *EPO,* erythropoietin; *NAC,* N-acetylcysteine.

restriction and diuretics to maintain lower central venous pressure in patients with acute respiratory distress syndrome, the conservative treatment led to fewer ventilatory days.[390] These results suggest that strategies to limit volume overload may affect mortality. Beginning and Ending Supportive Therapy for Kidney (BEST) was a large, multicenter, randomized prospective epidemiological study in ICUs from 54 centers and 23 countries.[442] In this study, 70% of the patients were treated with diuretics. Their results could not confirm findings of Mehta's study.[44] Instead, they found that diuretics were not associated with an increase in mortality in critically ill patients in the ICU.[442] Analysis of the data from the FACTT for the treatment of acute lung injury revealed that higher post-AKI furosemide doses had a protective effect on 60-day mortality, but this significant effect was lost after adjustment for post-AKI fluid balance. However, the authors noted that the benefit derived from diuretics may be due to reduction in fluid balance and that adjustment for fluid balance in the statistical analysis may not be appropriate.[339] Thus, although diuretics should not be used to prevent or treat AKI, their use should be included as part of the pharmacological management of fluid overload in AKI as well as renal replacement therapy.[337]

Antioxidants: N-Acetylcysteine, Vitamin C

N-Acetylcysteine (NAC) is a thiol-containing antioxidant with experimental evidence of improved renal function in mouse (and rat) renal IRI.[48-50] Because of positive early reports, it has been used as an intervention to prevent radiocontrast-induced AKI in high-risk populations.[51,52] Several randomized controlled clinical trials have been done subsequently to investigate the role of NAC in contrast-induced CI-AKI and in the setting of prolonged hypotension (e.g., abdominal aortic surgery).[53-55] Results of many of these do not support those early reports of benefit, and controversy still exists on the efficacy of NAC in this setting. A recent metaanalysis[56] of 41 randomized controlled trials (RCTs) with 6379 patients evaluated multiple therapeutic agents in high-risk patients who received radiocontrast. This metaanalysis found that, compared with hydration alone, NAC was the most effective agent at preventing radiocontrast-induced AKI of all the agents examined (theophylline, fenoldopam, dopamine, furosemide, mannitol, and bicarbonate). However, the authors noted this conclusion to be "debatable," with several limitations of the study, mainly the inconsistent definition of "radiocontrast-induced nephropathy" as primary outcome in most of the trials.

Recently, Hoffmann and colleagues[57] found that in healthy volunteers without AKI, NAC can reduce serum creatinine concentration (and eGFR) independent of an effect on true GFR as assessed by cystatin C (cys-C). This effect may be accomplished through an effect of NAC affecting creatinine metabolism[58] or altering the tubular secretion of creatinine. Despite this suggestion, not all studies support the concept that NAC alters serum creatinine independent of GFR.[59]

The Acetylcysteine for Contrast-Induced Nephropathy Trial (ACT) randomly assigned 2308 patients to receive 1200 mg NAC twice daily or placebo for 2 days to investigate the effect of NAC on the incidence of CI-AKI after coronary angiography. There was no difference in the incidence of CI-AKI between NAC and placebo arms (12.7% vs. 12.7%, $P = 0.97$). Also, a subgroup analysis of 367 patients revealed no benefit of NAC in reducing 30-day mortality or the need for renal replacement therapy.[356] The ACT trial had some shortcomings—predominantly that it included low-risk patients (only 15.7% patients had a serum creatinine of more than 1.5 mg/dL); in addition, high-risk agent (high osmolar contrast media) was used in 20% of the procedures; the baseline serum creatinine was obtained 3 months pre-procedure; and periprocedural fluid management was not standardized. Although the ACT trial does not prevent small increases in serum creatinine or serious 30-day outcomes in low-risk patients, there remains clinical equipoise on the use of NAC for the prevention of CI-AKI.[313] The results of the Prevention of Serious Adverse Events Following Angiography (PRESERVE) trial were recently published.[448] Using a two-by-two factorial design, the investigators randomly assigned 5177 patients at high risk for renal complications who were scheduled for angiography to receive intravenous (IV) 1.26% sodium bicarbonate or IV 0.9% sodium chloride and 5 days of oral acetylcysteine or oral placebo; of these patients, 4993 were included in the modified intention-to-treat analysis. The primary endpoint was a composite of death, the need for dialysis, or a persistent increase of at least 50% from baseline in the serum creatinine level at 90 days. Contrast-associated AKI was a secondary endpoint. Notably, the sponsor stopped the trial after a prespecified interim analysis. The primary endpoint occurred in 110 of 2511 patients (4.4%) in the sodium bicarbonate group compared with 116 of 2482 (4.7%) in the sodium chloride group (OR, 0.93; 95% CI, 0.72 to 1.22; $P = 0.62$) and in 114 of 2495 patients (4.6%) in the acetylcysteine group compared with 112 of 2498 (4.5%) in the placebo group (OR, 1.02; 95% CI, 0.78 to 1.33; $P = 0.88$). There was no interaction between sodium bicarbonate and acetylcysteine with respect to the primary endpoint ($P = 0.33$). There were no significant between-group differences in the rates of contrast-associated AKI.

Evidence does not support the use of NAC to reduce mortality or renal outcomes (such as AKI or AKI requiring renal replacement therapy) without radiocontrast administration. A metaanalysis of 10 RCTs with 1193 patients cumulatively undergoing major surgery evaluated the effectiveness of NAC in reducing mortality and renal outcomes. NAC was not associated with a reduction in mortality (OR, 1.05; 95% CI, 0.58 to 1.92), AKI requiring RRT (OR, 1.04; 95% CI, 0.45 to 2.37), or increase in serum creatinine by 25% more than baseline (OR, 0.84; 95% CI, 0.64 to 1.11).[346] In addition, use of NAC does not prevent development of AKI after off-pump cardiac surgery[427] and new-onset hypotension.[331] The results of the PRESERVE trial also confirmed these findings. The overall conclusion that can be reached with these studies and systematic reviews is that NAC is not of any benefit in prevention of radiocontrast- or ischemia-induced AKI.[60-63]

Ascorbic acid (vitamin C), a scavenger of reactive oxygen species (ROS), is another antioxidant that has shown some promise in animal experiments.[48-50,64] Human studies using ascorbic acid to prevent radiocontrast-induced AKI are less conclusive. Spargias and associates[65] randomly assigned 238 patients with a serum creatinine of 1.2 mg/dL and receiving nonemergent coronary angiography or intervention to receive 3 g of ascorbic acid or placebo about 2 hours before such procedures and then a second and third dose later in the day and the next morning. Mean serum creatinine concentration increased significantly in the control group versus the intervention group (difference of 0.09 mg/dL; 95% CI, 0 to 0.17; $P = 0.049$). These differences, however, did not seem to be clinically significant. More recently, a large trial (the REMEDIAL trial) found that the combination of ascorbic acid and NAC was no better than NAC and saline.[66] Also, high-dose NAC was compared with ascorbic acid in an RCT of 212 CKD patients who underwent coronary angiography. The incidence of CI-AKI was greater in the ascorbic acid group compared with NAC (4.4% vs. 1.2%, $P = 0.370$). Notably, among patients with diabetes, NAC significantly reduced CI-AKI rates compared with ascorbic acid (0% vs. 12.5%, $P = 0.039$).[358] In addition, ascorbic acid administration revisited in a metaanalysis of nine RCTs with 1536 patients suggested a 33% lesser risk for CI-AKI in patients treated with ascorbic acid compared with placebo or an alternative pharmacological treatment (relative risk [RR] by random-effects model, 0.672; 95% CI, 0.466 to 0.969, $P = 0.034$) However, there was heterogeneity in the route of administration of vitamin C (six orally and three intravenously) and another neutral or negative small RCT ($n = 250$), which could invalidate the positive results of the metaanalysis in the future.[417] A large RCT to address the clinical efficacy of vitamin C in CI-AKI is needed.

Thus the evidence does not support the use of ascorbic acid in the prevention of radiocontrast-induced AKI.

Insulin

Insulin resistance and hyperglycemia are common in critically ill patients, and intensive insulin therapy targeting blood glucose levels between 80 and 110 mg/dL reduced mortality[67] and the incidence of AKI.[67,68] It is well known that IRI is greater in chronic hyperglycemia[69] and thought to be related to increased oxidative stress.[70,71] Furthermore, acute hyperglycemia exacerbates myocardial[72] and renal IRI.[73] The effects of insulin may relate to improved glycemic control or be due to direct cellular effects of insulin. The relationship of hyperglycemia and adverse outcome in critically ill patients with AKI was also observed in subgroup analysis of the PICARD study.[74] The mechanism for clinical benefit may relate to the direct metabolic and nonmetabolic effects of hyperglycemia. Endothelial dysfunction and subsequent hypercoagulation and dyslipidemia, commonly observed in critically ill patients, can also be partially corrected by insulin independent of its blood glucose–lowering effect.[75,76] However, despite these promising results, the effect of intensive insulin treatment in the setting of critically ill patients is still controversial.[77,78]

The Normoglycemia in Intensive Care Evaluation—Survival Using Glucose Algorithm Regulation (NICE-SUGAR) study was the largest randomized control trial evaluating the question about intensive therapy or conventional therapy. The study enrolled 6100 patients to assess the risk-benefit ratio of tight glycemic control. The intensive glucose control group was associated with increased mortality compared with conventional glucose control (27.5% vs. 24.9%, $P = 0.02$). Also, there was no significant difference between the two groups in the incidence of RRT (15.4% vs. 14.5%).[330]

Intensive insulin therapy is associated with an adverse event of severe hypoglycemia. The Efficacy of Volume Substitution and Insulin Therapy in Severe Sepsis (VISEP) trial was a multicenter randomized trial in 537 patients with severe sepsis who were divided into an intensive insulin therapy group and a conventional insulin therapy group; the volume resuscitation was either 10% pentastarch or a modified Ringer's lactate solution. This trial was stopped early because of the safety signal of severe hypoglycemia in the intensive therapy group compared with the conventional treatment group (17% vs. 4.1%, $P < 0.01$).[309] Intensive insulin therapy is not recommended for the management of AKI and is associated with a severe hypoglycemia.

Dopamine, Dopamine Analogs, and Natriuretic Peptides

Exogenous dopamine can bind to at least three types of receptors: the dopamine receptor, the ß-adrenoreceptor, and the α-adrenoreceptor.[79] Differences in these receptors' affinity for dopamine account for its distinct dose-response profile. Dopamine is a selective renal vasodilator at low doses (1 to 3 mcg/kg/min).[79] Cardiac output and renal perfusion pressure are also improved at different doses of dopamine.[80,81] The ability to improve RBF provided the rationale for its use in the prevention and treatment of AKI.[82] Many clinical studies have been done to investigate the effect of dopamine on the natural history of AKI. The results of many of these studies have been conflicting and also complicated by the frequent use of surrogate endpoints that are sometimes not clinically relevant. A few systematic reviews and metaanalyses have also been undertaken.[82-87] The overall conclusion is that low-dose dopamine has no proven role in prevention and treatment of AKI.[82-88]

Why has dopamine failed in clinical trials? This has been examined in several reports. Low-dose dopamine consistently causes renal vasodilatation in healthy adults, but this effect is often attenuated or absent in ill patients.[89,90] In other reports, dopamine reduced renal vascular resistance in patients without AKI but paradoxically increased resistance indices in patients with AKI.[87] Several factors may account for this, including unpredictable pharmacokinetics in critically ill patients, hypertensive arteriopathy, or counterregulatory effects of other vasoactive hormones, such as activity of the renin-angiotensin-aldosterone system (RAAS) or sympathetic nervous system. Both extracellular volume depletion and hypoxemia have been found to abrogate the renal effects of dopamine.[91] Based on many studies, low-dose dopamine should not be used in the prevention of AKI.

Fenoldopam is a selective dopamine-1 receptor (DA1) agonist that has been found, like dopamine, to cause renal arteriolar vasodilatation, leading to an increase in RBF and improvement in renal function while attenuating the decline in RBF and function in animals exposed to radiocontrast.[92,93] Fenoldopam results in peripheral and renal vasodilation and diuresis and natriuresis via stimulation of vascular and renal tubular DA1 receptors.[94,95] Studies in healthy, salt-replete participants have confirmed dose-dependent increases in renal plasma flow, urine flow rate, and urinary sodium excretion without changes in GFR.[94,96-101] The lack of increase in the GFR is secondary to parallel vasodilation of both afferent and efferent renal arterioles, rendering intraglomerular pressure constant.[102] Animal studies have demonstrated fenoldopam to be markedly more potent than dopamine in decreasing renal vascular resistance and augmenting RBF.[95] Its relative potency, in conjunction with the absence of the potentially deleterious cardiac side effects characteristic of dopamine as a result of ß-adrenoreceptor stimulation, were the impetus for trials examining its potential to prevent and treat renal ischemia.

The clinical benefit in humans is inconclusive. Randomized controlled trials and metaanalyses of clinical trials concluded that there is no proven role for fenoldopam in prevention and treatment of AKI.[93,103-114]

For prevention of AKI, there are several underpowered studies and metaanalyses with inconclusive results as a result of heterogeneity among participants, inconsistent definitions of AKI, and lack of placebo arms.[370] Fenoldopam has mixed results in metaanalysis and systematic reviews.

The largest secondary prevention RCT to investigate the effect of fenoldopam in 667 patients after cardiac surgery was stopped early after a planned interim analysis revealed a safety signal of hypotension in the treatment arm compared with placebo. In addition, fenoldopam did not significantly reduce the need for RRT or risk for mortality at

30 days.[306] Of note, this was a secondary prevention trial in which patients were randomly allocated after the development of AKI (defined by 50% rise in serum creatinine). Also, the therapeutic intervention happened after a median of 32 hours (interquartile range of 26 to 52 hours) after initiation of surgery. A rising serum creatinine represents an already decreased level of GFR, and the delay in intervention may have contributed to the adverse results of the study. Besides, this trial suggested alternative pathophysiological mechanisms (e.g., inflammation) other than renal hypoperfusion in AKI after cardiac surgery.

Finally, a systematic review and metaanalysis of six RCTs with 507 surgical patients (cardiovascular surgery, partial nephrectomy, post–liver transplant) demonstrated a significant reduction in postoperative AKI but without any benefit on reduction in RRT or hospital mortality. It is an underpowered metaanalysis with heterogeneity in the criteria of AKI. Extrapolating the data to other surgical patients would be difficult.[335] In conclusion, clinical equipoise remains about the use of fenoldopam in the management of AKI.

Atrial natriuretic peptide (ANP) is not recommended for prevention and treatment of AKI based on the evidence, although it does exert pleiotropic effects (via guanylyl cyclase A activation) such as natriuresis, suppression of the renin-angiotensin system, vasodilation, and renoprotective effects.[303] Multiple large and multicenter RCTs have failed to find such clinical benefit, however.[152-154] A systematic review and metaanalysis of ANP in AKI found 19 RCTs (11 for prevention and 8 for treatment).[156] The studies were described as low to moderate quality and mostly underpowered, and as such no definitive statements could be made about ANP use in AKI prevention or therapy.[156] Also, data regarding potential confounders such as remote ischemic preconditioning and the use of isoflurane anesthesia were lacking.[391] After this metaanalysis, a few RCTs were conducted. Sezai et al.[425] studied the effect of low-dose ANP (carperitide) on postoperative serum creatinine in 303 CKD patients undergoing on-pump coronary artery bypass graft in a single-center RCT. The investigators reported a lower serum creatinine in the treatment group compared with placebo on the first day after surgery, and this effect persisted 1 year postoperatively ($P = 0.00665$, $P < 0.0001$).[425] Subsequently, the Acute Study of Clinical Effectiveness of Nesiritide in Decompensated Heart Failure (ASCEND) randomly assigned 7141 patients admitted with decompensated heart failure to receive nesiritide or placebo in addition to standard of care. The study reported a moderate symptomatic benefit of dyspnea in heart failure patients treated with nesiritide compared with placebo. However, there were no differences in rehospitalization rates or 30-day mortality between the two study arms. In addition, incidence of AKI defined by 25% change in serum creatinine from baseline was not different in the two groups (31.4% vs. 29.5%; OR, 1.09; 95% CI, 0.98 to 1.21; $P = 0.11$).[394] Continuous low-dose infusion of ANP needs to be performed in larger clinical trials before it can be recommended for routine use.

Norepinephrine

AKI is often associated with hypotension in patients with concurrent clinical problems like sepsis or liver failure, especially in ICUs. Attempts to maintain systemic blood pressure within limits that allow visceral organ perfusion (including autoregulation of RBF) are usually done with systemic vasoconstrictors.[116-118]

Norepinephrine effectively raises the systemic mean arterial blood pressure to greater than 80 mmHg in many hypotensive states associated with vasodilation by stimulation of both α- and β-adrenergic receptors.[116] This effect on mean arterial pressure is dose related, and, as such, the dosage of the drug can be titrated for desired effect. Some studies have found, however, that despite this desirable effect, there is often a less desirable decrease in splanchnic and vital organ blood flow (including kidneys).[119-121] Most of these older studies, together with experimental data, indicate that norepinephrine can be used to induce a reversible model of AKI—an observation that has discouraged its clinical use for AKI.[122,123] Some authors have argued that norepinephrine-induced renal hypoperfusion may not necessarily occur in sepsis or other vasodilated states, and they cite various animal experiments that support that mixed α- and β-adrenergic stimulation can increase RBF in such situations.[124-128] Anderson and colleagues[129] used infusions of norepinephrine at clinically relevant doses of 0, 0.1, 0.2, and 0.4 mcg/kg/min in conscious dogs and measured the RBF with an electromagnetic flow probe. Their findings indicated that mean arterial pressure, RBF, and GFR all increased with increasing dosage of norepinephrine, and renal vascular resistance decreased accordingly.[129] There is a need for clinical trials in humans that will give a reliable answer to the question of whether norepinephrine and the kidneys are "friends or foes."[117]

Vasopressin and Analogs

Arginine vasopressin (AVP) is an endogenous peptide hormone with vasopressor and antidiuretic properties historically used to treat bleeding from esophageal varices in cirrhotic patients and for diabetes insipidus.[130] Arginine vasopressin receptor 1A (AVPR1A), the first of three major receptor types for AVP, is found in vascular smooth muscle (and the brain, liver, and kidney). A relative deficiency of AVP has been reported in patients with septic shock.[131] This has led to the use of low-dose AVP infusions (about 0.01 to 0.03 units/min) as adjunctive support to catecholamines for vasoconstrictor effect in sepsis-related hypotension. The Vasopressin and Septic Shock Trial (VASST), a multicenter, randomized, double-blind study, assigned patients with septic shock and who were receiving a minimum of 5 mcg/min norepinephrine (open label) to receive, in addition, either low-dose vasopressin (0.01 to 0.03 units/min) or norepinephrine (5 to 15 mcg/min) with protocol titration to maintain a target blood pressure. The study found no significant difference in the primary endpoint (mortality rate at 28 days) or any of the secondary outcomes when low-dose vasopressin (0.3 units/min) was used along with catecholamine vasopressors.[132] In a subgroup analysis, vasopressin may have been beneficial in patients with less severe septic shock; the mortality rate was lower in the vasopressin group than in the norepinephrine group at 28 days (26.5% vs. 35.7%, $P = 0.05$).[132]

Terlipressin, a glycine vasopressin, is a 12-amino acid synthetic analog of AVP that is currently being considered by the US Food and Drug Administration (FDA) as an orphan drug for the treatment of type 1 hepatorenal syndrome (HRS). Consequently, it is not yet available for clinical use in the United States (or elsewhere in North America), but it is already in use in Europe. Its major advantage is the long half-life of the drug that makes intermittent dosing (every 6 hours) possible, rather than a continuous infusion.[116] Two recent clinical trials have had good results in cohorts of patients with AKI, specifically type 1 HRS.[133,134] Sanyal and associates[134] evaluated the safety and efficacy of terlipressin for reversal of type 1 HRS in patients with cirrhosis in a prospective, randomized, double-blind, placebo-controlled clinical trial. The treatment group ($n = 56$) received terlipressin 1 mg intravenously every 6 hours (vs. placebo, $n = 56$) plus albumin in both groups. The results indicated that terlipressin was superior to placebo for HRS reversal (34% vs. 13%, $P = 0.008$), and HRS reversal significantly improved survival at day 180.[134] Martin-Llahi and coworkers[133] found similar results in HRS when IV terlipressin was added to IV albumin.[133]

Angiotensin II

Septic AKI is associated with hypotension and reduced RBF.[295,320,423] However, during the hyperdynamic phase of sepsis, RBF is increased in experimental animals[371,372] and in humans,[322] which may be due to a greater increase in dilation of the efferent arteriole compared with the increase in dilation of the afferent arteriole.[445] When angiotensin II was infused in septic animals, arterial pressure was restored. RBF was reduced but urine output and creatinine clearance were increased, consistent with an effect to improve efferent arteriolar tone.[445] Recently, angiotensin II was infused in patients with vasodilatory shock and increased blood pressure when conventional vasopressors failed. Whether there was an improvement in renal function was not reported.[365]

Adenosine Analogs

Locally produced adenosine in the kidney controls renal circulation and metabolic cellular activity.[135] Four subtypes of adenosine receptors (A_1, A_{2A}, A_{2B}, and A_3) are characterized by having seven putative transmembrane-spanning domains, and they mediate a multitude of physiological responses.[136] Adenosine acts on these receptors in organs such as brain, heart, and skeletal muscle and induces vasodilation to allow matching of oxygen delivery and work.[135] Adenosine has been found to be involved in the renal hemodynamic response to radiocontrast agents and the immune response to renal IRI.[137,138] Theophylline, an adenosine A1 receptor antagonist, has been used successfully in several RCTs to prevent radiocontrast-induced AKI (as reviewed in references 139 to 141). Theophylline has been used in several case-control and randomized controlled studies as a potential prophylactic agent against radiocontrast-induced AKI.[139–144] A metaanalysis of these six studies indicated discordant results, with only four out of six studies finding some evidence of reduction of relative risk for radiocontrast-induced AKI.[56] Other systemic reviews and opinions agree that the results have been discordant, mainly with some consideration that it may be more useful in the cohort of preexisting decompensated cardiac failure.[56,140,145-150] There is little convincing evidence for recommending theophylline in the prevention of radiocontrast-induced AKI.

A single dose of theophylline may be given in postterm neonates who are at high risk for AKI.[364a] There is evidence of a reduction in AKI in postterm neonates with severe perinatal asphyxia in a recent metaanalysis of RCTs of 197 patients comparing theophylline to placebo. The pooled RR reduction of AKI = 0.38; 95% CI, 0.25 to 0.57, $P < 0.001$. However, we have to be cautious with the clinical use of theophylline because the long-term renal outcomes, neurodevelopmental outcomes, and adverse effects related to theophylline levels were not reported.[291]

Calcium Channel Antagonists

Calcium channel antagonists relieve afferent arteriolar vasoconstriction, among other actions, and have been found to be protective against radiocontrast-associated AKI in animals.[157,158] Calcium channel blockers have been used in different randomized controlled studies to assess ability to prevent AKI from radiocontrast and in renal allografts.[159-163] The preservation of GFR by day 2 in patients treated with nitrendipine versus placebo and exposed to radiocontrast study seems promising[163]; however, the others do not indicate any benefit of calcium channel blockers in this setting.[161,162]

Identification of effective pharmacological agents for the prevention and treatment of AKI remains a subject of intense focus for many investigators. None of the agents discussed have had enough impact to be considered sole and effective intervention for the prevention or treatment of AKI. Further, large clinical trials may give more information on these agents.

Recombinant Erythropoietin

Erythropoietin is a glycoprotein with a molecular weight of 30.4 kDa. Binding of erythropoietin to its receptor on target tissue leads to homodimerization of the receptor and initiation of complex intracellular signaling pathways.[210-212] Exogenously administered erythropoietin, before or at the time of reperfusion, reduced kidney injury by reducing tubular necrosis and apoptosis.[213-215] Recombinant erythropoietin has additional cell survival properties such as induction of phosphatidylinositol 3 kinase (PI3K)/Akt pathway[216] or heat shock protein 70.[217] Recombinant erythropoietin enhanced tubular proliferation in cisplatin-induced AKI[218] and also mediated mobilization and proliferation of endothelial progenitor cells (EPCs) from the bone marrow, which has been reported to participate in tissue repair.[219,220] The tissue-protective effects of recombinant erythropoietin appear to require a physical association between the common β-receptor chain subunit

(CD131) and erythropoietin receptor.[221] The helix B (amino acid residues 58 to 82) of erythropoietin and an 11-aa peptide composed of adjacent amino acids of helix B were found to be tissue protective and without erythropoietic activity.[222] These results indicate that nonerythropoietic peptides of erythropoietin that simulate a portion of erythropoietin receptor's three-dimensional structure possess tissue-protective properties. Thus recombinant erythropoietin or nonerythropoietic peptides are agents that have promise in the treatment of AKI. Early-phase clinical trials using erythropoietin in cardiac surgery have reported inconsistent results, some finding no clinical benefit[319,367,366] and others finding some benefit.[436,428,396] Endre and coworkers[324] performed a double-blind placebo-controlled trial to examine the early treatment with erythropoietin to prevent the development of AKI in ICU patients. To avoid the concerns of using a late marker of AKI such as serum creatinine, these investigators used two urinary biomarkers to trigger intervention (IV erythropoietin 500 U/kg to a maximum of 50,000 U), urinary proximal tubular brush border enzymes c-glutamyl transpeptidase and alkaline phosphatase. Allocation occurred within 3.5 ± 1.6 hours after obtaining urine samples. However, 64% were randomly allocated 6.3 ± 4.2 hours after admission to the ICU. Early intervention with high-dose erythropoietin was well tolerated but did not alter the outcome. The discordance between preclinical and clinical results may in part be explained by the design of preclinical studies. De Caestecker and coworkers[318] recently performed a careful analysis of 36 preclinical studies examining the efficacy of erythropoietin in various models of AKI, including toxin-associated, ischemic, and sepsis-associated AKI. Despite the performance of experiments in multiple models in different species (genetically inbred mice, pigs, macaques, and outbred rat strains), performance in humans have been inconclusive. Testing in models with common clinical morbidities and sex heterogeneity would improve preclinical testing,[407,318,398] and improved clinical trial design may facilitate translation to human AKI.[398] Thus, despite the potential for erythropoietin to prevent or treat AKI, the results remain inconclusive. An ongoing study on the use of erythropoietin in the prevention of AKI in cardiac surgery patients is near completion (NCT03007537).

Statins

Statins are not recommended for the prevention of AKI. A recent single-center RCT of 199 patients demonstrated no difference in the incidence of AKI among postoperative patients when high-dose atorvastatin was compared with placebo (RR, 1.06; 95% CI, 0.78 to 1.46). In addition, subgroup analysis in patients with CKD (eGFR <60 mL/min/1.73 m^2) noted a higher incidence of AKI in atorvastatin group compared with placebo. Hence, we do not recommend the use of statins for the prevention of AKI.[301]

Corticosteroids

Steroids have diminished the inflammatory response to cardiopulmonary bypass in a small-scale RCT.[450] However, methylprednisone was ineffective compared with placebo in decreasing the incidence of new renal failure, one of the composite primary outcomes, in a large-scale RCT of patients undergoing cardiac surgery (4% vs. 4%; RR, 0.87; 95% CI, 0.69 to 1.08).[449]

The proven preventive clinical strategies of good hydration and volume expansion with isotonic saline before exposure to radiocontrast agents; discontinuation of nonsteroidal antiinflammatory agents, metformin, and angiotensin-converting enzyme (ACE) inhibitors; limitation of nephrotoxin exposure; and efforts to maintain renal perfusion still remain very useful clinical strategies.

BOX 48.1 Emerging Pharmacological Agents for Treatment of Acute Kidney Injury

1. Antiapoptosis/necrosis agents
    a. Alpha melanocyte stimulating hormone
    b. Minocycline
    c. p53 siRNA
2. Antisepsis
    d. Soluble thrombomodulin
3. Growth factors
    e. Hepatocyte growth factor (HGF)
    f. Bone morphogenic protein 7
4. Vasodilators
    g. Levosimendan
5. Antiinflammatory drugs
    h. Sphingosine 1 phosphate analogs
    i. Adenosine 2A agonists
    j. Alkaline phosphatase
    k. Adenosine analogs
    l. Inducible nitric oxide synthase (iNOS) inhibitors
6. Mitochondrial agents
    m. MitoQ (mitoquinone mesylate)
    n. Szeto-Schiller (SS) peptides
7. Iron metabolism agents
    o. Deferoxamine
    p. Hepcidin
8. Mesenchymal stem cells
9. Volatile anesthetic agents

WHAT DRUGS ARE ON THE HORIZON?

A number of novel investigational compounds and established drugs (for other indications) are being explored, some in preclinical studies and others in early-phase clinical trials (Box 48.1). The goal of these agents is to either prevent AKI, treat and improve outcomes in established AKI, or halt or mitigate progression to ESRD.[326,363] They have been grouped by their known main mechanism of action; some of the compounds involve more than one mechanism; for example, an agent could be an antiapoptotic and an antiinflammatory at the same time.

Antiapoptotic Drugs

α-Melanocyte–Stimulating Hormone

α-Melanocyte–stimulating hormone (α-MSH) is a melanocortin agonist with antiapoptotic and antiinflammatory effects.[287,429] Early animal studies found that α-MSH decreased risk for AKI in IRI and sepsis and in nephrotoxin exposures.[363] A more potent analog of α-MSH, AP214, was licensed as ABT-719. It protected against AKI in animal models of sepsis and IRI. It has advanced to phase II trials in humans, where it was used in a randomized, double-blind, placebo-controlled study to prevent AKI in high-risk cardiac surgery patients. In this phase IIb study, ABT-719 analog did not decrease the incidence of AKI using AKIN criteria or change outcomes at 90 days after cardiac surgery, nor did it reduce the increase in novel biomarkers of AKI: serum neutrophil gelatinase–associated lipocalin (NGAL) and urine NGAL, IL-18, and kidney injury molecule 1 (KIM-1).[383]

Minocycline

Minocyclines are second-generation tetracycline antibiotics with proven human safety data. Minocycline is known to have antiapoptotic and antiinflammatory effects. When administered 36 hours before renal ischemia, minocycline reduced tubular cell apoptosis and mitochondrial release of cytochrome C, p53, and Bax.[172] Furthermore, minocycline reduced kidney inflammation and also microvascular permeability.[173] Minocycline has been used in clinical trials for rheumatoid arthritis[174] and amyotrophic lateral sclerosis.[175] Minocycline has been tested in treatment of AKI after cardiac surgery, acute spinal cord injury, and acute stroke (see www.clinicaltrials.gov). In a randomized, double-blind, and placebo-controlled trial to prevent AKI after cardiac surgery in 40 patients, minocycline or placebo was given in at least 4 doses (200 mg initially, then 100 mg every 12 hours until surgery) with a maximum of 14 doses. In this small underpowered study, the primary outcome, AKI (a 0.3 mg/dL or more rise in serum creatinine concentration within 5 days after surgery), was no different in both groups.[338]

p53 Small Interfering RNA

The tumor suppressor protein p53 is a homotetrameric transcription factor and regulates cell cycle and apoptosis by inducing cell cycle arrest or apoptosis in response to DNA damage. A variety of factors induce activation of p53, including irradiation, hypoxia, and nucleotide depletion.[176] Additional activities regulated by p53 are supported by studies, including regulation of autophagy, glycolysis, repair of genotoxic damage, cell survival, regulation of oxidative stress, motility, cellular senescence, and differentiation.[176] Once activated, p53 induces apoptosis by activating proapoptotic Bax, which triggers apoptosis via the intrinsic pathway. Pharmacological inhibition of p53 downregulates activation of Bax and inhibits the translocation of p53 to mitochondria,[177] decreases tubule cell apoptosis, and preserves renal function.[178] In p53-deficient mice, AKI was attenuated in cisplatin-induced AKI[179] but not in a model of renal IRI.[433]

QPI-1002 targeted at p53 is a synthetic antiapoptotic agent that has received "orphan drug" designation from the US Food and Drug Administration, the first small interfering RNA (siRNA) drug to be administered to humans (NCT00554359); after preclinical studies, siRNA for p53 showed a dose-dependent attenuation of apoptotic signaling in IRI, delayed graft function, and nephrotoxic (cisplatin)–related AKI.[385,354] Using two-photon microscopy, Cy3-labeled siRNA is rapidly filtered and taken up by proximal tubules, significantly reducing p53 gene expression for up to 24 to 48 hours.[385] Subsequent clinical studies are in phase II (NCT02610283) to examine the efficacy and safety of QPI-1002 in patients at high risk for AKI after cardiac surgery and in phase II (NCT00802347) and III (NCT02610296) targeting delayed graft function after kidney transplantation.

Antisepsis Drugs

Endocannabinoid Receptors

The endocannabinoids are an endogenous signaling system that modulates a variety of functions, including the immune system. Cannabinoid 1 (CB1) and cannabinoid 2 (CB2) are linked to the G-protein–coupled receptors Gi, which inhibit adenylyl cyclase and intracellular cyclic adenosine monophosphate (cAMP) accumulation.[421] CB2 receptors are expressed on leukocytes and regulate the immune system.[387,369,400] CB2 receptor agonists decrease leukocyte endothelial cell interaction and inflammation[368,414,415,420] and increase microcirculatory flow by intravital microscopy.[440] CB2 receptor–deficient mice had increased mortality, lung injury, and neutrophil recruitment at the site of infection after sepsis.[441] A highly selective CB2 receptor agonist, *N*-(piperidin-1-yl)-1-(2,4-dichlorophenyl)-1,4-dihydro-6-methylindeno[1,2-*c*]pyrazole-3-carboxamide (GP1a), reduced inflammation and bacterial colony count and improved survival time.[441]

Soluble Thrombomodulin

The thrombomodulin–protein C system is important for healthy endothelial cells that maintain regional microcirculation and prevent thrombosis.[380] Thrombomodulin (TM), a 557–amino acid glycoprotein expressed broadly on the surface of endothelial cells, exerts thromboresistance resulting in anticoagulation.[380] On the cell surface, cleavage of protein C by thrombin requires TM as a cofactor generating activated protein C (APC). APC is an important modulator of coagulation and inflammation associated with sepsis by inactivating factor Va and VIIIa, thereby promoting fibrinolysis and inhibiting thrombosis. In addition, soluble thrombomodulin (sTM) independent of its ability to generate APC reduced ischemia-reperfusion injury.[199] In this study an aortic clamp model was used; sTM not only attenuated the rise in creatinine after reperfusion, but it also improved microvascular erythrocyte flow, reduced microvascular endothelial leukocyte adhesion, and minimized endothelial permeability. A mutant, F376L, in which a point mutation was made in sTM, reduced IRI, suggesting that the protective effect of sTM is independent of its ability to generate APC.

APC, in addition to its effect on coagulation, has been found to have direct cellular effects via endothelial cell protein C receptors (EPCRs), including antiinflammatory and antiapoptotic activities, leukocyte activation, and stability of barrier function.[198,200-205] Through genetic engineering of wild-type APC, mutants have been created that have the cytoprotective effects of APC and anticoagulant activity.[206,207] After endotoxemia, these molecules with preserved cytoprotective properties are effective in preserving RBF, attenuating acute kidney injury,[207] and reducing mortality.[208] On the other hand, an APC mutant with potent antithrombotic activity but minimal cytoprotection was less effective in reducing endotoxin-induced murine mortality.[209] Although the data suggest that the protective effect is independent of its anticoagulant effect, sTM may exert its effect by several means. sTM may have antiinflammatory effects; studies using *N*-terminal lectin-like domain of TM, which lacks anticoagulant function, have found that it blocks leukocyte adhesion to endothelial cells.[315] In addition, sTM may have cytoprotective and anti-inflammatory effects through activating EPCR/protease activated receptor (PAR) signaling. Lastly, sTM inactivates C3a or C5a and blocks inflammation.[380] Thus additional studies are necessary to delineate the mechanism of action of sTM while clinical studies are ongoing to demonstrate its efficacy in sepsis (see Box 48.1).

Growth Factors

Hepatocyte Growth Factor

Hepatocyte growth factor (HGF) is a mesenchyme-derived polypeptide that is a potent mitogen for hepatocytes (reviewed in Brines et al.[222]). Mature HGF is a heterodimeric molecule consisting of a 69-kDa α chain and a 34-kDa β chain. HGF is synthesized and secreted as a 728-aa single-chain precursor processed by specific serine proteases to generate a biologically active form that is made up of two chains.[223] HGF can promote cell growth, motility, and morphogenesis and act as a cell survival factor.[224-227] Renal expression of HGF and its receptor, c-Met, increases after IRI, and exogenous administration of HGF reduces renal injury and accelerates renal regeneration in a murine model of AKI.[228-230] The mechanism of protection includes a decrease in leukocyte–endothelial interaction with reduced inflammation; promoting tubular regeneration; upregulating cell survival proteins, including Bcl-2; and decreasing in tubular cell apoptosis.[231,364,348,360,453,381] BB3 is a small molecule with hepatocyte-like growth factor activity that has been found to be effective in focal cerebral ischemia[312] and renal IRI. BB3 was administered to rats 24 hours after IRI and improved survival and renal function, while decreasing KIM-1, NGAL, and apoptosis. BB3 enhanced phosphorylation of cMET and Akt and upregulated Bcl-2.[389] BB3 is being tested in a phase II study (Guard Against Renal Damage [GUARD]), a multicenter, randomized, placebo-controlled, double-blind study of ~100 patients in the United States with risk factors for AKI (NCT02771509). BB3 was also tested in a phase II study in renal transplant patients for delayed graft function (NCT01286727). The interim analysis found that BB3 increased urine output, lowered serum creatinine, reduced the need for dialysis, and shortened length of hospitalization. A phase III study (Graft Improvement Following Transplantation [GIFT]) is being conducted in which BB3 or placebo is administered within 30 hours of transplantation to determine its effect on duration of dialysis or other measure of kidney function (NCT02474667).

Bone Morphogenic Protein

Bone morphogenetic proteins (BMP-7) are members of the transforming growth factor β superfamily, which has been found to be essential for cell growth, migration, and differentiation during development skeletal, kidney, and ocular development.[236] Renal IRI leads to decreased levels of BMP-7 messenger RNA in the rat kidney, primarily in the outer medulla and glomeruli at 6 hours, which is more pronounced at 16 hours.[237] Administration of exogenous BMP-7 at 1 hour and 16 hours after onset of reperfusion attenuates the severity of the injury.[238] BMP-7–treated proximal tubule cells block basal and TNF-α–stimulated expression of the proinflammatory cytokines IL-6 and IL-1β, the chemokines monocyte chemotactic protein 1 (MCP-1) and IL-8, and endothelin 2 (ET-2).[239] A phase II multicenter clinical trial using THR-184 in the prevention of AKI in at-risk patients undergoing cardiac surgery has been completed (NCT01830920). This study randomly allocated 140 patients undergoing high-risk cardiac surgery to either placebo or one of three THR-184 doses, given intravenously before surgery (and repeated postoperatively) and examined outcome of AKI in 7 days. There was a decrease in incidence of AKI in patients treated with the highest dose of THR-184. The drug was well tolerated and deemed safe and most effective in patients with CKD.

Vasodilators

The traditional concept that global ischemia is a major cause of AKI formed the basis for vasodilator therapy. The absence of benefit from dopamine, fenoldopam, and natriuretic peptides (see earlier) suggests that therapeutic interventions must consider the complexity of glomerular hemodynamics and its variability in response to different mechanisms of AKI. For example, prerenal azotemia from volume depletion leads to decrease in renal plasma flow, single-nephron GFR, and ultrafiltration coefficient (Kf).[302] On the other hand, in sepsis, RBF may be decreased, unchanged, or increased.[371] The decrease in GFR, primarily caused by a decrease in intraglomerular pressure, is governed by pressure in Bowman space as a result of a decrease in renal plasma flow, balance of afferent and efferent tone, downstream tubule obstruction, and decreased K_F.[412] Furthermore, in addition to factors that govern RBF and GFR, it is important to determine the contribution of peritubular microcirculation and tissue oxygenation.[382] The peritubular microcirculation may be altered by glycocalyx, adhesion molecule expression, leukostasis, inflammation, complement, and others.[382] The inability to measure continuously human RBF and GFR, as well as tissue microcirculatory flow, is a barrier to advancement of therapies targeting renal hemodynamics.

Adenosine Triphosphate–Sensitive K Channel Agonists

Adenosine triphosphate–sensitive K (K_{ATP}) channels are expressed on vascular smooth muscle, are characterized by a single channel conductance of 15 pS to 258 pS, and are inhibited by intracellular ATP and activated by adenosine diphosphate (ADP).[378,419] In vitro studies on isolated rabbit afferent arterioles constricted by K_{ATP} channel inhibitor glibenclamide were dilated by the K_{ATP} channel opener diazoxide.[378] K_{ATP}

channels also contribute to the myogenic response, and this response is attenuated in renal hypoxia, which may be important in controlling medullary circulation where oxygen tension is low.[419] Levosimendan is an K_{ATP} channel opener and myocardial sensitizer[404] and has antiinflammatory properties that may improve myocardial dysfunction and renal perfusion while reducing inflammation[403] during sepsis.[451] In a sepsis model, levosimendan conferred complete protection, had no effect on inflammation, and attenuated mesangial cell contraction in response to angiotensin II, suggesting that its vasoactive properties led to tissue protection. Furthermore, the lack of direct effect on hypoxic tubules suggest its potential role in sepsis or cardiorenal syndrome. Levosimendan is in a phase III study examining the effect of levosimendan versus dobutamine on renal function in patients with cardiorenal syndrome (NCT02133105), a phase IV study examining the effect of levosimendan versus placebo in patients with AKI after cardiac surgery (NCT02531724), and a phase II study examining the effect of levosimendan to reduce postoperative AKI in pediatric patients undergoing cardiac surgery (NCT02232399).

Antiinflammatory Drugs

Inflammatory cells, including polymorphonuclear cells, monocytes, macrophages, and T cells, have received considerable attention as important contributors to ischemic acute renal failure. Several new compounds appear to be effective in reducing injury for ischemia-reperfusion through direct action on leukocytes.

Sphingosine 1 Phosphate Analogs

Sphingosine 1 phosphate (S1P) is a specific ligand for a family of G-protein–coupled endothelial differentiation gene receptors (also referred to as S1PRs 1 to 5) that evoke diverse cellular signaling responses. S1PRs regulate different biological processes depending on their pattern of expression and the diverse G proteins present. S1P binds to receptors or acts as a second messenger to stimulate cell survival, inhibit cell apoptosis, and inhibit cell adhesion and movement.[256] An S1P analog, FTY720, acts as an agonist at four S1P receptors, which leads to sequestration of lymphocytes in secondary lymphatic tissue.[257] In studies of kidney IRI, FTY720 or similar compounds produced lymphopenia and renal tissue protection.[258,259] Activation of S1P1 on endothelial cells improves vascular integrity to protect from AKI and permit recovery.[408] Furthermore, activation of S1P1 on proximal tubule cells improves mitochondrial function to protect kidneys from IRI.[296] FTY720 reduced the number of lesions detected on magnetic resonance imaging and clinical disease activity in patients with multiple sclerosis,[261] and in 2010, FTY720 was approved by the FDA to treat relapsing forms of multiple sclerosis. With discovery of new S1P analogs, more potent and selective agents will be available for preclinical and clinical studies.[260]

A_{2A} Agonists and Other Adenosine Analogs

Adenosine binds to receptors that are members of the G-protein–coupled receptor family, which includes four subtypes: A_1R, $A_{2A}R$, $A_{2B}R$, and A_3R.[262] Selective activation of $A_{2A}Rs$ reduces parenchymal injury in nonrenal tissue, including heart, liver, spinal cord, lung, and brain.[263-265] The selective A_{2A} agonist, ATL146e, is highly protective against IRI of kidney and reduces injury by 70% to 80%.[266-268] After administration either before or immediately at the onset of reperfusion, ATL146e alone or in combination with a phosphodiesterase inhibitor reduced renal injury.[269] ATL146e is in human clinical studies for cardiac imaging, and efforts are directed toward human clinical studies in AKI. Additional studies demonstrate that strategies using A_1 agonists or A_3 blockers may be effective in AKI.[270,271] Although there are no trials in AKI, $A_{2A}R$ agonists (regadenoson) are being studied in a phase II study examining the effectiveness in reducing inflammation by its ability to reduce invariant natural killer T-cell activation (NCT0108520). Furthermore, a phase I trial will soon be underway to examine its tolerability in patients undergoing transplantation (NCT03072589). Both these studies are supported by preclinical studies demonstrating the potent effect of $A_{2A}R$ agonists in blocking inflammation in models of kidney[376] and lung ischemia-reperfusion[373] and occlusive vascular disease in sickle cell crises.[328,329]

Alkaline Phosphatase

In preclinical and clinical studies, systemic alkaline phosphatase administration as an antiinflammatory strategy demonstrated protection in sepsis-associated AKI.[411,409] The mechanism by which alkaline phosphatase protects from inflammation and tissue injury is thought to be due to direct dephosphorylation of endotoxin and neutralization of endotoxin activity. Alkaline phosphatase may also act as a nonselective phosphatase and catalyzes the conversion of ATP into adenosine. Adenosine may then act on adenosine receptors, of which there are four subtypes (A_1, A_{2a}, A_{2b}, and A_3). Activation of A_{2a} receptors has potent antiinflammatory actions,[431,377] and selective adenosine 2a analogs attenuate AKI[317,376] and improve survival in sepsis.[430] In phase IIa studies, administration of bovine alkaline phosphatase resulted in reduced inflammation and decreased sepsis-associated AKI, although there were no changes in mortality.[411,409] Recombinant human alkaline phosphatase was tested in a phase I study and found to be safe and tolerable while demonstrating favorable pharmacological properties and enzyme activity. A large phase II study is ongoing to test the safety, tolerability, efficacy, and quality of life in patients with sepsis-associated AKI (STOP-AKI) (NCT02182440).

Mitochondrial Agents

Mitochondria are dynamic organelles that have a critical role in cellular energy production, metabolism, calcium homeostasis, and programmed cell death. Mitochondria are abundant in proximal tubules and supply ATP from oxidative phosphorylation (OXPHOS) necessary for tubular function.[357] During renal ischemia, mitochondrial function diminishes[342]; during reperfusion, ultrastructural analysis reveals fragmented mitochondria associated with mitochondrial dysfunction, ATP depletion, generation of mitochondrial-derived ROS, and activation of cell death pathways.[307,357] These morphological and functional changes that occur contribute to AKI, and evidence supports the concept that preserving the integrity of mitochondria and enhancing mitochondrial biogenesis may promote recovery from AKI.[307,357]

Mitoquinone mesylate (MitoQ) is a mitochondria-targeted antioxidant that selectively accumulates in the mitochondrial matrix because of its positive charge.[316] In the mitochondrial matrix, MitoQ is reduced to the active antioxidant form, ubiquinol, by the respiratory chain, preventing oxidative damage–lipid peroxidation. MitoQ given to mice intravenously 15 minutes before ischemia protected mouse kidneys from injury.

SS-31 is a member of the Szeto-Schiller (SS) peptides. It selectively targets the inner mitochondrial membrane.[434] SS-31 carries a positive charge and binds to anionic phospholipid cardiolipin (CL). CL-phospholipid expressed on the inner mitochondrial membrane has an important structural role in the organization of the respiratory complexes for optimal OXPHOS. The interaction between CL and cytochrome c is vital for mitochondrial function because it dictates whether cytochrome c acts as an electron carrier or peroxidase. CL peroxidation is associated with energy deficiency. SS-31 protects electron carrying function by cytochrome c by preventing CL from converting cytochrome c into a peroxidase. SS-31 protects the structure of mitochondrial cristae and promotes OXPHOS. Remarkably, in a study of rats subjected to 45 minutes of bilateral renal ischemia and followed for 9 months, SS-31 arrested progression of kidney disease.[435] In control animals, glomerular and peritubular capillary rarefaction, macrophage infiltration, and fibrosis were observed, and there were marked morphological abnormalities of mitochondria. In animals treated with SS-31 for 6 weeks, beginning 1 month after ischemia, there was preserved glomerular capillary, podocyte, and mitochondrial structure with attenuated kidney fibrosis.

Iron Metabolism Agents

Deferoxamine and Hepcidin

Catalytic iron (or labile) iron damages cells through its ability to induce oxidative radicals,[341] and, in addition, mitochondrial function, and cell cycle and DNA repair are iron dependent.[418] Iron chelation with deferoxamine decreases injury after bleomycin- or cisplatin-induced nephrotoxicity.[297,298] Iron sequestration can be achieved through the release of hepcidin, an antimicrobial peptide released from the liver. Hepcidin is an endogenous acute-phase hormone that downregulates iron export protein, ferroportin, to induce reticuloendothelial iron sequestration.[323] Swaminathan and coworkers[424] tested whether hepcidin, by blocking iron export, can protect kidneys from IRI. Hepcidin administration decreased kidney injury, which was associated with decreased kidney ferroportin expression and increased expression of H-ferritin.[424] H-ferritin has been found to play a cytoprotective protective role in the proximal tubule after AKI.[452] These results suggest that a novel compound hepcidin through targeting ferroportin holds promise as a novel therapeutic target in the treatment of AKI.

Hypoxia-Inducible Factor 1 Inducing Agents

Hypoxia-inducible factor 1 (HIF1) is an evolutionary conserved transcription factor that consists of an oxygen-sensitive α subunit and a constitutively expressed β subunit that allows cellular adaption to hypoxia.[388] Prolyl hydroxylase hydroxylates HIF and targets the protein for degradation.[308] HIF prolyl hydroxylase inhibitors contribute to organ protection, including brain, heart, liver, and kidney.[299,447,289,340] Analogs of oxoglutarate inhibit prolyl hydroxylase and stabilize HIF.[422] Prolyl hydroxylase uses oxoglutarate as a cosubstrate, and 2-oxoglutarate analogs have been found to protect kidneys from IRI.[422] Daprodustat (GSK1278863) is an orally available prolyl hydroxylase inhibitor in clinical trials for other indications.

Mesenchymal Stem Cell Therapy

AKI resulting from toxins, ischemia, or sepsis is characterized by complex series of overlapping pathways that may necessitate a broad approach in combining multiple targets.[399,444,359] For example, in severe sepsis, critically ill patients require multiple vasopressors and fluid regimens because of marked hypotension and multiorgan dysfunction. Marked dysregulation of innate immunity contributes to the pathophysiological events in sepsis.[446,399,294,349] Mesenchymal stem cells (MSCs), derived from bone marrow, can differentiate into osteocytes, chondrocytes, and adipocytes. In preclinical studies, infused MSCs demonstrate protection and enhanced recovery in cisplatin- and glycerol-induced AKI and ischemia-reperfusion injury[344,437,300,345,386] and reduce inflammation and AKI in experimental sepsis.[379,406]

MSC-mediated tissue protection likely is due to paracrine mechanisms, including growth factors, cytokines that modulate mitogenesis, apoptosis, inflammation, and vasculogenesis and angiogenesis, rather than transdifferentiation.[437,410,438,336,439] MSCs have been found to enhance proliferation of tubule epithelial cells through growth factors and cytokines.[300] MSC microvesicles have been found to shuttle mRNA to injured cells to enhance survival.[310] The use of pulsed ultrasound improved MSC homing to diseased organs and enhanced the protection observed with MSCs alone.[311]

Because of their pluripotency, hypoimmunogenicity, easy accessibility from bone marrow, and rapid ex vivo expansion, MSCs have been used in clinical trials. AC607 are expanded bone marrow–derived MSCs obtained from healthy adult donors, and their efficacy and safety have been tested in a phase II study in at-risk patients undergoing cardiac surgery, but trials were terminated because of the lack of efficacy (NCT01602328). MSCs are in use in a pilot study examining the feasibility and safety of ex vivo expanded MSCs to repair kidneys and improve function in patients with solid organ cancer who develop AKI from cisplatin (NCT01275612). In another study, SBI0-101 is a combination product that combines MSCs with a bloodfiltration device used for continuous renal replacement therapy (CRRT). This phase I/II study seeks to determine the safety and tolerability of combining MSCs with CRRT in patients with AKI necessitating renal replacement therapy (NCT03015623). In donor after cardiac death transplantation, allogeneic bone marrow–derived MSCs are being examined in a phase I/II study to determine their efficacy and safety. Renal allograft function, patient/graft survival, and adverse events within 12 months will be monitored (NCT02561767).

Anesthetic Agents

Studies have demonstrated that volatile anesthetic agents have important protective effects on multiple organs in ischemic and inflammatory conditions.[332] Both in vitro and in vivo results indicate that volatile anesthetic agents attenuate IRI and inflammation. In ischemic AKI, volatile anesthetic agents have protective effects by decreasing inflammatory cell infiltration and proinflammatory cytokines[375,343,395] and through effects on endothelial and epithelial cells.[443] Importantly, the newer volatile anesthetic agents such as sevoflurane, isoflurane, desflurane, and halothane possess a triflourocarbon (CF3) molecule, which appears to exert immunomodulatory effects.[332] Of these new volatile anesthetic agents, desflurane is the least lipid soluble and is less potent in kidney protection in rats subjected to IRI compared with the other agents with greater lipid solubility (sevoflurane, isoflurane, and halothane).[375] A prospective randomized study compared the effect of sevoflurane versus desflurane on kidney function after living donation transplantion.[361] On postoperative days 1 and 7 there was no difference in creatinine, estimated GFR, NGAL, or IL-18 between the two groups.[361] In a related study, sevoflurane versus propofol on the incidence of acute rejection in recipients of living donation after circulatory death and donation after brain death, donor kidneys will be examined (NCT02727296). Additional studies will be necessary to establish whether certain volatile anesthetic agents confer greater kidney protection.

DISCLOSURES

Consultant or Scientific Advisory Board member for Astellas, Pfizer/AM Pharma, Mitobridge, and Merck. Dr. Okusa is a share holder of Adenosine Therapeutics, LLC.

ACKNOWLEDGMENTS

The authors are grateful to Dawn Kidd (University of Virginia) for helpful comments. This work was supported in part by funds from NIH (1R01DK105133, R01DK62324 1R01 DK085259 U18EB021787 to MDO).

A full list of references are available at www.expertconsult.com.

49

Renal Replacement Therapy for Acute Kidney Injury

Ashita J. Tolwani, MD, MS, Michael J. Connor, Jr., MD, and Paul M. Palevsky, MD

OUTLINE

The incidence of acute kidney injury (AKI) in hospitalized patients varies from 5% to 20%, depending on the definition of AKI used and clinical setting.[1–4] Most critically ill patients develop AKI as part of multiple organ failure (MOF) and have an increased risk for morbidity and reported mortality rates of 40% to 70% when renal replacement therapy (RRT) is required.[2,4–9] Since intermittent hemodialysis (IHD) became a common clinical tool for patients with severe AKI in the 1960s, options for RRT have expanded considerably. Biocompatible membranes, bicarbonate dialysate, and dialysis machines with volumetric ultrafiltration control have improved the ability to provide IHD to patients in the intensive care unit (ICU). Along with advances in methods of IHD, continuous renal replacement therapies, including hemofiltration and hemodiafiltration, and hybrid forms of prolonged intermittent RRT have gained widespread acceptance in the treatment of dialysis-requiring AKI.[4,10–13]

The indications, timing of initiation, and choice of modality and intensity of delivered therapy are factors that must be considered in prescribing RRT to patients with AKI. This chapter outlines current concepts in the use of RRT for AKI.

GOALS OF AND INDICATIONS FOR RENAL REPLACEMENT THERAPY

The treatment of AKI with RRT has several interrelated goals: (1) to maintain fluid and electrolyte, acid–base, and solute homeostasis; (2) to prevent complications of uremia; and (3) to allow other supportive measures (e.g., antibiotics, nutrition support) to proceed without limitation. Ideally, therapeutic interventions should be designed to achieve those goals while minimizing the risk for further insults to the kidney and facilitating recovery of kidney function. In practice, the use of RRT is commonly based on physician preferences and experience. No evidence-based criteria have been established to guide modality choice, thereby making comparisons among centers or strategies at the same or different institutions difficult. An important consideration is to recognize that patients with AKI are distinct from those with end-stage renal disease (ESRD). The rapid decline of kidney function in AKI does not permit the adaptive responses that characterize the course of the patient with chronic kidney disease (CKD). Consequently, the traditional indications for renal replacement, developed for patients with advanced CKD, are not necessarily valid in this context (Box 49.1). For instance, massive volume overload, resulting from volume resuscitation, a common strategy used for MOF, may be an indication for dialysis, even in the absence of significant elevations in blood urea nitrogen (BUN) or plasma creatinine. In this instance, it may be more appropriate to consider RRT in the ICU patient as a form of renal support as opposed to "replacement." Indeed, some of the traditional indications for dialysis (e.g., uremic pericarditis, pleuritis, or other serositis) would be considered "rescue indications" suggesting undue delay in initiation of RRT.

MODALITIES OF RENAL REPLACEMENT THERAPY

The most common RRT modalities used for AKI include IHD, prolonged intermittent renal replacement therapy (PIRRT), continuous renal replacement therapy (CRRT), and peritoneal dialysis (PD) (Tables 49.1 and 49.2). IHD, PIRRT,

BOX 49.1 Indications for Renal Replacement Therapy

Conventional Indications for Renal Replacement Therapy
Volume overload
Hyperkalemia
Metabolic acidosis
Drug intoxications
Uremic manifestation
Progressive azotemia in the absence of overt uremia

Potential Expanded Criteria for Renal Support
Volume management in heart failure, sepsis, and multisystem organ failure
Acid–base management in respiratory failure with low-tidal-volume ventilation
Nutrition management

TABLE 49.1 Renal Replacement Therapy Modalities for Acute Kidney Injury

Modality	Usual Duration	Access
Intermittent hemodialysis	<6 hours	Vascular
Prolonged intermittent renal replacement therapy	8–16 hours	Vascular
Continuous renal replacement therapies*	Continuous	Vascular
Slow continuous ultrafiltration		
Continuous venovenous hemofiltration		
Continuous venovenous hemodialysis		
Continuous venovenous hemodiafiltration		
Peritoneal dialysis	Variable	Peritoneal

*Most commonly provided as pump-driven venovenous therapies; may also be provided as arteriovenous therapy.

and CRRT are extracorporeal therapies that require vascular access in the form of a large-bore, double-lumen central venous catheter, whereas PD requires the placement of an intraabdominal dialysis catheter.

The various modalities of RRT use varying proportions of diffusion and convection for solute transport and ultrafiltration, driven either by hydrostatic or osmotic gradients, for volume management. With extracorporeal therapies, some solutes may also be removed by adsorption onto the membrane. The relative contributions of diffusion, convection, and adsorption depend on the solute, the membrane, the geometry of the dialyzer, and operating conditions such as blood and dialysate flow rates and ultrafiltration rate. Ultrafiltration, which is used for volume management and which drives convective clearance, occurs by application of a hydrostatic pressure across the membrane from the blood to effluent side in IHD, PIRRT, and CRRT and by an osmotic gradient in PD. In diffusion, blood is exposed to dialysate across a semipermeable membrane and solute transfer across the membrane is driven by the concentration gradient between blood and dialysate. With extracorporeal therapies, the concentration gradient is maximized and maintained throughout the length of the membrane by running the dialysate countercurrent to the blood flow. Solute clearance is dependent on molecular size, membrane characteristics such as pore size, charge, water permeability, and extracorporeal circuit factors such as dialysate and blood flow rates. Small molecular weight solutes (<500 Daltons) are cleared efficiently by diffusion because their mobility in solution is high. As molecular weight increases, the mobility of solutes in solution diminish and diffusive clearance decreases. Convective clearance occurs when application of a hydrostatic pressure or osmotic gradient across a semipermeable membrane forces solvent (i.e., plasma water) across the membrane by ultrafiltration and "drags" with it small- and middle-molecular-weight solutes by bulk flow. The size of solutes that can be removed by convection is determined primarily by the size selectivity and charge characteristics of

TABLE 49.2 Comparison of Key Characteristics of Modalities of Renal Replacement Therapy Used for Management of Acute Kidney Injury

Characteristic	IHD	PIRRT	CRRT	PD
Access	Vascular	Vascular	Vascular	Peritoneal
Duration	<6 hours	8–16 hours	Continuous	Continuous
Mode of solute removal	Diffusion	Diffusion	Diffusion (CVVHD, CVVHDF) and convection (CVVH, CVVHDF)	Diffusion
Hemodynamic tolerability	Low	High	High	High
Rate of solute removal	Rapid	Intermediate	Slow	Slow
Ultrafiltration rate	Rapid	Intermediate	Slow	Slow
Ultrafiltration control	Yes	Yes	Yes	No
Risk of membrane clotting	Low	Intermediate	High	None
Need for anticoagulation	Variable	Variable	Often	None
Treatment of intoxication or severe hyperkalemia	Rapid	Intermediate	Slow	Slow

CRRT, Continuous renal replacement therapy; *CVVH,* continuous venovenous hemofiltration; *CVVHD,* continuous venovenous hemodialysis; *CVVHDF,* continuous venovenous hemodiafiltration; *IHD,* intermittent hemodialysis; *PD,* peritoneal dialysis; *PIRRT,* prolonged intermittent renal replacement therapy.

the membrane. For solutes that are smaller than the size cutoff of the membrane, the major determinant of convective clearance is the rate at which ultrafiltration occurs.

Intermittent Modalities

Intermittent Hemodialysis

IHD primarily uses diffusion for small-solute clearance and ultrafiltration for volume removal. However, high-flux dialyzers can provide convective clearance of larger solutes through increased membrane porosity, enhanced transport capacity, and internal filtration and backfiltration.[14] IHD is typically delivered 3 or more days per week, 3 to 5 hours per session, with a blood flow rate of 300 to 500 mL/min and a dialysate flow rate of 500 to 800 mL/min. The duration and frequency of IHD sessions are determined by the patient's specific metabolic and volume requirements and degree of hemodynamic stability. Because IHD allows for rapid solute and volume removal, it is preferred for rapid correction of severe electrolyte disturbances, such as hyperkalemia, and treatment of amenable drug intoxications. The higher blood flow rate and shorter duration of therapy allows IHD to be performed with less or no anticoagulation compared with other extracorporeal RRT modalities. However, the rapid solute and fluid removal predispose to intradialytic hypotension, which occurs in 30% to 50% of acute IHD treatments.[15–18] Strategies for improving hemodynamic stability include cooling the dialysate, sodium modeling, increasing the dialysate calcium concentration, performing intermittent ultrafiltration, and prolonging the duration of therapy to slow the rate of ultrafiltration.[19] Despite this, approximately 10% of patients with AKI cannot tolerate IHD because of hypotension.[15,19–22] Furthermore, as the result of rapid intracellular fluid and solute shifts that may cause disequilibrium between the brain and extracellular compartments, IHD can increase intracranial pressure and exacerbate cerebral edema in patients with fulminant hepatic failure and acute brain injury.[23]

Prolonged Intermittent Renal Replacement Therapies

Prolonged intermittent renal replacement therapies are hybrid therapies used as an alternative to CRRT in critically ill patients with AKI.[24,25] Significant heterogeneity exists in practice with regard to PIRRT technology, prescription, and anticoagulation.[26] These techniques attenuate the hemodynamic effects of IHD by prolonging therapy duration and adapting conventional hemodialysis machines to provide lower blood-pump speeds (100 to 300 mL/min) and dialysate flow rates (100 to 300 mL/min). Treatment sessions may range from 6 hours every other day to greater than 12 hours daily. Diffusion-based PIRRTs have been described as sustained low efficiency (daily) dialysis (SLEDD), extended daily dialysis (EDD), slow continuous dialysis (SCD), and "go slow dialysis."[27–29] When both convective and diffusive therapy are used together, they have been described as low-efficiency daily diafiltration (SLEDD-f) and sustained hemodiafiltration (S-HDF)[30,31]; the term *accelerated venovenous hemofiltration (AVVH)* has been used to describe solely convective therapy.[32] PIRRT can also be provided using CRRT equipment, delivering treatment for 8 to 16 hours per day with proportionally augmented dialysate or replacement fluid flow rates.

PIRRTs combine advantages of both CRRT and IHD. They allow for improved hemodynamic stability by removing solute and fluid over a longer period while avoiding the need for 24-hour therapy and expensive CRRT machines and solutions. At the same time, they provide high solute clearances as in IHD and allow for scheduling of required diagnostic and therapeutic patient procedures without interruption of therapy. Furthermore, the therapy can be delivered at night to allow for patient mobilization during the day. Studies have indicated that PIRRTs provide comparable hemodynamic control to CRRT.[33–36] Appropriate adjustment of dosing of medications, especially antibiotics, is complicated by the significant variation in practice of delivery of PIRRT and the extended time of dialysis and small-solute clearance. For example, with IHD a given antimicrobial may be removed and reach subtherapeutic levels the last 2 hours of a given session and the medication can be redosed immediately after dialysis in 1 to 2 hours. However, with PIRRTs, a given antimicrobial may reach subtherapeutic concentrations after 2 to 3 hours of the session with another 6 to 10 hours remaining, and a midtreatment dose may be needed. Clear data do not exist on how to approach these dosing questions in PIRRT, and decisions must be individualized with close coordination with clinical pharmacy experts.

Continuous Modalities

Peritoneal Dialysis

In PD the peritoneum is used as a semipermeable membrane for diffusive removal of solutes. Dialysate consisting of a sterile, lactate-buffered electrolyte solution is instilled into the peritoneal cavity through a catheter, where it dwells for a prescribed period to allow solutes to diffuse from the blood into the dialysate. The saturated dialysate is then drained and discarded, and fresh dialysate reintroduced. Varying high concentrations of dextrose (or other nonelectrolyte solutes) are used in the dialysate to create an osmotic gradient for ultrafiltration. Acute PD can be performed intermittently or continuously and either manually or by an automated cycler. PD techniques for AKI include acute intermittent peritoneal dialysis (IPD), continuous equilibrated peritoneal dialysis (CEPD), tidal peritoneal dialysis (TPD), continuous flow peritoneal dialysis (CFPD), and high-volume peritoneal dialysis (HVPD). IPD is characterized by frequent short exchanges using volumes of 1 to 2 L and dialysate flows of 2 to 6 L/h.[37] It can be done manually or by using an automated cycler. CEPD is characterized by long dwells of 2 to 6 hours with up to 2 L of dialysate each. It is similar to continuous ambulatory PD used for chronic outpatient PD, except that the patients are not ambulatory.[38,39] TPD consists of an initial infusion of dialysate (typically 3 L) followed by a variable dwell and partial drain of the solution, leaving a residual amount of dialysate in constant contact with the peritoneal membrane until the final drain.[38] This approach is thought to enhance clearance of small solutes by reducing the loss of dialytic time that is associated with the drainage and reinfusion of dialysate; however, clinical experience with TPD has not confirmed any advantage over other PD techniques in terms of clearance or ultrafiltration.[40] In CFPD, inflow and outflow of dialysate occurs simultaneously through two access routes with maintenance of a fixed intraperitoneal volume. This technique is performed with high dialysate flow rates (150 to 300 mL/min) and produces greater small-solute clearance than conventional automated PD.[41] HVPD uses a cycler to provide continuous therapy with frequent exchanges (18 to 48 exchanges per 24 hours, 2 L per exchange) with dialysate volume ranging from 36 to 70 L per day and high small-solute clearance.[37]

Advantages of PD include technical simplicity, hemodynamic stability, lack of need for anticoagulation or vascular access, and lower cost. Because solute and fluid removal is gradual, it may be a safer modality among patients at risk for increased intracranial pressure. Disadvantages include the need for specialized training for catheter insertion, complications of PD catheter placement, risk for peritonitis, potential inability to provide sufficient solute clearance in hypercatabolic patients, unpredictable ultrafiltration rates, hyperglycemia, excessive protein loss across the peritoneal membrane, and potential respiratory compromise from increased abdominal pressure. PD is contraindicated in patients with recent abdominal surgery, abdominal drains, postoperative or traumatic diaphragm incompetence, or ileus. Acute PD is useful in AKI patients with hemodynamic instability or difficult vascular access issues or in AKI patients located in regions with limited resources or access to hemodialysis techniques.[42,43]

Continuous Renal Replacement Therapy

Continuous renal replacement therapy (CRRT) encompasses various modalities developed specifically to manage critically ill patients with AKI who cannot tolerate IHD because of hemodynamic instability. CRRT allows for better hemodynamic tolerance than IHD by providing slower solute and fluid removal per unit time. It is designed to be performed 24 hours a day with typical blood flow rates of 100 to 300 mL/min.[44–46] Potential advantages of CRRT over IHD include better hemodynamic tolerance, more continuous solute clearance, and better control of volume status.[47] The main disadvantages of CRRT include vascular access and filter clotting, greater need for anticoagulation, decreased patient mobility, and increased costs and demands on ICU nurse time compared with IHD.

CRRT employs diffusion, convection, or a combination of both for solute clearance. The different modalities of CRRT for solute removal include continuous venovenous hemofiltration (CVVH), continuous venovenous hemodialysis (CVVHD), and continuous venovenous hemodiafiltration (CVVHDF). In CVVH, solute clearance occurs by convection and is augmented by increasing the volume of ultrafiltrate produced. A “replacement” or “substitution” fluid is infused in the blood before the hemofilter (prefilter or predilution) or after the hemofilter (postfilter or postdilution) in varying amounts to replace the excess volume and electrolytes lost across the membrane from the high ultrafiltration rates. The use of postfilter replacement fluid is limited by the filtration fraction, which is the fraction of plasma water that is removed from blood during ultrafiltration and is defined as the ratio of ultrafiltration rate to plasma water flow rate.[48] Filtration fraction should be kept <0.25 to prevent increased risk of clotting because of hemoconcentration and protein-membrane interactions. Although adding some of the replacement fluid prefilter reduces the filtration fraction, it also dilutes the concentration of solutes entering the hemofilter, thereby decreasing solute clearance at a fixed ultrafiltration rate.[49] This reduction in clearance can be offset by increasing the ultrafiltration rate, which again increases filtration fraction, albeit to a value that is lower than before predilution. In CVVHD, solute removal occurs primarily by diffusion. In contrast to IHD, the dialysate flow rates (typically 0.5 to 3 L/h, or 8 to 50 mL/min) in CVVHD are significantly slower than the blood flow rates (100 to 300 mL/min), resulting in complete or near-complete saturation of the dialysate. Ultrafiltration is used only for volume control with rates much lower than required for convective solute clearance. CVVHDF uses a combination of convection and diffusion for solute removal and requires use of both dialysate and replacement fluid.

Despite increased clearance of middle-molecular-weight molecules with convective techniques, no study has found that CVVH or CVVHDF improves patient survival compared with CVVHD. In a metaanalysis comparing the outcomes of hemofiltration to hemodialysis for the treatment of AKI, the authors found no difference in patient survival or clinical outcomes such as organ dysfunction, vasopressor use, or renal recovery.[50] Hemofiltration was associated with an increased clearance of larger molecules but also a shorter CRRT filter and circuit life. Although cytokines can be removed by convective therapy, most controlled studies have failed to demonstrate an improvement in outcome.[51–56] High-volume hemofiltration (HVHF) with ultrafiltration rates >50 mL/kg/h has been attempted to augment the clearance of cytokines in AKI patients with sepsis and septic shock. However, a metaanalysis of four randomized controlled trials comparing HVHF to standard volume CVVH did not find any survival benefit with HVHF.[57] The High Volume Veno-venous Hemofiltration Versus Standard Care for Post-cardiac Surgery Shock (HEROICS) Study[58] was a randomized controlled trial in which patients with severe cardiogenic shock requiring high-dose catecholamines 3 to 24 hours after cardiac surgery were randomly assigned to early HVHF at 80 mL/kg/h for 48 hours followed by standard-volume CVVHDF versus standard care. Standard care involved initiating CVVHDF for conventional indications in the setting of AKI. Early HVHF did not lower 30-day mortality (odds ratio [OR], 1.00; 95% confidence interval [CI], 0.64 to 1.56; $P = 1.00$) or improve any other clinical outcomes. Multiple reasons may underlie this failure of augmented middle molecule clearance with convective clearance to improve clinical outcomes, including the fact that achieved cytokine clearances are still relatively low compared with their biological half-lives and that both pro- and antiinflammatory mediators are nonselectively removed.[59] Given insufficient data to recommend one type of CRRT modality over another, the choice of CRRT modality should be based on clinician preference and expertise.

TIMING OF INITIATION OF RENAL REPLACEMENT THERAPY

Although whether or not to provide dialytic support with RRT and when to start are two of the most fundamental questions facing nephrologists and intensivists in caring for patients with AKI, the optimal timing of acute RRT for AKI is not defined. An improvement in survival associated with early initiation of RRT was first suggested by case series with historical controls conducted in the 1960s and 1970s.[60–63] However, given that BUN concentrations at the start of dialysis in the "early" treatment groups in these studies were high by modern standards, their relevance to current practice is limited. Moreover, over the last 30 years, the severity of illness of hospitalized patients continues to increase, especially among the critically ill population, and life support technologies have rapidly progressed, allowing for improving survival, which further limits comparisons of distantly historical studies. More recent single-center observational studies that were restricted to AKI after trauma[64] and coronary artery bypass surgery[65,66] suggested a benefit to dialysis initiation at lower BUN concentrations. A prospective multicenter observational cohort study[67] performed by the Program to Improve Care in Acute Renal Disease (PICARD) analyzed dialysis initiation—as inferred by BUN concentration—in 243 patients from five geographically and ethnically diverse clinical sites. Survival rates were slightly lower for patients who started dialysis at higher BUN concentrations, despite a lesser burden of organ system failure. Adjusting for age, hepatic failure, sepsis, thrombocytopenia, and serum creatinine and stratified by site and initial dialysis modality, initiation of dialysis at higher BUN was associated with an 85% increased relative risk (RR) for death (RR = 1.85; 95% CI, 1.16 to 2.96).

Although the maintenance of BUN concentrations below arbitrarily set levels is usually a reference for starting dialysis treatment, BUN reflects factors not directly associated with kidney function, such as catabolic rate, nutritional intake (especially protein intake), and volume status. Plasma creatinine is influenced by age, race, muscle mass, and catabolic rate, and its concentration is also affected by changes in extracellular volume status (decreasing as total body volume increases). In a prospective multicenter observational study[68] conducted at 54 ICUs in 23 countries, timing of RRT was stratified into "early" or "late" by median urea at the time RRT started and also categorized temporally from ICU admission into early (less than 2 days), delayed (between 2 and 5 days), or late (more than 5 days). Timing by serum urea indicated no significant difference in mortality (63.4% for urea ≤ 24.2 mmol/L vs. 61.4% for urea > 24.2 mmol/L).[68] However, when timing was analyzed relative to ICU admission, late RRT was associated with greater crude mortality (72.8% late vs. 62.3% delayed vs. 59% early; $P = 0.001$) and covariate-adjusted mortality (OR, 1.95; 95% CI, 1.30 to 2.92; $P = 0.001$). Overall, late RRT was associated with a longer duration of RRT and a longer stay in hospital and greater dialysis dependence, which was attributed to accumulation of volume, worsening acidemia, and/or life-threatening electrolyte derangements. In addition, timing of initiation of RRT relative to ICU admission may also reflect differences with regard to whether AKI was present at ICU admission or developed as a complication during ICU admission, which may also influence these outcomes.

An important methodological flaw underlies these observational studies and limits their interpretation. By only including patients who actually received RRT rather than all patients in whom AKI was present and might have been considered as candidates for early RRT, these observational cohorts excluded patients with early AKI who either recovered kidney function or died without ever receiving RRT.[69] Because the clinical question is not early versus late initiation of RRT, but early initiation of RRT versus a delayed approach to management, failure to include these patients who do not receive RRT may provide a biased assessment of the benefits of early initiation of RRT.

Several randomized controlled trials have attempted to address this issue (Table 49.3). In an older study of critically ill patients, Bouman et al.[70] randomly assigned 106 critically ill patients with AKI to early or late initiation of dialysis. The early initiation group started CVVH within 12 hours of developing a low urine output (less than 30 mL/h for 6 hours, not responding to diuretics or hemodynamic optimization) or a creatinine clearance less than 20 mL/min. CVVH was started in the late initiation group when classic indications were met. Although underpowered to detect survival differences, the study did not find differences in ICU or hospital mortality between the early and late groups or in renal recovery among survivors.

Two more recent clinical trials—Artificial Kidney Initiation in Kidney Injury (AKIKI)[71] and Early Versus Late Initiation of Renal Replacement Therapy in Critically Ill Patients with Acute Kidney Injury (ELAIN)[72]—reached divergent conclusions. The AKIKI trial was a multicenter randomized controlled trial conducted in France that assigned 620 patients who reached Kidney Disease: Improving Global Outcomes (KDIGO) stage 3 AKI to either immediate initiation of RRT or a delayed initiation strategy in which RRT was not begun until specific metabolic parameters or life-threatening indications developed. Ninety-eight percent of the patients in the early arm received RRT compared with only 51% of the patients randomized to the delayed therapy arm. The median time from development of stage 3 AKI to initiation of RRT was 4.3 hours in the early treatment arm and 57 hours in the delayed arm; the predominant modality of RRT used was IHD. There was no difference in survival at 60 days between the early and delayed RRT groups (48.5% vs. 49.7%; $P = 0.79$).[71] Comparing the patients who received RRT, early RRT was associated with lower mortality compared with the patients initiated late (48.5% vs. 61.8% at 60 days); however, those patients in the delayed initiation arm who did not receive RRT had a substantially lower mortality (37.1% at 60 days) than those patients who received RRT.[71] Although these patients represented a lower risk population, with lower severity of illness at randomization, the inability to prospectively identify patients who ultimately do not receive RRT illustrates the need to include them in analyses of early versus delayed strategies of initiation.[73]

TABLE 49.3 Randomized Controlled Trials Evaluating Timing of Renal Replacement Therapy in Acute Kidney Injury

Study	Number of Patients	Study Setting	Study Design	RRT Modality	Criteria for Initiation of RRT: Early	Criteria for Initiation of RRT: Late	Percentage of Patients Receiving RRT: Early	Percentage of Patients Receiving RRT: Late	Mortality: Early	Mortality: Late	Mortality: *P* value
Bouman, 2002[70]	106	ICU	Two centers	CRRT	12 h from enrollment	BUN >112 mg/dL K > 6.5 mmol/L Pulmonary edema	70/70 (100%)	30/36 (83%)	28.6%	25%	0.80
Jamale, 2013[249]	208	Community-acquired AKI	Single center	IHD	BUN > 70 mg/dL Cr > 7 mg/dL	Usual care Mean BUN 101 ± 33 mg/dL Mean Cr 10.4 ± 3.3	93/102 (91%)	88/106 (83%)	20.6%	12.3%	0.20
Combes, 2015[58]	224	Post–cardiac surgery	Multicenter	CRRT	Post–cardiac surgery shock	Usual care	111/112 (99%)	64/112 (57%)	46%	38%	0.72
Wald, 2015[74]	100	ICU	Multicenter	IHD and CRRT	Stage 2 AKI	K > 6 mmol/L HCO_3< 10 mmol/L >72 h from enrollment	48/48 (100%)	33/52 (63.4%)	37.5%	36.5%	0.92
Zarbock, 2016[72]	231	Surgical ICU	Single center	CRRT	Stage 2 AKI	Stage 3 AKI	112/112 (100%)	108/119 (91%)	39.3%	54.7%	0.03
Gaudry, 2016[71]	319	ICU	Multicenter	IHD and CRRT	Stage 3 AKI	BUN > 112 mg/dL K > 6 mmol/L pH < 7.15 Oliguria > 72 h pulmonary edema	305/311 (98%)	157/308 (51%)	48.5%	49.7%	0.79

AKI, Acute kidney injury; *BUN,* blood urea nitrogen; *Cr,* creatinine; *CRRT,* continuous renal replacement therapy; *ICU,* intensive care unit; *IHD,* intermittent hemodialysis; *RRT,* renal replacement therapy.

The ELAIN trial was a single-center study[72] that randomly assigned 231 patients with KDIGO stage 2 AKI to either immediate RRT or delayed initiation until they reached KDIGO stage 3 AKI or developed life-threatening indications. CVVHDF was the modality of RRT used in all patients and only 9 of 118 in the delayed group did not receive RRT. The median time from reaching KDIGO stage 2 AKI to initiation of RRT was 6.0 hours in the early RRT arm compared with 25.5 hours in the late arm. Mortality at 90 days was 39.3% in the early RRT group versus 54.7% in the delayed group ($P = 0.03$) with a hazard ratio (HR) for death of 0.66 (95% CI, 0.45 to 0.97) in the early group. Two additional multicenter trials (Standard Versus Accelerated Initiation of Renal Replacement Therapy in AKI [STARRT-AKI; ClinicalTrial.gov #NCT01557361] and Initiation of Dialysis Early Versus Delayed in Intensive Care Unit [IDEAL-ICU; ClinicalTrial.gov #NCT01682590]) are ongoing. Pilot data from 100 participants enrolled in the pilot phase of the STARRT-AKI trial indicated a separation in time from eligibility in the two arms of approximately 24 hours with no significant difference in mortality between the two treatment groups (38% in the accelerated arm vs. 37% in the standard arm).[74]

The role of volume overload as an independent criterion for initiation of RRT in critically ill patients with AKI should be noted. Over the last 10 to 15 years, multiple studies in critically ill patients have demonstrated that volume overload is detrimental to critically ill patients both with and without AKI, contributing to mortality[47,75–81] and to other morbidities such as duration of ICU length of stay, time on mechanical ventilation,[82] and intraabdominal hypertension.[83,84] Almost all patients requiring acute RRT, especially in the ICU, have some degree of volume accumulation or frank volume overload, and there is a strong association between volume overload at time of RRT initiation and increased risk for death in both adults[47,76] and pediatric populations.[85,86] Furthermore, retrospective data suggest that the excess hospital mortality seen in AKI seems primarily driven by fluid overload, hyperkalemia, and metabolic acidosis rather than by azotemia.[75]

Much of the uncertainty regarding timing of initiation of RRT rests with difficulty that is often present in assessing the trajectory of AKI in an individual patient. Will oliguria be transient or prolonged? Will kidney function begin to recover in a matter of hours or days, or will the AKI be prolonged? Novel biomarkers of kidney injury such as neutrophil gelatinase-associated lipocalin (NGAL), tissue inhibitor of metalloproteinase-2 (TIMP-2), and insulin-like growth factor–binding protein 7 (IGFBP7) have been proposed as prognostic markers; however, further validation is required for widespread adoption in clinical decision-making.[87–90] The role of functional testing, such as the furosemide stress test, also has potential but requires further validation.[91,92]

In considering the optimal timing of initiation of RRT in AKI, safety concerns associated with RRT need to be considered. Whether blood based or peritoneal membrane based, acute RRT requires access insertion and maintenance, both of which can cause visceral and vascular injury, including bleeding, vascular laceration, acute arteriovenous fistula formation, pneumothorax, and abdominal wall or mesenteric injury, as well as infection, although the risks associated with vascular catheter insertion have been reduced with the adoption of bedside ultrasound guidance for insertion. In addition, RRT is associated with risks of hypotension and leukocyte and platelet activation from exposure to the extracorporeal circuit, both of which may delay recovery of kidney function.[93–96]

Thus the clinical decision to initiate RRT must balance both uncertainty regarding risks and benefits for the individual patient. The KDIGO Clinical Practice Guidelines for AKI have encapsulated this uncertainty in the ungraded recommendations to "initiate RRT emergently when life-threatening changes in fluid, electrolyte, and acid-base balance exist;" but to also "consider the broader clinical context, the presence of conditions that can be modified with RRT, and trends of laboratory tests—rather than single BUN and creatinine thresholds alone—when making the decision to start RRT."[97]

SELECTION OF MODALITY OF RENAL REPLACEMENT THERAPY

Multiple factors need to be taken into consideration in the selection of modality of RRT, including clinical setting, hemodynamic status, volume status, medication dosing, nutritional needs and the nursing and medical expertise and resources and available. Based on randomized controlled trials[17,98–101] and metaanalyses,[102–104] CRRT and IHD are generally considered to be complementary therapies with no clear evidence that either modality provides a survival advantage.[97] However, CRRT may be preferable to IHD in specific clinical settings.[105] In the setting of significant acute brain injury or fulminant hepatic failure, CRRT may better protect cerebral perfusion by avoiding the rapid shifts in blood osmolality which are associated with the more rapid solute clearance during IHD and may lead to increased intracranial pressure and decreased cerebral perfusion pressure.[106] Furthermore, CRRT has been associated with less need for escalation of vasopressors[102] and with achievement of greater net negative fluid balance.[47] Therefore CRRT may be better suited for some critically ill AKI patients who cannot not tolerate fluid shifts and fluctuations in metabolic parameters.[97,105]

The effect of modality of RRT on recovery of kidney function has been debated. Although observational studies have found CRRT to be associated with higher rates of renal recovery, the evidence is insufficient and most studies only evaluated renal recovery in patients who survived.[107,108] Studies analyzing combined mortality and nonrecovery of renal function between groups have found no difference in recovery of kidney function.[96,109] In a retrospective propensity matched cohort, Wald et al.[110] compared CRRT with IHD as the initial RRT modality in critically ill adults with AKI and found that CRRT was associated with a lower likelihood of chronic dialysis (HR 0.75; 95% CI, 0.65 to 0.87). However, a subsequent retrospective cohort study of 638 critically ill patients who received RRT for AKI and survived to hospital discharge or 90 days found no difference in renal recovery based on initial RRT modality.[111] Multiple randomized controlled trials have analyzed recovery of kidney function as a secondary endpoint and have found no difference in recovery of kidney function, based on dialysis independence, as a function of modality of RRT.[17,98–101] A metaanalysis of predominantly observational studies reported CRRT as the initial RRT modality to be associated with higher rates of renal recovery among survivors; however, when the analysis was limited to randomized controlled trials, no benefit with regard to renal recovery was observed.[112]

It has been postulated that continuous hemofiltration might have immunomodulatory benefits based on removal of proinflammatory mediators such as interleukin (IL)-6, IL-8, IL-1, and tumor necrosis factor by convection[113] or by adsorption to the membrane.[51] Despite some encouraging results, the clinical benefit of conventional CRRT in sepsis has been disappointing[114] and the preferential use of convective as opposed to diffusive modalities cannot be supported by the data.[50] A number of factors may contribute to this absence of benefit, including concomitant removal of both pro- and antiinflammatory mediators and relatively low extracorporeal cytokine clearance compared with endogenous clearance rates.[59]

Efforts at further augmenting cytokine clearance have used higher hemofiltration volumes,[58,115] high-cutoff membranes (with a molecular weight range of up to 60 kDa),[116,117] and coupled plasma filtration and adsorption (CPFA).[118,119] In a pilot study using a high-cutoff membrane for hemofiltration in septic AKI, clearance rates for IL-6 and IL-1 were found to be augmented and vasopressor requirements decreased[116,117]; however, benefits with regard to patient survival could not be demonstrated. Similarly, compared with conventional CRRT, CPFA in septic shock improves hemodynamics and decreases need for vasopressor support but has not been found to reduce mortality or other important clinical outcomes.[118,119] Similarly, the High Volume in Intensive Care (IVOIRE) and HEROICS trials were unable to demonstrate benefit to high-volume (70 to 80 mL/kg/h) hemofiltration in either sepsis-associated AKI or post–cardiac surgery cardiogenic shock compared with conventional management.[58,115] Thus use of these novel approaches to CRRT cannot be recommended for clinical practice.

There are limited data comparing other modalities of RRT in AKI. The few studies comparing IHD with PIRRT have not found a clear modality benefit.[120–122] Studies comparing PIRRT with CRRT have found that PIRRT provides comparable hemodynamic stability and solute control to CRRT with no significant differences in mortality.[28,34–36,123,124] A metaanalysis of studies comparing CRRT and PIRRT indicated no difference in mortality, recovery of kidney function, fluid removal, days in the intensive care unit, or solute control.[124]

Several small randomized controlled trials have compared PD with other RRT modalities in AKI. In a prospective study performed in Vietnam, 70 patients with AKI caused by either malaria or sepsis (48 and 22 individuals, respectively) were randomly assigned to either PD or CVVH. PD was associated with significantly increased risk for death (47% vs. 15%, OR 5.1, 95% CI, 1.6 to 16).[125] In this study the mortality rate for patients on CVVH was unusually low and PD was not performed using the most recent technological advances such as use of bicarbonate-based dialysate and soft catheters. In contrast, a prospective randomized controlled trial performed in Brazil[126] compared the effect of HVPD and daily hemodialysis (DHD) on AKI patient survival. A total of 120 patients with acute tubular necrosis (ATN) were assigned to HVPD or DHD. The delivered dose, assessed as weekly Kt/V, was 3.67 in HVPD and 4.77 in DHD (P = 0.01). Metabolic control, mortality rate (58% and 53%), and renal function recovery (28% and 26%) were similar in both groups, whereas HVPD was associated with a significantly shorter time to the recovery of renal function.[126] Another randomized controlled trial comparing high-volume PD to PIRRT found no difference in mortality.[127] A metaanalysis of seven cohort studies and four randomized trials studies comparing PD with extracorporeal therapies in the setting of AKI suggested there were no significant differences in outcomes between patients treated with PD and IHD or hemodiafiltration (HDF).[43]

Because studies comparing modalities of RRT for AKI have not demonstrated superiority of any individual modality with regard to survival or recovery of renal function, selection of RRT modality should be tailored to specific needs of the patient. Most clinicians choose IHD for AKI patients who are hemodynamically stable and CRRT or PIRRT for AKI patients who are hemodynamically unstable, are fluid overloaded, and/or have sepsis and multiorgan failure.[10, 13,97,128] Data suggest that given slower rates but more prolonged duration of fluid removal, CRRT may provide more effective volume management than conventional IHD,[47] whereas volume control with CRRT and PIRRT are comparable.[124] Similarly, the slower solute and volume removal with CRRT provides better preservation of cerebral perfusion, making it the preferred treatment compared with IHD in patients with fulminant hepatic failure or cerebral edema.[23,106] In contradistinction, IHD is favored in patients who need rapid solute removal, such as patients with marked hyperkalemia or drug intoxications. Pragmatically, CRRT and PIRRT require more continuous patient observation and are generally restricted to patients in critical care units. Given the continuous nature of CRRT, treatment interruptions are necessary if the patient needs to be moved for diagnostic imaging or surgical procedures. Breaks in time on treatment with PIRRT and IHD may also facilitate earlier initiation of physical therapy and minimize periods of prolonged immobilization. Transitions between modalities of therapy are common, reflecting the changing needs of patients during their hospital course. Finally, choice of RRT modality must also reflect the modalities available and physician and nursing expertise at the individual hospital as well as considerations of resources, cost, and provider preference.

DOSE OF RENAL REPLACEMENT THERAPY

Assessment of dose of acute RRT is complex and can be considered as a multidimensional construct encompassing clearance of small solutes (most often modeled based on urea clearance), larger solutes (so-called "middle" molecules), ultrafiltration, treatment duration, and treatment frequency. The relative significance of these factors varies based on the modality of RRT. For example, although treatment duration and frequency are important parameters for intermittent modalities such as IHD and PIRRT, their significance only relates to unplanned interruptions of therapy in the continuous therapies. There are also important interrelationships between duration and frequency of treatment and solute clearance and ultrafiltration: When an intermittent treatment is provided more frequently (e.g., daily IHD), less solute and volume removal during each treatment is required to achieve the same overall dose of therapy than if provided on a less frequent schedule (e.g., every other day or three times per week). In addition, when solute clearance is primarily provided by diffusion, clearance of larger solutes is more dependent on duration and membrane surface area and can be dissociated from clearance of smaller solutes such as urea. Similarly, ultrafiltration may be completely dissociated from solute clearance. Despite this multidimensional complexity, the majority of studies evaluating the relationship between delivered dose of therapy and outcomes have focused primarily on small-solute clearance, primarily modeled as urea clearance (Table 49.4).

Intermittent Hemodialysis and Prolonged Intermittent Renal Replacement Therapy

The intensity of IHD and PIRRT is a function of both the dose of dialysis provided during each individual treatment and the frequency of treatments. In the chronic dialysis setting, the dose of small-solute clearance during treatment is usually quantified in terms of urea removal, using either formal urea kinetic modeling or approximated by regression equations incorporating fractional urea reduction and ultrafiltration.[129–131] The standard parameter used to quantify dialysis dose in terms of the kinetics of urea clearance is the dimensionless term Kt/V, where K is the dialysis urea clearance, t is the duration of dialysis and V is the volume of distribution of urea. Calculation of Kt/V is based on the assumption that patients are in a relative steady state, with a stable rate of urea generation and renal and extrarenal urea clearance, and a relatively constant volume status with little variation in estimated dry weight and ultrafiltration volumes between treatments. During AKI, these assumptions are often violated; total body water and urea generation rates may vary widely over time in an individual patient, as may renal and extrarenal urea clearance.[132,133] In the chronic dialysis setting, Kt/V is often based on single-pool variable volume models of

TABLE 49.4 Randomized Controlled Trials Evaluating Intensity of Renal Replacement Therapy in Acute Kidney Injury

				DOSE OF RRT		MORTALITY		
Study	Number of Patients	Study Design	RRT Modality	Less Intensive	More Intensive	Less Intensive	More Intensive	*P* value
Ronco, 2000[147]	425	Single center	CRRT	CVVH at 20 mL/kg/h	CVVH at 35 or 45 mL/kg/h	59%	42%	<0.005
Schiffl, 2002[140]	160	Single center	IHD	IHD with Kt/V 0.94 ± 0.11 delivered every other day	IHD with Kt/V 0.92 ± 0.16 delivered daily	46%	28%	0.01
Bouman, 2002[70]	106	Two centers	CRRT	24–36 L per 24 h	5	28%	25%	0.80
Saudan, 2006[148]	206	Single center	CRRT	CVVH at 25 ± 5 mL/kg/h	CVVHDF at 24 ± 6 mL/kg/h UF and 15 ± 5 mL/kg/h dialysate	61%	46%	<0.001
Tolwani, 2008[149]	200	Single center	CRRT	CVVHDF at 20 mL/kg/h	CVVHDF at 35 mL/kg/h	60%	64%	0.56
Palevsky, 2008[16]	1124	Multicenter	IHD PIRRT CRRT	IHD and PIRRT with delivered Kt/V1.32 ± 0.37 delivered three times per week CVVHDF at 20 mL/kg/h	IHD and PIRRT with delivered Kt/V of 1.31 ± 0.33 delivered six times per week CVVHDF at 35 mL/kg/h	52%	54%	0.47
Bellomo, 2009[150]	1508	Multicenter	CRRT	CVVHDF at 25 mL/kg/h	CVVHDF at 40 mL/kg/h	45%	45%	0.99
Faulhaber-Walter, 2009[142]	156	Single center	PIRRT	Target BUN 48–70 mg/dL	Target BUN < 42 mg/dL	39%	44%	0.47

BUN, Blood urea nitrogen; *CRRT,* continuous renal replacement therapy; *CVVH,* continuous venovenous hemofiltration; *CVVHDF,* continuous venovenous hemodiafiltration; *IHD,* intermittent hemodialysis; *PIRRT,* prolonged intermittent renal replacement therapy; *RRT,* renal replacement therapy.

urea distribution, although multiple compartment and equilibrated models may provide a more accurate assessment.[130] In addition, assessment of Kt/V across modalities using differing schedules is complex, because it is not a simple arithmetic function. For example, reducing the delivered Kt/V per treatment by half while doubling the frequency of treatment (e.g., from every other day to daily hemodialysis) results in an increased effective weekly dose of therapy.[130,134] As a result, various models have been developed to relate the dose of therapy delivered on different schedules, normalizing based on the peak predialysis urea concentration,[135] the mean predialysis urea concentration,[130,134] or the time-averaged urea concentration.[136] None of these models have been rigorously validated in clinical practice. Despite these limitations, urea kinetics have been successfully used in the AKI setting[16,137,138] and serve as the basis for clinical practice guidelines for IHD delivery in AKI.[97]

There have been no prospective randomized controlled trials evaluating the optimal delivered dose of dialysis on a standard every other day or thrice weekly schedule. A single-center observational study[139] performed more than two decades ago evaluated survival in 844 critically ill patients with AKI requiring RRT, 417 of whom received only IHD and another 242 who received a combination of IHD and CRRT. Although there was no correlation between the delivered dose of dialysis and outcomes among patients with either very low or very high severity of illness, delivery of a $Kt/V > 1$ per treatment three times per week was associated with better survival than a lower delivered dose of dialysis among patients with intermediate severity of illness. Thus in the absence of more robust data, it is generally suggested that when IHD is provided to patients with AKI on a three-times-per-week schedule that the dose per treatment be at least equivalent to the minimum accepted dose for a patient with ESRD.[97]

The effect of increasing the frequency of IHD was assessed in a single-center study[140] that assigned 160 critically ill patients in alternating order to daily or every-other-day IHD. Although the prescribed Kt/V was 1.2 per treatment, the delivered Kt/V was only 0.94 ± 0.11 per treatment in the alternate-day group and 0.92 ± 0.16 in the daily IHD group. All-cause mortality 14 days after the last IHD session was 28% in the daily treatment group compared with 46% in patients receiving alternate-day IHD ($P = 0.01$) and the duration of IHD was 9 ± 2 days in the daily treatment arm compared with 16 ± 6 days in the alternate-day treatment arm.[140] Although suggesting a benefit to more frequent dialysis, the low delivered dose of dialysis per treatment in the alternate-day arm may have been inadequate, resulting in a high rate of complications, including infection, gastrointestinal bleeding, and altered mental status.[141] Thus, although more frequent IHD may improve clinical outcomes when the delivered dose of therapy is low, this study is not informative regarding the need for more frequent IHD when a higher delivered dose per treatment is achieved.

The Hanover Dialysis Outcome Study randomly assigned 148 critically ill patients with AKI to two different intensities of PIRRT: a standard-dose arm in which the target BUN level was 56 to 70 mg/dL or a more intensive strategy in which the frequency of treatment was increased to maintain the BUN level < 42 mg/dL.[142] The more intensive strategy was not associated with either decreased mortality at 28 days (44.4% in the intensive arm vs. 38.7% in the less-intensive arm; $P = 0.47$) or improved recovery of kidney function (60% vs. 63%; $P = 0.77$).

The VA/NIH Acute Renal Failure Trial Network (ATN) study was a multicenter randomized controlled trial that compared strategies of more-intensive and less-intensive RRT in 1124 critically ill patients with AKI.[16] Unlike the previously described trials, which restricted patients to a single modality of RRT, patients in the ATN study moved between modalities of RRT as their hemodynamic status changed, receiving IHD when hemodynamically stable and CRRT or PIRRT when hemodynamically unstable. In the more-intensive arm, IHD and PIRRT were provided 6 days per week and CRRT at an effluent flow rate of 35 mL/kg/h; in the less-intensive arm IHD and PIRRT were provided on a thrice weekly schedule and CRRT at an effluent flow rate of 20 mL/kg/h. The median delivered Kt/V during IHD was 1.3 per treatment in both study arms. More-intensive therapy was not associated with better outcomes (60-day mortality of 53.6% with more-intensive therapy vs. 51.5% with less-intensive therapy; $P = 0.47$)[16] with no difference between treatment arms when stratified by the percentage of time treated with IHD.[143] Although there was no difference in recovery of kidney function overall, in the subset of patients who only received IHD, more-intensive therapy was associated with delayed time to recovery of kidney function.[144]

Continuous Renal Replacement Therapy

During continuous hemofiltration, the concentration of urea and most non–protein-bound small solutes in the ultrafiltrate approximates that of plasma water.[145] Similarly, during continuous hemodialysis, with blood flow rates much higher than dialysate flow rates, urea and other small solutes achieve near complete equilibration between blood and dialysate.[49] Thus, during CRRT, so long as clotting or excessive protein layering is not contributing to membrane fouling, the clearance of urea and other low-molecular-weight solutes approximates effluent flow rate.[146] Thus the dose of CRRT is generally expressed in terms of effluent flow rate normalized to body weight (Q_E). The daily delivered Kt/V can be estimated as $Q_E \times 24/V_{urea}$, where V_{urea} is the volume of distribution of urea. Approximating V_{urea} as 600 mL/kg, the daily delivered Kt/V can be estimated as $0.04 \times Q_E$. Thus at a continuous effluent flow of 20 mL/kg/h, the delivered Kt/V will be approximately 0.8 per day, and at 35 mL/kg/h, the delivered Kt/V will be approximately 1.4 per day.

A series of studies published between 2000 and 2009 evaluated the relationship between the delivered dose of CRRT and outcomes in critically ill patients. In the first of these studies, 425 patients at a single center were randomly assigned to CVVH at an effluent flow of 20, 35 or 45 mL/kg/h with postfilter infusion of replacement fluid.[147] Individuals receiving

CVVH at the two higher doses experienced lower mortality rates assessed 14 days after discontinuation of RRT than those receiving the lower dose of CVVH (42% and 43% vs. 59%; $P < 0.005$). In a subsequent single-center study, 206 critically ill patients with AKI were randomly assigned to receive CVVH, with a mean effluent flow of 25 ± 5 mL/kg/h, or CVVHDF delivered with a similar ultrafiltration rate (24 ± 6 mL/kg/h) augmented by the addition of dialysate flow (18 ± 5 mL/kg/h).[148] Survival at both 28 days and 90 days was higher among patients who received augmented clearance with CVVHDF (90-day survival of 34% in the CVVH arm vs. 59% in the CVVHDF arm; $P = 0.005$). However, the benefits of higher doses of CRRT were not seen across all studies. In a two-center study[70] of 106 patients assigned to early, HVHF (median 48.2 [interquartile ratio (IQR) 42.3 to 58.7] mL/kg/h), early low-volume hemofiltration (median 20.1 [IQR 17.5 to 22.0] mL/kg/h), or late low-volume hemofiltration (median 19.0 [IQR 16.6 to 21.1] mL/kg/h), the augmented dose of continuous hemofiltration was not associated with improved survival at 28 days (74.3% vs. 71.8%; $P = 0.80$). Similarly, in a single-center trial[149] in which 200 critically ill patients with AKI were randomly assigned to CVVHDF with prefilter administration of replacement fluid at a total effluent flow of either 20 mL/kg/h or 35 mL/kg/h, survival to earlier of either ICU discharge or to day 30 was 49% in the higher-dose arm compared with 56% in the lower-dose arm (OR 0.75; 95% CI, 0.43 to 1.32; $P = 0.32$). The Randomized Evaluation of Normal Versus Augmented Level (RENAL) Replacement Therapy Study was a multicenter randomized controlled trial conducted at 35 intensive care units in Australia and New Zealand that randomly assigned 1508 patients to CVVHDF with postfilter administration of replacement fluid at a total effluent flow of either 25 mL/kg/h or 40 mL/kg/h.[150] Overall mortality at 90 days was 44.7% in both treatment arms ($P = 0.99$). Similarly, in the ATN study, no difference in survival was identified between the more-intensive strategy of RRT that used CVVHDF at 35 mL/kg/h and the less-intensive strategy that used CVVHDF at 20 mL/kg/h.[16] Several studies have used even higher doses of CVVH, up to 70 mL/kg/h, in patients with sepsis-associated AKI without finding a benefit to more intensive CRRT.[57,115]

Effect of Dose on Recovery of Kidney Function

Although recovery of kidney function was comparable between the more-intensive and less-intensive management strategies in each of the individual trials described earlier, more intensive RRT was associated with delayed recovery of kidney function in a patient-level metaanalysis pooling data from the majority of the individual studies.[151] In a subgroup analysis, delayed recovery of kidney function was observed in patients initially managed using CRRT but not in patients initially managed using intermittent renal replacement therapy, although the latter finding may reflect the smaller number of intermittent dialysis patients included in the analysis. In a separate analysis of patients in the ATN study who were treated exclusively with IHD, six times per week dialysis was also associated with delayed recovery of kidney function.[144] The reason for delay in recovery of kidney function is not understood. Although this may reflect the effect of more episodes of intradialytic hypotension among patients treated with more frequent IHD, intensity of therapy is not associated with hypotension during CRRT. More aggressive solute control may diminish the solute load and contribute to lower urine output associated with more intensive RRT,[152] which may mask early recovery of kidney function.

Volume Management

Volume management needs to be considered as an independent aspect in the dosing of acute RRT. Fluid excess has been found to be independently associated with increased mortality in observational studies of AKI in both adult and pediatric populations, where fluid excess is defined as a percentage of premorbid weight.[47,76,86] In the largest pediatric study the percentage fluid excess at dialysis initiation correlated with mortality risk, even after adjustment for severity of illness.[86] Ultrafiltration must be tailored to individual patient needs, with a goal of reversing severe volume overload without causing intravascular volume depletion and hypotension, which might adversely affect recovery of kidney function.

Summary and Recommendations

Although the data from recent trials indicate that augmented intensity of RRT is not associated with clinical benefit in patients with AKI, these data should not be interpreted as demonstrating that the delivered dose of RRT does not matter. Although a minimum dose of RRT is not clearly established, using the data from these multiple trials, and drawing analogies to accepted minimum doses of RRT in ESRD, general recommendations regarding dosing can be made.[97,128] Although these general recommendations apply to the vast majority of patients, individualization of treatment prescription for each patient is appropriate.

For patients receiving IHD, a thrice weekly treatment schedule is generally sufficient if an $spKt/V_{urea}$ of at least 1.2 per treatment (corresponding to a urea reduction ratio [URR] of ≥0.67) is achieved. In patients who are hypercatabolic, have severe electrolyte disturbances (e.g., hyperkalemia) or persistent metabolic acidosis, or have severe volume overload or require obligate administration of large volumes of fluids, a more frequent hemodialysis schedule may be necessary. In addition, treatment frequency may need to be increased if the targeted dose of therapy per treatment cannot be achieved. In patients receiving dialysis for AKI there may be a marked discrepancy between the prescribed and delivered dose of dialysis, with delivered Kt/V as much as 30% lower than prescribed as the result of hypotension, dialyzer clotting, and catheter dysfunction.[140,153,154] Monitoring of the delivered dose of therapy is therefore necessary to ensure adequacy of treatment.

For patients being treated with CRRT, a total effluent flow of 20 to 25 mL/kg/h is generally appropriate; however, more intensive treatment may be required for patients who are very hypercatabolic or for control of electrolytes or acid–base status. As with IHD, the delivered dose of therapy may be less than prescribed as the result of system clotting and time off of therapy for diagnostic tests or surgical procedures.[155] Thus a prescribed dose of 25 to 30 mL/kg/h may be necessary to achieve the target delivered dose.

TECHNICAL ASPECTS OF MANAGEMENT OF RRT IN AKI

Vascular Access

The availability of appropriate venous angioaccess is crucial for IHD and CRRT (CVVH, CVVHD, or CVVHDF); an intraperitoneal catheter is required for PD. A variety of vascular catheters are available that can be placed in the jugular, subclavian, or femoral vessel and can sustain blood flows consistently greater than 300 mL/min, though it may be difficult to achieve and maintain these flow rates in hemodynamically unstable patients. If vascular access cannot be obtained, PD may be the only alternative, particularly in the pediatric patient.

The type of catheter and the technique of insertion are important to minimize complications. Access-placement–related complications depend on the expertise of the operator and may be exacerbated by underlying coagulopathy.[156] The use of real-time ultrasound guidance is recommended for the placement of dialysis catheters to minimize complications from insertion, including arterial puncture, catheter misplacement, and hematoma formation from repeated attempts at cannulation.[157] Late complications associated with vascular catheters include infection, thrombosis, and stenosis. These complications are associated with site of insertion and properties of catheter material. Although there generally is a higher risk for bacteremia with femoral compared with jugular or subclavian venous catheters,[158] in a randomized controlled trial of 750 patients with AKI requiring RRT, there were comparable rates of catheter colonization, bacteremia, and thrombosis between the jugular and femoral access sites.[159] In this study the relative risk for catheter colonization between the jugular and femoral sites appeared to depend on patient body mass index (BMI): At higher BMIs (>28.4 kg/m^2), femoral catheters had higher rates of colonization, whereas at lower BMIs, jugular venous catheters appeared to have higher rates of colonization.

Venous thrombosis and stenosis has been increasingly recognized as a serious complication associated with catheter use, particularly with cannulation of the subclavian vein.[160,161] The incidence of this complication is difficult to establish, because only a few studies have been systematically performed. Stricture in the subclavian vein previously used for temporary dialysis is a particular concern for patients who fail to recover after AKI and subsequently require long-term dialysis. In a retrospective study involving 52 patients, after 2 years of catheterization, venograms indicated a 50% incidence of long-term venous stricture. No significant venous stricture was found along the course of the cannula in patients with previous internal jugular vein catheters.[162–164] The right internal jugular vein is generally preferred over the left internal jugular vein based on anatomical considerations, with a straighter course from the vein to the right atrium. Based on these considerations, the KDIGO Clinical Practice Guidelines for AKI recommend the right jugular vein as the preferred choice for access placement, with the femoral cannulation as the second choice, the left jugular vein as the third choice, and the subclavian vein as the least preferred site,[97] although this recommendation is ungraded and does not reflect that depth of catheter tip insertion is a key component of internal jugular vein insertion sites. When the catheter tip is positioned at the vena cava–atrial junction or right atrium rather than more proximally in the SVC, access and dialysis circuit function is improved.[165] The position of the catheter is often inadequate when inserted in the left internal jugular vein if care is not taken to individualize catheter length based on patient height, with most adults requiring a catheter longer than 20 cm internal length from the left internal jugular vein.[166] Although tunneled catheters are not routinely recommended, they are associated with decreased risk for infection, higher blood flows, and lower complication rates and should be considered when the need for RRT is expected to exceed 1 to 3 weeks.[97,167]

Blood recirculation in venous catheters is an important factor that contributes to a lower delivered dialysis dose in AKI patients. The proximal (arterial) port of the catheter can extract part of the blood that was just returned through the distal (venous) port. This recirculation is accentuated in short catheters, where up to 23% of the blood flow may recirculate.[168] Thus, as previously discussed, it is important that the catheter length be appropriate for the site of insertion. For jugular catheters, the catheter tip should be at the junction of the superior vena cava and right atrium or in the right atrium, depending on catheter type; for femoral catheters, the longest possible catheter should be used, with a goal of having the catheter tip in the inferior vena cava.

Anticoagulation

Most types of extracorporeal RRT require anticoagulation to prevent clotting of the extracorporeal circuit. The contact of blood with the foreign surface of the extracorporeal circuit results in activation of both the intrinsic and the extrinsic pathway of coagulation and activation of platelets.[169] Clotting of the extracorporeal circuit leads to decreased solute and fluid removal and blood loss in the extracorporeal circuit. The most commonly used anticoagulant is unfractionated heparin (UFH). UFH has several significant advantages, including its wide availability, low cost, ease of administration and monitoring, and reversibility with protamine. Disadvantages include its unpredictable pharmacokinetics, risk for heparin-induced thrombocytopenia (HIT), heparin resistance because of low patient antithrombin levels, and increased risk for bleeding.[170] For IHD, UFH can be given as a bolus at the start of the dialysis treatment with a midtreatment dose or an initial bolus followed by a constant fixed infusion of heparin.

Although IHD and PIRRT can be generally performed without anticoagulation given their shorter durations of treatment and higher blood flow rates, CRRT often requires anticoagulation. Adequate CRRT filter survival without anticoagulation has been described in critically ill patients at a high risk for bleeding as a result of coagulopathy, platelet dysfunction, liver dysfunction, and invasive procedures.[171–174] Placement of a well functioning vascular access is essential for maintaining CRRT circuit patency. Strategies to prolong filter survival in CRRT without anticoagulation include using saline flushes, predilution replacement fluid, and high blood flow rates; reducing the blood–air contact in the bubble trap; and reacting promptly to machine alarms.[175,176]

The most common anticoagulants for CRRT include UFH and regional citrate anticoagulation (RCA). Less common strategies include UFH with protamine reversal, low-molecular-weight heparin (LMWH), thrombin antagonists, and platelet-inhibiting agents. UFH is typically administered as a bolus of 2000 to 5000 IU (30 IU/kg), followed by a continuous infusion of 5 to 10 IU/kg/h into the arterial limb of the dialysis circuit. The optimal activated partial thromboplastin time (aPTT) is not known with certainty, and the therapeutic benefit of preventing clotting in the extracorporeal circuit must be balanced with the risk for systemic bleeding.[170,177,178] Generally, aPTT between 45 to 60 seconds or 1.5 to 2.0 times normal is targeted. The incidence of bleeding episodes with heparin as an anticoagulant for CRRT ranges from 10% to 50%, with mortality from bleeding as high as 15%.[177,179,180] As a result, regional anticoagulation with citrate has been gaining wider acceptance in CRRT, and multiple RCA protocols for CRRT have been described in the literature.[181–194]

Citrate is infused into the blood at the beginning of the extracorporeal circuit where it chelates ionized calcium and inhibits the coagulation cascade.[195] Coagulation is adequately inhibited with an ionized calcium level less than 0.35 mmol/L in the extracorporeal circuit, which correlates with a citrate blood concentration of 3 to 6 mmol/L.[195,196] Because the majority of the formed calcium-citrate complex is freely filtered across the hemofilter, calcium has to be infused to replace the calcium lost in the effluent and titrated to maintain a normal serum ionized calcium concentration. The remaining calcium-citrate complex that is not removed by the hemofilter enters the patient's systemic circulation and is metabolized by the liver, kidney, and skeletal muscles to bicarbonate. Each citrate molecule potentially yields three bicarbonate molecules. Calcium released from the calcium-citrate complex helps restore the serum ionized calcium levels back to normal. Advantages of RCA include avoidance of HIT and decreased risk for bleeding because only the CRRT circuit is anticoagulated. Relative drawbacks include the risk for metabolic alkalosis, hypernatremia (when hypertonic citrate solutions are used), hypomagnesemia, and hypocalcemia. Thus frequent monitoring of acid–base status, electrolytes, and ionized calcium in the systemic circulation is necessary. Citrate accumulation may occur in patients who cannot metabolize citrate, such as those with liver failure or severe lactic acidosis, leading to severe hypocalcemia and metabolic disorders.[197–200] However, if properly monitored, complications associated with RCA are uncommon. In fact, RCA has been used safely and successfully in patients with advanced liver disease,[201] as well as in perioperative liver transplant patients.[202] Furthermore, in recent years, new commercially available citrate solutions together with adapted CRRT machines have rendered the technique safer and easier to use.

Overall, studies of RCA, compared with UFH, report better filter survival times and less bleeding.[181–188,190–192,203–211] Based on the evidence, the KDIGO guideline for AKI recommends RCA over systemic heparin for most patients who require CRRT.[97] Furthermore, in a recent metaanalysis of 11 randomized controlled trials comparing RCA with UFH, RCA significantly increased CRRT circuit life span, decreased circuit failure, and lowered bleeding risk.[212] Based on high-quality evidence that has accumulated, RCA can be strongly recommended in most patients who require CRRT.

Regional anticoagulation of the circuit can also be achieved by infusing UFH continuously prefilter via the arterial line and reversing its effects with a constant infusion of protamine administered postfilter on the return line of the extracorporeal circuit. This approach requires measurement of both circuit and systemic aPTT. The advantage of this method is that the anticoagulant effects of UFH are restricted to the extracorporeal circuit, thereby lowering the risk for systemic patient bleeding. For CRRT, UFH is usually infused at 1000 to 1500 IU/h prefilter and neutralized with protamine infused at 10 to 12 mg/h infused postfilter with subsequent adjustment according to the aPTT. However, the amount of protamine needed to neutralize heparin varies substantially, and the protocols are cumbersome and difficult to standardize.[172,177,206,213–216] Protamine infusion can be associated with hypotension, anaphylaxis, cardiac depression, leukopenia, and thrombocytopenia.[217] Although several small studies have reported that regional heparinization with protamine is feasible and safe, its efficacy in prolonging filter life span has been variable.[172,214,216]

LMWHs have higher anti-Xa/anti-IIa activity than UFH.[170] LMWHs have a more reliable anticoagulant response and a lower incidence of HIT compared with UFH. Nadroparin and dalteparin are administered at a loading dose of 15 to 25 IU/kg followed by a maintenance dose of 5 IU/kg/h. Anticoagulation is monitored using anti-Xa levels with target levels between 0.25 to 0.35 units/mL.[218–221] Higher anti-Xa levels between 0.45 and 0.8 units/mL have been associated with bleeding complications.[222] The disadvantages associated with LMWH include prolonged anticoagulation effect in patients with renal failure, less effective reversal with protamine because of stronger anti-Xa effect, requirement of special assays to measure anti-Xa activity, and increased cost compared with UFH. Randomized controlled trials have found that fixed-dose LMWHs are as effective as but not superior to standard heparin in prolonging circuit life.[218–221]

The most common thrombin antagonists used for anticoagulation of the CRRT circuit in the setting of HIT are argatroban and bivalirudin. Argatroban is metabolized in the liver and has a short half-life of 35 minutes even in patients on chronic dialysis.[223] It is administered as a loading dose of 100 mcg/kg followed by an infusion to achieve a target aPTT 1.5 to 3.0 times normal.[224] Dosing can range between 0.7 and 1.7 μg/kg/min. A dose reduction is needed in hepatic failure and most critically ill patients even with intact liver function. Disadvantages include bleeding risks and absence of an antidote. Bivalirudin is used as an alternative to argatroban in patients who have both liver and renal failure because it has extrarenal and extrahepatic clearance. It has a short half-life with reversible thrombin binding. One study comparing bivalirudin anticoagulation with heparin anticoagulation in CVVH found longer filter survival time associated with bivalirudin.[225] Bivalirudin was administered at an initial rate of 2 mg/h and titrated to maintain the prefilter aPTT to 1.5 to 2.5 times the patient's baseline aPTT.

Prostacyclin (PGI2) and its synthetic derivative epoprostenol act by inhibiting platelet aggregation and adhesion. Clinical experience is limited, with few published reports about its safety and efficacy. Prostacyclin is infused prefilter at 2 to 8 ng/kg/min and can be used in combination with low-dose UFH at a rate of 5 to 6 IU/kg/h.[179,226–231] Its main disadvantages are its expensive cost and potential to cause hypotension.

Membrane Composition

Interactions between the dialysis membrane and the blood may lead to complement activation, activation of the coagulation cascade, and neutrophil sequestration and has been postulated to impair recovery of kidney function.[232,233] Clinical trials comparing dialysis with less biocompatible cellulosic dialysis membranes and more biocompatible synthetic membranes have yielded variable results, with some studies finding better recovery of kidney function with more biocompatible membranes.[93,94,232,234,235] The issue of membrane composition has become less relevant, however, as synthetic membranes have generally replaced cellulosic membranes in clinical practice. The use of a proprietary acrylonitrile-sodium methallyl sulfonate membrane (AN69) in patients concomitantly treated with angiotensin-converting enzyme inhibitors has been associated with anaphylactoid reactions, thought to be mediated by increased bradykinin generation.[236,237] Thus this membrane, which is often used for CRRT, should be avoided in patients being treated with angiotensin-converting enzyme inhibitors.

Procedure-Related Complications

The most common complication during IHD is hypotension, occurring in 30% to 50% of patients.[16–18] A variety of strategies can be employed to minimize the development of intradialytic hypotension, including ultrafiltration control, increasing the dialysate sodium concentration, decreasing the dialysate temperature, and prolonging the treatment duration to allow for more gradual ultrafiltration and solute removal[17,18,22] (Table 49.5). The use of sodium modeling (beginning at a dialysate sodium of 160 mmol/L and gradually decreasing the concentration to 140 mmol/L over the duration of the treatment) and ultrafiltration profiling (50% ultrafiltration in the first hour and 50% over the remainder of the dialysis session) produced improved hemodynamic stability compared with the use of a constant dialysate sodium of 140 mmol/L and a linear ultrafiltration profile in critically ill patients undergoing IHD.[22] Similarly, in another study[18] the use of biocompatible membranes, low temperature dialysate, and a dialysate sodium of 145 mmol/L as part of a bundle of interventions significantly decreased the development of intradialytic hypotension during IHD. In the Hemodiafe study,[17] in which the majority of patients undergoing IHD were vasopressor dependent, hemodynamic instability was minimized by using prolonged treatment times (median of 5.2 hours) combined with isovolemic connection, use of a dialysate temperature of 35°C, and a sodium of 150 mmol/L.

TABLE 49.5 Strategies to Minimize Complications of Intermittent Hemodialysis

Complication	Interventions
Hypotension	Extend dialysis time
	Decrease dialysate temperature
	Increase dialysate sodium
	Decrease ultrafiltration rate
	Use ultrafiltration modeling
	Reassess ultrafiltration target (end dialysis weight)
	Use isovolemic connection
	Increase dialysate calcium
	Hold vasodilators
Hypoxemia	Use noncellulosic dialyzer
	Use bicarbonate dialysate
	Provide supplemental oxygen
Arrhythmia	Use higher dialysate potassium concentration
	Provide supplemental oxygen
	Minimize intradialytic hypotension
Muscle cramps	Extend dialysis time
	Decrease ultrafiltration rate
	Treat symptoms with hypertonic saline
Dialysis disequilibrium	Attenuate solute clearance by limiting time, dialyzer surface area, blood flow and dialysate flow
Pyrogen reaction	Ensure water quality
	Use ultrapure dialysate

The risk for hypotension as a treatment complication with CRRT is generally perceived to be lower than during IHD as a result of the slower rates of solute removal and ultrafiltration with prolonged treatment times. In the Hemodiafe study,[17] however, rates of hypotension were similar during both IHD and CRRT.[17] CRRT, particularly when higher clearances are used, may result in hypophosphatemia, hypokalemia, and micronutrient depletion.[16] Close monitoring of serum electrolytes is therefore necessary. Hypokalemia can be avoided by using higher potassium concentrations in dialysate and/or replacement fluids. Phosphate replacement is most often provided using intravenous phosphate; however, regimens with oral phosphate have been employed.[238] Alternatively, phosphate can be added to the dialysate and replacement fluids to prevent the development of significant phosphate depletion.[239] Hypocalcemia and metabolic alkalosis may develop as a complication of citrate anticoagulation.[197–200]

Hypoxemia has been described as a complication during hemodialysis, particularly in the past when cellulosic membranes and acetate-buffered dialysate were commonly employed. Consumption of CO_2 during acetate metabolism from an acetate-buffered dialysate or alkalinization of the blood caused by diffusion from a bicarbonate-based dialysate can induce hypoventilation and worsening hypoxia.[240,241] This effect is more pronounced in patients with underlying lung disease and those with chronic obstructive pulmonary disorder during or after hemodialysis. Hypothermia may develop as a result of heat loss from the extracorporeal circuit and may necessitate the use of blood warmers.

Medication Dosing

The effect of RRT on drug dosing is of particular importance in patients with AKI, particularly when associated with sepsis. Drug removal during dialysis may result in subtherapeutic levels, particularly when higher doses of RRT are used.[242–244] It has been suggested that inadequate drug dosing during more intensive RRT may have contributed to the lack of observed benefit. Factors that affect drug clearance during RRT include the drug's molecular weight (smaller molecules are more readily cleared across the dialysis membrane), the degree of protein binding (which inhibits clearance), and the drug's volume of distribution (the larger the volume of distribution, the smaller the fractional removal that will occur via RRT). For medications whose clinical response can be readily assessed, such as pain medications, sedatives, and vasopressors, dosing should be titrated based on the clinical response. For medications whose clinical response cannot be readily observed, such as antibiotics, plasma drug levels should be monitored and dosing adjusted accordingly. If medication dosage cannot be titrated to clinical response and plasma drug levels are not readily obtained, dosing needs to be based on RRT clearances, using published dosing guides as reference.

OUTCOMES

Renal replacement for AKI is based on the premise that eventually there will be a return of kidney function allowing discontinuation of dialysis. Although this is the desired outcome, it does not always occur. This is particularly true for the patient with AKI complicating MOF, wherein the ultimate prognosis depends on recovery of other organ systems. Traditional teaching suggests that most patients with AKI who survive the acute illness will recover sufficient kidney function to achieve dialysis independence within 4 to 6 weeks, and dialysis dependence beyond 8 to 12 weeks likely represents the development of ESRD. In rare circumstances, recovery of kidney function may be substantially delayed. The majority of studies addressing renal recovery include only critically ill patients requiring dialysis and consider renal recovery as freedom from dialysis at hospital discharge[245]; however, recovery of kidney function may be incomplete, and patients who survive their episode of AKI are at increased risk for subsequent progression to ESRD.[246] The duration of dialytic support may need to be predefined in some patients with AKI when other organ system failure accompanies AKI. For instance, a time-limited course of RRT (days to 1 to 2 weeks) should be considered for a patient with respiratory, cardiac, and liver failure secondary to sepsis requiring dialytic support for AKI, with continued provision of dialytic support reassessed based on evidence of improvement in all organ systems.[247] Withdrawal or withholding of RRT should be considered in selected patients with severe AKI accompanying MOF who are extremely unlikely to recover nonrenal organ function.[248]

SUMMARY

Multiple methods of RRT are available for the management of patients with severe AKI. Rational use of these techniques requires an understanding of factors influencing the choice of a modality and appreciation of the advantages and disadvantages of each technique. Management of AKI is different from that of ESRD, and the RRT prescription should incorporate the unique characteristics of each patient. Therapeutic alternatives to traditional IHD permit flexibility in the modality and dosing used to meet the individual needs of the patient.

A full list of references is available at www.expertconsult.com.

INDEX

Note: Page numbers followed by "f" indicate figures, "t" indicate tables, "b" indicate boxes.

D

O